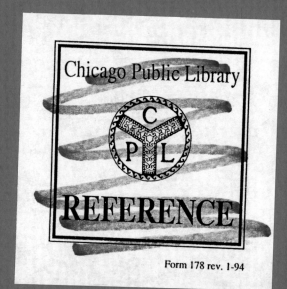

DIET
AND
HEALTH

Implications for Reducing
Chronic Disease Risk

Committee on Diet and Health
Food and Nutrition Board
Commission on Life Sciences
National Research Council

NATIONAL ACADEMY PRESS
Washington, D.C.   1989

NATIONAL ACADEMY PRESS • 2101 CONSTITUTION AVENUE, NW • WASHINGTON, DC 20418

NOTICE: The project that is the subject of this report was approved by the Governing Board of the National Research Council, whose members are drawn from the councils of the National Academy of Sciences, the National Academy of Engineering, and the Institute of Medicine. The members of the committee responsible for the report were chosen for their special competences and with regard for appropriate balance. This report has been reviewed by a group other than the authors according to procedures approved by a Report Review Committee consisting of members of the National Academy of Sciences, the National Academy of Engineering, and the Institute of Medicine.

The National Academy of Sciences is a private, nonprofit, self-perpetuating society of distinguished scholars engaged in scientific and engineering research, dedicated to the furtherance of science and technology and to their use for the general welfare. Upon the authority of the charter granted to it by the Congress in 1863, the Academy has a mandate that requires it to advise the federal government on scientific and technical matters. Dr. Frank Press is president of the National Academy of Sciences.

The National Academy of Engineering was established in 1964, under the charter of the National Academy of Sciences, as a parallel organization of outstanding engineers. It is autonomous in its administration and in the selection of its members, sharing with the National Academy of Sciences the responsibility for advising the federal government. The National Academy of Engineering also sponsors engineering programs aimed at meeting national needs, encourages education and research, and recognizes the superior achievements of engineers. Dr. Robert M. White is president of the National Academy of Engineering.

The Institute of Medicine was established in 1970 by the National Academy of Sciences to secure the services of eminent members of appropriate professions in the examination of policy matters pertaining to the health of the public. The Institute acts under the responsibility given to the National Academy of Sciences by its congressional charter to be an adviser to the federal government and, upon its own initiative, to identify issues of medical care, research, and education. Dr. Samuel O. Thier is president of the Institute of Medicine.

The National Research Council was organized by the National Academy of Sciences in 1916 to associate the broad community of science and technology with the Academy's purposes of furthering knowledge and advising the federal government. Functioning in accordance with general policies determined by the Academy, the Council has become the principal operating agency of both the National Academy of Sciences and the National Academy of Engineering in providing services to the government, the public, and the scientific and engineering communities. The Council is administered jointly by both Academies and the Institute of Medicine. Dr. Frank Press and Dr. Robert M. White are chairman and vice chairman, respectively, of the National Research Council.

The study summarized in this publication was supported by funds from the National Research Council Fund, a pool of private, discretionary, nonfederal funds that is used to support a program of Academy-initiated studies of national issues in which science and technology figure significantly. The NRC Fund consists of contributions from a consortium of private foundations including Carnegie Corporation of New York, Charles E. Culpeper Foundation, William and Flora Hewlett Foundation, John D. and Catherine T. MacArthur Foundation, Andrew W. Mellon Foundation, Rockefeller Foundation, and Alfred P. Sloan Foundation; the Academy Industry Program, which seeks annual contributions from companies that are concerned with the health of U.S. science and technology and with public policy issues with technological content; and the National Academy of Sciences and National Academy of Engineering endowments. The study was also supported by W.K. Kellogg Foundation, The Henry J. Kaiser Family Foundation, Pew Charitable Trusts, Fannie E. Rippel Foundation, and Occidental Petroleum Corporation.

Library of Congress Cataloging-in-Publication Data

National Research Council (U.S.). Committee on Diet and Health.
   Diet and health : implications for reducing chronic disease risk /
Committee on Diet and Health, Food and Nutrition Board, Commission
on Life Sciences, National Research Council.
      p. cm.
   Includes bibliographies and index.
   ISBN 0-309-03994-0
   1. Chronic diseases—Nutritional aspects. I. Title.
   [DNLM: 1. Chronic Disease. 2. Diet. 3. Health. 4. Risk Factors.
QU 145 N2761d]
RC108.N38 1989
613.2—dc20
DNLM/DLC
for Library of Congress   89-3261
                                                            CIP

Printed in the United States of America

Cover photographs:
Paul Robert Perry/UNIPHOTO (*black-eyed peas*); Peter Beck/UNIPHOTO (*fish*); Hanley and Savage/UNIPHOTO (*milk*); Peter Beck/UNIPHOTO (*fruits; vegetables*); Gordon E. Smith/UNIPHOTO (*bread*); Renee Comet/UNIPHOTO (*basket*).

Dedication

The Committee on Diet and Health dedicates this report to the late Lucille Hurley, a diligent and enthusiastic member of the committee who made an invaluable contribution to this study, and to the American people, whose demonstrated interest and concerns about how diet affects their health inspired us to undertake this effort. We hope that this detailed assessment of the data will facilitate an understanding of the complex interrelationship between diet, chronic diseases, and health, and enhance the potential for reducing the risk of chronic diseases.

COMMITTEE ON DIET AND HEALTH

FOOD AND NUTRITION BOARD

COMMISSION ON LIFE SCIENCES

Preface

In the first half of the twentieth century, research in human nutrition was concerned primarily with the role of essential nutrients, particularly vitamins, in human deficiency diseases. It was not until the end of World War II that nutrition research in human populations in the United States focused on the role of diet in chronic diseases, such as coronary heart disease and cancer. The link forged by these later epidemiologic studies was strengthened by complementary evidence from laboratory studies. In the last decade, the wealth of information provided by these studies has been used by U.S. government agencies and other expert groups to propose dietary guidelines aimed at reducing the risk of one or more chronic diseases among North Americans.

Although there has been increasing consensus among various groups on many of the dietary guidelines, there remains a lack of agreement on several specific points. Our incomplete knowledge about the multiple environmental and genetic factors that determine chronic disease risk, specifically dietary and nutritional risk factors, the imprecision in methods for assessing nutrient and dietary status, and the differences among target groups and the objectives of recommendations proposed by many expert groups have all contributed to the variability in dietary guidelines. Furthermore, there has been insufficient documentation of the scientific bases underlying the conclusions and recommendations and the criteria used to derive them.

In recent years, the public has been confronted with a plethora of information on diet and its association with chronic diseases without guidance on how to separate fact from fallacy. The National Research Council's Food and Nutrition Board in the Commission on Life Sciences recognized this dilemma and the need to address the important issue of the role of diet in the etiology and prevention of the major causes of morbidity and mortality in the United States. In 1984, the Board established the Committee on Diet and Health to undertake a comprehensive analysis of the scientific literature on diet and the spectrum of major chronic diseases and to evaluate the criteria used to assess the strength of the evidence on associations of diet with health. This report is the result of this critical and detailed analysis and is the first of a systematic series of reports to be issued in a pattern similar to the Board's *Recommended Dietary Allowances* (RDAs)—a periodic review that provides guidelines on the desirable amounts of essential nutrients in the diet.

The three major objectives of this study were:

• to develop criteria for systematically evaluating the scientific evidence relating dietary components, foods, food groups, and dietary patterns to the maintenance of health and to the reduction of risk of chronic disease;

• to use these criteria to assess the scientific evidence relating these same factors (dietary components, foods, food groups, and dietary patterns) to health and to the reduction of chronic disease risk; and

• on the basis of this assessment, to propose dietary guidelines for maintaining health and reducing chronic disease risk, to suggest directions for future research, and to provide the basis for periodic updates of the literature and guidelines as new information on diet and health is acquired.

The 19-member interdisciplinary committee appointed to conduct the study was assisted by one adviser and two Food and Nutrition Board liaison members. Collectively, the Committee on Diet and Health included expertise in such disciplines as biochemistry, biostatistics, clinical medicine, epidemiology, foods and food consumption patterns, human genetics, metabolism, various aspects of nutrition, public health, and toxicology. During the course of the study, the committee examined data on the association between diet, health, and chronic disease, focusing on coronary heart disease, peripheral arterial disease, stroke, hypertension, cancer, obesity, osteoporosis, diabetes mellitus, hepatobiliary disease, and dental caries. Whenever possible, the committee looked directly at primary sources of data contained in the literature. Works of other evaluative bodies, for example, the *Surgeon General's Report on Nutrition and Health* published in 1988 and *Dietary Guidelines for Americans* published in 1985 by the Departments of Agriculture and Health and Human Services, were important secondary sources of information. By drawing from the vast and diverse epidemiologic and laboratory data base, the committee has attempted to ensure a comprehensive and critical review. Thus, the conclusions and recommendations throughout this report are supported by a detailed discussion of the basis underlying them.

The committee held 13 meetings during which it evaluated the literature and prepared its general review and summary. A public meeting convened at the outset of the study served as a forum for open discussion and presentation of views and information by the public and by representatives of the food industry, consumer groups, and scientists.

In the early stages of the study, the committee conducted five workshops during which it interacted with and shared the expertise and research findings of a larger community of scientists. These workshops provided committee members an opportunity to consider new or controversial data and all valid scientific points of view and to identify gaps in knowledge. The subjects considered in the workshops included the role of vitamins, minerals, and trace elements in chronic disease risk; the importance of genetic factors in selected diet-related chronic diseases; the association of energy, fiber, and carbohydrates with chronic disease; pediatric diet and the risk of adult chronic disease; and criteria for formulating dietary guidelines.

The committee's report is presented in four parts. Part I (Introduction, Definitions, and Methodology) offers four introductory chapters in addition to the Executive Summary (Chapter 1). These chapters highlight the methods and criteria used by the committee as well as the major conclusions and dietary recommendations, their bases, and their implications. Chapter 2 presents the criteria for evaluating the evidence linking diet and chronic disease. The strengths and weaknesses of methodologies for assessing dietary intake as well as those of specific kinds of studies (both human and animal) designed to assess diet–health relationships are reviewed. Trends in, and assessment of, food consumption patterns and the nutritional status of the U.S. population are discussed in Chapter 3. In Chapter 4, the committee discusses the role of genetics in nutrition and how genetic and environmental factors interact to influence diet-associated risks of chronic disease. Chapter 5 presents the rationale for selecting the major diet-related chronic diseases addressed in this report and provides an overview of the extent and distribution of those diseases in the United States. In Part II of this report (Evidence on Dietary Components and Chronic Diseases), the criteria described in Chapter 2 provide the basis of a review of the evidence by *nutrients*. The 13 chapters in that section (6 through 18) summarize the epidemiologic, clinical, and laboratory data pertaining to each nutrient or dietary factor and the chronic diseases identified by the committee. Nutrient interactions and mechanisms of action are discussed where applicable. Part III (Impact of Dietary Patterns on Chronic Diseases) briefly reassembles the evidence relating nutrients to specific chronic diseases or conditions and comments on the importance of diet relative to nondietary risk factors in the etiology of those diseases. Part IV (Overall Assessment, Conclusions, and Recommendations) contains two chapters. Chapter 27 presents the committee's conclusions, along with a summary of the process, criteria, and scientific bases underlying them. Chapter 28 presents the committee's dietary recommendations and the rationales for each, as well as a detailed discussion of how the recommendations compare to those issued in the past by other expert groups and the bases for similarities and dissimilarities among these. Also contained in this section is an in-depth discussion of the potential risks and public health benefits of the committee's dietary recommendations.

The committee hopes this report will be a useful resource document for scientists in academia and industry, for the general public, and for policymakers. Furthermore, it believes that the nine dietary recommendations presented in Chapter 28 and in the Executive Summary (Chapter 1) can be implemented within the framework of the current U.S. lifestyle. Collaboration among government agencies, the food industry, health professionals (physicians, nutritionists, dietitians, and public health personnel), educational institutions, leaders in mass media, and the general public is encouraged to attain this goal.

The committee greatly appreciates the hard work and organization provided by the Food and Nutrition Board staff headed by Dr. Sushma Palmer and consisting of Drs. Christopher Howson, Farid Ahmed, and Susan Berkow, Mrs. Frances Peter, Mr. Aldon Griffis, Ms. Marian Millstone, Ms. Dorothy Majewski, Ms. Avis Harris, Ms. Michelle Smith, and Mrs. Elsie Sturgis.

The committee is also greatly indebted to Dr. Charles Lieber of the Bronx Veterans Administration Medical Center for his major contribution to the chapter on alcohol and to the many people who served as consultants, as advisers, and in other resource capacities. Many of these people drafted manuscripts for consideration by the committee, presented their views at the public meeting, or upon request, commented on drafts, presented data, or engaged in discussions during committee meetings, conferences, or workshops. Specifically, the committee expresses its thanks to Dr. Norman Bell, Veterans Administration Medical Center, Charleston; Dr. Peter Bennett, National Institutes of Health; Dr. Gerald Berenson, Louisiana State University Medical School; Dr. Jan Breslow, Rockefeller University; Dr. Raymond Burk, University of Texas Health Sciences Center; Dr. Ritva Butrum, National Institutes of Health; Dr. Tim Byers, State University of New York; Dr. T. Colin Campbell, Cornell University; Dr. James Carlos, National Institute of Dental Research; Dr. Marie Cassidy, George Washington University; Dr. George Christakis, University of Miami School of Medicine; Dr. Charles Davidson, Massachusetts

Institute of Technology; Dr. William Dietz, New England Medical Center; Dr. Jean Durlach, Hospital Cochin; Dr. Johanna Dwyer, Francis Stern Nutrition Center; Dr. S. Boyd Eaton, Emory University; Dr. R. Curtis Ellison, University of Massachusetts Medical Center; Dr. Gail Eyssen, University of Toronto; Dr. L. Jack Filer, Jr., Executive Director of the International Life Sciences Institute–Nutrition Foundation; Dr. Michael Goldblatt, McDonald's Corporation; Dr. Clifford Grobstein, University of California, San Diego; Dr. Scott Grundy, University of Texas Health Sciences Center; Dr. Suzanne Harris, Deputy Assistant Secretary for Food and Consumer Services; Dr. Robert Heaney, Creighton University; Dr. Dwight Heath, Brown University; Dr. D. Mark Hegsted, Harvard University; Dr. Richard Hillman, Washington University Medical School; Dr. Paul Hochstein, University of California; Dr. Michael Holick, Tufts Human Nutrition Research Center; Dr. Paul Hopper, General Foods Corporation; Dr. Edward Horton, University of Vermont; Dr. Thomas Hostetter, University of Minnesota; Dr. Michael Jacobson, Center for Science in the Public Interest; Dr. Norman Kaplan, University of Texas; Dr. Carl Keen, University of California, Davis; Dr. Ahmed Kissebah, University of Wisconsin; Dr. Leslie Klevay, USDA–Human Nutrition Research Center; Dr. David Klurfeld, Wistar Institute; Dr. William Knowler, National Institutes of Health; Dr. Stephen Krane, Harvard University Medical School; Dr. Peter Kwiterovich, Johns Hopkins University; Dr. Orville Levander, USDA–Human Nutrition Research Center; Dr. A. Harold Lubin, American Medical Association; Dr. Lawrence Machlin, Hoffman–La-Roche, Inc.; Dr. Aaron Marcus, New York Veterans Administration Medical Center; Dr. Alvin Mauer, University of Tennessee; Dr. Paul McCay, Oklahoma Medical Research Foundation; Dr. Janet McDonald, Food and Drug Administration; Dr. J. Michael McGinnis, Department of Health and Human Services; Dr. Donald McNamara, University of Arizona; Dr. Judy Miller, Indiana University School of Medicine; Dr. John Milner, University of Illinois; Dr. William Mitch, Emory University School of Medicine; Dr. Curtis Morris, University of California, San Francisco; Dr. Janice Neville, Case Western Reserve University; Dr. Ralph Paffenberger, Stanford University; Mr. Richard Peto, University of Oxford; Dr. Ernesto Pollitt, University of California, Davis; Dr. Gerry Reaven, Stanford University; Dr. Floyd Rector, University of California, San Francisco; Dr.

Lawrence Resnick, New York Hospital–Cornell Medical Center; Dr. Irwin Rosenberg, Tufts University; Dr. Paul Saltman, University of California, San Diego; Dr. Raymond Schucker, Food and Drug Administration; Dr. William Schull, University of Texas; Dr. Noel Solomons, Institute of Nutrition of Central America and Panama; Dr. Charles Sing, University of Michigan Medical School; Dr. Michael Stern, University of Texas Health Science Center; Dr. Ira Tabas, Columbia University; Dr. Paul R. Thomas, Institute of Medicine; Dr. Michael Tuck, University of California, Los Angeles; Dr. Myron Weinberger, Indiana University; Dr. Sidney Weinhouse, Temple University School of Medicine; Ms. Clair Wilson, Council for Research Planning in Biological Sciences and the Vegetarian Society of D.C.; Dr. Richard Wurtman, Massachusetts Institute of Technology; and Dr. Catherine Woteki, National Center for Health Statistics.

Finally, the committee would like to thank the staff of the library of the National Academy of Sciences for their invaluable assistance in preparing this report and the staff of the National Academy Press, especially Chief Manuscript Editor Richard Morris, who herded this volume through production. Special acknowledgment is due to Dr. Richard J. Havel, Chairman of the Food and Nutrition Board, and other board members for their expert advice, oversight, and constant encouragement over the course of this 3.5-year study.

ARNO G. MOTULSKY
Chairman
Committee on Diet and Health

Contents

PART III:
IMPACT OF DIETARY PATTERNS ON CHRONIC DISEASES

PART IV:
OVERALL ASSESSMENT, CONCLUSIONS,
AND RECOMMENDATIONS

DIET

AND

HEALTH

PART I

Introduction, Definitions, and Methodology

1

Executive Summary

The twentieth century has witnessed noticeable shifts in the direction of nutrition programs, policy, and research in industrialized nations—from identification and prevention of nutrient deficiency diseases in the first three decades of the century to refinement and application of knowledge of nutrient requirements in the subsequent two decades. In the second half of the century, emphasis on nutrient deficiency diseases decreased as the major causes of mortality shifted from infectious to chronic diseases. Attention then turned to investigating the role of diet in the maintenance of health and the reduction of the risk of such chronic diseases as heart disease and cancer. Subsequently, epidemiologic, clinical, and laboratory research demonstrated that diet is one of the many important factors involved in the etiology of these diseases. During the past few decades, scientists have been faced with the challenge of identifying dietary factors that influence specific diseases and defining their pathophysiological mechanisms. Simultaneously, public health policymakers, the food industry, consumer groups, and others have been debating how much and what kind of evidence justifies giving dietary advice to the public and how best to mitigate risk factors on which there is general agreement among scientists.

PURPOSE, APPROACH, AND SCOPE OF THE STUDY

This study on diet, chronic diseases, and health was launched in an effort to address the scientific issues that are fundamental to nutrition policy on reducing the risk of these diseases. The Committee on Diet and Health was appointed to conduct the study within the Food and Nutrition Board of the National Research Council's Commission on Life Sciences. The committee began with the understanding that lack of consensus on the role of diet in the etiology of chronic diseases derived partly from incomplete knowledge and partly from the absence of generally accepted criteria for interpreting the evidence. It also noted that the totality of the evidence relating dietary components to the entire spectrum of major chronic diseases had yet to be examined systematically. Several reports issued to date have addressed many issues of public health importance. However, most have not been sufficiently comprehensive and have not crossed the boundary separating the simple assessment of dietary risk factors for single chronic diseases from the complex task of determining how these risk factors influence the entire spectrum of chronic diseases—atherosclerotic cardiovascular diseases, cancer, diabetes, obesity, osteoporosis, dental caries, and chronic liver and kidney diseases.

3

This report attempts to cross that boundary. It complements the recent *Surgeon General's Report on Nutrition and Health* and other efforts of government agencies and voluntary health and scientific organizations by providing an in-depth analysis of the overall relationship between diet and the full spectrum of major chronic diseases.

In this report, the committee reviews the evidence regarding all major chronic public health conditions that diet is believed to influence. It draws conclusions about the effects of nutrients, foods, and dietary patterns on health, proposes dietary recommendations that have the potential for diminishing risk, and estimates their public health impact.

The committee focuses on risk reduction rather than on management of clinically manifest disease. It recognizes, however, that the distinction between *prevention* or *risk reduction* and *treatment* may be blurred in conditions where dietary modification might delay the onset of clinical diseases (e.g., the cardiovascular complications in diabetes mellitus) or might slow the progression of impaired function; therefore, conditions such as these are addressed, but only briefly. The committee defined risk reduction broadly to include decreased morbidity as well as mortality from chronic diseases and believes that consideration should be given to dietary modification to reduce the risk for both. The difficulty of quantifying the role of diet in the etiology of chronic diseases and the potential public health impact of dietary modification are discussed in Chapters 2 and 28.

In Chapter 2, the committee presents criteria for assessing the data from single studies and explains its procedure for evaluating the overall evidence. Special attention is given to the role of nutrient interactions and to the assessment of benefits and risks in arriving at conclusions and formulating dietary recommendations. Throughout the report, the committee recognizes that genetically dependent variability among individuals, and variability due to age, sex, and physiological status, may all affect physiological requirements for nutrients, responses to dietary exposures, the risk of chronic diseases, and consequently the effectiveness of dietary recommendations in reducing the risk of chronic diseases. The report addresses in detail the risks that apply to the general population and comments on the feasibility of defining risks for subpopulations and individuals with different susceptibilities. Finally, the committee discusses the limitations of data on diet-disease relationships, emphasizes the necessarily interim nature of its

conclusions and recommendations, and proposes directions for research.

CRITERIA FOR ASSESSMENT

The strengths and weaknesses of different kinds of clinical, epidemiologic, and laboratory studies and the methodologies for dietary assessment are reviewed in Chapter 2. To the extent possible, the committee evaluated data from studies in humans as well as in animals. It noted that ecological correlations of dietary factors and chronic diseases among human populations provide valuable data but cannot be used alone to estimate the strength of the association between diet and diseases. The effect of diet on chronic diseases has been most consistently demonstrated in comparisons of populations with substantially different dietary practices, possibly because it is more difficult to identify such associations within a population whose diet is fairly homogeneous. Thus in general, associations within populations based on case-control and prospective cohort studies underestimate the association. In intervention studies, long exposure is usually required for the effect of diet on chronic disease risk to be manifested. Furthermore, the strict criteria for selecting participants in such studies may result in more homogeneous study samples, which limit the applicability of results to the general population. Despite the limitations of various types of studies in humans, the committee concluded that repeated and consistent findings of an association between certain dietary factors and diseases are likely to be real and indicative of a cause-and-effect relationship.

Experiments on dietary exposure of different animal strains can take genetic variability into account and permit more intensive observation. However, extrapolation of data from animal studies to humans is limited by the ability of animal models to simulate human diseases and the comparability of absorption and metabolic phenomena among species. The committee placed more confidence in data derived from studies on more than one animal species or test system, on results that have been reproduced in different laboratories, and on data that indicate a dose-response relationship.

The committee concluded that assessments of the strength of associations between diet and chronic diseases cannot simply be governed by criteria commonly used for inferring causality in other areas of human health. Faced with the special characteristics of studies on nutrients, dietary patterns, and chronic diseases, the committee first assessed the strengths and weaknesses of each kind of study and then evaluated the total evidence against six criteria: strength of association, dose-response relationship, temporally correct association, consistency of association, specificity of association, and biologic plausibility. Finally, it assessed the overall strength of the evidence on a continuum from highly likely to very inconclusive. Overall, the strength, consistency, and preponderance of data and the degree of concordance in epidemiologic, clinical, and laboratory evidence determined the strength of the conclusions in this report.

Integration of the Overall Evidence

In Section II of this report, Evidence on Dietary Components and Chronic Diseases (Chapters 6 through 18), the committee uses the approach described briefly above and more fully in Chapter 2. Throughout this section, the committee considers the epidemiologic, clinical, and experimental data pertaining to each nutrient or dietary factor and specific chronic diseases, including cardiovascular diseases, specific cancers, diabetes, hypertension, obesity, osteoporosis, hepatobiliary disease, and dental caries. Nutrient interactions and mechanisms of action are discussed where applicable.

In Section III, Impact of Dietary Patterns on Chronic Diseases, the evidence relating nutrients to specific chronic diseases and diet-related conditions is briefly reassembled and leads to the committee's conclusions on the role of dietary patterns in the etiology of the diseases and assessment of the potential for reducing their frequency and severity. These conclusions are drawn directly from the research data, where the evidence pertains to dietary patterns or foods and food groups, or from extrapolations from the evidence on individual nutrients. In its overall review and integration of the evidence, the committee moved from a consideration of individual nutrients to foods, to food groups, and then to dietary patterns as they relate to the spectrum of chronic diseases.

CRITERIA AND PROCESS FOR FORMULATING DIETARY RECOMMENDATIONS

Absolute proof is difficult to obtain in any branch of science. As evidence accumulates, however, it often reaches the point of proof in an operational sense, even though proof in an abso-

lute sense may be lacking. In law, proof beyond a reasonable doubt is generally accepted as a standard for making decisions and taking action. The degree of evidence as well as the severity of the crime are the bases for the relative intrusiveness of legal actions taken, e.g., issuing a warning for a misdemeanor compared to the imposition of severe penalties for a felony.

A similar paradigm can be applied to evidence on dietary patterns and associated health risks. For example, public education might be sufficient to warn against the potential hazard of excess caffeine intake, whereas evidence on the toxicity and carcinogenicity of aflatoxin warrants government regulation to curtail aflatoxin contamination of grains and milk. The strength of the evidence might not be the only relevant criterion for determining the course of action; other factors include the likelihood and severity of an adverse effect, potential benefits of avoiding the hazard, and the feasibility of reducing exposure.

Much remains to be learned about the impact of diet on chronic disease risk. Nonetheless, in accordance with this paradigm, the committee concluded that the overall evidence regarding a relationship between certain dietary patterns (e.g., a diet high in total fat and saturated fat) and chronic diseases (e.g., cardiovascular diseases and certain cancers) supports (1) a comprehensive effort to inform the public about the likelihood of certain risks and the possible benefits of dietary modification and (2) the use of technological and other means (e.g., production of leaner animal products) to facilitate dietary change.

Assessing Risks and Benefits

The committee hopes to contribute to knowledge about the process of arriving at dietary recommendations by documenting the considerations and the logic that underlie its dietary recommendations. An essential step in developing dietary recommendations for overall health maintenance is the synthesis of recommendations pertaining to single diseases into a single coherent set of recommendations to reduce the overall risk of diet-related chronic diseases. For example, recommendations to enhance calcium intake for possible protection against osteoporosis might, in isolation, be viewed as conflicting with recommendations for coronary heart disease, because dairy products—which contribute the most calcium to the U.S. diet—are also rich sources of saturated fats, which increase coronary heart disease risk. Thus, recommendations for maintaining adequate bone mass as well as for preventing coronary disease would logically stress consumption of low-fat dairy products.

The committee also considered the synergistic and antagonistic effects of dietary interactions. For example, the potential benefits of encouraging adequate trace element intake for reducing the risk of certain cancers could in principle be offset by a recommendation to increase vegetable intake for the possible prevention of colon cancer, because high plant food diets are also high in fiber, which could initially inhibit absorption of certain trace elements. To a large extent, the task of assessing such potential competing risks and benefits and nutrient interactions was simplified by an inherent consistency in dietary recommendations to maintain good health. For example, the advisability of consuming a diet low in saturated fatty acids, total fat, and cholesterol is supported by strong evidence of potential benefit in reducing the risk of cardiovascular diseases as well as comparatively weaker evidence that low-fat diets decrease the risk of certain kinds of cancers.

Other Considerations

The committee also considered whether to base recommendations on individual nutrients, on single foods or food groups, or on overall pattern of dietary intake. Although recommendations based on nutrients or food groups are of value, in the committee's experience guidelines directed toward overall dietary patterns are the most useful because they address the total diet and are more easily interpreted by the general public. Moreover, because many studies on diet and chronic diseases in humans have focused on foods rather than on single nutrients, food-based recommendations may more accurately reflect current understanding about the relationship between chronic diseases and diet. Nonetheless, many of the diet-disease relationships examined required consideration of single foods, food groups, and specific nutrients. This is reflected in the committee's recommendations.

The committee agreed that quantitative guidelines should be proposed when warranted by the strength of the evidence and the potential importance of recommendations to public health. Such guidelines can take into account nutrient interactions, they are less susceptible to misinterpretation when translated into food choices, and they provide specific targets that can serve as a basis for

nutrition programs and policy. The committee has attempted to explain the degree of certainty warranted by the evidence and to make quantitative recommendations to the extent justified.

Recommendations for Individuals as Opposed to Populations

There are two complementary approaches to reducing risk factors in the target population. The first, the public health or population-based approach, is aimed at the general population, and the second, the high-risk or individual-based approach, is aimed at individuals with defined risk profiles. Most chronic diseases etiologically associated with nutritional factors (e.g., atherosclerotic cardiovascular diseases, hypertension, obesity, many cancers, osteoporosis, and diabetes mellitus) also have genetic determinants, and genetic-environmental interactions play an important role in determining disease outcome. For most diseases, however, it is not yet possible to identify susceptible genotypes and thus risks to specific individuals. Furthermore, the variability in nutrient requirements among individuals is not well defined. Therefore, it is usually not possible to make recommendations for individuals. On the other hand, because the major chronic disease burden falls on the general population (approximately 70% of all deaths in the U.S. population are due to cardiovascular diseases and cancer), the most benefit is likely to be achieved by a public-health prevention strategy to shift the distribution of dietary risk factors by means of dietary recommendations to reduce chronic disease risk in the general population.

The public health approach to prevention recognizes that even though reduction of risk for individuals with average risk profiles (e.g., an average serum cholesterol level) might be small or negligible, because these people represent the great majority of the population, the benefit for the total population is likely to be paradoxically large (e.g., because most coronary deaths occur among those who have only moderate elevations in serum cholesterol levels). However, when it is possible to identify high-risk persons, such as those with certain hyperlipidemias, special attention can be directed to their management. Therefore, in the committee's judgment, an effective prevention strategy should be aimed at the general public and, where knowledge permits, it should be complemented with recommendations for those at high risk.

MAJOR CONCLUSIONS AND THEIR BASES

The committee analyzed trends in the major chronic diseases as well as in eating patterns (Chapters 3 and 5). It reviewed the epidemiologic, clinical, and laboratory evidence pertaining to dietary factors and chronic diseases (Chapters 6 through 26) and attempted to put into perspective the role of diet as it relates to other environmental and genetic factors in the etiology of these diseases (Chapters 4 and 5).

Following are the general conclusions drawn from the committee's in-depth review, as well as the specific conclusions pertaining to the major dietary components and specific chronic diseases.

General Conclusions

• A comprehensive review of the epidemiologic, clinical, and laboratory evidence indicates that diet influences the risk of several major chronic diseases. The evidence is very strong for atherosclerotic cardiovascular diseases and hypertension and is highly suggestive for certain forms of cancer (especially cancers of the esophagus, stomach, large bowel, breast, lung, and prostate). Furthermore, certain dietary patterns predispose to dental caries and chronic liver disease, and a positive energy balance produces obesity and increases the risk of noninsulin-dependent diabetes mellitus. However, the evidence is not sufficient for drawing conclusions about the influence of dietary patterns on osteoporosis and chronic renal disease.

• Most chronic diseases in which nutritional factors play a role also have genetic and other environmental determinants, but not all the environmental risk factors have been clearly characterized and susceptible genotypes usually have not been identified. Furthermore, the mechanisms of genetic and environmental interactions involved in disease are not fully understood. It is evident that dietary patterns are important factors in the etiology of several major chronic diseases and that dietary modifications can reduce such risks. Nevertheless, for most diseases, it is not yet possible to provide quantitative estimates of the overall risks and benefits.

Fats, Other Lipids, and High-Fat Diets

The following conclusions derive from the committee's extensive review of the data described in Chapters 6 (Calories), 7 (Fats and Other Lipids), 19 (Atherosclerotic Cardiovascular Diseases), 21 (Obesity and Eating Disorders), 22 (Cancer), and 25 (Hepatobiliary Disease).

General Conclusion

• There is clear evidence that the total amounts and types of fats and other lipids in the diet influence the risk of atherosclerotic cardiovascular diseases and, to a less well-established extent, certain forms of cancer and possibly obesity. The evidence that the intake of saturated fatty acids and cholesterol are causally related to atherosclerotic cardiovascular diseases is especially strong and convincing.

Total Fats

• In several types of epidemiologic studies, a high-fat intake is associated with increased risk of certain cancers, especially cancers of the colon, prostate, and breast. The epidemiologic evidence is not totally consistent, but it is supported by experiments in animals. The combined epidemiologic and laboratory evidence suggests that a reduction of total fat intake is likely to decrease the risk of these cancers.

• High-fat intake is associated with the development of obesity in animals and possibly in humans. In short-term clinical studies, a marked reduction in the percentage of calories derived from dietary fat has been associated with weight loss.

• Although gallbladder disease is associated with obesity, there is no conclusive evidence that it is associated with fat intake.

• Intake of total fat per se, independent of the relative content of the different types of fatty acids, is not associated with high blood cholesterol levels and coronary heart disease. A reduction in total fat consumption, however, facilitates reduction of saturated fatty acid intake; hence, in addition to reducing the risk of certain cancers, and possibly obesity, it is a rational part of a program aimed at reducing the risk of coronary heart disease.

Saturated Fatty Acids

• Clinical, animal, and epidemiologic studies demonstrate that increased intakes of saturated fatty acids (12 to 16 carbon atoms in length) increase the levels of serum total and low-density-lipoprotein (LDL) cholesterol and that these higher levels in turn lead to atherosclerosis and increase the risk of coronary heart disease. Saturated fatty acid intake is the major dietary determinant of the serum total cholesterol and LDL cholesterol levels in populations and thereby of coronary heart disease risk in populations. Lowering saturated fatty acid intake is likely to reduce serum total and LDL cholesterol levels and, consequently, coronary heart disease risk.

• The few epidemiologic studies on dietary fat and cancer that have distinguished between the effects of specific types of fat indicate that higher intakes of saturated fat as well as total fats are associated with a higher incidence of and mortality from cancers of the colon, prostate, and breast. In general, these findings are supported by data from animal experiments.

Polyunsaturated Fatty Acids

• Clinical and animal studies provide firm evidence that omega-6 polyunsaturated fatty acids when substituted for saturated fatty acids result in a lowering of serum total cholesterol and LDL cholesterol and usually also some lowering of high-density-lipoprotein (HDL) cholesterol levels.

• Laboratory studies in rodents suggest that diets with high levels of vegetable oils containing omega-6 polyunsaturated fatty acids promote certain cancers more effectively than diets with high levels of saturated fats, whereas there is some evidence that diets with a high content of omega-3 polyunsaturated fatty acids may inhibit these same cancers. However, these findings are not supported by the limited number of epidemiologic studies that have distinguished between the effects of different types of fat. There are no human diets that naturally have very high levels of total polyunsaturated fatty acids, and there is no information about the long-term consequences of high polyunsaturated fatty acid intakes.

• Fish oils containing large amounts of omega-3 polyunsaturated fatty acids reduce plasma triglyceride levels and increase blood clotting time. Their effects on LDL cholesterol vary, and data on the long-term health effects of large doses of omega-3 polyunsaturated fatty acids are limited. Limited epidemiologic data suggest that consumption of one or two servings of fish per week is associated with a lower coronary heart disease risk, but the evidence is not sufficient to ascertain whether the association is causal or related to the omega-3 polyunsaturated fatty acid content of fish.

Monounsaturated Fatty Acids

• Clinical studies indicate that substitution of monounsaturated for saturated fatty acids results in a reduction of serum total cholesterol and LDL cholesterol without a reduction in HDL cholesterol.

Dietary Cholesterol

• Clinical, animal, and epidemiologic studies indicate that dietary cholesterol raises serum total cholesterol and LDL cholesterol levels and increases the risk of atherosclerosis and coronary heart disease. There is substantial inter- and intra-individual variability in this response. High dietary cholesterol clearly seems to contribute to the development of atherosclerosis and increased coronary heart disease risk in the population.

Trans Fatty Acids

• Clinical studies indicate that trans fatty acids and their cis isomers have similar effects on plasma lipids. Animal studies do not indicate that trans fatty acids have a greater tumor-promoting effect than their cis isomers.

Carbohydrates, Vegetables, Fruits, Grains, Legumes, and Cereals and Their Constituents

The committee's conclusions on carbohydrates and foods containing complex carbohydrates—i.e., vegetables, fruits, grains, legumes, and cereal products—derive from a review of direct and indirect evidence throughout the report, especially in Chapters 9 (Carbohydrates), 10 (Dietary Fiber), 11 (Fat-Soluble Vitamins), 12 (Water-Soluble Vitamins), and 22 (Cancer).

• Diets high in plant foods—i.e., fruits, vegetables, legumes, and whole-grain cereals—are associated with a lower occurrence of coronary heart disease and cancers of the lung, colon, esophagus, and stomach. Although the mechanisms underlying these effects are not fully understood, the inverse association with coronary heart disease may be largely explained by the usually low saturated fatty acid and cholesterol content of such diets. Such diets are also low in total fat, which is directly associated with the risk of certain cancers, but rich in complex carbohydrates (starches and fiber) and certain vitamins, minerals, trace elements, and nonnutritive constituents, and these factors probably also confer protection against certain cancers and coronary heart disease.

• Compared to nonvegetarians, complete vegetarians and lacto-ovovegetarians have lower serum levels of total and LDL cholesterol and triglycerides. These lower levels may be the combined result of lower intakes of saturated fatty acids and total fat and higher intakes of water-soluble fiber (e.g., pectin and oat bran). In clinical and animal studies, such fiber has been found to produce small reductions in serum total cholesterol independently of the effect due to fat reduction.

• Populations consuming high-carbohydrate diets, which are high in plant foods, have a comparatively lower prevalence of noninsulin-dependent diabetes mellitus, possibly because of the higher proportion of complex carbohydrate intake and lower prevalence of obesity—a risk factor for noninsulin-dependent diabetes mellitus. In clinical studies, such diets have been shown to improve glucose tolerance and insulin sensitivity.

• Epidemiologic studies indicate that consumption of carotenoid-rich foods, and possibly serum carotene concentration, are inversely associated with the risk of lung cancer.

• Laboratory studies in animals strongly and consistently indicate that certain retinoids prevent, suppress, or retard the growth of chemically induced cancers at a number of sites, including the esophagus, pancreas, and colon, but especially the skin, breast, and bladder. However, most epidemiologic studies do not show an association between preformed vitamin A and cancer risk or a relationship between plasma retinol level and cancer risk.

• Epidemiologic studies suggest that vitamin C-containing foods such as citrus fruits and vegetables may offer protection against stomach cancer, and animal experiments indicate that vitamin C itself can protect against nitrosamine-induced stomach cancer. The evidence linking vitamin C or foods containing that vitamin to other cancer sites is more limited and less consistent.

• Some investigators have postulated that several other vitamins (notably vitamin E, folic acid, riboflavin, and vitamin B_{12}) may block the initiation or promotion of cancer, but the committee judged the evidence too limited to draw any conclusions.

• Epidemiologic and clinical studies indicate that a diet characterized by high-fiber foods may be associated with a lower risk of coronary heart disease, colon cancer, diabetes mellitus, diverticulosis, hypertension, or gallstone formation, but there is no conclusive evidence that it is dietary fiber, rather than the other components of vegetables, fruits, and cereal products, that reduces the risk of those diseases. Although soluble fibers can decrease serum cholesterol and glucose levels, and certain insoluble fibers inhibit chemically induced tumorigenesis, it is difficult to compare the effects of specific dietary fibers tested in the laboratory

with the effects of fiber-containing foods or of other potentially protective substances present in these foods.

• Although human and animal studies indicate that all fermentable carbohydrates can cause dental caries, sucrose appears to be the most cariogenic. The cariogenicity of foods containing fermentable carbohydrates is influenced by the consistency and texture (e.g., stickiness) of the food as well as by the frequency and sequence of consumption. Sugar consumption (by those with an adequate diet) has not been established as a risk factor for any chronic disease other than dental caries in humans.

Protein and High-Protein Diets

Studies of the association of protein and high-protein diets with chronic diseases are reviewed in Chapters 8 (Protein), 13 (Minerals), 19 (Atherosclerotic Cardiovascular Diseases), 22 (Cancer), and 23 (Osteoporosis) and form the basis of the following major conclusions.

• In intercountry correlation studies, diets high in meat—a major source of animal protein—have a strong positive association with increased atherosclerotic coronary artery disease and certain cancers, notably breast and colon cancer. Such diets are often characterized by a high content of saturated fatty acids and cholesterol, which probably accounts for a large part of the association with coronary heart disease, and by a high content of total fat, which is directly associated with the risk of these cancers. However, these diets also tend to have low levels of plant foods, the consumption of which is inversely associated in epidemiologic and animal studies with the risk of heart disease and certain cancers. Total serum cholesterol can be reduced in people with high blood cholesterol by replacing animal foods in their diet with plant foods.

• High protein intake can lead to increased urinary calcium excretion. The impact of this finding on the development of osteoporosis in the general population is unclear.

• The data linking elevated intakes of animal protein to increased risk of hypertension and stroke are weak, and no plausible mechanisms have been posited for either effect.

Energy

The following conclusions are based on assessment of the roles of energy intake and expenditure in chronic disease risk as described in Chapters 6 (Calories) and Chapter 21 (Obesity and Eating Disorders).

• Positive energy balance can result from increased energy intake, reduced energy expenditure, or both, and over the long term, can lead to obesity and its associated complications.

• Although data from clinical and animal studies demonstrate that overfeeding leads to obesity, increased body weight in cross-sectional and longitudinal population surveys of adults cannot be accounted for by increased energy intake. Thus, it is likely that obesity develops in adult life either because of reduced physical activity, or overfeeding, or both. Obesity is enhanced not only by this energy imbalance but also by a genetic predisposition to obesity and altered metabolic efficiency.

• Epidemiologic studies indicate that increased energy expenditure is inversely associated with the risk of coronary heart disease.

• Epidemiologic and clinical studies and some experiments in animals demonstrate that obesity is associated with an increased risk of noninsulin-dependent diabetes mellitus, hypertension, gallbladder disease, endometrial cancer, and osteoarthritis. It may also be associated with a higher risk of coronary heart disease and postmenopausal breast cancer.

• Studies in humans suggest that fat deposits in the abdominal region pose a higher risk of noninsulin-dependent diabetes mellitus, coronary heart disease, stroke, hypertension, and increased mortality than do fat deposits in the gluteal or femoral regions.

• Experience in long-term management of obesity indicates that neither frequent fluctuations in body weight nor extreme restrictions of food intake are desirable.

• Long-term follow-up studies indicate that extreme leanness is associated with increased mortality and that the causes of mortality are different from those associated with excess weight.

• The specific causes of obesity are not well known, although some obese people clearly consume more energy compared to people of normal weight, whereas others are very sedentary or may have increased metabolic efficiency. Compared to maintenance of stable weight, weight gain in adult life is associated with a greater risk of cardiovascular disease, noninsulin-dependent diabetes mellitus, hypertension, gallbladder disease, and endometrial cancer. Certain risk factors—e.g., high serum cholesterol, elevated serum glucose, and high blood pressure—can be curtailed by weight reduction in overweight adults.

Alcoholic Beverages

The extensive data on the health effects of alcohol consumption are examined in Chapters 16 (Alcohol), 19 (Atherosclerotic Cardiovascular Diseases), 20 (Hypertension), 22 (Cancer), and 25 (Hepatobiliary Disease). Following are the committee's major conclusions related to alcohol.

• When consumed in excess amounts, alcohol replaces essential nutrients including protein and micronutrients and can lead to multiple nutrient deficiencies.

• Sustained, heavy intake of alcoholic beverages leads to fatty liver, alcoholic hepatitis, and cirrhosis. It also increases the risk of cancers of the oral cavity, pharynx, esophagus, and larynx, especially in combination with cigarette smoking, whereupon the effects on cancer risk become synergistic. There is some epidemiologic evidence that alcohol consumption is also associated with primary liver cancer and that moderate beer drinking is associated with rectal cancer. The association of alcohol consumption with increased risk of pancreatic or breast cancer is less clear.

• Excessive alcohol consumption is associated with an increased incidence of coronary heart disease, hypertension, stroke, and osteoporosis.

• Alcohol consumption during pregnancy can damage the fetus, cause low infant birth weight, and lead to fetal alcohol syndrome. No safe level of alcohol intake during pregnancy has been determined.

Salt and Related Compounds

The following conclusions derive from the evidence on salt and related compounds and their relation to chronic diseases. This evidence is reviewed in Chapters 15 (Electrolytes), 20 (Hypertension), and 22 (Cancer).

• Blood pressure levels are strongly and positively correlated with the habitual intake of salt. In populations with a sustained salt intake of 6 g or more per day, blood pressure rises with age and hypertension is frequent, whereas in populations consuming less than 4.5 g of salt per day, the age-related rise in blood pressure is slight or absent and the frequency of hypertension is uniformly low. Clinical studies demonstrate that once hypertension is established, it cannot always be fully corrected by resumption of a moderately low (<4.5 g/day) salt intake.

• Although clinical and epidemiologic studies indicate that some people are more susceptible to salt-induced hypertension than others, there are no reliable markers to predict individual responses. Epidemiologic evidence suggests that blacks, people with a family history of hypertension, and all those over age 55 are at a higher risk of hypertension.

• Epidemiologic and animal studies indicate that the risk of stroke-related deaths is inversely related to potassium intake over the entire range of blood pressures, and the relationship appears to be dose dependent. The combination of a low-sodium, high-potassium intake is associated with the lowest blood pressure levels and the lowest frequency of stroke in individuals and populations. Although the effects of reducing sodium intake and increasing potassium intake would vary and may be small in some individuals, the estimated reduction in stroke-related mortality for the population is large.

• A high salt intake is associated with atrophic gastritis in epidemiologic and animal studies, and there is also epidemiologic evidence that a high salt intake and frequent consumption of salt-cured and salt-pickled foods are associated with an elevated incidence of gastric cancer. The specific causative agents in these foods have not been fully identified.

Minerals and Trace Elements

The conclusions listed below are based on a review of the evidence on calcium, magnesium, trace elements, and chronic diseases discussed in Chapters 13 (Minerals), 14 (Trace Elements), 20 (Hypertension), 22 (Cancer), and 23 (Osteoporosis).

• Epidemiologic, clinical, and animal studies suggest that sustained low calcium intake is associated with a high frequency of fractures in adults, but the role of dietary calcium in the development of osteoporosis and the potential benefits of calcium supplements—in amounts that exceed the Recommended Dietary Allowances (RDAs)—in decreasing the risk of osteoporosis are unclear.

• Some epidemiologic studies have shown an association between calcium intake and blood pressure, but a causal association between low calcium intake and high blood pressure has not been established.

• A few data from epidemiologic and animal studies suggest that a high calcium intake may

protect against colon cancer, but the evidence is preliminary and inconclusive.

• Unequivocal evidence from epidemiologic and clinical studies indicates that fluoridation of drinking water supplies at a level of 1 ppm protects against dental caries. Such concentrations are not associated with any known adverse health effects, including cancer.

• Low selenium intake in epidemiologic and animal studies and low selenium levels in human sera have been associated with an increased risk of several cancers. Moreover, some studies in animals suggest that diets supplemented with large doses of selenium offer protection against certain cancers. These data should be extrapolated to humans with caution, however, because high doses of selenium can be toxic.

• The data on most trace elements examined in this report (e.g., copper and cadmium) are too limited or weak to permit any conclusions about their effects on chronic disease risk.

Dietary Supplements

Claims for the health benefits of dietary supplements have drawn substantial attention in recent decades. The committee has reached the following conclusion on the basis of the evidence reviewed in Chapter 18 (Dietary Supplements).

• A large percentage of people in the United States take dietary supplements, but not necessarily because of nutrient needs. The adverse effects of large doses of certain nutrients (e.g., vitamin A) are well documented. There are no documented reports that daily multiple vitamin-mineral supplements, equaling no more than the RDA for a particular nutrient, are either beneficial or harmful for the general population. The potential risks or benefits of the long-term use of small doses of supplements have not been systematically examined.

Coffee, Tea, and Other Nonnutritive Dietary Components

The following major conclusions pertaining to coffee, tea, and other nonnutritive dietary components are based on a review of the evidence in Chapter 17 (Coffee, Tea, and Other Nonnutritive Dietary Components).

• Coffee consumption has been associated with slight elevations in serum cholesterol in some epidemiologic studies. Epidemiologic evidence linking coffee consumption to the risk of coronary heart disease and cancer in humans is weak and inconsistent.

• Tea drinking has not been associated with an increased risk of any chronic disease in humans.

• The use of such food additives as saccharin, butylated hydroxyanisole, and butylated hydroxytoluene does not appear to have contributed to the overall risk of cancer in humans. However, this lack of evidence may be due to the relatively recent use of many of these substances or to the inability of epidemiologic techniques to detect the effects of additives against the background of common cancers from other causes. The association between food additives and cancer is also complicated by the long latency period between initial exposure to a carcinogen and the subsequent development of cancer.

• A number of environmental contaminants (e.g., some organochlorine pesticides, polychlorinated biphenyls, and polycyclic aromatic hydrocarbons) cause cancer in laboratory animals. The committee found no evidence to suggest that any of these compounds *individually* makes a major contribution to the risk of cancer in humans; however, the risks from simultaneous exposure to several compounds and the potential for adverse effects in occupationally exposed people have not been adequately investigated.

• Certain naturally occurring contaminants in food (e.g., aflatoxins and *N*-nitroso compounds) and nonnutritive constituents (e.g., hydrazines in mushrooms) are carcinogenic in animals and thus pose a potential risk of cancer in humans. Naturally occurring compounds shown to be carcinogenic in animals have been found in small amounts in the average U.S. diet. There is no evidence thus far that any of these substances *individually* makes a major contribution to cancer risk in the United States.

• Most mutagens detected in foods have not been adequately tested for carcinogenic activity. Although mutagenic substances are generally suspected of having carcinogenic potential, it is not yet possible to assess their contribution to the incidence of cancer in the United States.

• Overall, there is a shortage of data on the complete range of nonnutritive substances in the diet. Thus, no reliable estimates can be made of the most significant exposures. Exposure to nonnutritive chemicals individually, in the minute quantities normally present in the average diet, is unlikely to make a major contribution to the overall cancer risk to humans in the United States. The risk from simultaneous exposure to many such compounds cannot be quantified on the basis of current evidence.

THE COMMITTEE'S DIETARY RECOMMENDATIONS

The dietary recommendations of the Committee on Diet and Health, given below, are directed to healthy, North American adults and children. Wherever evidence permits, the committee attempts to identify the special dietary needs of population subgroups at high risk for specific diseases or with different dietary requirements because of age, sex, or physiological status. The special dietary needs of the elderly are largely unknown.

As discussed in Chapter 28, the quantities proposed in the committee's recommendations are goals for intake by *individuals*. To achieve these goals, the mean intake by the *population* (the public health goal) would have to be higher or lower than the recommended intake for individuals, depending on the direction of the proposed dietary modification. For example, a recommendation that all *individuals* should reduce their fat intake to 30% or less of calories can be expected to lead to a population mean intake substantially *below* 30% of calories from fat. Similarly, a recommendation that individuals increase their carbohydrate intake to more than 55% of total calories can be expected to lead to a population mean intake clearly above 55% of calories from carbohydrates. Thus, the guidelines for individuals differ somewhat from the public health (population) goals, which need to be more stringent in order to achieve the goals for individuals.

The extent to which the public health goal for a nutrient differs from the goal for individuals in the population will depend on the distribution of intake for that nutrient in the population. In most cases, however, the variation in nutrient intakes in the population is not well known.

The recommendations in this report are the product of a systematic and extensive analysis of the literature by a multidisciplinary committee that considered the criteria and the process for arriving at recommendations and documented the extensive literature on which they are based. They are generally in agreement with the advice provided by other expert panels in the United States and abroad, although in most cases they include more specific quantitative recommendations. These recommendations are appropriate for current patterns of dietary intake and disease morbidity and mortality in the United States and are based on conclusions regarding the association of dietary factors with the entire spectrum of chronic diseases. They take into account competing risks for different diseases as well as nutrient interactions. These recommendations should be reexamined as new knowledge is acquired and as the patterns of morbidity and mortality change over the next decades.

The committee's recommendations are presented in a logical sequence that also reflects a general order of importance. For example, all dietary macrocomponents are addressed first. Among these, highest priority is given to reducing fat intake, because the scientific evidence concerning dietary fats and other lipids and human health is strongest and the likely impact on public health the greatest. Lower priority is given to recommendations on other dietary components, because they are derived from weaker evidence or because the public health impact is likely to be comparatively less. Where the evidence is strongest, the committee presents quantitative recommendations. It recognizes that setting specific quantitative goals is somewhat arbitrary and is based on informed judgment rather than on scientifically derivable formulas; however, quantification facilitates translation of goals into dietary patterns and food choices. Goals are needed to develop and evaluate programs aimed at achieving dietary changes and serve as the basis for regulatory actions such as those relating to food labeling and the validity of health claims for foods and nutrients.

The committee's recommendations derive from an assessment of the evidence on chronic diseases, but should be used in combination with the RDAs to achieve an optimal and highly desirable dietary pattern for the maintenance of good health. In the committee's judgment, these recommendations have the potential for a substantial reduction in the risk of diet-related chronic diseases in the general population.

• *Reduce total fat intake to 30% or less of calories. Reduce saturated fatty acid intake to less than 10% of calories, and the intake of cholesterol to less than 300 mg daily. The intake of fat and cholesterol can be reduced by substituting fish, poultry without skin, lean meats, and low- or nonfat dairy products for fatty meats and whole-milk dairy products; by choosing more vegetables, fruits, cereals, and legumes; and by limiting oils, fats, egg yolks, and fried and other fatty foods.*

A large and convincing body of evidence from studies in humans and laboratory animals shows that diets low in saturated fatty acids and choles-

terol are associated with low risks and rates of atherosclerotic cardiovascular diseases. High-fat diets are also linked to a high incidence of some types of cancer and, probably, obesity. Thus, reducing total fat and saturated fatty acid intake is likely to lower the rates of these chronic diseases. Fat intake should be reduced by curtailing the major sources of dietary fats rather than by eliminating whole categories of foods. For example, by substituting fish, poultry without skin, lean meats, and low- or nonfat dairy products for high-fat foods, one can lower total fat and saturated fatty acid intake while ensuring an adequate intake of iron and calcium—two nutrients of special importance to women. Dietary fat can also be reduced by limiting intake of fried foods, baked goods containing high levels of fat, and spreads and dressings containing fats and oils.

Different types of fatty acids have different effects on health. Saturated fatty acids and dietary cholesterol tend to increase total and LDL serum cholesterol and, consequently, the risk of cardiovascular disease. The extent of this activity differs among saturated fatty acids; palmitic, myristic, and lauric acids have the greatest cholesterol-raising effect. The main dietary sources of these cholesterol-raising saturated fatty acids are dairy and meat products and some vegetable oils, such as coconut, palm, and palm-kernel oils. Dietary cholesterol is found mainly in egg yolks, certain shellfish, organ meats, and, to a lesser extent, in other meats and dairy products. Thus, the intake of these foods should be curtailed.

Monounsaturated fatty acids are found in a variety of foods but are especially abundant in olive oil and canola oil. Polyunsaturated fatty acids are of two types—omega-6 and omega-3; both are essential nutrients and cannot be synthesized endogenously. Omega-6 polyunsaturated fatty acids are common in several plant oils, including corn, safflower, soybean, and sunflower oils. Omega-3 polyunsaturated fatty acids are found in cold-water marine fish (such as salmon and mackerel) and in some plant oils (e.g., soybean and canola oils). Omega-6 polyunsaturated fatty acids and monounsaturated fatty acids (and carbohydrates) lower LDL cholesterol when substituted for saturated fatty acids. Omega-3 polyunsaturated fatty acids also lower LDL-cholesterol when substituted for saturated fatty acids, but they are more effective in lowering elevated serum triglyceride levels. Although consumption of fish one or more times a week has been associated with a reduced risk of coronary heart disease, the committee does not recommend the use of concentrated fish oil supplements, because there is insufficient evidence that they are beneficial and the absence of long-term adverse effects has not been established.

The evidence linking high-fat diets to increased cancer risk is less persuasive than that associating saturated fatty acids and dietary cholesterol to coronary heart disease, but the weight of evidence indicates that high-fat diets are associated with a higher risk of several cancers, especially of the colon, prostate, and breast. Most evidence from studies in humans suggests that total fat or saturated fatty acids adversely affect cancer risk. No studies in humans have yet examined the benefits of changing to low-fat diets; however, such evidence exists from experiments in animals. The combined evidence from epidemiologic and laboratory studies suggests that reduction of total fat is likely to reduce the risk of these cancers.

Epidemiologic data on the possible association of low serum cholesterol levels with an increased incidence of and mortality from cancer in general or colon cancer in men in particular are inconsistent and do not suggest a causal association. Rather, they indicate that the lower serum cholesterol levels in some of these studies were in part the consequence of undetected cancers. The overall evidence indicates that dietary modification to lower serum total cholesterol and coronary heart disease risk is likely to reduce the risk of colon cancer without increasing the risk of other cancers.

Animal studies also suggest that high-fat diets may lead to obesity, possibly because dietary fat is converted to body fat more efficiently than are other sources of calories. Short-term clinical studies in humans indicate that a substantial reduction in fat intake may be accompanied by weight loss; however, reduced caloric intake was observed in some of these reports and although not specifically noted is likely to have occurred in others. This indicates that a substantial reduction in fat intake may result in overall caloric reduction, perhaps because of the caloric density of dietary fat. From a public health perspective, this phenomenon may be important, regardless of whether fat reduction per se results in weight loss or whether weight loss results from an overall reduction in caloric intake.

In the committee's judgment, concerns that reduced fat intake may curtail intake of meats and dairy products and thus limit intakes of iron and calcium by women and children or that young children on reduced-fat diets might not obtain adequate calories to support optimal growth and development are not justified. Fat intake can be reduced to approximately 30% of calories without risk of nutrient deficiency, and this level of fat intake after infancy has not been associated with any detrimental effects. Furthermore, adequate caloric intake can readily be maintained in children on diets containing 30% of calories from fat.

Although the committee recommends that the total fat intake of individuals be 30% or less of calories, there is evidence that further reduction in fat intake may confer even greater health benefits. However, the recommended levels are more likely to be adopted by the public because they can be achieved without drastic changes in usual dietary patterns and without undue risk of nutrient deficiency. Furthermore, they permit gradual adaptation to lower-fat diets as more lower-fat foods become available on the market. The committee recommends that people who should not lose weight should compensate for the caloric loss resulting from decreased fat intake by consuming greater amounts of foods containing complex carbohydrates (e.g., vegetables, certain fruits, legumes, and whole-grain cereal products).

Although the committee recommends that saturated fatty acid intake be maintained at less than 10% of total calories by individuals, it is highly likely that further reduction, to 8 or 7% of calories or lower, would confer greater health benefits. Such further reductions can best be achieved by substituting additional complex carbohydrates and monounsaturated for saturated fatty acids in the diet. Larger reductions in cholesterol intakes—e.g., to 250 or 200 mg or even less per day—may also confer health benefits.

The committee recommends that the polyunsaturated fatty acid intake of individuals not exceed 10% of total calories and that polyunsaturated fatty acid intake in the population be maintained at current levels in the U.S. diet, i.e., an average of approximately 7% of total calories. (The requirement for omega-6 polyunsaturated fatty acids can be met by 1 to 2% of calories as linoleic acid.) Concern that an increase in polyunsaturated fatty acid intake may increase risk of certain cancers derives primarily from studies of animals on very-high-polyunsaturated fatty acid diets. Given the absence of human diets naturally very high in total polyunsaturated fatty acids and the lack of information about the long-term consequences of high polyunsaturated fatty acid intake (see Chapter 7), it seems prudent to recommend that polyunsaturated fatty acid intake not be increased above the current average in the U.S. population. However, since most of the polyunsaturated fatty acids in the current U.S. diet are of the omega-6 rather than the omega-3 type, and since the committee's recommendation is directed mainly at omega-6 polyunsaturated fatty acids, any increase in total polyunsaturated fatty acid resulting from an increase in foods containing omega-3 polyunsaturated fatty acids (e.g., by eating more fish containing such fatty acids) is reasonable.

• *Every day eat five or more servings* of a combination of vegetables and fruits, especially green and yellow vegetables and citrus fruits. Also, increase intake of starches and other complex carbohydrates by eating six or more daily servings of a combination of breads, cereals, and legumes.*

The committee recommends that the intake of carbohydrates be increased to more than 55% of total calories by increasing primarily complex carbohydrates. Fats and carbohydrates are the two major sources of calories in the diet. National food consumption surveys indicate that the content of the average U.S. diet is high in fat and low in complex carbohydrates (e.g., starches, vegetables, legumes, breads, cereals, and certain fruits). Green and yellow vegetables; fruits, especially citrus fruits; legumes; and whole-grain cereals and breads, which constitute a small portion of the present U.S. diet, generally contain low levels of fat; thus, they are good substitutes for fatty foods and good sources of several vitamins, minerals, complex carbohydrates, and dietary fiber. The recommended number of servings is derived from experience in planning nutritionally balanced diets that would meet the committee's dietary recommendations. The amounts recommended would facilitate an increase in the total carbohydrate and complex carbohydrate content of the diet, make up for the caloric deficit due to fat reduction, and supply sufficient quantities of essential vitamins and minerals. The committee does not recommend increasing the intake of added sugars, because their consumption is strongly associated with dental caries, and, although they are a source of calories for those who may need additional calories, they provide no nutrients. Furthermore, foods high in added sugars (e.g., desserts and baked goods) are generally also high in fat.

Studies in various parts of the world indicate that people who habitually consume a diet high in

plant foods have low risks of atherosclerotic cardiovascular diseases, probably largely because such diets are usually low in animal fat and cholesterol, both of which are established risk factors for atherosclerotic cardiovascular diseases. Some constituents of plant foods, e.g., soluble fiber and vegetable protein, may also contribute—to a lesser extent—to the lower risk of atherosclerotic cardiovascular diseases. The mechanism for the link between frequent consumption of vegetables and fruits, especially green and yellow vegetables and citrus fruits, and decreased susceptibility to cancers of the lung, stomach, and large intestine is not well understood because the responsible agents in these foods and the mechanisms for their protective effect have not been fully determined. However, there is strong evidence that a low intake of carotenoids, which are present in green and yellow vegetables, contributes to an increased risk of lung cancer. Fruits and vegetables also contain high levels of fiber, but there is no conclusive evidence that the dietary fiber itself, rather than other nutritive and nonnutritive components of these foods, exerts a protective effect against these cancers. The committee does not recommend the use of fiber supplements.

Vegetables and fruits are also good sources of potassium. A diet containing approximately 75 mEq of potassium (i.e., approximately 3.5 g of elemental potassium) daily may contribute to reduced risk of stroke, which is especially common among blacks and older people of all races. Potassium supplements are neither necessary nor recommended for the general population.

• *Maintain protein intake at moderate levels.*

Protein is an essential nutrient, and protein-containing foods are important sources of essential amino acids in the diet. However, because there are no known benefits and possibly some risks in consuming diets with a high animal protein content, the committee recommends that protein intake not be increased to compensate for the caloric loss that would result from the recommended reduction in fat intake. In general, average protein intake by adults in the United States considerably exceeds the RDA, which is 0.8 g/kg of desirable body weight for adults. The committee recommends maintaining total protein intake at levels lower than twice the RDA for all age groups (e.g., less than 1.6 g/kg body weight for adults).

Increased risks of certain cancers and coronary heart disease have been associated in some epidemiologic studies with diets high in meat and, as a

---

*An average serving is equal to a half cup for most fresh or cooked vegetables, fruits, dry or cooked cereals and legumes, one medium piece of fresh fruit, one slice of bread, or one roll or muffin.

consequence, in animal protein, and with high protein intake alone in laboratory studies. It is not known whether these adverse effects are due solely to the usually high total-fat, saturated fatty acid, and cholesterol content of diets that are rich in meat or animal protein, or to what extent protein per se or other factors also contribute. High protein intake may also lead to increased urinary calcium loss.

The committee is aware of concerns among some scientists that animal protein restriction might curtail the ability of some population subgroups with habitually lower protein intakes (e.g., women and the elderly) to meet the RDA for certain other essential nutrients such as iron. However, the recommendation to maintain intake below twice the RDA for all age groups would require no reduction of current average intakes in the United States. The committee does not recommend against eating meat; rather, it recommends consuming lean meat in smaller and fewer portions than is customary in the United States.

- *Balance food intake and physical activity to maintain appropriate body weight.*

Excess weight is associated with an increased risk of several chronic disorders, including noninsulin-dependent diabetes mellitus, hypertension, coronary heart disease, gallbladder disease, osteoarthritis, and endometrial cancer. The risks appear to decline following a sustained reduction in weight. Increased abdominal fat carries a higher risk for these disorders than do comparable fat deposits in the hips and thighs. New standards for healthy body composition take into account such differences in regional body fat distribution as well as weight-to-height ratios. Neither large fluctuations in body weight nor extreme restrictions in food intake are desirable.

In the U.S. population and other westernized societies, body weight and body mass index are increasing while the overall caloric intake of the population is decreasing. These trends as well as the association of moderate, regular physical activity with reduced risks of heart disease lead to the committee's recommendation that the U.S. population increase its physical activity level and that all healthy people maintain physical activity at a moderately active level, improve physical fitness, and moderate their food intake to maintain appropriate body weight. For adult men and women of normal weight, this will also allow the ingestion of adequate calories to meet all known nutrient needs. Overweight people should increase their physical activity and reduce their caloric intake, and people with a family history of obesity should avoid calorically dense foods and select low-fat foods.

- *The committee does not recommend alcohol consumption. For those who drink alcoholic beverages, the committee recommends limiting consumption to the equivalent of less than 1 ounce of pure alcohol in a single day. This is the equivalent of two cans of beer, two small glasses of wine, or two average cocktails. Pregnant women should avoid alcoholic beverages.*

Excessive alcohol drinking increases the risk of heart disease, high blood pressure, chronic liver disease, some forms of cancer, neurological diseases, nutritional deficiencies, and many other disorders. Even moderate drinking carries some risk in circumstances that require neuromotor coordination and judgment, e.g., driving vehicles, working around machinery, and piloting airplanes or boats. Consumption of even small amounts of alcohol can lead to dependence. Approximately 10% of those who consume alcoholic beverages in the United States are alcoholics. Pregnant women and women who are attempting to conceive should avoid alcoholic beverages because there is a risk of damage to the fetus and no safe level of alcohol intake during pregnancy has been established.

Although several studies show that moderate alcohol drinking is associated with a lower coronary heart disease risk, it would be unwise to recommend moderate drinking for those who do not drink because, in the committee's judgment, a causal association has not been established and because even moderate drinking poses certain other risks, including the risk of alcohol addiction.

- *Limit total daily intake of salt (sodium chloride) to 6 g or less. Limit the use of salt in cooking and avoid adding it to food at the table. Salty, highly processed salty, salt-preserved, and salt-pickled foods should be consumed sparingly.*

Studies in human populations in different parts of the world show that a diet containing more than 6 g of salt per day is associated with elevated blood pressure, and many Americans habitually exceed this level. It is probable that susceptibility to salt-induced hypertension (salt sensitivity) is genetically determined, but no reliable genetic marker has yet been identified. Thus, those who are most susceptible to developing salt-induced hypertension, and therefore likely to benefit most from this recommendation, cannot yet be identified. In salt-sensitive people, the recommended level of salt intake is unlikely to contribute to blood pressure elevation and may even lead to blood pressure reduction. In the general population, the recommended level will have no detrimental effect. The committee is aware that a greater reduction in salt intake (i.e., to 4.5 g or less) would probably confer greater health benefits than its present recommendation, but chose 6 g as an initial goal that can be achieved more readily. This does not preclude a subsequent recommendation for further reduction.

The evidence linking salt intake per se to stomach cancer is less persuasive than that for salt and hypertension. There is consistent evidence, however, that frequent consumption of salt-preserved or salt-pickled foods increases the risk of stomach cancer. The specific causative agents in those foods have not been identified.

• *Maintain adequate calcium intake.*

Calcium is an essential nutrient; it is necessary for adequate growth and skeletal development. Certain segments of the population, especially women, because of their low caloric intake, and adolescents, because of their higher nutrient requirements, need to make careful food choices to obtain adequate calcium from the food supply. The committee recommends consumption of low- or nonfat dairy products and dark-green vegetables, which are rich sources of calcium and can assist in maintaining calcium intake at approximately RDA levels. Although low calcium intake is associated with a higher frequency of fractures and possibly with high blood pressure, the potential benefits of calcium intakes above the RDAs to prevent osteoporosis or hypertension are not well documented and do not justify the use of calcium supplements.

• *Avoid taking dietary supplements in excess of the RDA in any one day.*

A large percentage of the U.S. population consumes some vitamin or mineral supplement daily. The supplements are often self-prescribed and not based on known nutrient deficiencies. It is not known what, if any, benefits or risks accrue to individuals or the general population from taking small doses of supplements. Some population subgroups (e.g., those suffering from malabsorption syndromes) may require supplements, but they should take them only under professional supervision. A single daily dose of a multiple vitamin-mineral supplement containing 100% of the RDA is not known to be harmful or beneficial; however, vitamin–mineral supplements that exceed the RDA and other supplements (such as protein

powders, single amino acids, fiber, and lecithin) not only have no known health benefits for the population but their use may be detrimental to health. The desirable way for the general public to obtain recommended levels of nutrients is by eating a variety of foods.

Thus, the committee supports the general scientific opinion and the opinions of several other expert panels that have recently commented specifically on supplement use. It emphasizes, however, that the long-term health effects (risks and benefits) of supplements have not been adequately studied.

• *Maintain an optimal intake of fluoride, particularly during the years of primary and secondary tooth formation and growth.*

There is convincing evidence that consumption of optimally fluoridated water (i.e., 0.7 to 1.2 ppm fluoride, depending on ambient temperature) significantly reduces the risk of dental caries in people of all ages, especially in children during the years of primary and secondary tooth formation and growth. There is no evidence that such fluoride concentrations have any adverse effects on health, including cancer risk. In the absence of optimally fluoridated water, the committee supports the use of dietary fluoride supplements in the amounts generally recommended by the American Dental Association, the American Academy of Pediatrics, and the American Academy of Pediatric Dentistry.

IMPLICATIONS OF RECOMMENDATIONS FOR FOOD CHOICES

What do the committee's recommendations imply with regard to selection of foods and food groups? To some extent, this issue is addressed under each recommendation. Therefore, only a synthesis is provided here. Principles of food selection will also be explained in more detail in the committee's forthcoming report to the general public.

In summary, the diet recommended by the committee should contain moderately low levels of fat, with special emphasis on restriction of saturated fatty acids and cholesterol; high levels of complex carbohydrates; only moderate levels of protein, especially animal protein; and only low levels of added sugars. Caloric intake and physical activity should be balanced to maintain appropriate body weight. The recommendation to maintain total fat intake at or below 30% of total caloric intake and saturated fatty acid intake at less than 10%, combined with the recommendation to maintain protein intake only at moderate levels, means that for most North Americans it will be necessary to select leaner cuts of meat, trim off excess fat, remove skin from poultry, and consume fewer and smaller portions of meat and poultry. Fish and many shellfish are excellent sources of low-fat protein. By using plant products (e.g., cereals and legumes) instead of animal products as sources of protein, one can also reduce the amount of saturated fatty acids and cholesterol in the diet.

Dairy products are an important source of calcium and protein, but whole milk, whole-milk cheeses, yogurt, ice cream, and other milk products are also high in saturated fatty acids. Therefore, low-fat or skim milk products should be substituted. Furthermore, it is desirable to change from butter to margarine with a low saturated fatty acid content, to use less oils and fats in cooking and in salad dressings, and to avoid fried foods.

For most people, the recommended restriction of fat intake, coupled with the recommendation for moderation in protein intake, implies an increase in calories from carbohydrates. These calories should come from an increased intake of whole-grain cereals and breads rather than from foods or drinks containing added sugars. For example, bakery goods, such as pies, pastries, and cookies, although they provide complex carbohydrates also tend to contain high levels of total fat, saturated fatty acids, and added sugars, all of which need to be curtailed to meet the committee's recommendations.

In general, vegetables and fruits are unlikely to contribute substantially to caloric intake but are major sources of vitamins, minerals, and dietary fiber. The committee places special emphasis on increasing consumption of green and yellow vegetables as well as citrus fruits, particularly since their consumption in North America is relatively low. The committee's recommendations would lead to a substantial increase in consumption frequency and portion sizes, especially of vegetables, for the average person. Thorough washing of fresh vegetables (especially leafy ones) and fruits will minimize the consumption of pesticide residues in the diet.

The need for restriction of certain dietary components—such as egg yolks; salt; salty, smoked, and preserved foods; and alcoholic beverages—is clearly explained in the recommendations. Further considerations include methods of preparation, cooking, and processing, which can have impor-

tant effects on the composition of foods. The committee emphasizes the need to read the labels on prepared, formulated, and other processed foods to identify their contribution of nutrients in general and of salt, fats and cholesterol, and sugars in particular. With regard to the risk of chronic diseases, maximum benefit can be attained and any unknown, potentially harmful effects of dietary constituents minimized by selecting a variety of foods from each food group, avoiding excessive caloric intake (especially excessive intake of any one item or food group), and engaging regularly in moderate physical exercise.

IMPACT ON PUBLIC HEALTH: BENEFITS AND RISKS OF DIETARY MODIFICATION

The committee used several approaches and lines of evidence to assess potential adverse consequences of its dietary recommendations for the general population (see Chapter 28). For example, it examined the degree of concordance in death rates and mortality trends between the two leading diet-related causes of death—i.e., coronary heart disease and cancer—to assess the degree to which common dietary risk and protective factors may be operating. It also analyzed the possible adverse consequences of reducing the intake of total fat, saturated fatty acids, and cholesterol, which would lead to a reduction in serum cholesterol levels and in the risk of atherosclerotic cardiovascular disease.

In some studies, low serum cholesterol is associated with increased colon cancer mortality. However, this finding is inconsistent and the data do not suggest that lowering serum cholesterol by dietary modification would increase the risk of any cancer. Furthermore, the committee considered the effect of reducing total serum cholesterol on increasing risk of hemorrhagic stroke in hypertensives; the possible adverse effects of increased intakes of polyunsaturated fatty acids, carbohydrates, vegetables, and carotene and of moderate intakes of alcohol (as opposed to total avoidance); the effect of potential increases in exposure to pesticides; and the potential for nutrient deficiencies or toxicity among population subgroups (see Chapter 28). It concluded that despite using the worst-case hypothetical scenarios, the benefits of dietary modification far outweigh the potential for adverse effects, which is minimal if any, as summarized below.

The lines of evidence examined in Chapter 28 indicate that risk factors and protective characteristics for the major diet-related chronic diseases and causes of death are concordant. In general, dietary intervention to reduce the risk of one disease (e.g., coronary heart disease) is also likely to reduce the risk of other diseases (e.g., several cancers).

Central to the committee's deliberations was the extent to which the overall risk of chronic diseases in the general U.S. population might be reduced by dietary modification. Because the role of dietary factors in the etiology of chronic diseases differs by factor and disease (see Major Conclusions), the impact of dietary modification on the risk of different diseases is likely to vary considerably.

As discussed in Chapter 28, the committee used several approaches in developing quantitative estimates of the potential public health impact if its dietary recommendations were to be fully adopted by the public. It recognized at the outset that the accuracy of such estimates is determined by the strength, consistency, and congruence of the evidence from a variety of sources, especially from extensive, long-term observations and dietary interventions in human populations, which provide the most reliable estimates of association. The best of these data pertain to serum cholesterol levels and the risk of coronary heart disease; those on dietary factors as they relate to coronary heart disease, cancer, and other major causes of mortality are not as extensive.

Estimates of the reduction of coronary heart disease risk in human populations can be derived by extrapolating the effects of a downward shift in average serum cholesterol levels, by comparing coronary heart disease risk in populations with greatly different saturated fatty acid or total fat intakes or wide ranges in mean serum cholesterol levels, or by examining the results of serum-cholesterol-lowering trials on cardiovascular disease incidence. The many drawbacks to these approaches are explained in Chapter 28. In general, however, by using these approaches, the committee estimates that its recommendations for reducing intake of saturated fatty acids, dietary cholesterol, and total fat could lead to at least a 10% reduction in serum cholesterol levels and a 20% reduction in coronary heart disease risk in the United States beyond the 1987 levels. More stringent dietary modification provides the potential for even greater reduction in coronary disease risk in the future. This underestimates the potential benefits of dietary modification because it only focuses on certain lipids and does not take into account

the potential benefits of reductions in body weight and blood pressure in the population.

The picture is less clear for the risk of cancer and other chronic diseases. Some epidemiologists estimate that as much as 90% of all cancer in humans can be attributed to various environmental factors, including diet. Others attribute 30 to 40% of cancers in men and 60% of cancers in women to diet. Still others have estimated that 10 to 70% of the deaths from cancer could be prevented by dietary modifications, especially for cancers of the stomach, the large bowel, and to a lesser extent, the breast, the endometrium, and the lung.

The conclusions of the Committee on Diet and Health are in general agreement with those of the National Research Council's Committee on Diet, Nutrition, and Cancer, which in 1982 concluded that cancers of most major sites are influenced by dietary patterns. The data are not sufficient, however, to quantify the contribution of diet to the overall cancer risk or to determine the quantitative reduction in risk that might be achieved by dietary modifications. The committee notes that several countries with dietary patterns similar to those recommended in this report have about half the U.S. rates for diet-associated cancers. This suggests that the committee's dietary recommendations could have a substantial impact on reducing the risk of cancer in the United States.

For the other chronic diseases and conditions considered in this report (i.e., hypertension, obesity, osteoporosis, diabetes mellitus, hepatobiliary disease, and to a lesser extent, dental caries), the magnitude of risk reduction expected through full implementation of the committee's guidelines on diet and health cannot be reliably estimated at this time due to limitations in the data. Nevertheless, on the basis of its overall assessment of the data, the committee concludes that implementation of its dietary recommendations through readily available natural diets is likely to greatly reduce the overall risk of these chronic diseases without discernibly increasing the risk of any cause of death or disability.

In Chapter 28, the committee categorizes dietary factors according to the strength of the evidence and relates each to the risk of chronic diseases and the potential public health benefit of dietary modification. In the committee's judgment, modification of the total diet along the lines recommended in this report is necessary to achieve the maximum public health benefit; and among dietary factors, reduced intakes of total fat, saturated fatty acids, and cholesterol are likely to have the greatest impact.

IMPLEMENTATION OF DIETARY RECOMMENDATIONS

What strategies are needed to implement the committee's dietary recommendations, and what are their implications for different sectors of society? These issues are the subject of a separate study by the Food and Nutrition Board. Therefore, they only receive brief consideration below and in Chapter 28 of this report.

It is apparent to the committee and the Food and Nutrition Board that if one of our national goals is to reduce the risk of chronic diseases and if dietary modification is likely to assist in achieving that goal, then various sectors of society need to collaborate in implementing dietary recommendations of the type proposed by the committee. The committee is aware that many nutrition programs and regulatory actions that are already in place or under way under the auspices of government agencies and in the private sector are consistent with implementing the proposed recommendations. Nevertheless, it wishes to draw special attention to the following general issues.

A concerted effort will be needed to make the changes in the food supply and in nutrition policy and programs that will be required to increase the availability of low-fat and low-salt foods in supermarkets and in public eating facilities such as school cafeterias and restaurants. Consideration needs to be given to the most effective means of achieving such modification: through technological changes, massive public education efforts, legislative measures such as food labeling, or a combination of such strategies. Although the committee's report to the public, which will be issued in the near future, will explain its major conclusions and recommendations in lay terms, leaders in government agencies, the health professions, the food industry, and the mass media face the challenge of interpreting the committee's nine recommendations for the general public as well as for high-risk groups. They will need to convey in practical terms the concept of certainty or uncertainty of benefit, competing risks, dietary interactions, and target populations. There is a need to develop adequate educational tools and to identify the best means of educating and motivating the public. Health professionals, government agencies, and the industry must also undertake additional research to identify ways of effecting dietary change.

In the committee's judgment, it is feasible to implement the proposed recommendations within the framework of the average lifestyle in the United States, and the committee is encouraged by the knowledge that dietary habits in this country have already changed markedly in many ways that are consistent with these recommendations. To convey a full understanding of these recommendations to the public and to implement them will require close collaboration among government agencies, the food industry, health professionals (physicians, nutritionists, dietitians, and public health personnel), educational institutions, leaders in mass media, and the general public.

RESEARCH DIRECTIONS

Fundamental scientific discoveries generally occur in completely unexpected ways. Thus it is impossible to predict where the major discoveries will be made or which research directions will prove to be the most fruitful. Therefore, the committee does not wish to stifle creativity by specifying experimental protocols or directing research. Nevertheless, it is possible and desirable to propose a scheme for organizing research to seek more definitive data on the associations between diet and chronic diseases. The committee's conclusions and dietary recommendations reflect its assessment of current knowledge and actions justified now; they can be made more definitive only through additional research of the kind recommended in this section.

The seven categories of research proposed below are not presented in order of priority. Rather, taken together, they reflect a conceptual framework for interdisciplinary collaborative research that encompasses different kinds of investigations: short- and long-term experiments in vitro and in vivo, food consumption surveys, food composition analyses, descriptive and analytical epidemiologic studies, metabolic studies and clinical trials in humans, and social and behavioral research. More detailed and specific research recommendations are summarized in Chapter 28 and presented in Chapters 4 and 6 through 26.

• *Identification of foods and dietary components that alter the risk of chronic diseases and elucidation of their mechanisms of action.*

Much needed research falls in this category. Many dietary constituents are already known to play a role in the etiology of chronic diseases, but additional and more specific knowledge, especially concerning mechanisms of action, will lead to more definitive conclusions and provide more precise guidance about ways to reduce the risk of different chronic diseases.

• *Improvement of the methodology for collecting and assessing data on the exposure of humans to foods and dietary constituents that may alter the risk of chronic diseases.*

Methodological shortcomings inhibit the interpretation and analysis of data and often prevent the derivation of precise conclusions about the association of diet and chronic diseases. Thus, the committee recommends that high priority be given to development of better methods for data collection, quantification of dietary exposures and effects, and data analysis.

• *Identification of markers of exposure and early indicators of the risk of various chronic diseases.*

This category of research is designated for two purposes: first, to circumvent the shortcomings of using the disease itself as the sole end point—i.e., because of the long latency period of many chronic diseases evidenced by the delay between dietary exposure and disease expression; and second, to circumvent problems due to exposure misclassification when dietary recall methods are used. In the committee's judgment, there is a pressing need to identify biochemical/biological markers of dietary exposure, early biological markers that can forecast the emergence of clinical disease, and genetic markers that can identify high-risk subgroups in the population. In addition, the committee proposes greater use of the techniques of molecular biology to study gene–nutrient interactions that can help characterize individual variability in nutrient requirements and response to various chronic diseases.

• *Quantification of the adverse and beneficial effects of diet and determination of the optimal ranges of intake of dietary macro- and microconstituents that affect the risk of chronic diseases.*

Although most dietary constituents are known to have some effect on the risk of certain chronic diseases, much less is known about the magnitude of this effect. The committee believes that there is a strong need to quantify these effects in order to estimate the contribution of diet to the risk of chronic diseases. These efforts should include a study of nutrient interactions, competing risks, and dose-response relationships. The ultimate aim of such research should be to determine the opti-

mal ranges of intake of various dietary components for health maintenance, keeping in mind the desirability of identifying their effects and the shape of the dose-response curve.

• *Through intervention studies, assessment of the potential for chronic disease risk reduction.*

Carefully designed intervention studies should be conducted to assess the public health impact of dietary modification. Although many such studies have been conducted for heart disease, hypertension, dental caries, and obesity, and a few have focused on osteoporosis, no such long-term studies have yet been completed for cancer. The committee has considered whether priority should be given to additional large-scale trials or whether current knowledge is sufficient to undertake dietary interventions in the population and subsequently to assess their effectiveness by carefully monitoring trends in disease incidence and mortality.

Intervention trials should be undertaken only when a substantial body of data indicates a high likelihood of benefit without discernible risk. Such trials might be warranted to obtain more definitive data, especially because the kinds of diets tested in such trials might yield data about potential benefits of dietary intervention to simultaneously reduce the risk of multiple chronic diseases, but they should not be used as a basis for delaying prudent dietary modifications warranted by current knowledge. Any intervention studies should be accompanied by effective monitoring to assess disease incidence, prevalence, and mortality rates.

• *Application of knowledge about diet and chronic diseases to public health programs.*

Social and behavioral research should be undertaken to achieve a better understanding of factors that motivate people to modify their food habits. This knowledge is indispensable for designing effective public health programs to reduce the risk of chronic diseases. Furthermore, improved technologies are needed to increase the availability of foods that conform to the committee's dietary recommendations.

• *Expansion of basic research in molecular and cellular nutrition.*

The six categories described above focus on research to enhance knowledge of the interrelationship among dietary factors, chronic diseases, and health, and this research includes an understanding of the underlying mechanisms. The committee wishes to emphasize the need for such fundamental research to advance our knowledge of basic cellular and molecular mechanisms. Research in disciplines ranging from the physical sciences, to biochemistry, physiology, applied biology, nutrition, medicine, epidemiology, biophysics, cellular and molecular biology, and genetics is needed to fill the gaps in our understanding of how dietary, environmental, and genetic factors interact to influence the risk of chronic diseases.

The committee hopes that the findings contained in this report will be as widely disseminated as possible and urges that all those with an interest in and responsibility for public health participate in this effort. Recognizing the limitations of current knowledge, it strongly believes that periodic updates of its findings will be necessary as new data emerge to shed more light on associations between diet and chronic diseases.

2

Methodological Considerations in Evaluating the Evidence

Many factors affect the validity of scientific data on the effects of diet on human health. The most straightforward way to study such relationships is to select a group of subjects, collect relevant data on dietary intake and health indications for each person in the group, and attempt to determine causal relations between the two based on clues from such other sources as feeding studies in animals. This direct approach is rarely possible because of limitations in our ability to accurately quantify dietary intake and because of the many unknowns about the direct effect of diet on health and chronic diseases relative to the effects of other environmental and genetic variables. Thus, indirect approaches are commonly required. The first part of this chapter addresses various approaches to the assessment of dietary intake by humans. The second part deals with the evaluation of all types of single studies relevant to assessing the impact of dietary intake on health. In the third part of the chapter, the committee considers criteria for drawing inferences about causality from the evidence as a whole.

ASSESSMENT OF DIETARY INTAKE OF HUMANS

Methods for Assessing Dietary Intake

A major impediment in studying the effects of diet on health is the difficulty of assessing dietary intake of humans (Bazzarre and Myers, 1980; Bingham, 1987; Block, 1982; Burk and Pao, 1976; Dwyer, 1988; Marr, 1971; Medlin and Skinner, 1988; Pekkarinen, 1970; Sorenson, 1982; Young and Trulson, 1960). Each of the assessment methods in use has its weaknesses. The choice of method depends on whether the assessment pertains to the average intake of a group or to the habitual intakes of individuals within a group, the level of detail (e.g., food groups, foods, or nutrients) desired, and the degree of precision needed in determining amounts of foods consumed. Additional considerations include the costs, burden on respondents, and availability of critical resources such as trained interviewers and accurate food composition tables. The chosen dietary intake assessment method must be tested to ensure its accuracy and reliability in the study population, and adequate training of personnel involved in collecting and analyzing data is essential. In certain circumstances, dietary survey methods can be combined to improve accuracy (Dwyer, 1988). Methods commonly used in epidemiologic research to assess dietary intake are discussed below, along with their advantages, disadvantages, and problems of validation.

Group Dietary Data

In most nations, average dietary intake is estimated from national food supply data or from

23

national surveys of food intake by households or individuals. Food supply is estimated by adding the quantity of food imported to the quantity produced within a country and then subtracting the sum of food exported, destroyed by pests during storage, and put to nonfood use (e.g., in the production of industrial alcohol). The final figure is divided by the total population to obtain the average per-capita food availability. The results are estimates of foods that disappear into wholesale and retail markets; they fail to account for food wasted before consumption, food fed to pets, and home-grown foods (when the latter is not included in production data). Nutrients available in the food supply are usually estimated from standard food composition tables.

Data on per-capita food availability provide useful leads for further research on the relationship of diet to disease, because they enable investigators to compare rates of chronic diseases among countries with marked differences in mortality rates from chronic diseases and in the availability of specific nutrients in their food supply. These cross-sectional comparisons do not control for confounding factors, nor can they be used to show associations between diet and disease in individuals. The food supply in the United States has been monitored by the U.S. Department of Agriculture (USDA) since 1909, and the information gathered has been used to estimate trends in food use (see Chapter 3).

In household food inventories, food consumed is estimated by recording the difference between inventories of foods on hand at the beginning and end of the study period—usually 1 week—and accounting for food purchased or otherwise brought into the house. Average per-capita intake is estimated by dividing total household food intake by the number of people in that home.

Per-capita intakes by different age–sex groups in U.S. households are provided by national surveys conducted by USDA (USDA, 1984, 1987) and the U.S. Department of Health and Human Services (Carroll et al., 1983). These are also discussed in Chapter 3.

Individual Dietary Data

Food supply data and household food inventories supply only rough estimates of foods available and cannot be used to determine intakes of individuals. Methods most often used to assess individual intakes are food records and dietary recalls, both of which include diet histories and food frequency questionnaires.

The *food record* method requires participants to measure and record types and amounts of all foods and drinks consumed over a specified time. In some studies, all foods are weighed. In others, measuring cups and spoons and a ruler are used to assess dimensions. Food models, volume models, and photographs have also been used.

The *24-hour recall* method requires that respondents report the types and amounts of foods they consumed over the previous 24-hour period. Information is obtained by face-to-face (in-person) interview or by telephone.

Diet history methods rely on interviewers or questionnaires to estimate the usual diet (or certain aspects of the diet) of subjects over a long period. The objective is to obtain a picture of habitual intake, which is more likely to be related to slowly developing diseases than is the intake over a time as short as 24 hours, which cannot represent the customary or usual intake. The classic diet history method used by Bertha Burke (1947) included a 3-day food intake record, a 24-hour recall, and an accounting of the frequency of food intakes over a period of 1 to 3 months. This method is rarely used today in its entirety. A less intensive version consists of two steps. First, an interviewer obtains detailed information about usual diet and portion sizes, e.g., what is usually consumed for each meal and for snacks. Then, to improve recall and obtain a more complete picture of habitual food practices, the interviewer helps the respondent review a detailed list of foods and adds anything omitted (Fehily, 1984).

Some diet histories are obtained through questionnaires, administered by an interviewer or completed independently by the respondent, that ask about the number of times each listed food is consumed (and sometimes the amounts) over a specified period, such as a few weeks or a year. This is often called the *food frequency* method. Few or many food items may be listed on the questionnaire. For example, in studies of the association between diet and cancer, the questionnaire may focus only on foods that provide a nutrient of particular interest.

In most case-control studies to determine the etiology of chronic diseases, investigators have recognized the difficulty of determining past dietary intake and have assumed that the current diet (or the diet prior to the onset of symptoms of the disease) reflects past intake sufficiently well to identify associations of dietary factors with disease (Morgan et al., 1978). However, recall of a diet from the distant past (17 to 25 years ago) or the more recent past (3 years ago) can be influenced by current diet (Byers et al., 1983; Garland et al., 1982; Møller Jenson et al., 1984; Rohan and Potter, 1984; Van Leeuwen et al., 1983).

Accuracy

The most accurate methods are in large part free of random and systematic errors (Bingham, 1987). The accuracy of a particular data set (or, more generally, of a method) is defined as the degree to which recorded estimates of intake approximate actual intake. Accuracy can be reduced by many factors, such as poor memory of past dietary practices, inaccurate recall of amounts, wishful thinking, and a desire to please an interviewer. Thus, true intake can generally be known only if actual intake is observed and measured or weighed surreptitiously. This has been feasible in only a few studies of small numbers of subjects conducted for a short time. Since true dietary intake can rarely be determined, investigators often try to assess the accuracy of a new method by comparing results not with true intake but with results from some other accepted but possibly flawed method.

Following is a list of the errors that may occur in methods to assess intake. These include sampling errors, reporting errors, and errors due to wide day-to-day variation in dietary intake.

- *Sampling Errors:* Because of interindividual variation in usual diet, small samples may provide highly unrepresentative estimates of food intakes by populations even when individual data items are accurate.
- *Nonresponse Bias:* When randomly selected samples are meant to represent an entire population, high refusal rates will introduce a serious bias if those who refuse differ from respondents in important ways.
- *Reporting Errors:* Respondents must be motivated to cooperate. Most people have little reason to remember exactly what they ate in the recent past as well as at times long past. In recall methods, subjects may fail to remember accurately all foods eaten. In general, recall is more accurate if respondents have been alerted to the requirements of the recall method. Some groups, such as very old people and young children, may be poor subjects for recall methods.

Subjects may report intakes of foods and amounts they believe the investigator approves instead of their actual intakes. They may also be reluctant to admit to such habits as binge eating or high alcohol consumption. Many subjects do not correctly estimate portion sizes when they recall or record food intake.

If respondents are required to weigh or measure their foods to determine their exact intake, they may alter their usual dietary habits to make recording easier or to provide answers they think will please the investigator.

- *Errors Relative to Day-to-Day Dietary Variability:* Individuals vary widely from day to day in their intake of foods and nutrients. Indeed, even an accurate 24-hour recall will not include the most common foods if they were not consumed on the day of recall. In homogeneous populations, the variability within a given subject's intake may be much greater than that between subjects (Liu et al., 1978).

The number of days of dietary intake data needed for moderately accurate estimates of the usual or habitual intake of individuals varies from one nutrient to another and can sometimes exceed 30 days (to account for day-to-day variability).

- *Interviewer Bias:* Poorly trained interviewers may introduce errors by suggesting answers or by leading respondents.
- *Errors Due to Use of Food Composition Tables:* A given food item may vary in nutrient composition because of genetic variation, growing conditions, pest control measures, and conditions of storage, processing, or preparation for consumption. Single values in food composition tables are averages of representative samples of a given food and do not indicate the nutrient content of any specific sample.

Some food composition data are biased, because they are based on inappropriate analytical methods or because nutrient values are imputed. Nutrient data currently available in U.S. food composition tables are far from complete (Beecher and Vanderslice, 1984; Hepburn, 1987). Food composition tables do not account for incomplete bioavailability of nutrients in individual foods. They also do not include data on nutrients inadvertently added to food during preparation, such as calcium from tap water or iron from utensils (Bazzarre and Myers, 1980).

A few investigators have weighed and chemically analyzed samples of food identical to those actually consumed to determine actual intake of nutrients as calculated from food composition tables. Some of them have found general agreement of analyzed values with published tables (Bazzarre and Myers, 1980), but others report errors ranging from 2 to 20%, depending on the nutrient studied (Bingham, 1987).

A dietary intake method need not necessarily determine exact quantities of nutrients consumed (Block, 1982). For example, if data are to be used only to place individuals within upper and lower categories of a distribution, the assessment method might be tested for its ability to do this accurately rather than for its quantitative precision. Interest is increasing in the use of biologic markers to check the accuracy of food intake assessment methods; some possible markers are discussed below in the section on Biologic Markers.

The investigator must be cautious, however, in concluding that one method of assessing some dietary risk factor is fully interchangeable with another. Analyses comparing two methods commonly make use of some combination of group means, correlation coefficients, and regression slopes. Two methods used to measure the same risk factor may not agree on all three of these parameters. In the strictest sense, two methods are interchangeable only if the slope of the linear regression of one method on the other is unity (Lee, 1980; Lee and Kolonel, 1982; Lee et al., 1983).

Another important concept is that of *reliability*—the ability of a method to produce the same results when used repeatedly under the same conditions. While good reliability generally means that any bias is constant and random variability is not serious, failure to obtain the same results may be due either to actual changes in dietary intake or to an unreliable instrument. It may be necessary, therefore, to use biologic markers or other information about changes in food choices to determine whether or not dietary changes have occurred over time (Block, 1982).

Strengths and Weaknesses of Dietary Intake Assessment Methods

Each method of ascertaining dietary intake has its strengths and weaknesses. None of them is suitable for every purpose.

Food Records

Many investigators believe that records of food weights provide the most accurate estimation of food intake. Consequently, they are often used as the standard against which other methods are validated (Bazzarre and Myers, 1980). However, this method requires highly cooperative, motivated, and literate respondents as well as trained personnel to supervise them and to code and calculate their nutrient intakes. As noted above,

respondents may alter their diets to facilitate recording, thereby producing records that fail to reflect their usual intakes. Some subjects may be unable to weigh foods consumed away from home. Consequently, their recall of those foods and amounts may be inaccurate. Because of the burden placed on respondents who are asked to weigh their foods, cooperation rates are low—from 35 to 75% (Bazzarre and Myers, 1980). The large burden placed on the investigative staff by this method results in high costs, thus making it difficult for the investigator to obtain a sample that is both representative and sufficiently large. Because of the high costs and low cooperation rates, epidemiologists generally find that weighed or measured food intake records are useful chiefly to validate less costly and more easily applied methods.

Respondent cooperation may be improved if household measures rather than weights are used to determine amounts. Pilot studies in the target population may be undertaken to determine whether estimated weights of food are sufficiently free of bias (Bingham, 1987). Actual intake may be underreported with this method (Mertz and Kelsay, 1984).

The number of days during which food records should be kept depends on the research objectives (e.g., whether individual or group means are desired), the nutrients of interest, and the sample size. More extensive food records are required to estimate individual intake of highly variable nutrients such as vitamin A than to estimate less variable ones such as food energy. In one study, 29 adults kept daily food intake records for 1 year (Basiotis et al. 1987). An average of 31 days of intake data was required to predict an individual's usual intake of food energy, whereas an average of 433 days would have been needed to predict usual intake of vitamin A with the same degree of accuracy. In contrast, mean food energy intake of the group could be estimated from only 3 days of data, and mean vitamin A intake could be estimated from 41 days of data. Other investigators have also concluded that to estimate the mean intake of a group, 3-day records are adequate, provided that day-of-week variations are taken into account [intake on weekends may differ from that on weekdays (Sorenson, 1982)] and that the sample size is sufficiently large (Bingham, 1987).

The 24-Hour Recall

This method is popular because the respondent burden is small, the time required for administration is short, and costs generally are low. Limitations include inaccurate reporting due to failure to recall all foods and the portion sizes consumed, high day-to-day variability in nutrient intake, and bias due to a desire to please the interviewer or reluctance to report large intakes of alcohol, sweets, and other items that might draw disapproval. Even accurate 24-hour recall data cannot represent the habitual intake of individuals and cannot be used to identify individuals in the sample whose intakes are consistently high or low in the nutrients studied (Beaton et al., 1979; Block, 1982; Todd et al., 1983). Most investigators agree that a single 24-hour recall is valuable for assessing the mean intake of a group (Gersovitz et al., 1978; Madden et al., 1976; Sorenson, 1982; Young et al., 1952), but systematic errors may result in serious misclassification of respondents. It may be worthwhile to assess the accuracy of this method (perhaps in a subsample) by comparing 24-hour recall data with diet records (Bingham, 1987). Validity checks against biologic markers (such as 24-hour urinary nitrogen as a reflection of protein intake) can increase confidence that the 24-hour recall accurately reflects intake of certain nutrients in the past 24 hours (Bingham, 1987; Block, 1982). Several 24-hour recalls obtained periodically from the same people over several months or more can increase the accuracy of estimates of their usual intakes; this may be especially important for nutrients that are highly variable in the diet (Bazzarre and Myers, 1980; Liu et al., 1978; Rush and Kristal, 1982). A common misuse of data from a single 24-hour recall is the designation of cutoff points below which dietary intakes of individuals are considered to be inadequate (see Chapter 3).

Diet Histories

In the diet history method, which covers longer periods, seasonal and other dietary variations can be taken into account and usual diet is not altered. However, a complex diet history requires a highly skilled interviewer and takes 1 to 2 hours of respondent time, followed by extensive checking and coding of records. Thus, costs are high. An alternative approach to estimating usual intakes, called the food frequency assessment method, often ignores portion sizes, so that questionnaires are easier to standardize, more rapidly administered (some are self-administered by the study subjects), and less expensive. Methods that provide information on the frequency of food consumption but not on the amounts consumed may be useful in ecological studies that do not require high accuracy, but may not be suitable for case-control or cohort

studies (Chu et al., 1984). Because of validation problems, investigators often place greater confidence in the accuracy of a diet history method if it produces results consistent from one experimental situation or one study group to another.

Diet histories tend to produce higher estimates of intakes than do food records (Bazzarre and Myers, 1980; Bingham, 1987; Block, 1982; Dwyer, 1988; Jain et al., 1980; Sorenson, 1982; Young et al., 1952). The reproducibility of the diet history method based on repeated administration has been fairly good (Dawber et al., 1962; Hankin et al., 1983; Nomura et al., 1976; Reshef and Epstein, 1972).

Both the full diet history and the food frequency method are subject to recall errors and the possibility that respondents may report a diet of better quality than they have actually consumed. The survey instrument may need to be complex if the study population contains two or more groups with distinctly different dietary patterns.

Willett et al. (1985) and Block et al. (1986) developed semiquantitative food frequency questionnaires. Block and colleagues used dietary data from adult respondents in the Second National Health and Nutrition Examination Survey, whereas Willett and co-workers obtained information from a large sample of nurses. These questionnaires are promising but they have not yet been adequately studied in groups that may differ sharply from the general U.S. population, nor have they been sufficiently evaluated to determine how well they assess the dietary intakes of individuals (Dwyer, 1988).

Recall bias occurs when study subjects consistently remember their intake of a food as higher or lower than it really was. This bias is a special concern when different study groups have different degrees of recall bias. For example, patients with cancer of the gastrointestinal tract may seek to explain their disease in terms of dietary factors and consequently overestimate or underestimate a particular food component that they believe may be responsible, or they may think harder about their past diet and report more accurately than the rest of the population. Recall biases can be large, either positive or negative, and very difficult to detect.

Incompleteness of Food Composition Tables

Another problem in assessing nutrient intakes is the limited accuracy and completeness of standard food composition tables. There are sufficiently accurate data on the occurrence of protein and fat in most foods; but for dietary fiber, some vitamins, and trace minerals, for example, the data are much more limited. Furthermore, the tables give average values and do not reflect variability among samples of the same food, nor do they reflect differences over time or geographic location, such as might be introduced by new strains of food animals or plants or by new methods of food preservation and storage (Beecher and Vanderslice, 1984; Hepburn, 1987).

Biologic Markers

Because of difficulties in validating dietary intake assessment methods, biologic markers are receiving more and more attention as independent validity checks. Such markers can indicate dietary intake, but the complexities of nutrient metabolism and genetic and environmental factors may affect their usefulness. For example, disease may affect nutrient intake (rather than vice versa), and it may also directly affect levels of a given marker in blood or urine. It is also important to know the length of time for which a marker can estimate dietary intake. To date, little has been done to establish the accuracy of dietary markers.

Possible markers include 24-hour urinary sodium excretion as a measure of sodium intake (Fregly, 1985) and 24-hour urinary nitrogen as an estimate of protein intake (Bingham and Cummings, 1985; Isaksson, 1980). The value of markers depends on the completeness of 24-hour urine collections, which can be assessed by measuring the urinary recovery of orally administered *para*-aminobenzoic acid (Bingham and Cummings, 1983). Creatinine excretion has often been used to check completeness of urine collections, but the coefficient of variation of 24-hour creatinine excretion is as high as 25%, and excretion is increased when meat is consumed (Bingham, 1987).

Other possible markers include toenail levels of selenium to assess selenium intake (Morris et al., 1983) and adipose tissue concentrations of fatty acids to assess types of fatty acids consumed (Beynen et al., 1980). Standard energy output equations, which include adjustment for the weight and age of subjects, can provide an approximate check on stated energy intake (Schofield et al., 1985).

EVALUATING SINGLE STUDIES FOR QUALITY AND RELEVANCE

The research methods used to gain reliable scientific knowledge, particularly knowledge about biologic phenomena, and the criteria used to evaluate their results have been developed over many years by a combination of intuition; biologic, statistical, and mathematical reasoning; and practical experience. A strong impetus for developing better methods of research design and statistical analysis came originally from the needs of agricultural research (Fisher, 1935). Many of those techniques are applicable to research in nutrition.

Knowledge about the relationship of diet to health is based on many thousands of reports of experimental and observational research published during the past century. In order to evaluate such a large amount of research, it is useful to distinguish between the accuracy of data (internal quality control that can generally be judged by others only if the research report is sufficiently complete) and the accuracy of conclusions (which often requires a broad range of additional knowledge for evaluation).

Scientists can agree that data are accurate even while they dispute conclusions. Furthermore, data remain accurate even when interpretations change. Although any valid scheme for combining information from separate studies would depend, in part, on their individual strengths and weaknesses, the committee has attempted to ensure adequate standards of quality by giving emphasis to peer-reviewed studies.

The criteria used by the committee in evaluating conclusions from individual studies are common to evaluation of all scientific evidence and can be divided into two major categories:

• those related to study design and execution, including observational research and true experiments; and
• those related to interpretation, which depends heavily on the concepts and sometimes on the mathematical techniques of statistics as well as a broad understanding of biologic phenomena.

Investigations in humans include cross-sectional, case-control, cohort, and intervention studies, including clinical and community trials. Observational studies, in which the investigator must make use of situations that arise without intervening in them, differ in many critical ways from experiments in which the investigator controls both the assignment of subjects to treatments and the treatments themselves. Many studies of nutrition in humans are by necessity observational, and the general criteria for the quality of such work are similar to those for other observational investigations. Such criteria are discussed in textbooks on epidemiologic methods (e.g., Lilienfeld and

Lilienfeld, 1980; Mausner and Kramer, 1985). Likewise, experiments in humans and animals can be evaluated against general criteria for good experimental design, execution, and analysis that apply in all scientific disciplines and are described in many textbooks.

The following sections address the special problems encountered in meeting these criteria in studies of diet and health.

Problems Common to Observational Studies

Assessment of Dietary Intakes

Most knowledge about the relationship of diet to human health and disease, particularly chronic disease, has been derived from observational studies of people who selected their own food and drink over a lifetime. The strengths and weaknesses of different methods of measuring dietary intakes of groups and individuals are discussed earlier in this chapter.

Assessment of Disease Incidence and Prevalence

It is difficult to measure the prevalence or incidence of some diseases. Most cancers are detected efficiently and are diagnosed and reported accurately. Some other medical conditions of considerable consequence, such as hypertension and loss of bone density, require special techniques for detection, since they may become clinically apparent only when there is a catastrophic complication.

Mortality rates for demographic groups (e.g., nations) and subgroups (e.g., adults) are reliable indicators of the incidence of diseases that are detected clinically with accuracy and thoroughness and have a high case-fatality rate. Such diseases include severe myocardial infarction, cancer of the lung, and cirrhosis of the liver. Mortality rates are not reliable indicators of the incidence of diseases that are often not detected clinically and do not commonly cause death. Diseases in this category are bone loss and cholelithiasis. For these, later disease manifestations (i.e., disease sequelae) may be used as proxy indicators of disease. For example, hip fracture in an elderly person is often used as an indicator of osteoporotic bone. Otherwise, disease rates must be measured by surveys of population samples.

Biologic markers can sometimes be used to estimate past exposures, as when blood lead levels are used to assess intake of lead. They can also serve as markers of a developing disease, as when

serum cholesterol concentrations and, more recently, serum lipoprotein concentrations are used to predict the risk of atherosclerosis and its sequelae. Much of the evidence relating nutrition to atherosclerosis is based on observational and experimental studies of associations between diet and serum lipid or lipoprotein levels. The relevance of this evidence depends directly on the strength of the association of serum lipoprotein levels with atherosclerosis and related diseases.

Hypertension is a diet-related characteristic that is easy to measure in a large population sample. It also has a variety of serious sequelae (cardiac hypertrophy, congestive heart failure, stroke), although these also have other causes. Osteoporosis is an example of a disease for which new technology can measure a biologic marker (bone density) easily and accurately. Indeed, bone density measurements are so readily available and so closely linked to underlying pathophysiology that they are refining our definition of osteoporosis.

Autopsy results can be used to determine the presence of some diseases and conditions with great accuracy, but such information must be used with caution because the combined clinical observations and autopsy findings are available for only a small and highly selected (and thus potentially highly biased) proportion of the population. Only about 15% of all deaths in the United States are now investigated by autopsy, and in recent years the rate has declined by approximately 1% per year (Council on Scientific Affairs, 1987). Furthermore, autopsy findings are rarely used to revise the cause of death that is recorded on death certificates. In some studies of diet and health that include detailed, long-term individual nutritional assessments, such as the Honolulu Heart Program (McGee et al., 1984) and the Puerto Rico Heart Health Program (Garcia-Palmieri et al., 1980), autopsy findings have been valuable both for improving the accuracy of the assigned cause of death and for assessing other conditions of nutritional interest that did not contribute to the death.

Another valuable use of the autopsy is to study early stages of a disease that has a long natural history by examining the tissues of children and young adults who die of other causes. The most frequent cause of death between the ages of about 2 and 40 years in industrialized countries is accidents, which affect a cross-section of the population that in general is not seriously biased by the late complications of chronic diseases. Thus, autopsies of accident victims are useful for detecting early, subclinical stages of atherosclerosis, osteoporosis, gallbladder disease, and obesity in the population from which they were drawn. Unfortunately, it is extremely difficult to obtain accurate and detailed nutritional data for people who die from accidental causes. Thus, even when the investigator uses great caution, data from autopsies could lead to erroneous conclusions about associations among diseases and between diseases and environmental exposures such as diet.

When the prevalence or incidence of or mortality from disease is correlated with food intakes and compared among specific populations (i.e., ecological correlations), problems of interpretation are encountered. For example, in industrialized countries, compared to those less technically developed, death reporting and assignment of causes of deaths on death certificates are usually more accurate. The criteria for diagnosing a disease may vary among regions, and there may be local biases in diagnosing certain diseases. Thus, there are many opportunities for errors or differences in disease measurement and classification that could bias ecological correlations. Intensive studies of death certificate data have shown that the accuracy of disease rates based on conventional death certificates varies greatly among cities, countries, and causes of death (Puffer and Griffith, 1967).

In summary, accurate assessment of disease end points is critical in the evaluation of nutrition-related causes of disease. Each disease presents different problems, and each study must be evaluated in light of the best knowledge about the disease in question.

Effects of Misclassification

The effect of misclassifying individuals with regard to dietary exposure or disease end point depends on the type of study. In ecological correlations, in which group rates and means are used, random misclassification of a small proportion of subjects may increase variance in study results and make it more difficult to detect diet–disease correlations; however, such errors do not ordinarily introduce serious bias when they affect all subgroup means to about the same degree. However, if the misclassifications are systematic, and vary from group to group, they may bias the means in different ways and thus bias the comparisons of interest. For example, if certain diseases are underreported in countries or regions with both poor medical services and low intakes of a nutrient, a spurious correlation of the disease with high nutrient intake may be introduced or a correlation in the other direction obscured.

In studies of individuals, random misclassification with regard to diet or disease can seriously attenuate correlations and thus reduce the power to detect associations when they are present.

Temporal Relationships

A special type of misclassification of exposure arises if dietary intake data are collected at a time when diet could not have caused the disease in question. Dietary intake after a disease is established may not be an index of the relevant exposure since the disease may have affected the diet, rather than vice versa. Misclassification of this type is especially serious in studies of chronic diseases, most of which develop over long periods during which they do not produce readily detectable signs or symptoms. For example, atherosclerosis begins in childhood but usually does not produce clinically manifest disease until middle age or later. Sometimes the error is obvious, but the temporal relationship of diet to the critical stages of pathogenesis is often unknown, and misclassification of this type may sometimes be undetectable. Similarly, in some diseases, exposure to a dietary factor may be important only during certain periods, such as the hypothesized effect of fat intake early in life on breast cancer. In a few long-term prospective epidemiologic studies, investigators have measured disease outcome 10 to 20 years after the dietary assessment—a useful approach for many chronic diseases with a long latency—but the opportunities for such long follow-up are rare.

Confounding

Confounding refers to associations that are real but do not indicate a causal link. A confounding factor, or *confounder*, must be associated with both the exposure of interest and the effect. For example, absence of teeth is associated with the consumption of large quantities of milk, but milk is certainly not a cause of the condition; edentulous infants drink a lot of milk, and age (correlated with both milk consumption and absence of teeth) is a critical confounder. More subtle, and hence more serious, confounding often results because of correlations among food or nutrient intakes (is it sodium or chloride—whose occurrence in foods is highly correlated—that is more harmful?) and bias in determining dietary exposure, health outcomes, or both.

It may be impossible to control for known sources of confounding, much less for those unrecognized and unsuspected. The great strength of randomized clinical studies is that the randomization of study subjects reduces bias and provides a basis for such valid statistical measures as p values and confidence limits. It can never be entirely certain that nonrandomized subjects in the comparison groups are sufficiently similar to ignore possible confounding.

Confounding must be considered in attempts to relate nutrition to chronic diseases, because most chronic diseases have multiple causes and because nutrition is also greatly influenced by social, cultural, economic, and geographic factors. For example, differences among countries in the incidence of coronary heart disease (CHD) are correlated with differences in fat and cholesterol intake, but they are also correlated with many other aspects of life. Other evidence—such as that derived from experimental research on possible causal mechanisms—must be considered in order to determine which dietary correlates of disease are causal and, hence, what dietary changes are likely to be beneficial.

Discrepancies Between Ecological and Individual Correlations

Correlations between disease rates and dietary intake levels can be computed by using group rates or means or values for individuals. However, there are many examples of diet–disease correlations that are strong when based on population means (e.g., dietary and serum cholesterol levels) but weak or nonexistent when based on values for individuals. Prominent examples are the strong ecological correlations found between dietary fats and CHD, and between dietary fats and breast cancer, and the weak or absent individual correlations for the same pairs of variables. Each type of correlation has strengths not present in the other, and both may be important in gaining an understanding of specific relationships. Ecological correlations are less affected by random variability and can exploit large interpopulation differences in diet, whereas individual correlations can be used more effectively in dealing with bias and confounding.

Different correlation coefficients obtained with these two approaches are not necessarily contradictory. In ecological correlations, averaging across individuals to determine the mean dietary intake or disease occurrence of a population greatly reduces the effects of variation among individuals and of random errors in classification. Furthermore, there is often an opportunity to select populations representing high and low extremes of exposure and disease rates. Both effects tend to

increase the precision of the correlation coefficient, so that causal associations are more readily detectable. In contrast, in individual correlations, variation among subjects in exposure or response, as well as in genetic variability, are not masked by averaging across subjects. Furthermore, variation in diet among subjects within a population is usually much less than variation among populations. Both of these effects attenuate the correlation coefficient computed from individual values. On the other hand, studies of individuals can more often be designed and conducted to reduce the effects of bias.

Case-Control Studies

In a case-control study, subjects with the disease in question are compared with disease-free control subjects with regard to suspected causative agents. Thus, subjects are enrolled on the basis of their outcome (diseased or healthy) rather than on the basis of their exposure (with or without some dietary factor) (White and Bailar, 1956). The case-control study is a valuable epidemiologic method for identifying causes of diseases, because it can be rapid (even when critical exposure data refer to times long past) and inexpensive. However, it has potentially severe limitations when used to examine dietary causes of chronic diseases. The major limitation is the difficulty of sorting out the time of exposure and the time of disease origin, as discussed previously. Another limitation of case-control studies is that the choice of control subjects (e.g., hospital-based versus neighborhood-based controls) can influence study findings, especially in studies of chronic diseases with subclinical forms whose prevalence is high. Atherosclerosis is a prominent example. Almost every adult has some degree of atherosclerosis; many have severe atherosclerosis without clinical manifestations. Consequently, atherosclerosis in apparently healthy control subjects may be almost as extensive as in subjects with clinically manifest CHD. Thus, associations are likely to be weakened by classification of disease as present or absent (implicit in the differentiation of cases from controls), rather than as a graded condition.

Misclassification of dietary exposures can be serious in case-control studies, even with unambiguous health outcomes such as cancer. When bias is not serious, positive findings from case-control studies are likely to give conservative estimates of the strength of the association. When bias is likely to be strong, neither positive nor negative results of case-control studies are reliable.

Longitudinal (Cohort) Studies

In some epidemiologic studies, a group of apparently healthy people (a cohort) is characterized and then followed for a long time for occurrence of disease. The Framingham Study (Dawber, 1980) is an example of this. Since information on relevant risk factors must be collected at the outset of the study, however, cohort studies have usually focused on the confirmation of suspected risk factors, as well as on estimation of magnitude of effects, identification of subgroups at especially high or low risk, and other refinements of exposure–outcome relationships. In cohort studies, it is common to measure all independent variables at one time, which may not represent usual exposures over a prolonged period. Furthermore, as in case-control studies, misclassifications of dietary exposure can occur. Nevertheless, cohort studies have been very successful in the investigation of suspected risk factors for chronic disease, e.g., associations of serum cholesterol concentration and dietary components with cardiovascular diseases (Shekelle et al., 1981).

Problems Common to Intervention Studies

Experimental Design

Experimental design is discussed thoroughly in many textbooks (e.g., Lilienfeld and Lilienfeld, 1980; Mausner and Kramer, 1985). A variety of techniques can be used to increase and improve the quality of the information provided by experiments. In experiments with a small number of subjects and considerable individual variability, the crossover design is useful. In that type of study, each subject is exposed to two or more dietary treatments (Bailar and Mosteller, 1986). When applied to disease end points, however, the crossover design is strongest when the disease or its marker is temporary and readily reversible. This approach is not often applicable to the study of long-term or permanent effects of diet.

Duration of Exposure

The long exposure required for diet to produce the common chronic diseases of adults is probably the greatest single handicap to the use of experimental methods in nutrition research. It is difficult to control the diets of noninstitutionalized people for any length of time and, as a practical matter, impossible to control diets for months or years, much less decades, as would be required to test dietary hypotheses regarding CHD, certain cancers, osteoporosis, and certain other chronic diseases. One useful stratagem to balance what is ideal with what is feasible is to study the effect of diet on intervening variables rather than on disease occurrence.

This approach is illustrated by one of the most ambitious nutrition research projects ever conducted—the National Diet–Heart Study (AHA, 1968) of approximately 1,000 men in each of five centers in the United States. This was designed as a feasibility study for a definitive trial of diet and heart disease. A central laboratory prepared foods with different amounts and types of fats and different amounts of cholesterol, but with similar appearances and using similar methods of food preparation, so that treatments were blinded. Foods were provided to participants at costs competitive with those of ordinary foods for 1 year. The results demonstrated conclusively that fat-modified diets lowered serum cholesterol concentrations in noninstitutionalized men. There was no attempt to assess CHD. With the results of this study in hand, the possibility of conducting a diet trial with CHD as an end point was examined by an independent body of experts. They concluded that such a project was not feasible, in view of the number of people (up to 100,000), length of time (10 years), and enormous cost required to achieve reasonable statistical power (NHLBI, 1971).

Clinical Trial Design

The design of clinical trials has been developed extensively over the past 20 years (Peto et al., 1976, 1977; Shapiro and Louis, 1983). Such trials have been used to great advantage in comparing drugs, devices, and operative procedures (including placebos) but to only a limited extent in testing hypotheses about nutrition and chronic diseases. As shown in the National Diet–Heart Study (AHA, 1968), it is difficult and expensive to conduct a study using a double-blind design involving manipulation of diet, but the difficulty and expense may well be justified in light of the potential value of the findings—that is, when compared to the cost of *not* doing such a study. As discussed above, duration of exposure is also a major obstacle.

The problems that have affected some of the intervention (experimental) trials in humans include (Bailar and Mosteller, 1986):

• incomplete compliance of the study group assigned to treatment;

• dilution of effect by control subjects who decide on their own to adopt the intervention (a strong possibility with high-risk subjects properly informed of the risks of nonintervention at the outset of a study);

• secular changes in intercurrent illness and death, especially when the changes (good or bad) may be influenced by the treatment; and

• uncertainty about the optimal timing of the intervention in relation to the outcomes of interest.

Because of these problems, few questions of nutrition and chronic diseases are suitable for rigorously controlled, double-blind clinical trials.

Clinical Investigations

Most experiments concerned with nutrition and chronic diseases in human subjects are short-term studies of small numbers of people and include manipulation of dietary variables and measurement of physiological responses that may illuminate disease mechanisms or may be predictors of chronic diseases. Some of these are conducted with tightly controlled formula diets prepared in a laboratory kitchen and fed to subjects residing in a metabolic ward; others are conducted with noninstitutionalized subjects who are instructed to eat more or less of certain foods. In metabolic ward studies, dietary control and information collection are maximized, but since the costs of such studies tend to be very high, exposure periods and numbers of subjects are limited. In studies involving noninstitutionalized people, larger study populations and longer exposures are possible, but control of the diet is limited, blinding is rarely possible, and assessment of actual diet is difficult, as discussed above for observational studies.

Strengths and Weaknesses of Laboratory Experiments

Studies in Animals

Historically, experiments in animals have played an important role in research on nutrition, even though there are considerable differences among species in their needs for various nutrients and in their responses to specific dietary manipulations. Experiments in dogs were used to determine the relationship of niacin to pellagra, and rats and other animals were used in research on vitamin D. Much has been accomplished with rodents in defining essential amino acids and identifying complete proteins. Even though scurvy was identified and preventive diets were designed from

observations and therapeutic trials on sailors, much additional information was gained by feeding vitamin C-deficient diets to guinea pigs—one of the few nonhuman species unable to make this vitamin. However, most of these studies were designed to induce deficiencies of single nutrients for relatively brief periods, usually not more than a few months, and the physiological derangements or tissue lesions produced were easily measurable.

In contrast, experiments in animals to investigate the relationship of nutrition to chronic diseases are more complex, but nevertheless have provided useful leads. The first evidence that dietary cholesterol was related to heart disease was the observation that feeding cholesterol to rabbits caused hypercholesterolemia and arterial lesions simulating atherosclerosis in humans. Human-like hypercholesterolemia and atherosclerosis have been produced by fat and cholesterol feeding in a variety of other species, including swine, dogs, and nonhuman primates. These models have confirmed and amplified the observations on dietary fats and cardiovascular disease in humans and have yielded considerable insight into the pathogenesis of the underlying atherosclerotic lesions (see Chapters 7 and 19). The induction of hypertension in rats by dietary salt supports the suspected relationship of salt intake to hypertension in humans (see Chapters 15 and 20). Animal models have confirmed the epidemiologic association of alcohol to liver injury and cirrhosis (see Chapters 16 and 25). Animal experiments are essential in screening foods and food additives for possible carcinogenic effects (see Chapter 17), and they have provided an important data base for evaluation of the role of dietary factors in carcinogenesis (NRC, 1982).

Variability among species is a more severe problem when research is directed toward diet and chronic disease relationships that are more likely to be unique to humans or to depend on uniquely human exposures. The more complex the physiological mechanisms involved in the pathogenesis of a human disease, the more difficult it is to ensure that the disease is (or can be) adequately simulated in animal models. The rat, for example, does not respond to diets enriched with cholesterol and fats by elevations in serum lipoproteins, whereas the rabbit, in which the effects of dietary cholesterol were discovered, is extraordinarily sensitive to such diets. There is no satisfactory animal model for testing the effects of dietary calcium on postmenopausal osteoporosis, perhaps because few animals undergo the spontaneous ovarian failure in middle age that humans experience. Extensive reviews of animal models for each of the major chronic diseases have included assessments of their advantages and limitations (NRC, 1981, 1982).

Problems related to the interpretation of results of studies in animals are complex, and only a few general principles apply. When manipulation of nutritient composition in such studies produces a disease whose pathogenesis and pathology resemble those of a disease in humans and when the intervening variables are nearly identical, observations in animal studies support inferences of causation derived from studies in humans. However, a failure to induce the human disease in animals does not necessarily disprove a causal relationship in humans. Conversely, the existence of a diet-induced disease in one or more animal species does not prove its existence in humans, unless the relationship is also supported by evidence derived from studies in humans.

The advent of molecular biology has made possible the study of dietary effects at fundamental levels of cellular metabolism. These studies may explain differences among species in response to diet in terms of gene expression.

The most valuable role of animal models in research on nutrition and chronic diseases in humans is in the study of mechanisms and pathogenesis. Studies of the effects of diet on serum lipids and lipoproteins, calcium absorption and metabolism, tumor initiation and growth, blood pressure, and other physiological processes in selected animals have been useful in testing and refining hypotheses regarding mechanisms. In evaluating data obtained from animals and other laboratory studies, the committee gave greater weight to data derived from studies in more than one animal species or test system, on results reproduced in different laboratories, and on data demonstrating increases in response with increases in exposure.

Short-Term Tests

Short-term tests are used primarily to prescreen chemical compounds for their possible carcinogenic or mutagenic potential (de Serres and Ashby, 1981). They can detect DNA-reactive or genotoxic agents (Weisburger and Williams, 1981) and can be used in a variety of biological systems such as microorganisms, mammalian cells, insects, and whole animals (de Serres and Ashby, 1981). In addition, these tests have high statistical power, are easily replicated, are relatively inexpensive, can be performed under different sets of experimental conditions, and have the ability to detect

several end points relevant to carcinogenesis (Brockman and DeMarini, 1988).

A battery of these tests is usually used, with or without metabolic activation of the parent compound. These include tests for gene mutations in microorganisms, yeast, fungi, insects, or mice; structural chromosome aberrations; and other genotoxic effects such as numerical chromosome aberrations, DNA damage and repair, mammalian cell transformation, and target organ/cell analysis (EPA, 1982).

Short-term tests for mutagenicity have yielded useful data in investigation of the role of diet in carcinogenesis (see Chapter 17, and NRC, 1982). However, there are a number of drawbacks to the use of short-term tests in prediction of carcinogenicity: They are unable to detect carcinogens that do not interact with DNA (often called epigenetic carcinogens) such as some hormones and promoters (Weisburger and Williams, 1981); they cannot take into account metabolic effects of absorption, transportation, activation, detoxification, and excretion; and it is difficult to make quantitative risk assessments based only on the results of these tests (NRC, 1982).

EVALUATING THE EVIDENCE AS A WHOLE

The first step in assessing the evidence on diet and chronic diseases is to evaluate the quality and relevance of individual studies in light of the criteria discussed above. The second step involves assembling and evaluating all the evidence. In this step, the committee paid particular attention to the criteria for assessing inferences of causality and to the relative weights ascribed to each category of evidence reviewed.

Categories of Research Subjects and Methods

The committee considered both the subjects and the methods in each study. Most data reviewed by the committee were from studies in humans or animals. Other evidence obtained from short-term experiments in bacteria, cultured cells, or organs applied primarily to mutagenicity and cancer. In reviewing studies in animals, the committee considered whether or not experimental diets were within physiological ranges of intake or represented more extreme variations, whether the animal species selected for study were sufficiently similar to humans in responses to dietary modification, and whether duration of exposures and periods of observation were appropriate.

Underlying Assumptions

To evaluate the aggregate data on diet and chronic diseases, the committee considered some a priori assumptions about the relative weights or degrees of importance ascribed to each category of evidence considered. For example, which categories of studies provide the strongest and weakest evidence for the associations in question? Specifically, does a well-controlled study of laboratory animals provide more or less convincing evidence about diet and human health than a weaker but more relevant epidemiologic study? The committee concluded, however, that such an approach is naive and would lead to ignoring important data or giving undue emphasis to certain studies because, as described above, no single category of study is perfect. Each has strengths and weaknesses. Therefore, the committee did not rely solely on any one category of evidence (e.g., relative risks in epidemiologic studies or responses in animal studies) but, rather, based its evaluation on the strength of the overall combined evidence.

Furthermore, there is no universally valid hierarchy or weighting of categories of studies and hence no comprehensive procedure for leaping from results to conclusions. Each putative association between diet and chronic disease must be evaluated on a case-by-case basis, taking into account such factors as the natural history of the disease under review and the inherent strengths and weaknesses of each category of study.

Common Problems in the Weighting of Studies

Studies in Humans

In evaluating the various types of studies in humans, the committee considered the traditional hierarchy based on the supposed degree of causal inference that can be derived from each. According to this hierarchy, for example, ecological studies may be useful in pointing to hypotheses but often provide the weakest evidence for causation, whereas case-control studies, cohort studies, metabolic studies, and randomized clinical and community trials provide increasingly stronger evidence for causation. Although the committee recognized that such an a priori weighting scheme could be helpful in evaluating many types of health-related data, its application to studies on

diet and chronic diseases did not seem appropriate because of such problems as variable or unknown exposure levels and long disease latency periods.

The complex, interrelated nature of research on the association of diet with human health may sometimes diminish the generalizability of findings of metabolic ward studies in which only a few dietary components are altered and hence may weaken the inferences of causality derived from such data. In general, therefore, the committee accorded more weight to the findings of observational studies of noninstitutionalized individuals.

Studies in Animals

Evidence from animal experiments regarding nutrition and chronic diseases must be evaluated in light of all knowledge about the disease in question, the host, and the diet itself. The obvious advantages of experimental control over such matters as genetics and diet, and the opportunities for more intensive observation, are counterbalanced by the uncertainties of interspecies variability and by the highly uniform experimental conditions. Animal models are most valuable in studying the physiological and molecular mechanisms involved in nutritional effects; modern molecular biology has made them even more useful. Results from studies in animals cannot be used alone either to affirm or negate relationships between human diet and chronic diseases, nor can they be used to estimate accurately the size of the effects in humans.

Studies in Humans Compared to Studies in Animals and Other Experimental Models

In general, the committee accorded greater weight to studies in humans than to studies in animals and other experimental models. Studies in humans provide the most direct means for investigating the possible dietary causes of human diseases and thus circumvent the problem of species specificity in response and the need to extrapolate findings from animals to humans. In addition, more realistic dose–response relationships can be deduced from data on human populations than from data on animals, since the exposures (as well as the outcomes) are those that actually occur among people.

Studies in animals can play a critical role, however, by confirming findings in humans and going beyond proof of causation to examine such factors as mechanisms of action, determinants of individual susceptibility or resistance, and dose–response curves. Where human evidence suggests an association, consistent laboratory findings can provide strong confirmation. Similarly, when animal data are not consistent with human data favoring an association, confidence in that association is diminished.

The committee had more difficulty in assessing the few cases in which a putative association was supported by strong evidence from laboratory animals but confirmatory evidence in humans was lacking. One such example is the evidence on polycyclic aromatic hydrocarbons—a class of naturally occurring food contaminants that are carcinogenic in animal experiments but not in dietary studies of humans. In such circumstances, the possibilities suggested by the animal experiments cannot be ignored but neither can they be taken as conclusive proof of human risk.

Experimental Studies Compared to Observational Studies

Experimental studies have several advantages: the investigator assigns exposure including randomization, observations are structured, controls are internal, and study subjects are deliberately selected. Such factors tend to increase the strength and precision of inferences of causality. However, because experimental studies tend to be based on small selected samples, their findings are not easily generalizable to noninstitutionalized populations. When the results of an experiment were judged not to be applicable to the general population, the committee gave greater consideration to observational studies.

Inferring Causality in Associations Between Diet and Chronic Diseases

Empirical Criteria for Inferring Causality

The committee used six general criteria, patterned after those adopted by Hill (1971), for inferring causality in associations between diet and chronic diseases: strength of association, dose–response relationship, temporally correct association, consistency of association, specificity of association, and biologic plausibility. All criteria were accorded roughly equal weight, with the exception of biologic plausibility, which in practice was given a little less weight since it is more dependent on subjective interpretation. Only the probability that an association is causal was considered, since complete proof of causality is rarely obtainable.

Three of the criteria used by the committee (strength of association, dose–response relationship, and temporally correct association) may be applied to the findings of single studies and can therefore be regarded in part as measures of internal validity. Any of these criteria may be satisfied in some, but not in all, studies testing the same or similar hypotheses. The other three criteria (consistency of association, specificity of association, and biologic plausibility) are not necessarily study specific and depend to a large degree on a priori knowledge.

Strength of Association

This is usually expressed as relative risk, i.e., the ratio of disease rates for people exposed compared to those not exposed to the hypothesized causal factor. Generally, the larger the relative risk, the greater the likelihood that a risk factor is causally related to outcome, i.e., the less likely it is due to confounding or other systematic error.

In applying this criterion, the committee recognized that weak associations, common in studies of diet and chronic diseases, may still be causal and may even have quite large population-wide effects. Furthermore, if most members of a population are similarly exposed to a suspected dietary risk factor—a common situation in the U.S. population—relative risks may show small differences in disease rates among population subgroups.

Dose–Response Relationship

The existence of a dose–response relationship (that is, greater effects with greater exposures) strengthens an inference that an association is causal. However, one high relative risk in the high-exposure category might provide evidence of a strong nonlinear dose–response trend or even of a threshold below which the effect does not occur. Conversely, there may be an upper limit on the size of an effect; i.e., little or no additional effect of increasing doses will be observed if most people studied are exposed to levels above the threshold for the risk factor. This upper limit may also explain why some studies of diet and chronic diseases show no association within the U.S. population. In studies of carcinogenic agents and cancer in laboratory animals, dose–response relationships are sometimes attenuated and even reversed at high doses (Bailar et al., 1988).

Temporally Correct Association

If an observed association is causal, exposure to the putative risk factor must precede the onset of disease by at least the duration of disease induction and latency. The committee interpreted the lack of appropriate time sequence in an association as strong evidence against causation, but recognized that insufficient knowledge about the natural history and pathogenesis of chronic diseases may limit the effectiveness of using this criterion to infer causality.

Consistency of Association

This criterion requires that an association be found in a variety of studies, for example, in more than one study population and with different study methods. However, some studies have low statistical power and in certain cases can be systematically biased toward a no-effect finding. Similarly, many consistent findings limited to a particular category of evidence (e.g., from observational studies in humans) were, in general, given less weight than findings that are consistent across several categories of evidence. For example, in comparing ecological and individual correlations, more weight could be given to one or two ecological studies supported by a technically strong study of individual correlations than to a larger number of ecological studies without that support.

Specificity of Association

This is the degree to which one factor predicts the frequency or magnitude of a single outcome (disease). The more specific an association, the greater the likelihood that the association is causal. However, perfect specificity is rare, given the complex nature of most chronic diseases, the overlapping and often ill-defined nutrient composition of the human diet, and the effects of many dietary components on a variety of organ systems and pathogenic processes. Thus, the committee generally regarded lack of specificity in diet–disease associations with less importance than clear evidence of substantial specificity.

Biologic Plausibility

Biologic plausibility requires that a putatively causal association fits existing biologic or medical knowledge. The committee therefore recognizes that interpretation of this criterion depends to a large degree on current knowledge of the natural history of a given disease or of its pathophysiological mechanisms. Sufficient biologic evidence contradictory to a postulated association is, however, strong evidence against causality.

The committee did not find it possible to develop an algorithm or decision matrix to apply these six criteria to specific problems. Such an approach would require grading the causal criteria for their relative importance, assigning quantitative weights to the various categories of evidence considered, and standardizing the judgments that are implicit in such models for inferring cause and effect. The validity and utility of standardization in the present report would be severely restricted by the multifactorial etiology of the diseases under review and the limited ability to define, observe, and measure the causal processes involved. As a result, hypotheses about causation were examined case by case, and for each case the application of the criteria depended on the extent and nature of evidence examined.

SUMMARY

The strengths and weaknesses of different kinds of clinical, epidemiologic, and laboratory studies and the methodologies for dietary assessment are reviewed above. Accurate assessment of most diet–chronic disease relationships requires that data from studies in humans as well as in animals be evaluated. Ecological correlations of dietary factors and chronic diseases among human populations provide valuable data but cannot be used alone to estimate the strength of the association between diet and diseases. The effect of diet on chronic diseases has been most consistently demonstrated in comparisons of populations with substantially different dietary practices, possibly because it is more difficult to identify such associations within a population whose diet is fairly homogeneous. Thus in general, associations within populations based on case-control and prospective cohort studies underestimate the association. In intervention studies, long exposure is usually required for the effect of diet on chronic disease risk to be manifested. Furthermore, the strict criteria for selecting participants in such studies may result in more homogeneous study samples, which limit the applicability of results to the general population. Despite the limitations of various types of studies in humans, repeated and consistent findings of an association between certain dietary factors and diseases are likely to be real and indicative of a cause-and-effect relationship.

Experiments on dietary exposure of different animal strains can take genetic variability into account and permit more intensive observation. However, extrapolation of data from animal studies to humans is limited by the ability of animal models to simulate human diseases and the comparability of absorption and metabolic phenomena among species. More confidence should therefore by placed in data derived from studies on more than one animal species or test system, on results that have been reproduced in different laboratories, and on data that indicate a dose–response relationship.

Assessments of the strength of associations between diet and chronic diseases cannot simply be governed by criteria commonly used for inferring causality in other areas of human health. Faced with the special characteristics of studies on nutrients, dietary patterns, and chronic diseases, this committee first assessed the strengths and weaknesses of each kind of study and then evaluated the total evidence against six criteria: strength of association, dose–response relationship, temporally correct association, consistency of association, specificity of association, and biologic plausibility. It assessed the overall strength of the evidence on a continuum from highly likely to very inconclusive. Overall, the strength, consistency, and preponderance of data and the degree of concordance in epidemiologic, clinical, and laboratory evidence determined the strength of the conclusions in this report.

REFERENCES

AHA (American Heart Association). 1968. National Diet–Heart Study: Final Report. AHA Monograph No. 18. National Diet–Heart Study Research Group, Executive Committee on Diet and Heart Disease, National Heart Institute. American Heart Association, New York. 428 pp.

Bailar, J.C., III, and F. Mosteller. 1986. Medical Uses of Statistics. Massachusetts Medical Society, Waltham, Mass. 425 pp.

Bailar, J.C., III, E. Crouch, R. Shaikh, and D. Spiegelman. 1988. One-hit models of carcinogenesis: conservative or not? Risk Analysis 8:485–498.

Basiotis, P.P., S.O. Welsh, F.J. Cronin, J.L. Kelsay, and W. Mertz. 1987. Number of days of food intake records to estimate individual and group nutrient intakes with defined confidence. J. Nutr. 117:1638–1641.

Bazzarre, T.L., and M.P. Myers. 1980. The collection of food intake data in cancer epidemiology studies. Nutr. Cancer 1:22–45.

Beaton, G.H., J. Milner, P. Corey, V. McGuire, M. Cousins, E. Stewart, M. de Ramos, D. Hewitt, P.V. Grambsch, N. Kassim, and J.A. Little. 1979. Sources of variance in 24-hour dietary recall data: implications for nutrition study design and interpretation. Am. J. Clin. Nutr. 32:2546–2559.

Beecher, G.R., and J.T. Vanderslice. 1984. Determination of nutrients in foods: factors that must be considered. Pp. 29–55 in K.K. Stewart and J.R. Whitaker, eds. Modern Methods of Food Analysis: IFT Basic Symposium Series. Avi Publishing Co., Westport, Conn.

Beynen, A.C., R.J. Hermus, and J.G. Hautvast. 1980. A mathematical relationship between the fatty acid composition of the diet and that of the adipose tissue in man. Am. J. Clin. Nutr. 33:81–85.

Bingham, S.A. 1987. The dietary assessment of individuals: methods, accuracy, new techniques and recommendations. Nutr. Abstr. Rev. 57:705–741.

Bingham, S., and J.H. Cummings. 1983. The use of 4-aminobenzoic acid as a marker to validate the completeness of 24 h urine collections in man. Clin. Sci. 64:629–635.

Bingham, S.A., and J.H. Cummings. 1985. Urine nitrogen as an independent validatory measure of dietary intake: a study of nitrogen balance in individuals consuming their normal diet. Am. J. Clin. Nutr. 42:1276–1289.

Block, G. 1982. A review of validations of dietary assessment methods. Am. J. Epidemiol. 115:492–505.

Block, G., A.M. Hartman, C.M. Dresser, M.D. Carroll, J. Gannon, and L. Gardner. 1986. A data-based approach to diet questionnaire design and testing. Am. J. Epidemiol. 124:453–469.

Brockman, H.E., and D.E. DeMarini. 1988. Utility of short-term tests for genetic toxicity in the aftermath of the NTP's analysis of 73 chemicals. Environ. Mol. Mutagenesis 11:421–435.

Burk, M.C., and E.M. Pao. 1976. Methodology for Large-Scale Surveys of Household and Individual Diets. Home Economics Research Rep. No. 40. Agriculture Research Service, U.S. Department of Agriculture, Hyattsville, Md. 88 pp.

Burke, B.S. 1947. The dietary history as a tool in research. J. Am. Diet. Assoc. 23:1041–1046.

Byers, T.E., R.I. Rosenthal, J.R. Marshall, T.F. Rzepka, K.M. Cummings, and S. Graham. 1983. Dietary history from the distant past: a methodological study. Nutr. Cancer 5:69–77.

Carroll, M.D., S. Abraham, and C.M. Dresser. 1983. Dietary Intake Source Data: United States, 1976–1980. Vital and Health Statistics, Series 11, No. 231. DHHS Publ. No. (PHS) 83-1681. National Center for Health Statistics, Public Health Service. U.S. Department of Health and Human Services, Hyattsville, Md. 483 pp.

Chu, S.Y., L.N. Kolonel, J.H. Hankin, and J. Lee. 1984. A comparison of frequency and quantitative dietary methods for epidemiologic studies of diet and disease. Am. J. Epidemiol. 119:323–334.

Council on Scientific Affairs. 1987. Autopsy: a comprehensive review of current issues. J. Am. Med. Assoc. 258:364–369.

Dawber, T.R. 1980. The Framingham Study: The Epidemiology of Atherosclerotic Disease. Harvard University Press, Cambridge, Mass. 257 pp.

Dawber, T.R., G. Pearson, P. Anderson, G.V. Mann, W.B. Kannel, D. Shurtleff, and P. McNamara. 1962. Dietary assessment in the epidemiologic study of coronary heart disease: the Framingham Study. II. Reliability of measurement. Am. J. Clin. Nutr. 11:226–234.

de Serres, F.J., and J. Ashby, eds. 1981. Evaluation of Short-Term Tests for Carcinogens: Report of the International Collaborative Program. Progress in Mutation Research, Vol. I. Elsevier/North-Holland, New York. 827 pp.

Dwyer, J.T. 1988. Assessment of dietary intake. Pp. 887–905 in M.E. Shils and V.R. Young, eds. Modern Nutrition in Health and Disease, 7th ed. Lea & Febiger, Philadelphia.

EPA (Environmental Protection Agency). 1982. Pesticide Assessment Guidelines. Subdivision F, Hazard Evaluation: Human and Domestic Animals. Hazard Evaluation Division, Office of Pesticide Programs, Office of Pesticides and Toxic Substances, U.S. Environmental Protection Agency. National Technical Information Service, U.S. Department of Commerce, Springfield, Va. 157 pp.

Fehily, A.M. 1984. Epidemiology for nutritionists. 4. Survey methods. Hum. Nutr. Appl. Nutr. 37:419–425.

Fisher, R.A. 1935. The Design of Experiments, 1st ed. Oliver and Boyd, Edinburgh, Scotland. 252 pp.

Fregly, M.J. 1985. Attempts to estimate soduim intake in humans. Pp. 93–112 in M.J. Horan, M. Blaustein, J.B. Dunbar, W. Kachadorian, N.M. Kaplan, and A.P. Simopoulos, eds. NIH Workshop on Nutrition and Hypertension: Proceedings from a Symposium. Biomedical Information Corp., New York.

Garcia-Palmieri, M.R., P. Sorlie, J. Tillotson, R. Costas, Jr., E. Cordero, and M. Rodriguez. 1980. Relationship of dietary intake to subsequent coronary heart disease incidence: the Puerto Rico Heart Health Program. Am. J. Clin. Nutr. 33:1818–1827.

Garland, B., M. Ibrahim, and R. Grimson. 1982. Assessment of past diet in cancer epidemiology. Am. J. Epidemiol. 116:577.

Gersovitz, M., J.P. Madden, and H. Smiciklas-Wright. 1978. Validity of the 24-hr. dietary recall and seven-day record for group comparisons. J. Am. Diet. Assoc. 73:48–55.

Hankin, J.H., A.M. Nomura, J. Lee, T. Hirohata, and L.N. Kolonel. 1983. Reproducibility of a diet history questionnaire in a case-control study of breast cancer. Am. J. Clin. Nutr. 37:981–985.

Hepburn, F.N. 1987. Food Consumption/Composition Interrelationships. Report No. 382. Human Nutrition Information Service, U.S. Department of Agriculture, Hyattsville, Md.

Hill, A.B. 1971. Principles of Medical Statistics, 9th ed. Oxford University Press, New York.

Isaksson, B. 1980. Urinary nitrogen output as a validity test in dietary surveys. Am. J. Clin. Nutr. 33:4–5.

Jain, M., G.R. Howe, K.C. Johnson, and A.B. Miller. 1980. Evaluation of a diet history questionnaire for epidemiologic studies. Am. J. Epidemiol. 111:212–219.

Lee, J. 1980. Alternate approaches for quantifying aggregate and individual agreements between two methods for assessing dietary intakes. Am. J. Clin. Nutr. 33:956–958.

Lee, J., and L.N. Kolonel. 1982. Nutrient intakes of husbands and wives: implications for epidemiologic research. Am. J. Epidemiol. 115:515–525.

Lee, J., L.N. Kolonel, and J.H. Hankin. 1983. On establishing the interchangeability of different dietary-intake assessment methods used in studies of diet and cancer. Nutr. Cancer 5:215–218.

Lilienfeld, A.M., and D.E. Lilienfeld. 1980. Foundations of Epidemiology, 2nd ed. Oxford University Press, New York. 375 pp.

Liu, K., J. Stamler, A. Dyer, J. McKeever, and P. McKeever. 1978. Statistical methods to assess and minimize the role of intra-individual variability in obscuring the relationship between dietary lipids and serum cholesterol. J. Chronic Dis. 31:399–418.

Madden, J.P., S.J. Goodman, and H.A. Guthrie. 1976. Validity of the 24-hr. recall. Analysis of data obtained from elderly subjects. J. Am. Diet. Assoc. 68:143–147.

Marr, J.W. 1971. Individual dietary surveys: purposes and methods. World Rev. Nutr. Diet. 13:105–164.

Mausner, J.S., and S. Kramer. 1985. Mausner & Bahn Epidemiology—An Introductory Text, 2nd ed. W.B. Saunders, Philadelphia. 361 pp.

McGee, D.L., D.M. Reed, K. Yano, A. Kagan, and J. Tillotson. 1984. Ten-year incidence of coronary heart disease in the Honolulu Heart Program. Relationship to nutrient intake. Am. J. Epidemiol. 119:667–676.

Medlin, C., and J.D. Skinner. 1988. Individual dietary intake methodology: a 50-year review of progress. J. Am. Diet. Assoc. 88:1250–1257.

Mertz, W., and J.L. Kelsay. 1984. Rationale and design of the Beltsville one-year dietary intake study. Am. J. Clin. Nutr. 40 suppl. 6:1323–1326.

Møller-Jenson, O., J. Wahrendorf, A. Rosenqvist, and A. Geser. 1984. The reliability of questionnaire-derived historical dietary information and temporal stability of food habits in individuals. Am. J. Epidemiol. 120:281–290.

Morgan, R.W., M. Jain, A.B. Miller, N.W. Choi, V. Matthews, L. Munan, J.D. Burch, J. Feather, G.R. Howe, and A. Kelly. 1978. A comparison of dietary methods in epidemiologic studies. Am. J. Epidemiol. 107:488–498.

Morris, J.S., M.J. Stampfer, and W. Willett. 1983. Dietary selenium in humans: toenails as an indicator. Biol. Trace Element Res. 5:529–537.

NHLBI (National Heart, Lung and Blood Institute). 1971. Arteriosclerosis: A Report by the National Heart, Lung and Blood Task Force on Arteriosclerosis, Vol. 1. DHEW Publ. No. (NIH) 72-219. National Institutes of Health, Public Health Service, U.S. Department of Health, Education, and Welfare, Bethesda, Md. 365 pp.

Nomura, A., J.H. Hankin, and G.G. Rhoads. 1976. The reproducibility of dietary intake data in a prospective study of gastrointestinal cancer. Am. J. Clin. Nutr. 29:1432–1436.

NRC (National Research Council). 1981. Mammalian Models for Research on Aging. Report of the Committee on Animal Models for Research on Aging, Assembly of Life Sciences. National Academy Press, Washington, D.C. 587 pp.

NRC (National Research Council). 1982. Diet, Nutrition, and Cancer. Report of the Committee on Diet, Nutrition, and Cancer, Assembly of Life Sciences. National Academy Press, Washington, D.C. 478 pp.

Pekkarinen, M. 1970. Methodology in the collection of food consumption data. World Rev. Nutr. Diet. 12:145–171.

Peto, R., M.C. Pike, P. Armitage, N.E. Breslow, D.R. Cox, S.V. Howard, N. Mantel, K. McPherson, J. Peto, and P.G. Smith. 1976. Design and analysis of randomized clinical trials requiring prolonged observation of each patient. I. Introduction and design. Br. J. Cancer 34:585–612.

Peto, R., M.C. Pike, P. Armitage, N.E. Breslow, D.R. Cox, S.V. Howard, N. Mantel, K. McPherson, J. Peto, and P.G. Smith. 1977. Design and analysis of randomized clinical trials requiring prolonged observation of each patient. II. Analysis and examples. Br. J. Cancer 35:1–39.

Puffer, R.R., and G.W. Griffith. 1967. Patterns of Urban Mortality: Report of the Inter-American Investigation of Mortality. Sci. Publ. No. 151. Pan American Health Organization, Pan American Sanitary Bureau, Regional Office of the World Health Organization, Washington, D.C. 353 pp.

Reshef, A., and L.N. Epstein. 1972. Reliability of dietary questionnaire. Am. J. Clin. Nutr. 25:91–95.

Rohan, T.E., and J.D. Potter. 1984. Retrospective assessment of dietary intake. Am. J. Epidemiol. 120:876–887.

Rush, D., and A.R. Kristal. 1982. Methodologic studies during pregnancy: the reliability of the 24-hour dietary recall. Am. J. Clin. Nutr. 35:1259–1268.

Schofield, W.N. 1985. Predicting basal metabolic rate, new standards and review of previous work. Human Nutr. Clin. Nutr. 39 suppl. 1:5–41.

Shapiro, S.H., and T.A. Louis, eds. 1983. Clinical Trials: Issues and Approaches. Statistics, Textbooks and Monographs, Vol. 46. Marcel Dekker, New York. 209 pp.

Shekelle, R.B., A.M. Shryock, O. Paul, M. Lepper, J. Stamler, S. Liu, and W.J. Raynor, Jr. 1981. Diet, serum cholesterol, and death from coronary heart disease: the Western Electric Study. N. Engl. J. Med. 304:65–70.

Sorenson, A.W. 1982. Assessment of nutrition in epidemiologic studies. Pp. 434–474 in S. Schottenfeld and J.F. Fraumeni, eds. Cancer Epidemiology and Prevention. W.B. Saunders, Philadelphia.

Todd, K.S., M. Hudes, and D.H. Calloway. 1983. Food intake measurement: problems and approaches. Am. J. Clin. Nutr. 37:139–146.

USDA (U.S. Department of Agriculture). 1984. Nationwide Food Consumption Survey. Nutrient Intakes: Individuals in 48 States, Year 1977–78. Report No. I-2. Consumer Nutrition Division, Human Nutrition Information Service, Hyattsville, Md. 439 pp.

USDA (U.S. Department of Agriculture). 1987. Nationwide Food Consumption Survey. Continuing Survey of Food Intakes of Individuals. Women 19–50 Years and Their Children 1–5 Years, 4 Days, 1985. Report No. 85–4. Nutrition Monitoring Division, Human Nutrition Information Service, Hyattsville, Md. 182 pp.

Van Leeuwen, F.E., H.C.W. de Vet, R.B. Hayes, W.A. van Staveren, C.E. West, and J.G.A.J. Hautvast. 1983. An assessment of the relative validity of retrospective interviewing for measuring dietary intake. Am. J. Epidemiol. 118:752–758.

Weisburger, J.H., and G.M. Williams. 1981. Carcinogen testing: current problems and new approaches. Science 214:401–407.

White, C., and J.C. Bailar. 1956. Retrospective and prospective methods of studying association in medicine. Am. J. Public Health 46:35–44.

Willett, W.C., L. Sampson, M.J. Stampfer, B. Rosner, C. Bain, J. Witschi, C.H. Hennekens, and F.E. Speizer. 1985. Reproducibility and validity of a semiquantitative food frequency questionnaire. Am. J. Epidemiol. 122:51–65.

Young, C.M., and M.F. Trulson. 1960. Methodology for dietary studies in epidemiological surveys. II. Strengths and weaknesses of existing methods. Am. J. Public Health 50:803–814.

Young, C.M., G.C. Hagan, R.E. Tucher, and W.D. Foster. 1952. A comparison of dietary study methods. 2. Dietary history vs. seven-day record vs. 24-hour recall. J. Am. Diet. Assoc. 28:218–221.

3

Dietary Intake and Nutritional Status: Trends and Assessment

Throughout most of history, the quest for sufficient food was the chief occupation of the earth's people. The diet of Paleolithic hunter–gatherers, before the development of agriculture, is believed to have consisted of approximately 35% meat and 65% plant foods; no dairy products and practically no cereal grains were consumed. Meat from wild animals contains low levels of fats (4% in this early diet compared to 25 to 30% fat in today's domesticated animals), and the plant foods in this early diet consisted of a variety of vegetables and fruits (Eaton and Konner, 1985). The high-meat diet resulted in a high protein intake, but dietary fat was relatively low and contained more polyunsaturated fats than saturated fats. The intake of cholesterol, dietary fiber, calcium, and ascorbic acid is believed to have been high, but sodium intake was remarkably low. The accuracy of these estimates of the diet of hunter–gatherers cannot be established, however.

Two notable revolutions caused major changes in food supplies. The first occurred around 10,000 B.C., when people began to give up their nomadic ways in favor of living on specific plots of land, existing chiefly on plants they grew and animals they domesticated. For the first time, dairy products and cereal grains became a part of the diet. Agricultural innovations evolved slowly at first, but accelerated greatly with the onset of the second important revolution—the Industrial Rev-

olution of the 1800's. Industrialization gave rise to two new socioeconomic classes: a new middle class of merchants and managers, who demanded a variety of socially desirable foods, and a new class of industrial workers, who could afford only the cheapest foods. Although the poverty, poor sanitary conditions, malnutrition, and disease that prevailed among workers in the industrial cities and towns was a blight on the Industrial Revolution, resources were soon mobilized to meet the food demands of the middle classes. Eventually the poor also benefited, as increased production and new techniques made cheaper foods available to them (Tannahill, 1973).

When large numbers of people left farming to work for wages in factories or to become entrepreneurs, there was a marked change in the kinds and quantities of food that were readily accessible. In the years since the Industrial Revolution, the U.S. diet has again undergone very large changes. In 1800, 95% of all Americans consumed minimally processed foods produced chiefly on their own small farms, but by 1900, only 60% of the population remained on farms (Hampe and Wittenberg, 1964). In less than 175 years, nearly all Americans have become dependent on others to produce and distribute food to supermarkets where their ability to obtain items they desire is determined largely by their financial resources.

The construction of railroads across the country in the mid-1880s was responsible for changes in

41

the character of the food supply. Foods were no longer strictly seasonal in nature, because they could be shipped from different climates. This trend accelerated with the advent of refrigerated railcars and trucks. Innovations in food processing were also important. In 1869, processed foods consisted chiefly of milled flour and cornmeal, refined sugar, cured meats, and processed dairy products. Today, in addition to these foods, the consumer finds canned, frozen, fermented, and dehydrated foods, as well as foods fabricated in the laboratory to resemble traditional foods. These include drinks resembling fruit juices, but containing no fruit juice, and analogs of meat or fish made from soybeans or wheat gluten. Innovations such as sugared breakfast cereals and a variety of snack items were unheard of before World War II. Hampe and Wittenberg (1964) estimate that 60% of the items on supermarket shelves in 1960 came into existence during the 15 years after the end of World War II. Home refrigerators and freezers also increased the homemaker's ability to select and store a variety of foods. Today's large supermarkets carry as many as 15,000 different items from which consumers must choose, complicating the task of nutrition educators.

The next section focuses on changes in the food supply during the twentieth century and describes national surveys to determine the U.S. population's intake of foods, nutrients, and, to a limited extent, pesticides and industrial chemicals. This is followed by a discussion of the limitations of the studies and a section on consumption trends.

NATIONAL SURVEYS OF DIETARY INTAKE AND NUTRITIONAL STATUS

Surveys Conducted by the U.S. Department of Agriculture (USDA)

The Food Supply: Historical Data

Changes in foods available to the public from 1909 to the present have been ascertained from USDA data based on the disappearance of foods into wholesale and retail markets. Annually, foods available to the civilian population are estimated by subtracting data on exports, year-end inventories, nonfood use, and military procurement from data on total production, imports, and beginning-of-the-year inventories. These quantities are larger than those actually consumed, because they fail to take into account losses that occur during processing, marketing, and home use. Since they do not represent actual consump-

tion, they are referred to here as *availability* or *use* of foods or nutrients.

The USDA estimates per-capita use of foods or food groups by dividing total available food by the population of the 50 states and the District of Columbia. The nutritive value of the food supply is calculated from per-capita use by using nutritive values found in food composition tables. Although these data provide no information on how foods are distributed among individuals or population groups, or on changes in patterns of waste and other losses, they nevertheless reflect changes in overall patterns of foods available over time. Furthermore, these data are similar to data produced in many other countries, and they have been useful in epidemiologic research across countries, such as studies of dietary lipids and atherosclerotic diseases (Stamler, 1979).

The Nationwide Food Consumption Surveys (NFCS)

NFCS focuses on the food use of households and the dietary intakes and patterns of individuals. These surveys have been conducted approximately every 10 years since 1935 by USDA's Human Nutrition Information Service (HNIS), but the first four surveys (in 1935, 1942, 1948, and 1955) obtained information only on household food use over a 7-day period. These data reflect food use in an economic sense only and do not take into account food waste or how food is distributed among household members. Beginning in 1965, data have been collected on intakes by individuals. Surveys were conducted in 1965–1966 and in 1977–1978; separate surveys were conducted in 1977–1978 in Puerto Rico, Alaska, and Hawaii, and among low-income and elderly populations. The most recent NFCS, 1985 and 1986, were the Continuing Surveys of Food Intakes of Individuals (CSFII), designed to be conducted annually. The household screening procedures for CSFII were designed to provide three separate samples: (1) women 19 to 50 years of age and their children 1 to 5 years of age—the core group; (2) a similar age sample of low-income women and children; and (3) men 19 to 50 years of age. Data have been published on both the 1985 and 1986 surveys (USDA, 1985, 1986a,b, 1987a,b,c, 1988).

Surveys Conducted by the U.S. Department of Health and Human Services (DHHS)

In the Ten-State Nutrition Survey conducted during 1968–1970, DHHS studied low-income populations in 10 states (DHEW, 1972). In the biennial Food Label and Package Survey (Woteki, 1986), DHHS studies a statistically representative sample of packaged food products to obtain information on ingredients and on the extent of nutrient labeling. Two other DHHS studies—the Total Diet Study, conducted by the Food and Drug Administration (FDA), and the National Health and Nutrition Examination Survey (NHANES), conducted by the National Center for Health Statistics (NCHS)—are of greatest interest in the present report.

Total Diet Study

The only national system for studying average intakes of pesticides, toxic substances, radionuclides, and industrial chemicals is FDA's Total Diet Study. That study also provides estimates of dietary intakes of certain essential elements: iodine, iron, sodium, potassium, copper, magnesium, and zinc. The extent to which selected age–sex groups (males and females age 6 to 11 months, 2 years, 14 to 16 years, 25 to 30 years, and 60 to 65 years) are exposed to harmful substances and to essential minerals through diet can be determined from the results of this annual study.

Four times a year, foods representative of U.S. diets are purchased in grocery stores across the nation and are individually analyzed in FDA laboratories for the constituents mentioned above. The food items used in the Total Diet Study through April 1982 were based on data from the 1965 NFCS. Since 1982, the food items have been based on data from the 1977–1978 NFCS and the Second National Health and Nutrition Examination Survey (NHANES II), conducted during 1976–1980 and described below. Revisions to the list of food items have been described by Pennington (1983).

An example of findings from the Total Diet Study was the observation that iodine was present in the food supply in larger-than-recommended amounts, chiefly because of a higher-than-usual iodine content of milk and cereal grain products (Park et al., 1981). These findings are discussed in greater detail in the Minerals subsection of Trends in the Food Supply and Dietary Intakes, below.

Another important finding of that study in the early 1970s was that polychlorinated biphenyls (PCBs) were migrating into foods through paperboard packaging. Such packaging materials were immediately banned. Since that time, PCBs have been detected in this study only in minute amounts and then only sporadically (E. Gunderson, FDA, personal communication, 1987).

A 1987 survey conducted by the Food Marketing Institute indicated that 76% of the food shoppers questioned believed that pesticides in foods constitute a "serious hazard" (Food Marketing Institute, 1987). No pesticide examined in the Total Diet Study as far back as 1961 has been found in the diet above tolerance levels. However, the FDA's laboratory methods did not permit analyses of all pesticides that might contaminate foods, and so few samples were taken that rare but high contamination levels could be missed entirely. According to a National Research Council (NRC) report, 71 to 80% of pesticides on U.S. markets have been insufficiently tested for carcinogenesis, 90% have never been tested for damage to the nervous system, and 50 to 61% have not been tested for teratogenicity (NRC, 1984).

A 1987 report from the NRC Board on Agriculture pointed out that government regulation of herbicides, fungicides, and insecticides needs to be greatly improved to protect consumers from cancer risks due to the presence of these contaminants in food. Consistent standards are not applied to old and new pesticides, with the result that continued use of some pesticides is permitted, despite the fact that newer alternative compounds posing smaller cancer risks are available (NRC, 1987).

National Health and Nutrition Examination Survey (NHANES)

NHANES is conducted by NCHS, in part to monitor the overall nutritional status of the U.S. population through health and medical histories, dietary interviews, physical examinations, and laboratory measurements. Information is obtained about many medical conditions, including nutrition-related disorders. Among these are obesity, growth retardation, anemia, diabetes, atherosclerotic cardiovascular diseases, hypertension, and deficiencies of vitamins or minerals. NHANES I was conducted between 1971 and 1974, NHANES II between 1976 and 1980, and the Hispanic HANES (HHANES) between 1982 and 1984. NHANES III, which began in 1988, includes a potential for following people throughout their lives, surveying them at regular intervals, and using a national death certificate system to establish cause and date of death. It may also be possible in NHANES III to reexamine respondents to earlier studies. During 1982–1984, reexamination of respondents who were 25 to 74 years old during NHANES I provided a unique research opportunity for epidemiologists (Madans et al., 1986).

Nutrition Monitoring in the United States

National Nutrition Monitoring System (NNMS)

In 1977, Congress directed USDA and DHHS to integrate their surveys, and by 1981, the two departments had developed a Joint Implementation Plan for a National Nutrition Monitoring System (NNMS). The plan was to design a system for coordinating survey methods and reporting survey findings to Congress through reports from the Joint Nutrition Monitoring Evaluation Committee (JNMEC) established by the two departments in 1983. In the first report, issued in 1986 (DHHS/USDA, 1986), food intake data from the 1977–1978 NFCS, biochemical analyses from NHANES II (1976–1980), and USDA's historical food supply data were used to determine food components of public health importance. That report categorizes some food components as "warranting public health monitoring priority status." Those components are discussed below in the section on Trends in the Food Supply and Dietary Intakes. Additional details on certain aspects of NNMS were recently published (DHHS/USDA, 1987), and the second JNMEC report will be published in 1989. USDA and DHHS are also working together to coordinate their survey methods, to publish results promptly, to conduct the NFCS more frequently, and to add longitudinal aspects to data collection in NHANES.

Coordinated State Surveillance System (CSSS)

The Centers for Disease Control (CDC) contribute to nutrition monitoring through CSSS, in which the nutritional status of the high-risk pediatric population and pregnant women is monitored on the basis of information obtained from service delivery programs operated by selected state and metropolitan health jurisdictions. The CSSS provides information about the prevalence of overweight, underweight, retarded growth, and anemia among high-risk children. Among pregnant women, data are gathered on anemia, abnormal weight changes, fetal survival, birth weights, and infant feeding practices. In 1986, 34 states, the District of Columbia, and Puerto Rico participated in the pediatric survey, and 14 states, the District of Columbia, and Puerto Rico participated in the pregnancy survey.

Limitations of NFCS AND NHANES

NFCS and NHANES systematically provide valuable data on the dietary and nutritional status of Americans. Through them, desirable and undesirable trends in dietary patterns can be monitored, and data can be used to evaluate the need for group interventions. The limitations in methods used and differences in the design of the two surveys, however, influence the interpretations and conclusions that can be drawn from the data.

Populations Represented by NFCS and NHANES

The sampling units in NFCS and NHANES are households and individuals within those households; the samples are designed to represent the civilian, noninstitutionalized population. Excluded are the homeless and residents of hotels, rooming or boarding houses, dormitories, Indian reservations, military posts, prisons, hospitals, and residential treatment centers for drug addiction, alcoholism, and obesity. Clearly these surveys were not designed to represent the entire U.S. population. Omission of homeless and noninstitutionalized people underrepresents the population at greatest risk of nutritional deficiencies, but the magnitude of this bias has yet to be determined (NRC, 1986).

Data from NFCS generally are drawn from the 48 conterminous states; data from Alaska and Hawaii, when obtained, have come from separate surveys and are reported separately. NHANES II, on the other hand, included Alaska and Hawaii. NHANES oversamples low-income groups, but in the past included no respondents over age 75. A recent NFCS of low-income women and their children has been completed as part of CSFII.

How well do NFCS and NHANES represent the civilian, noninstitutionalized population? The 1977–1978 NFCS was based on a stratified area probability sample of households in the 48 conterminous states. Of the 20,812 households in the original sample, 14,930 (72%) completed the household questionnaire. Furthermore, of eligible individuals in participating households, 81% provided 3 days of dietary information. It is important to know whether nonparticipating households (28% of the original sample) differ greatly from participating households. Similarly, there would be reason for concern if the additional 19% of eligible people in participating households who failed to contribute 3-day food intake data were (for example) less educated or had lower incomes (NRC, 1986). Weighting factors were applied to make the sample more representative; however, in the absence of studies to determine the bias of nonresponders, the extent to which the 1977–

1978 NFCS is representative of the noninstitutionalized population cannot be known.

The 1985 CSFII was designed to include a stratified area probability sample in the 48 conterminous states. The first sample of women was obtained from 1,893 households containing at least one age-eligible woman (19 to 50 years old); 1,341 households (71%) provided usable data. For men 19 to 50 years old, one sample was drawn from all income levels, and an independent sample was drawn to represent households containing at least one man in that age group whose income was at or below 130% of the poverty guidelines. Of the 744 all-income sample households, 71% participated, compared with 67% of the 149 low-income sample households. USDA interviewed neighbors to determine whether people who did not participate in the 1985 CSFII differed from participants (R. Rizek, USDA, personal communication, 1987). Weighting factors were applied to adjust for nonresponders.

The response rate for NHANES is tabulated for people who participated in the initial interview held in the home, when medical histories and sociodemographic data were obtained, and who furnished dietary information and were physically examined in mobile examination centers. In NHANES I (1971–1974), 74% of the original sample completed both parts of the survey. Two reinterview surveys were conducted to determine reasons for nonparticipation (Forthofer, 1983). Of 27,801 people in the original NHANES II sample, 25,286 (91%) participated in the initial interview and 20,322 (73%) completed all aspects of the study. The investigation of potential nonresponse bias was more extensive than for NHANES I and indicated that the poststratification and nonresponse adjustments made by NCHS removed most factors that were potential sources of bias (Carroll et al., 1983; Forthofer, 1983). It was possible to do only a limited analysis of the characteristics of the 9% of the original sample who failed to participate in even the first interview. Even when studies of nonrespondents indicate minimal bias, individual users of these data should be aware that data are missing on 27 and 28% of the samples in NHANES II and the 1977–1978 NFCS, respectively, and 29 to 33% of the sample in the 1985 CSFII (NRC, 1986).

Comparability of NFCS and NHANES Data

Data from these two surveys are difficult to compare because of differences in the survey de-signs and methods of data collection. These differences lie chiefly, but not exclusively, in methods of estimating dietary intake, food composition data used to estimate nutrient intake, and standards used for determining dietary adequacy.

Methods of Estimating Dietary Intake

The 1-day (24-hour) dietary recall method has been used in NFCS and in NHANES. In the 1965–1966 NFCS, food intake data were recalled, not necessarily by the specific individual identified to respond to the questions, but by one designated respondent in each household, usually the person who shopped for and prepared the food. In the 1977–1978 NFCS, all eligible people in a household (except for their small children whose intakes were reported by adults) recalled their intake on the day before the interview and then recorded their intake on the day of the interview and on the following day, thus providing information on intake for 3 consecutive days. Standard measuring cups, spoons, and a ruler were used as aids in estimating quantities of foods consumed. Interviews were conducted on all days of the week; therefore, the data for some people included weekend days. Studies show that dietary intake on weekends may differ from that on weekdays (Acheson et al., 1980; Beaton et al., 1979; Richards and Roberge, 1982).

In the 1985 CSFII, data were collected by using the 1-day dietary recall only. Data on women and their children were obtained on 6 separate days throughout the year at intervals of approximately 2 months. The initial 1-day recall was obtained by in-person interview; later, recall data were obtained by telephone. At the time of this writing, data on only 4 nonconsecutive days of intake have been published. Men in the 1985 CSFII supplied recall data by in-person interview for only 1 day.

Respondents in the 1965–1966 and the 1985 NFCS were not notified in advance about the interviews, but they were notified by letter in the 1977–1978 NFCS. Notification ahead of time may have resulted in more accurate recalls or in modification of dietary intake, since the letter suggested that respondents should begin to keep records of foods purchased for the household. This could have affected some people's ability to recall their food intake.

An important change in method was introduced in the 1985 CSFII. Interviewers probed specifically to learn brand names of processed foods; whether fat on meat or skin on poultry was consumed; whether salt or butter was added to food during cooking or at the table; whether food items were eaten during cooking or cleaning up; and if snack items or beverages had been forgotten. Although these changes were made for appropriate reasons, one needs to keep these differences in mind when attempting to use NFCS data to study changes in food consumption over time. In addition, we do not know the extent to which differences in NFCS and NHANES estimates of nutrient intake are due to differences in the extent to which interviewers probed for specific information.

In both NHANES I and NHANES II, 1-day recalls were obtained through in-person interviews conducted in a mobile unit, where laboratory measures (e.g., blood pressure) were also obtained. Three-dimensional food models were used as aids in estimating quantities consumed. Dietary interviews were conducted in such a way that 1-day intakes were for weekdays only, and the method of obtaining intakes was the same for NHANES I and II. Respondents supplied information on the frequency with which foods had been consumed during the preceding 3-month period. This was an attempt to ascertain the usual pattern of food consumption. In both NHANES I and II, a letter announcing the survey was sent to each household 1 week before the first interview, but the letter informed respondents only of the general purpose of the survey and said nothing about the plan to obtain information on food intake.

Research is needed on the extent to which differences in methods used by NFCS and NHANES affect the results reported. These differences include days of the week for which data are collected; the use of probing questions and methods to aid respondents in estimating portion sizes; assignment of food codes; and privacy during the interview. In NFCS, other household members could have been present. In NHANES, only the respondent was present with the interviewer (Woteki, 1985).

Limitations of Food and Nutrient Intake Assessment Methods

One of the most difficult tasks in nutrition research is documenting the actual or habitual food and nutrient intake of individuals or groups. A single 24-hour recall cannot be used to estimate the habitual intake of a person, although it can be used to estimate the average intake of a group. Problems involved in estimating food intake are discussed at length in Chapter 2 and are not repeated here.

A recent publication comments on errors in reporting dietary intake and on differences in the

distributions of intakes reported in several recent large surveys (NRC, 1986). These differences were inconsistent across nutrients and suggested bias in either food intake estimates or food composition data. Systematic biases can affect estimates of nutrient intake; for example, the failure of the 1977–1978 NFCS to record supplement use resulted in underestimating the intake of vitamins and minerals.

Limitations of Food Composition Data

In both NHANES and NFCS, food composition data (discussed below) are used to calculate the nutritive value of food consumed by respondents. The nutrients and dietary fiber reported by the major national surveys are shown in Table 3–1.

The major repository of nutrient composition data for individual foods in the United States is USDA's Nutrient Data Bank (NDB), sections of which have been published in a revision of USDA Agriculture Handbook No. 8, *Composition of Foods— Raw, Processed, and Prepared.* Sources of data for the NDB include studies in the scientific literature, unpublished reports from federal government and university laboratories, studies contracted by USDA, and data from industry for foods bearing nutrition labels. Generally, NDB data used in the 1977–1978 NFCS pertained to nutrients in food as purchased (not as actually consumed) and therefore did not account for losses or modifications due to preparation or processing. In addition to the NDB data, NHANES has also used data from industry on the composition of new food products and brand-name products of unique formulation. The data bases of both surveys are updated as new information is obtained. For example, for the 1985 and 1986 CSFII, corrections were made for changes in moisture and fat and for retention of nutrients during preparation (F.N. Hepburn, USDA, personal communication, 1987).

Little is known about the quantity of some nutrients and nonnutrients in foods because of inadequate analytical methods. The presence of nonnutrients, such as dietary fiber, in foods has sparked scientific interest, but data on these food constituents are not yet complete. Table 3–2 makes it clear that there are large gaps in food composition data. When possible, amounts of nutrients in foods noted in the tables come from actual chemical analyses, but if such data are unavailable, the amounts in the table are imputed. For nutrients that have been tracked for a long time, such as calcium and protein, the proportion of analytical data in the tables, as opposed to

TABLE 3–1 Nutrients and Other Food Constituents Reported by National Studies[a]

Nutrient or Food Constitutent	Data Source							
	Historical Food Supply[b]	1977–1978 NFCS[c]		1985 CSFII[d]	NHANES[e]		Total Diet Study[f]	Food Composition[g]
		House-hold	Indivi-dual		I	II		
Water	−	−	−	−	−	−	−	+
Energy (kcal)	+	+	+	+	+	+	−	+
Protein, total	+	+	+	+	+	+	−	+
Amino acids	−	−	−	−	−	−	−	*,**
Carbohydrates, total	+	+	+	+	−	+	−	+
Sugars	+	−	**	−	−	−	−	−
Lipids								
Total fat	+	+	+	+	−	+	−	+
Saturated fat	+	−	−	+	−	+	−	*
Oleic acid	+	−	−	−	−	+	−	*
Total monounsaturated fat	−	−	−	+	−	−	−	*
Linoleic acid	+	−	−	−	−	+	−	*
Total polyunsaturated fat	−	−	−	+	−	−	−	*
Cholesterol	+	−	**	+	−	+	−	*
Vitamins								
A, IU	+	+	+	+	+	+	−	+
A, RE	−	−	−	−	−	−	−	*
Carotene	−	−	−	+	−	−	−	−
E	−	−	−	+	−	−	−	*,**
Thiamin (B₁)	+	+	+	+	+	+	−	+
Riboflavin (B₂)	+	+	+	+	+	+	−	+
Niacin (preformed)	+	+	+	+	+	+	−	+
Pantothenic acid	**	−	−	−	−	−	−	*,**
B₆	+	+	+	+	−	−	−	+
Folate	**	−	−	−	−	−	−	*,**
B₁₂	+	+	+	+	−	−	−	+
C	+	+	+	+	+	+	−	+
Minerals								
Calcium	+	+	+	+	+	+	+	+
Phosphorus	+	+	+	+	−	+	+	+
Magnesium	+	+	+	+	−	−	+	+
Iron	+	+	+	+	+	+	+	+
Iodine	−	−	−	−	−	−	+	−
Sodium	+	−	**	+	−	+	+	+
Potassium	+	−	−	+	−	+	+	+
Copper	−	−	−	+	−	−	+	*,**
Zinc	+	−	−	+	−	−	+	*
Manganese	−	−	−	+	−	−	+	*,**
Selenium	−	−	−	−	−	−	+	−
Chromium	−	−	−	−	−	−	+	−
Fiber, crude	+	−	−	−	−	−	+	+
Dietary	−	−	−	+	−	−	−	**
Alcoholic beverages	−	+	+	+	−	+	+	+

NOTE: +, Data reported; −, data not reported; *, nutrient data will be available in revised USDA Agriculture Handbook No. 8 (USDA, in press); **, data incomplete or questionable.
[a]Table based on information from USDA (1987a) and Woteki (1986).
[b]USDA's food supply data indicating disappearance of food into consumer channels.
[c]Nationwide Food Consumption Survey (USDA, 1984).
[d]Continuing Survey of Food Intakes of Individuals (USDA, 1985, 1986b).
[e]National Health and Nutrition Examination Survey I (1971–1974) and II (1976–1980).
[f]Total Diet Study of Food and Drug Administration (unpublished data).
[g]Woteki (1986).

TABLE 3–2 Percentage of Analytical Data for a Given Nutrient in USDA Primary Data Set (PDS)[a]

Nutrient	Percentage		Nutrient	Percentage	
	All Foods	Best Sources		All Foods	Best Sources
Calcium	97		Cholesterol	80	
Protein	97		Magnesium	75	72
Fat	96		Zinc	73	79
Thiamin	91		Copper	67	71
Riboflavin	91		Vitamin B$_6$	64	72
Niacin	91		Vitamin B$_{12}$	64	70
Sodium	90		Vitamin A (RE)	61	73
Potassium	90		Folate	56	69
Phosphorus	90		Carotene	54	88
Iron	90		Dietary fiber	29	40
Vitamin C	83	92	α-Tocopherol	28	39
Vitamin A (IU)	80	89			

[a]From Hepburn (1987). The USDA Primary Data Set contains data on basic foods, including ingredients of foods, such as flour.

imputed data, is high, but the proportion is low for nutrients recently added to USDA surveys, such as dietary fiber and α-tocopherol (Hepburn, 1987). Table 3–2 indicates, for example, that only 64% of the data on vitamin B$_6$ in all foods in the data set are analytical values, but a higher proportion (72%) of the data on foods that are best sources of vitamin B$_6$ represent analytical as opposed to imputed data.

Although there are ample data on nutrients in commodities, there is little information on highly processed or manufactured foods such as snack foods, baked products, convenience foods, restaurant meals, fast foods, and frozen dinners. In addition, knowledge is limited regarding the amounts of vitamin B$_6$, pantothenic acid, folacin, vitamin E, zinc, copper, magnesium, manganese, chromium, and selenium in foods (Beecher and Vanderslice, 1984). Information on other substances of interest, such as carotenoids and dietary fiber, is rapidly accumulating. Lack of information on nonnutrients is of particular concern for those studying the relationship between diet and cancer.

Food composition tables necessarily show typical values, but the nutrient composition of a specific food portion depends on many factors; for example, the composition of fresh fruits and vegetables depends on the variety, extent of exposure to sun, maturity, and transport and storage conditions. Biases in food composition data may result when inappropriate analytical methods are used (e.g., such as certain methods used in gathering data on fiber) and when a food item is incorrectly identified (e.g., as skim milk instead of whole milk) (NRC, 1986).

In both NHANES and NFCS, the nutrient values are calculated by matching each reported food to a description in the survey's food composition data base, then selecting and assigning the appropriate food code. In NHANES II, interviewers coded the responses on site. In NFCS, coding was done at a central location by persons other than the interviewers. The extent to which this methodological difference in assigning the codes resulted in different estimates of nutrient intakes in the two surveys is unknown (Woteki, 1985).

Use and Misuse of Standards of Dietary Adequacy

Standards used in national surveys to judge dietary adequacy differ. In NFCS, the 1980 Recommended Dietary Allowances (RDAs) were used. NHANES has its own set of standards that are developed by an ad hoc advisory group and differ from the RDAs in several ways; in particular, standards for vitamin A and calcium are lower.

RDAs have been set for protein, certain vitamins (A, D, E, B$_6$, B$_{12}$, thiamin, riboflavin, niacin, and folacin), and certain minerals (calcium, phosphorus, magnesium, iron, zinc, and iodine). Because data were inadequate in 1980 to set RDAs for other nutrients, ranges of Estimated Safe and Adequate Daily Dietary Intakes (ESADDI) were given for three vitamins (biotin, pantothenic acid, and vitamin K) and for several minerals (copper, manganese, fluoride, chromium, selenium, molybdenum, sodium, potassium, and chloride).

The RDAs have been often used to interpret survey data on food intake obtained by a single

24-hour recall or by 1- to 3-day food intake records. In discussing the results of such studies, investigators may use cutoff points to report the number or percentage of respondents whose intakes fall within specific percentiles or cutoff points of the RDA, e.g., two-thirds or 70% of the RDA for a nutrient, implying that certain segments of the respondent population have inadequate intakes of the nutrient, or that they are "at nutritional risk." Because these cutoff points are arbitrary, this practice leads to incorrect estimates of the frequency of adequate and inadequate intakes in the population and is based on misunderstandings of the appropriate uses of the RDAs and of a single 24-hour recall or 3-day record in food intake studies.

The RDAs are *not requirements* below which deficiency diseases are apt to develop. Rather, for many nutrients they are set at sufficiently high levels to cover the needs of practically all healthy people. Since individuals differ in their requirements for specific nutrients, however, it is impossible to know from a dietary survey which person requires at least the RDA and which one requires less or possibly even more. Therefore, all cutoff points are misleading, even if the dietary method used provides accurate data on the customary intake of each person. Many people who rank below the cutoff point actually have adequate intakes because they require less, whereas some above the cutoff point have too low an intake to meet their needs. The magnitude and direction of the errors involved in the misuse of the RDAs are not known (NRC, 1986).

As pointed out in Chapter 2, because of the enormous day-to-day variation in the amounts and kinds of foods eaten by one person, 1 or 3 consecutive days of intake are not representative of usual or customary intake over an extended period. Thus, although a single 24-hour recall or 1- to 3-day record, if carefully done, may be useful in assessing the average or median intake of a population group, their use in ranking individuals is inappropriate (Garn et al., 1978; Hegsted, 1972).

In summary, NFCS and NHANES dietary data obtained at different times must be compared cautiously and with full knowledge of the differences in methods used to gather and summarize data. Food intake data can be compared with somewhat less difficulty than nutrient intake data.

NFCS and NHANES samples are sufficiently large to detect major public health problems but not to uncover clinical illness scattered throughout the population. A deficiency or other nutritional disorder would have to affect approximately 1% of the population—about 2 million people—to be reasonably sure of being detected by these surveys (DHHS/USDA, 1986).

USDA and DHHS recognize the problems described and are attempting to devise solutions to improve comparability of the two surveys. NHANES III, to be conducted between 1988 and 1994, will oversample (i.e., sample more people in a subgroup than warranted by their percentage in the general population) the elderly, blacks, Hispanics, and the very young. Data for the 1987–1988 NFCS are currently being gathered, and CSFII will cover all sex and age groups beginning in 1989. In planned nutrition monitoring activities, data on dietary intakes will be collected through 1996. Efforts will be made to expedite publication of data from these surveys (DHHS/USDA, 1987).

Problems in Assessing Nutritional Status

Nutritional status has been defined as an individual's health condition as it is influenced by the intake and utilization of nutrients (Todhunter, 1970). In theory, optimal nutritional status should be attained by consuming sufficient, but not excessive, sources of energy, essential nutrients, and other food components (such as dietary fiber) not containing toxins or contaminants.

Traditionally, efforts to detect poor nutritional status have centered on nutritional deficiencies in populations, since defining or assessing optimal health is difficult. Nutritional deficiency follows a pattern starting with low intake or utilization of one or more nutrients, then progressing to biochemical abnormalities, abnormal growth, abnormal body mass, and, eventually, to full-blown deficiency. Poor nutritional status is not confined to undernutrition. It may also result from excessive intake or inadequate expenditure of food energy, or from excessive intakes of specific nutrients, resulting in acute toxicity or chronic diseases.

A major problem in interpreting national dietary surveys and their relationship to nutritional assessment for populations, especially with regard to chronic diseases, is the use of fixed cutoff points, such as a fixed percentage of the RDAs, as criteria for judging the adequacy of dietary intakes. The Food and Nutrition Board Subcommittee on Criteria for Dietary Evaluation (NRC, 1986) proposed that multiple criteria be used for assessing adequacy of dietary intake contingent on the intended outcome. Thus, adequate intake levels might range progressively from those required to maintain high tissue concentrations of a nutrient to lower levels needed to just maintain normal metabolic functions or to still lower levels required to prevent clinical deficiency (NRC, 1986). Clinical or laboratory indicators would be developed for each level of nutriture so that they could be used in population assessments.

Cutoff points frequently are used in nutritional assessment studies, but as noted earlier in relation to dietary intake, no single cutoff can separate adequately nourished people from those with nutritional deficiencies. As Figure 3–1 illustrates, regardless of the cutoff used, the nutritional status of some people will be erroneously classified as deficient, whereas some individuals with nutritional deficiencies will be classified as adequately nourished. The Food and Nutrition Board Subcommittee on Criteria for Dietary Evaluation proposed that problems stemming from use of a cutoff point might be overcome if the distribution of nutrient requirements was compared with the distribution of nutrient intakes in a sample population (NRC, 1986). This probability approach would allow investigators to make better estimates of the prevalence of inadequate intakes in a population, but would still not permit the identification of people with adequate nourishment. The success of this method will depend on development of more accurate estimates of the mean requirement for each nutrient and its variability in the population, as well as the improvement of methods of assessing dietary intakes. Analogous conceptual approaches may be used for biochemical assessment of nutritional status (Beaton, 1986).

Many investigators have used regression or correlation analyses to examine the relationship of dietary intake to biochemical or other indicators of nutritional status within populations, and some have reported no relationship or only a weak one. Beaton (1986) identified several possible causative factors for this. First is the failure to determine usual dietary intake, which cannot be accomplished by obtaining only one 24-hour recall from each respondent (as was done in NHANES I and II) because of the large day-to-day variability in intake by individuals (Block, 1982). Second is the known biologic variability in nutrient requirements and laboratory indicators at a given level of nutritional status. Third is the variable sensitivity of some nutritional status indicators across different levels of nutriture. For example, as iron stores increase with high iron intakes, hemoglobin is no longer a sensitive indicator of iron nutritional status. Thus, only if nutritional status among

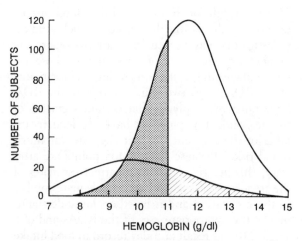

FIGURE 3–1 Difficulties when cutoff points are used to assess nutritional status. Eleven grams of hemoglobin per deciliter is an arbitrary cutoff for assessing iron status. The lower left-hand curve represents the distribution of hemoglobin levels among individuals known to respond to increased iron intake. The upper right-hand curve represents the distribution among those known to have adequate iron intakes. The cross-hatched area above 11 g represents individuals who are anemic but classified as normal by this cutoff point; the stippled area below 11 g represents those classified as anemic by this cutoff, but who are not responsive to increased iron intakes. Since the two distributions overlap, no single cutoff point can separate adequately from inadequately nourished individuals. From Beaton (1986).

subjects varies greatly would it be possible to demonstrate a strong relationship between intake and the laboratory indicator. If all subjects are adequately nourished with respect to some nutrient, the variability in amounts of the nutrient required and the normal physiological variability that subjects show in the laboratory indicator may obscure any association between intake and the laboratory indicator. Beaton (1986) notes that much of the controversy regarding relationships between dietary intake and nutritional status is due to flawed concepts, which can obscure relationships when they exist and produce spurious evidence of relationships when they do not. New conceptual frameworks are needed to overcome these problems.

In the past, evaluations of nutritional status have focused chiefly on criteria for prevention of nutrient deficiencies. Today, there is substantial interest in the association of nutrition with chronic diseases. Excessive intakes of nutrients can work through normal biologic or metabolic functions to produce some chronic diseases or risk factors for disease. The Food and Nutrition Board Subcommittee on Criteria for Dietary Evaluation

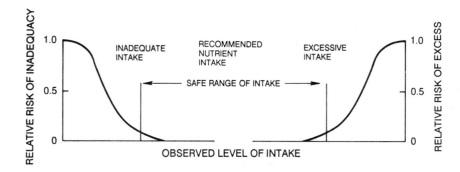

FIGURE 3–2 The curve on the left, based on a cumulative distribution of requirements, indicates increasing risk of inadequate intake. The curve on the right indicates increasing risk of excess. The safe range of intake is between these levels. From Beaton (1986).

(NRC, 1986) noted that the probability approach can be used to analyze excessive intakes of nutrients or food components just as it can be used to assess inadequate intakes (Figure 3–2). To date, little attention has been paid to the frequency distribution of intakes that are or may be detrimental; this must be remedied before this method can be used. Other relationships between diet and disease may not fit into this conventional conceptual view, because metabolic functions—which form the basis of the conceptual framework described above—may not be involved (Beaton, 1986).

Data gathered to assess nutritional status, as in NHANES, are of limited value in evaluating possible relationships between diet and many cancers because of the long latency periods between exposure and clinical manifestation. In most cancers—for example, breast cancer—information about intake during the distant past, rather than present intake, is needed. Problems in obtaining such information are discussed in Chapter 2. Furthermore, causative or protective dietary constituents—such as nonessential trace elements (cadmium), contaminants (aflatoxins, pesticides), and carotenoids with no vitamin A activity—may be among many substances that are included in surveys and current food composition tables. Methods by which foods are stored or prepared may play a role in the causation of cancer, but such data are not generally collected through NFCS or NHANES.

Objectives and priorities for research on diet and cancer have been identified by a National Research Council committee in its report *Diet, Nutrition, and Cancer: Directions for Research* (NRC, 1983). Among other priorities, that committee noted a pressing need for short-term tests to identify early biologic indicators of exposure to dietary constituents that affect carcinogenesis. The complexities of studying the relationships of diet to cancer are just beginning to be appreciated, but it is already obvious that studies must be designed specifically to test hypotheses regarding this relationship.

NHANES and Nutritional Assessment

NHANES is the only national survey providing information on the nutritional status of the population. Four types of NHANES data are of importance in studies of diet and health: dietary intake, to determine kind and amount of food consumed and its nutrient quality; anthropometry, to describe growth and body weight patterns; biochemical tests, to determine nutrient levels in blood and urine; and clinical examinations, to detect signs of nutritional problems. NHANES data have been used to evaluate the proportion of the population at risk for deficiencies of vitamin A, vitamin C, folate, iron, zinc, and protein.

Experience gained in NHANES I led to changes in the collection of biochemical data in NHANES II. For example, because vitamin A deficiency was judged not to be a problem among older age groups in NHANES I, biochemical values for this vitamin were obtained only for children 3 to 11 years of age in NHANES II. The current interest in vitamin A relative to cancer risk had not yet emerged. Blood levels of zinc and copper were obtained in NHANES II but not in NHANES I, and assessment of anemia was intensified in NHANES II by adding several biochemical tests and gathering additional information in the medical history and physical examination. No attempt was made in either NHANES to gather data on toxins and contaminants in the diet.

Problems in Using NHANES Data to Study Diet–Chronic Disease Relationships

Although NHANES was designed to examine nutrition and health status in the United States—not to study hypotheses regarding diet and chronic diseases—some investigators have used NHANES data to evaluate dietary intake and certain risk factors for cardiovascular diseases (e.g., blood pressure and serum cholesterol levels) (Harlan et al., 1983, 1984; McCarron et al., 1984; Sempos et al., 1986). Although NHANES data are extensive and derive from a broad range of measurements, there are some limitations, which affect attempts to use NHANES data in the study of chronic diseases. The following discussion of limitations is based on publications by Yetley and Johnson (1987) and by Murphy and Michael (1982).

NHANES provides only cross-sectional, periodic data, which are not suitable for studying causal relationships. Only longitudinal studies can supply data appropriate for determining causality. Furthermore, because many respondents are under treatment for medical conditions at the time of the survey, they may have altered their dietary habits and thereby certain biochemical parameters. In a longitudinal study, their prediagnostic dietary and biochemical data would be known, making possible more accurate tracking of the influence of dietary intake on the disease under study. Such people must be excluded from analyses of relationships between diet and disease when using NHANES data.

Certain measurements needed for such studies of diet and chronic diseases may not have been made in NHANES, or the methods used may have been inappropriate. Furthermore, biochemical measurements are usually evaluated in NHANES according to specified cutoff points, which are as inappropriate for studies of chronic diseases as they are for judging dietary adequacy. Erroneous estimates of nutritional risk can result if there are substantial differences in physiological status at a given biochemical level (e.g., blood level of nutrients).

Investigators who use NHANES data in studies of chronic diseases need to evaluate carefully whether the potential nonresponse bias (discussed above) and measurement bias will affect their application of the data. In addition, the complex sample designs and weighting factors must be taken into account when data are analyzed. The use of statistical programs that assume simple random sampling is rarely appropriate; NHANES investigators have developed computer programs that are appropriate for the data gathered.

TRENDS IN THE FOOD SUPPLY AND DIETARY INTAKES

Changes in dietary patterns since the turn of the century have been extensive and include changes in sources of calories; the composition of foods;

consumption of specific food groups, including nonalcoholic and alcoholic beverages; and eating patterns, such as snacking and eating away from home and the selection of diets that differ from those of the average American. A discussion of these changes, below, is based on historical food supply data, results from NFCS and NHANES, and other sources.

Food Energy

Total caloric intake is of interest in epidemiologic studies not only because of its association with body weight, but also because of implications that it may be involved in the relationship between nutrients and chronic diseases. Whether or not an individual gains, loses, or maintains body weight depends on the balance between caloric intake and physical activity, body size, body composition, and probably metabolic efficiency (Sims et al., 1973) (see Chapter 6). These factors largely explain the differences in energy intake among individuals.

Because individuals vary in their energy needs, there is no satisfactory dietary standard for assessing adequacy of energy intake. Fully recognizing this fact, investigators in the 1977–1978 NFCS chose the midpoints of the ranges of the Recommended Energy Intakes (REIs) given by the Food and Nutrition Board in 1980 (NRC, 1980). Food energy intakes reported in that survey averaged 84% of the REI midpoints. Approximately 25% of the respondents had intakes of the REI midpoints or greater, and 52% had at least 80% of the REI midpoints.

A comparison of data from national surveys indicates that reported caloric intakes have decreased over time, whereas body weights have increased. A comparison of 1971–1974 NHANES I data with data from the 1960–1962 Health and Examination Survey shows average weight increases of 3 lb for females and 6 lb for males. Heights also increased over the same period (Abraham, 1979). The 1977–1978 NFCS data obtained by 24-hour recall showed a decline in caloric intake for men and women 19 to 50 years of age when compared with 1965 NFCS data (USDA, 1984). The reported energy intakes for males 9 to 64 years old were 10 to 17% lower in 1977–1978 than in 1965; for females 23 to 50 years old, energy intakes were 9% lower. The average intake reported for females (1,500 to 1,600 kcal/day) is of concern because of the difficulty in incorporating all nutrients at recommended levels in a diet so low in calories (Mertz and Kelsay, 1984).

TABLE 3–3 Nutrients Available for Consumption Per Capita Per Day, 1909 to 1985

Nutrient	Unit	1909–1913	1947–1949	1967–1969	1977–1979	1984	1985	Percent Change[a] 1967–1969 to 1985	1984 to 1985
Food energy	kcal	3,500	3,200	3,300	3,300	3,400	3,600	9	3
Protein	g	99	93	97	98	101	102	5	1
Fats	g	124	140	156	158	164	172	10	5
Cholesterol	mg	500	570	520	480	480	480	−8	0
Carbohydrates	g	493	403	378	391	401	413	9	3
Calcium	mg	750	980	900	880	920	920	3	0
Phosphorus	mg	1,480	1,490	1,470	1,470	1,510	1,510	3	1
Magnesium	mg	380	340	310	310	320	320	3	1
Iron	mg	14.8	15.9	16.2	16.4	18.0	18.3	13	1
Zinc	mg	12.7	11.4	12.1	12.0	12.2	12.3	2	1
Vitamin A	IU	7,200	8,100	7,300	9,100	9,800	9,900	37	2
Vitamin E	mg α-TE[b]	11.2	12.5	14.3	16.0	16.4	17.6	23	7
Ascorbic acid	mg	101	110	98	108	110	114	16	4
Thiamin	mg	1.6	2.0	2.0	2.1	2.1	2.2	10	1
Riboflavin	mg	1.8	2.3	2.3	2.3	2.4	2.4	5	0
Niacin	mg	19	20	23	25	26	26	14	2
Vitamin B_6	mg	2.2	1.9	1.9	2.0	2.0	2.1	8	2
Vitamin B_{12}	μg	7.9	8.6	9.2	9.0	8.9	8.8	−5	−1

[a]The last two columns (percent change) are based on rounded quantities of nutrients from foods available for consumption per capita per day. Data from Marston and Raper (1987).
[b]α-TE = α-tocopherol equivalents.

As pointed out above, some differences in survey data over time may reflect differences in methods of obtaining data, yet the reported decline in caloric intake accompanied by weight gain requires some explanation. Decline in physical activity may have occurred but was not monitored in these surveys. In addition, studies indicate that there may have been some underreporting of food intake. For example, the USDA's Beltsville Human Nutrition Research Center reported that subjects in nutrition studies conducted over the past 10 years generally required more calories to maintain body weight on a controlled dietary regimen (as encountered in the studies) than they reported in dietary records of their usual self-selected diets collected for 7 days before they entered the studies (Mertz and Kelsay, 1984). Hallfrisch et al. (1982) reported that compared with caloric intake reported on 7-day records of self-selected diets, male subjects required an average of 500 additional calories and females 900 additional calories to maintain constant weight on an 18-week controlled diet. The observed differences may have been due to differences in physical activity, although subjects were cautioned to maintain usual activity. Subjects in this study were fed in a "modified gorging" pattern, receiving 25% of calories at breakfast and 75% at the evening meal—a definite change in eating pattern; the influence of this pattern on caloric need, if any, is unknown. Another possible explanation of the observed difference in caloric intake is that portion sizes were underestimated on the records or that the requirement to record intake resulted in modification of usual eating patterns (see Chapter 2).

In the 1977–1978 NFCS, the average daily food energy intake for all survey participants was estimated to be 1,826 kcal based on a 3-day intake. The group with the highest average daily intake, 2,568 kcal, was 15- to 18-year-old males. Men 75 years and older averaged 1,866 kcal. The highest average intake for females was 1,849 kcal for 9- to 11-year-olds. This declined with age to a low of 1,417 kcal for women 75 years and older based on a 3-day intake. The intake of women 19 to 50 years of age averaged 1,588 kcal/day in the 1986 CSFII based on a 1-day intake, compared with 1,528 kcal/day based on a 4-day intake in the 1985 CSFII and 1,573 kcal/day in the 1977–1978 NFCS.

Sources of Food Energy

As noted above, historical food supply data represent amounts of foods that disappear into the food distribution system. These data have provided a way to assess trends in the availability of foods

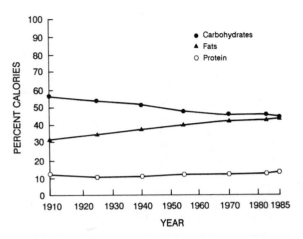

FIGURE 3–3 Percentage of calories from protein, carbohydrates, and fat from 1909–1913 to 1985. These data fail to present the entire picture, since food supply data do not include alcohol or grains used in production of alcoholic beverages. From R.M. Marston, USDA/HNIS, unpublished data, 1986.

and nutrients in the food supply since early in this century.

The distribution of food energy between carbohydrates and fats in the food supply has changed since the first decades of this century. The availability of fats has steadily increased (Table 3–3), whereas carbohydrate levels fell from 1909 to 1969 but have increased by approximately 9% since then. Of the percentages of calories provided by the macronutrients, protein has contributed approximately 11% from 1909 to 1985, while the percentage from fats increased from 32 to 43% and the percentage available from carbohydrates fell from 57 to 46% (Figure 3–3).

Food groups consisting of grain products and of meat, poultry, or fish supply the largest share of calories in the U.S. diet. Fats, sweets, and beverages combined contribute about as many calories as fruits plus vegetables or milk plus milk products, and substantially more than the combination of eggs, legumes, nuts, and seeds (Figure 3–4; see figure caption for definitions of groups).

Fats, Fatty Acids, and Cholesterol

Dietary fat is of concern in relation to coronary heart disease (CHD), cancer, and possibly obesity. The associations of saturated, monounsaturated, and polyunsaturated fatty acid intakes with CHD have received particular attention.

The per-capita availability of fatty acids in the food supply increased from 1909 to 1985. This increase was markedly greater for linoleic acid (which increased 19 g/day) and oleic acid (a 20-g/day increase) than for saturated fatty acids (a 7-g/day increase) (Figure 3–5). In 1985, linoleic acid in the food supply accounted for 7% of total calories, oleic acid for 17%, and saturated fatty acids for 15% (Figure 3–6). Changes since 1909 resulted in a large increase in the percentage of total fat calories from linoleic acid and a decline in the percentage of fat calories from saturated fatty acids (Figure 3–7). Nevertheless, saturated fatty acids and oleic acid still make up the highest percentage of calories from fats and of total calories from fatty acids in the food.

Fat Intake

Does actual fat consumption reflect these food supply changes? Data from NFCS indicate that mean fat intakes by individuals were lower during 1977–1978 (40.3% of calories) than in 1965 (42.1% calories). The 1985 CSFII for women and men 19 to 50 years of age indicated that fat intakes continued to decline. As shown in Table 3–4, however, data from NHANES contradict these results. These data indicate that for women 19 to

TABLE 3–4 Mean Percentage of Total Calories from Fats, Derived from Five Surveys of Women 19 to 50 Years Old in the United States from 1971 to 1986[a]

Age Groups (years)	Fat (% of total calories)				
	1971–1974 NHANES I, 1-day intake	1976–1980 NHANES II, 1-day intake	1977–1978 NFCS, 3-day intake	1985 CSFII, 4-day (non-consecutive) intake	1986 CSFII, 1-day intake
19–34	36.1	35.9	40.4	36.6	36.1
35–50	37.0	36.8	41.3	37.0	36.7
All	36.5	36.3	40.8	36.8	36.4

[a]From C.E. Woteki, DHHS/NCHS, unpublished data, 1986.

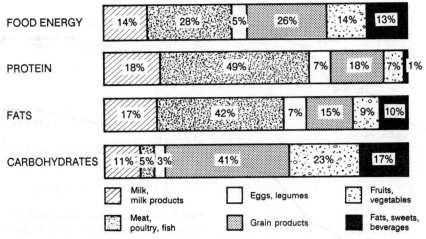

FOOD ENERGY — 14% | 28% | 5% | 26% | 14% | 13%

PROTEIN — 18% | 49% | 7% | 18% | 7% | 1%

FATS — 17% | 42% | 7% | 15% | 9% | 10%

CARBOHYDRATES — 11% | 5% | 3% | 41% | 23% | 17%

Milk, milk products   Eggs, legumes   Fruits, vegetables

Meat, poultry, fish   Grain products   Fats, sweets, beverages

Milk and milk products exclude butter, soy-based imitation milk and baby formulas, and nondairy creamers. They include ice cream and other milk desserts, as well as cheeses, including imitation cheese.

Meats, poultry, and fish include mixtures such as soup, stews, hash, frozen meats, and sandwiches reported as a single item.

Legumes, nuts, and seeds include soy-based formulas and milk substitute.

Grain products include breads, crackers, pasta, grits and other cooked cereals, breakfast cereals, pancakes, cakes, pies, cookies, pastries, and main-dish items such as pizza, quiche, and rice and pasta mixtures.

Fruits include fruits, fruit juices, tomatoes, and products made with tomatoes such as tomato sauce and catsup. Citrus fruit drinks and ades are reported under beverages.

Vegetables include potatoes, starchy Puerto Rican vegetables, pickles, olives, relishes, vegetable juices and soups, and baby food vegetables.

Fats and oils include solid and liquid shortenings, meat drippings, nondairy creamers, butter, margarine, and sauces that are chiefly fat.

Sugars and sweets include candy, icings, jellies, jams, ices, gelatin desserts, toppings, and sweet sauces.

Beverages include all types of coffee, tea, soft drinks, and fruit drinks and ades.

FIGURE 3–4 Food sources of energy and energy nutrients in percentages per person per day, as indicated in the 1977–1978 NFCS. Based on data from USDA (1984).

50 years of age, no difference in fat intake occurred between the 1971–1974 and 1976–1980 surveys (NHANES I and II). On the other hand, data from NFCS show a higher intake of fat in 1977–1978 than NHANES data indicated in 1976–1980 and a decline in intakes in the 1985 and 1986 CSFII. Thus, all surveys except the 1977–1978 NFCS seem to provide similar values. The discrepancies between NFCS and NHANES may be explained by systematic biases inherent in methods used in NHANES, NFCS, and CSFII (Jacobs et al., 1985). Differences in fat intake observed in the 1977–1978 NFCS and 1985 and 1986 CSFIIs may have been due to differences in the type and depth of questions asked in the two surveys. For example, the CSFII included specific questions concerning the type of fat (e.g., meat fat, poultry skin) consumed, but the 1977–1978 NFCS did not. Thus, the national surveys fail to tell us whether or not fat intake has really decreased over time.

At this writing, the most recent estimates of usual intake are those from the 1985 CSFII survey of women 19 to 50 years old and their children

between the ages of 1 and 5. In this survey, estimates of usual intake were based on 4 nonconsecutive days of intake obtained by 24-hour recall rather than on only one 24-hour recall (USDA, 1987b). Women consumed a mean of 36.8% of their calories as fat—13.3% from saturated fat, 13.6% from monounsaturated fat, and 7.4% from polyunsaturated fat. Children consumed a mean of 34.7% of their calories as fat—13.7% from saturated fat, 12.7% from monounsaturated fat, and 5.9% from polyunsaturated fat. These are mean values; many respondents consumed higher or lower percentages.

Dietary Food Sources of Fat

Changes in levels of specific fatty acids in the food supply can be attributed to several changes in the availability of foods. The increase in linoleic acid supplies was due chiefly to the remarkable increase in the use of salad and cooking oils from 2 to 25 lb per capita from 1909 to 1985 (Table 3–5). The increased use of margarine and shortening containing vegetable fat also contributed to supplies of linoleic acid as well as to oleic acid.

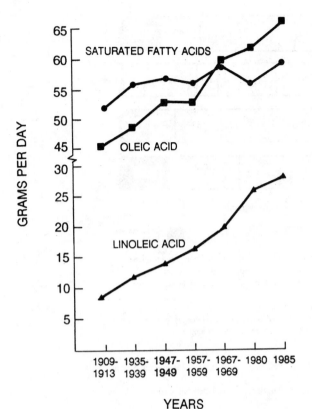

FIGURE 3–5 Trends in per-capita intake of oleic acid, saturated fatty acids, and linoleic acid in the U.S. food supply from 1909–1913 to 1985. From R.M. Marston, USDA/HNIS, unpublished data, 1986.

The contribution of poultry to fat intake greatly increased after 1940. In the meat, poultry, and fish group, however, pork has contributed the most fat since 1909–1913; beef contributed the second highest amount. Fluid whole milk was the major source of fat in the dairy products group until 1980, when cheese became the chief source. Table 3–5 indicates that consumption of fluid whole milk declined by almost 50% since 1967–1969, whereas the consumption of low-fat milk almost doubled.

Data from the 1977–1978 NFCS and the 1976–1980 NHANES show that the meat, poultry, and fish group is the primary source of dietary fats. Sources of fats reported in the 1977–1978 NFCS are shown in Figure 3–4. Fats contributed by grain products come chiefly from added fats or oils in cakes, pies, pastries, and other baked products. Because the two surveys differed in the ways foods were assigned to food groups and in the data bases used for calculating nutrients, detailed direct comparisons cannot be made.

NHANES II data for the total adult population surveyed indicate that on the 1 day surveyed,

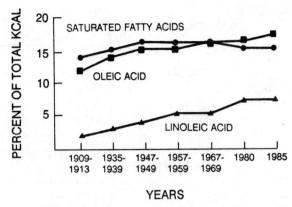

FIGURE 3–6 Trends in percentage of total calories from selected fatty acids in the U.S. food supply. From R.M. Marston, USDA/HNIS, unpublished data, 1986.

13% of total fat and 16% of saturated fat came from a food group made up of hamburgers, cheeseburgers, meat loaf, hot dogs, ham, and luncheon meats (Block et al., 1985). Beef items furnished more than 15% of total fat. Approximately one-third of the saturated fat reported came from meats, and about one-fourth was provided by milk, milk products, and nondairy creamers. Mayonnaise and salad dressings contributed approximately 15% of the linoleic acid reported; margarine contributed 10%. French fries and other forms of fried potatoes supplied almost 8% of the linoleic acid consumed (Block et al., 1985).

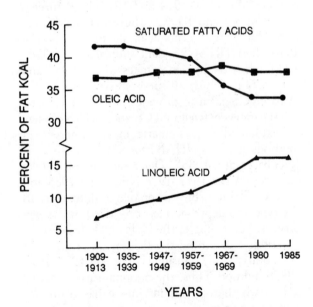

FIGURE 3–7 Trends in contribution of selected fatty acids to percentage of calories from fat in U.S. food supply. From R.M. Marston, USDA/HNIS, unpublished data, 1986.

TABLE 3–5 U.S. Food Supply: Trends in Quantities of Foods Available for Consumption per Capita[a]

Foods	Lb/Year			Foods	Lb/Year		
	1909-1913	1967-1969	1985		1909-1913	1967-1969	1985
Meat, poultry, and fish				Vegetables			
Beef	54	81	79	Tomatoes	46	36	38
Pork	62	61	62	Dark green and	34	25	31
Poultry	18	46	70	yellow[g]			
Fish	12	15	19	Other			
Total[b]	171	221	224	Fresh	136	87	96
Eggs	37	40	32	Processed	11	35	29
				Total	227	183	194
Dairy products							
Whole milk	223	232	122	Potatoes, white			
Low-fat milk	64	44	112	Fresh	182	67	55
Cheese[c]	5	15	26	Processed	0	15	28
Other[d]	28	100	86	Total[h]	182	82	83
Total[e]	339	440	450	Dry beans, peas,	16	16	18
				nuts, and soybeans			
Fats and oils							
Butter	18	6	5	Grain products			
Margarine	1	10	11	Wheat products	216	116	122
Shortening	8	16	23	Corn products	56	15	7
Lard and beef tallow	12	5	4	Other grains	19	13	26
Salad and cooking oil	2	16	25	Total	291	144	155
Total[f]	41	54	67	Sugar and sweeteners			
Fruits				Refined sugar	77	100	63
Citrus	17	60	72	Syrups and other	14	22	90
Noncitrus				sweeteners			
Fresh	154	73	87	Total	91	122	153
Processed	8	35	34	Miscellaneous[i]	10	17	14
Total	179	168	193				

[a]Based on unpublished data from R. Marston, USDA, 1986.
[b]Also includes veal, lamb, mutton, and offal.
[c]Product weight, not calcium equivalents.
[d]Includes cream; canned, evaporated, and dry milk; whey; yogurt; ice cream and other frozen desserts.
[e]Total given in calcium equivalents, in which cheese and other dairy products are expressed in terms of fluid whole cow's milk having the same quantity of calcium as the milk product in question.
[f]Totals may not appear accurate due to rounding.
[g]Includes sweet potatoes.
[h]Data before 1960 not comparable with data after 1960.
[i]Includes coffee, tea, cocoa, and spices.

Dietary Trans Fatty Acids

Unsaturated fatty acids in natural foods exist chiefly in the *cis* form, in which the hydrogen atoms are on the same side of the double bond. When fats and oils are partially hydrogenated during commercial processing, varying amounts of *trans* isomers form. In this form, the hydrogen atoms are on opposite sides of the double bond. Although small amounts of *trans* isomers occur naturally in milk and butter, the large increase in usage of partially hydrogenated vegetable oils has resulted in increases in *trans* isomers in foods during past decades, raising questions concerning possible adverse effects of these isomers (see Chapter 7).

As yet there are no reliable data on the *trans* fatty acid intake by the U.S. population, but Hunter and Applewhite (1986) estimate, based on market share and product composition data, that per-capita availability (not actual consumption) is about 7.6 g/person per day. An Ad Hoc Review Panel of the Federation of American Societies for Experimental Biology estimated 8.3 g/person per day based on USDA food supply data and published analytical values (Senti, 1985). A higher estimate of 12.1 g/person per day (8% of total fat) was based on 1972 food supply data (Enig et al., 1978).

Since estimates of fatty acids available in the food supply are higher than amounts actually consumed, studies of actual consumption are of interest. In one such study, the fatty acid content of the diet as reported by 7-day food intakes of eight adolescent females were quantitated by using gas chromatography to analyze duplicate meals. The average daily consumption of *trans* fatty acids was estimated to be 3.1 g (6.5% of total fatty acids) (van den Reek et al., 1986). In another study based on gas chromatographic analysis, Aitchison et al. (1977) found that in the self-selected diets of 11 women 25 to 35 years of age, *trans* isomers accounted for an average of 5% of total fatty acids. Since the numbers of subjects were small in these studies and fails to represent the U.S. population, further research is needed to ascertain the usual intake of these isomers.

Trans-octadecanoic acid (18:1t) is the predominant *trans* isomer in foods. In an analysis of 220 samples of 35 food types, Enig et al. (1983) found that most samples of mayonnaise, salad dressings, and salad and cooking oils contained no 18:1t, unless the label indicated partial hydrogenation of the oil. Margarines varied in 18:1t content as follows (by weight of fat): stick margarines, 16 to 31%; tub margarines, 7 to 18%; and diet margarines, 11 to 13%. In contrast, cakes, candies, and frostings varied from 3 to 33%; cream substitutes, from 0.4 to 12%; cookies and crackers, from 2 to 34%; breads and rolls, from 0.2 to 24%; and puddings, from 28 to 35%. Van den Reek et al. (1986) observed that approximately two-thirds of the 18:1t consumed by their eight adolescent subjects could be calculated using the analyses of Enig et al. (1983).

Dietary Cholesterol

The association of dietary cholesterol with CHD is also of interest. Cholesterol in the food supply increased from 500 mg during 1909–1913 to its highest point, 570 mg, during 1947–1949, but declined by 16% to 480 mg/person per day during 1977–1979, where it has remained (Table 3–3). The decline in the availability of cholesterol was due chiefly to reduced use of eggs—from a peak of 49 lb/person per year in 1951 (Welsh and Marston, 1982) to 32 lb/person in 1985 (Table 3–5). The 1985 food supply data show that equal amounts of cholesterol (40%) came from eggs and from the meat, poultry, and fish group; 14% came from dairy products (excluding butter); and 5% from fats and oils (including butter) (Marston and Raper, 1987). Beef contributes more cholesterol to the food supply than do other meats (Marston and Raper, 1987).

The average cholesterol intake found in the 1977–1978 NFCS (USDA, 1984) was 385 mg/day, or 214 mg per 1,000 calories. In terms of caloric intake, cholesterol levels were lowest for respondents under age 19; higher for blacks than for whites; higher for those below the poverty level; and highest in the South and West. The relationship of dietary fats and cholesterol to blood cholesterol levels is discussed in Chapter 7.

Carbohydrates and Caloric Sweeteners

Carbohydrates are often categorized as complex carbohydrates (polysaccharides, consisting chiefly of starches), dietary fiber, and mono- and disaccharides (sugars). The major sugars relevant to this discussion are sucrose (table sugar) and fructose.

Food Supply Data

Carbohydrate availability has declined since 1909–1913, both in absolute amounts (Table 3–3) and as a percentage of total calories (Figure 3–3). A striking change occurred in the relative proportions of total carbohydrates available from starches and from sugars. In 1909–1913, the proportion was approximately two-thirds starch and one-third sugar. By 1980, sugars furnished a little more than one-half the carbohydrates in the food supply. The decline in starches was due to the marked decrease in use of grain products and potatoes; at the same time, the use of refined sugars, syrups, and other sweeteners dramatically increased (Table 3–5).

The availability of specific sugars also changed. Sucrose peaked at 102 lb/person per year in 1971–1972 (Glinsmann et al., 1986), but declined to 63 lb in 1985 (Table 3–5). This decline is attributable to the replacement of sucrose in soft drinks and other products by corn sweeteners, which increased in the food supply from 21 lb/person per year in 1972 to 58 lb/person in 1984 (Glinsmann et al., 1986). This increase was due chiefly to the greater availability of high-fructose corn syrup (HFCS)—from 1 lb/person per year in 1972 to 36 lb/person by 1984 (Glinsmann et al., 1986). By 1985, HFCS in the food supply had increased another 20% (Marston and Raper, 1987). Thus, over the century, sugar use has changed—from primarily sucrose to a mixture of sucrose, glucose (largely from corn syrup), and fructose (from HFCS).

TABLE 3-6 Summary of Intake of Sugars[a]

Sugars	Mean[b]		90th Percentile[c]	
	Total Population	14 Age–Sex[d] Group Range	Total Population	14 Age–Sex[d] Group Range
	Daily per-capita intake (g/day)			
Added[e]	53	10–84	104	30–155
Naturally occurring	42	33–59	74	60–99
Total minus lactose	80	31–116	139	65–193
Total	95	62–143	160	93–230
	Daily intake as a percentage of caloric intake			
Added[e]	11	5–14	20	15–24
Naturally occurring	10	7–27	16	12–38
Total minus lactose	18	15–20	27	25–31
Total	21	18–32	31	27–43

[a]From Glinsmann et al. (1986).
[b]Total may not be equal to the sum of added and naturally occurring sugars due to rounding.
[c]Data represent the 90th percentile value for each category of sugars. Thus, the values of added and naturally occurring sugars cannot be summed to give the 90th percentile value of total sugars.
[d]Fourteen individual age–sex groups as identified in the 1980 RDAs (NRC 1980).
[e]Excludes lactose added to infant formulas.

Because of concern about possible effects of increased fructose use on certain chronic diseases or on carbohydrate metabolism, the FDA established a Sugars Task Force to review and interpret recent scientific studies relative to the health effects of sugars and sweeteners added to foods. In its report (Glinsmann et al., 1986), the task force pointed out that the true increase in fructose availability over the past 10 years is more than the food supply data suggest, because approximately 60% of sucrose added to acidic beverages is converted to glucose and fructose. Such beverages consequently contain more fructose and less sucrose than food supply data indicate.

Carbohydrate Intake

The 1977–1978 NFCS found that carbohydrate intakes averaged 43% of calories. (These estimates do not include calories from alcohol.) For children 1 to 8 years of age, carbohydrates averaged 47% of calories, whereas for males and females 9 to 18 years old, they averaged 45 and 46%, respectively. Individuals below poverty levels had higher carbohydrate intakes than those above (DHHS/USDA, 1986).

Caloric Sweetener Intake

Using intake data from the 1977–1978 NFCS and a specially developed data base on the sugar content of foods, the FDA's Sugars Task Force estimated the intake of added, naturally occurring, and total sugars (Glinsmann et al., 1986). Sum-

maries of the task force's estimates appear in Tables 3–6 and 3–7. Since lactose was not a part of the safety evaluation, figures are given for total sugars minus lactose, as well as for total sugars including lactose. The 14 age–sex groups chosen were those used in the Food and Nutrition Board's report *Recommended Dietary Allowances* (NRC, 1980).

The average daily intake of total sugars (minus lactose) within age–sex groups ranged from 31 to 116 g/day (mean, 80 g/day). As a percentage of calories, total sugars (minus lactose) averaged 18% of calories, about half of which was contributed by sugars added to foods. The 90th percentile level of daily intake of total sugars (minus lactose) was 139 g/day (range, 65 to 193 g), or a mean of 27% of calories.

The mean and the 90th percentile values for added sugars were 53 g/day and 104 g/day, respectively, or 11 and 20% of caloric intake, respectively. Table 3–7 indicates that the mean percentage of total calories from added sugars for all age–sex groups was 2% for fructose, 6% for sucrose, and 4% for HFCS. The average daily intake of added sugars was highest (13 to 14% of caloric intake) for children 4 to 10 years old, for males 11 to 18 years, and females 11 to 22 years (Glinsmann et al., 1986).

Dietary Sources of Carbohydrates

The 1977–1978 NFCS data indicate that grain products provide more carbohydrates than other food groups. Grain products include cereals and

TABLE 3–7 Summary of Intake of Specific Sugars[a]

Specific Sugar	Mean[b]		90th Percentile[c]	
	Total Population	14 Age–Sex[d] Group Range	Total Population	14 Age–Sex[d] Group Range
	Daily per-capita intake (g/day)			
Fructose				
Added	10	2–17	23	5–35
Naturally occurring	7	6–8	14	12–16
Total	16	8–24	37	16–43
Sucrose				
Added	28	6–43	56	19–80
Naturally occurring	13	9–17	23	18–28
Total	41	14–60	73	31–101
Sugars from corn sweeteners				
HFCS	19	3–33	43	10–66
Others	6	1–8	11	3–15
Total	24	4–41	52	13–79
	Daily intake as a percentage of caloric intake			
Fructose				
Added	2	1–3	5	2–7
Naturally occurring	2	1–3	3	2–7
Total	4	3–4	7	5–8
Sucrose				
Added	6	3–8	11	9–13
Naturally occurring	3	3–4	5	4–9
Total	9	7–11	14	13–16
Sugars from corn sweeteners				
HFCS	4	2–6	9	5–13
Others	1	1–1	2	2–2
Total	5	2–7	11	7–14

[a]From Glinsmann et al. (1986).
[b]Totals may not equal the sum of the numbers above them due to rounding.
[c]Data represent the 90th percentile value for each category of specific sugar. Thus, the values above the totals cannot be summed to give the 90th percentile value for total specific sugars.
[d]Fourteen individual age–sex groups as identified in the 1980 RDAs (NRC, 1980).

pasta as well as baked products, which contribute both starch and sugar. The sweets group contributed only half the amount of carbohydrates supplied by either fruits or vegetables, but sugars are added to foods in the grain products, fruit, and beverage groups (Figure 3–4). Beverages and fruits contribute similar proportions to carbohydrate intake.

Beverage Consumption

One of the most striking changes in food consumption patterns in the past two decades is the increased consumption of soft drinks, citrus juices, beer, and wine, accompanied by decreased consumption of coffee and milk. Data in Table 3–8 indicate that over the past 20 years, the availability of citrus juices and soft drinks increased by 138% each, wine by 123%, and beer by 23%.

Coffee availability declined by 29% and milk by 18%. Data from the 1977–1978 NFCS indicate that on the 3 days surveyed, coffee was consumed by 51% of the respondents, tea by 39%, fruit ades and drinks by 14%, and decaffeinated coffee by 7% (Pao et al., 1982).

Alcohol Consumption

The data in Table 3–8 on alcohol availability overestimate actual consumption, because they are based on industry production data and fail to account for wasted beverages due to bottle breakage, spillage, alcohol evaporation when beverages are used in cooking, and other losses. On the other hand, data from NFCS are underestimates due to underreporting by some individuals and the inability to assess usual intake over long periods, which results in underreporting by heavy drinkers. The

TABLE 3–8 Per-Capita Availability of Beverages from 1965 to 1985[a]

	Per-Capita Availability (gal)				
Beverage	1965	1970	1975	1980	1985
Nonalcoholic Beverages					
Milk					
Whole	28.6	24.8	20.6	16.7	14.0
Other	4.3	6.7	9.5	11.4	13.1
Total	33.1	31.4	30.1	28.0	27.1
Tea[b]	6.3	6.7	7.5	7.3	6.8
Coffee[c]	36.3	33.4	31.3	27.0	25.9
Soft drinks	19.2	23.7	27.3	37.8	45.6
Juices					
Citrus	2.4	3.7	5.3	5.2	5.7
Noncitrus	0.8	0.9	.8	1.1	1.6
Total	3.2	4.6	6.1	6.3	7.3
Total, excluding alcohol	98.1	99.9	102.1	106.4	112.7
Alcoholic Beverages					
Resident population					
Beer	16.6	19.2	22.2	25.2	23.4
Wine	1.0	1.3	1.7	2.1	2.5
Distilled spirits	1.5	1.8	2.0	2.0	1.7
Total	19.1	22.4	25.9	29.3	27.6
Adult population[d]					
Beer	28.0	31.6	35.1	38.3	34.5
Wine	1.7	2.2	2.7	3.2	3.8
Distilled spirits	2.6	3.0	3.1	3.0	2.5
Total	32.2	36.7	41.0	44.5	40.8
Total, including alcohol[e]	117.3	122.4	128.2	135.2	140.3

[a]From Bunch (1987). Soft drink and alcoholic beverage per-capita figures are constructed by the USDA Economic Research Service on the basis of industry data. Milk, soft drinks, and alcoholic beverages are based on the resident population; coffee and tea are based on the total population; and fruit juices are based on the civilian population.

[b]Fluid equivalent conversion factor is 200 6-oz cups per pound of tea leaf equivalent.

[c]Includes instant and decaffeinated coffee. Converted to fluid equivalent on the basis of 60 6-oz cups per pound of roasted coffee.

[d]Adult population includes all those 21 years old and older.

[e]Total includes consumption of alcohol based on resident population.

1977–1978 NFCS indicated that 8% of individuals reported consuming beer or ale at least once in the 3 days surveyed; 5% reported wine intake; and 3%, distilled liquor (Pao et al., 1982). On the other hand, NHANES II data indicated that on the day surveyed, a higher proportion of the population consumed alcohol and in larger amounts than were reported by the 1977–1978 NFCS. One possible reason for the discrepancy may be that respondents felt more comfortable disclosing their alcohol consumption during NHANES interviews because family members were not present (Woteki, 1985). Furthermore, intake on 1 day does not reflect the usual intake of individuals.

In the Alcohol and Health Practices Survey—a component of the National Health Interview Survey by DHHS—investigators gathered data on consumption of alcoholic beverages during a 2-week period by adults 20 years of age and older (Schoenborn and Cohen, 1986). Fifty percent of males and 23% of females reported they had consumed five or more drinks in 1 day at least once during the year. Thirty percent of the respondents were classified as "lighter" drinkers (0.01 to 0.21 oz of ethanol/day), 21% were "moderate" drinkers (0.22 to 0.99 oz of ethanol/day), while 10% were "heavier" drinkers (1 or more oz of ethanol/day). "Moderate" drinkers, by this definition, consumed between 5.5 and 24 oz of beer, between 1.5 and 6.5 oz of wine, or 0.5 to 2 oz of distilled liquor/day. Men were four times more likely to be "heavier" drinkers than women. About one-third of respondents were abstainers.

Whites were less likely to be abstainers than blacks and other racial minorities. Younger people were more likely to be drinkers, and they drank more heavily than older people. The more highly educated and those with higher incomes were more apt to drink and apt to drink more than those with less education and income except that 43% of those in the lowest income group—<$7,000 year—had consumed five drinks or more on at least 1 day in the past year, compared with 36% of those whose income was $40,000 or more (Schoenborn and Cohen, 1986).

Heavy alcohol consumption can drastically alter the proportion of calories obtained from carbohydrates, fats, and protein. An individual who drinks a fifth of a gallon of whiskey daily derives 2,120 kcal from ethanol or 58% of a 3,600 kcal diet (Scheig, 1970). A study of the alcohol intake of respondents in the 1977–1978 NFCS indicated that on the 3 days surveyed, alcohol supplied an average of 19% of total calories consumed by drinkers (Windham et al., 1983). There is a need for better documentation of actual alcohol consumption through national surveys. The present estimates of the percentage of calories from macronutrients in the diet are in error because of inadequate estimates of alcohol intake.

Alcohol was among the food components given high-priority monitoring status by the Joint Nutrition Monitoring Evaluation Committee (DHHS/USDA, 1986). Chapter 16 discusses the health aspects of alcohol consumption.

Drinking Water

Respondents in the 1977–1978 NFCS (USDA, 1984) reported drinking an average of 3.3 cups (8 fl oz/cup) of water per day on the 3 days surveyed. The median intake was 2.8 cups.

Dietary Fiber

Dietary fiber is composed of complex plant substances that resist digestion by secretions of the human intestinal tract. The chief difficulty in relating dietary fiber to the occurrence of chronic diseases in populations is the paucity of data on the amount and kinds of dietary fiber in foods. Until the recent past, data were available in food composition tables only for "crude fiber"—the residue resulting after foods are treated with acids and alkalies. Since this method of analysis destroys many components of dietary fiber, crude fiber is an inadequate indicator of dietary fiber in foods.

There are few data on dietary fiber in the food supply or in diets consumed by respondents in 1977–1978 NFCS or 1976–1980 NHANES. The first surveys to include an estimate of dietary fiber were the 1985 and 1986 CSFIIs, but USDA data are as yet limited regarding dietary fiber in foods. In these surveys, dietary fiber included both the insoluble fraction (neutral detergent fiber) and soluble fraction (such as gums in cereal grains and pectin in fruits and vegetables). The values for these fractions were based chiefly on the method of Englyst et al. (1982) and to a lesser extent on that of Prosky et al. (1985). In 1985, average intake of dietary fiber per day for women 19 to 50 years of age was 10.9 g, for children 1 to 5 years old, 9.8 g (both based on 4 days of intake), and for men 19 to 50 years old, 18 g (based on a 1-day intake). The 1986 CSFII (USDA, 1987c) indicated that women in the West and Midwest had higher intakes of dietary fiber than those in the South or Northeast.

Information on dietary fiber in foods is building rapidly as the USDA data base expands. The new USDA Agriculture Handbook No. 8 when completed will provide more up-to-date data on dietary fiber. Foods highest in dietary fiber include whole (unrefined) grains and breads made from them, legumes, vegetables, fruits, nuts, and seeds.

Protein

As mentioned above, Figure 3–3 indicates that the food supply has provided about 11% of calories as protein since 1909–1913, or about 100 g of protein per person per day (Table 3–3). A major change over the years in the food supply is the increased use of animal over plant protein sources. During 1909–1913, about 52% of protein came from animal sources compared with about 68% in 1982. This change was a result of increased use of meats, poultry, fish, dairy products, and eggs, accompanied by decreased use of flour, cereal products, and potatoes. Animal products provide almost three-fourths of the eight essential amino acids in the food supply and contributed 70% of the total protein in the 1977–1978 NFCS (USDA, 1984). Protein available in the food supply is much higher than the RDA for protein, which is 56 g/day for males 15 years and older weighing 70 kg and 44 g/day for females in the same age group weighing 55 kg (NRC, 1980).

Protein Intakes

According to the 1977–1978 NFCS, protein intakes averaged 74.3 g/day for all respondents and exceeded the RDA for all 22 age–sex groups. Race, poverty status, region, urbanization, and season had little influence on dietary protein levels. Protein contributed an average of 17% of total calories

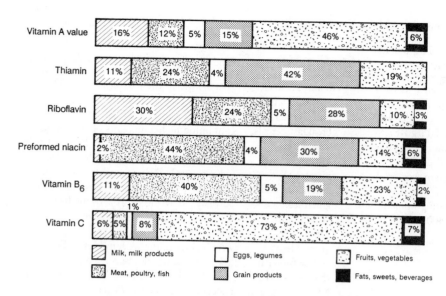

FIGURE 3–8 Food sources of vitamins in percentage per individual per day. Data from the 1977–1978 NFCS (USDA, 1984).

in both males and females in the 1977–1978 NFCS and in the 1985 and 1986 CSFII. Annual per-capita consumption of beef and veal changed from 32 kg in 1960 to 36 kg in 1982; consumption of pork remained stable; and poultry consumption increased from 16 kg in 1960 to 29 kg in 1982 (USDA, 1981, 1983). Other surveys, such as the CSFII (USDA, 1986b), have found slightly different results based on a 1-day recall. For example, 42% of males 19 to 50 ate beef on a 1-day recall in 1977 whereas 28.3% of this same population ate beef during this period in 1985. The intake of poultry remained the same while fish intake increased from 8.5% in 1977 to 11.4% in 1985. In 1985, as compared to 1977, meat intakes decreased as income increased. Low-income people eat more meat than high-income people.

In the 1977–1978 NFCS, meats, poultry, and fish contributed by far the largest amount of dietary protein (49%); dairy products and grain products each supplied 18%. The largest part of the food dollar was used to purchase meat, poultry, and fish; however, lower income households obtained more protein per dollar than higher income households.

Vitamins

Vitamins most often reported in food supply data and in food consumption surveys include vitamins A and C, thiamin, riboflavin, preformed niacin, vitamin B_6, and vitamin B_12 (Table 3–1). Data regarding amounts of vitamin E and folic acid in foods are at present incomplete and of doubtful validity.

Table 3–9 summarizes the 1980 RDAs for specific vitamins, major food sources, availability in the food supply, intakes by survey populations, and

conclusions by the JNMEC regarding the adequacy of intakes and current knowledge of the vitamin status of the population. In Tables 3–9 and 3–10, average intakes are expressed as percentages of the RDAs; the intent is to indicate the relative amount. Intakes below the RDA should not to be construed as inadequate. Figure 3–8 presents food sources of vitamins reported in the 1977–1978 NFCS.

As summarized in Table 3–9, the JNMEC accorded priority status to only one vitamin—vitamin C—due to low serum levels among some segments of the population in NHANES II. The group also concluded that vitamin A, thiamin, riboflavin, and niacin warrant continued monitoring and that further investigation of the relationship between dietary intake and nutritional status is needed relative to vitamin B_6 and folacin.

Minerals

Minerals included in the 1977–1978 NFCS were calcium, phosphorus, magnesium and iron, whereas NHANES II included all these except magnesium. CSFII included those in the 1977–1978 NFCS as well as sodium, potassium, copper, and zinc. The Total Diet Study is the only national study at present that includes all those plus iodine, manganese, selenium, and chromium.

Table 3–10 summarizes information about minerals, including the 1980 RDAs, major food sources, availability in the food supply, intakes by survey populations, and nutritional status. Figure 3–9 shows food sources of minerals reported in the 1977–1978 NFCS.

Among national surveys, only the Total Diet Study included manganese, selenium, and iodine

TABLE 3–9 Vitamins: A Summary of Major Food Sources, Availability, Intake, and Nutritional Status

Vitamin	Alternative Names	1980 RDA, amount per day[a]	Major Food Sources	Food Supply, Intakes, and Nutritional Status
Vitamin A (plus carotenoids)	Retinol (vitamin A alcohol)	Children 1 to 10 years, 400–700 µg RE[b] Males 11–>51 years, 1,000 µg RE Females 11–>51 years, 800 µg RE Pregnant women, +200 µg RE Lactating women, +400 µg RE	Vitamin A: liver, egg yolk, whole milk, butter, breakfast cereals, margarines fortified with vitamin A. Carotenoids: dark-green leafy vegetables, yellow vegetables, yellow fruits. In the 1977–1978 NFCS, fruits and vegetables furnished 46% of the vitamin A intake; milk and grain products furnished about 15% each.[e]	Availability in the *food supply* rose 37% during the last 20 years due chiefly to new varieties of vegetables, such as carrots, containing higher amounts of carotenoids.[c] In the 1985 CSFII, 81% of children 1 to 5 years old and 46% of women 19 to 50 years old consumed 100% or more of the RDA (mean of 4 nonconsecutive days). Men 19 to 50 years old averaged 122% of the RDA on the 1 day surveyed. Intakes were lower among low- compared to high-income groups and were highest in the western United States and lowest in the northeastern region.[d] In the 1977–1978 NFCS, 50% of the survey population (infancy to 75 years and older) consumed at least 100% of the RDA, and more than 66% had intakes of at least 70% of the RDA. Intakes were highest in the western region and lowest in the South.[e] JNMEC concluded that the vitamin A intake and nutritional status of the U.S. population appear to be adequate but that public health monitoring should continue. Mean serum vitamin levels in NHANES II were within normal ranges, regardless of economic level, race, or sex.[f]
Carotenoids	β-Carotene (most plentiful)	No RDA has been set; measured in RE	See above.	Intakes reported for the first time in the 1985 and 1986 CSFIIs. Mean intakes for children 1 to 5 years old were 254 RE, and for women 19 to 50 years old were 342 RE in 1985 (based on a 4-day intake). Mean intake by men 19 to 50 years old in 1985 was 429 RE (based on a 1-day intake). Intakes by women and men but not by children were lower in low- than in high-income groups.
Vitamin D	D₃ (chole-calcif-erol) D₂ (ergo-calcif-erol)	Birth to 18 years, 10 µg Males and females 19–22 years, 7.5 µg 23–>51 years, 5 µg	Fatty fish and fish oils, eggs, butter, liver, milk fortified with vitamin D. Vitamin D also obtained by the action of ultra-violet light on 7-dehydrocho-lesterol in skin.	National surveys do not report vitamin D intakes, since little information is available on vitamin D in foods. JNMEC did not discuss vitamin D.[f]
Vitamin E	α-Toco-pherol α-TE	Infants, 3–4 mg α-TE[g] Children 1–10 years, 5–7 mg α-TE Males 11–14 years, 8 mg α-TE	Oils from soybeans, sunflower, corn, and cottonseed; germ of whole grains; fish liver oils; nuts.	*Availability* in the food supply increased from 11.2 mg α-TE in 1909–1913 to 17.6 mg α-TE in 1985 (Table 3-3) due to increased use of cooking and salad oils.

65

TABLE 3–9 *continued*

Vitamin	Alternative Names	1980 RDA, amount per day[a]	Major Food Sources	Food Supply, Intakes, and Nutritional Status
Vitamin E (*continued*)		Females 11–>51 years, 8 mg α-TE Males 15–>51 years, 10 mg α-TE Pregnant women, 10 mg α-TE Lactating women, 11 mg α-TE		The 1985 CSFII reported vitamin E intakes for the first time, despite the fact that a high percentage of values in food composition data banks are imputed.[d] Children 1 to 5 years old averaged 5.5 mg α-TE, men 19 to 50 years old averaged 9.8 mg α-TE, and women 19 to 50 years old consumed an average of 7.1 mg α-TE. Intakes were higher among those with higher compared with lower incomes. JNMEC did not discuss vitamin E.[f]
Thiamin	Vitamin B₁	Generally 0.5 mg/1,000 kcal Infants, 0.3–0.5 mg Children 1–10 years, 0.7–1.2 mg Males 11–>51 years, 1.2 mg Females 11–>51 years, 1.0–1.1 mg Pregnant women, +0.4 mg Lactating women, +0.5 mg	Whole grains, dried legumes, pork muscle, liver, products made with enriched flour. Highest proportion in 1978 (1977–1978 NFCS) came from grain products (42%) and from meats, poultry, and fish (24%) (USDA, 1984).	The *availability* of thiamin in the food supply has increased since 1909–1913 due to the addition of thiamin to highly refined flours and cereal products (Table 3-3). In the 1985 CSFII, women and men 19 to 50 years old consumed a mean of 0.70 mg/1,000 kcal, children 1 to 5 years old had a mean intake of 0.79 mg/1,000 kcal. In the 1977–1978 NFCS, the mean intake for all age and sex groups was 112% of the RDA. Dietary intakes were highest for children up to 8 years of age and were higher for people 9 to 18 years old than for older people of the same sex. Intakes differed little by poverty status or region.[e] JNMEC concluded that thiamin intake appears to be adequate but continuing public health monitoring is recommended. Health indicators of thiamin status were not available from national surveys.[f]
Riboflavin		Generally 0.6 mg/1,000 kcal Infants, 0.4–0.6 mg Children 1–10 years, 0.8–1.4 mg Males 11–>51 years, 1.4–1.7 mg Females 11–>51 years, 1.2–1.3 mg Pregnant women, +0.3 mg Lactating women, +0.5 mg	Milk and milk products; whole and enriched grain products; meat, liver, poultry, fish; dark-green vegetables. The highest proportions of intakes in the 1977–1978 NFCS[e] came from milk and milk products (30%), grain products (28%), and meat, poultry, and fish (24%).	The *availability* of riboflavin in the food supply has increased since 1909–1913 chiefly because of the enrichment of grain products (Table 3-3). In the 1985 CSFII, the mean intake for children 1 to 5 years old was 1.12 mg/1,000 kcal, for women 19 to 50 years old, 0.88 mg/1,000 kcal, and for men 19 to 50 years old, 0.82 mg/1,000 kcal.[d] In the 1977–1978 NFCS, the mean intake for all age and sex groups was 132% of the RDA; 66% consumed at least 100% of the RDA. Intakes were lowest for females 19 to 64 years of age; only one-half had intakes of at least the RDA. Intakes differed little by poverty status, but were lower in the South and highest in the West.[e] JNMEC concluded that dietary intakes appear to be adequate but continuing public health monitoring is recommended. Health indicators of riboflavin status were not available from national surveys.[f]

TABLE 3–9 *continued*

Vitamin	Alternative Names	1980 RDA, amount per day[a]	Major Food Sources	Food Supply, Intakes, and Nutritional Status
Niacin (only preformed niacin— not that formed in metabolism of tryptophan— is reported in national surveys.)	Nicotinic acid Nicotinamide	Generally 6.6 mg NE[h]/1,000 kcal Infants, 6–8 mg NE Children 1–10 years, 9–16 mg NE Males 11–>51 years, 16–19 mg NE Females 11–>51 years, 13–15 mg NE Pregnant women, +2 mg NE Lactating women, +5 mg NE	Preformed niacin: meats, poultry, fish; whole and enriched grain products; legumes; nuts. In addition, some of the tryptophan present in meats, poultry, fish, cheese, legumes, and seeds can be converted in the body to niacin. The highest proportion of preformed niacin intakes in the 1977–1978 NFCS came from meat, poultry, and fish (44%) and grain products (30%).	*Availability* of preformed niacin in the food supply has increased since 1909–1913, partly because of the enrichment of flour and cereal products (Table 3-3). In the 1985 CSFII, mean intake of preformed niacin per 1,000 kcal was 10.8 mg NE for men 19 to 50 years old and 9.6 mg NE for children 1 to 5 years old.[d] In the 1977–1978 NFCS, the mean intake for all age and sex groups was 124% of the RDA. For the same age groups, intake levels were higher for males than for females. Intake levels were lowest for those 9 to 18 years of age and highest for those ages 19 to 64 years. Those below poverty level had lower intakes than those of higher income groups.[e] JNMEC concluded that the dietary intakes of the U.S. population appear to be adequate in niacin but that public health monitoring should continue. Health indicators of nutritional status have not been obtained in national surveys.[f]
Vitamin B_6 (food composition data for B_6 are less reliable than is desirable.)	Pyridoxine Pyridoxal Pyridoxamine	Generally 0.02 mg/g of protein consumed. The RDA for vitamin B_6 assumes that the usual daily protein intake for women is 100 g and for men 110 g. Infants, 0.3–0.6 mg Children 1–10 years, 0.9–1.6 mg Males 11–>51 years 1.8–2.2 mg Females 11–>51 years, 1.8–2.0 mg Pregnant women, 2.0 mg +0.6 mg Lactating women, 2.0 mg +0.5 mg	Meat, poultry, fish; bananas; and nuts. The highest proportion of vitamin B_6 intakes in the 1977–1978 NFCS came from meat, poultry, and fish (40%); fruits and vegetables (23%); and grain products (19%).	*Availability* of vitamin B_6 in the food supply appears to have decreased from 1909–1913 to 1967–1968, but increased by 8% in the past two decades (Table 3-3). In the 1985 CSFII, mean intakes of women 19 to 50 years old were 57% of the RDA, whereas mean intakes for men 19 to 50 years old were 85% of the RDA. For children 1 to 5 years old, mean intakes were 119% of the RDA. Intakes were somewhat higher among higher income groups. The mean intake in terms of mg B_6/g protein for women was 0.019 and for chldren, 0.023.[d] In the 1977–1978 NFCS, the mean intake of all people was 75% of the RDA, but females over 14 years old were between 58 and 63% of the RDA. The percentage of the population having at least the recommended B_6-to-protein ratio was about 33% higher than the percentage of the population having at least the RDA.[e] JNMEC concluded that both the B_6 intake and the status of the population require further investigation. Health indicators of vitamin B_6 status have not been assessed in national surveys.[f]

TABLE 3–9 *continued*

Vitamin	Alternative Names	1980 RDA, amount per day[a]	Major Food Sources	Food Supply, Intakes, and Nutritional Status
Vitamin B_{12}	Cobalamin	Infants, 0.5–1.5 μg Children 1–10 years, 2.0–3.0 μg Males and females 11–>51 years, 3.0 μg Pregnant women, +1.0 μg Lactating women, +1.0 μg	Only foods of animal origin supply B_{12}. Liver, muscle meats, fish, eggs, and milk and milk products supply varying amounts.	*Availability* of vitamin B_{12} in the food supply increased up to 1967–1969 but declined 5% by 1985 (Table 3-3). In the 1985 CSFII, the mean intake in the age group 19 to 50 years was 4.85 μg for women, 7.84 μg for men, and 3.80 μg for children 1 to 5 years old. Dietary intakes were positively associated with economic status and were highest in the northeastern region.[d] In the 1977–1978 NFCS, among all age and sex groups, 67% consumed 100% or more of the RDA. Intakes were higher for males than for females and were higher generally for young adults than for older people.[e] JNMEC concluded that vitamin B_{12} intake is adequate. Nutritional surveys have not assessed vitamin B_{12} nutritional status.[f]
Folacin	Folic acid Folate	Infants, 30–45 μg Children 1–10 years, 100–300 μg Males and females 11–>51 years, 400 μg Pregnant women, +400 μg Lactating women, +100 μg	Liver, dark-green leafy vegetables, dry beans, peanuts, wheat germ, whole grains. Ability to utilize folacin depends on the chemical form in food. Losses in cooking and canning can be very high due to heat destruction.	*Availability* of folacin in the food supply reached a peak between 1940 and 1950 and has declined somewhat since that time. The current RDA for adults is higher than the availability in the food supply. In the 1985 CSFII, average intakes for men and women 19–50 years of age averaged 305 μg/day and 189 μg/day, respectively. Children 1 to 5 years old averaged 185 μg/day.[d] Folacin intake was not determined in the 1977–1978 NFCS because data were unavailable on many foods consumed.[e] JNMEC[f] concluded that folacin intake and status need to be investigated further. The folacin RDA may be higher relative to population requirements than is the case for other nutrients. On the basis of limited data from NHANES II, females 20 to 44 years of age were judged to be at greatest risk of developing folacin deficiencies. *Comment:* The current method used to analyze for folacin in foods fails to give reproducible results from laboratory to laboratory. A relatively high percentage of values for folacin in the USDA data base are imputed rather than measured.[d]
Vitamin C	Ascorbic acid	Infants, 35 mg Children 1–10 years, 45 mg Males and females 11–>51 years, 60 mg	Citrus fruits, dark-green leafy vegetables, tomatoes, potatoes, liver. The 1977–1978	*Availability* of vitamin C in the food supply was 13% higher in 1985 than in 1909–1913 (Table 3-5). Fortification of fruit drinks and other foods increased the supply. In the 1985 CSFII, the mean daily intakes were: for children, 84 mg; for women, 77 mg; and for

TABLE 3-9 *continued*

Vitamin	Alternative Names	1980 RDA, amount per day[a]	Major Food Sources	Food Supply, Intakes, and Nutritional Status
Vitamin C (*continued*)		Pregnant women, +20 mg Lactating women, +40 mg	NFCS indicated that 73% of the vitamin C intake came from fruits and vegetables.	men 19 to 50 years old, 104 mg.[d] In the 1977–1978 NFCS, the mean intake (82 mg/day) for the entire survey population was above the RDA. Dietary levels were positively associated with economic status.[e] JNMEC noted that the 1976–1980 NHANES found that 3% of the survey population 3 to 74 years of age had low serum vitamin C levels. Subpopulations of adults who were at high risk of poor vitamin C status included consumers of diets low in vitamin C, cigarette smokers, and the very poor. A higher proportion of males than females had low serum vitamin C levels. Vitamin C is accorded public health monitoring priority because of low serum vitamin C levels and low intakes in some population groups.[f]

[a]From NRC (1980). Comparisons with the RDA are intended to indicate relative amounts; intakes below the RDA should not be construed as inadequate.

[b]RE = retinol equivalents. One RE = 1 µg of retinol; 6 µg of β1-carotene; 12 µg of other provitamin A carotenoids; 3.33 IU of vitamin activity from retinol; 10 IU of vitamin A activity from β-carotene.

[c]Historical food supply data from USDA (see Table 3-3).

[d]USDA (1986b, 1987a).

[e]USDA (1984).

[f]DHHS/USDA (1986).

[g]α-TE = α-tocopherol equivalent; 1 mg d-α-tocopherol = 1α-TE.

[h]NE = niacin equivalents. 1 NE = 1 mg niacin or 60 mg of dietary tryptophan.

TABLE 3–10 Minerals: A Summary of Major Food Sources, Availability, Intake, and Nutritional Status

Mineral	1980 RDA, amount per day[a]	Major Food Sources	Food Supply, Intakes, and Nutritional Status
Calcium	Infants, 360–540 mg Children 1–10 years, 800 mg Children 11–18 years, 1,200 mg Males and females 19–>51 years, 800 mg Pregnant women, +400 mg Lactating women, +400 mg	Milk, cheese, broccoli, dark-green leafy vegetables such as collard, turnip, and mustard greens. In the 1977–1978 NFCS, 50% of the calcium intake came from milk and milk products, and 22% from grain products (which contain milk and milk products).	*Availability* of calcium in the food supply was 23% higher in 1985 than in 1909–1913 (Table 3-3). Today's food supply furnishes more skim and low-fat milk, yogurt, and cheese, and less whole milk than in 1909–1913. In the 1985 CSFII, 22% of women 19 to 50 years old consumed 100% or more of the RDA. The mean intake was 74% of the RDA. Among children 1 to 5 years old, 45% consumed 100% and more of the RDA. The mean intake of men 19 to 50 years old was 115% of the RDA. For women, the mean intake per 1,000 kcal was 397 mg, a higher intake than for men (360 mg/1,000 kcal). Black women had a mean intake of only 55% of the RDA compared with 77% for white men. Calcium intakes were lower among men and women 35 to 50 years, among those living in poverty, and among those living in the northeastern and southern United States.[b] In the 1977–1978 NFCS, the mean intake for the entire survey population was 87% of the RDA. The mean intake for blacks was 71% of the RDA compared with 89% for whites. Black females between 12 and 64 years old averaged 58% of the RDA, compared with 72% for white females in the same age groups. Mean intakes per 1,000 kcal were higher for females 19 to 50 years of age (374 mg/1,000 kcal) than for males the same age (343 mg/1,000 kcal). Calcium intakes were positively associated with income and were lower in the northeastern and southern United States than in the north-central and western regions.[c] JNMEC noted that NHANES has not investigated calcium status because clinical and biochemical indicators for assessing calcium status are not applicable to survey populations. Although postmenopausal white women are at greater risk of developing osteoporosis than men, and women consume less calcium than do men, factors other than calcium intake are related to osteoporosis. These include genetic susceptibility, age, sex, body weight, hormonal status, and physical activity. However, calcium merits public health monitoring priority status because of the possible association of low calcium intakes among women with osteoporosis in later life.[d]

TABLE 3–10   *continued*

Mineral	1980 RDA, amount per day[a]	Major Food Sources	Food Supply, Intakes, and Nutritional Status
Phosphorus	Infants, 240–260 mg Children 1–10 years, 800 mg Children 11–18 years, 1,200 mg Males and females 19–>51 years, 800 mg Pregnant women, +400 mg Lactating women, +400 mg	Meats, milk products, grains, phosphate, food additives. In the 1977–1978 NFCS, milk products and meat, poultry, and fish each contributed 29% of the intake; grain products contributed 20%.	*Availability* of phosphorus in the food supply has remained fairly steady throughout the century (Table 3-3). In the 1985 CSFII, mean intakes per day by men and women 19 to 50 years old were 1,536 mg and 966 mg, respectively. Children 1 to 5 years old consumed a mean of 992 mg/day. Among women, 63% consumed the RDA more.[b] In the 1977–1978 NFCS, the mean intake of all people was 134% of the RDA. Intakes were higher for males than for females, but the average intakes of females were above the RDA. Intakes were somewhat higher among whites than among blacks and were positively associated with economic status. Mean intakes of these groups were above the RDA, however. Intakes were lowest in the South and highest in the West.[c] JNMEC reported no biochemical or other health indicators for assessing phosphorus status in national surveys. The phosphorus intake appears to be adequate.[d]
Magnesium	Infants, 50–70 mg Children 1–10 years, 150–250 mg Males 11–14 years, 350 mg Males 15–18 years, 400 mg Males 19–>51 years, 350 mg Females 11–>51 years, 300 mg Pregnant women, +150 mg Lactating women, +150 mg	Green vegetables (chlorophyll contains magnesium), nuts, seeds, dried beans, whole grains, and meats. Refining of cereals results in large losses. In the 1977–1978 NFCS, food groups contributing the largest amounts were dairy products, meats, grain products, and fruits and vegetables.	*Availability* in the food supply has declined since 1909–1913 (Table 3-3), and today it is 320 mg/person/day. The decline is due to decreased use and refinement of grains and flour. In the 1985 CSFII, mean daily intakes were 193 mg/day for children 1 to 5 years old, 207 mg for women (69% of the RDA) 19 to 50 years old, and 329 mg (94% of the RDA) for men 19 to 50 years old. In the 1977–1978 NFCS, the avergae intake for all people was 83% of the RDA; 25% had intakes of at least the RDA. Children under 9 years of age had higher intakes than did older people. For all age groups, males had higher intakes than females. Intakes were higher for whites than for blacks; for both racial groups, intakes were somewhat higher for those above the poverty line. Intakes were higher in the West and lowest in the South.[c] JNMEC concluded that the magnesium intake and status of the U.S. population require further investigation. National surveys have not included biochemical or other health indicators of magnesium status.[d]
Iron	Infants, 10–15 mg Children 1–3 years, 15 mg Children 4–10 years, 10 mg Children 11–18 years, 18 mg	Liver, red meat, whole-grain and enriched grain products, beans,	*Availability* of iron in the food supply has risen considerably since 1909–1913 (Table 3-3), largely due to enrichment of flour and other grain products beginning in the 1940s.

TABLE 3–10 *continued*

Mineral	1980 RDA, amount per day[a]	Major Food Sources	Food Supply, Intakes, and Nutritional Status
Iron (continued)	Males 11–18 years, 18 mg Females 11–>51 years, 18 mg Males 19–>51 years, 10 mg	nuts, and dark-green leafy vegetables. In the NFCS 1977–1978, 35% of iron in diets came from meats, poultry, and fish and 33% came from grain products. Absorption of the iron in meats, poultry, and fish is greater than in plant foods. The presence of vitamin C in a meal also increases iron absorption. Some forms of iron used in enriching or fortifying foods are poorly absorbed. Neither the RDA nor national surveys take into account the extent to which iron in food is absorbable.	In the 1985 CSFII, the mean daily intake for children 1 to 5 years old was 9.7 mg (78% of the RDA); for women 19 to 50 years old, 10.1 mg (56% of the RDA); and for men the same age, 15.9 mg (159% of the RDA). Only 4% of women met or exceeded the RDA. In the 1977–1978 NFCS, the average intake was 103% of the RDA, but average intakes were below the RDA for children 1 to 8 years old, for males and females 9 to 18 years old, and for females 19 to 64 years old. Females 9 to 64 years had the lowest intakes in terms of the RDA; less than 20% of this group had intakes that reached the RDA. Intakes were higher among those in higher income groups.[b] Clinical and biochemical tests of iron status in the 1976–1980 NHANES indicate that the highest prevalence of impaired iron status occurred among children 1 to 5 years old, black females 12 to 17 years old, and females below poverty level in the age groups 25 to 54. A slightly higher prevalence of impaired iron status was observed in blacks than in whites and in children 1 to 5 years old and females 25 to 54 years old who were below the poverty level.[c] About 80% of females 19 to 64 years of age, compared with only 10% of males in this age group, reported iron intakes that failed to reach their RDA for iron. The iron RDA for women in their reproductive years is quite high—clearly, an amount not required by all women. Thus, assessments of iron status are more important than assessments of dietary intake alone. JNMEC concluded that high priority should be given to public health monitoring of iron status.[d]
Zinc	Infants, 3–5 mg Children 1–10 years, 10 mg Males and females 11–>51 years, 15 mg Pregnant women, +5 mg Lactating women, +10 mg	Shellfish (oysters), meat, poultry, cheese, whole grains, dry beans, nuts. The biologic availability of zinc depends on the food source and the presence of other food components in the diet. Zinc from animal foods is more	*Availability* of zinc in the food supply dropped between 1909–1913 and 1947–1949 but then slowly increased to the present level of 12.3 mg/person per day (Table 3-3). In the 1985 CSFII, as percentages of their RDA, children 1 to 5 years old consumed an average of 73% and women and men 19 to 50 years old consumed 56%.[b] In the Total Diet Study, men 19 to 30 years old and teenage boys consumed on average somewhat more than the RDA. In percentages of the RDA, girls 14 to 15 years old consumed an average of 66%; women 25 to 30 years, 64%; women 60 to 65 years, 57%; and men 60 to 65 years, 84%.[f]

TABLE 3–10   *continued*

Mineral	1980 RDA, amount per day[a]	Major Food Sources	Food Supply, Intakes, and Nutritional Status
Zinc (continued)		absorbable than zinc from plants.	In the 1977–1978 NFCS, zinc intakes were not evaluated due to insufficient data on the zinc content of foods.[c] JNMEC concluded that zinc intake and nutritional status merit further investigation.[d] A study of serum zinc levels reported in NHANES II concluded that data were inadequate to determine whether low serum zinc levels observed in 2% of males and 3% of females were related to low dietary intake.[g] The RDA for zinc is higher than levels in the food supply, and studies of adults on self-selected diets indicate that average intakes are below the RDA.[h]
Copper	ESADDI[i] Infants, 0.5–1.0 mg Children 1–6 years, 1.0–2.0 mg Children 7–10 years, 2.0–2.5 mg Males and females 11–>51 years, 2.0–3.0 mg	Crab meat, fresh vegetables and fruits, nuts, seeds, legumes.	*Availability* in the food supply has not been estimated. In the 1985 CSFII, mean intakes for children 1 to 5 years old were 0.8 mg/day; for women and men 19 to 50 years old, they were 1.0 and 1.6 mg/day, respectively.[b] In the Total Diet Study, highest daily intakes were 1.18 mg for boys 14 to 15 years old, 1.24 mg for men 25 to 30 years old, and 1.17 mg for men 60 to 65 years old. Earlier studies covering 1974–1982 also indicated intakes below the ESADDI.[f,i] Copper intakes were not estimated in the 1977–1978 NFCS. JNMEC did not evaluate copper intakes or status.[d] Although overt signs of copper deficiency are not seen in the general population, research is needed to determine whether the ESADDI is unrealistically high and whether there are any problems related to copper status in the population.
Sodium (to convert mg of sodium to sodium chloride [salt] multiply sodium by 2.5. To convert mg of salt to sodium, multiply salt by 0.40.)	ESADDI[i] Infants, 115–705 mg Children 1–3 years, 325–975 mg Children 4–6 years, 450–1,350 mg Children 7–10 years, 600–1,800 mg Adolescents, 900–2,700 mg Adults, 1,100–3,300 mg (The upper level of 3,300 mg equates to 1,600 mg per 1,000 kcal based on the midpoint of the Recommended Energy Intake range for adult females of 2,000 kcal.)	Salt (sodium chloride); cured meats (ham, bacon, sausage, frankfurters, luncheon meats); cheeses, olives; pickles; condiment sauces; frozen and canned meat and fish entrees and dinners; canned and dried soups; commercial pasta, noodle,	*Availability* in the food supply has not been reported. Data obtained from table-salt purchasers, from the use of salt in food production and processing, from national surveys, and from urinary sodium excretion studies suggest a total daily intake of salt in the United States ranging from 10 to 14.5 g per capita (4,000 to 5,800 mg of sodium). About one-third of this is estimated to occur naturally in foods, one-third is added during food processing, and one-third is added at home during cooking or at the table.[k] In the 1985 CSFII, sodium intake in mg/1,000 kcal averaged 1,415 for children 1 to 5 years old, and for women and men 19 to 50 years old, 1,569 and 1,470, respectively (excludes sodium added during

TABLE 3–10 *continued*

Mineral	1980 RDA, amount per day[a]	Major Food Sources	Food Supply, Intakes, and Nutritional Status
Sodium (*continued*)		and potato dishes; salted snacks; commercial mixes for waffles, muffins, and cakes; canned vegetables; frozen vegetables with sauces; baking powder; baking soda; certain emulsifiers and other food additives; drinking water in some locations; softened water; drugs such as some antacids.	cooking or at the table, in drinking water, and in medications).[b] In the 1977–1978 NFCS, the mean for all sex and age groups was 1,540 mg/1,000 kcal. One-third of the respondents reported intakes above 1,600 mg/1,000 kcal; 9% had intakes above 2,000 mg/1,000 kcal. Blacks had lower intakes than did whites. This survey underestimated sodium intake for the same reason as did the CSFII (above).[c] JNMEC found that dietary intakes of sodium appeared to be high, particularly since surveys underestimate intakes. National surveys have not included health indicators directly related to sodium intakes. Sodium merits priority in consideration of diet and public health.[d]
Potassium	ESADDI Infants, 350–1,275 mg Children 1–3 years, 550–1,650 mg Children 4–6 years, 775–2,325 mg Children 7–10 years, 1,000–3,000 mg Adolescents, 1,525–4,575 mg Adults, 1,875–5,525 mg (The upper limit of 5,625 mg relative to an energy intake of 2,000 kcal provides a standard of comparison of 2,800 mg/1,000 kcal.)	Milk, fruits (especially oranges, prunes, apples, pears, peaches, bananas, and grapefruit), vegetables (especially fresh broccoli, carrots, tomatoes, and potatoes), fish, shellfish, turkey, chicken, and cooked oatmeal.	*Availability* in the food supply has not been reported. In the 1985 CSFII, intakes of women and men 19 to 50 years old averaged 1,378 mg/1,000 kcal and 1,351 mg/1,000 kcal, respectively, well below the ESADDI. Mean intakes per 1,000 kcal were 100–200 mg higher in sodium than in potassium. Mean intakes of children 1 to 5 years old were 1,349 mg/1,000 kcal.[b] In the 1977–1978 NFCS, potassium intakes were not reported.[c] In NHANES, 98–99% of respondents had potassium intakes below the standard of 2,800 mg/1,000 kcal.[i] JNMEC did not consider potassium.[d]

[a]When intakes are expressed in terms of the RDA, the intent is merely to indicate relative amounts. Intakes below the RDA are not to be construed as inadequate.
[b]USDA (1986b, 1987b).
[c]USDA (1984).
[d]DHHS/USDA (1986).
[e]LSRO (1984b).
[f]Pennington et al. (1986).
[g]LSRO (1984c).
[h]Patterson et al. (1984); Smith et al. (1983).
[i]Estimated safe and adequate daily dietary intake (NRC 1980).
[j]Carroll et al. (1983).
[k]Fregly (1985).

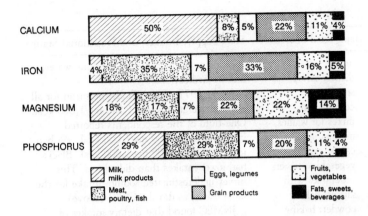

FIGURE 3–9 Food sources of minerals shown as percentage per person per day. Data from the 1977–1978 NFCS (USDA, 1984).

(Pennington et al., 1986). The iodine content of foods purchased in grocery stores between 1982 and 1984 was sufficient to provide dietary intakes markedly higher than the iodine RDA for all age–sex groups. For example, infants 6 to 11 months of age consumed 400%, 2-year-olds, 657%, and boys 14 to 16 years old, 473% of the RDA for iodine.

Although no evidence of adverse effects of present iodine intakes have been observed, the Food and Nutrition Board's report *Recommended Dietary Allowances* states that "any additional increases should be viewed with concern" (NRC, 1980). The report also contains a recommendation that iodophors used in the dairy industry, dough conditioners containing iodine, alginates, and certain coloring dyes be replaced, if possible, with substances not containing iodine (NRC, 1980).

Iodine is present in seafoods and in foods grown on high iodine soils. During the past 15 years or so, dairy products have become the chief iodine source in U.S. diets due to the use of iodine-containing substances to clean and disinfect equipment and to the addition of iodine to the feed of dairy cows. Some dough conditioners used in breadmaking and Red Dye No. 3 used in candies, breakfast cereals, and vitamin pills contain high levels of iodine. However, the iodine in Red Dye No. 3 is believed not to be absorbed. Many fast foods are also high in iodine (Taylor, 1981). Iodized table salt also contributes to iodine intake.

Selenium intakes were judged to be within the Estimated Safe and Adequate Daily Dietary Intake (ESADDI) in the Total Diet Study (Pennington et al., 1986). Manganese intakes were judged to be high in 6- to 11-month-old infants and low in teenage girls and women up to age 65.

Fluoride is important in the prevention of dental caries, but fluoride intakes have not been determined in any of the large surveys. Dietary fluoride is provided by seafood and tea leaves, but occurs in relatively small amounts in other foods. The fluoride content of drinking water, either naturally or artificially fluoridated, is probably the best indicator of dietary exposure. Not all Americans live in areas where the water supply is fluoridated, however. JNMEC concluded that fluoride should receive public health monitoring status, because not everyone in the U.S. population may consume amounts adequate to prevent dental caries (DHHS/USDA, 1986).

In summary, JNMEC listed sodium, calcium, iron, and fluoride among the nutrients that merit priority in considerations of diet and public health. It also noted that magnesium and zinc warrant further investigation (DHHS/USDA, 1986).

Fortification and Enrichment of Foods

The term *fortification* is usually used to designate the addition of nutrients not naturally present in a food (e.g., the fortification of milk with vitamin D), whereas the term *enrichment* generally means the addition of nutrients already present in a food. Often the terms are used interchangeably, however (Quick and Murphy, 1982).

The FDA sets standards specifying the nutrients and their amounts to be added to enrich flour, cereals, and bread products; standards are also set for the addition of vitamins A and D to milk products and of vitamin A to margarine. State agencies, not the FDA, are responsible for requiring that specific foods be enriched or fortified. Enrichment of bread and white flour is mandatory in about two-thirds of the states, but in fact, nearly all white flour in the United States is enriched with certain B vitamins and iron.

In 1980, the FDA published guidelines to promote the rational fortification of food. Sugars, candies, carbonated beverages, and other snack foods were considered to be inappropriate for fortification. Fortification was considered to be appropriate (1) to correct a dietary inadequacy recognized by the scientific community to result in a deficiency disease; (2) to restore nutrient levels to those present in a food before conventional processing and storage; (3) to adjust the protein, vitamin, and mineral content of the food to meet specific caloric requirements (i.e., a food must furnish a specific number of calories per serving); and (4) to ensure that a substitute food is nutritionally similar to the traditional food it replaces (Quick and Murphy, 1982).

USDA prohibits the direct fortification of meat and poultry, taking the view that these are highly nutritious foods that do not need additional nutrients. Enriched flour or cereals may be used in meat mixtures, however.

A direct relationship between food fortification and improved nutritional status is difficult to establish because of problems in controlling all the factors that may contribute to such improvements. Some attempts have been made to assess the influence of enrichment and fortification on nutrient intake. A survey covering 1966 to 1970 (Friend, 1972) indicated that nutrients added to the food supply increased the availability of thiamin by 40%, iron by 25%, niacin by 20%, riboflavin by 15%, and 10% each for vitamin A and ascorbic acid. Among foods supplemented at that time were flour and baked products, cereal products, beverages, milk, infant formulas, margarine, and formulated meal replacements.

In a recent study, Cook and Welsh (1987) used food consumption data from the 1977–1978 NFCS to study the effect of enriched and fortified grain products on nutrient intake. Enrichment and fortification of grain products were found to provide 32, 18, 20, and 19% of the total intakes of thiamin, riboflavin, niacin, and iron, respectively (Cook and Welsh, 1987). Grain enrichment led to thiamin intakes averaging 110% of the RDA, rather than the former level of 74%. Fortified breakfast cereals provided approximately 20% of the added thiamin, niacin, and iron, and about 25% of the added riboflavin for all respondents.

Fortification and enrichment clearly have made important contributions to the nutrient intake of the U.S. population. Nevertheless, many nutrition scientists have warned against indiscriminate fortification of foods (Mertz, 1984).

CHANGES IN EATING PATTERNS

Marked changes in the availability and nutrient content of foods in the food supply have occurred in parallel with lifestyle changes affecting the kinds and amounts of foods consumed. The 1977–1978 NFCS (USDA, 1984) assessed eating patterns only on 3 consecutive days, and the 1986 NFCS (USDA, 1987c) was based on 1 day of reported intake. The resulting data are inadequate to assess the habitual eating patterns of individuals, but can be used to assess eating patterns of groups.

Eating Occasions

The 1977–1978 NFCS (USDA, 1984) indicated that fewer males and females 19 to 34 years old ate breakfast at least once in 3 days than did people in other age groups. Children under 12 and adults 65 years old and over were most likely to eat breakfast. In 1985, 53% of women 19 to 50 years of age and 85% of children 1 to 5 years old ate breakfast on all 4 days of the survey (USDA, 1987a).

Respondents ate alone on 29% of eating occasions, primarily breakfasts and snacks (USDA, 1984). Nine percent of respondents packed lunches to eat away from home. Twenty percent of all eating occasions away from home (food obtained and eaten away from home) were at restaurants, 19% at work, 16% at school, 16% at someone else's home, and 13% at fast-food places (USDA, 1984).

Eating Away from Home

In the United States, people have been eating away from home at an increasing rate for many years. Data based on a 1-day intake obtained in 1986 (USDA, 1987c) indicated that 57% of women ages 19 to 50 obtained and ate some food away from home, compared with 45% in 1977 to 1978. On the basis of a 4-day intake in 1985, 88% of women 19 to 50 years of age reported eating some food away from home on at least 1 of the 4 days (USDA, 1987b). Forty-five percent of children 1 to 5 years old consumed some food away from home in 1986, compared with 30% in 1977 (USDA, 1987c). A larger proportion of men also reported obtaining and eating food away from home in 1985 than in 1977 (69 vs 53%).

Compared to the foods prepared and eaten at home, the nutrient densities (amount of a given nutrient per 1,000 kcal) of foods eaten away from home during the 3 days surveyed were lower for nearly all nutrients (USDA, 1984). Ries et al. (1987) reported the nutritive value of foods consumed at restaurants, fast-food places, and snack bars in grocery or drug stores by respondents 15 years of age and older who were interviewed in the 1977–1978 NFCS. Nutrient densities were lower for practically all nutrients in these foods than in food eaten at home except for fat, which was higher in the foods eaten "out." This survey did not determine the habitual behavior of individual respondents. The authors concluded that the respondents did not eat outside the home frequently enough to significantly diminish the adequacy of their diets, but cautioned that individuals who do eat frequently in such places (particularly teenagers and the elderly) are at risk of low intakes of calcium, vitamin A, vitamin B_6, and vitamin C (Ries et al., 1987).

Snacking

Eating defined by respondents as "a snack, a coffee break, or a beverage break" was practiced by 77% of all respondents at least once during the 3 days reported in the 1977–1978 NFCS (USDA, 1984). Such snacks provided an average of 18% of the day's calories and a higher proportion of carbohydrates (23%) than fats (15%) or protein (11%). Preschoolers and teenagers obtained about 20% of their total caloric intake from snacks. The increased frequency of eating away from home and increased snacking practices appear to have affected the nutritive quality of diets in a negative way.

Dieting

Respondents in the 1977–1978 NFCS were asked whether or not their food intake on the day of the interview differed from their usual intake. If so, they were asked whether or not they were on a diet to lose weight. Among females, 11% of those 15 to 18 years old and 16 to 19% of those 19 to 64 years old answered "yes" to this question. Twelve percent of women 65 to 74 years of age reported they were on weight-reduction diets.

Alternative Diets

The surveys discussed in this chapter indicate that the U.S. population consumes relatively large amounts of meat and sugar, more refined than whole-grain products, and larger amounts of commercially processed than fresh foods. In contrast, most of the world's population today subsists on vegetarian or near-vegetarian diets for reasons that are economic, philosophical, religious, cultural, or ecological. Indeed, humans appear to have sub-

sisted for most of their history on near-vegetarian diets (ADA, 1980).

During the 1960s and 1970s, interest in diets other than the usual intakes heightened in the United States. Some young people for the first time became vegetarians. Others following alternative diets include users of whole (minimally processed) foods or organically grown foods, as well as those who simply try to avoid food additives. Many obtain a large percentage of their food from health food stores or from small food cooperatives, rather than from supermarkets. Wolff (1973) noted that such a group in Hawaii avoided such foods as refined sugar, bread and other products made with white flour, white rice, processed foods containing additives, soft drinks, processed meats and cereals, and coffee. Instead, they bought (in descending order of frequency) whole-grain products, whole-wheat bread, fresh vegetables and fruits, raw nuts, wheat germ, brown rice, honey, yogurt, dried fruit, brewer's yeast, and seeds (Wolff, 1973). Their chief reason for adhering to their alternative diet was that they believed it to be healthier. Today, increased demand for these kinds of foods has prompted many large supermarkets to offer such foods as brown rice, whole-grain flour, unsalted nuts, seeds, and dried fruit, often in bulk, as well as additive-free whole-grain breads.

People who call themselves vegetarians vary from those who avoid only red meat, but eat poultry or fish, to lacto-ovovegetarians (who eat milk and eggs but no flesh foods), to total vegetarians (who eat no foods of animal origin). Vegetarian organizations generally do not classify as vegetarian those who avoid only red meat. Technically, vegans are those who not only avoid all animal foods, but use no other kinds of animal products such as wool, silk, or leather.

The first national survey to recognize the increasing interest in vegetarianism was the 1977–1978 NFCS in which respondents were asked: "Are you a vegetarian?" Of the 37,135 people surveyed, 464 (1.2%) answered "yes," but since some of these people reported consumption of flesh foods during the 3 days on which dietary information was obtained, it is not clear how vegetarianism was defined by the respondents. Data from this survey indicated that vegetarians obtained 15.5% of their calories from protein, 37.6% from fats, and 47.3% from carbohydrates, whereas nonvegetarians obtained 16.6, 40.6, and 42.6% of calories from protein, fats, and carbohydrates, respectively (USDA, 1984). The nutritive values of the food intakes of vegetarians and nonvegetarians are shown in Tables 3–11 and 3–12 as percentages of the 1980 RDAs for various nutrients.

Vegetarians had higher caloric intakes than nonvegetarians, except for women 35 years of age and older, who consumed 72% of the energy requirements for their subgroup, which is 2,000 kcal for women ages 35 to 50; 1,840 kcal for those ages 51 to 64; 1,800 kcal for those ages 65 to 74; and 1,600 kcal for those 75 and over (NRC, 1980). Although mean heights of vegetarians were similar to their nonvegetarian counterparts, mean weights tended to be lower in vegetarians.

A comparison of Tables 3–11 and 3–12 indicates that vegetarians had lower intakes of protein, preformed niacin, and vitamin B_{12} than nonvegetarians, but that their average intakes of all three nutrients were above the RDAs. All other nutrients were, on average, at the same level or higher in vegetarian than in nonvegetarian diets. Average intakes of vitamin B_6 and magnesium were below the RDA for vegetarians and nonvegetarians, but the nutrient data base used to estimate these nutrients is less well established than that for other nutrients. Intakes of calcium, vitamin A, and vitamin C averaged 20 to 24% higher, and magnesium 14% higher, in vegetarian than in nonvegetarian diets.

Since the RDA for iron is highest (18 mg/day) for females in their reproductive years, it is instructive to compare average intakes of vegetarian women 19 to 34 years of age with the comparable group of nonvegetarians women. Although these two groups had comparable energy intakes (78% of the RDA) and comparable iron intakes (60% and 61% of the RDA), vegetarian women had higher mean intakes of calcium, magnesium, phosphorus, vitamin A, riboflavin, vitamin B_{12}, and vitamin C and slightly higher intakes of vitamin B_6 and thiamin. Nonvegetarians had higher mean intakes of protein and preformed niacin, but these nutrients still met or exceeded the RDA in vegetarian diets.

It is possible that the iron in vegetarian diets (all inorganic, if no flesh foods are consumed) is less well absorbed than iron in nonvegetarian diets, which include heme iron in meat. However, the absorption of inorganic iron is enhanced by the simultaneous consumption of vitamin C. Iron deficiency anemia appears to be no more prevalent among vegetarian women than among nonvegetarian women, but further study of iron bioavailability in vegetarian diets is needed.

Groups with the lowest caloric intakes were female vegetarians 35 years of age and older whose energy intake averaged 72% of the RDA. The diets of vegetarian women 65 years old and above were nutritionally inferior to those of nonvegetarian women of similar age (Tables 3–11 and 3–12). In this age group, vegetarians had lower intakes of protein, iron, magnesium, phosphorus, thiamin, preformed niacin, vitamin B_6, vitamin B_{12}, and vitamin C than did nonvegetarians. However, each of these nutrients met or exceeded 88% of the RDA in vegetarian diets except magnesium (68%) and vitamin B_6 (52%) for which the intake was also below the RDA for nonvegetarians (75 and 62%, respectively.)

DO FOOD CHOICES IN THE UNITED STATES REFLECT A CONCERN ABOUT HEALTH?

Scholars of dietary behavior have long recognized that although biologic functioning is related to one's lifetime food intake, complex economic, social, political, and cultural factors govern food choices. Specialists who seek the cooperation of designated respondents in nutrition surveys or who endeavor to change food habits to provide good health must appreciate fully the fact that food choices have strong symbolic, emotional, and cultural meanings (Sanjur, 1982).

One of many factors affecting food choices is the individual's belief about the health or nutritional benefits or harm associated with specific choices. Investigators working in the area of diet and chronic diseases consequently have focused their attention on ways to modify belief systems to effect desired changes in food choices. In recent years, national campaigns have been launched to inform the public about the association between dietary salt/sodium and hypertension; between dietary fat/saturated fat and cholesterol and heart disease; and between dietary fats and fiber-containing foods and certain cancers. The National High Blood Pressure Education Program began at the National Heart, Lung, and Blood Institute (NHLBI) in 1972, and major efforts to inform the public about the link between sodium/salt and hypertension began in 1981. The NHLBI's National Cholesterol Education Program was launched in 1984 to educate the public about the relationship of dietary fat/saturated fat and cholesterol to high blood cholesterol—a major risk factor for CHD. The National Cancer Institute began a program in fall 1984 to encourage the public to reduce fat intake and increase fiber intake in an effort to reduce the risks for breast and colorectal cancer.

TABLE 3-11 Vegetarians: Nutritive Value of Food Intake as a Percentage of the 1980 RDA. Average per Individual per Day, 1977–1978[a]

Sex and Age (years)	N	Daily Intake, % of RDA												
		Food Energy	Protein	Calcium	Iron	Magnesium	Phosphorus	Vitamin A	Thiamin	Riboflavin	Preformed Niacin[b]	Vitamin B6	Vitamin B12	Vitamin C
Males and females														
>3	18[c]	99	192	138	105	176	164	277	192	257	122	138	279	209
3–8	34	91	209	112	103	120	147	176	124	153	114	97	127	164
Males														
9–18	20	98	203	107	121	97	151	182	166	171	150	123	191	225
19–34	49	90	162	166	163	124	216	189	128	154	122	97	201	277
35–64	45	92	166	106	179	106	185	174	129	136	149	86	173	214
≥65	25	89	134	120	145	92	174	126	125	143	116	73	151	196
Females														
9–18	31	91	170	87	90	115	129	121	143	118	118	81	142	172
19–34	113	78	133	103	61	87	138	101	123	100	100	62	150	144
35–64	83	72	130	72	80	74	114	154	101	109	110	55	138	141
≥65	47	72	110	78	88	68	107	166	95	110	92	52	114	141
All	464	83	150	104	103	95	146	163	117	136	114	76	156	176

[a]From 1977–1978 NFCS for 48 conterminous states (USDA, 1984); based on 3 consecutive days of dietary intake.
[b]Based on RDAs as preformed niacin rather than niacin equivalents.
[c]Excludes breast-fed infants.

TABLE 3-12 Nonvegetarians: Nutritive Value of Food Intake as a Percentage of the 1980 RDA. Average per Individual per Day, 1977–1978[a]

Sex and Age (years)	N	Daily Intake, % of RDA												
		Food Energy	Protein	Calcium	Iron	Magnesium	Phosphorus	Vitamin A	Thiamin	Riboflavin	Preformed Niacin[b]	Vitamin B6	Vitamin B12	Vitamin C
Males and females														
>3[c]	1,438	95	193	120	82	149	154	193	174	236	120	124	210	180
3–8	3,526	89	209	105	98	100	136	155	128	171	126	93	166	171
Males														
9–18	3,462	86	193	97	91	80	133	123	121	149	122	94	205	173
19–34	3,697	88	176	109	158	86	185	114	109	127	130	80	214	142
35–64	4,686	86	164	93	155	88	168	130	113	126	136	78	206	145
≥65	1,490	83	139	88	142	80	149	144	129	125	125	71	192	152
Females														
9–18	3,600	82	160	74	76	103	115	112	134	111	111	72	148	150
19–34	5,082	78	145	74	60	69	121	109	99	111	119	58	134	119
35–64	6,609	72	147	67	84	76	118	140	103	112	127	61	157	135
≥65	2,080	83	136	71	108	75	115	163	104	119	120	62	151	150
All	35,671	84	165	87	102	83	136	132	113	124	124	75	176	147

[a] From 1977–1978 NFCS for 48 conterminous states (USDA, 1984); based on 3 consecutive days of dietary intake.
[b] Based on RDAs as preformed niacin rather than niacin equivalents.
[c] Excludes breast-fed infants.

PUBLIC OPINION SURVEYS ABOUT DIET AND HEALTH

FDA and the National Institutes of Health (NIH) periodically have conducted public opinion surveys to evaluate the effectiveness of these public information programs. These telephone surveys reach a sample of approximately 4,000 consumers chosen to be representative of the U.S. population. These results indicate that by 1986, two-thirds of adults in the United States had heard about a relationship between salt/sodium and hypertension; 44% reported that they studied package ingredient lists to avoid or limit salt/sodium; and 61% reported purchasing low-sodium products at least once. Many food manufacturers responded to consumer demands not by lowering salt/sodium in their basic line of products, but by introducing new sodium-reduced products (Heimbach, 1985).

Public perceptions that risks for heart disease may be affected by diet also grew: from 58% of the respondents in 1982 to 76% in 1986. Furthermore, beliefs that dietary fats and cholesterol are related to heart disease risks became widespread among the respondents: from 29% for fats and 26% for cholesterol in 1982 to 43 and 40%, respectively, in 1986. In response to the question, "What things that people eat and drink might make them more likely to get cancer?" 19% named fats or fat-containing foods in 1986, compared with only 12% two years earlier. To the question, "What things that people eat or drink are likely to prevent cancer?" 22% in 1986 compared with 10% in 1984 answered vegetables/fruits; 32% in 1986 compared with 9% in 1984 answered fiber/bran/roughage/whole grains. The latter response was attributed to the $75 million advertising campaign for high fiber breakfast cereals launched in fall 1984 (Heimbach, 1985).

Although self-reports of behavior are apt to be misstated, sales data show declining use of red meats, butter, whole milk, and eggs and increased sales of fresh produce and high-fiber cereals (but not whole-wheat bread). In addition, 61% of respondents in the FDA and NIH public opinion surveys (Health and Diet Surveys) reported major dietary changes between 1984 and 1986 in an effort to prevent heart disease or cancer. Reported changes included reducing fat intake, primarily by eating less meat, and reducing intakes of salt, cholesterol, and sugar. At the same time, the respondents reported consuming more fresh vegetables, fruits, fish, poultry, grain products, and bran. The survey indicated that those most knowl-edgeable and most apt to avoid or limit consumption of substances believed to be linked to health problems were better educated, had higher incomes, and were between 30 and 45 years of age (Heimbach, 1985).

A recent study of NHANES II data (1976–1980) indicates that on the 1 day surveyed, a relatively small percentage of respondents consumed foods recommended as possibly protective against cancer by a committee of the National Research Council (NRC, 1982) and the American Cancer Society (ACS, 1984). Only 18% of the respondents reported they consumed cruciferous vegetables (e.g., cabbage, Brussels sprouts, cauliflower), 21% reported eating fruits and vegetables high in vitamin A, and 16% reported the consumption of breads and cereals high in dietary fiber (Patterson and Block, 1988). A larger percentage reported they consumed red meats (55%); 43% reported eating bacon and luncheon meats. Diets of females were closer to the recommended guidelines than those of males. Older people were closer to the guidelines than younger people, and blacks were closer than whites, because blacks consumed more vegetables, fruits, fish, and poultry than did whites. These data do not represent the usual dietary intake of individual respondents, since only 1 day of dietary intake was obtained. Surveys being conducted by USDA and DHHS will provide additional data on food choices relative to dietary recommendations.

SUMMARY

In the United States, food patterns have changed significantly since 1909, when USDA began to collect data on the food supply. These data represent foods, excluding alcohol, that disappear into civilian markets—not actual consumption—but they reflect changes in overall patterns of food use by the population over time. Between 1909 and 1985 the percentage of calories available in the food supply from fats increased from 32 to 43%, the percentage from carbohydrates declined from 57 to 46%, and the percentage from protein remained unchanged at 11%.

Saturated and monounsaturated fatty acids provide the highest percentage of calories from fat in the food supply, although the availability of polyunsaturated fatty acids greatly increased over the years due to wider use of oils and margarines. Compared to 1909–1913, the food supply in 1985 furnished larger amounts of beef, poultry, fish, dairy products, fats, oils, fruits, sugars, and sweeteners, but furnished lower amounts of eggs, vegetables, potatoes, and grain products.

Public health agencies and several expert groups concerned with diet and health in the United States have urged the public to decrease total fat intake to approximately 30% of total calories. Whether or not actual consumption has decreased over the years is uncertain, however, because data from NFCS and NHANES fail to agree on this point.

NHANES monitors the overall nutritional status of the U.S. population, whereas NFCS determines the food use of households and the dietary intakes and patterns of individuals. Although these surveys have provided valuable data regarding the dietary intake and nutritional status of the population, some limitations in methods used and differences in design of the two surveys must be taken into account when interpreting their results and drawing conclusions. Furthermore, cross-sectional data traditionally provided by these surveys are unsuitable for studying causal relationships between dietary factors and chronic diseases. Data appropriate for studying causality can be supplied only by longitudinal studies, which are included in plans for NHANES III.

JNMEC was established by USDA and DHHS in 1983 to coordinate the survey methods used by the two departments to report their findings. The first report, issued in 1986, provides food intake data from the 1977–1978 NFCS and information on nutritional status based on biochemical analyses from NHANES II (1976–1980). JNMEC concluded that food components deserving high-priority monitoring status because of high consumption by a considerable portion of the population include food energy, total fats, saturated fat, cholesterol, sodium, and alcohol. Nutrients deserving high-priority monitoring because some portions of the population appear to have low intakes are vitamin C, calcium, iron, and fluoride. The group concluded that protein, vitamin A, thiamin, riboflavin, niacin, total carbohydrates, vitamin B_{12}, and phosphorus should continue to be monitored. In addition, added caloric sweeteners, fiber, vitamin B_6, folacin, magnesium, and zinc were judged to require further investigation since data regarding intake and nutritional status are inadequate at present.

Information on food composition and criteria for assessing nutritional status are incomplete for most nutrients. JNMEC noted that the most complete information exists for food energy, vitamin C, iron, protein, and vitamin A. For all other nutrients listed above, there is a need for more accurate information about the occurrence of the nutrient in foods and methods of nutritional assessment.

Women in their reproductive years constitute a group at risk for nutritional inadequacies because their total caloric intakes tend to be low, while their needs for certain nutrients may be high because of menstrual losses and increased requirements during pregnancy and lactation. Consequently, USDA surveys (NFCS and CSFII) in 1985 and 1986 focused on women 19 to 50 years of age and their children 1 to 5 years of age.

The USDA used the 1980 RDAs as a standard of comparison in reporting their data, fully recognizing that failure to reach this standard does not indicate inadequate intake, since the RDAs for many nutrients are deliberately set to exceed the requirements of most individuals. According to the 1985 survey (based on 4 nonconsecutive days of intake), women's mean caloric intake was only 1,528 kcal, but their mean intakes were above the RDA for eight nutrients (protein, vitamin A, ascorbic acid, thiamin, riboflavin, preformed niacin, vitamin B_{12}, and phosphorus). Their mean intakes were below the RDA for vitamin E (87%), calcium (74%), magnesium (67%), vitamin B_6 (57%), iron (56%), zinc (56%), and folacin (46%). On the basis of only one 24-hour dietary recall, male respondents 19 to 50 years of age reported a mean caloric intake of 2,838 kcal and intakes equal to 98% or more of the RDA for all nutrients listed above except magnesium (94%), zinc (94%), vitamin B_6 (85%), and folacin (76%). Clearly, a major reason that the diets of women are relatively lower in many nutrients than the diets of males is that total caloric intake by women is lower.

Although better-educated, higher-income people appear to be altering their diets in the direction advocated by public health experts, national surveys and other studies indicate that intakes of total fats and saturated fats generally are higher than recommended. White bread is by far the favorite kind of bread, and sweet baked products such as cookies and cakes are very popular. Carbonated soft drinks containing either caloric or noncaloric sweeteners are consumed in large amounts. Alcoholic beverages also contribute calories to the diet, but the extent of actual consumption is uncertain at present because of reporting methods. Fruits, vegetables, and other foods high in dietary fiber are consumed in relatively low amounts. Consumption of cruciferous vegetables such as cabbage, Brussels sprouts, broccoli, and cauliflower is relatively low as are intakes of carotenoid-containing foods such as carrots, sweet potatoes, and winter squash.

Extensive changes in eating patterns have occurred over the century, including marked increases in eating away from home and in snacking. Dieting to lose weight is practiced by many people, especially females. Deviations from recommended dietary guidelines have persisted, and in some instances increased, despite the overall growth in variety of commonly available food, improved transportation and storage of fresh foods, increased disposable income, and greater public and professional knowledge about dietary needs to maintain good health and nutrition.

REFERENCES

Abraham, S., C.L. Johnson, and M.F. Najjar. 1979. Weight and Height of Adults 18–74 Years of Age: United States, 1971–74. Vital and Health Statistics, Ser. 11, No. 211. DHEW Publ. No. PHS-79-1659. National Center for Health Statistics, Public Health Service, U.S. Department of Health, Education, and Welfare, Hyattsville, Md. 49 pp.

Acheson, K.J., I.T. Campbell, O.G. Edholm, D.S. Miller, and M.J. Stock. 1980. The measurement of food and energy intake in man—an evaluation of some techniques. Am. J. Clin. Nutr. 33:1147–1154.

ACS (American Cancer Society). 1984. Nutrition and Cancer: Cause and Prevention. American Cancer Society Special Report. American Cancer Society, New York. 10 pp.

ADA (American Dietetic Association). 1980. Position paper on the vegetarian approach to eating. J. Am. Diet. Assoc. 77:61–69.

Aitchison, J.M., W.L. Dunkley, N.L. Canolty, and L.M. Smith. 1977. Influence of diet on *trans* fatty acids in human milk. Am. J. Clin. Nutr. 30:2006–2015.

Beaton, G.H. 1986. Toward harmonization of dietary, biochemical, and clinical assessments: the meanings of nutritional status and requirements. Nutr. Rev. 44:349–358.

Beaton, G.H., J. Milner, P. Corey, V. McGuire, M. Cousins, E. Stewart, M. de Ramos, D. Hewitt, P.V. Grambsch, N. Kassim, and J.A. Little. 1979. Sources of variance in 24-hour dietary recall data: implications for nutrition study design and interpretation. Am. J. Clin. Nutr. 32:2546–2559.

Beecher, G.R., and J.T. Vanderslice. 1984. Determination of nutrients in foods: factors that must be considered. Pp. 29–55 in K.K. Stewart and J.R. Whitaker, eds. Modern Methods of Food Analysis. Avi Publishing Co., Westport, Conn.

Block, G. 1982. A review of validations of dietary assessment methods. Am. J. Epidemiol. 115:492–505.

Block, G., C.M. Dresser, A.M. Hartman, and M.D. Carroll. 1985. Nutrient sources in the American diet: quantitative data from the NHANES II survey. II. Macronutrients and fats. Am. J. Epidemiol. 122:27–40.

Bunch, K. 1987. Food Consumption, Prices, and Expenditures, 1985. Bulletin No. 749. Economic Research Service, U.S. Department of Agriculture, Washington, D.C. 128 pp.

Carroll, M.D., S. Abraham, and C.M. Dresser. 1983. Dietary Intake Source Data: United States, 1976–80. Vital and

Health Statistics, Ser. 11, No. 231. DHHS Publ. No. (PHS) 83-1681. National Center for Health Statistics, Public Health Service, U.S. Department of Health and Human Services, Hyattsville, Md. 483 pp.

Cook, D.A., and S.O. Welsh. 1987. The effect of enriched and fortified grain products on nutrient intake. Cereal Foods World 32:191–196.

DHEW (Department of Health, Education, and Welfare). 1972. Ten-State Nutrition Survey 1968–1970, Vols. I–VI. DHEW Publ. No. HSM-72-8130, 72-8131, 72-8132, 72-8133, 72-8134. Center for Disease Control, Health Services and Mental Health Administration, Atlanta. (various pagings)

DHHS/USDA (Department of Health and Human Services/U.S. Department of Agriculture). 1986. Nutrition Monitoring in the United States—A Progress Report from the Joint Nutrition Monitoring Evaluation Committee. DHHS Publ. No. (PHS) 86-1255. National Center for Health Statistics, Public Health Service, U.S. Department of Health and Human Services, Hyattsville, Md. 356 pp.

DHHS/USDA (Department of Health and Human Services/U.S. Department of Agriculture). 1987. Operational Plan for the National Nutrition Monitoring System: Report to Congress. Public Health Service, U.S. Department of Health and Human Services, Bethesda, Md. 47 pp.

Eaton, S.B., and M. Konner. 1985. Paleolithic nutrition: a consideration of its nature and current implications. N. Engl. J. Med. 312:283–289.

Englyst, H., H.S. Wiggins, and J.H. Cummings. 1982. Determination of the non-starch polysaccharides in plant foods by gas-liquid chromatography of constituent sugars as alditol acetates. Analyst 107:307–318.

Enig, M.G., R.J. Munn, and M. Kenney. 1978. Dietary fat and cancer trends—a critique. Fed. Proc. 37:2215–2220.

Enig, M.G., L.A. Pallansch, J. Sampugna, and M. Keeney. 1983. Fatty acid composition of the fat in selected food items with emphasis on *trans* components. J. Am. Oil. Chem. Soc. 60:1788–1795.

Food Marketing Institute. 1987. Trends: Consumer Attitudes and the Supermarket. Food Marketing Institute, Washington, D.C. 50 pp.

Forthofer, R.N. 1983. Investigation of nonresponse bias in NHANES II. Am. J. Epidemiol. 117:507–515.

Fregly, M.J. 1985. Attempts to estimate sodium intake in humans. Pp. 33–112 in M.J. Horan, M. Blaustein, J.B. Dunbar, W. Kachadorian, N.M. Kaplan, and A.P. Simopoulos, eds. NIH Workshop on Nutrition and Hypertension. Proceedings from a Symposium, Bethesda, Md., March 12–14, 1984. Biomedical Information Corp., New York.

Friend, B. 1972. Enrichment and Fortification of Foods, 1966–70. National Food Situation (142):29–33.

Garn, S.M., F.A. Larkin, and P.E. Cole. 1978. The real problem with 1-day diet records. Am. J. Clin. Nutr. 31:1114–1116.

Glinsmann, W.H., H. Irausquin, and Y.K. Park. 1986. Evaluation of health aspects of sugars contained in carbohydrate sweeteners: report of Sugars Task Force, 1986. J. Nutr. 116:S1–S216.

Hallfrisch, J., P. Steele, and L. Cohen. 1982. Comparison of seven-day diet record with measured food intake of twenty-four subjects. Nutr. Res. 2:263–273.

Hampe, E.C., Jr., and M. Wittenberg. 1964. The Lifeline of America; Development of the Food Industry. McGraw-Hill, New York. 390 pp.

Harlan, W.R., A.L. Hull, R.P. Schmouder, F.E. Thompson,

F.A. Larkin, and J.R. Landis. 1983. Dietary Intake and Cardiovascular Risk Factors, Part II. Serum Urate, Serum Cholesterol, and Correlates. Vital and Health Statistics, Ser. 11, No. 227. DHHS Publ. No. (PHS) 83-1677. National Center for Health Statistics, Public Health Service, U.S. Department of Health and Human Services, Hyattsville, Md. 94 pp.

Harlan, W.R., A.L. Hull, R.L. Schmouder, Jr., J.R. Landis, F.E. Thompson, and F.A. Larkin. 1984. Blood pressure and nutrition in adults. The National Health and Nutrition Examination Survey. Am. J. Epidemiol. 120:17–28.

Hegsted, D.M. 1972. Problems in the use and interpretation of the recommended dietary allowances. Ecol. Food Nutr. 1: 255–265.

Heimbach, J.T. 1985. Cardiovascular disease and diet: the public view. Public Health Rep. 100:5–12.

Hepburn, F.N. 1987. Food Consumption/Food Composition Interrelationships. Human Nutrition Information Service, U.S. Department of Agriculture, HNIS Report No. Adm-382. Hyattsville, Md. 77 pp.

Hunter, J.E., and T.H. Applewhite. 1986. Isomeric fatty acids in the U.S. diet: levels and health perspectives. Am. J. Clin. Nutr. 44:707–717.

Jacobs, D.R., Jr., P.J. Elmer, D. Gorder, Y. Hall, and D. Moss. 1985. Comparison of nutrient calculation systems. Am. J. Epidemiol. 121:580–592.

LSRO (Life Sciences Research Office). 1984a. Assessment of the Folate Nutritional Status of the U.S. Population Based on Data Collected in the Second National Health and Nutrition Examination Survey, 1976–1980. Federation of American Societies for Experimental Biology. Bethesda, Md. 96 pp.

LSRO (Life Sciences Research Office). 1984b. Assessment of the Iron Nutritional Status of the U.S. Population Based on Data Collected in the Second National Health and Nutrition Examination Survey, 1976–1980. Federation of American Societies for Experimental Biology. Bethesda, Md. 120 pp.

LSRO (Life Sciences Research Office). 1984c. Assessment of the Zinc Nutritional Status of the U.S. Population Based on Data Collected in the Second National Health and Nutrition Examination Survey, 1976–1980. Federation of American Societies for Experimental Biology. Bethesda, Md. 82 pp.

Madans, J.H., J.C. Kleinman, C.S. Cox, H.E. Barbano, J.J. Feldman, B. Cohen, F.F. Finucane, and J. Cornoni-Huntley. 1986. 10 Years after NHANES I: report of initial followup, 1982–84. Public Health Rep. 101:465–473.

Marston, R., and N. Raper. 1987. Nutrient content of the U.S. food supply. National Food Review, Winter–Spring, NFR-36:18–23.

McCarron, D.A., C.D. Morris, H.J. Henry, and J.L. Stanton. 1984. Blood pressure and nutrient intake in the United States. Science 224:1392–1398.

Mertz, W. 1984. Foods and nutrients. J. Am. Diet. Assoc. 84: 769–770.

Mertz, W., and J.L. Kelsay. 1984. Rationale and design of the Beltsville one-year dietary intake study. Am. J. Clin. Nutr. 40 suppl. 6:1323–1326.

Murphy, R.S., and G.A. Michael. 1982. Methodologic considerations of the National Health and Nutrition Examination Survey. Am. J. Clin. Nutr. 35 suppl. 5:1255–1258.

NRC (National Research Council). 1980. Recommended Dietary Allowances, 9th ed. Report of the Committee on Dietary Allowances, Food and Nutrition Board, Division of Biological Sciences, Assembly of Life Sciences. National Academy Press, Washington, D.C. 185 pp.

NRC (National Research Council). 1982. Diet, Nutrition, and Cancer. Report of the Committee on Diet, Nutrition, and Cancer, Assembly of Life Sciences. National Academy Press, Washington, D.C. 478 pp.

NRC (National Research Council). 1983. Diet, Nutrition, and Cancer: Directions for Research. Report of the Committee on Diet, Nutrition, and Cancer, Commission on Life Sciences. National Academy Press, Washington, D.C. 74 pp.

NRC (National Research Council). 1984. Toxicity Testing: Strategies to Determine Needs and Priorities. Report of the Steering Committee on Identification of Toxic and Potentially Toxic Chemicals for Consideration by the National Toxicology Program, Board on Toxicology and Environmental Health Hazards, Commission on Life Sciences. National Academy Press, Washington, D.C. 382 pp.

NRC (National Research Council). 1986. Nutrient Adequacy: Assessment Using Food Consumption Surveys. Report of the Subcommittee on Criteria for Dietary Evaluation, Coordinating Committee on Evaluation of Food Consumption Surveys, Food and Nutrition Board, Commission on Life Sciences. National Academy Press, Washington, D.C. 146 pp.

NRC (National Research Council). 1987. Regulating Pesticides in Food: The Delaney Paradox. Report of the Committee on Scientific and Regulatory Issues Underlying Pesticide Use Patterns and Agricultural Innovation, Board on Agriculture. National Academy Press, Washington, D.C. 272 pp.

Pao, E.M., K.H. Fleming, P.M. Guenther, and S.J. Mickle. 1982. Foods Commonly Eaten by Individuals: Amount Per Day and Per Eating Occasion. Home Economics Research Report No. 44. Human Nutrition Information Service, U.S. Department of Agriculture, Hyattsville, Md. 431 pp.

Park, Y.K., B.F. Harland, J.E. Vanderveen, F.R. Shank, and L. Prosky. 1981. Estimation of dietary iodine intake of Americans in recent years. J. Am. Diet. Assoc. 79:17–24.

Patterson, B.H., and G. Block. 1988. Food choices and the cancer guidelines. Am. J. Public Health 78:282–286.

Patterson, K.Y., J.T. Holbrook, J.E. Bodner, J.L. Kelsay, J.C. Smith, Jr., and C. Veillon. 1984. Zinc, copper, and manganese intake and balance for adults consuming self-selected diets. Am. J. Clin. Nutr. 40 suppl. 6:1397–1403.

Pennington, J.A.T. 1983. Revision of the total diet study food list and diets. J. Am. Diet. Assoc. 82:166–173.

Pennington, J.A.T., B.E. Young, D.B. Wilson, R.D. Johnson, and J.E. Vanderveen. 1986. Mineral content of foods and total diets: the selected minerals in foods survey, 1982 to 1984. J. Am. Diet. Assoc. 86:876–891.

Prosky, L., N.G. Asp, I. Furda, J.W. DeVries, T.F. Schweizer, and B.F. Harland. 1985. Determination of total dietary fiber in foods and food products: collaborative study. J. Assoc. Off. Anal. Chem. 68:677–679.

Quick, J.A., and E.W. Murphy. 1982. The Fortification of Foods: A Review. Agriculture Handbook No. 598. Food Safety and Inspection Service. U.S. Department of Agriculture, Washington, D.C. 39 pp.

Richards, L., and A.G. Roberge. 1982. Comparison of caloric and nutrient intake of adults during week and weekend days. Nutr. Res. 2:661–668.

Ries, C.P., K. Kline, and S.O. Weaver. 1987. Impact of

commercial eating on nutrient adequacy. J. Am. Diet. Assoc. 87:463–468.

Sanjur, D. 1982. Food and food intake patterns—central issues in their conceptualization and measurement. Mass. Agric. Exp. Stn. Bull. (675):73–103.

Scheig, R. 1970. Effects of ethanol on the liver. Am. J. Clin. Nutr. 23:467–473.

Schoenborn, C.A., and B.H. Cohen. 1986. Trends in Smoking, Alcohol Consumption, and Other Health Practices Among U.S. Adults, 1977 and 1983: Advance Data from Vital and Health Statistics of the National Center for Health Statistics, No. 118. DHHS Publ. No. (PHS) 86-1250. Public Health Service, U.S. Department of Health and Human Services, Hyattsville, Md. 16 pp.

Sempos, C., R. Cooper, M.G. Kovar, C. Johnson, T. Drizd, and E. Yetley. 1986. Dietary calcium and blood pressure in National Health and Nutrition Examination Surveys I and II. Hypertension 8:1067–1074.

Senti, F.R., ed. 1985. Health Aspects of Dietary trans Fatty Acids. Federation of American Societies for Experimental Biology, Bethesda, Md. 148 pp.

Sims, E.A.H., E. Danforth, Jr., E.S. Horton, G.A. Bray, J.A. Glennon, and L.B. Salans. 1973. Endocrine and metabolic effects of experimental obesity in man. Recent Prog. Horm. Res. 29:457–496.

Smith, J.C., Jr., E.R. Morris, and R. Ellis. 1983. Zinc: requirements, bioavailabilities and recommended dietary allowances. Pp. 147–169 in A.S. Prasad, A.O. Çavdar, G.J. Brewer, and P.J. Aggett, eds. Progress in Clinical and Biological Research, Vol. 129: Zinc Deficiency in Human Subjects. Alan R. Liss, New York.

Stamler, J. 1979. Population studies. Pp. 25–88 in R.I. Levy, B.M. Rifkind, B.H. Dennis, and N. Ernst, eds. Nutrition, Lipids, and Coronary Heart Disease. Raven Press, New York.

Tannahill, R. 1973. Food in History. Stein and Day, Briarcliff Manor, N.Y. 448 pp.

Taylor, F. 1981. Iodine: going from hypo to hyper. FDA Consumer 15:14–18.

Todhunter, E.N. 1970. A Guide to Nutrition Terminology for Indexing and Retrieval. National Institutes of Health, Public Health Service, U.S. Department of Health, Education, and Welfare, Bethesda, Md. 270 pp.

USDA (U.S. Department of Agriculture). 1981. Food Consumption, Prices, and Expenditures, 1960–1980. Statistical Bulletin No. 672. Economic Research Service, U.S. Department of Agriculture, Washington, D.C. 106 pp.

USDA (U.S. Department of Agriculture). 1983. Food Consumption, Prices and Expenditures, 1962–1982. Statistical Bulletin No. 102. Economic Research Service, U.S. Department of Agriculture, Washington, D.C. 103 pp.

USDA (U.S. Department of Agriculture). 1984. Nationwide Food Consumption Survey. Nutrient Intakes: Individuals in 48 States, Year 1977–78. Report No. I-2. Consumer Nutrition Division, Human Nutrition Information Service, Hyattsville, Md. 439 pp.

USDA (U.S. Department of Agriculture). 1985. Nationwide Food Consumption Survey. Continuing Survey of Food Intakes of Individuals. Women 19–50 Years and Their Children 1–5 Years, 1 Day, 1985. Report No. 85-1. Nutrition Monitoring Division, Human Nutrition Information Service, Hyattsville, Md. 102 pp.

USDA (U.S. Department of Agriculture). 1986a. Nationwide Food Consumption Survey. Continuing Survey of Food Intakes of Individuals. Low-Income Women 19–50 Years and Their Children 1–5 Years, 1 Day, 1985. Report No. 85-2. Nutrition Monitoring Division, Human Nutrition Information Service, Hyattsville, Md. 186 pp.

USDA (U.S. Department of Agriculture). 1986b. Nationwide Food Consumption Survey. Continuing Survey of Food Intakes of Individuals. Men 19–50 Years, 1 Day, 1985. Report No. 85-3. Nutrition Monitoring Division, Human Nutrition Information Service, Hyattsville, Md. 94 pp.

USDA (U.S. Department of Agriculture). 1987a. Nationwide Food Consumption Survey. Continuing Survey of Food Intakes of Individuals. Low-Income Women 19–50 Years and Their Children 1–5 Years, 1 Day, 1986. Report No. 86-2. Nutrition Monitoring Division, Human Nutrition 106 pp.

USDA (U.S. Department of Agriculture). 1987b. Nationwide Food Consumption Survey. Continuing Survey of Food Intakes of Individuals. Women 19–50 Years and Their Children 1–5 Years, 1 Day, 1986. Report No. 86-1. Nutrition Monitoring Division, Human Nutrition Information Service, Hyattsville, Md. 98 pp.

USDA (U.S. Department of Agriculture). 1987c. Nationwide Food Consumption Survey. Continuing Survey of Food Intakes of Individuals. Women 19–50 Years and Their Children 1–5 Years, 4 Days, 1985. Report No. 85-4. Nutrition Monitoring Division, Human Nutrition Information Service, Hyattsville, Md. 182 pp.

USDA (U.S. Department of Agriculture). 1988. Nationwide Food Consumption Survey. Continuing Survey of Food Intakes of Individuals. Low-Income Women 19–50 Years and Their Children 1–5 Years, 4 days, 1985. Report No. 85-5. Nutrition Monitoring Division, Human Nutrition Information Service, Hyattsville, Md. 220 pp.

USDA (U.S. Department of Agriculture). In press. USDA Agricultural Handbook No. 8. Comparison of Foods—Raw, Processed, and Prepared. Nutrient Data Research, Human Nutrition Information Service, United States Department of Agriculture. Hyattsville, Md. (various pagings)

van den Reek, M.M., M.C. Craig-Schmidt, J.D. Weete, and A.J. Clark. 1986. Fat in the diets of adolescent girls with emphasis on isomeric fatty acids. Am. J. Clin. Nutr. 43:530–537.

Welsh, S.O., and R.M. Marston. 1982. Review of trends in food use in the United States, 1909 to 1980. J. Am. Diet. Assoc. 81:120–125.

Windham, C.T., B.W. Wyse, and R.G. Hansen. 1983. Alcohol consumption and nutrient density of diets in the Nationwide Food Consumption Survey. J. Am. Diet. Assoc. 82:364–373.

Wolff, R.J. 1973. Who eats for health? Am. J. Clin. Nutr. 26:438–445.

Woteki, C.E. 1985. Improving estimates of food and nutrient intake: applications to individuals and groups. J. Am. Diet. Assoc. 85:295–296.

Woteki, C.E. 1986. Dietary survey data: sources and limits to interpretation. Nutr. Rev. suppl. 44:204–213.

Yetley, E., and C. Johnson. 1987. Nutritional applications of the Health and Nutrition Examination Surveys (HANES). Annu. Rev. Nutr. 7:441–463.

4

Genetics and Nutrition

Studies have demonstrated remarkable genetic diversity among humans. No two individuals on this planet are alike genetically, except for identical twins, and even they vary because of somatic mutations in the immune system. The well-known individual uniqueness of physiognomic features extends to a variety of genetically determined biochemical and immunologic characteristics. Such traits include blood groups and tissue histocompatability antigen (HLA) types as well as enzymatic and other proteins. More recently, extensive variability in noncoding DNA has been described.

The variability of enzyme levels within the normal range in a population often has a simple genetic basis—different structural alleles at a gene locus that specify slightly different mean enzyme levels (Harris, 1975). The widely variable but unimodal distribution of activity for a given enzyme in a normal population may be the sum of overlapping curves, each characteristic of its underlying allele.

No *general* predictions regarding the impact of genetic variation on nutrition, health, and disease can be made. Every genetic system has a different evolutionary background and must be investigated separately.

APPLICABILITY TO NUTRITION

Assessments of human nutrition are not complete without consideration of the underlying genetic variability, which may be reflected as differences in nutritional processes such as absorption, metabolism, receptor action, and excretion (Velazquez and Bourges, 1984). Inborn differences in the activity of enzymes and other functional proteins contribute to variations in nutritional requirements and to the differential interaction of certain nutrients with genetically determined biochemical and metabolic factors. This inborn variation is quite different from epigenetic variation under conditions of growth, pregnancy, and old age. Genetic variation may also affect food likes and dislikes and, as a consequence, nutrition. For example, the inability to taste the synthetic chemical phenylthiocarbamide is a common monogenic trait that makes a large portion of the population unable to taste this chemical that others find quite bitter (Harris and Kalmus, 1941). Other examples, such as variability in the tasting of artificial sweeteners, are less well studied.

A key question of significance to nutrition is the extent of variation for a given gene product. Small variation can often be disregarded when making recommendations on nutrition, whereas wide variation cannot be ignored. The number of people affected by the variation is also important for policy setting. In the case of a monogenic variant, common genetic polymorphisms become important, especially when many people are affected. Rare variants affecting only a few people may pose a problem if their health would be placed at risk under circumstances conferring benefits to the health of most of the population.

Nutritional factors may have played a role in human evolution by selecting for certain genotypes (Neel, 1984). Thus, periods of starvation may have favored genotypes predisposing to hyperlipidemia and non-insulin-dependent diabetes by allowing more ready mobilization of lipids and glucose that provided a slightly better chance of survival and reproduction. A similar reasoning applies to genotypes predisposing to obesity. Such a hypothesis would explain the relatively high frequency of these traits.

INBORN ERRORS OF METABOLISM AS A MODEL

Even though inborn errors of metabolism are rare, their mechanisms may illustrate the role that more common genes may play in nutrition. The intrinsic processes required for proper nutrition, such as digestion, absorption, and excretion, are affected selectively by many different inborn errors of nutrient metabolism (Rosenberg, 1984). More than 200 such disorders have already been described. Among them are lactose intolerance (the inability to digest lactose); glucose–galactose malabsorption (the inability to absorb these nutrients); familial hypercholesterolemia, which develops in people who lack the receptors necessary to remove low-density lipoproteins (LDLs) from plasma; ornithine transcarbamylase deficiency, in which people lack an enzyme involved in the detoxification of ammonia; and hypophosphatemic rickets, in which the renal reabsorption of phosphorus and the intestinal absorption of phosphorus are impaired (Rosenberg, 1980). These disorders vary with regard to nutrients involved, frequency of occurrence, ethnic distribution, clinical severity, and disease manifestations (Holtzman et al., 1980). They may produce an internal or functional deficiency of an essential macro- or micronutrient despite adequate dietary intake; they may lead to chemical toxicity by blocking a catabolic pathway needed to metabolize an ingested nutrient; they may interfere with the formation of a needed product from an ingested nutrient; they may disrupt feedback regulatory pathways; or they may lead to pathological accumulation of macromolecules. Many of these metabolic disorders can be managed by modifying nutrient intake. For example, deficient intestinal absorption of a nutrient can be remedied by high oral intakes or parenteral administration; toxicity resulting from a blocked catabolic pathway of an essential amino acid can be relieved by restricting intake; vitamin supplementation may help to ameliorate a disturbance due to deficiency of an enzyme that requires the vitamin as a cofactor (Rosenberg, 1980).

Uptake of a variety of nutrients and other critical metabolites by cells is carried out by receptor-mediated endocytosis. The receptor that facilitates the uptake of LDLs (LDL receptor) has been studied in detail in the normal state and is an excellent model for receptor function in general (Goldstein and Brown, 1985). Some mutations of this receptor lead to defective transfer of LDLs into cells and increased LDL and cholesterol levels in the blood; this in turn predisposes to coronary heart disease (CHD). Mutations for the heterozygote state of familial hypercholesterolemia are found in approximately 1 in 500 people and predispose to premature coronary arteriosclerosis. Homozygotes are very rare (one in a million) and often develop CHD before 20 years of age (Goldstein and Brown, 1983).

These rare genetic disorders affecting enzymes and receptors illustrate how a severe genetic defect may lead to malnutrition or specific damage to a given organ system. They can serve as models for the study of milder but more common genetic variations in their effect on nutrition.

Possible Effects of Heterozygosity

The expression of most inborn errors of metabolism requires the presence of two identical mutant genes—each contributed by the carrier parent of an affected patient. The most common genetic disease of this sort is phenylketonuria, an autosomal recessive disease with a maximum frequency of 1 in 10,000 births. Most other inborn errors of metabolism have frequencies between 1 in 40,000 and 1 in 250,000 (Vogel and Motulsky, 1986). These rare inborn errors are not usually considered in making nutritional recommendations for the population as a whole, but carriers of the relevant mutant gene are quite common in the population. For example, 2% of the population are carriers of the mutant gene for phenylketonuria. In patients with inborn errors of metabolism, the involved enzyme has very little normal activity. Normal people have approximately 100% activity; carriers have about 50%. Under most conditions, a 50% level of enzyme activity is sufficient for adequate function. Thus, carriers are in good health. Under conditions of growth, stress, illness, or malnutrition, however, even 50% of enzyme activity may not be sufficient, and specific abnormalities related to the underlying enzyme activity might result (Vogel and Motulsky, 1986). Familial hypercholesterolemia is a relatively common heterozygous condition (1 in 500), which in the homozygous state is very rare (1 in 1 million) (Goldstein and Brown, 1983). More research is required to define whether the carrier heterozygotes for rare inborn errors are at risk for disease.

RESEARCH METHODS IN MEDICAL GENETICS

The number of genes shared by family members depends on their degree of relatedness (Vogel and Motulsky, 1986). First-degree relatives (full siblings or parents and their children) share an average of 50% of their genes; second-degree relatives share an average of 25% of their genes. Unrelated members of an ethnic group or race with common ancestry share a common gene pool and, hence, may resemble one another (biochemically and physically) more than they resemble people from other groups.

Generally, proof that a trait is genetically determined comes initially from a demonstration of familial aggregation, i.e., the trait is more frequent among relatives of affected persons than it is in the general population. However, familial aggregation by itself does not prove the involvement of genetic factors. Environmental exposures and lifestyle are also shared by family members and may cause a higher frequency of a particular trait among relatives. Absence of correlation for a given trait among spouses living in the same household and among children and their adoptive parents or siblings (who share no genes) argues against common environmental factors when positive correlations for the trait are obtained for biologic relatives. Higher correlations among identical twins (who share all their genes) than among nonidentical twins (who share half their genes) also argue for genetic factors. However, because identical twins are likely to select similar environments, ideal studies attempt to assess identical twins reared apart. Since such twin pairs are not found frequently, study sizes are necessarily small (Vogel and Motulsky, 1986; see also Chapter 7).

Biometrically analyzed studies of identical twins reared separately may suggest the operation of genetic factors for a given trait, but they provide no information regarding the number of genes involved or the mechanisms of their action. Obe-

sity is a good example. Studies of adoptive families and twins suggest that genetic factors are operative (see section on Obesity), but their mechanisms remain unknown.

The inheritance of single genes can be inferred from the nature of their segregation in families. Appropriate genetic–statistical techniques such as segregation analysis are available to test for the mode of inheritance. The principle of such methods is to test family data against various models of genetic transmission and find the best-fitting model (MacLean et al., 1985).

When the nature of the genetic abnormality is known for a monogenic or Mendelian trait, the abnormal or variant gene product can be studied in families, and appropriate segregation studies can be conducted. Where the specific structural defect in a protein or enzyme has been identified, the corresponding alteration in DNA can be inferred.

Much biologic insight into the role of genetics in humans has come from investigations of the role of specific genes and gene products. These approaches are reductionistic in nature, and their results ultimately need to be integrated with other observations of complex interaction of several genes. Furthermore, the role of special environmental factors in modifying gene action must be considered (see section on Gene–Environment Interaction, below).

Another approach to monogenic action is based on linkage analysis, the study of cosegregation of a common (or marker) gene with a physiologically or pathobiologically important gene in which the close physical apposition of these two genes on a given chromosome is studied. This type of study requires investigations of families in which an informative marker gene occurs in various related family members. Many DNA variants distributed over every one of the 23 chromosomes in humans are already known, and marker genes for closely spaced chromosomal sites are rapidly being elucidated. Because most DNA does not code for proteins, the variability of DNA is usually not expressed phenotypically, but DNA variants can be used as genetic markers to detect closely linked genes of physiological or pathological importance (Botstein et al., 1980).

Recently, some DNA mutations have been detected by linking harmless DNA variants to the diseased gene before any information about the nature of the defect was known. This approach has been referred to as *reverse genetics* (Orkin, 1986).

Population studies demonstrate different frequencies of genetic traits in various ethnic groups (Vogel and Motulsky, 1986). If the genetic trait is of physiologic or clinical significance, the total impact of a given gene's variation may differ in different populations.

GENE–ENVIRONMENT INTERACTION

Genes do not act in a vacuum; the action of one gene may depend not only on other genes, but also on the environment. This principle is well illustrated by the field of pharmacogenetics. Certain inherited enzyme variants are harmless by themselves but may cause untoward effects in the presence of a drug that requires the normal variety of that enzyme for its inactivation. The presence of the enzyme variant without the drug and the administration of the drug to a person with the normal enzyme are harmless. If the drug is given to the carrier of the enzyme variant, however, a reaction to the drug ensues. Examples include hemolytic anemia from glucose-6-phosphate dehydrogenase deficiency, prolonged apnea from pseudocholinesterase variation, and various drug reactions associated with defective acetylation of drugs such as isoniazid (Stanbury et al., 1983).

The concept of pharmacogenetics has been widened to ecogenetics, i.e., the interaction of specific genetic traits with any environmental agent to produce a given effect. There are three ecogenetic examples with relevance to nutrition: (1) severe flushing of the skin after exposure to alcohol in many Orientals, who often lack an isozyme of aldehyde dehydrogenase, which is involved in the metabolism of alcohol (NIAAA, 1987); (2) hypertension in genetically predisposed persons who migrate from a primitive environment to a more westernized one (Page, 1979); and (3) gastrointestinal distress after moderate milk consumption by many people with genetically determined lactase insufficiency (see section on Lactose Malabsorption, below) (Lisker, 1984). There are many more examples. As more is learned about the nature and extent of genetic variability, its interaction with the environment, and its effect on disease resistance and susceptibility, it will become increasingly possible to advise genetically susceptible individuals about environmental factors (including diet) that will prevent various diseases determined by genetic-environmental interaction.

OTHER GENETIC FACTORS THAT AFFECT NUTRITION

In the central nervous system, genetic variation probably affects perception of taste, degree of satiation, and other factors likely to affect food intake. However, no critical data on humans exist in this area. Absorption can also be affected. Examples include increased iron absorption in hemochromatosis (see section on Hemochromatosis, below) and genetically determined absence of gastric intrinsic factor, which leads to defective vitamin B_{12} absorption and pernicious anemia (Velazquez and Bourges, 1984).

Ethnic and racial factors also require consideration. Relatives share common ancestors and therefore are more likely to share similar genes derived from that ancestor. In a sense, an ethnic group is an extended family, and similar considerations apply. Often, therefore, frequencies of genetically determined traits or diseases will differ among races (e.g., Caucasians, blacks, or Orientals), and even among ethnic groups of the same race. It may not be apparent whether an ethnic or racial difference for a given trait or disease is caused by the existence of different genes or because the unequally affected racial group lives in a different environment. However, if the presence of a gene or genes can be demonstrated, the differentiation between genetic and environmental factors usually becomes clear. Thus, although we strongly suspect that genetic factors cause the difference between Pima Indians and Caucasians in the frequency of obesity, we cannot be absolutely sure since we have no gene marker. On the other hand, there is little question that the difference in frequency of hypolactasia in blacks and whites has a genetic cause, since tests for hypolactasia exist.

Such ethnic or racial differences may have policy implications; a nutritional policy may be desirable for one population group but would cause health problems in another.

GENETIC FACTORS IN SOME CHRONIC DISEASES

Coronary Heart Disease and Lipids

Hypercholesterolemia, high LDL levels, low levels of high-density lipoprotein (HDL), and low apolipoprotein A1 levels have all been implicated as risk factors for CHD, and all are influenced by both genetic and environmental factors. The presence of two different but common alleles at the apolipoprotein E locus has a large effect on cholesterol and apolipoprotein B levels (Sing and Davignon, 1985). The transmission of familial hypercholesterolemia due to various LDL receptor defects is Mendelian (Goldstein and Brown, 1983), and genetic factors seem to play a role in most hyperlipidemias. A common condition known as familial combined hyperlipidemia appears to be transmitted as a monogenic autosomal dominant trait and is usually associated with elevation of apolipoprotein B (Brunzell and Motulsky, 1984). The etiology of this condition appears to be heterogenous. Various DNA markers of the apolipoprotein loci have been associated with hyperlipidemia, or CHD, or both, but findings are not entirely consistent (Deeb et al., 1986). Considerable research is under way in these areas and is likely to help in clarifying the exact contribution of genetic factors to the hyperlipidemias.

A crucial issue is the relevance of such data in the development of nutritional advice for the population. Some argue that regardless of genetic variation, a lowering of the cholesterol level of Western populations by dietary modification would substantially reduce the frequency of CHD. Those with the lowest blood cholesterol levels have the lowest mortality from CHD, which increases progressively with higher cholesterol levels (Martin et al., 1986). Most CHD deaths and most excess coronary events related to elevated cholesterol levels do not occur at the upper end but in the center of the distribution curve (see Chapter 7). What will be the effects of lowering cholesterol levels in the population? For example, reducing an individual's cholesterol level from 226 to 210 mg/dl (which could be achieved through dietary modification) decreases the absolute risk of coronary mortality only slightly. However, a small reduction in absolute risk for an individual may translate into a major effect in the large number of people who constitute the population. In a hypothetical example, one can assume that by dietary modification, a person can reduce his or her risk of having a myocardial infarct within a given time span from 1 in 80 to 1 in 100. Applied to 100,000 persons, the expected frequency of 1,250 myocardial infarcts (1/80) would be reduced to 1,000 heart attacks (1/100). This 20% reduction (or prevention of 250 heart attacks) would be of significant public health importance.

Little is known about the effect of nutrition–genetic interactions on lipids. The role of the LDL receptor, structural variation in apolipoproteins B and E, the regulation of hepatic apolipoprotein B synthesis, and many other factors need to be studied to resolve these issues. Further knowledge in this important area is required to assess the role of diet in reducing lipid levels in individuals. It is certain, however, that genetic factors play an important role in determining cholesterol levels.

Response to dietary restriction of saturated fats and cholesterol or lipid levels will be variable, and not everyone will benefit equally from dietary moderation. Some people will be sensitive, whereas lipid levels in others may be resistant to control by dietary changes.

Hypertension and Salt

Blood pressure levels are under strong genetic control, as shown by studies in families, adopted children, and twins (Burke and Motulsky, 1985). There is good evidence for the role of sodium in the causation and maintenance of high blood pressure. In populations, the frequency of high blood pressure is related to average sodium intake. However, sodium loading does not cause elevation of blood pressure in all people, and sodium restriction lowers blood pressure in many but not all hypertensives. Hypertension is an ecogenetic trait in that so-called primitive populations have little hypertension. High blood pressure develops in some people when they translocate to a Western-type environment that includes a high salt intake. Populations of African origin in the United States have a higher mean blood pressure and a higher frequency of hypertension than those of European origin. Recently discovered differences between black and white hypertensive populations include the absence of elevated red-cell sodium/lithium countertransport in blacks—a finding that is common among white hypertensives. This transport trait appears to be under monogenic control (Motulsky, 1987a). This and other evidence suggests that hypertension is a heterogeneous entity with different genetic mechanisms.

Salt restriction has been advocated to reduce the frequency of high blood pressure but may not be equally helpful for all individuals (see Chapters 15, 20, and 28). In addition, clinical or laboratory criteria needed to characterize the degree of salt-sensitivity among people are lacking.

Diabetes Mellitus

Most cases of diabetes mellitus in humans fall into one of two categories: noninsulin-dependent diabetes mellitus (NIDDM) and insulin-dependent diabetes mellitus (IDDM). Twin and family studies strongly indicate the existence of genetic factors in both varieties, but the exact mechanisms remain unknown. More is known about some of the specific genes involved in IDDM (e.g., HLA-related genes) than in the more common NIDDM variety. The very high concordance of identical twins for NIDDM suggests that genes play a more central role in this disease (Barrett et al., 1981). Although nutrition and dietary components are important in the treatment of clinical diabetes, they do not appear to be involved in the pathogenesis of either form of the disease (Glinsmann et al., 1986), aside from the clear relationship of NIDDM to total caloric intake.

Obesity

The development of obesity is not simply a matter of caloric intake but involves genetic factors as well. This has been shown in studies of humans and of animals.

Epidemiologic Studies

It has been known for many decades that obesity is a familial trait. Most obese patients have at least one obese parent; however, members of a family or relatives share many common aspects of nutrition and environment. For example, in the analysis of the Ten State Nutrition Survey (Garn and Clark, 1976), other factors such as socioeconomic class, age, and sex were prominent predictors of obesity (Garn and Clark, 1976). More recently, Garn (1985) noted that most children of obese parents become overweight, whereas those of lean parents are thinner.

The most compelling evidence for genetic factors comes from studies of monozygotic and dizygotic twins (Borjeson, 1976; Bouchard et al., 1985; Fabsitz et al., 1980; Feinleib et al., 1977; Medlund et al., 1977; Stunkard et al., 1986a,b). Borjeson (1976) studied 40 monozygotic twin pairs and 61 same-sex dizygotic twin pairs and estimated heritability of obesity to be 88%. (Heritability may range from 0%, i.e., no genetic factors, to 100%, indicating that a trait is determined entirely by genetics). A similar conclusion was reached by Brook et al. (1975). A much larger twin study based on the large Swedish Twin Registry showed a high concordance of body fatness in monozygotic but not in dizygotic twins (Fabsitz et al., 1980). A potent interaction between genetic predisposition and environment is suggested by a recent feeding and exercise challenge study in monozygotic and dizygotic twins (Poehlman et al., 1986).

The relative roles of genetics and the environment have also been examined by comparing obesity among adoptees to obesity in their adoptive and biologic parents. In several early adoption studies, no clear trends were found (Annest et al.,

1983; Withers, 1964). In at least one study, obesity was found among children with obese adoptive parents (Annest et al., 1983). In most of these studies, no information on biologic parents was available. Children may have spent an extended period with a biologic parent before adoption, and adoptive placement may have been based on physical similarity between adoptive parents and the adopted child—a common practice several decades ago. However, two recent studies, one based on a Danish adoption registry (Stunkard et al., 1986a) and another on fatness data from Iowa (Price et al., 1987), included information on biologic parents as well as adoptive parents. These show a stronger correlation in body mass index (BMI) between adoptees and their biologic parents than between adoptees and their adoptive parents. In the Iowa study, the correlation of BMI was independent of height and applied to the full range of obesity. In stepwise multiple regression analyses, the best correlations were predicted by a model in which genetic and nonfamily environmental factors were both considered. Even so, much of the variance was unexplained. Additional studies examining biologic parents and siblings have shown a variable genetic and genetic–environmental contribution (Bouchard, 1988). Nevertheless, taken together, the results of such studies suggest that multifactorial polygenic factors play a role in human obesity. This formulation does not rule out the involvement of major genes that have yet to be identified.

Ethnic differences also are consistent with, but do not prove, the role of genes in obesity. The higher frequency of overweight among black women compared to white women may at least partially be caused by genetic factors (Van Itallie, 1985). This may also apply to Mexican-American children, who are fatter than either white or black children (Mueller, 1988). The high prevalence of obesity among several Native American tribes and Pacific Island populations is difficult to explain by excess calories alone.

There is evidence from a study of twins (Bouchard, 1988) and from several studies of ethnic groups (Mueller, 1988) that patterns of body fat distribution are inherited. This is especially apparent among children. For example, Mexican-American children have a pronounced upper body fat distribution, which is sometimes independent of adiposity per se (Mueller, 1988), whereas children of European origin seem to have a more peripheral distribution of fat (Mueller, 1988).

The nature of the specific genes causing such phenomena is still unknown.

Animal Studies

Obesity in mice and rats can be caused by several different single-gene mutations (Bray and York, 1971). Some strains of pigs and rats become obese under some feeding circumstances in which control animals do not. The exact biochemical or metabolic defects responsible for this have not yet been discovered. Intensive research is under way to clone relevant candidate genes.

It is unlikely that any of the animal models of monogenic obesity will fully explain the genetic factors operative in human obesity, since the genetic mechanism of human obesity does not appear to be monogenic. It is likely, however, that some of the genes involved in monogenic animal obesity may play some role in human obesity. Information on the nature of the genes involved in animal obesity will allow direct testing of the involvement of similar genes in humans by using techniques of molecular genetics.

Cancer

Certain types of cancer appear to be inherited. It is becoming increasingly apparent, however, that most cancers can be attributed to interactions between genetic (hereditary, or endogenous) factors and environmental (exogenous) factors.

It is helpful to consider causes of cancers in three broad groups: genetic, genetic–environmental, and environmental alone. The first group consists of cancers that appear to be determined largely by genetic factors with little or no environmental influence. One example is the high risk for colon cancer in people with familial polyposis of the colon. Other cancers in this group appear to be associated with impaired DNA repair mechanisms, such as in xeroderma pigmentosum and Bloom's syndrome. These examples illustrate a merging with the second group; for example, the development of malignancies in people with xeroderma pigmentosum requires exposure to an environmental agent (ultraviolet light) in predisposed individuals.

For the second group of cancers, genetic and environmental factors appear to be important—independently or synergistically. Examples include cancers that tend to run in families, such as some cancers of the stomach, colon, and breast. There is evidence that in colon cancer and possibly other cancers in this category, the pathogenic mechanism may involve the genetic transmission of a recessive gene that is present in all body cells and by itself does not cause cancer (Bodmer et al.,

1987). A somatic mutational event of the allelic partner in a single colon cell causes homozygosity at this locus and frees this cell of growth restraint, ultimately causing clinical colon cancer. Different environmental agents, including metabolites derived from food, could cause the second somatic mutation (Knudson, 1985; Solomon et al., 1987).

Cancers in the third group are produced largely by environmental agents, which in general are independent of genetic variation. This category includes most malignant neoplasms. For some of these, however, genetic variation may affect cancer risks, for example, by altering the metabolism of carcinogens. Such mechanisms may affect individual risks of some of the smoking-related cancers (Ayesh et al., 1984; Mulvihill, 1976).

No studies of cancer risk in humans have yet indicated a relationship between dietary factors and genetic factors; however, such a relationship may be responsible for the increased cancer risk in genetically predisposed individuals. Therefore, there is some reason to postulate that dietary changes could have at least as much effect on cancers dependent on a genetic mechanism as they have on cancers that are free of genetic influence.

Lactose Malabsorption

At the time of birth, all humans (and all other mammals) produce the intestinal enzyme lactase to metabolize lactose—the main constituent of milk—into glucose and galactose. In most humans, the ability to digest lactose disappears after weaning due to progressive decline in intestinal lactase activity; such individuals are often referred to as lactose malabsorbers. Undigested lactose in the gastrointestinal tract of such people is decomposed by bacteria, causing bloating, diarrhea, intestinal rushes, flatulence, and even nausea and vomiting in severe cases. However, some people—particularly those of European origin—do not lose this ability and have persistent intestinal lactase activity (Lisker, 1984). This persistence of lactose absorption is controlled by a gene for persistence of intestinal lactase activity (L). People who do not carry this gene, and therefore cannot digest lactose after weaning, are homozygotes (ll) at this locus—the usual status for the majority of the world population. Milk drinking does not induce intestinal lactase activity in those who no longer have this capacity, nor will lactose restriction reduce the intestinal lactase activity among those who never lost it. Lactose absorption or malabsorption is an inborn genetic trait. Acute or chronic gastrointestinal disease may cause secondary hypolactasia among people with persistent lactase activity, but such activity returns after the illness. Most populations throughout the world have hypolactasia of the genetic variety. Only populations from central and northwestern Europe and from areas in Africa with a long history of dairy farming have high frequencies of persistent lactase activity. Presumably, the gene for lactase persistence had a survival advantage in dairy farming cultures and over the generations increased in frequency because people who were able to absorb milk as children and young adults were either more fertile or less likely to die early.

Milk is not consumed widely in populations where lactose malabsorption is common. Since milk is an important source of protein, calcium, and riboflavin, the existence of the lactase polymorphism has policy implications for the use of milk as a supplement for the world's lactose malabsorbers. However, most lactose malabsorbers can drink at least 250 ml of milk without much difficulty. Further studies are required to define more fully the amounts of lactose tolerated by malabsorbers.

Hemochromatosis

The clinical manifestations of primary hemochromatosis (including liver and heart damage, arthritis, diabetes, and skin discoloration) are caused by the toxic effects of excessive iron stores in many organs following increased iron absorption over many years. Nonspecific symptoms such as weakness and fatigue are frequent.

Affected persons are homozygotes for a gene that facilitates increased iron absorption and is carried on the short arm of chromosome 6, closely linked to HLA Locus A (Bothwell et al., 1983). The homozygous state affects from 1 in 600 to 1 in 1,000 people in the United States and western Europe, indicating that approximately 7% of the population are heterozygotes or gene carriers for the condition. Clinically apparent disease is more common among males, since females can eliminate some excess iron in their menses. The increasing practice of measuring serum iron and iron saturation is leading to the detection of cases who are not yet affected clinically but who will develop clinically apparent disease at a later stage. The extent of increased iron storage in hemochromatosis can be estimated by serum ferritin measurements.

Since iron deficiency is common among the general population, additional supplementation of

flour with iron has been recommended by public health authorities and is practiced in Sweden. The onset of clinical hemochromatosis in homozygotes presumably would be hastened by such a process. However, since the homozygous hemochromatosis genotype is found in, at most, 1 in 500 people, some observers believe that iron supplementation benefits a much larger fraction of the population (primarily women and children) and outweighs the damaging effects of iron for homozygotes. A crucial issue in this connection is related to the iron absorption status of the very common hemochromatosis heterozygotes (i.e., close to 1 in 10 persons). However, although liver iron stores increase somewhat among male heterozygotes as they get older, there is no evidence that heterozygotes are at risk for clinically apparent iron toxicity. Furthermore, there is currently no test for detecting heterozygotes in population studies.

The benefits of iron supplementation should be considered in the context of possible risk to occasional hemochromatosis homozygotes, especially since the health effects of mild to moderate iron deficiency are not as fully defined as desirable (Cook and Lynch, 1986).

Alcoholism

It has been known for many years that alcoholism is a familial occurrence, but the role of genetic and environmental factors within the family have been difficult to separate. Evidence accumulated over the past two decades suggests that alcoholism results from the interaction of heredity and the environment (NIAAA, 1987; Motulsky, 1987a; Omenn, 1987). Data on the genetic contribution comes from studies of familial alcoholism (Cloninger et al., 1978; Winokur et al., 1970), twins (Kaij, 1960; Loehlim, 1972), adoptees separated from their biologic parents at an early age (Bohman, 1978; Goodwin 1987), and animal breeding studies (Crabbe et al., 1981; Thurman, 1980).

The phenotype of "alcoholism" is heterogeneous. Alcohol-seeking behavior must be differentiated from alcohol dependence and alcohol tolerance. Target organ damage, such as that seen in Korsakoff's syndrome or alcoholic cirrhosis, poses genetic problems that are different from alcoholism (see Chapter 16).

Several studies of adopted children indicate that natural sons of alcoholics are three to four times more likely to be alcoholic than are natural sons of nonalcoholics, regardless of whether the sons were raised by their alcoholic biologic parents or by nonalcoholic adoptive parents (Goodwin, 1987). Studies of adoptees in Sweden identify two types of genetic disposition to alcoholism: milieu limited and male limited. Milieu-limited susceptibility occurs in both sexes and needs environmental challenge for its expression. The alcoholism is usually not severe, has a late onset, and is often associated with minor law violations. Male-limited susceptibility occurs in the biologic fathers of adoptees, is highly heritable, is reflected in severe, early-onset alcoholism that often requires extensive treatment, and is often associated with major law violations.

Studies of twins have not provided as clear evidence for genetic factors as have the adoption studies. Several studies have shown higher concordance in identical twins than in nonindentical twins, whereas others have not (NIAAA, 1987).

Efforts are under way to identify neurophysiological, neuropsychological, and biochemical markers of genetic susceptibility to alcoholism. Characteristic electrical brain patterns have been found in nonalcoholic offspring of alcoholic fathers (Mendelson and Mello, 1979). Fast electroencephalographic (EEG) activity and deficiencies in alpha, theta, and delta EEG activity have been reported in sons of alcoholics (Gabrielli et al., 1982). Studies of event-related potentials in the nonalcoholic sons of alcoholic fathers showed that they had a decreased amplitude in their P_3 wave similar to that found in abstinent alcoholics (Begleiter et al., 1980). Evidence suggests that decreased P_3 amplitude precedes the onset of alcohol abuse and may be a genetic marker of susceptibility (NIAAA, 1987). Tests of abstracting, problem solving, perceptual-motor functioning, and stimulus augmenting showed that nonalcoholic men with a family history of alcoholism performed less well than controls with no such family history (Schaeffer et al., 1984).

Research on biochemical markers has included the study of genetic variation in alcohol-metabolizing enzymes, especially alcohol dehydrogenase and aldehyde dehydrogenase. These enzymes help to eliminate alcohol from the body, mainly by oxidative metabolism in the liver. However, markers for these enzymes have not been associated with predisposition to alcoholism (NIAAA, 1987).

Oriental populations have a much higher frequency of the aldehyde dehydrogenase polymorphism. Carriers of this genetic trait flush more readily on exposure to alcohol. It is likely that this flushing reaction is a deterrent to excess alcohol consumption (NIAAA, 1987).

POLICY IMPLICATIONS OF GENETIC VARIATIONS

Public health policies generally focus on the average human being, without considering genetic variation. Thus, dietary recommendations usually provide a sufficient nutrient intake even for those with the highest requirements. This policy appears sound when variation for a given nutrient is small. If special dietary requirements affect only very few people with an inborn error of metabolism, policy recommendations could legitimately ignore such outliers, since such people can be identified and treated by physicians. In many instances, however, the true extent of genetic variation is unknown. The frequency of genetic variants in enzymes and proteins and their effect on enzyme activity suggest that there may be great variations in nutritional requirements or in gene–nutrition interaction.

Genetic factors as they relate to nutrition must be considered individually. The role of genetics in relation to dietary lipids and CHD is one example. High-fat intake constituting 40% of the calories in many Western diets and with a high saturated fat content leads to relatively high lipid levels and high frequencies of CHD. Serum cholesterol at all levels has been correlated with CHD frequency, but approximately 40% of all coronary events occur in the population with the highest 25% of cholesterol levels, including many genetic hyperlipidemias (see Chapter 7).

Many coronary events could be prevented if the entire population would reduce its cholesterol levels by decreasing saturated fat intake. Although individual risk reduction for those with "normal" cholesterol levels is relatively small, the total effect on the population would be considerable, because even small reductions in risk lead to a large public health benefit when the entire population is considered. This phenomenon of small effects in individuals, but a large impact on the population, has been termed the *prevention paradox*. A double-pronged strategy of case detection and individual management of those at high risk, together with a public health strategy to reduce cholesterol levels in the population as a whole, could therefore have large effects.

Currently, the adverse public health effects of obesity are well known. Thus it is appropriate to advise everyone to avoid obesity. In the future, it may be possible to identify those at particular risk of obesity from excess caloric intake and to focus special preventive efforts on this group (i.e., help them to avoid gaining weight).

For many diseases, there are substantial racial or ethnic differences in frequencies. Thus, a recommendation for a population subgroup may need to differ from that for the racial majority, though this may raise difficult policy questions because the recommendation can be easily misunderstood. However, there are precedent examples unrelated to nutrition including greater screening for Tay–Sachs disease among Ashkenazi (Eastern European) Jews, thalassemia among Mediterranean and Southeast Asian populations, and sickle-cell disease among blacks.

Problems can arise when a small group of persons is placed at high risk by a policy decision that would benefit the majority. An especially poignant example relates to iron supplementation and its effect on people with hemochromatosis (see section on Hemochromatosis).

Public health policy designed to benefit the population without discernible risk to certain individuals or subgroups has many merits: it is simple to implement, may cost less to society, and may benefit many people. Examples of such policies are vaccination against poliomyelitis even though some are genetically susceptible to paralysis (Motulsky, 1987b) or fluoridation of the entire water supply to prevent caries even though there are genetic differences in caries susceptibility. As knowledge of genetic variation and its impact grows, it may be possible to direct recommendations to individuals, and it may no longer be necessary to assume the existence of an average person who can respond to general recommendations. A more sophisticated form of disease prevention based on biologic variation will then be desirable.

SUMMARY

Genetic variability in biochemical processes is ubiquitous; every person is genetically unique. The relevance of this genetic individuality for nutrition and for the role of certain nutrients in disease causation requires much greater understanding. Processes of absorption, enzyme digestion, biosynthesis, catabolism, transport across cell membranes, uptake by cell receptors, storage, and excretion all vary extensively, and the variation is often known to be genetically determined, at least in part. The importance of such variation for nutrition needs to be determined by further studies in families. Inborn errors of metabolism affecting these processes are genetic diseases that cause nutritional disorders of various kinds. Their rarity makes them medical problems; they are not usually viewed as problems of nutrition that affect public health. Heterozygotes, or carriers, of these inborn errors are much more common in the population. The possible role of the carrier state in

causing clinically manifest disease during periods of stress, infection and malnutrition, for example, requires more study.

Most chronic diseases whose etiology and pathogenesis are influenced by nutritional factors have genetic determinants. High blood pressure, obesity, hyperlipidemia, atherosclerosis, and various cancers appear to aggregate in families for genetic reasons rather than merely because of a common environment. Recommendations to avoid nutrient excesses that predispose to these diseases are therefore unlikely to apply to everyone in the same way, and poorly understood interactions between genetics and the environment often govern the outcome of suboptimal nutrition. For most diseases, we lack the knowledge needed to identify susceptible genotypes by appropriate tests. For other conditions, however, such as the hyperlipidemias, we can already identify persons at high risk and concentrate specific medical efforts on this subpopulation. For conditions where specific tests are lacking but there is a strong family history of a given disease, appropriate preventive approaches can be tried for family members who have not yet been affected.

With advances in knowledge, an increasing number of population subgroups will be found to be at higher, or lower, risk for one or another chronic disease because of their genetic makeup. Specific recommendations directed at high-risk populations therefore will become possible and desirable. In the meantime, dietary recommendations directed at the entire population are appropriate for many conditions, even though different people will benefit unequally from such advice. As an example, a diet low in both fat and salt is likely to reduce disease incidence in the general population even though the beneficial effects for a given person may be small or nil. This paradox explains some of the controversies between those who promote an approach based on attention to persons at high risk and those who support a more global public health approach. Both approaches are needed. The high-risk approach is most appropriate in medical practice. The population approach requires support by the media, the food industry, nutritionists and dietitians, the public health profession, and the medical profession. When using the population approach, however, one must guard against harming certain genetically variant persons.

As we acquire a better understanding of genetics and it becomes increasingly possible to investigate genetic phenomena at a fundamental level, we will be able to conduct better studies to elucidate the exact role of genetic factors for each nutrient and for various diseases. As these roles become understood, the associations between genetic factors and the interactions between heredity and the environment will become clearer and may lead to the modification of current policies.

DIRECTIONS FOR RESEARCH

- Investigate the extent of genetic variability in requirements for a given nutrient and whether there are racial or ethnic differences.
- Determine whether the heterozygous state for certain inborn errors of metabolism is a marker for increased risk for disease.
- Define the interaction between heredity and the environment for nutrients, e.g., whether persons with certain common genotypes react in unusual ways to certain foods.
- Define salt sensitivity in hypertensives and simple methods for its detection.
- Learn how various ions (e.g., those of sodium, potassium, and chlorine) affect blood pressure and the role of genetic variation.
- Study why blacks have a higher frequency of high blood pressure, i.e., the role of genetic–environmental variation.
- Elucidate the role of genetics in dietary responsiveness to lipids.
- Define genes that affect parameters of lipid metabolism (e.g., HDL, LDL) and their interactions among themselves and with various nutrients.
- Conduct family studies to learn about mechanisms of racial differences in osteoporosis.
- Determine the basic genetic defect responsible for hemochromatosis.
- Study genetics of taste and olfaction.
- Delineate specific genes involved in NIDDM.
- Delineate genes involved in alcoholism.
- Define genes involved in human obesity.
- Conduct research on genetic variability and responsiveness to given dietary nutrients.
- Conduct research on the molecular basis of specific disorders responsive to diet. For example, the basis of salt sensitivity in hypertension, hyperlipidemia, osteoporosis, hemochromatosis, NIDDM, alcoholism, and obesity are currently amenable to further study.

REFERENCES

Annest, J.L., C.F. Sing, P. Biron, and J.G. Mongeau. 1983. Family aggregation of blood pressure and weight in adoptive families. III. Analysis of the role of shared genes and shared household environment in explaining family resemblances for height, weight, and selected height/weight indices. Am. J. Epidemiol. 117:492–506.

Ayesh, R., J.R. Idle, J.C. Richie, M.J. Chrothers, and M.R. Hetzel. 1984. Metabolic oxidation phenotypes as markers for susceptibility to lung cancer. Nature 312:169–170.

Barrett, A.H., C. Eff, R.D.G. Leslie, and D.A. Pyke. 1981. Diabetes in identical twins: a study of 200 pairs. Diabetologia 20:87–93.

Begleiter, H., B. Porjesz, and M. Tenner. 1980. Neuroradiological and neurophysiological evidence of brain deficits in chronic alcoholics. Acta Psychiatr. Scand. 286:3–13.

Bodmer, W.F., C.J. Bailey, J. Bodmer, H.J.R. Bussey, A. Ellis, P. Gorman, F.C. Lucibello, V.A. Murday, S.H. Rider, P. Scambler, D. Sheer, E. Solomon, and N.K. Spurr. 1987. Localization of the gene for familial adenomatous polyposis on chromosomes. Nature 328:614–616.

Bohman, M. 1978. Some genetic aspects of alcoholism and criminality. A population of adoptees. Arch. Gen. Psychiatry 35:269–276.

Borjeson, M. 1976. The aetiology of obesity in children. Acta Paediatr. Scand. 65:279–287.

Bothwell, T.H., R.W. Charton, and A.G. Motulsky. 1983. Idiopathic hemochromatosis. Pp. 1269–1298 in J.B. Stanbury, J.B. Wyngaarden, D.S. Fredrickson, J.L. Goldstein, and M.S. Brown, eds. The Metabolic Basis of Inherited Disease, 5th ed. McGraw-Hill, New York.

Botstein, D., R.L. White, M. Skolnick, and R.W. Davis. 1980. Construction of a genetic linkage map in man using restriction fragment length polymorphisms. Am. J. Hum. Genet. 32:314–331.

Bouchard, C. 1988. Inheritance of human fat distribution. Pp. 103–125 in C. Bouchard and F.E. Johnson, eds. Fat Distribution During Growth and Later Health Outcomes. Alan R. Liss, New York.

Bouchard, C., R. Savad, J.-P. Depus, A. Tremblay, and C. Leblanc. 1985. Body composition in adopted and biological siblings. Hum. Biol. 57:61–75.

Bray, G., and D.A. York. 1971. Genetically transmitted obesity in rodents. Physiol. Rev. 51:598–646.

Brook, C.G.D., R.M.C. Huntley, and J. Slack. 1975. Influence of heredity and environment in determination of skinfold thickness in children. Br. Med. J. 2:719–721.

Brunzell, J.D., and A.G. Motulsky. 1984. Status of "familial combined hyperlipidemia." Pp. 541–548 in D.C. Rao, R.C. Elston, L.H. Kuller, M. Feinleib, C. Carter, and R. Havlik, eds. Genetic Epidemiology of Coronary Heart Disease: Past, Present, and Future. Alan R. Liss, New York.

Burke, W., and A.G. Motulsky. 1985. Hypertension—some unanswered questions. J. Am. Med. Assoc. 253:2260–2261.

Cloninger, C.R., K.O. Christiansen, T. Reich, and I.I. Gottesman. 1978. Implication of sex differences in the prevalences of antisocial personality, alcoholism, and criminality for familial transmission. Arch. Gen. Psychiatry 35:941–951.

Cook, J.D., and S.R. Lynch. 1986. Review: the liabilities of iron deficiencies. Blood 68:803–809.

Crabbe, J.C., D.K. Gray, E.R. Young, J.S. Janowsky, and H. Rigter. 1981. Initial sensitivity and tolerance to ethanol in mice: correlations among open field activity, hypothermia, and loss of righting reflex. Behav. Neurol. Biol. 33:188–203.

Deeb, S., A. Failor, B.G. Brown, J.C. Brunzell, J.J. Albers, and A.G. Motulsky. 1986. Molecular genetics of apolipoproteins and coronary heart disease. Pp. 403–409 in Cold

Spring Harbor Symposia on Quantitative Biology, Vol. LI. Molecular Biology of Homo Sapiens. Cold Spring Harbor, New York.

Fabsitz, R., M. Feinleib, and Z. Hrubec. 1980. Weight changes in adult twins. Acta Genet. Med. Gemellol. 29:273–279.

Feinleib, M., R.J. Garrison, R. Fabsitz, J.C. Christian, Z. Hrubec, N.O. Borhani, W.B. Kannel, R. Rosenman, J.T. Schwartz, and J.O. Wagner. 1977. The NHLBI twin study of cardiovascular disease risk factors: methodology and summary of results. Am. J. Epidemiol. 106:284–295.

Gabrielli, W.F., Jr., S.A. Mednic, J. Volavka, V.E. Pollock, F. Schulsinger, and T.M. Itil. 1982. Electroencephalograms in children of alcoholic fathers. Psychophysiology 19:404–407.

Garn, S.M. 1985. Continuities and changes in fatness from infancy through adulthood. Curr. Prob. Pediatr. 15:1–47.

Garn, S.M., and D.C. Clark. 1976. Trends in fatness and the origins of obesity: Ad Hoc Committee to Review the Ten-State Nutrition Survey. Pediatrics 57:443–456.

Glinsmann, W.H., H. Irausquin, and Y.K. Park. 1986. Evaluation of health aspects of sugars contained in carbohydrate sweeteners: report of Sugars Task Force, 1986. J. Nutr. 116:S1–S216.

Goldstein, J.L., and M.S. Brown. 1983. Pp. 672–712 in J.B. Stanbury, J.B. Wyngaarden, D.S. Fredrickson, J.L. Goldstein, and M.S. Brown, eds. The Metabolic Basis of Inherited Disease, 5th ed. McGraw-Hill, New York.

Goldstein, J.L., and M.S. Brown. 1985. The LDL receptor and the regulation of cellular cholesterol metabolism. J. Cell Sci. 3:131–137.

Goodwin, D.M. 1987. Adoption studies of alcoholism. Pp. 3–20 in H.W. Goedde and D.P. Agarwal, eds. Genetics and Alcoholism. Alan R. Liss, New York.

Harris, H. 1975. The Principles of Human Biochemical Genetics, 2nd ed. North-Holland, Amsterdam. 473 pp.

Harris, H., and H. Kalmus. 1941. The measurement of taste sensitivity to phenylthiocarbamide. Ann. Eugen. 15:24–31.

Holtzman, N.A., M.L. Batshaw, and D.L. Valle. 1980. Genetic aspects of human nutrition. Pp. 1193–1219 in R.S. Goodhard and M.E. Shils, eds. Modern Nutrition in Health and Disease, 6th ed. Lea & Febiger, Philadelphia.

Kaij, L. 1960. Alcoholism in Twins: Studies on the Etiology and Sequels of Abuse of Alcohol. Almqvist and Wiksell, Stockholm. 144 pp.

Knudson, A.G. 1985. Hereditary cancer, oncogenes and antioncogenes. Cancer Res. 45:1437–1443.

Lisker, R. 1984. Lactase Deficiency. Pp. 93–104 in A. Velazquez and H. Bourges, eds. Genetic Factors in Nutrition. Academic Press, Orlando, Fla.

Loehlim, J.C. 1972. An analysis of alcohol-related questionnaire items from the National Merit Twin Study. Ann. N.Y. Acad. Sci. 197:117–120.

MacLean, C.J., N.E. Morton, and R. Lew. 1985. Efficiency of lod scores for representing multiple locus linkage data. Genet. Epidemiol. 2:145–154.

Martin, M.J., S.B. Hulley, W.S. Browner, L.H. Kuller, and D. Wentworth. 1986. Serum cholesterol, blood pressure, and mortality: implications for a cohort of 361,662 men. Lancet 2:934–936.

Medlund, P., R. Cederlöf, B. Floderus-Myrhed, L. Friberg, and S. Sörensen. 1977. A new Swedish twin registry containing environmental and medical baseline data from about 14000 same sexed pairs born 1926–1958. Acta Med. Scand. Suppl. (600):1–111.

Mendelson, J.H., and N.K. Mello. 1979. Biologic concomitants of alcoholism. N. Engl. J. Med. 301:912–921.

Motulsky, A.G. 1987a. Genetics and environment. Pp. 327–329 in H.W. Goedde and D.P. Agarwal, eds. Genetics and Alcoholism. Alan R. Liss, New York.

Motulsky, A.G. 1987b. Human genetic variation and nutrition. Am. J. Clin. Nutr. 45:1108–1113.

Mueller, W.H. 1988. Ethnic differences in fat distribution during growth. Pp. 127–145 in C. Bouchard and F.E. Johnson, eds. Fat Distribution During Growth and Later Health Outcomes. Alan R. Liss, New York.

Mulvihill, J.J. 1976. Host factors in human lung tumors: an example of ecogenetics in oncology. J. Natl. Cancer Inst. 57:3–7.

Neel, J.V. 1984. Genetics and nutrition: an evolutionary perspective. Pp. 3–16 in A. Velazquez and H. Bourges, eds. Genetics Factors in Nutrition. Academic Press, Orlando, Fla.

NIAAA (National Institute on Alcohol Abuse and Alcoholism). 1987. The Sixth Special Report to the U.S. Congress on Alcohol and Health from the Secretary of Health and Human Services. DHHS Publ. No. (ADM) 87-1519. National Institutes of Health, Public Health Service, U.S. Department of Health and Human Services. U.S. Government Printing Office, Washington, D.C. 147 pp.

Omenn, G.S. 1987. Heredity and environmental interactions. Pp. 333–341 in H.W. Goedde and D.P. Agarwal, eds. Genetics and Alcoholism. Alan R. Liss, New York.

Orkin, S.H. 1986. Reverse genetics and human disease. Cell 47:845–850.

Page, L.B. 1979. Hypertension and atherosclerosis in primative and acculturating societies. Pp. 1–12 in J.C. Hunt, ed. Hypertension Update: Mechanisms, Epidemiology, Evaluation and Management. Health Learning Systems, Bloomfield, N.J.

Poehlman, E.T., A. Tremblay, J.P. Depres, E. Fontaine, L. Perusse, G. Theriault, and C. Bouchard. 1986. Genotype-controlled changes in body composition and fat morphology following overfeeding in twins. Am. J. Clin. Nutr. 43:723–731.

Price, A., R. Cadoret, A.J. Stunkard, and B.A. Troughton. 1987. Genetic contributions to human fatness: an adoption study. Am. J. Psychiatry 144:1003–1008.

Rosenberg, L.E. 1980. Inborn errors of metabolism. Pp. 73–103 in P.K. Bondy and L.E. Rosenberg, eds. Metabolic Control and Disease, 8th ed. W.B. Saunders, Philadelphia.

Rosenberg, L.E. 1984. Inborn errors of nutrient metabolism: Garrod's lesson and legacies. Pp. 61–77 in A. Velazquez and H. Bourges, eds. Genetic Factors in Nutrition. Academic Press, New York.

Schaeffer, K.M., O.A. Parsons, and J.R. Yohman. 1984. Neuropsychological differences between male familial and nonfamilial alcoholics and nonalcoholics. Alcohol. Clin. Exp. Res. 8:347–351.

Sing, C.F., and J. Davignon. 1985. Role of the apolipoprotein E polymorphism in determining normal plasma lipid and lipoprotein variation. Am. J. Hum. Genet. 37:268–285.

Solomon, E., R. Voss, V. Hall, W.F. Bodmer, J.R. Jass, A.J. Jeffrey, F.C. Lucibello, I. Patel, and S.H. Rider. 1987. Chromosome 5 allele loss in human colorectal carcinomas. Nature 328:616–619.

Stanbury, J.B., J.B. Wyngaarden, D.S. Fredrickson, J.L. Goldstein, and M.S. Brown, eds. 1983. The Metabolic

Basis of Inherited Disease, 5th ed. McGraw-Hill, Trenton, N.J. 1048 pp.

Stunkard, A.J., T.I.A. Sorenson, C. Hanis, T.W. Teasdale, R. Chakraborty, W.J. Schull, and F. Schulsinger. 1986a. An adoption study of human obesity. N. Engl. J. Med. 314:193–198.

Stunkard, A.J., T.T. Foch, and Z. Hrubec. 1986b. A twin study of human obesity. J. Am. Med. Assoc. 256:51–54.

Thurman, R.G. 1980. Ethanol elimination rate is inherited in the rat. Pp. 655–667 in R.G. Thurman, ed. Alcohol and Aldehyde Metabolizing System. IV. Advances in Experimental Medicine and Biology. Plenum Publishing Corp., New York.

Van Itallie, T.B. 1985. Health implications of overweight and obesity in the United States. Ann. Intern. Med. 103:983–988.

Velazquez, A., and H. Bourges, eds. 1984. Genetic Factors in Nutrition. Academic Press, Orlando, Fla. 434 pp.

Vogel, F., and A.G. Motulsky. 1986. Human Genetics: Problems and Approaches, 2nd ed. Springer-Verlag, Berlin. 807 pp.

Winokur, G., J. Reich, J. Rimmer, and F.N. Pitts, Jr. 1970. Alcoholism. III. Diagnosis and familial psychiatric illness in 259 alcoholic probands. Arch. Gen. Psychiatry 23:104–111.

Withers, R.F.J. 1964. Problems in the genetics of human obesity. Eugen. Rev. 56:81–90.

5

Extent and Distribution of Chronic Disease: An Overview

There are subtle, but important, differences between health and the absence of disease and between health promotion and disease prevention. The Constitution of the World Health Organization states in its preamble that "health is a state of complete physical, mental, and social well-being and not merely the absence of disease or infirmity." Definitions of health and of disease prevention promulgated by the Office of Disease Prevention and Health Promotion of the U.S. Department of Health and Human Services (DHHS) stress the differences in terms of personal behavior, level of prevention, and sense of well-being:

Health promotion = personal, environmental, or social interventions that facilitate behavioral adaptations conducive to improved health, level of function, and sense of well-being.

Disease prevention = personal, environmental, or social interventions that impede the occurrence of disease, injury, disability, or death—or the progression of detectable but asymptomatic disease (J. Michael McGinnis, DHHS, personal communication, 1988).

The committee carefully considered these definitions and decided that any attempt to address the association between diet and health in its broadest sense would necessarily be superficial, incomplete, and so diffuse as to be ineffective. Thus, it opted to focus on specific diet-related chronic diseases and conditions related to them.

The definition of diet is straightforward: Diet comprises all food and drink consumed by people. It is characterized by the average and the distribution of nutrients and foods consumed by an individual or by a defined group.

The committee gave special attention to major diet-related chronic diseases and conditions of adulthood, including atherosclerotic cardiovascular diseases (i.e., coronary heart disease, stroke, and peripheral arterial diseases), hypertension and related diseases, obesity and related diseases, cancers, osteoporosis, diabetes mellitus, hepatobiliary disease, and dental caries. It selected these because, according to current evidence, they are the most common diet-associated causes of death and disability among U.S. adults.

This chapter presents the descriptive epidemiologic features of those eight chronic diseases and conditions.

ATHEROSCLEROTIC CARDIOVASCULAR DISEASES

Coronary Heart Disease

Coronary heart disease (CHD) affects the cardiac muscle, mainly as a result of atherosclerotic disease of the coronary arteries and its complications. Atheromas and thrombosis combine to interrupt blood flow to the heart, producing clinical

99

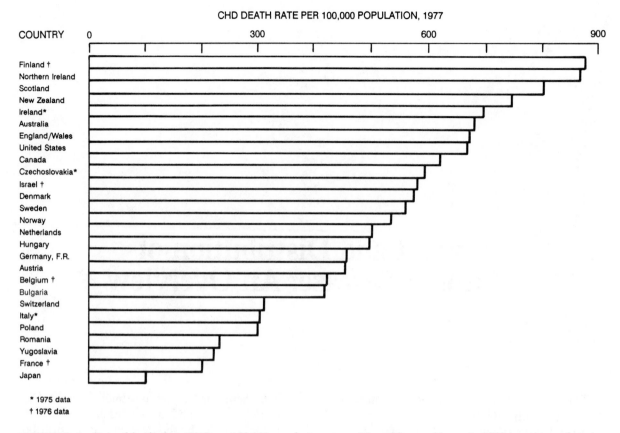

FIGURE 5-1 Rate of deaths from CHD per 100,000 population among 35- to 74-year-old men in 1977 (except as otherwise noted) by country. Adapted from the report of the Inter-Society Commission for Heart Disease Resources (1984).

events that may include sudden death. Morbidity from CHD, measured by population-based surveys and hospital records, includes clinical syndromes of myocardial infarction with damage to and scarring of the myocardium; coronary insufficiency, including angina pectoris and other symptoms of inadequate blood supply; complex arrhythmias, which may lead to sudden coronary death; and chronic heart disease characterized by heart failure or arrhythmias. Mortality from CHD is defined as the number or proportion of death certificates that are coded as International Classification of Disease (ICD) categories 410–411 (myocardial infarction) or 412–414 (angina pectoris and other chronic heart disease manifestations).

Population Differences In Frequency

Among Countries

Figure 5–1 depicts wide differences among countries in the vital statistics on CHD death among 35- to 74-year-old men in the 1970s. The highest reported CHD death rates occurred in Finland and the English-speaking countries, including the

United States; the lowest rates were in Japan (Inter-Society Commission for Heart Disease Resources, 1984).

CHD death rates for women in the same year (not shown) were highest in Northern Ireland, Scotland, and the United States and lowest in Japan (Inter-Society Commission for Heart Disease Resources, 1984). These large geographic differences in CHD death rates were confirmed by studies comparing geographic differences in CHD incidence rates, such as the Seven Countries Study, in which the 10-year incidence rate among men 40 to 59 years old at the beginning of the study was about 200 per thousand in Finland as compared to about 40 per thousand in Japan and the Greek Islands (Keys, 1980).

Geographic differences in trends of reported deaths from CHD have been equally dramatic (see Figure 5–2). The largest decline among men from 35 to 74 years old occurred in the United States, followed closely by Australia and Canada, whereas rates rose strongly in Northern Ireland, Poland, and Bulgaria. Similar changes in death rates were also reported for women (not shown)—the largest

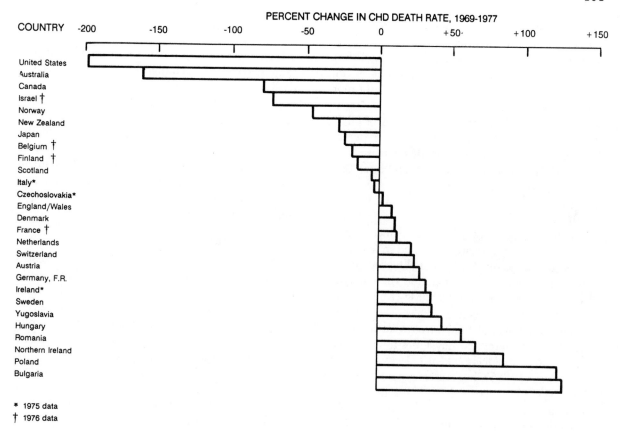

FIGURE 5–2 Percent change in rates of death from CHD from 1969 through 1977 among 35- to 74-year-old men by country. Adapted from the report of the Inter-Society Commission for Heart Disease Resources (1984).

declines again occurring in the United States and Australia, smaller decreases in other countries, and increases in several Eastern European countries (Inter-Society Commission for Heart Disease Resources, 1984).

Within the United States

In the United States, there are substantial regional differences in CHD death rates. In 1980, rates were highest in the East and Southeast (290–305 deaths per 100,000), intermediate (210–249) in the Midwest, and lowest (149–209) in the West and Southwest (DHHS, 1987).

Time Trends in the United States

From the 1950s to the mid-1960s, CHD rates in the United States rose 1 to 2% per year among men and women, whites and nonwhites. Subsequently, death rates declined by 2 to 3% per year. This decline has affected all ages, but has been especially evident in younger groups and was observed a few years earlier in women than in men.

From 1973 through 1979, CHD death rates again increased, but since 1980, they have re-

turned to the 1965–1973 rate of decline. Unadjusted data suggest that the decline has continued through 1986 and early 1987, but with a slowing of rate (DHHS, 1987). This decline was greater in better educated, more affluent groups (DHHS, 1987) and is characterized by fewer out-of-hospital deaths, sudden unexpected deaths, and acute nonfatal myocardial infarction (Anastasiou-Nana et al., 1982; Elveback et al., 1986; Folsom et al., 1987; Gillum et al., 1984; Goldberg et al., 1986; Goldman et al., 1982; Gomez-Marin et al., 1987; Kuller et al., 1986; Pell and Fayerweather, 1985). These findings have been attributed to the increased availability of more sophisticated cardiac care and more effective emergency services (Gillum et al., 1984; Goldman and Cook, 1984). In addition, the decline in CHD deaths was generally accompanied by, and probably preceded by, decreased CHD incidence and by lowered average levels of factors associated with increased CHD risk in the population (e.g., cigarette smoking, hypertension, and high serum cholesterol levels) (Inter-Society Commission for Heart Disease Resources, 1984;

Pell and Fayerweather, 1985). A decline in severity of atherosclerotic lesions at autopsy has also been noted (Solberg and Strong, 1983), although current evidence is insufficient to link this to the concomitant decrease in CHD mortality rates.

Similarly, in long-term cohort studies of CHD, decreases in sudden and out-of-hospital deaths, in-hospital proportion of cases dying (case fatality), and discharge diagnoses of CHD have been reported (Inter-Society Commission for Heart Disease Resources, 1984). The decrease in CHD case fatality rates may reflect improved medical care. With the exception of an increased incidence of nonfatal myocardial infarction noted in a study of women in Rochester, Minnesota (Elveback et al., 1981), there is much evidence that the incidence of first coronary events is declining (Kuller et al., 1986; Pell and Fayerweather, 1985). The evidence for improved survival from myocardial infarction over the short term (30 days) is strong (Folsom et al., 1987; Goldberg et al., 1986; Pell and Fayerweather, 1985), but not consistent (Elveback et al., 1986; Goldman et al., 1982). One study has shown an improvement in 4-year survival after myocardial infarction, but much of that was due to improved survival in hospital (Gomez-Marin et al., 1987).

In the United States, there have been large regional differences in the trends of CHD death rates between 1960 and 1980 (DHHS, 1987). For example, age- and sex-adjusted CHD mortality rates (ages 35 to 74) declined 48 to 53% in Maryland, Delaware, Illinois, and Nevada and 40 to 44% in Connecticut, Washington, and California. Smaller declines have been noted throughout the western, midwestern, southern, and south-central states including Appalachia. The smallest changes were observed in Oklahoma, Mississippi, Tennessee, and Kentucky, where there were declines of only 12 to 21%.

Associations Between Risk Factors in Individuals and CHD

Age

CHD prevalence, incidence, and mortality rates rise steeply with age, approximately doubling in each 5-year age class past age 24. The decline in age-specific CHD death rates between 1968 and 1978 in the United States occurred across all age groups; it was 40 to 50% for those in the 35- to 44-year-old age group and 15 to 20% among those over age 70 (DHHS, 1987).

Sex

CHD death rates in men are three times greater than in women in such high-incidence countries as the United States, the United Kingdom, northern European countries, New Zealand, and Australia (Inter-Society Commission for Heart Disease Resources, 1984). These sex differences are smaller after women pass menopause and in such low-CHD-incidence countries as France and Japan. In countries where CHD deaths have declined, percentage declines have generally been steeper among women than among men.

Ethnic, Racial, and Migrant Differences

Ethnic and racial differences in CHD deaths within countries are closely associated with socioeconomic level. In the United States, CHD death rates are highest for white males, followed in descending order by black males, other nonwhite males, black females, white females, and nonwhite (other than black) females. The greatest rate of decline in CHD deaths between 1968 and 1978—almost 50%—occurred among nonwhite (but not black) women, followed by white women. Black women had the smallest decline (DHHS, 1987).

Differences among migrants were systematically documented in the Ni-Hon-San study conducted among Japanese living in Japan, Honolulu, and San Francisco. In that study, investigators observed that CHD prevalence and incidence rates tripled among Japanese within a generation of their migration to the West Coast of the United States and doubled in Japanese who migrated to Hawaii (Marmot et al., 1975; Robertson et al., 1977). This change was generally paralleled by changes in average levels of risk factors, including saturated fat in the diet and serum cholesterol levels. Similar changes occurred in Boston men who were born in Ireland compared to their brothers who stayed in Ireland (Kushi et al., 1985) and in South Pacific islanders who settled in New Zealand (Beaglehole et al., 1977; Prior and Stanhope, 1980). In all these groups, rates among migrants were near those of the newly adopted culture within 10 to 20 years.

Socioeconomic, Occupational, and Psychosocial Factors

The relationship of socioeconomic class and occupation to CHD risk differs among cultures. For example, a social classification based primarily on occupation was positively associated with CHD mortality in the United Kingdom in the 1950s and 1960s. Since 1960, this picture has changed; the social classification is now inversely related to CHD deaths in England and Wales (Marmot et al., 1978). In the United States, hourly wage earners now have greater CHD mortality and incidence rates than do salaried employees, although there appear to be no specific occupational exposures that exacerbate CHD risk (Pell and Fayerweather, 1985).

Other relationships are found between psychosocial factors and CHD risk. Generally, better educated people are nonsmokers and have healthier patterns of eating, lower serum cholesterol levels, leaner body mass index, and greater physical activity. Numerous studies have indicated slight to moderately strong associations between CHD risk and other psychosocial and behavioral characteristics, but the existence of coronary-prone behavior and personality has been increasingly questioned because few of those studies controlled for social networks, physical activity, diet, and alcohol intake (Inter-Society Commission for Heart Disease Resources, 1984; Jenkins, 1983).

Familial and Genetic Factors

Family history of early-onset CHD is an independent risk indicator in high-risk populations (Inter-Society Commission for Heart Disease Resources, 1984); however, familial hypercholesterolemia accounts for only a small percentage of the people with relatively high serum cholesterol levels in affluent cultures.

It is likely that individual differences in biologic risk factors such as serum lipoprotein levels and in responses to dietary factors (e.g., dietary cholesterol) are determined in large part by genetic factors. However, the absence of specific genetic markers limits the power of family studies to separate the genetic components. New findings concerning cell receptors for lipoproteins hold promise for improving understanding of the differences in individual responses to diet and susceptibility to CHD.

Other Risk Factors

The relationship of specific dietary components to serum lipoprotein levels is discussed throughout this report (e.g., Chapters 6–10, 14, 16, 17, and 19), as are relative risk, attributable risk, and the population risk attributable to elevated blood lipoproteins.

CHD is a classic model of a disease with multiple causes. Evidence indicates that a diet high in saturated fatty acids and cholesterol along with relatively high levels of serum cholesterol are the greatest contributors to elevated *population* risk of atherosclerosis and CHD; population risk differences are largely explained by these related factors. However, within populations with a significant burden of atherosclerosis, several factors interact to determine an individual's risk. The most prominent of these, after age, sex, diet, and blood lipoproteins, are the level of arterial blood pressure and the number of cigarettes smoked. Peripheral arterial disease is one of the strongest independent predictors of CHD, stroke, and all causes of death (Criqui et al., 1985a). Numerous other factors, including lack of habitual physical activity, relative body weight (see section below on Obesity and Related Diseases), and diabetes, contribute to CHD (Inter-Society Commission for Heart Disease Resources, 1984).

Stroke

Stroke is the abrupt onset of neurological disability due to infarction of the area of brain served by an artery that is clogged by atherosclerotic plaque, blocked by an embolus, or ruptured, with destruction of brain tissue by hemorrhage. Transient ischemic attacks (TIAs) are episodes of temporary neurological disability due to insufficient arterial blood supply to the brain. In the United States, most strokes result from cerebral infarction, followed in frequency by the two major forms of cerebral hemorrhage—intracerebral and subarachnoid.

Stroke is a major cause of death among adults worldwide. In industrial countries, it is usually third among causes of death, following heart diseases and cancer.

Population Differences in Frequency

Among Countries

There are large differences in reported mortality rates for stroke. For example, age-adjusted 1970 estimates of prevalence rates for stroke per 100,000 people were 556 in Rochester, Minnesota, and 363 in the United Kingdom (Kurtzke, 1976). Studies in Japan suggest that the distribution of the types of stroke (e.g., infarction and hemorrhage) also varies widely (Omae et al., 1976). In populations, death rates from cerebral infarction generally parallel those from atherosclerosis and CHD, whereas rates of intracerebral hemorrhage usually parallel the frequency of hypertension. For example, stroke is the leading cause of deaths among adults in Japan, where hypertension is prevalent but CHD is uncommon (Komachi, 1977).

In past years, accurate assessment of stroke incidence and mortality has been hampered by frequent misdiagnosis. The descriptive epidemiology of stroke should improve, however, as diagnosis is enhanced by computed tomography (CT), which allows differentiation among the several basic causes of the stroke syndrome.

Within the United States

Strokes of all types were reported as the cause of death for approximately 182,000 persons in the United States in 1977; limitations in death certification do not permit reliable estimates by type of stroke. The American Heart Association (AHA, 1983) estimated the 1981 prevalence of residual damage from strokes at 1.87 million and of coronary disease at 4.6 million. Fatality shortly after the stroke occurs in about 15% of those affected, another 16% require institutional care, and 50% are permanently disabled (Kannel and Wolf, 1983). The average annual incidence of stroke in a 20-year follow-up of 45- to 74-year-old subjects in Framingham, Massachusetts, was 340 per 100,000 among men and 290 among women. Two-thirds of these cases had cerebral infarction (Kannel and Wolf, 1983). Rates were about equal for men and women from age 65 onward, and the rates climbed precipitously with age—1 per thousand at ages 45 to 54, 3.5 at ages 55 to 64, 9.0 at ages 65 to 74, 20.0 at ages 75 to 84, and 40.0 at age 85 and over.

In the United States, approximately 50% of the strokes are attributed to atherosclerosis and thrombosis, 12% to cerebral hemorrhage, 8% to subarachnoid hemorrhage, and 8% to embolism. The remainder are ill-defined (Kurtzke, 1976).

Time Trends in Mortality and Morbidity

Stroke deaths have declined for the past 50 years. In the 1940s and 1950s the rate of decline was 1% per year. Since 1972, the rate of decline has increased to 5% per year (Levy, 1979; Soltero et al., 1978). Between 1968 and 1981, the age-adjusted death rate from stroke fell 46% (Inter-Society Commission for Heart Disease Resources, 1984). The decline has been especially notable among nonwhites, especially nonwhite females. Population-based data on stroke incidence in the United States are rare, but in Rochester, Minnesota, the average annual incidence for all types of stroke declined from 190 per 100,000 during 1945–1949 to 104 during 1970–1974 (Garraway and

Whisnant, 1987; Garraway et al., 1979). The Rochester data also documented that the decline in death rates ascribed to intracerebral hemorrhage began well before better diagnoses became possible through the use of more widely available CT scans and continued to 1979.

There is evidence that fatality among hospitalized stroke patients has not declined much. This indicates that the drop in deaths overall is attributable to out-of-hospital stroke deaths and suggests strongly that incidence must therefore have declined (Gillum et al., 1985).

The underlying causes of the long-term decline in stroke deaths are not well established. It is clear, however, that there has been improved control of the major risk factor—hypertension—as well as effective prevention of stroke in cases experiencing TIA. Nevertheless, computer modelling by Bonita and Beaglehole (1986) suggests that drug treatment of hypertension contributed less to reduced stroke mortality than reduction in levels of population risk factors (e.g., serum cholesterol).

Associations Between Risk Factors in Individuals and Stroke

Age

Stroke deaths and incidence rates are very low until age 45. After that, they rise precipitously, more than doubling for each decade (Kannel and Wolf, 1983).

Sex

Stroke deaths, prevalence, and incidence rates are generally similar for men and women after age 55, in contrast to the much larger and more persistent sex differential for CHD. Cerebral atherosclerosis and stroke begin later in life. In postmenopausal women this is presumed to be due to the loss of protection afforded by their hormonal status (Kannel and Wolf, 1983). The downward trend in stroke deaths, which started earlier and was greater among women, can be explained in part by more effective hypertension control (Garraway and Whisnant, 1987).

Ethnic, Racial, and Migrant Differences

In the United States, stroke deaths and incidence rates are higher among blacks than among whites (Kannel and Wolf, 1983). However, Ni-Hon-San data suggest that environment exerts an even greater influence, since stroke rates were substantially greater among Japanese living in Japan than among Japanese migrants living in Hawaii and California (Kagan et al., 1976, 1980). Because there is little difference in the prevalence of hypertension in migrant Japanese populations, the difference in stroke rates was an early clue to the possibility that habitual diet and serum cholesterol levels play a role in hemorrhagic stroke (Kagan et al., 1976; Komachi, 1977; Takeya et al., 1984; Ueshima et al., 1980). Other studies confirm the role of acculturation in the rise and fall of stroke risk (Bonita and Beaglehole, 1982).

Socioeconomic, Occupational, and Psychosocial Factors

There are few systematic data on the relationship of socioeconomic, occupational, or psychosocial characteristics to stroke death or incidence.

Familial and Genetic Factors

Close relatives of a stroke patient are at slightly greater risk of stroke than genetically unrelated persons (Heyden et al., 1969). Results of a study conducted in Göteborg, Sweden (Welin et al., 1987), suggest that maternal history is more important than paternal history in determining risk.

Other Risk Factors

Hypertension has been consistently, strongly, continuously, and independently related to risk of stroke in individuals within populations at high risk for stroke (Dyken, 1984; Kannel and Wolf, 1983; Welin et al., 1987). Because of the great prevalence of hypertension in the United States, the population risk of stroke attributable to hypertension, as well as the risk for stroke for individuals, is high. The risk associated with elevated blood pressure increases continuously with increases in diastolic and systolic levels. It increases with increases in systolic blood pressure levels even when the diastolic level remains constant. In the Framingham 24-year follow-up study, for example, the 2-year incidence of stroke among men and women ages 50 to 79 was progressively greater as systolic blood pressure levels increased from below 140 to above 160 mm Hg, regardless of level of diastolic pressure. This finding suggests that an elevated systolic blood pressure even in the presence of normal diastolic blood pressure (i.e., isolated systolic hypertension) constitutes a risk for stroke (Kannel and Wolf, 1983).

Age-adjusted annual incidence of cerebral infarction was more than twice as great in people with *diabetes* as in those without the disease (Kannel and Wolf, 1983). This differential applied to both sexes and was independent of the associated risk factors:

blood pressure, serum cholesterol, cigarette smoking, and electrocardiographic findings.

Cigarette smoking was positively and independently associated with cerebral infarction in men below age 65 in the Honolulu and Framingham studies (Abbott et al., 1986; Kannel and Wolf, 1983), but only a weak relationship was found in the Chicago Stroke Study (Ostfeld et al., 1974).

In the Framingham Study, stroke incidence was negatively related to relative *body weight* in men over age 65, but positively related under age 65 (Kannel and Wolf, 1983). Excessive abdominal fat was positively related in Göteborg men (Welin et al., 1987).

Several surveys link self-reported *alcohol* intake to risk of stroke, including cerebral hemorrhage and cerebral infarction. Age-adjusted incidence rose steadily from the level of nondrinkers to those drinking more than 30 ounces of alcohol per month in populations followed in Japan (Omae et al., 1976), Honolulu (Kagan et al., 1980), Alabama (Peacock et al., 1972), Framingham (Marshall, 1971), and Chicago (Gill et al., 1986).

The presence of CHD, *peripheral arterial disease* (PAD), or *hypertensive heart disease* is strongly associated with stroke risk (Ostfeld et al., 1974).

Peripheral Arterial Disease (PAD)

The term PAD is used here to refer to a specific entity of peripheral vascular disease (PVD) and includes clinical syndromes of arterial insufficiency in the lower extremities. These syndromes are characterized by pain, inflammation, and ischemic damage to soft tissues from occlusion of the arteries. The characteristic syndrome of PAD is intermittent claudication—i.e., cramping, aching, and numbness of the extremities—which is induced by exercise but resolves promptly when exercise ceases. Arterial aneurysms, an advanced form of PAD, lead to swelling, tissue separation, or rupture of major arteries in the abdomen or pelvis. Arteriosclerosis obliterans is the most common clinical form, constituting the majority of cases of public health concern. Its basic pathology is obliteration of the arterial lumen due to the formation of atherosclerotic plaques with or without thrombosis.

PAD is diagnosed by a combination of clinical history (e.g., history of pain in the extremities upon exertion) and changes in the color, temperature, and appearance of the skin; arterial pulsations or abnormalities of blood flow; and blood pressure or pulse transmission or reappearance time. Angiography is the reference method for assessing type and severity of the arterial disease, but ultrasound promises to provide effective, non-invasive diagnoses.

There are few systematic data for comparing frequency of PAD among or within populations, and few studies of risk characteristics have been conducted within populations. In addition, mortality data for PAD are unreliable because of the variety of syndromes involved, their low relative frequency as a direct cause of death, and uncertainties pertaining to cause of death, which is usually ascribed to associated cardiac, brain, or kidney disease. Furthermore, there is no reliable information on trends in prevalence, incidence, or deaths from PAD. An exception is one population-based study, predominantly of whites with an average age of 66, which provided evidence that large-vessel PAD was present in 11.7% of the subjects (Criqui et al., 1985b).

Peripheral venous disease is not considered here because of its remote relationship to diet and nutrition.

Associations Between Risk Factors in Individuals and PAD

Age

PAD is characteristically, but not exclusively, a disease of older age. In a California study, there was a dramatic increase in PAD prevalence by age (Criqui et al., 1985b). Framingham data also showed a steady rise in the average annual incidence of intermittent claudication by age, mainly from age 55 onward (Kannel and McGee, 1985). Clinical onset may be delayed to older ages by the large caliber of the arteries involved and, thus, the extreme degree of obstructive atherothrombotic disease that is required before blood flow is sufficiently impaired to produce symptoms.

Sex

There are few systematic data on the distribution of PAD by sex. An older Mayo Clinic series conducted in the 1940s indicated that the prevalence of PAD was six times higher in males than in females (Allen et al., 1946). In California, the prevalence of intermittent claudication was greater in men (2.2%) than in women (1.7%) (Criqui et al., 1985b). In Framingham, the incidence of intermittent claudication in men was approximately twice that in women up to age 65 (11.6 vs 5.3%); at older ages, the incidence was similar (Kannel and McGee, 1985).

Ethnic, Racial, and Migrant Differences

There are no systematic population data on ethnic, racial, and migrant differences in PAD, but a clinical series in the United States suggest no large ethnic or racial differences (Juergens et al., 1959).

Socioeconomic, Occupational, and Psychosocial Factors

Systematic data are not available.

Familial and Genetic Factors

There is apparently no strong familial or genetic role in PAD. However, diabetes mellitus, which is associated with PAD as described below, does aggregate in families and could thus lead to a similar familial association for PAD.

Other Risk Factors

Clinical observations suggest a strong concentration of PAD risk among people with *diabetes* (Schadt et al., 1961). This was confirmed by the greater annual incidence of intermittent claudication in diabetic men and women in the Framingham Study. The attributable fraction—i.e., the excess cases of intermittent claudication due to diabetes (at ages 45 to 74)—affects more men (13.6%) than women (2.7%) (Kannel and McGee, 1985).

Elevation of blood sugar, urinary sugar, or clinical diabetes increases the risk for intermittent claudication about four- or fivefold. In a population-based cohort of diabetics in Rochester, Minnesota, the cumulative incidence of PAD was 15% at 10 years and 45% at 20 years after diagnosis of diabetes (Melton et al., 1980). Diabetes and glucose intolerance are consistently associated with PAD in these and other studies (Bothig et al., 1976; Keen et al., 1965; Reunanen et al., 1982).

The incidence of intermittent claudication increases steadily and steeply at all ages with the number of *cigarettes smoked* (Kannel and McGee, 1985). Even beyond age 65, women smokers in Framingham were at greater risk. Some clinical series some years ago indicated that 90% of all PAD cases were cigarette smokers (Juergens et al., 1960). The strong relationship of PAD to smoking was confirmed by autopsy studies in which the incidence of aortic atheromatous plaque in white males was much greater in smokers than in nonsmokers (Strong and Richards, 1976).

The relationship between systolic *blood pressure* and annual incidence of intermittent claudication in the Framingham 14-year followup was positive in both sexes. Ratios between hypertensives and normotensives were 2 or 3 to 1 (Kannel and Sorlie, 1979).

In the Framingham study, there was an inverse relationship between *physical activity* and intermittent claudication, but it was not statistically significant (Kannel and Sorlie, 1979). In Framingham, there was also a strong curvilinear relationship between the incidence of intermittent claudication and a coronary risk index of CHD risk characteristics including age, blood cholesterol level, electrocardiographic (ECG) findings, systolic blood pressure, relative weight, hemoglobin, and cigarette use (Kannel and McGee, 1985). The strongest relationships were observed for cigarette smoking and hypertension for both sexes and for impaired glucose tolerance, which was stronger for women than for men. Serum total cholesterol and relative weight were only weakly significant risk factors. Clustering of intermittent claudication with other atherosclerotic and cardiovascular diseases was also pronounced in the Framingham Study. Overt coronary disease, cerebrovascular disease, or congestive heart failure was found in one out of three cases of intermittent claudication at the time it was initially diagnosed, suggesting common risk characteristics. The relative risk of developing intermittent claudication in Framingham patients with CHD was four times the standard risk in the cohort, whereas people with angina pectoris had three times greater risk (Kannel and Shurtleff, 1971).

In the most recent systematic study of *multiple risk factors* for PAD, Criqui used objective diagnostic criteria for large- and small-vessel diseases (Michael Criqui, University of California, San Diego, personal communication, 1988). For large-vessel disease, they showed that age, smoking, fasting plasma glucose, and systolic blood pressure were strongly associated with the prevalence of PAD and that obesity, LDL, and HDL were marginally related. Small-vessel PAD was only weakly related to atherosclerotic cardiovascular disease risk factors.

In general, the risk factors for PAD are similar to those for CHD and stroke, although their relative importance differs. For example, diabetes and smoking are the preeminent risk factors for PAD but not for CHD, followed by triglycerides, VLDL, and blood glucose tolerance, and to a lesser extent LDL, HDL, and serum total cholesterol, which strongly predict CHD.

HYPERTENSION AND HYPERTENSION-RELATED DISEASES

Hypertension is defined as elevated arterial blood pressure measured indirectly by an inflatable cuff and pressure manometer. Blood pressure is a continuous or graded phenomenon, and the risk of hypertension increases steadily with blood pressure level—either systolic (SBP) or diastolic (DBP). Therefore, any definition of elevated blood pressure is arbitrary and is done primarily to facilitate decisions regarding pharmacological therapy.

Traditionally, physicians diagnose hypertension using DBP, which is the lower value found during the resting phase of the cardiac cycle. DBP levels have been closely associated in clinical studies with manifest diseases or complications associated with high blood pressure (e.g., stroke, hypertensive heart disease, CHD, and kidney disease) and are used as the basis of most treatment decisions. Systematic population studies indicate, however, that systolic blood pressure, the higher value recorded during cardiac systole, is not only a more reliable measurement but also a more precise indicator of the risk of future complications in hypertension.

For practical treatment purposes and for population comparisons, the following criteria developed by the World Health Organization (WHO, 1978) are often used: *normotension*, systolic ≤140 and diastolic ≤90 mm Hg; *borderline hypertension*, systolic 141–159 and diastolic 91–94 mm Hg; and *hypertension*, systolic ≥160 and diastolic ≥95 mm Hg. Severe hypertension is often defined as diastolic levels of 115 mm Hg and above. The Joint National Committee on Detection, Evaluation, and Treatment of High Blood Pressure (JNC, 1988) added classifications for high normal, mild, moderate, severe, and isolated systolic hypertension (see Table 20–1, Chapter 20).

Deaths related to hypertension have been variously classified over recent years. They have either been considered as a separate entity or combined with such classes of atherosclerotic cardiovascular diseases as CHD and stroke. Thus, it is not useful to consider vital statistics alone in discussing the epidemiology of hypertension. Hypertension is treated here primarily as a risk characteristic for atherosclerotic cardiovascular diseases rather than as a disease entity in itself.

Population Differences in Blood Pressure and Hypertension

Among Countries

Surveys comparable to those of the U.S. National Center for Health Statistics (DHEW, 1963) have not been conducted outside the United States. However, many smaller-scale surveys attest to the fact that hypertension is prevalent in industrialized nations throughout the world. The prevalence in England (Hamilton et al., 1954), Western Europe (Keys, 1980), and Australia (MacMahon and Leeder, 1984) is similar to that in the United States. Data from China (Wu et al., 1982), Japan (Komachi and Shimamoto, 1980), and Korea (Kesteloot et al., 1976) show prevalence rates in urban populations equal to or greater than those in United States.

A low prevalence of hypertension has often been found in studies of traditional rural populations outside Western culture. More than 20 societies, representing a variety of races, diets, habitats, and modes of life, have been found to have virtually no hypertension and little or no tendency for blood pressure to rise with age. Social and anthropological characteristics of these populations are similar: they are relatively isolated, subsistence cultures; their salt intake is less than 4.5 g daily; there is an absence of obesity; and they remain physically active throughout life (Page, 1979). For more detailed data on the geographic distribution of blood pressure, see Epstein and Eckoff (1967).

Within Countries

There have been reports of regional differences in the frequency of hypertension and in mean blood pressure values. People in the southeastern United States tend to have higher pressures (DHHS, 1986) as do people in the northern provinces of Japan (Komachi, 1977; Omae et al., 1976) and in the French-speaking areas of Belgium (Kesteloot et al., 1980). Regional differences are not well explained, but they appear to be independent of race and socioeconomic status.

Time Trends in Frequency and Mortality

In the United States, average trends in blood pressure for people between the ages of 25 and 74 have been examined in surveys conducted by the National Center for Health Statistics—the Nationwide Health Examination Survey (NHES I) of 1960–1962 (DHEW, 1963) and the Nationwide Health and Nutrition Examination Surveys of 1971–1975 (NHANES I) (Abraham et al., 1983) and 1976–1980 (NHANES II) (Carroll et al., 1983). Assuming comparability of methods and design (DHEW, 1963; DHHS, 1986), one can see no significant trend in the population means or the distribution of average blood pressures for given ages between the first two surveys. However, the third survey, NHANES II, shows markedly lower average systolic blood pressures at all ages above 30. A much lower prevalence of hypertension is also apparent in people over 40 in that survey compared to those in the earlier two. When NHANES II data (DHHS, 1986) are used, the prevalence of definite hypertension is 17.7% in adults as defined by the World Health Organization (WHO, 1978) or 29.7% as defined by the criteria of the third Joint National Committee on Detection, Evaluation, and Treatment of High Blood Pressure (JNC, 1988).

Concurrent with the decline in hypertension prevalence and in mean blood pressure indicated in these U.S. national surveys, there has been an improvement in the status of medical detection and control of high blood pressure. Previously undetected hypertension (i.e., cases newly diagnosed at screening) was halved—from 51.1% during 1960–1962 to 26.6% during 1976–1980. The proportion of hypertension controlled by medication doubled—from 16% during 1960–1962 to 34.1% during 1976–1980.

Data are insufficient to attribute these changes with certainty to medical detection and control or to primary prevention in the general population. Both have occurred as modelled by Bonita and Beaglehole (1986), but there is as yet no direct evidence of a decrease in mean population blood pressure independent of medical treatment. There is also evidence that trends in high blood pressure are not an indirect result of changes in average relative weight or alcohol intake—both of which have risen in recent years in the United States while mean blood pressure has fallen.

The increased risk of morbidity and mortality from cardiovascular diseases associated with hypertension has been repeatedly demonstrated in epidemiologic studies throughout the industrialized world (Stamler et al., 1975). The risk of hypertension varies markedly with age, sex, race, and the total burden imposed by associated risk factors, including socioeconomic status, occupation, obesity, family history, psychosocial stresses, and other factors (as discussed below). The American Heart Association (AHA, 1973) has published multiple risk calculations for different age and sex groups based on major risk factors using Framingham study data. In general, the risk for major coronary disease events increases by 30% for each 10 mm Hg increase in systolic blood pressure in both men and women of all ages (Dawber and Kannel, 1972). Interaction of hypertension with other risk factors may alter their risk as much as sixfold.

A striking feature of the epidemiology of hypertension is the remarkable decrease in hypertension-related deaths, i.e., from all cardiovascular disease, cerebrovascular disease, renal disease, hypertensive heart disease, and CHD (DHHS, 1987). This trend is so consistent and strong that it must represent a real change, independent of improved classification in death certification. The beginning of the decline in hypertension-related mortality clearly antedated the widespread use of effective antihypertensive drugs, but it accelerated in the early 1970s when such products came into wide use. Population-based surveys in the U.S. Southwest (Franco et al., 1985) and in Minnesota (Folsom et al., 1983) indicate that 85 to 90% of high blood pressure cases are now detected and under therapeutic control in urban areas.

Estimating the proportion of cases of hypertension in the population attributed to a known risk factor (the population-attributable fraction) indicates the potential impact that effective reduction in the risk factor could have in reducing hyperten-

sion-associated mortality in the population. Calculation of the attributable fraction for all known risk related to hypertension suggests that effective control of hypertension in the population could result in a 20% reduction in all-cause mortality among whites along with a 30% reduction among black men and a 45% reduction among black women based on mortality rates among nonhypertensives. The estimated decline in death rates is similar to the observed decline in the age-adjusted U.S. mortality from 1968 to 1975. It is therefore likely that part of the decline in cardiovascular deaths as well as in all-cause deaths since 1972 is attributable to the improved medical control of hypertension. However, the actual contribution of control may be less than this estimation (Bonita and Beaglehole, 1986).

Associations Between Risk Factors in Individuals and Hypertension

Age

As shown in Figure 5–3, systolic blood pressure rises steeply from infancy to adulthood (Voors et al., 1978) and levels off once adult height is reached. The age-related upward trend in mean systolic pressure occurs across most adult populations. Cross-sectional and cohort data from the Framingham Study (Kannel, 1980) give a somewhat different picture of the relationship of systolic and diastolic blood pressure to age in adults (Figure

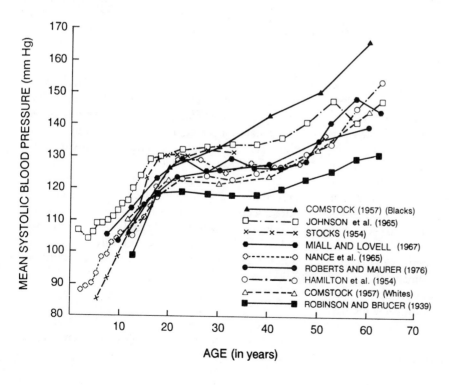

FIGURE 5–3 Changes in mean systolic blood pressures from infancy to age 70 in nine studies—Comstock, 1957; Hamilton et al., 1954; Johnson et al., 1965; Miall and Lovell, 1967; Nance et al., 1965; Roberts and Maurer, 1976; Robinson and Brucer, 1939; Stocks, 1954. From Voors et al. (1978).

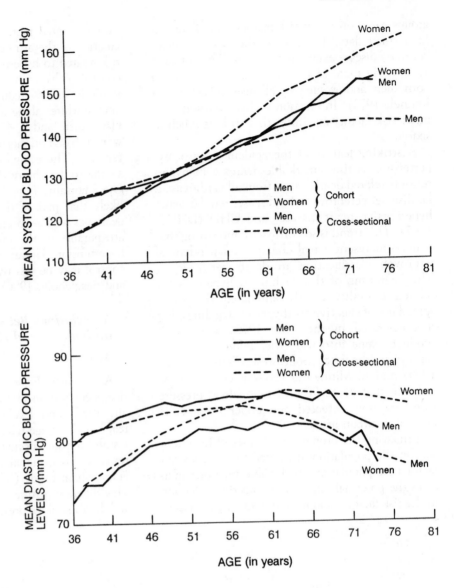

FIGURE 5–4 Cohort and cross-sectional age trends in systolic and diastolic blood pressures by sex. From Kannel (1980).

5–4). The cross-sectional data show systolic pressure starting lower in women than in men but rising more steeply, crossing over in the fifth decade, and continuing upward with age into the 80s, whereas pressures in men level off after age 70. Cohort data show systolic pressure starting lower in women, but rising to meet that of men by age 60, after which systolic pressure rises in men and women at the same rate. With respect to diastolic blood pressure, the cross-sectional data show a higher level in men than in women in their early decades and the reverse during the middle 50s when levels decrease in men and further increase in women. The cohort data show that diastolic pressures are consistently lower in women than in men of all ages, increase in both sexes in the early decades, flatten in the 50s, and decline after age 65.

On average, longitudinal studies show that sys-tolic pressure increases about 20 mm Hg between ages 20 and 60 and an additional 20 mm between ages 60 and 80. Diastolic blood pressure, on the other hand, rises approximately 10 mm between the ages of 20 and 60 and gradually declines thereafter (Kannel, 1980).

The dramatic age trends in blood pressure observed in the Framingham data are characteristic of those seen in most Western societies. A notable feature of this age-related rise is the phenomenon called tracking, i.e., where elevated blood pressures tend to persist from youth to adulthood (Berenson et al., 1980).

Sex

A consistent finding among industrialized societies is a higher mean blood pressure and higher prevalence of hypertension among males from

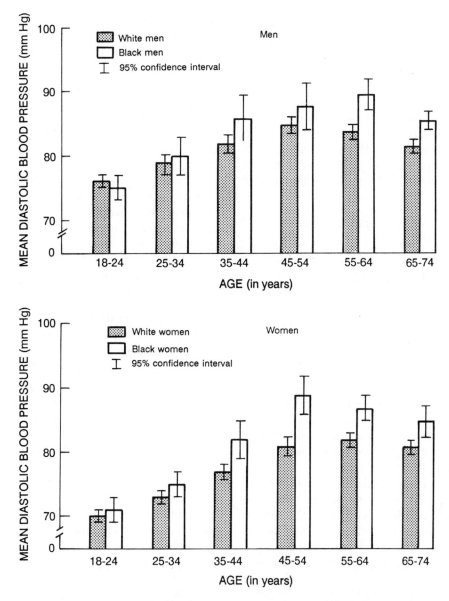

FIGURE 5–5   Mean diastolic blood pressure in U.S. whites and blacks by age and sex from data collected from 1976 to 1980. From DHHS (1986).

adolescence through age 45. After age 45, mean blood pressure values are higher in women (DHHS, 1986).

Ethnic, Racial, and Migrant Differences

An excess of hypertension and its complications has been found in black adults in the U.S. population (DHHS, 1986) and in most other societies that have been systematically studied. Among U.S. blacks there is a stronger upward age trend than among whites and a higher prevalence of hypertension at all ages (Figure 5–5). The point at which the average blood pressure of women crosses that of men (the cut point) is about 5 years earlier

for blacks than for whites. In the Hypertension Detection and Follow-Up Program (HDFP, 1979) and in the Evans County Study (Heyman et al., 1971), blacks also had a higher prevalence of hypertension-related complications (such as cerebrovascular, cardiovascular, and renal events) than whites at all blood pressure levels (HDFP, 1979). Data on young people are inconsistent, but in Bogalusa, Louisiana, where automated instruments were used to reduce observer bias, higher blood pressure levels were demonstrated in blacks as early as age 5 (Berenson, 1980).

Migrant studies emphasize the effects of cultural and environmental factors on the expression of hypertension in individuals, and hence on population differences. Average blood pressure and the frequency of hypertension and its complications rise rapidly when people move from rural to urban settings. The effects of migration are evident as early as 1 month after changing location, and the proportionate increase in blood pressure is greater among older adults. These findings suggest that trends in blood pressure with age as well as mean levels of blood pressure are very sensitive to diet and other environmental influences (see Chapter 20).

Socioeconomic, Occupational, and Psychosocial Factors

The prevalence of hypertension varies inversely with educational attainment and with occupational, social, and economic status for blacks as well as whites. However, the higher blood pressure levels in blacks persist after control for socioeconomic variables (HDFP, 1979).

In the few occupational studies conducted, data on blood pressure differences are confounded by relative weight and alcohol intake, among other factors, and no specific occupations are known to be associated with excess hypertension. Physical activity associated with occupation is not consistently related to average blood pressure level (Leon and Blackburn, 1982).

Migrant population studies confirm that blood pressure is affected by the transition from traditional to urban societies (see Chapter 20), but it is difficult to separate the effects of psychosocial change from the changed physiological exposures that accompany migration. Life events, social behaviors, cultural dissonance, and related factors have been associated with blood pressure differences, but these studies have rarely controlled for physiological or nutritional confounders.

Familial and Genetic Factors

Within cultures where average blood pressure is elevated and the prevalence of hypertension is substantial, studies of families show a genetic effect relatively stronger than environmental variables, including relative body weight and sodium intake. First-degree genetic relatives have similar systolic and diastolic pressures. Relatives in the same household may share environmental factors as well as genes that may influence blood pressure; however, the similarity of blood pressure among genetic relatives is greater than among nongenetic relatives, greater for monozygotic than dizygotic twins, greater for first-degree genetic relatives, and

greater among natural than among adopted children (Folkow, 1982). All these point to an influence of genetic factors on blood pressure. But these are weak predictors, and genetic susceptibility of individuals is not now measurable.

Blood pressure is a result of interaction between environmental and host factors. Phenotypic expression is modified by changing the environment, but this does not negate the overall importance of genes in etiology. The large variation in the frequency of hypertension among populations, the rapid changes in blood pressure levels and frequency of hypertension in migrant populations, and the ability to modify blood pressure levels experimentally without drugs all suggest that susceptibility is widespread and that the environment is the prominent factor in the expression of hypertension (Prineas and Blackburn, 1985).

Associations of Blood Pressure with Relative Body Weight and Obesity

The evidence associating dietary factors with hypertension is summarized in Chapter 20. Obesity has also been associated with hypertension, but in one study when body build was taken into consideration, total fatness was no longer related to blood pressure (Weinsier et al., 1985). Thus, hypertension may be affected by body build as well as by fatness. Weight reduction has also been associated with a decrease in blood pressure, independent of a decrease in sodium intake (Reisin et al., 1978). Evans County data show that overweight and a weight gain of 10 pounds or more are associated with the occurrence of new hypertension (≥ 95 mm Hg), and that blood pressure rises stepwise according to the level of overweight or weight gain (Tyroler et al., 1975). Those overweight at the outset of the study, and those who gained 10 pounds or more, were 8 to 10 times more likely to develop new hypertension than those who were neither overweight nor had gained weight. The absolute effect was somewhat greater among blacks, but the gradient of relative risk was somewhat steeper among whites.

Associations of Blood Pressure and Hypertension with Atherosclerotic Cardiovascular Diseases and Death

Blood pressure is a strong and independent risk predictor for CHD—a relationship that was thoroughly reviewed in the report of Inter-Society Commission for Heart Disease Resources (1984). CHD patients have higher average blood pressure than controls. Atherosclerosis in laboratory ani-

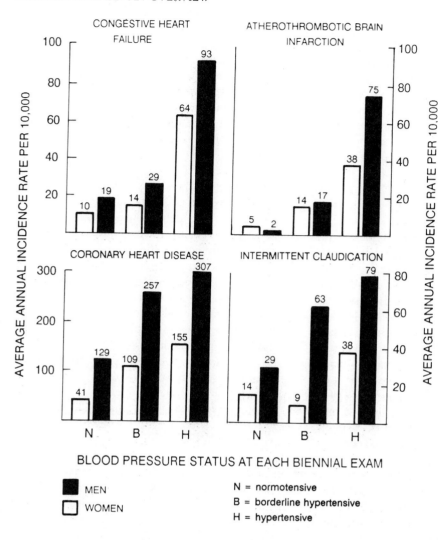

FIGURE 5–6 Average annual incidence of cardiovascular disease according to blood pressure status at each biennial examination for men and women between the ages of 55 and 64, as observed during the 16-year follow-up of a population in Framingham, Massachusetts. From Kannel (1974).

mals is directly related to pressure within the arterial system. Short-term and long-term follow-up studies indicate that both systolic and diastolic blood pressure predict CHD risk; this observation was strongest for systolic blood pressure, but it is not clear whether this resulted from more precise measurement or whether systolic pressure is closer in the chain of causation leading to atherosclerosis and CHD. The relationship between elevated blood pressure and risk of cerebral vascular accidents (CVA) and congestive heart failure (CHF) is even stronger than that between blood pressure and CHD. These relationships are consistent and widely confirmed (Inter-Society Commission for Heart Disease Resources, 1984).

Despite the strong individual correlations between blood pressure level and CHD risk within populations, the frequency of hypertension does not account for much of the variation of CHD incidence between populations. Nevertheless, estimates of the number of population events attribut-

able to blood pressure suggest that changes in CHD incidence rates related to relatively small average blood pressure differences (reductions) hold a great potential for the prevention of CHD (Rose, 1981).

For men and for women, there is a strong and consistent relationship between systolic and diastolic blood pressure levels and death from all causes, including CHD and stroke, and the incidence of first coronary events.

More relevant to the public health importance of hypertension are the Framingham data on 55- to 64-year-old men and women (see Figure 5–6). These data show a doubling of risk for coronary and peripheral vascular disease, a quintupling of risk for heart failure, and a 10- to 20-fold higher risk of cerebral infarction in hypertensives (Kannel, 1974). The proportion of increased risk attributable to elevated blood pressure ranges from 57% (coronary events) to 89% (brain infarction). Thus, hypertension has a large impact on two leading causes of death—CHD and brain infarction.

OBESITY AND RELATED DISEASES

Obesity is defined as excessively high body fat in relation to lean body mass. *Overweight* refers to a deviation in body weight above some standard of acceptable weight, which is usually defined in relation to height. Because obesity and overweight are both continuous variables, any cut point is arbitrary. A rational basis for a cut point is the relative weight causally associated with the lowest mortality (see Chapter 21).

Techniques for measuring body fat are needed to distinguish between obesity and overweight resulting from increases in lean body mass. For most people, overweight is associated with increases in body fat stores. Professional athletes and body builders may be overweight despite low body fat stores. Overweight can be expressed in several ways, as shown below, and the varied use of these measurements confounds interpretation among studies. Relative weight refers to the ratio or percentage of actual weight to some standard or desirable weight. The most widely used standards are the Metropolitan Life Insurance Tables; actual weights-for-height compared to them are called Metropolitan Relative Weights. Weight and height can also be related by ratios such as weight divided by height, height divided by the cube root of weight (ponderal index), or weight divided by height to some power. When this power is 2, the ratio (weight/height^2) is called the body mass index (BMI) or Quetelet Index (QI). Degrees of excess weight can also be defined in terms of the Broca Index, in which desirable weight in kilograms equals height in centimeters minus 100. Weights 20% higher than the Broca desirable weight are considered excessive in most European studies. Relative weight and the BMI are used most frequently in the United States and are becoming widely used internationally.

Obesity is measured by a number of techniques. Skinfold measurements are widely used in epidemiologic studies; however, comparisons of skinfold measurements to BMI by the National Center for Health Statistics (Abraham et al., 1983) indicated that a substantial proportion of people in the top 15% of BMI are not included in the top 15% of skinfolds, and vice versa. When only the top 5% for each measurement were compared, however, there was almost complete congruence, indicating that overweight (BMI) and obesity (skinfolds) are synonymous at this level. Thus, definitions of obesity can be based on either skinfold measurements or body weight in relation to height (BMI) as follows: (1) a BMI above 30 kg/m^2, (2) a triceps plus subscapular skinfold above 45 mm in males and 65 mm in females, or (3) body fat more than 25% of body weight in males or 30% in females. Overweight, on the other hand, has been defined as follows: (1) a BMI between 25 and 30 kg/m^2, (2) body weight 20 to 40% above the median weight for normal frame size according to the Metropolitan Life Insurance Tables, or (3) weight 20% above the calculated Broca Index.

In addition to definitions of total body fat, considerable evidence suggests that regional fat distribution influences the risk of mortality from atherosclerotic cardiovascular diseases and diabetes mellitus. The most widely used techniques for assessing regional fat distribution involve determining the ratio of abdominal (waist) circumference to gluteal region (hip) circumference, measuring subscapular skinfolds, or determining the ratio of skinfolds on the trunk to those on the extremities (see Chapter 21).

Population Differences in Frequency

Between Countries

In a survey of selected European countries, Kluthe and Schubert (1985) showed that the prevalence of obesity among females ranged from 2 to more than 50%, and among males, from 2 to more than 40%. These differences were partly related to the different measurements used.

Bray (1985) compared the percent of overweight (BMI between 25 and 30) and obese (BMI over 30) people in Australia, the United States, Canada, Great Britain, and the Netherlands (Table 5–1). The overall percentage of males and females with a BMI between 25 and 30 is similar in the five countries. The percentages for those with a BMI above 30 kg/m^2 is similar in Australia and Britain, but nearly twice as great in the United States and Canada.

Within the United States

On the basis of the evidence described above, approximately 34 million adults in the United States were overweight between 1976 and 1980. Of these, about 12.4 million were severely overweight (Abraham et al., 1983).

In Migrants

Japanese migrants living in Hawaii or California have a higher relative body weight compared to

TABLE 5-1 Percentage of People with a Given Body Mass Index in Several Affluent Countries[a]

Country	Age	Overweight (BMI 25–30 kg/m^2)		Obese (BMI >30 kg/m^2)	
		M	F	M	F
United States	20–74	31	24	12	12
Canada	20–69	40	28	9	12
Great Britain	16–65	34	24	6	8
Netherlands	20+	34	24	4	6
Australia	25–64	34	24	7	7

[a]Adapted from Bray (1985). Data Sources: Abraham et al. (1983); Black et al. (1983); Millar and Stephens (1987); National Heart Foundation of Australia (1981); Seidell et al. (1986).

native Japanese living in Japan. Similarly, Irish immigrants living in Boston tend to be heavier than brothers of the same height and age remaining in Ireland (Brown et al., 1970).

Time Trends in Frequency

Several studies suggest that there has been a progressive increase in relative weight throughout the past hundred years in industrial societies (Abraham et al., 1983; Bray, 1979). For example, the weight of men 5 feet, 8 inches tall inducted into U.S. military service rose from 147 pounds in 1863 to 168 pounds in 1962. Life insurance data and NCHS data also show a small age-related increase in average relative body weight. Increases in the percentage of overweight men and women are greatest in the younger age groups. A comparison of the three sets of NHANES data (1960–1962, 1971–1974, 1976–1980) (Harper, 1987) based on the same criteria for overweight in men is shown in Figure 5–7. Overall, there was no change over the three surveys. In the 25- to 54-year age groups, however, there was an increase in the percentage of overweight men and women. Be-

yond age 54, the percentage of overweight men and women decreased.

Associations Between Risk Factors in Individuals and Obesity

Age

Relative body weight increases with age in both men and women, but there is a greater proportional increase among women (Figure 5–8). The percentage of overweight among black women is higher than among white women at all ages. The percentage of overweight among white men is higher than among black men until age 35 when the proportion of overweight black men begins to exceed that of white men. After age 55, the percentage of overweight among white and black men is similar (Abraham et al., 1983).

Sex

Women tend to weigh more than their male counterparts. A higher percentage of women are obese in almost all reported studies (Kluthe and Schubert, 1985; Van Itallie, 1985) (see Figure 5–8).

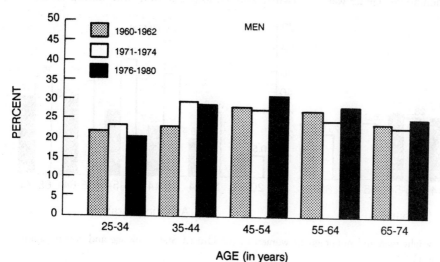

FIGURE 5–7 Percentage of overweight men in the United States, by age, 1960–1962, 1971–1974, and 1976–1980. From Harper (1987).

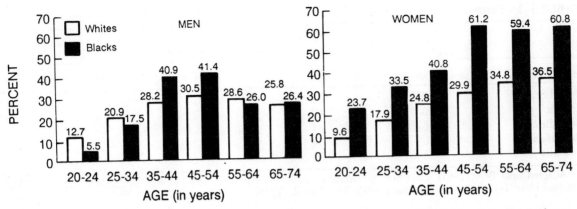

FIGURE 5–8 Percentage of overweight men and nonpregnant women in the United States, by age and race, during 1976–1980. From Van Itallie (1985).

Racial and Ethnic Differences

The prevalence of obesity differs among races (Figure 5–8). For men between 20 and 34 years of age, more whites than blacks are obese, but between the ages of 35 and 54, the frequency of obesity is higher among black men than among white men. After age 55, these race differences for men vanish. The data for women are more uniform: a higher percentage of black women (solid bars) are overweight between ages 20 and 74. Between the ages of 45 and 54, for example, 29.9% of white women compared to 61.2% of black women are obese.

Socioeconomic, Occupational, and Psychosocial Factors

Studies of obesity have almost uniformly demonstrated the importance of socioeconomic status in females and, to a much smaller degree, in males (Moore et al., 1962). As Figure 5–9 indicates, the percentage of overweight women above age 25 was highest in the poverty group. The differences among males were small and not statistically significant. There is no clear evidence that occupation plays an important role in the development of obesity. Although a number of studies have purported to show personality or behavioral patterns associated with obesity, other more methodologically rigorous studies have, in general, shown no association. Thus, no psychological risk factors for the development of obesity have been identified (Wadden and Stunkard, 1985).

Familial and Genetic Factors

There is a high familial association with obesity. If both parents are overweight, approximately 80% of the offspring are overweight. When neither parent is overweight, fewer than 10% of the children are overweight (Bray, 1987). The separation of genetic from environmental factors has relied on studies of twins and adopted children. Using path analysis to evaluate data on identical twins, nonidentical twins, and various parental and sibling relation-

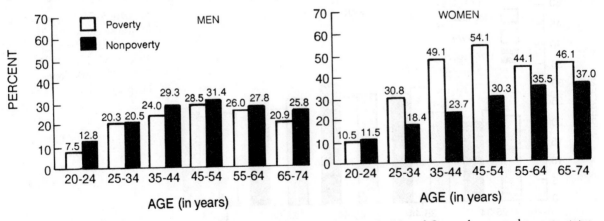

FIGURE 5–9 Percentage of overweight men and nonpregnant women in the United States, by age and poverty status, during 1976–1980. From Van Itallie (1985).

ships, Bouchard et al. (1988) concluded that approximately 50% of the variation in body fatness is transmissible to offspring, and of this amount, approximately half is under genetic control. This is lower than the estimates of heritability published by Stunkard et al. (1986), who compared BMI among identical and nonidentical twins and estimated heritability of body weight to be between 50 and 80%.

From these studies in affluent countries, it can be concluded that there is an important genetic component in the development of obesity. This genetic component interacts with environmental agents, primarily diet and level of physical activity, to produce obesity in susceptible people.

Obesity as a Risk Factor for Chronic Diseases

There is evidence that obesity is an independent risk factor for the development of atherosclerotic cardiovascular diseases, hypertension, diabetes mellitus, gallbladder disease, and some cancers, but opinions about the relative importance of these associations differ. In five prospective studies, fat distribution was found to be more strongly related to risk of total deaths, stroke, heart disease, and diabetes mellitus than was BMI or total body fat. The risk doubled in people with an increased ratio of abdominal to hip fat and showed a graded relationship at higher levels (Donahue et al., 1987; Ducimetiere et al., 1986; Lapidus et al., 1984; Larsson et al., 1984; Stokes et al., 1985).

Using BMI or relative weight, studies with small populations or of short duration usually fail to find an independent association of overweight with cardiovascular deaths (Keys et al., 1972; Pooling Project Research Group, 1978). Some longer studies (Hubert et al., 1983; Rabkin et al., 1977) or studies with more subjects (Lew and Garfinkel, 1979; Society of Actuaries, 1980; Waaler, 1984) have led to the conclusion that overweight is an independent predictor of risk of atherosclerotic cardiovascular diseases. This may be due to the strong association of obesity with risk of hypertension, diabetes mellitus, and lowered levels of HDL cholesterol, which are in themselves important risk factors for atherosclerotic cardiovascular diseases (Manson et al., 1987).

Diabetes mellitus is the disease most strongly associated with obesity. Mortality among people with a BMI of 35 kg/m² or greater is eightfold higher than that of people with a normal BMI (20 to 25 kg/m²) (Lew and Garfinkel, 1979; Waaler, 1983).

The next strongest association of obesity is with gallbladder disease. Those with a BMI of 33 kg/m² had four times the death rate from gallbladder disease as those with normal BMI (Lew and Garfinkel, 1979).

Obesity and possibly body build are also related to risk of hypertension (Weinsier et al., 1985; see Chapter 20). Weight reduction is associated with reduced blood pressure levels (Reisen et al., 1978).

Obesity is a risk factor for endometrial cancer (Lew and Garfinkel, 1979) and for postmenopausal breast cancer (Lubin et al., 1985). Further considerations of these associations and of possible associations with other cancer sites (e.g., ovary and prostate) are discussed in Chapter 21.

CANCERS

Cancers are populations of cells that have acquired the ability to multiply and spread without the usual biologic restraints (NRC, 1982). There are at least as many different cancers as there are tissues of the body. It is important to consider the distribution and determinants of cancers according to the individual cancer sites. This section focuses on cancers that are common in the United States today and are associated with dietary factors.

Cancers are diagnosed by many different procedures but are usually confirmed by histological examination of resected tissue. They are classified by the International Classification of Diseases (ICD) largely by site, such as lung cancer and breast cancer. A few cancers are classified according to their histologic characteristics, e.g., melanomas and leukemias.

The cancers discussed in this report fall within ICD-9 categories 140 through 208 for malignant tumors (ICD, 1977). ICD-9 categories 210 through 239 apply to tumors of uncertain nature or to those known to be benign (i.e., not infiltrating into tissues or spreading to other parts of the body).

There are major differences in the occurrence of cancers among countries. In general, rates are high in North America and low in parts of Africa and Asia. For certain cancer sites (e.g., esophagus, stomach, and liver), however, this general tendency is reversed. Within the United States, there tends to be a slightly higher incidence of all cancers in the industrial Northeast and slightly lower rates in rural areas. But for stomach cancers, the reverse is true. Most cancers occur with greater frequency as people age. Some tumors, however, are relatively frequent in children. These include leukemia—especially acute leukemia—bone tumors, and brain tumors.

Esophageal Cancer (ICD 150)

There is substantial international variation in incidence of esophageal cancer. High rates are found across most of middle Asia, from northern Iran and southern USSR around the Caspian Sea to northern China. In Europe, high rates occur in the Calvados region of France. Even within these areas, however, there is a large variation in incidence. For example, age-adjusted annual incidence rates in the Caspian region of Iran ranged from a high of 165.5 and 195.3 per 100,000 for males and females, respectively, in the northeast region of Gonbad to a low of 17.9 and 4.9 in the north-central region of Gilan (Mahboubi et al., 1973).

Incidence rates in the United States, a relatively low-risk area for esophageal cancer, vary considerably by race and sex. For example, rates among blacks in the San Francisco Bay Area are 11.7 for males and 3.6 for females; the corresponding rates for Chinese and whites in the same area are 6.9 and 2.1, and 4.0 and 1.9, respectively (Waterhouse et al., 1982). The higher incidence among males in all three groups has been observed in other U.S. populations as well and is a characteristic common to low-risk populations (Day and Munoz, 1982).

The disproportionately high incidence of esophageal cancer in Bay Area blacks relative to whites mirrors the higher rates of the disease seen in U.S. blacks in general. Annual age-adjusted esophageal cancer mortality rates for U.S. blacks from 1976 to 1980 exceeded those for whites by approximately threefold (14.0 and 4.2 per 100,000 among males; 3.4 and 1.2 among females). The excess mortality in blacks relative to whites was greater at younger ages; a more than sixfold difference in rates was noted in males under age 55. From 1950 to 1980, mortality rates for blacks nearly doubled, whereas rates among whites have remained fairly constant. Annual age-specific mortality rates among blacks have also risen sharply over time, but current data suggest that the rate of increase is less in people born after 1925 (Blot and Fraumeni, 1987).

The influence of migration on esophageal cancer rates is uncertain. Polish immigrants in the United States have been reported to have higher mortality rates than either U.S. whites or Poles living in Poland (Staszewski, 1974). Mortality rates among U.S. residents who migrated from Italy, Germany, Sweden, Norway, and Ireland have also been higher

than those among natives of the host country or the country of origin (Haenszel, 1961).

Stomach Cancer (ICD 151)

In the United States, there has been a striking decrease in both incidence of and mortality from stomach cancer over the past 40 to 50 years (Howson et al., 1986). U.S. rates are now among the lowest in the world. Fifty years ago, stomach cancer was the most important cause of cancer death in both sexes and is now ranked fifth to sixth in importance among cancer deaths. This decline has occurred among all age groups, but stomach cancer remains more common in older people.

The mortality rate for stomach cancer is approximately twice as high for males as for females. This form of cancer tends to be more common among lower socioeconomic groups and people who migrate to the United States, compared to native-born Americans. Rates among immigrant populations tend to change to levels of the adopted country relatively slowly over one to two generations.

Stomach cancer is more frequent in Asia, particularly in Japan, but incidence rates in that country have also fallen substantially in recent years (Waterhouse et al., 1982).

Colorectal Cancer (ICD 153, 154)

Although there are differences between colon and rectal cancer, both cancers are often considered together. Colorectal cancers tend to be more common in countries where breast cancer is common and relatively rare in countries where breast cancer is also relatively rare (Waterhouse et al., 1982). There is also a strong international association between colorectal cancer rates and rates for endometrial, ovarian, and to a lesser extent prostate cancer. Within the United States, rates tend to be higher in the northern part of the country and in urban areas. The male-to-female ratio for colon cancer is close to 1; for rectal cancer, it is 1.4. Migrants to the United States from eastern Europe and Asia have an increased incidence, resembling that of the host country within 10 to 15 years. There are still differences in incidence among racial groups, but these are narrowing. There is familial aggregation of colon cancer, and the disease is common in those with certain rare genetic disorders, particularly familial polyposis and Gardner's syndrome.

Both incidence and mortality from colorectal cancer have been relatively stable for the past 30 to

40 years. Recently, however, there has been an indication that mortality is decreasing among females in North America and, possibly, among males in the United States.

Liver Cancer (ICD 155.0)

Liver cancer is relatively rare in the United States but is common in Africa and Asia (Waterhouse et al., 1982), where it has been associated with hepatitis B infection as well as aflatoxin contamination of foods (see Chapter 22). Primary liver cancer is more common in men than in women (ratio, about 3 or 4 to 1), among persons of low socioeconomic groups and among blacks and Hispanics, compared to whites. Genetic or familial aggregation has not been noted. Like most other cancers, incidence increases progressively with age.

Pancreatic Cancer (ICD 157)

The incidence of pancreatic cancer in the United States has apparently increased in the past 20 to 30 years, but it has been relatively stable in the past 10 years. Some of these increases may have been due to better diagnosis. Pancreatic cancer is more common among men (ratio, approximately 1.5 to 1) and occurs more frequently in the United States than in Africa and Asia. High rates are also found among Polynesians in New Zealand and in Hawaii (Waterhouse et al., 1982). In the United States, rates seem to be higher for blacks than for whites. In general, pancreatic cancer occurs more commonly in higher socioeconomic groups and does not appear to have a familial association. Changes with migration have not been studied.

Lung Cancer (ICD 162)

Some of the highest lung cancer rates in the world are found in the United States—among whites living in Hawaii and blacks in Los Angeles (Waterhouse et al., 1982). In the past, rates were lower for blacks than for whites, but this has been reversed in some areas, especially among males at ages below 55. Rates are generally lower in other ethnic groups, particularly Hispanics and people of Asian origin, but are increasing rapidly. When the data within individual birth cohorts are considered, lung cancer is found to increase progressively with increasing age, particularly at older ages. In the United States, lung cancer began to increase

for males early in this century and for females, shortly after World War II. The overall rates are beginning to stabilize for males and to fall for those under 55 years old. In 1983, the male age-standardized rate was lower than in any year since 1977 (Horm and Kessler, 1986). For females, however, rates are continuing to increase, and deaths from lung cancer currently surpass deaths from breast cancer in many states. If present trends continue, there will be a 1-to-1 sex ratio for lung cancer by about the year 2000 (in comparison to the current ratio of 3 or 4 to 1 and the ratio 20 years ago of 6 or 8 to 1). Historically, rates have tended to be higher in the highest socioeconomic group, but these groups now have rates below average (Devesa et al., 1987).

Breast Cancer (ICD 174)

Breast cancer incidence in females is much greater than in males (ratio, 100 to 1). For this reason, the following discussion concentrates on breast cancer in females.

Breast cancer is more common in the United States than in other parts of the world, but rates are beginning to rise in many other countries. In recent tabulations, the highest incidence rate in the world is found among Caucasians living in Hawaii. Other high rates in the United States are found in the northern parts of the mainland, particularly in affluent areas (Waterhouse et al., 1982).

Breast cancer risk increases with age, but the slope of the age-specific incidence curve is different before and after menopause. Thus, risk rises rapidly up to about the age of 50 to 55. There is then a slowing of the rate of increase, or even a reversal in some populations, followed by another rise in high-risk populations. Breast cancer tends to be more common among higher socioeconomic groups and among Caucasians. Recently, however, rates have been rising among blacks, Hispanics, and people of Asian origin. Women who migrate to the United States from Europe, particularly eastern Europe, and from Asia generally have a lower incidence of breast cancer, which over the next one or two generations generally rises to approximate that of the United States.

There is a clear familial aggregation for 10 to 25% of breast cancer cases. In a rare subset of these, breast cancer behaves as a dominantly inherited characteristic from either the maternal or paternal side. Most cases of breast cancer appear to be spontaneous, but if genetic variation is widely distributed and its effect weak, it would be extremely difficult to determine with current epidemiologic methods the percentage of genetically induced breast cancers. Attempts are under way to identify genetic markers of transmission. One marker, the enzyme glutamic-6-pyruvate transaminase, was found to be linked to a number of families (King et al., 1983), but further study has not shown this to be a general phenomenon. Mortality from breast cancer has been stable in the United States for the past 40 years. Recently, however, there appears to be a slight reduction of deaths among women under age 50 and a slight increase in deaths among women over age 50. The incidence of breast cancer as reported by most cancer registries over the past 20 to 30 years has been rising, first in premenopausal women and then in postmenopausal women, but this increase may be spurious. Some of these changes may be related to changes in reproductive practices and to earlier diagnoses prompted by an increased awareness of the importance of breast cancer. A particularly dramatic example of the latter occurred during the 1970s: After breast cancer was diagnosed in the wives of the President and Vice-President of the United States, reported incidence rates in the United States rose by more than 10% in a single year and then subsided, without a detectable effect on mortality rates. This reflects an increased awareness by women, their subsequent visits to physicians for breast examinations, and the diagnosis of very early lesions with good prognosis.

Endometrial Cancer (ICD 182.0)

Endometrial cancer is correlated internationally with the incidence of breast, colorectal, and ovarian cancers, but tends to be more common in the United States than in other parts of the world (Waterhouse et al., 1982) and is found most frequently in higher socioeconomic groups and among whites. U.S. incidence rates have increased in the past 10 to 15 years, particularly in the western part of the country, without a corresponding increase in mortality. This rise was followed by a fall after demonstration of an association between the occurrence of endometrial cancer and administration of noncontraceptive estrogens after menopause (Austin and Roe, 1982).

Ovarian Cancer (ICD 183.0)

Ovarian cancer is the major cause of death from cancer of the reproductive system in women in North America. It is relatively common in the United States and other western countries compared to Asia and tends to occur more frequently in countries with high rates for cancer of the breast, colon, and endometrium (Waterhouse et al., 1982). The age-specific curve shows an earlier increase in incidence than for many other cancer sites, with a tendency for incidence to stabilize in middle years and then possibly to decline at older ages. Ovarian cancer tends to be more common in higher socioeconomic groups and aggregates in some families, suggesting that it may have a genetic basis. In general, however, ovarian cancer has only a weak association with familial association.

Bladder Cancer (ICD 188)

Cancer of the urinary bladder is relatively frequent in the United States compared to other parts of the world (Waterhouse et al., 1982). In some areas in North Africa, however, bladder cancer associated with schistosomiasis is common. Bladder cancer occurs more frequently in men than in women (ratio, approximately 2 to 1) and in lower socioeconomic groups, but does not appear to aggregate in families. There are no major ethnic or racial variations in bladder cancer. Changes upon migration have not been studied.

Prostate Cancer (ICD 185)

Cancer of the prostate is common in the United States and in other western countries (Waterhouse et al., 1982). Among U.S. blacks, it is particularly common and is increasing. It is relatively rare in males under the age of 45; the highest incidence is found among men in their seventies and eighties. Although incidence is increasing, there seems to be no corresponding trend in mortality, perhaps because part of the increase is a diagnostic artifact from more frequent detection of early-stage prostate cancer.

OSTEOPOROSIS

Osteoporosis (see Chapter 23) is a multifactorial, complex disorder characterized by an absolute decrease in bone mass per unit volume. Defining osteoporosis is difficult, since for a specific age and sex there is a wide, continuously distributed amount of bone mass (Mazess, 1983; Newton-John and Morgan, 1970; Riggs et al., 1981). Studies based on radiological techniques have demonstrated unequal rates of bone loss in different parts of the skeleton (Genant et al., 1982; Riggs et al., 1981, 1982). Bone mass tends to decrease after the fourth or fifth decade of age. As it becomes too low, structural integrity and mechanical support are not maintained and fractures occur after minimal trauma. The major sites of fracture are the hip, vertebrae, distal forearm (Colles' fracture), humerus, and pelvis. In clinical research, the diagnosis of osteoporosis is frequently applied only to patients in whom one or more fractures have already occurred (NIH, 1984).

Population Differences in Frequency

Among Countries

Age- and sex-adjusted hip fracture incidence rates in the United States are higher than those in any other region on which data have been published (Lewinnek et al., 1980; Nordin, 1966). Residents of New Zealand and western Europe as well as Israelis from western Europe also have high rates. The lowest reported rates are found among the South African Bantu (Bloom and Pogrund, 1982; Lewinnek et al., 1980).

Within the United States

Osteoporosis afflicts 24 million Americans (half of the women over 45 years of age and 90% of the women over 75 years of age). It is associated with an estimated 1.3 million fractures of the vertebrae, hips, forearms, and other bones per year (NIAMS, 1988).

In Migrants

The committee found no data on osteoporosis in migrants.

Time Trends

In Nottingham in the United Kingdom, the number of patients with fractures of the proximal femur more than doubled between 1971 and 1981. From 1971 to 1977, the rate of increase in fracture incidence was approximately 6% per year; after 1977, it rose to 10% per year (Wallace, 1983). In this same population, the rate of femoral fractures in women increased from 8 per 1,000 in 1971 to 16 per 1,000 in 1981. Similar trends have been reported for Denmark (Jensen and Tøndevald, 1980).

At the present rates of population change, by the year 2030 approximately 20% of the population in the United States will be 65 years of age or older (NIH, 1984). Thus, the proportion of individuals predisposed to fractures of the hip, femur, forearm, or vertebrae is expected to increase.

Associations Between Risk Factors in Individuals and Osteoporosis

The demographic characteristics associated with osteoporosis and osteoporosis-related fractures are age over 40, female sex, and Caucasian race. Loss of bone mass begins at approximately 40 years of age in men and women and in blacks and whites. The most rapid decrease in bone density occurs among white women, particularly around 50 years of age (Garn, 1975).

Age and Sex

Osteoporotic fractures are more common in elderly women than in men of the same ages, but the degree of female predominance depends on the type of fracture. Less than 20% of the women between 45 and 49 years of age have x-ray evidence of osteoporosis in their dorsolumbar spines; however, almost all women age 75 years and older have evidence of osteoporosis in this region (Iskrant and Smith, 1969). Females are two to three times more likely than males to suffer hip fractures (Gallagher et al., 1980). Incidence rates for Colles' fractures and fractures of the proximal humerus, vertebrae, and pelvis are six to eight times higher in women than in men (Owen et al., 1982; Rose et al., 1982).

Because women tend to live longer than men, the absolute incidence is even higher. One-third of women 65 years of age and older have vertebral fractures—the most common break caused by osteoporosis. By extreme old age, one-third of all women and one-sixth of all men will have suffered hip fractures, leading to death in 12 to 20% of the cases. For half of those who survive, the fracture leads to long-term nursing care (Cummings et al., 1985). Studies of postmenopausal women suggest that the number of years since menopause may be more important than chronological age as a determinant of bone mass (Lindquist et al., 1979; Richelson et al., 1984).

Osteoporosis most commonly found in men and women after middle life may consist of two distinct syndromes called Type I and Type II. Type I osteoporosis occurs in a relatively small subset of postmenopausal women between 51 and 65 years of age. It is characterized by excessive and disproportionate trabecular bone loss and is associated with vertebral fractures and decreased sex hormone production. Type II occurs in a large proportion of women or men who are more than 75 years of age. This is characterized by a proportionate loss of both cortical and trabecular bone and is associated with hip or vertebral fractures. Osteoporosis occurring between 66 and 75 years of age may represent a combination of these types (Riggs et al., 1982).

Racial and Ethnic Differences

White women are about twice as likely as black women to suffer hip fractures. Most studies, but not all, indicate that the risk for hip fractures is higher among white men than black men (Bollett et al., 1965; Farmer et al., 1984). The incidence of hip and other osteoporotic fractures in Asian or Hispanic populations in the United States has not been reported, but Asian-Americans appear to have somewhat less cortical bone mass than whites of similar age (Garn et al., 1964; Yano et al., 1984).

Socioeconomic, Occupational, and Psychosocial Factors

Socioeconomic status has not been associated with osteoporosis, except possibly through poor diet. Gross malnutrition stunts growth and reduces bone mass. No occupational, social, behavioral, or psychological factors have been associated with osteoporosis.

Familial and Genetic Factors

Genetically determined differences in bone mass are illustrated by differences between races. In comparison to whites, blacks in the United States have higher bone mass, greater bone density, thicker bone cortex, and greater vertebral density (Cohn et al., 1977; Garn et al., 1972; Smith and Rizek, 1966; Trotter et al., 1960).

DIABETES MELLITUS

Diabetes mellitus, a disorder of carbohydrate utilization secondary to a relative or absolute deficiency of insulin, is the seventh leading underlying cause of death in the United States. Diabetes mellitus is characterized by high blood glucose levels. It can be diagnosed by the presence of classical signs and symptoms, including elevated blood glucose levels, by a fasting plasma glucose ≥ 140 mg/dl, or by an abnormal oral glucose tolerance test (Harris, 1985). Two distinct primary forms of diabetes mellitus are Type I, or insulin-dependent (IDDM), and Type II, or non-insulin dependent (NIDDM). This classification replaces the older terminology, juvenile-onset and adult-onset diabetes. IDDM is usually the result of the destruction of the insulin-secreting β cells in the pancreatic islets of Langerhans. It is

believed to be an immune-linked disorder, and there seems to be an increased risk of IDDM in subjects with certain traits associated with the HLA (human leukocyte group A) or histocompatibility immune response genes. In contrast, NIDDM is associated with aging and genetic traits and is closely linked to the insulin resistance associated with adiposity.

Other forms of diabetes include gestational diabetes. This transient condition occurs in approximately 2 to 5% of pregnancies and is believed to be a marker for future development of NIDDM. Diabetes mellitus can also be secondary to or associated with other conditions. This accounts for approximately 2% of all cases of diabetes (Melton et al., 1983; Merkatz et al., 1980). Although some data on the distribution of IDDM are presented for contrast, this report is concerned primarily with NIDDM, which is the only form of diabetes associated with diet as a risk factor. Except where indicated, the data on NIDDM (and IDDM) presented below are taken from two comprehensive reviews (Everhart et al., 1985; LaPorte and Cruickshanks, 1985), which appeared in a publication of the National Institutes of Health *Diabetes in America* (National Diabetes Data Group, 1985).

Population Differences in Frequency

Among Countries

Statistics on NIDDM are available for less than 2% of the world's population (LaPorte et al., 1985) and most probably underestimate the true magnitude of disease. Population surveys of blood glucose levels suggest that undiagnosed (occult) disease is common and increases with age. Data do suggest, however, that age-adjusted incidence rates of NIDDM vary considerably. Rates per 1,000 people age 40 and older range from 9.4 among male Israeli civil servants, to 16.8 and 11.3 among male and female Nauruans (in the South Pacific), and to 55.3 and 45.8 in U.S. males and females, respectively.

Within the United States

Approximately 6 million people in the United States have been diagnosed by a physician as being diabetic, and each year, approximately 500,000 new cases are diagnosed. An additional 4 million to 5 million people may have diabetes without knowing it. Since IDDM accounts for only 5% of known cases of diabetes and only an additional 2% of diabetes is secondary to or associated with other disorders, it is clear that the vast majority of diabetics have NIDDM.

In 1982, diabetes was identified as the underlying cause of almost 35,000 deaths in the United States. It was the seventh leading cause of death that year and was listed as a contributing cause in an additional 95,000 deaths. Reliable mortality rates for NIDDM alone are not available; however, there are estimates that the 20-year survival for people with NIDDM is 50 to 80% of survival in the general adult population.

In Migrants

The prevalence of NIDDM in Japanese who migrated to Hawaii is higher (12.3 per 100 people) than in Japanese residing in Hiroshima, Japan (6.9 per 100 people) (Kawate et al., 1979). The age-adjusted prevalence rates in Japanese residents of Hawaii appear to be intermediate between those of Caucasians and native Hawaiians (Sloan, 1963). Asian-Indian migrants to high-risk countries also exhibit higher prevalence rates than their native counterparts and the same or even higher rates than those for natives of their adoptive country (Taylor and Zimmet, 1983). This increase in risk has also been observed in Yemenite migrants to Israel (Cohen et al., 1979).

Time Trends

NIDDM incidence rates in the United States have increased from 3.8 per 10,000 people in 1935–1936 (Spiegelman and Marks, 1946) to 22.7 per 10,000 people in 1979–1981. It is unlikely that improved screening and diagnosis alone can account for the increase in NIDDM.

Associations Between Risk Factors in Individuals and Diabetes Mellitus

Age

The median age of people with diabetes (61) is higher than that of the general U.S. population (42). Approximately 9% of people 65 years old and older are believed to have NIDDM (Drury et al., 1985).

NIDDM mortality rates are difficult to ascertain, because this disease is a major contributor to cardiovascular and cerebrovascular deaths and is often a contributing cause (sometimes not even listed) rather than the certified underlying cause of death from these diseases. Approximately 76% of diabetes-related deaths (most presumed to be NIDDM) occur among people 65 years of age and older; 45% of those deaths occur after age 74 (Harris and Entmacher, 1985).

Sex

There are no clear sex differences in IDDM and NIDDM incidence rates. Rates are slightly higher among U.S. females, possibly reflecting more frequent use of physicians and, presumably, higher rates of NIDDM detection.

Racial and Ethnic Differences

Prevalence rates of NIDDM among adult blacks, Hispanics, and Asian-Americans appear to be higher than those among whites. For blacks, the rates are 50% higher than those for whites. The incidence rates for diabetes in some Native American tribes, such as the Pimas, are among the highest recorded in the world, their age–sex-adjusted incidence rates being more than 40 times higher than comparable rates in Rochester, Minnesota (Knowler et al., 1978).

Socioeconomic Factors

The U.S. data linking NIDDM rates to socioeconomic status are inconsistent with international data. Unlike rates in economically developing countries, which are positively associated with socioeconomic status, NIDDM rates in the United States are highest among the poor (Everhart et al., 1985).

Familial and Genetic Factors

There is some degree of familial aggregation for NIDDM. It is two to four times more common among the parents of children 20 years old or older with diabetes; nearly 33% of persons with diabetes compared to 4% of those without report having a sibling with the disease, and concordance rates of NIDDM are higher among monozygotic than among dizygotic twins. There are no known genetic markers to identify people at high risk of NIDDM. However, adiposity, a risk factor for NIDDM, appears to be at least partly determined by genetic predisposition.

Other Risk Factors

Adiposity is the major risk factor for NIDDM. It is consistently correlated with NIDDM prevalence rates in intercountry, migrant, and other epidemiologic studies. A high waist-to-hip ratio, indicating a more central distribution of body fat, may also increase NIDDM risk in nondiabetics.

Diabetes as a Risk Factor for Other Chronic Diseases

The primary causes of death among diabetics are varied, since NIDDM is associated with a host of complications. These complications include ketoacidosis, kidney and renal disorders, accelerated arteriosclerosis leading to CHD, peripheral vascular and cerebrovascular diseases, blindness, hypertension, infections, complications of pregnancy, and neuropathy. Death among diabetics below age 20 (presumably with IDDM) is caused primarily by acute diabetic complications (e.g., ketoacidosis), but at older ages, renal disease accounts for nearly half of diabetic deaths and coronary atherosclerosis is responsible for most of the remainder.

HEPATOBILIARY DISEASE

Because of its many functions, the liver is subject to injury from a variety of causes, including nutritional imbalance. In industrialized Western countries, however, nutritional causes of chronic liver disease are uncommon and are related primarily to intake of alcoholic beverages. The prevalence of alcohol-induced liver disease, commonly called alcoholic cirrhosis, is quite high in most industrialized countries, including the United States. The major disease of the biliary system, gallstones (cholelithiasis), also is believed to be associated with nutritional factors, but the evidence is not as conclusive and the responsible nutrients have not been identified precisely.

Another liver disease is viral hepatitis—a frequent cause of acute hepatic inflammation and necrosis that occasionally becomes a chronic infection and produces one variety of cirrhosis. A few inherited disorders include hemochromatosis, which involves iron metabolism; Wilson's disease, which involves copper metabolism; and α_1-antitrypsin deficiency. The liver is frequently injured by circulatory disorders, metastatic cancer, and obstruction of the biliary system by gallstones. These are not discussed here because nutrition is not a major contributor to their causes.

Effects of Alcohol on the Liver

Three distinct, but often overlapping, types of liver damage are found in chronic alcoholics: fatty liver, alcoholic hepatitis, and cirrhosis (Galambos, 1972; Mezey, 1980, 1982). Fatty liver occurs in most heavy drinkers (Bhathl et al., 1975) and is an immediate metabolic consequence of ethanol. It has been observed in animals (Lieber et al., 1963, 1975) as well as in humans (Rubin and Lieber, 1968) after ingestion of ethanol. Fatty liver, however, is not specific for alcohol ingestion; it may also result from a variety of other toxic, nutri-

tional, and circulatory injuries. Alcoholic hepatitis (hepatic necrosis and inflammation) and cirrhosis occur less frequently than fatty liver among chronic alcoholics, but they are more advanced stages of liver disease. Alcoholic hepatitis, a life-threatening complication of heavy chronic alcohol consumption, may be a precursor to alcoholic cirrhosis (Rubin and Lieber, 1974). The metabolic processes involved in the effects of alcohol on the liver are described in detail in Chapter 16 of this report.

Both fatty liver and hepatitis due to alcohol ingestion are reversible when alcohol is withdrawn, and they leave no permanent stigmata. However, repeated episodes of fatty liver and hepatitis, and possibly other direct effects of alcohol on the liver, cause progressive scarring, which begins in the portal triads and extends to encircle the liver lobules. Some liver cells may regenerate in a disorganized pattern to form nodules, but the total liver mass is markedly decreased and the effective functioning liver mass is reduced even more.

There is no universally accepted definition of cirrhosis of the liver, but a committee of the World Health Organization defined it as a diffuse process characterized by fibrosis, loss of normal liver architecture, and the development of structurally abnormal nodules of liver tissue (Anthony et al., 1977). The essential features of cirrhosis also include fatty degeneration and necrosis of liver cells, regeneration of liver cells in abnormal patterns, proliferation of connective tissue, and alterations in the vascular supply. These changes eventually result in liver cell failure and portal hypertension (O'Brien et al., 1979).

Cirrhosis has been classified on the basis of anatomic characteristics, clinical history, and presumed etiology, with these various classifications differing in frequency according to age, sex, and geography. The most commonly encountered type in the United States is alcoholic cirrhosis, also referred to interchangeably as portal cirrhosis and Laennec's cirrhosis. Diagnoses of these cases are based on a history of chronic alcoholism together with the characteristic clinical manifestations and pathological findings. They must be differentiated from cirrhosis due to other causes, such as chronic viral hepatitis, hemochromatosis, obstructive lesions of the biliary tract, congestive heart failure, and congenital malformations (O'Brien et al., 1979). In their terminal stages, as in chronic renal disease, the different types of cirrhosis have many features in common, and clinical history often provides the most decisive information in determining its etiology. Morbidity and mortality due to alcoholic cirrhosis are related principally to the loss of liver function, to derangements in the vascular system of the liver, or to both.

Cholelithiasis is often associated with cholecystitis. Gallstones form most frequently in the gallbladder but may infrequently occur in other portions of the biliary system. Most gallstones (80% or more) are composed predominantly of cholesterol combined with small amounts of calcium salts. Less frequently, gallstones are composed of calcium bilirubinate and related heme pigments derived from the degradation of hemoglobin. Gallstones may range from less than 1 mm up to several centimeters in diameter. Radiopacity is determined by their calcium content.

Because cholesterol-containing gallstones are more frequent, most research efforts have focused on their etiology and pathogenesis. The conditions that contribute to the formation of these gallstones are complex. The major factor is the ratio of cholesterol to bile acids and phospholipids, which stabilize cholesterol in an aqueous solution by forming micelles with a hydrophilic shell around a core of cholesterol. The proportions of cholesterol and solubilizing materials are determined by intake and absorption of dietary cholesterol, efficiency of evacuation of the gallbladder, endogenous synthesis of cholesterol, efficiency of the enterohepatic circulation of bile acids, rates of bile acid synthesis, drugs and hormones (particularly estrogens), and probably by many other factors. Nutrition is likely to affect many of these processes (reviewed by Bennion and Grundy, 1978a,b, and by Low-Beer, 1985).

Alcoholic Cirrhosis

Population Differences in Frequency

Among Countries

Rates of mortality from alcoholic cirrhosis vary greatly among countries. In the early 1970s, France, Italy, and Portugal had the highest rates, averaging between 50 and 60 deaths per 100,000 people 25 years and older. The United States ranked eighth out of 26 countries with an annual rate of approximately 29 deaths per 100,000 people over age 25. Similar rates were found in Japan, Switzerland, and Czechoslovakia. The United Kingdom had the lowest rate (5.7 deaths/ 100,000 over age 25) of the 26 countries (Schmidt, 1977). The rates of few other chronic diseases in the technologically developed Western countries vary as widely from country to country as do rates of alcoholic cirrhosis of the liver.

Within Countries

Rates of mortality from alcoholic cirrhosis are approximately twice as high for men as for women in the United States and Canada (Schmidt, 1977), and the ratio of rates for men to those for women have increased gradually since World War II. The highest mortality is concentrated in the 25- to 64-year-old range, particularly in the 35- to 44-year-old group. Since alcoholic cirrhosis is associated most strongly and consistently with alcohol consumption, it shares the many socioeconomic and ethnic correlates of alcoholism.

In Migrants

There are few data on alcoholic cirrhosis in migrants. Rates of alcoholism vary greatly among Hispanics from various countries, and Asian-Americans tend to have lower frequencies of alcohol abuse than does the general population, but there are no specific data on alcoholic cirrhosis (NIAAA, 1985).

Time Trends in Mortality and Morbidity

Rates of death from alcoholic cirrhosis in the United States rose from 1959 to 1971 by an average of 3.8% per year in men and 3.4% per year in women (Schmidt, 1977). The rate of annual increase during the same period was much higher among men in Czechoslovakia (9.2%), Sweden (7.5%), and Italy (7.1%) and was somewhat higher in several other countries. In none of the 18 countries examined did the rate of change in men decrease. Since 1950, alcoholic cirrhosis has ranked consistently among the 10 leading causes of deaths in the U.S. population between the ages of 25 and 64. In some years, it has ranked much higher among middle-aged people. In 1977, for example, alcoholic cirrhosis was the fourth leading cause of death among 45- to 64-year-old people. At a rate of 39.2 per 100,000, it was just behind stroke (52.4) and ahead of motor vehicle accidents (25.5) (DHEW, 1979b). In general, consistent with the gradual but steady increase from year to year, alcoholic cirrhosis moved from seventh to fifth place among leading causes of death in the United States between 1950 and 1973 (Schmidt, 1977). However, mortality from alcoholic cirrhosis began to decline shortly thereafter and in 1983 reached the lowest level recorded since 1959. In that year, it was the ninth leading cause of death for all ages, accounting for 28,000 deaths (NIAAA, 1985).

In other countries, marked fluctuations in mortality from alcoholic cirrhosis have accompanied drastic changes in the availability of beverage alcohol. The most dramatic example occurred in France, where the rates fell from approximately 35 per 100,000 before World War II to about 6 per 100,000 during the war, and then increased to 35 or more per 100,000 after the war (Terris, 1967). Less dramatic but similar changes over time have been observed in other countries.

Associations Between Risk Factors in Individuals and Alcoholic Cirrhosis

Alcoholic cirrhosis has consistently been correlated predominantly with the per-capita consumption of alcohol on a national basis (Gordis et al., 1983). In turn, alcohol consumption and alcoholic cirrhosis have been correlated positively with the availability and the ease of access to alcohol as stated above, and inversely with cost (Terris, 1967).

Rates of mortality from alcoholic cirrhosis are twofold higher in males than in females, are negligible under 25 years of age, are appreciable in the 25- to 44-year age group (8.6/10,000), peak from age 45 to 64 (39.2/100,000), and decline slightly after age 65 (36.7/100,000) (DHEW, 1979b).

The risk of alcoholic cirrhosis from lifetime alcohol consumption was expressed in a mathematical model by Skog (1984). Most alcoholics develop cirrhosis only after many years of alcohol abuse, and the risk increases as a function of any suitable measure of consumption. More than 50% of the risk is determined by current intake plus the preceding 5 years of consumption. Consumption rates during the preceding 6 to 25 years contribute to the balance of the risk, but the weight of the predictive power for each of those years is much less. This model of risk is consistent with observations that mortality due to most chronic progressive diseases decreases rapidly when the causative agent is removed.

Gallbladder Disease and Gallstones

Population Differences in Frequency

Among Countries

The prevalence of gallstones also varies widely among countries, but reliable data are difficult to obtain because gallstones are difficult to detect in population surveys. Furthermore, although they are frequent causes of morbidity, they do not often cause death. Thus, mortality rates cannot be used as indices of occurrence.

The prevalence of gallstones at autopsy is high (affecting 10% or more of all adults) in the industrialized countries—in the United States, Australia, and Europe. It is lower (5% or less) in the nonindustrialized countries of Asia and Africa (Brett and Barker, 1976). However, there have been no systematic population surveys using similar methods in different areas to compare gallstone prevalence among countries or morbidity related to gallstones.

Within Countries

In most countries, the prevalence of gallstones is two to three times higher in women than in men (Brett and Barker, 1976). In the United States, Native Americans and people descended from an admixture of New World natives (such as Latin Americans or Mexican Americans) have a much higher prevalence of gallstones than those with a West European heritage (Arevalo et al., 1987; Comess et al., 1967; Hesse, 1959; Sampliner et al., 1970; Weiss et al., 1984). Three-fourths of middle-aged Pima Indian women had evidence of gallbladder disease when surveyed by cholecystography, and approximately 80% of those with abnormal cholecystograms were found to have gallstones at surgery or at autopsy (Sampliner et al., 1970). Thus, the prevalence of gallstones in adult Pima women exceeds 50%, compared to estimates of 10 to 20% for comparable U.S. whites and blacks.

In Migrants

Information comparing the frequency of gallstones and gallbladder disease in migrants with that in their countries of origin is limited. Data do suggest, however, that environmental factors (e.g., diet) may influence risk. A survey of hospital admissions in Hawaii showed that Chinese had the highest admission rate for gallbladder disease. In contrast, gallbladder disease is reported to be rare among native Chinese living in China (Yamase and McNamara, 1972).

Time Trends in Mortality and Morbidity

There is no information regarding changes in prevalence of gallstones or gallbladder disease over time in the United States. In Japan, evidence suggests that the prevalence of gallstones at autopsy increased about threefold between 1950 and 1970 (Nagase et al., 1978).

Associations Between Risk Factors in Individuals and Gallbladder Disease and Gallstones

Being a female and being obese are most consistently associated with gallstones (reviewed by Bennion and Grundy, 1978a,b, and by Low-Beer, 1985). Obesity is also related to supersaturation of gallbladder bile, and gallstones have been linked with high-calorie diets, but not with cholesterol intake, type of dietary fat, or dietary fiber (Bennion and Grundy, 1978a,b). In an analysis of the Framingham cohort after 10 years of observation, incidence of gallbladder disease (principally cholelithiasis) was twice as high in women as in men and was associated with an increase in weight and number of pregnancies, but was not related to serum cholesterol concentration, cigarette smoking, physical activity, CHD, or intakes of alcohol, cholesterol, fat, or protein (Friedman et al., 1966). In Japan, a review of surgical patients indicated that younger people had more cholesterol-containing gallstones (Nagase et al., 1978).

DENTAL CARIES

Dental caries is localized demineralization of the tooth surface caused primarily by organic acid metabolites of oral microorganisms. The disease leads to a chronic progressive destruction of the teeth. In epidemiologic studies, caries prevalence is expressed as decayed, missing, and filled teeth (dmft) for primary dentition and as DMFT for permanent teeth.

Population Differences in Prevalence

Among Countries

Sreenby (1982) compared the prevalence of dental caries in children ages 6 (in 23 countries) and 12 (in 47 countries) using data obtained from the World Health Organization's Global Oral Epidemiology Bank (Barmes and Sardo-Infirri, 1977). The dmft and DMFT values used by Sreenby (1982) are indices of the cumulative effect of dental caries over the life of the dentition. Thus, for the primary dentition in 6-year-olds, the exposure period was approximately 4 to 5 years; for permanent teeth in the 12-year-olds, the period was 4 to 6 years for the molars and anterior teeth. Prevalence of DMFT in the 6-year-olds surveyed ranged from 0.9 per child in Cameroon to 9.3 in Japan. Prevalence was highest in Asian countries

and lowest in the African countries surveyed except in South Africa, which had an intermediate level (4.4) similar to that of the United States (3.4) and the United Kingdom (4.5).

The prevalence of DMFT among 12-year-old children ranged from 0.1 in Zambia to 10.6 in Switzerland. Again, the mean DMFT tended to be lowest in African countries; however, unlike the prevalence for 6-year-olds, the DMFT prevalence for 12-year-olds was highest in Switzerland and in the northern European countries of Denmark and Finland. Rates for Asian countries tended to be intermediate like those of the United States (4.0) and the United Kingdom (5.5)

Within Countries

Striking differences in the prevalence of caries in the U.S. population by geographic area were noted in the 1980 national survey of caries in schoolchildren (NIDR, 1981). Caries prevalence was highest in the Northeast, lowest in the Southwest, and at intermediate levels elsewhere.

According to data derived from the the National Health Survey for 1971 to 1973 (NIDR, 1981), people of both sexes and all ages (1 to 74 years) had an average of 13 decayed, missing, and filled permanent teeth. A closer review of this figure indicates that there was an average of 1.3, 5.3, and 6.4 decayed, missing, and filled teeth, respectively. An estimated 14.7% of the adults (18 to 74 years old) had lost all their permanent teeth. In a study of the oral health of U.S. adults, completed in 1986, only 4% of people of ages 18 to 65 were edentulous (Miller et al., 1987).

In Migrants

No information on caries in migrants was found.

Time Trends

Until the 1970s, caries was most prevalent (affecting 95% of the population) in developed countries, especially in those with diets high in refined carbohydrates. The only exception occurred during and just after World War II, when the prevalence rates of caries dropped precipitously, although temporarily, in children living in Europe (Sognnaes, 1948; Toverud, 1957) and Japan (Takeuchi, 1961). During the 1970s, the prevalence of caries declined dramatically again among school-aged children not only in many countries of western Europe but also in North America (Glass, 1982). In contrast, the rate of caries is increasing in many Third World countries (Barmes and Sardo-Infirri, 1977).

In the 1971–1973 National Health Survey, children between the ages of 5 and 17 had decay or fillings in an average of 7.06 teeth (NIDR, 1981). By 1981, this number had dropped to 4.77 (NIDR, 1981). Likewise, as noted above, the prevalence of edentulia dropped from 14.7% in 18- to 74-year-old people during 1971–1973 (NIDR, 1981) to 4% in the 18- to 65-year age group in 1986 (Miller et al., 1987). There are reports that root surface caries is becoming more prevalent among older people—a result perhaps of decreased edentulia (Seichter, 1987). This is discussed in the next section.

Associations Between Risk Factors in Individuals and Dental Caries

Age

Caries of the tooth crown is predominantly a disease of children and adolescents. It begins as soon as teeth erupt; incidence remains high, and prevalence increases linearly up to ages 18 to 20. After age 25 or so, the incidence of coronal caries diminishes, but the disease may still occur. The epidemiologic study of caries in adults becomes increasingly complicated by the fact that it is often not possible to distinguish between teeth lost because of caries and those missing because of periodontal and other oral diseases. What is certain is that caries of the root surface of the teeth, secondary to exposure of the root by recession of the gingivae, becomes increasingly prevalent with advancing age. In a national survey of employed U.S. adults, completed in 1986 (Miller et al., 1987), root-surface caries had affected approximately 60% of the population by age 65; the average was about three lesions per person.

Sex

Caries prevalence is higher among females than among males at every age. This observation is only partly explained by the earlier eruption of teeth in females, leading to longer exposure to the oral environment. Root-surface caries is more common in males for reasons that are not yet clear (Carlos, 1984).

Racial, Ethnic, and Socioeconomic Differences

Chung et al. (1970) analyzed the relationship of race to caries prevalence in 9,912 12- to 18-year-old children in Hawaii. They noted that dental caries was most prevalent among children of Japanese origin, followed by children of Hawaiian origin. Children with Caucasian, Puerto Rican, or Filipino parentage had the lowest caries activity. In a subsequent survey of 910 eighth-grade students in Hawaii, Hankin et al. (1973) found that the prevalence of caries in Hawaiian children had surpassed that in children of Japanese ancestry. Caucasian children continued to enjoy the lower rates. A 1980 U.S. national survey (NIDR, 1981) showed no notable differences in caries prevalence with respect to color, ethnic group, or socioeconomic status. However, the HHANES (Hispanic Health and Nutrition Examination Survey) of 1982–1984 indicated that Mexican-American children residing in the Southwest had a dental caries distribution similar to that of other groups in the region, but that Mexican-American children from low-income families had nearly two times more decayed teeth than did Mexican-American children from high income families (Ismail et al., 1987).

Occupational and Psychosocial Risk Factors

No information on caries was found in these areas.

Familial and Genetic Factors

There is some evidence of genetic predisposition to caries (Witkop, 1962), but this appears to be a minor etiologic factor compared to the local influences of diet, bacterial deposits on teeth, and less than optimal ingestion of fluoride.

REFERENCES

Abbott, R.D., Y. Yin, D.M. Reed, and K. Yano. 1986. Risk of stroke in male cigarette smokers. N. Engl. J. Med. 315: 717–720.

Abraham, S., M.D. Carroll, M.F. Najjar, and R. Fulwood. 1983. Obese and overweight adults in the United States. Vital and Health Statistics, Series 11, No. 230. DHHS Publ. No. (PHS) 83–1680. National Center for Health Statistics. Public Health Service, U.S. Department of Health and Human Services, Hyattsville, Md. 93 pp.

AHA (American Heart Association). 1973. Coronary Risk Handbook: Estimating Risk of Coronary Heart Disease in Daily Practice. American Heart Association, New York. 35 pp.

AHA (American Heart Association). 1983. 1984 Heart Facts. Office of Communications, Dallas. 25 pp.

Allen, E.V., N.W. Barker, and E.A. Hines, Jr. 1946. Peripheral Vascular Diseases. W.B. Saunders, Philadelphia. 871 pp.

Anastasiou-Nana, M., S. Nanas, J. Stamler, J. Marquardt, R. Stamler, H.A. Lindberg, D.M. Berkson, K. Liu, E. Stevens, M. Mansour, and T. Tokich. 1982. Changes in rates of sudden CHD death with first vs. recurrent events,

Chicago Peoples Gas Co. Study, 1960–1980. Circulation, Suppl. 66:II-236.

Anthony, P.P., K.G. Ishak, N.C. Nayak, H.E. Poulsen, P.J. Scheuer, and L.H. Sobin. 1977. The morphology of cirrhosis: definition, nomenclature, and classification. Bull. W.H.O. 55:521–540.

Arevalo, J.A., A.O. Wollitzer, M.B. Corporon, M. Larios, D. Huante, and M.T. Ortiz. 1987. Ethnic variability in cholelithiasis: an autopsy study. West. J. Med. 147:44–47.

Austin, D.F., and K.M. Roe. 1982. The decreasing incidence of endometrial cancer: public health implications. Am. J. Public Health 72:65–68.

Barmes, D.E., and J. Sardo-Infirri. 1977. World Health Organization activities in oral epidemiology. Community Dent. Oral Epidemiol. 5:22–29.

Beaglehole, R., C.E. Salmond, A. Hooper, J. Huntsman, J.M. Stanhope, J.C. Cassel, and I.A. Prior. 1977. Blood pressure and social interaction in Tokelauan migrants in New Zealand. J. Chronic Dis. 30:803–812.

Bennion, L.J., and S.M. Grundy. 1978a. Risk factors for the development of cholelithiasis in man (first of two parts). N. Engl. J. Med. 229:1161–1167.

Bennion, L.J., and S.M. Grundy. 1978b. Risk factors for the development of cholelithiasis in man (second of two parts). N. Engl. J. Med. 229:1221–1227.

Berenson, G.S. 1980. Cardiovascular Risk Factors in Children: The Early Natural History of Atherosclerosis and Essential Hypertension. Oxford University Press, New York. 453 pp.

Berenson, G.S., A.W. Voors, and L.S. Webber. 1980. Importance of blood pressures in children: distribution and measurable determinants. Pp. 71–97 in H. Kesteloot and J.V. Joossens, eds. Epidemiology of Arterial Blood Pressure. Martinus Nijhoff, The Hague.

Bhathal, P.S., P. Wilkinson, S. Clifton, J.B. Rankin, and J.N. Santamaria. 1975. The spectrum of liver diseases in alcoholism. Aust. N.Z.J. Med. 5:49–57.

Black, D., W.P.T. James, G.M. Besser, C.G.D. Brook, D. Craddock, J.S. Garrow, T.D.R. Hockaday, B. Lewis, T.R.E. Pilkington, J.T. Silverstone, J.I. Mann, D.S. Miller, D.A. Pyke, D.G. Williams, and R.K. Skinner. 1983. A report of the Royal College of Physicians. J. R. Coll. Physicians London 17:5–65.

Bloom, R.A., and H. Pogrund. 1982. Humeral cortical thickness in female Bantu—its relationship to the incidence of femoral neck fracture. Skeletal Radiol. 8:59–62.

Blot, W.J., and J.F. Fraumeni, Jr. 1987. Trends in esophageal cancer mortality among U.S. blacks and whites. Am. J. Public Health 77:296–298.

Bollet, A.J., G. Engh, and W. Parson. 1965. Epidemiology of osteoporosis; sex and race incidence of hip fractures. Arch. Intern. Med. 116:191–194.

Bonita, R., and R. Beaglehole. 1982. Trends in cerebrovascular disease mortality in New Zealand. N.Z. Med. J. 95:411–414.

Bonita, R., and R. Beaglehole. 1986. Does treatment of hypertension explain the decline in mortality from stroke? Br. Med. J. 292:191–192.

Bothig, S., V.I. Metelitsa, W. Barth, A.A. Aleksandrov, I. Schneider, T.P. Ostrovskaya, E.V. Kokurina, I.I. Saposhinkov, I.P. Iliushina, and L.S. Gurevich. 1976. Prevalence of ischaemic heart disease, arterial hypertension, and intermittent claudication, and distribution of risk factors among middle-aged men in Moscow and Berlin. Cor Vasa 18:104–118.

Bouchard, E., L. Perusse, C. Leblanc, A. Tremblay, and G. Theriault. 1988. Inheritance of the amount and distribution of human body fat. Int. J. Obesity 12:205–215.

Bray, G.A., ed. 1979. Obesity in America. NIH Publ. No. 79–359. National Institutes of Health, Public Health Service, U.S. Department of Health, Education, and Welfare, Bethesda, Md. 285 pp.

Bray, G.A. 1985. Obesity: definition, diagnosis and disadvantages. Med. J. Aust. 142:S2-S8.

Bray, G.A. 1987. Obesity and the heart. Modern Concepts Cardiovasc. Dis. 56:67–71.

Brett, M., and D.J. Barker. 1976. The world distribution of gallstones. Int. J. Epidemiol. 5:335–341.

Brown, J., G.J. Bourke, G.F. Gearty, A. Finnegan, M. Hill, F.C. Heffernan-Fox, D.E. Fitzgerald, J. Kennedy, R.W. Childers, W.J.E. Jessop, M.F. Trulson, M.C. Latham, S. Cronin, M.B. McCann, R.E. Clancy, I. Gore, H.W. Stroudt, D.M. Hegsted, and F.J. Stare. 1970. Nutritional and epidemiologic factors related to heart disease. World Rev. Nutr. Diet. 12:1–42.

Carlos, J.P. 1984. Epidemiologic trends in caries: impact on adults and the aged. Pp. 131–148 in B. Guggenheim, ed. Cariology Today. S. Karger, Basel.

Carroll, M.D., S. Abraham, and C.M. Dresser. 1983. Dietary Intake Source Data: United States, 1976–1980. Vital and Health Statistics, Series 11, No. 231. DHHS Publ. No. (PHS) 83–1681. National Center for Health Statistics, Public Health Service, U.S. Department of Health and Human Services, Hyattsville, Md. 483 pp.

Chung, C.S., D.W. Runck, J.D. Niswander, S.E. Bilben, and M.C.W. Kau. 1970. Genetic and epidemiologic studies of oral characteristics in Hawaii's schoolchildren. I. Caries and periodontal disease. J. Dent. Res. 49:1374–1385.

Cohen, A.M., J. Fidel, B. Cohen, A. Furst, and S. Eisenberg. 1979. Diabetes, blood lipids, lipoproteins, and change of environment: restudy of the "new immigrant Yemenites" in Israel. Metabolism 28:716–728.

Cohn, S.H., C. Abesamis, S. Yasumura, J.F. Aloia, I. Zanzi, and K.J. Ellis. 1977. Comparative skeletal mass and radial bone mineral content in black and white women. Metabolism 26:171–178.

Comess, L.J., P.H. Bennet, and T.A. Burch. 1967. Clinical gallbladder disease in Pima Indians: its high prevalence in contrast to Framingham, Massachusetts. N. Engl. J. Med. 277:894–898.

Comstock, G.W. 1957. An epidemiologic study of blood pressure levels in a biracial community in the southern United States. Am. J. Hyg. 65:271–315.

Criqui, M.H., S.S. Coughlin, and A. Fronek. 1985a. Noninvasively diagnosed peripheral arterial disease as a predictor of mortality: results from a prospective study. Circulation 72:768–773.

Criqui, M.H., A. Fronek, E. Barrett-Connor, M.R. Klauber, S. Gabriel, and D. Goodman. 1985b. The prevalence of peripheral arterial disease in a defined population. Circulation 71:510–515.

Cummings, S.R., J.L. Kelsey, M.C. Nevitt, and K.J. O'Dowd. 1985. Epidemiology of osteoporosis and osteoporotic fractures. Epidemiol. Rev. 7:178–208.

Dawber, T.R., and W.B. Kannel. 1972. Current status of coronary prevention. Lessons from the Framingham Study. Prev. Med. 1:499–512.

Day, N.E., and N. Munoz. 1982. Esophagus. Pp. 596–623 in D. Schottenfeld and J.F. Fraumeni, Jr., eds. Cancer Epidemiology and Prevention. W.B. Saunders Co., Philadelphia.

Devesa, S.S., D.T. Silverman, J.L. Young, Jr., E.S. Pollack, C.C. Brown, J.W. Horm, C.L. Percy, M.H. Myers, F.W. McKay, and J.F. Fraumeni, Jr. 1987. Cancer incidence and mortality trends among whites in the United States, 1947–84. J. Natl. Cancer Inst. 79:701–770.

DHEW (U.S. Department of Health, Education, and Welfare). 1963. Origin, Program, and Operation of the U.S. National Health Survey. Vital and Health Statistics, Series 1, No. 1. PHS Publ. No. 1000. National Center for Health Statistics, Public Health Service, U.S. Department of Health, Education, and Welfare, Washington, D.C. 41 pp.

DHEW (U.S. Department of Health, Education, and Welfare). 1979a. Dietary Intake Source Data: United States, 1971–74. Vital and Health Statistics, DHEW Publ. No. (PHS) 79-1221. National Center for Health Statistics, Public Health Service, U.S. Department of Health, Education, and Welfare, Hyattsville, Md. 421 pp.

DHEW (U.S. Department of Health, Education, and Welfare). 1979b. Healthy People: The Surgeon General's Report on Health Promotion and Disease Prevention. DHEW (PHS) Publ. No. 79-55071, Office of the Assistant Secretary for Health and Surgeon General, Public Health Service. U.S. Government Printing Office, Washington, D.C. (various pagings).

DHHS (U.S. Department of Health and Human Services). 1986. Blood Pressure Levels in Persons 18–74 Years of Age in 1976–80, and Trends in Blood Pressure from 1960 to 1980 in the United States. Data from the National Health Survey, Series 11, No. 234. DHHS Publ. No. (PHS) 86-1684. National Center for Health Statistics, Public Health Service, U.S. Department of Health and Human Services, Hyattsville, Md. 68 pp.

DHHS (U.S. Department of Health and Human Services). 1987. Monthly Vital Statistics Report, Vol. 36: The Advance Report of Final Mortality Statistics, 1985. DHHS Publ. No. (PHS) 87-1120. National Center for Health Statistics, Public Health Service, U.S. Department of Health and Human Services, Hyattsville, Md. 48 pp.

Donahue, R.P., R.D. Abbott, E. Bloom, D.M. Reed, and K. Yano. 1987. Central obesity and coronary heart disease in men. Lancet 1:821–824.

Drury, T.F., K.M. Danchik, and M.I. Harris. 1985. Sociodemographic characteristics of adult diabetics. Pp. VII-1 to VII-37 in M.I. Harris and R.F. Hamman, eds. Diabetes in America: Diabetes Data Compiled 1984. Report of the National Diabetes Data Group. NIH Publ. No. 85-1468. National Institute of Arthritis, Diabetes and Digestive and Kidney Diseases, National Institutes of Health, Public Health Service. U.S. Department of Health and Human Services, Bethesda, Md.

Ducimetiere, P., J. Richard, and F. Cambien. 1986. The pattern of subcutaneous fat distribution in middle-aged men and the risk of coronary heart disease: the Paris Prospective Study. Int. J. Obes. 10:229–240.

Dyken, M.L., P.A. Wolf, H.J.M. Barnett, J.J. Bergan, W.K. Hass, W.B. Kannel, L. Kuller, J.F. Kurtzke, and T.M. Thoralf. 1984. Risk factors in stroke: a statement for physicians by the subcommittee on risk factors and stroke of the Stroke Council. Stroke 15:1105–1111.

Elveback, L.R., D.C. Connolly, and L.T. Kurland. 1981. Coronary heart disease in residents of Rochester, Minnesota. II. Mortality, incidence, and survivorship, 1950–1975. Mayo Clin. Proc. 56:665–672.

Elveback, L.R., D.C. Connolly, and L.J. Melton III. 1986. Coronary heart disease in residents of Rochester, Minnesota. VII. Incidence, 1950 through 1982. Mayo Clin. Proc. 61:896–900.

Epstein, F.H., and R.D. Eckoff. 1967. The epidemiology of high blood pressure—geographic distribution and etiologic factors. Pp. 155–161 in J. Stamler, R. Stamler, and T.M. Pullman, eds. Epidemiology of Hypertension. Grune and Stratton, New York.

Everhart, J., W.C. Knowler, and P.H. Bennett. 1985. Incidence and risk factors for noninsulin-dependent diabetes. Pp. IV-1 to IV-35 in M.I. Harris and R.F. Hamman, eds. Diabetes in America: Diabetes Data Compiled 1984. Report of the National Diabetes Data Group. NIH Publ. No. 85-1468. National Institute of Arthritis, Diabetes and Digestive and Kidney Diseases, National Institutes of Health, Public Health Service. U.S. Department of Health and Human Services, Bethesda, Md.

Farmer, M.E., L.R. White, J.A. Brody, and K.R. Bailey. 1984. Race and sex differences in hip fracture incidence. Am. J. Public Health 74:1374–1380.

Folkow, B. 1982. Physiological aspects of primary hypertension. Physiol. Rev. 62:347–504.

Folsom, A.R., R.V. Luepker, R.F. Gillum, D.R. Jacobs, R.J. Prineas, H.L. Taylor, and H. Blackburn. 1983. Improvement in hypertension detection and control from 1973–1974 to 1980–1981. The Minnesota Heart Survey experience. J. Am. Med. Assoc. 250:916–921.

Folsom, A.R., O. Gomez-Marin, R.F. Gillum, T.E. Kottke, W. Lohman, and D.R. Jacobs, Jr. 1987. Out-of-hospital coronary death in an urban population—validation of death certificate diagnosis. The Minnesota Heart Survey. Am. J. Epidemiol. 125:1012–1018.

Franco, L.J., M.P. Stern, M. Rosenthal, S.M. Haffner, H.P. Hazuda, and P.J. Cameaux. 1985. Prevalence, detection and control of hypertension in a biethnic community. The San Antonio Heart Study. Am. J. Epidemiol. 121:684–696.

Friedman, G.D., W.B. Kannel, and T.R. Dawber. 1966. The epidemiology of gallbladder disease: observations in the Framingham Study. J. Chron. Dis. 19:273–292.

Galambos, J.T. 1972. Alcoholic hepatitis: its therapy and prognosis. Prog. Liver Dis. 4:567–588.

Gallagher, J.C., L.J. Melton, B.L. Riggs, and E. Bergstrath. 1980. Epidemiology of fractures of the proximal femur in Rochester, Minnesota. Clin. Orthop. 150:163–171.

Garn, S.M. 1975. Bone-loss and aging. Pp. 39–57 in R. Goldman and M. Rockstein, eds. The Physiology and Pathology of Human Aging. Academic Press, New York.

Garn, S.M., E.M. Pao, and M.E. Rihl. 1964. Compact bone in Chinese and Japanese. Science 143:1439–1440.

Garn, S.M., S.T. Sandusky, J.M. Nagy, and M.B. McCann. 1972. Advanced skeletal development in low-income Negro children. J. Pediatr. 80:965–969.

Garraway, W.M., and J.P. Whisnant. 1987. The changing pattern of hypertension and the declining incidence of stroke. J. Am. Med. Assoc. 258:214–217.

Garraway, W.M., J.P. Whisnant, A.J. Furlan, L.H. Phillips II, L.T. Kurland, and W.M. O'Fallon. 1979. The declining incidence of stroke. N. Engl. J. Med. 300:449–452.

Genant, H.K., C.E. Cann, B. Ettinger, and G.S. Gordan. 1982. Quantitative computed tomography of vertebral spongiosa: a sensitive method for detecting early bone loss after oophorectomy. Ann. Intern. Med. 97:699–705.

Gill, J.S., A.V. Zezulka, M.J. Shipley, S.K. Gill, and D.G.

Beevers. 1986. Stroke and alcohol consumption. N. Engl. J. Med. 315:1041–1046.

Gillum, R.F., P.J. Hannan, R.J. Prineas, D.R. Jacobs, Jr., O. Gomez-Martin, R.V. Luepker, J. Baxter, T.E. Kottke, and H. Blackburn. 1984. Coronary heart disease mortality trends in Minnesota, 1960–1980: the Minnesota Heart Survey. Am. J. Public Health 74:360–362.

Gillum, R.F., O. Gomez-Marin, T.E. Kottke, D.R. Jacobs, Jr., R.J. Prineas, A.R. Folsom, R.V. Luepker, and H. Blackburn. 1985. Acute stroke in a metropolitan area, 1970 and 1980. The Minnesota Heart Survey. J. Chronic Dis. 38:891–898.

Glass, R.L., ed. 1982. The First International Conference on the Declining Prevalence of Dental Caries. J. Dent. Res. (sp. iss.) 61:1301–1383.

Goldberg, R.J., J.M. Gore, J.S. Alpert, and J.E. Dalen. 1986. Recent changes in attack and survival rates of acute myocardial infarction (1975 through 1981). The Worcester Heart Attack Study. J. Am. Med. Assoc. 255:2774–2779.

Goldman, L., and E.F. Cook. 1984. The decline in ischemic heart disease mortality rates: an analysis of the comparative effects of medical interventions and changes in lifestyle. Ann. Intern. Med. 101:825–836.

Goldman, L., F. Cook, B. Hashimoto, P. Stone, J. Muller, and A. Loscalzo. 1982. Evidence that hospital care for acute myocardial infarction has not contributed to the decline in coronary mortality between 1973–1974 and 1978–1979. Circulation 65:936–942.

Gomez-Marin, O., A.R. Folsom, T.E. Kottke, S.C. Wu, D.R. Jacobs, Jr., R.F. Gillum, S.A. Edlavitch, and H. Blackburn. 1987. Improvement in long-term survival among patients hospitalized with acute myocardial infarction, 1970 to 1980. The Minnesota Heart Survey. N. Engl. J. Med. 316:1353–1359.

Gordis, E., V.P. Dole, and M.J. Ashley. 1983. Regulation of alcohol consumption: individual appetite and social policy. Am. J. Med. 74:322–334.

Haenszel, W. 1961. Cancer mortality among the foreign-born in the United States. J. Natl. Cancer Inst. 26:37–132.

Hamilton, M., G.W. Pickering, J.A. Roberts, and G.S. Sowry. 1954. Aetiology of essential hypertension; arterial pressure in the general population. Clin. Sci. 13:11–35.

Hankin, J.H., C.S. Chung, and M.C. Kau. 1973. Genetic and epidemiologic studies of oral characteristics in Hawaii's school children: dietary patterns and caries prevalence. J. Dent. Res. 52:1079–1086.

Harper, A.E. 1987. Transitions in health status: implications for dietary recommendations. Am. J. Clin. Nutr. 45:1094–1107.

Harris, M.I. 1985. Classification and diagnostic criteria for diabetes and other categories of glucose intolerance. Pp. II-1 to II-10 in M.I. Harris and R.F. Hamman, eds. Diabetes in America: Diabetes Data Compiled 1984. Report of the National Diabetes Data Group. NIH Publ. No. 85–1468. National Institute of Arthritis, Diabetes and Digestive and Kidney Diseases, National Institutes of Health, Public Health Service. U.S. Department of Health and Human Services, Bethesda, Md.

Harris, M.I., and P.S. Entmacher. 1985. Mortality from diabetes. Pp. XXIX-1 to XXIX-48 in M.I. Harris and R.F. Hamman, eds. Diabetes in America: Diabetes Data Compiled 1984. Report of the National Diabetes Data Group. NIH Publ. No. 85–1468. National Institute of Arthritis, Diabetes and Digestive and Kidney Diseases, National In-

stitutes of Health, Public Health Service. U.S. Department of Health and Human Services, Bethesda, Md.

HDFP (Hypertension Detection and Follow-up Program Cooperative Group). 1979. Five-year findings of the Hypertension Detection and Follow-up Program. II. Mortality by race–sex, and age. J. Am. Med. Assoc. 242:2572–2577.

Hesse, F.G. 1959. Incidence of cholecystitis and other diseases among Pima Indians of Southern Arizona. J. Am. Med. Assoc. 170:1789–1790.

Heyden, S., A. Heyman, and L. Camplong. 1969. Mortality patterns among parents of patients with atherosclerotic cerebrovascular disease. J. Chronic Dis. 22:105–110.

Heyman, A., H.R. Karp, S. Heyden, A. Bartel, J.C. Cassel, H.A. Tyroler, and C.G Hames. 1971. Cerebrovascular disease in the biracial population of Evans County, Georgia. Arch. Intern. Med. 128:949–955.

Horm, J.W., and L.G. Kessler. 1986. Falling rates of lung cancer in men in the United States. Lancet 1:425–426.

Howson, C.P., T. Hiyama, and E.L. Wynder. 1986. The decline in gastric cancer: epidemiology of an unplanned triumph. Epidemiol. Rev. 8:1–27.

Hubert, H.B., M. Feinleib, P.M. McNamara, and W.P. Castelli. 1983. Obesity as an independent risk factor for cardiovascular disease: a 26-year follow-up of participants in the Framingham Heart Study. Circulation 67:968–977.

ICD (International Classification of Diseases). 1977. Manual of the International Statistical Classification of Diseases, Injuries, and Causes of Death, Vol. 1. Based on the Recommendations of the Ninth Revision Conference, 1975, and Adopted by the Twenty-Ninth World Health Assembly. World Health Organization, Geneva. 773 pp.

Inter-Society Commission for Heart Disease Resources. 1984. Optimal resources for primary prevention of atherosclerotic diseases. Circulation 70:153A–205A.

Iskrant, A. P., and R.W. Smith, Jr. 1969. Osteoporosis in women 45 years and over related to subsequent fractures. Public Health Rep. 84:33–38.

Ismail, A.L., B.A. Burt, and J.A. Brunelle. 1987. Prevalence of dental caries and periodontal disease in Mexican American children aged 5 to 17 years: results from southwestern NHANES, 1982–83. Am. J. Public Health 77:967–970.

Jenkins, C.D. 1983. Psychosocial and Behavioral Factors. Pp. 98–112 in N.M. Kaplan and J. Stamler, eds. Prevention of Coronary Heart Disease. W.B. Saunders, Philadelphia.

Jensen, J.S., and E. Tøndevald. 1980. A prognostic evaluation of the hospital resources required for the treatment of hip fractures. Acta Orthop. Scand. 51:515–522.

JNC (Joint National Committee on Detection, Evaluation, and Treatment of High Blood Pressure). 1988. The 1988 Report of the Joint National Committee on Detection, Evaluation, and Treatment of High Blood Pressure. Arch. Intern. Med. 148:1023–1038.

Johnson, B.C., F.H. Epstein, and M.O. Kjelsberg. 1965. Distributions and family studies of blood pressure and serum cholesterol levels in a total community—Tecumseh, Michigan. J. Chronic Dis. 18:147–160.

Juergens, J.L., N.W. Barker, and E.A. Hines, Jr. 1959. Arteriosclerosis obliterans: review of 520 cases with special reference to pathogenic and prognostic factors. Circulation 21:188–195.

Kagan, A., J. Popper, G.G. Rhoads, Y. Takeya, H. Kato, G.B. Goode, and M. Marmot. 1976. Epidemiologic studies of coronary heart disease and stroke in Japanese men living in Japan, Hawaii and California: prevalence of stroke. Pp.

267–277 in P. Scheinberg, ed. Cerebrovascular Diseases: Tenth Princeton Conference. Raven Press, New York.

Kagan, A., J.S. Popper, and G.G. Rhoads. 1980. Factors related to stroke incidence in Hawaiian Japanese men. The Honolulu Heart Study. Stroke 11:14–21.

Kannel, W.B. 1974. Role of blood pressure in cardiovascular morbidity and mortality. Prog. Cardiovasc. Dis. 17:5–24.

Kannel, W.B. 1980. Host and environmental determinants of hypertension: perspective from the Framingham Study. Pp. 265–295 in H. Kesteloot and J.V. Joossens, eds. Epidemiology of Arterial Blood Pressure. Martinus Nijhoff, The Hague.

Kannel, W.B., and D.L. McGee. 1985. Update on some epidemiologic features of intermittent claudication: the Framingham Study. J. Am. Geriatr. Soc. 33:13–18.

Kannel, W.B., and D. Shurtleff. 1971. The natural history of arteriosclerosis obliterans. Cardiovasc. Clin. 3:37–52.

Kannel, W.B., and P. Sorlie. 1979. Some health benefits of physical activity. The Framingham Study. Arch. Intern. Med. 139:857–861.

Kannel, W.B., and P.A. Wolf. 1983. Epidemiology of cerebrovascular disease. Pp. 1–24 in R.W.R. Russell, ed. Vascular Disease of the Central Nervous System. Churchill Livingstone, Edinburgh.

Kawate, R., M. Yamakido, Y. Nishimoto, P.H. Bennett, R.F. Hamman, and W.C. Knowler. 1979. Diabetes mellitus and its vascular complications in Japanese migrants on the Island of Hawaii. Diabetes Care 2:161–170.

Keen, H., G. Rose, D.A. Pyke, D. Boyns, C. Chlouverakis, and S. Mistry. 1965. Blood-sugar and arterial disease. Lancet 2:505–508.

Kesteloot, H., C.S. Song, J.S. Song, B.C. Park, E. Brems-Heyns, and J.V. Joossens. 1976. An epidemiological survey of arterial blood pressure in Korea using home reading. Pp. 141–148 in G. Rorive and H. Van Cauwenberge, eds. The Arterial Hypertensive Disease: A Symposium. Masson, New York.

Kesteloot, H., B.C. Park, C.S. Lee, E. Brems-Heyns, and J.V. Joossens. 1980. A comparative study of blood pressure and sodium intake in Belgium and in Korea. Pp. 453–470 in H. Kesteloot and J.V. Joossens, eds. Epidemiology of Arterial Blood Pressure. Martinus Nijhoff, The Hague.

Keys, A. 1980. Seven Countries: A Multivariate Analysis of Death and Coronary Heart Disease. Harvard University Press, Cambridge, Mass. 381 pp.

Keys, A., C. Arvanis, H. Blackburn, F.S.P. Van Buchem, R. Buzina, B.S. Djordjevic, F. Fidanza, M.J. Karvonen, A. Menotti, V. Puddi, and H.L. Taylor. 1972. Coronary heart disease: overweight and obesity as risk factors. Ann. Intern. Med. 77:15–27.

King, M.C., R.C. Go, H.T. Lynch, R.C. Elston, P.I. Terasaki, N.L. Petrakis, G.C. Rodgers, D. Lattanzio, and J. Bailey-Wilson. 1983. Genetic epidemiology of breast cancer and associated cancers in high-risk families. II. Linkage analysis. J. Natl. Cancer Inst. 71:463–467.

Kluthe, R., and A. Schubert. 1985. Obesity in Europe. Ann. Intern. Med. 103:1037–1042.

Knowler, W.C., P.H. Bennett, R.F. Hamman, and M. Miller. 1978. Diabetes incidence and prevalence in Pima Indians: a 19-fold greater incidence than in Rochester, Minnesota. Am. J. Epidemiol. 108:497–505.

Komachi, Y. 1977. Recent problems in cerebrovascular accidents: characteristics of stroke in Japan. Nippon Ronen Igakkai Zasshi 14:359–364.

Komachi, Y., and T. Shimamoto. 1980. Regional differences in blood pressure and its nutritional background in several Japanese populations. Pp. 379–400 in H. Kesteloot and J.V. Joossens, eds. Epidemiology of Arterial Blood Pressure. Martinus Nijhoff, The Hague.

Kuller, L.H., J.A. Perper, W.S. Dai, G. Rutan, and N. Traven. 1986. Sudden death and the decline in coronary heart disease mortality. J. Chronic Dis. 39:1001–1019.

Kurtzke, J.F. 1976. An introduction to the epidemiology of cerebrovascular disease. Pp. 239–253 in P. Scheinberg, ed. Cerebrovascular Diseases: Tenth Princeton Conference. Raven Press, New York.

Kushi, L.H., R.A. Lew, F.J. Stare, C.R. Ellison, M. el Lozy, G. Bourke, L. Daly, I. Graham, N. Hickey, R. Mulcahy, and J. Kevaney. 1985. Diet and 20-year mortality from coronary heart disease. The Ireland–Boston Diet–Heart Study. N. Engl. J. Med. 312:811–818.

Lapidus, L., C. Bengtsson, B. Larsson, K. Pennert, E. Rybo, and L. Sjöström. 1984. Distribution of adipose tissue and risk of cardiovascular disease and death: a 12-year follow up of participants in the population study of women in Gothenburg, Sweden. Br. Med. J. 289:1257–1261.

LaPorte, R.E., and K.J. Cruickshanks. 1985. Incidence and risk factors for insulin-dependent diabetes. Pp. III-1 to III-12 in M.I. Harris and R.F. Hamman, eds. Diabetes in America: Diabetes Data Compiled 1984. Report of the National Diabetes Data Group. NIH Publ. No. 85-1468. National Institute of Arthritis, Diabetes and Digestive and Kidney Diseases, National Institutes of Health, Public Health Service. U.S. Department of Health and Human Services, Bethesda, Md.

LaPorte, R.E., N. Tajima, H.K. Akerblom, N. Berlin, J. Brosseau, M. Christy, A.L. Drash, H. Fishbein, A. Green, R. Hamman, M. Harris, H. King, Z. Laron, and A. Neil. 1985. Geographic differences in the risk of insulin-dependent diabetes mellitus: the importance of registries. Diabetes Care 8 suppl. 1:101–107.

Larsson, B., K. Svärdsudd, L. Welin, L. Wilhelmsen, P. Björntorp, and G. Tibblin. 1984. Abdominal adipose tissue distribution, obesity, and risk of cardiovascular disease and death: 13-year follow-up of participants in the study of men born in 1913. Br. Med. J. 288:1401–1404.

Leon, A.S., and H. Blackburn. 1982. Physical activity and hypertension. Pp. 14–36 in P. Sleight and E. Freis, eds. Hypertension: Cardiology, Vol. 1. Butterworth Scientific, London.

Levy, R.I. 1979. Stroke decline: implications and prospects. N. Engl. J. Med. 300:490–491.

Lew, E.A., and L. Garfinkel. 1979. Variations in mortality by weight among 750,000 men and women. J. Chronic Dis. 32:563–576.

Lewinnek, G.E., J. Kelsey, A.A. White III, and N.J. Kreiger. 1980. The significance and a comparative analysis of the epidemiology of hip fractures. Clin. Orthop. (152):35–43.

Lieber, C.S., D.P. Jones, J. Mendelson, and L.M. DeCarli. 1963. Fatty liver, hyperlipemeia and hyperuricemia produced by prolonged alcohol consumption, despite adequate dietary intake. Trans. Assoc. Am. Physicians 76:289–301.

Lieber, C.S., L. DeCarli, and E. Rubin. 1975. Sequential production of fatty liver, hepatitis, and cirrhosis in subhuman primates fed ethanol with adequate diets. Proc. Natl. Acad. Sci. U.S.A. 72:437–441.

Lindquist, O., C. Bengtsson, T. Hansson, and B. Roos. 1979. Age at menopause and its relation to osteoporosis. Maturitas 1:175–181.

Low-Beer, T.S. 1985. Nutrition and cholesterol gallstones. Proc. Nutr. Soc. 44:127–134.

Lubin, F., A.M. Ruder, Y. Wax, and B. Modan. 1985. Overweight and changes in weight throughout adult life in breast cancer etiology. A case-control study. Am. J. Epidemiol. 122:579–588.

MacMahon, S.W., and S.R. Leeder. 1984. Blood pressure levels and mortality from cerebrovascular disease in Australia and the United States. Am. J. Epidemiol. 120:865–875.

Mahboubi, E., J. Kmet, P.J. Cook, N.E. Day, P. Ghadirian, and S. Salmasizadeh. 1973. Oesophageal cancer studies in the Caspian Littoral of Iran: the Caspian cancer registry. Br. J. Cancer 28:197–214.

Manson, J.E., M.J. Stampfer, C.H. Hennekens, and W.C. Willett. 1987. Body weight and longevity. A reassessment. J. Am. Med. Assoc. 257:353–358.

Marmot, M.G., S.L. Syme, A. Kagan, H. Kato, J.B. Cohen, and J. Belsky. 1975. Epidemiologic studies of coronary heart disease and stroke in Japanese men living in Japan, Hawaii and California: prevalence of coronary and hypertensive heart disease and associated risk factors. Am. J. Epidemiol. 102:514–525.

Marmot, M.G., A.M. Adelstein, N. Robinson, and G.A. Rose. 1978. Changing social-class distribution of heart disease. Br. Med. J. 2:1109–1112.

Marshall, J. 1971. Familial incidence of cerebrovascular disease. J. Med. Genet. 8:84–89.

Mazess, R.B. 1983. The noninvasive measurement of skeletal mass. Pp. 223–279 in W.A. Peck, ed. Bone and Mineral Research, Annual 1: A Yearly Survey of Developments in the Field of Bone and Mineral Metabolism. Excerpta Medica, Amsterdam.

Melton, L.J., III, K.M. Macken, P.J. Palumbo, and L.R. Elveback. 1980. Incidence and prevalence of clinical peripheral vascular disease in a population-based cohort of diabetic patients. Diabetes Care 3:650–654.

Melton, L.J., III, P.J. Palumbo, and C.P. Chu. 1983. Incidence of diabetes mellitus by clinical type. Diabetes Care 6:75–86.

Merkatz, I.R., M.A. Duchon, T.S. Yamashita, and H.B. Houser. 1980. A pilot community-based screening program for gestational diabetes. Diabetes Care 3:453–457.

Mezey, E. 1980. Alcoholic liver disease: roles of alcohol and malnutrition. Am. J. Clin. Nutr. 33:2709–2718.

Mezey, E. 1982. Alcoholic liver disease. Prog. Liver Dis. 7:555–572.

Miall, W.E., and H.G. Lovell. 1967. Relation between change of blood pressure and age. Br. Med. J. 2:660–664.

Millar, W.J., and T. Stephens. 1987. The prevalence of overweight and obesity in Britain, Canada, and United States. Am. J. Public Health 77:38–41.

Miller, A.J., J.A. Brunelle, J.P. Carlos, L.J. Brown, and H. Löe. 1987. Oral Health of United States Adults. The National Survey of Oral Health in U.S. Employed Adults and Seniors: 1985–1986, National Findings. NIH Publ. No. 87-2868. Epidemiology and Oral Disease Prevention, National Institute of Dental Research, National Institutes of Health, Public Health Service, U.S. Department of Health and Human Services, Bethesda, Md. 168 pp.

Moore, M.E., A. Stunkard, and L. Srole. 1962. Obesity, social class, and mental illness. J. Am. Med. Assoc. 181:962–966.

Nagase, M., H. Tanimura, M. Setoyama, and Y. Hikasa. 1978. Present features of gallstones in Japan. A collective review of 2,144 cases. Am. J. Surg. 135:788–790.

Nance, W.E., H. Krieger, E. Azevedo, and M.P. Mi. 1965. Human blood pressure and the ABO blood group system: an apparent association. Hum. Biol. 37:238–244.

National Diabetes Data Group. 1985. Diabetes in America: Diabetes Data Compiled 1984. NIH Publ. No. 85-1468. National Institute of Arthritis, Diabetes and Digestive and Kidney Diseases, National Institutes of Health, Public Health Service, U.S. Department of Health and Human Services, Bethesda, Md. (various pagings).

National Heart Foundation of Australia. 1981. Risk Factor Prevalence Study. No. 1. NHFA, Canberra, Australia. 136 pp.

Newton-John, H.F., and D.B. Morgan. 1970. The loss of bone with age, osteoporosis, and fractures. Clin. Orthop. 71:229–252.

NIAAA (National Institute on Alcohol Abuse and Alcoholism). 1985. Liver Cirrhosis Mortality in the United States: U.S. Alcohol Epidemiologic Data Reference Manual, Vol. II. Alcohol, Drug Abuse, and Mental Health Administration, Public Health Service, U.S. Department of Health and Human Services, Rockville, Md. 232 pp.

NIAMS (National Institute of Arthritis and Musculoskeletal and Skin Diseases). 1988. Arthritis, Rheumatic Diseases, and Related Disorders: Moyer Report. National Institutes of Health, Public Health Service, U.S. Department of Health and Human Services, Bethesda, Md. 23 pp.

NIDR (National Institute of Dental Research). 1981. The Prevalence of Dental Caries in United States Children, 1979–1980: The National Dental Caries Prevalence Survey. NIH Publ. No. 82-2245. National Caries Program, National Institutes of Health, Public Health Service, U.S. Department of Health and Human Services, Bethesda, Md. 159 pp.

NIH (National Institutes of Health). 1984. Osteoporosis: NIH Consensus Development Conference. National Institute of Arthritis, Diabetes, and Digestive and Kidney Diseases and the Office of Medical Applications of Research, Bethesda, Md. 87 pp.

Nordin, B.E. 1966. International patterns of osteoporosis. Clin. Orthop. 45:17–30.

NRC (National Research Council). 1982. Diet, Nutrition, and Cancer. Report of the Committee on Diet, Nutrition, and Cancer, Assembly of Life Sciences. National Academy Press, Washington, D.C. 478 pp.

O'Brien, M.J., M.R.C. Path, and L.S. Gottlieb. 1979. The liver and biliary tract. Pp. 1009–1091 in S.L. Robbins and R.S. Cotran, eds. Pathologic Basis of Disease, 2nd ed. W.B. Saunders, Philadelphia.

Omae, T., M. Takeshita, and Y. Hirota. 1976. The Hisayama Study and Joint Study on cerebrovascular diseases in Japan. Pp. 255–265 in P. Scheinberg, ed. Cerebrovascular Diseases: Tenth Princeton Conference. Raven Press, New York.

Ostfeld, A.M., R.B. Shekelle, H. Klawans, and H.M. Tufo. 1974. Epidemiology of stroke in an elderly welfare population. Am. J. Public Health 64:450–458.

Owen, R.A., L.J. Melton III, K.A. Johnson, D.M. Ilstrup, and B.L. Riggs. 1982. Incidence of Colles' fracture in a North American community. Am. J. Public Health 72:605–607.

Page, L.B. 1979. Hypertension and atherosclerosis in primitive and acculturating societies. Pp. 1–12 in J.C. Hunt, ed. Hypertension Update, Vol. 1. Health Learning Systems, Lyndhurst, N.J.

Peacock, P.B., C.P. Riley, T.D. Lampton, S.S. Raffel, and

J.S. Walker. 1972. The Birmingham Stroke, Epidemiology and Rehabilitation Study. Pp. 231–345 in G.T. Stewart, ed. Trends in Epidemiology: Application to Health Service Research and Training. C.C. Thomas, Springfield, Ill.

Pell, S., and W.E. Fayerweather. 1985. Trends in the incidence of myocardial infarction and in associated mortality and morbidity in a large employed population, 1957–1983. N. Engl. J. Med. 312:1005–1111.

Pooling Project Research Group. 1978. Relationship of blood pressure, serum cholesterol, smoking habit, relative weight and ECG abnormalities to incidence of major coronary events: final report of the Pooling Project. J. Chronic Dis. 31:201–306.

Prineas, R.J., and H. Blackburn. 1983. Clinical and epidemiologic relationships between electrolytes and hypertension. Pp. 63–85 in M.J. Horan, M. Blaustein, J.B. Dunbar, W. Kachadorian, N.M Kaplan, and A.P. Simopoulos, eds. NIH Workshop on Nutrition and Hypertension: Proceedings from a Symposium. Biomedical Information Corp., New York.

Prior, I.A.M., and J.M. Stanhope. 1980. Blood pressure patterns, salt use and migration in the Pacific. Pp. 243–262 in H. Kesteloot and J.V. Joossens, eds. Epidemiology of Arterial Blood Pressure. Martinus Nijhoff, The Hague.

Rabkin, S.W., F.A. Mathewson, and P.H. Hsu. 1977. Relation of body weight to development of ischemic heart disease in a cohort of young North American men after a 26 year observation period: the Manitoba Study. Am. J. Cardiol. 39:452–458.

Reisin, E., R. Abel, M. Modan, D.S. Silverberg, H.E., Eliahou, and B. Modan. 1978. Effect of weight loss without salt restriction on the reduction of blood pressure in overweight hypertensive patients. N. Engl. J. Med. 298:1–6.

Reunanen, A., H. Takkunen, and A. Aromaa. 1982. Prevalence of intermittent claudication and its effect on mortality. Acta Med. Scand. 211:249–256.

Richelson, L.S., H.W. Wahner, L.J. Melton III, and B.L. Riggs. 1984. Relative contributions of aging and estrogen deficiency to postmenopausal bone loss. N. Engl. J. Med. 311:1273–1275.

Riggs, B.L., H.W. Wahner, W.L. Dunn, R.B. Mazess, K.P. Offord, and L.J. Melton III. 1981. Differential changes in bone mineral density of the appendicular and axial skeleton with aging: relationship to spinal osteoporosis. J. Clin. Invest. 67:328–335.

Riggs, B.L., H.W. Wahner, E. Seeman, K.P. Offord, W.L. Dunn, R.B. Mazess, K.A. Johnson, and L.J. Melton III. 1982. Changes in bone mineral density of the proximal femur and spine with aging. Differences between the postmenopausal and senile osteoporosis syndromes. J. Clin. Invest. 70:716–723.

Roberts, J., and K. Maurer. 1976. Blood Pressure of Persons 6–74 Years of Age in the United States: Advance Data from Vital and Health Statistics of the National Center for Health Statistics, No. 1. Public Health Service, U.S. Department of Health, Education, and Welfare, Rockville, Md. 6 pp.

Robertson, T.L., H. Kato, G.G. Rhodes, A. Kagan, M. Marmot, S.L. Syme, T. Gordon, R.M. Worth, J.L. Belsky, D.S. Dock, M. Miyanishi, and S. Kawamoto. 1977. Epidemiologic studies of coronary heart disease and stroke in Japanese men living in Japan, Hawaii and California: incidence of myocardial infarction and death from coronary heart disease. Am. J. Cardiol. 39:239–243.

Robinson, S.C., and M. Brucer. 1939. Range of normal blood pressure: statistical and clinical study of 11,383 persons. Arch. Intern. Med. 64:409–444.

Rose, G. 1981. Strategy of prevention: lessons from cardiovascular disease. Br. Med. J. 282:1847–1851.

Rose, S.H., L.J. Melton III, B.F. Morrey, D.M. Ilstrup, and B.L. Riggs. 1982. Epidemiologic features of humeral fractures. Clin. Orthop. 168:24–30.

Rubin, E., and C.S. Lieber. 1968. Alcohol-induced hepatic injury in nonalcoholic volunteers. N. Engl. J. Med. 278:869–876.

Rubin, E., and C.S. Lieber. 1974. Fatty liver, alcoholic hepatitis and cirrhosis produced by alcohol in primates. N Engl. J. Med. 290:128–135.

Sampliner, R.E., P.H. Bennett, L.J. Comess, F.A. Rose, and T.A. Burch. 1970. Gallbladder disease in Pima Indians. Demonstration of high prevalence and early onset by cholecystography. N. Engl. J. Med. 283:1358–1364.

Schadt, D.C., E.A. Hines, Jr., J.L. Juergens, and N.W. Barker. 1961. Chronic atherosclerotic occlusion of the femoral artery. J. Am. Med. Assoc. 175:937–940.

Schmidt, W. 1977. Cirrhosis and alcohol consumption: an epidemiological perspective. Pp. 15–47 in G. Edwards and M. Grant, eds. Alcoholism: New Knowledge and New Responses. University Park Press, Baltimore.

Seichter, U. 1987. Root surface caries: a critical literature review. J. Am. Dent. Assoc. 115:305–310.

Seidell, J.C., K.C. Bakx, P. Deurenberg, H.J. van den Hoogen, J.G. Hautvast, and T. Stijnen. 1986. Overweight and chronic illness—a retrospective cohort study, with a follow-up of 6–17 years, in men and women of initially 20–50 years of age. J. Chronic Dis. 39:585–593.

Skog, O.J. 1984. The risk function for liver cirrhosis from lifetime alcohol consumption. J. Stud. Alcohol 45:199–208.

Sloan, N.R. 1963. Ethnic distribution of diabetes mellitus in Hawaii. J. Am. Med. Assoc. 183:419–424.

Smith, R.W., and J. Rizek. 1966. Epidemiologic studies of osteoporosis in women of Puerto Rico and southeastern Michigan with special reference to age, race, national origin and to other related or associated findings. Clin. Orthop. 45:31–48.

Society of Actuaries. 1980. Build Study of 1979. Society of Actuaries and Association of Life Insurance Medical Directors of America, Chicago. 255 pp.

Sognnaes, R.F. 1948. Analysis in wartime reduction of dental caries in European children with special regard to observations in Norway. Am. J. Dis. Child. 75:792–821.

Solberg, L.A., and J.P. Strong. 1983. Risk factors and atherosclerotic lesions. A review of autopsy studies. Arteriosclerosis 3:187–198.

Soltero, I., K. Kiu, R. Cooper, J. Stamler, and D. Garside. 1978. Trends in mortality from cerebrovascular diseases in the United States, 1960 to 1975. Stroke 9:549–555.

Spiegelman, M., and H.H. Marks. 1946. Age and sex variations in the prevalence and onset of diabetes mellitus. Am. J. Public Health 36:26–33.

Sreenby, L.M. 1982. Sugar availability, sugar consumption and dental caries. Community Dent. Oral Epidemiol. 10:1–7.

Stamler, J., D. Berkson, A. Dyer, M.H. Lepper, H.A. Lindberg, O. Paul, H. McKean, P. Rhomberg, J.A. Schoenberger, R.B. Shekelle, and R. Stamler. 1975. Relationship of multiple variables to blood pressure findings from four Chicago epidemiologic studies. Pp. 307–356 in O. Paul, ed.

Epidemiology and Control of Hypertension. Stratton Intercontinental Medical Book Co., New York.

Staszewski, J. 1974. Cancer of the upper alimentary tract and larynx in Poland and in Polish-born Americans. Br. J. Cancer 29:389–399.

Stocks, R. 1954. The etiology of essential hypertension. 1. The arterial pressure in the general population. Clin. Sci. 13:11–35.

Stokes, J., III, R.J. Garrison, and W.B. Kannel. 1985. The independent contributions of various indices of obesity to the 22-year incidence of coronary heart disease: the Framingham Heart Study. Pp. 49–57 in J. Vague, P. Bjorntorp, B. Guy-Grand, and M. Rebuffe-Scrive, eds. Metabolic Complications of Human Obesities. Elsevier, New York.

Strong, J.P., and M.L. Richards. 1976. Cigarette smoking and atherosclerosis in autopsied men. Atherosclerosis 23:451–476.

Stunkard, A.J., T.I.A. Sorensen, C. Hanis, T.W. Teasdale, R. Chakraborty, W.J. Schull, and F. Schulsinger. 1986. An adoption study of human obesity. N. Engl. J. Med. 314:193–198.

Takeuchi, M. 1961. Epidemiologic study on dental caries in Japanese children, before, during and after World War II. Int. Dent. J. 11:443–457.

Takeya, Y., J.S. Popper, Y. Shimizu, H. Kato, G.G. Rhoads, and A. Kagan. 1984. Epidemiologic studies of coronary heart disease and stroke in Japanese men living in Japan, Hawaii and California: incidence of stroke in Japan and Hawaii. Stroke 15:15–23.

Taylor, R., and P. Zimmet. 1983. Migrant studies in diabetes epidemiology. Pp. 58–77 in J.I. Mann, K. Pyorala, and A. Teuscher, eds. Diabetes in Epidemiological Perspective. Churchill Livingstone, Edinburgh.

Terris, M. 1967. Epidemiology of cirrhosis of the liver: national mortality data. Am. J. Public Health 57:2076–2088.

Toverud, G. 1957. The influence of war and post-war conditions on the teeth of Norwegian school children. III. Discussion of food supply and dental condition in Norway and other European countries. Milbank Mem. Fund Q. 35:373–459.

Trotter, M., G.E. Broman, and R.R. Peterson. 1960. Densities of bones of white and negro skeletons. J. Bone Jt. Surg. Am. Vol. 42A:50–58.

Tyroler, H.A., S. Heyden, and C.G. Hames. 1975. Weight and hypertension: Evans County studies of blacks and whites. Pp. 177–204 in O. Paul, ed. Epidemiology and Control of Hypertension. Stratton Intercontinental Medical Book Co., New York.

Ueshima, H., M. Iida, T. Shimamoto, M. Konishi, K. Tsujioka, M. Tanigaki, N. Nakanishi, H. Ozawa, S. Kojima, and Y. Komachi. 1980. Multivariate analysis of risk factors for stroke. Eight-year follow-up study of farming villages in Akita, Japan. Prev. Med. 9:722–740.

Van Itallie, T.B. 1985. Health implications of overweight and obesity in the United States. Ann. Intern. Med. 103:983–988.

Voors, A.W., L.S. Webber, and G.S. Berenson. 1978. Relationship of blood pressure levels to height and weight in children. Cardiovasc. Med. 3:911–918.

Waaler, H.T. 1984. Height, weight and mortality. The Norwegian experience. Acta Med. Scand. 679:1–56.

Wadden, T.A., and A.J. Stunkard. 1985. Social and psychological consequences of obesity. Ann. Intern. Med. 103:1062–1067.

Wallace, W.A. 1983. The increasing incidence of fractures of the proximal femur: an orthopaedic epidemic. Lancet 1:1413–1414.

Waterhouse, J., C. Muir, K. Shanmugaratnam, and J. Powell. 1982. Cancer Incidence in Five Continents, Vol. IV. IARC Scientific Publications No. 42. International Agency for Research on Cancer, Lyon, France. 811 pp.

Weinsier, R.L., D.J. Norris, R. Birch, R.S. Bernstein, J. Wang, M.U. Yang, R.N. Pierson, Jr., and T.B. Van Itallie. 1985. The relative contribution of body fat and fat pattern to blood pressure level. Hypertension 7:578–585.

Weiss, K.M., R.E. Ferrell, C.L. Hanis, and P.N. Styne. 1984. Genetics and epidemiology of gallbladder disease in New World native peoples. Am. J. Hum. Genet. 36:1259–1278.

Welin, L., K. Svärdsudd, L. Wilhelmsen, B. Larsson, and G. Tibblin. 1987. Analysis of risk factors for stroke in a cohort of men born in 1913. N. Engl. J. Med. 317:521–526.

WHO (World Health Organization). 1978. Arterial Hypertension: Report of a WHO Expert Committee. Technical Rep. Ser. 628. World Health Organization, Geneva. 58 pp.

Witkop, C.J., Jr., ed. 1962. Genetics and Dental Health: Proceedings of an International Symposium Held at the National Institutes of Health. McGraw-Hill, New York. 300 pp.

Wu, Y.K., C.Q. Lu, R.C. Gao, J.S. Yu, and G.C. Liu. 1982. Nation-wide hypertension screening in China during 1979–1980. Chin. Med. J. 95:101–108.

Yamase, H., and J.J. McNamara. 1972. Geographic differences in the incidence of gallbladder disease: influence of environment and ethnic background. Am. J. Surg. 123:667–670.

Yano, K., R.D. Wasnich, J.M. Vogel, and L.K. Heilbrun. 1984. Bone mineral measurements among middle-aged and elderly Japanese residents in Hawaii. Am. J. Epidemiol. 119:751–764.

PART II

Evidence on Dietary Components and Chronic Diseases

6

Calories: Total Macronutrient Intake, Energy Expenditure, and Net Energy Stores

Carbohydrates, protein, fats, and alcohol—the dietary macrocomponents—are the sources of energy in the diet. Under normal circumstances, more than 95% of this food energy is digested and absorbed from the gastrointestinal tract to provide the body's energy needs. Studies of normal and overweight subjects have not shown any significant differences in the proportion of food energy absorbed. In some underweight subjects, however, malabsorption of nutrients is an important factor. Food energy is used to meet the body's needs, including protein synthesis; maintenance of body temperature, cardiac output, respiration, and muscle function; and storage and metabolism of food sources of energy. When more energy is consumed than is needed for metabolism and physical activity, the excess is stored, primarily as adipose tissue.

Energy is the capacity to do work. In biologic systems it is usually measured in kilocalories (kcal) or kilojoules (kJ). One kilocalorie (equivalent to 4.184 kJ) is the amount of heat required to raise the temperature of 1 kg of water 1°C (e.g., from 15 to 16°C) at standard atmospheric pressure (760 mm Hg).

Energy balance refers to the relationship of energy intake to energy expenditure and energy storage. Less energy expenditure than energy intake results in a positive energy balance and storage of energy primarily as body fat. Increased fat storage is appropriate during pregnancy and lactation, during some periods of growth and de-

velopment, and during recovery from trauma or malnutrition, but it may not be desirable under other conditions. When energy expenditure exceeds energy intake, energy balance is negative and leads to weight loss. When intake equals expenditure, equilibrium results and body fat is maintained, regardless of whether the body weight is at, above, or below normal. Even at stable body weight, however, the percentage of body fat frequently increases with age unless regular physical activity is maintained. At the same body weight, some sedentary people have relatively more body fat than those who exercise. Thus even at normal weights, these individuals may have more adiposity than desirable.

Prolonged insufficient energy intake results in malnutrition, which is observed in many developing countries and is also a public health concern for a minority of the U.S. population. In most cases, insufficient food intake results from a lack of economic ability to obtain food, from an illness, or from physical or mental disorders that prevent sufficient ingestion or utilization of food to meet energy expenditure, or in some cases from voluntary restriction of food intake and dieting.

ENERGY INTAKE

In general, carbohydrates and fats are completely oxidized in the body. In contrast, protein is

139

only partially oxidized, resulting in the excretion of urea and other nitrogenous products. Oxidation of 1 g of dietary carbohydrate and 1 g of dietary protein (which is oxidized to urea) each yield approximately 4 kcal, whereas oxidation of 1 g of alcohol yields approximately 7 kcal and oxidation of 1 g of dietary fat yields approximately 9 kcal. The energy cost of storing dietary fats as triglycerides is lower than that of converting protein or carbohydrates into fat. Donato and Hegsted (1985) have suggested that in growing animals, dietary fat can be stored as body fat with little energy expenditure and, therefore, that dietary fat stored as adipose tissue fat still yields approximately 9 kcal per gram. In contrast, energy is required to store dietary carbohydrates as body fat and 4 kcal per gram of dietary carbohydrate yields only approximately 3.27 kcal when stored as fat and subsequently oxidized for energy. Therefore, the ratio of the energy required to store dietary fat as body fat relative to the energy cost to store dietary carbohydrates or protein as body fat may be close to 9 to 3.27. That is, the conversion of fats in food to body fat (triglycerides) is more efficient than the conversion of carbohydrates or protein in food to body fat.

Historical Trends

Food disappearance data indicate that energy available in the food supply had not changed from 1909 to 1982, averaging 3,500 kcal/day per person during 1909–1913 and 3,600 kcal/day per person in 1985 (see Table 3–3). However, these amounts are considerably higher than actual intakes reported by individuals (see below). The percentage of total calories available from carbohydrates decreased from 57% during 1909–1913 to 46% in 1985, whereas the proportion from fats increased from 32% during 1909–1913 to 43% in 1985 (see Figure 3–3).

Recent Surveys of Energy Intake

Caloric intake by men and women has been reported in several recent surveys (Beaton et al., 1979; Braitman et al., 1985; Goor et al., 1985; USDA, 1987). Using the 24-hour recall method, Beaton et al. (1979) found that the mean daily energy intake was 2,639 kcal/day for men and 1,793 kcal/day for women. Using data from the National Center for Health Statistics (NCHS), which were based on 24-hour recall, Braitman et al. (1985) reported intakes of 2,359 kcal/day for men and 1,639 kcal/day for women.

Data from the Nationwide Food Consumption Survey (NFCS) can be used to compare energy intakes in 1965 and in 1977. Data from a single 24-hour recall plus 2-day records indicate that the energy intakes of males 9 to 64 years of age in 1977 were 10 to 17% lower than in 1965. Females ages 23 to 50 consumed 8.5 to 9% fewer calories in 1977 than in 1965 (USDA, 1984). The highest intakes were found among younger people. In 1965, males ages 15 to 18 consumed 3,008 kcal/day compared to 2,698 kcal/day in 1977. The highest intake for females in 1965 was 2,146 kcal/day among 12- to 14-year-old girls. This declined to 1,903 kcal/day by 1977. With advancing age, the average caloric intake declines for men and women (Goor et al., 1985). Among 20-year-old men, the intake reported between 1972 and 1978 in the Lipid Research Clinics Prevalence Study (LRC, 1980) ranged from 2,800 to 3,500 kcal/day, but for 59-year-old men, this range was 1,900 to 2,600 kcal/day. Intakes for 20-year-old women during the same period ranged from 2,000 to 2,200 kcal/day. Intakes had fallen to a range of 1,500 to 1,700 kcal/day by age 59. These data suggest that energy intake has declined for both sexes by approximately 10% during the past 10 to 20 years.

Factors Influencing Energy Intake

Caloric intake is influenced by many variables, including age, sex, environmental temperature, energy expenditure, pregnancy, hormonal status, and dieting behaviors. Figure 6–1 shows the effect of age on caloric intake among Americans based on three studies: the NFCS (USDA, 1984), the Health and Nutrition Examination Survey (HANES I), and studies of the Lipid Research Clinics Prevalence Study (Braitman et al., 1985; Goor et al., 1985). For both sexes, caloric intake peaked in the second decade of life and declined thereafter. At all ages, males had higher total caloric intakes than females and higher intakes for all three classes of macronutrients—fats, carbohydrates, and protein.

Caloric intake is also modestly affected by environmental temperature: at high and low ambient temperature, energy intake increases. Energy expenditure also affects caloric intake. For example, long-distance runners have high caloric intakes. More moderate levels of physical activity may increase food intake by lean but not by obese subjects. In controlled metabolic ward studies, Woo et al. (1985) compared the effect of three levels of physical expenditure on food intake by

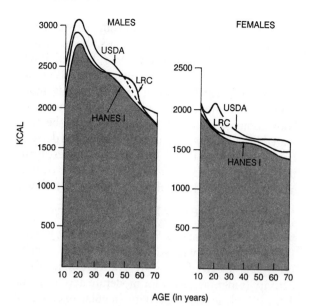

FIGURE 6-1 Relationship of caloric intake to age for males and females. Based on data from three studies—the Lipid Research Clinics Prevalence Study (LRC, 1980), the Nationwide Food Consumption Survey of the U.S. Department of Agriculture (USDA, 1980), and the Health and Nutrition Examination Survey (HANES I) of the National Center for Health Statistics (Carroll et al., 1983).

normal-weight and obese subjects. They noted that as energy expenditure was increased by increasing the time spent in physical activity, lean women increased their food intake in proportion to the increase in energy expenditure. Obese women, on the other hand, did not (Woo et al., 1985).

During pregnancy, a new life with its own energy stores is created. Thus, it is usually suggested that pregnant women should increase their food intake (NRC, 1980). Recent measurements from several countries indicate that increases in energy needs and food intake during pregnancy may be less than previously suggested (Durnin, 1986). (See section on Pregnancy, below, under Energy Balance in Special Situations.)

ENERGY EXPENDITURE

Measurement of Energy Expenditure

Energy expenditure can be measured in a variety of ways (McLean and Tobin, 1988). In the classic procedure, a calorimeter is used to measure heat production. In direct calorimetry, heat produced is measured as temperature changes through thermal gradients or as heat added to the ambient environment in an insulated chamber. Indirect calorimetry can be used to determine energy expenditure by measuring oxygen consumption and carbon dioxide production (e.g., in ventilated hoods) and then relating these measurements to the energy value of the oxygen consumed and the carbon dioxide produced. In ambulatory subjects, energy expenditure can be measured indirectly by collecting samples of expired air in which oxygen consumption and carbon dioxide production are determined and related to work activity. A recently developed technique is the use of doubly labelled water ($^2H_2^{18}O$ or $D_2^{18}O$) for measuring energy expenditure in ambulatory subjects. The heavy oxygen (^{18}O) can be incorporated into carbon dioxide $C^{18}O_2$ during metabolism or excreted as water ($H_2^{18}O$). Deuterium, on the other hand, can only be excreted as water (D_2O). Thus the rate at which ^{18}O declines relative to the decline in deuterium is a measurement of metabolic rate. This method holds promise for resolving issues related to the stoichiometry of energy expenditure and intake in ambulatory subjects (Lifson, 1966; Schoeller et al., 1986).

Other methods of estimating energy expenditure include diaries of physical activity, which are widely used in epidemiologic studies, and measurement of heart rate, because it varies directly with activity level. However, basal heart rate is a poor index of resting energy expenditure.

Components of Energy Expenditure

Energy expenditure can be subdivided into resting metabolic rate (RMR), thermic effects of food, physical activity, and growth. RMR is the quantity of energy needed to maintain body temperature, repair internal organs, support cardiac function, maintain ionic gradients across cells, and support respiration. This constitutes approximately two-thirds of total energy expenditure. The second largest component of energy expenditure is required for physical work. The energy expenditure required to move the body is related directly to body weight, to the distance that weight is moved, and to the state of physical fitness.

The heat produced following ingestion of a meal is usually termed the thermic effect of food (TEF) or diet-induced thermogenesis (DIT). (It was formerly called specific dynamic action.) This effect can be produced by any food, but the consumption of protein or carbohydrates results in much larger thermic effects than does consumption of fat.

There is an adaptive component to energy expenditure (adaptative thermogenesis). An acute large increase or decrease in energy intake lasting more than a few days is accompanied by a corresponding change in total energy expenditure. Thus, the overall RMR decreases during food restriction or starvation and increases with overfeeding; this may act in a counterregulatory way to decrease energy loss (Forbes, 1987; Garrow, 1978; Woo et al., 1985).

Historical Trends

The transition from an agricultural economy to a manufacturing economy and more recently to an information-gathering sedentary society has been associated with a steady decline in energy intake, presumably because of decreased caloric expenditure. Average energy intake has been used as a surrogate measurement for energy expenditure, since it is assumed that over time, individuals are in energy balance. Between 1965 and 1977, average caloric intake for all people dropped from 2,060 to 1,865 kcal/day. Protein intake dropped from 81.5 to 75.5 g/day, fat intake decreased from 99.3 to 85.3 g/day, and carbohydrates, from 209.8 to 195.7 g/day (USDA, 1984). In 1985, the mean daily energy intake by women over 4 days was 1,528 kcal (USDA, 1987). There are no direct surveys of trends in energy expenditure.

Factors Influencing Energy Expenditure

Resting energy expenditure is influenced by age, sex, body weight, pregnancy, and hormonal status. The highest rates of energy expenditure per unit of body weight occur during infancy and decline through childhood. In adult life, the decline continues at approximately 2% per decade because of a decline in lean body mass. Females have a lower energy expenditure per unit of weight than do males, probably because of the higher proportion of body fat in women. When expressed on the basis of fat-free mass, however, the differences between men and women and younger and older adults disappear. Resting energy expenditure is directly related to body weight and fat-free mass in men as well as women. People with high body weight on average also have high resting energy expenditure. Pregnancy increases energy expenditure to support fetal growth and the increase in maternal tissues. Several hormones, including thyroxin, catecholamines, and insulin, also increase energy expenditure.

Obese people have a modestly, but significantly, higher 24-hour energy expenditure than do normal-weight subjects (James, 1983). There is a positive and significant relationship between energy expenditure and fat-free mass, body surface area, or body weight (Garrow, 1978; Jequier, 1984; Owen et al., 1986, 1987; Ravussin et al., 1988; de Boer et al., 1987). Since body weight is more readily determined than specific components of body composition, basal energy needs can be estimated from body weight using the formulas derived by Owen et al. (1986, 1987). One can estimate total energy needs from an assessment of overall activity level (high, moderate, or low) as follows:

Basal energy needs = RMR × activity factor,

where RMR for men is $900 + 10 \times$ body weight (kg) and for women is $800 + 7 \times$ body weight (kg), and activity factors are 1.2 for low levels of activity (sedentary), 1.4 for moderate activity, and 1.6 for high levels of activity (regular exercise or manual labor).

The data of Bogardus et al. (1986) and Bouchard and his colleagues (1986) have shown a significant genetic component for resting metabolic rate (Fontaine et al., 1985) and endurance performance, although there is less evidence of a heredity effect on maximal oxygen consumption (VO_2 max) (Bouchard et al., 1986). This suggests that important genetic determinants influence metabolic activity. For example, a decreased metabolic rate may predict the onset of weight gain in some adults (Ravussin et al., 1988) and infants (Roberts et al., 1988).

Using time-lapse motion pictures, Bullen et al. (1964) showed lower levels of physical activity in obese as compared to nonobese adolescents swimming or playing volleyball or tennis. Others, however, have found little difference between the activity level of obese and control subjects (Stefanik et al., 1959; Tryon, 1987; Wilkinson et al., 1977). Brownell et al. (1980) observed that when confronted with a choice between escalators and stairs, more lean than obese subjects used the stairs.

Several, but not all, studies suggest that obese people are less physically active; however, to interpret this observation as an indication that obese subjects expend less energy, one must know the energy cost of the activity. Since overweight people must do more physical work to move their bodies, smaller total amounts of movements may add up to comparable or greater total energy expenditure.

Waxman and Stunkard (1980) compared activity levels of lean and obese boys within the same families. In this setting, total energy expenditure, when corrected for energy costs for specific activities, was comparable between the paired individuals. Bray (1983) observed that the efficiency of energy expenditure in muscles of obese and lean subjects is comparable, but because the obese subjects carry more weight, their total energy expenditure may be higher. One important difference in energy expenditure among individuals may be the extent and degree of fidgeting. Bogardus et al. (1986) in their studies of the Pima Indians observed important differences between different groups of people in the amount of time spent in fidgeting when they were studied in a metabolic chamber.

The efficiency of energy transfer from foods to adenosine triphosphate (ATP) and of ATP utilization may also influence energy needs. In some forms of obesity, the obese may be more efficient than lean subjects in utilizing nutrients for resting metabolic requirements and, thus, may have more energy to store as fat (Sims et al., 1973). A number of mechanisms have been suggested for this metabolic efficiency, including reduced sodium pump activity, lower protein turnover, altered nutrient partitioning, faulty thermogenic mediation by the sympathetic nervous system, impaired function of brown adipose tissue, and reduced efficiency of muscular contraction (Bray, 1983). The thermogenic effect of a meal usually amounts to approximately 10% of the caloric value of the ingested food (Jequier, 1984) and is higher for carbohydrates and protein than for fats. It may also differ with the type of food eaten (Forbes, 1987). It is not known if such thermogenesis is higher in obese people, but energy requirements do appear to decrease with weight loss (Geissler et al., 1987; Leibel and Hirsch, 1984). A number of biochemical changes, including alterations in oxygen consumption, increased lipoprotein lipase (LPL) levels in adipose tissue, and altered pancreatic insulin kinetics, have been demonstrated in the first week of life in genetically obese rodents, but definitive biochemical lesions have yet to be found in humans. There is increasing evidence, however, that metabolic mechanisms relevant to efficiency play a role in human energy balance as well.

ENERGY BALANCE

Measurement of Body Fat

Body fat is the primary energy store in humans. Because direct chemical analysis of fat is impossible in living human beings, indirect methods have been developed to assess body composition and thus measure body fat. These methods are summarized below. Anthropometric methods are noninvasive, are quick, and require inexpensive equipment. They include measurements of height, weight, body circumferences, body diameters, and skinfold thickness. The coefficient of variation for height and weight is very small (1 to 2%) but is greater for the other measures: 5 to 10% for circumferences and up to 20% for skinfold thickness of obese individuals, whose skinfolds are often too thick to be measured with commonly used calipers (Bray et al., 1978). Many equations have been developed for estimating body fat from measurements of skinfold thickness at one or more sites. These equations are usually influenced by the sex, age, and ethnic group from which they were developed. Skinfolds have frequently been used in epidemiologic studies of normal populations, but their limitations must be kept in mind. In general, circumference measures are less subject to investigator bias and are more helpful in assessing both total body fat and fat distribution.

Measurement of body density is one of the better and most widely accepted methods for estimating total body fat and is often used as the reference standard. By determining body weight in air and under water, and correcting for lung volume, the body can be subdivided into its fat and fat-free compartments. It is assumed that the density of the fat-free compartment does not vary, but this assumption may require modification for children, well-trained athletes, and the elderly. Various radioactive materials (^3H_2O, ^{40}K, ^{82}Br, ^{24}Na) and nonradioactive substances (stable isotopes, cyclopropane, krypton, and antipyrine) can also be used to estimate body compartments; several recent methods have extended the range of tools available for taking these measurements.

Following is a list of techniques used to determine body composition:

Direct Carcass Analysis

Indirect Analysis of Body Composition
- Visual Observation (somatotypes)
- Anthropomorphic Measurements
  Height and Weight
  Circumferences and Diameters
  Skinfold Thicknesses
- Isotope or Chemical Dilution
  Body Water (^3H_2O, antipyrine)
  Body Potassium (^{40}K, ^{42}K)
  Body Fat (cyclopropane, krypton)

- Body Density and Body Volume
- Conductivity
  Total Body Electrical Conductivity (TOBEC)
  Bioelectric Impedance Analysis (BIA)
- Neutron Activation
- Imaging Techniques
  Ultrasound
  Computed Tomography (CT)
  Nuclear Magnetic Resonance Spectroscopy
  (NMRS)

Using the differences in electrical conductivity between water and fat, one can estimate the fat and nonfat compartments by TOBEC or BIA. The latter method is likely to be particularly useful (Segal et al., 1988), since it correlates highly with body fat estimated by density and it is highly reproducible between laboratories. The thickness of fat can be measured with ultrasound, CT (Sjöström et al., 1986), and magnetic resonance imaging. All these methods can be used to assess body fat as a function of body weight as well as its regional and intraabdominal distribution.

As noted in Chapter 21, it is not only the total quantity of fat (high or low) that is associated with health risks but also the location of fat. Abdominal or central body fat carries a higher risk of coronary heart disease (CHD), diabetes mellitus, hypertension, stroke, endometrial cancer in women, and overall mortality compared to peripheral or lower-body gluteal fat. This risk can be assessed by determining the ratio of abdominal-to-gluteal circumference or by the ratio of central-to-peripheral skinfolds.

The Association of Caloric Intake with Body Weight and Energy Stores

Epidemiologic Data

There is little question that changes in food intake can produce corresponding changes in body weight (Bray, 1976; Forbes, 1987; Garrow, 1978). Increased body fatness during adult life has been observed with increasing frequency during this century. This appears to be associated primarily with a reduction in physical activity and a corresponding reduction in lean body mass. An increase in energy intake may also be associated with this phenomenon.

In studies of Army recruits, Edholm et al. (1970) observed a wide range of daily variations in food intake among normal-weight individuals. However, he also showed a correlation between energy intake and expenditure over 7 days. There was an intraindividual correlation between intake and expenditure only over periods longer than 7 days. Body composition and physical activity have been examined in "big eaters" and "small eaters" who have similar levels of fat-free mass. Male big eaters consumed 48.8 kcal per kilogram of body weight per day (204 kJ/kg per day) compared to 19.8 kcal/kg per day (83 kJ/kg per day) for the small eaters. Body fat, on the other hand, was 31.5% in the small eaters and 21.1% in the large eaters (George, in press).

In several cross-sectional studies, overweight subjects have often been found to eat the same or smaller amounts of food compared to normal-weight subjects (Baecke et al., 1983; Braitman et al., 1985; Keen et al., 1979; Kromhout, 1983b; Lincoln, 1972; Noppa, 1980; Romieu et al., 1988). (See Table 6–1.) In all cases, except the study of "research patients" by Beaudoin and Mayer (1953), the mean intake by the overweight subjects was less than that of the controls (for details on the control groups, see footnotes to Table 6–1). In the studies of females alone, this difference was statistically significant, but it was only significant in one of three studies of men. Keen et al. (1979) also found a negative correlation between energy intake and body mass index. Romieu et al. (1988) reported that obese women tended to be older, to exercise less, and to drink less alcohol than younger women. After correcting for these variables, the inverse correlation between energy intake and relative weight was significantly reduced from $R = -.11$ to $R = -.02$, showing almost no correlation between these two variables. Of particular interest is that in the obese women there was a positive correlation between relative weight and total fat intake as well with the intake of saturated fat.

These cross-sectional findings have been confirmed in longitudinal studies (Kromhout, 1983a; Lapidus et al., 1986). In a cohort study of 871 men in Zutphen, the Netherlands, energy intake decreased approximately 450 kcal/day over a 10-year period, during which body weight increased by 3.5 kg (Kromhout, 1983a). Food intake has declined over the past decade when body weight and presumably fat stores have, on average, increased. From the epidemiologic data, it appears that increased caloric intake in the population cannot explain the positive energy balance observed in adult life in the United States, the Netherlands, or Sweden.

Clinical Data

The clinical data on the effect of over- and undereating on changes in fat stores clearly show that overeating can increase body fat stores,

TABLE 6–1 Caloric Intake of Overweight and Normal-Weight (Control) Subjects

Control Subjects			Overweight Subjects				
N	Sex	(kcal/day)	N	Sex	(kcal/day)	p	Reference
58[a]	F	2,198±587[b]	59	F	1,964±594[b]	<.05	Beaudoin and Mayer (1953)
20[c]	F	2,201±475[b]	33	F	2,829±674[b]	<.01	
98[d]	M&F	3,319	101	M&F	3,144	NS[e]	Lincoln (1972)
47[f]	M	3,070±105[b]	27	M	2,983±167[b]	NS	Baecke et al. (1983)
50	F	2,280±65[b]	45	F	2,045± 64[b]	<.05	
202[g]	M	3,193±606[b]	202	M	2,916±652[b]	<.001	Kromhout (1983b)
708[h]	M	2,359	79	M	2,411	NS	Braitman et al. (1985)
1,246	F	1,639	245	F	1,525	<.001	
45[i]	F	1,684±315[j]	47	F	1,635±340[j]	NS	Romieu et al. (1988)

[a]A population-based study in New York.
[b]Mean±SEM.
[c]Women before pregnancy.
[d]An industrial population that responded to a questionnaire.
[e]NS = not significant.
[f]A young Dutch population; comparison of the lowest and highest quartile.
[g]Middle-aged Dutch men; comparison of the lowest and highest quartile.
[h]National Center for Health Statistics data comparing people <101% of optimum weight with those >149% optimum weight.
[i]Nurses Health Study comparing lowest and highest tertiles.
[j]Mean±SD.

whereas undereating can result in a decrease of body fat stores. (See Chapter 21 for details.)

Animal Studies

There are sex-specific responses to the effects of voluntarily increased food intake by animals. In general, female animals respond to calorie-dense diets with an increased intake and a higher percent increment of body fat than males (Jen et al., 1981). Whether this effect is related to the increment in total caloric intake or to the amount or type of fat in the diet is presently unclear. In pregnant and lactating animals of most species, food intake increases voluntarily during the latter part of pregnancy and throughout lactation. In animal studies, these are among the few times when increased voluntary intake of the usual diet occurs. During pregnancy, food efficiency—i.e., weight gained per gram of food eaten—is also enhanced. Much of the weight gain in later pregnancy is associated with growth of the fetus; during early pregnancy, the enhanced metabolic efficiency contributes to fat accumulation, which is regionally specific (in either the inguinal or omental region). One of the few natural examples of increased voluntary food intake with decreasing or stabilized weight gain is noted during lactation. Under these conditions, the nearly doubled or tripled caloric intake is utilized primarily for milk synthesis to supply the lactational demands of the suckling young. At the end of lactation, despite the large increase in food intake, the body fat stores of the rat are reduced below prepregnant and prelactating levels.

In spontaneously obese mutants, particularly among rodents, hyperphagia is a correlate of obesity. Thus, it appears that overeating is an important feature of the obesity; however, obesity in these mutants cannot be attributed solely to increased total caloric intake. Pair-feeding of the obese or preobese animal to a lean control leads to a reduction in the body weight of these spontaneously obese rodents but has little effect on body composition (Cleary et al., 1980; Cox and Powley, 1977). That is, genetically obese animals pair-fed to lean controls maintain as much as 60% body fat compared to 20% in lean animals of equivalent body weight. Thus, obesity in normal animals is induced primarily by overingestion, whereas in genetically obese animal models, hyperphagia is not a prerequisite for obesity.

Association Between Energy Expenditure and Net Energy Stores

Epidemiologic Data

Changes in net energy stores are a sensitive indicator of the relationship between energy intake and expenditure. The increase in body fat stores with age indicates imbalance. Since the data show that energy intake declines with age in adults, the most probable explanation is that energy expenditure declines as people grow older (Kromhout, 1983a).

Clinical Data

Physical exercise may reduce the total quantity of body fat and body weight. In a review of training programs lasting from 7 to 22 weeks, Wilmore (1983) found that changes in body composition were surprisingly small. On average, body fat decreased by only 1.6%, and in 5 of 55 studies there was actually an increase in body fat after training. Moreover, lean body mass dropped in 17 of these 55 studies.

A decrease in body fat after exercise can be demonstrated more readily in moderately obese subjects than in normal-weight subjects. In 12 studies of overweight men and women, the mean decrease in body weight ranged from 2.6 to 13.3 kg, most of which was accounted for by a decrease in body fat. In contrast to data on moderately obese people, a reduction in body fat after physical training is difficult to demonstrate in massively obese subjects. Frequently, this can be attributed to the fact that only modest amounts of weight are lost. Thus, the decrease in fat may not be readily detectable. Reduction in body fat content during physical training is accompanied by a decrease in the average size of fat cells. People with larger fat cells (hypertrophic obesity) may lose more fat during exercise program than those with a larger number of relatively small fat cells (Krotkiewski et al., 1977).

Both acute exercise and prolonged physical training modify the metabolism of glucose, insulin, and lipids in obese and normal subjects. During physical training, glucose tolerance is improved and insulin levels decrease, suggesting reduced resistance to insulin. Exercise by normal-weight subjects can be associated with an increase in levels of high-density lipoproteins (HDLs). In obese people, however, changes in lipid metabolism that occur with exercise are more complex (Bray and Gray, 1988).

Obesity is usually associated with reduced levels of HDL cholesterol. Brownell et al. (1982) reported that a 10.7 kg weight loss in men was associated with a 5% increase in HDL cholesterol, a 15.8% decrease in low-density lipoprotein (LDL) cholesterol, and, thus, a 30% increase in the ratio of HDL to LDL cholesterol. In women, on the

other hand, a weight loss of 8.9 kg produced no change in HDL cholesterol.

Animal Studies

The concept that some cases of obesity result from an energy imbalance related primarily to decreased caloric expenditure rather than to increased caloric intake has received much attention over the past decade. In rats spontaneously ingesting a cafeteria diet (mixed human food), thermogenesis increased to compensate for increased food intake (Stock and Rothwell, 1981). There has been considerable debate in the literature concerning the basis of this effect. Since many of these studies were conducted in rodents that possess brown adipose tissue (which is highly thermogenic), Himms-Hagen (1985) examined the ability of brown adipose tissue to uncouple the mitochondrial proton conductance pathway and thus to produce heat without producing equivalents for ATP synthesis. The effects on thermogenesis may be related to dietary effects on the sympathetic nervous system, which in turn may be related to other potentially thermogenic effects in tissues such as liver and muscle. This area requires further research.

It has been well demonstrated in several species of normally lean animals (males, not females) that increased physical activity in the absence of increased caloric intake leads to a decrease in body weight and a change in body composition. The amount of caloric expenditure is proportional to these effects. In addition, spontaneous or genetic inter- and intraspecies effects on RMR may underlie the animals' responsiveness to exercise. The concept has been advanced that there is a set point—a weight level that is maintained within a small margin—that regulates energy balance in animals. In support of this concept, Boyle et al. (1978), Keesey (1980), and Keesey and Powley (1986) have proposed that caloric consumption can be predicted from RMR. (See also Kleiber, 1947.)

Some investigators have reasoned that a thermogenic defect in genetically obese or experimentally manipulated obese animals provides evidence that defective themogenesis plays a role in the genesis of obesity (Himms-Hagen, 1985). In fact, genetically obese adult rodents of several species exhibit decreased overall thermogenesis, diet-induced thermogenesis, and poor responsiveness to cold. In addition, there is frequently decreased guanosine 5'-diphosphate (GDP) binding in their brown adipose tissue (Himms-Hagen, 1985); how-

TABLE 6-2 Energy Expenditure During Pregnancy in Four Different Countries[a]

Source of Energy Expenditure	Energy Cost (kcal)			
	Scotland	Holland	Thailand	Philippines
Fetus	8,110	8,230	7,140	6,900
Placenta	730	740	600	600
Uterus and blood volume	2,890	2,950	2,480	2,410
Maternal fat	25,230	14,300	15,400	14,300
Basal metabolic rate	30,100	34,500	24,000	19,000
TOTAL	67,060	60,720	49,620	43,210

[a]Adapted from Durnin (1986).

ever, extirpation of brown adipose tissue does not promote the development of obesity (Horwitz et al., 1985), and proliferation of such tissue as a consequence of exposure to cold does not promote leanness (Miller and Faust, 1982). In at least some species, alterations in body fat content clearly precede any changes in the metabolism of brown adipose tissue (Greenwood et al., 1981). In obese animals, alterations in substrate utilization lead to alterations in body composition (i.e., increased fatness and decreased lean tissue) and may reduce the thermogenic contribution of skeletal and other muscle tissue. Thus, it is not clear how thermogenic defects per se may contribute to the etiology of obesity, but it is becoming evident that they may be important factors to delineate in order to understand different types of obesity.

Energy Balance in Special Situations

As noted earlier in this chapter, positive energy balance occurs normally during growth and pregnancy. During lactation, food energy increases as does energy expenditure. This results in negative energy balance.

Periods of Rapid Growth

Estimated nutrient requirements for human growth are 117 kcal/kg body weight at 0 to 0.5 year of age, 108 kcal/kg at 0.5 to 1.0 year, and 1,300 kcal at 1 to 3 years (NRC, 1980). It is not yet possible to precisely specify the macronutrient composition of this caloric requirement. The best indication that an infant is growing properly is normal linear growth.

Energy requirements peak during adolescence—a time of rapid growth and changes in body composition. The adolescent growth spurt begins at about 10 years of age in girls and at about 12 years of age in boys. Energy requirements increase to support this rapid rate of growth. In boys,

estimated energy intake is 2,500 to 3,200 kcal/day between the ages of 10 and 20. Girls between the ages of 10 and 20 require an estimated 1,800 to 2,000 kcal/day (see Figure 6-1).

Pregnancy

The amounts of extra energy intake recommended during pregnancy vary from 240 to 285 kcal/day and are based on the classic calculations of Hytten and Leitch (1971). In a recent multinational study, Durnin (1986) reexamined these assumptions using measurements of changing body weight and basal metabolic rate during pregnancy. The energy cost of pregnancy from data on four countries in that study is shown in Table 6-2. All the values in the table are lower than the 80,000 kcal calculated by Hytten and Leitch (1971). The most unexpected finding by Durnin (1986) was that food intake increased little or not at all during pregnancy, suggesting that much of the net energy needed for pregnancy comes from altered metabolic efficiency.

Lactation

Approximately 900 kcal of energy are required to produce 1 liter of milk in women. The 2 to 4 kg of body fat that are stored during pregnancy can be mobilized to supply a portion of the additional energy needed for lactation. Additional energy needs during the first 3 months of lactation are derived by ingesting an additional 500 kcal/day.

The Elderly

Studies in several countries show that energy intake declines with advancing age (Figure 6-1). In a cross-sectional study of 20- to 93-year-old male executives in Baltimore, McGandy et al. (1966) found a steady decline in energy intake from 2,700 kcal/day at 30 years to 2,100 kcal/day at 80 years. Approximately 200 kcal of this decline was due to the decrease of lean body mass with advancing age; the remaining 400 kcal appears to be due to a decline in physical activity. The second National Health and Nutrition Examination Survey (NHANES II) showed that men reduce their daily energy intake from 2,700 kcal at 23 to 24 years of age to 1,800 kcal at 65 to 74 years and that women reduce their daily energy consumption from 1,600 kcal to 1,300 kcal over the same period (Carroll et al., 1983). The NFCS indicated that elderly men averaged 1,700 kcal/day, whereas elderly women averaged 1,330 kcal (USDA, 1980). The energy requirements estimated in the Food and Nutrition Board's *Recommended Dietary Allowances* for a 70-kg man are 2,400 kcal at 51 to 75 years and 2,050 for those over 75 years. For 55-kg women, the requirements are 1,800 and 1,600 kcal, respectively, for the same age groups (NRC, 1980). These estimated requirements are well above the measured values noted above. It is possible that the RDAs are too high or that elderly people are inactive.

EVIDENCE ASSOCIATING TOTAL ENERGY INTAKE WITH CHRONIC DISEASES

Atherosclerotic Cardiovascular Diseases

Epidemiologic Studies

The relationship of total energy intake to cardiovascular diseases has been examined in several studies. Subjects who develop heart disease have a history of lower total caloric intake on the average compared to those who remain free of the disease (Gordon et al., 1981). In the Honolulu Heart Study, crude caloric intake and the intake of 8 of 11 other nutrients were lower for those who subsequently developed CHD; for the remaining three nutrients, there were no associations with CHD (Willett and Stampfer, 1986). The authors proposed expressing the data in the form of the nutrient density of caloric intake. "Because coronary heart disease is associated with low caloric intake, nutrient density expressed as a percentage of total calories will tend to be positively associated with disease" (Willett and Stampfer, 1986, p. 21). However, for some nutrients there may be a negative association with CHD, and for others there may be no association. When this approach was used, the ratio of specific nutrients to total calories was positive for protein and for total, saturated, and monounsaturated fats but was negative for carbohydrates.

In the Göteborg longitudinal study, Lapidus et al. (1986) reported that energy intake was inversely correlated with death from all causes and with several variables, including age, systolic blood pressure, body mass index, and ratio of waist-to-hip circumference. Percentage of energy intake derived from fats was positively correlated with serum triglycerides. Although there was a negative relationship between energy intake and risk of myocardial infarction, there was no correlation between energy intake and 12-year overall mortality from or incidence of stroke. Energy intake was also inversely correlated with the risk of myocardial infarction when such factors as obesity, smoking habits, serum cholesterol concentration, serum triglyceride concentration, diabetes, systolic blood pressure, and physical activity were taken into account.

Clinical Studies

In studies of experimental overfeeding, Sims and his colleagues (1973) demonstrated an increase in plasma triglycerides, insulin, and glucose. These same factors are observed to change during spontaneous alterations in body weight (Ashley and Kannel, 1974). A reduction in food intake by obese subjects under experimental conditions is associated with a marked decrease in triglycerides and an initial reduction in serum total cholesterol, which may subsequently increase even though caloric intake remains reduced (Henry et al., 1986).

Therefore, although a direct relationship of total caloric intake with morbidity and mortality cannot be shown in population studies, it is possible to demonstrate that several salient cardiovascular disease risk factors can be manipulated in individuals by changing their overall caloric intake. In general, many studies have shown that short-term weight loss—however achieved—results in lowered blood lipids except for HDL cholesterol, which is increased, and lowered blood pressure, blood glucose, and insulin levels.

Animal Studies

In animals, it has been difficult to demonstrate any specific effect of total calories, other than their contribution to body weight and body composition as a correlate of cardiovascular diseases. Several species of animals with high levels of body fat have high cardiovascular risk indices. Although increased caloric intake in laboratory animals leads to increased adiposity, most of the effects of diet on cardiovascular risk factors, such as altered plasma lipid profiles, stroke, and hypertension, have been attributed to changes in the macronutrient composition of the diet rather than to the increments in total calories (see Chapter 7). In addition, overingestion, especially of carbohydrates, leads to increased blood insulin levels. This in turn leads to increased norepinephrine turnover in several tissues (Young and Landsberg, 1977), which may have direct effects on adipose tissue blood flow and blood pressure. Thus, increased total caloric intake by obese and nonobese animals may alter hemodynamics and blood pressure and may influence the development of hypertension.

In the spontaneously hypertensive rat (SHR), decreased overall caloric intake resulted in lower blood pressure, whereas overfeeding elevated it (Young and Landsberg, 1977). However, this effect may be related more to the intake of sucrose than to total caloric intake, since equicaloric intake of high-fat diets did not provoke the same response in the sympathetic nervous system. Furthermore, even moderate caloric restriction frequently can effect changes in blood pressure or blood lipids in animals already identified as being at risk.

Diabetes Mellitus

Epidemiologic Studies

Decreased death rates from diabetes were observed during World War I in Berlin, Paris, and London but not in New York or Tokyo (Himsworth, 1935). During World War II, there was a drop in the incidence of diabetes in Japan (Goto et al., 1958). After both wars, the incidence of and mortality from diabetes returned to prewar levels as caloric intake increased.

In contrast to the decline in diabetes incidence observed in epidemiologic studies of starvation, evidence that total caloric intake is related to the development of noninsulin-dependent diabetes mellitus (NIDDM) within a population with adequate supplies of food is weak. Himsworth (1935) analyzed dietary intakes in several countries and found that those with the highest death rates tended to have a relatively low proportion of dietary fats. Whether caloric intake, independent of obesity, plays a role in the development of NIDDM is unclear. West and Kalbfleisch (1971) established that there is a strong relationship between the prevalence of diabetes and relative weight, but they could not show a relationship with total caloric intake. Acculturation is often associated with a change in the quality of the diet

and with an increased incidence of diabetes, obesity, hypertension, and heart disease. Physical activity is also often reduced during acculturation, further confounding the interpretation of the relationship between diet and chronic diseases. In a cross-sectional study, Japanese living in Hiroshima have been compared with those who migrated to Hawaii (Kawate et al., 1979). Obesity was approximately seven times more prevalent among those living in Hawaii, and the incidence of diabetes was nearly double. The total quantity of calories consumed by these two groups did not differ, although more fats and more simple carbohydrates were consumed by those living in Hawaii. Over a 5-year period, investigators conducting the Israeli Heart Study also failed to find a relationship between energy intake and the risk of developing NIDDM (Medalie et al., 1975). In summary, there is no evidence to indicate that total caloric intake is related to the onset of NIDDM.

Clinical Studies

Restriction of caloric intake in both inpatient and outpatient settings improves glucose tolerance in most obese people (Arky, 1976). This effect and the detrimental consequences of subsequent weight regain were clearly shown by Drenick et al. (1972). (See Chapter 21 for more detail.)

Metabolic pathways, including those concerned with glucose metabolism, can be disturbed by overeating. Sims et al. (1973) found that glucose levels following an oral glucose load were higher after weight gain in normal-weight volunteers. Insulin was also slightly increased and associated with the development of insulin resistance in adipose tissue. These deleterious effects of forced overeating were reversed with weight loss.

Animal Studies

There is no evidence that total caloric intake is a cause of either NIDDM or insulin-dependent diabetes mellitus (IDDM) in animals (Glinsmann et al., 1986). However, there is little question that when animals increase their total food intake they develop adiposity (see Animal Studies subsection of The Relationship of Caloric Intake to Body Weight and Energy Stores, above), and adiposity is usually associated with the development of insulin resistance (Stern et al., 1975; Susini and Lavau, 1978). Accompanying the insulin resistance and impaired glucose tolerance are impaired pancreatic responses to oral glucose tolerance tests and hyperglycemia. Nonetheless, frank diabetes with marked hyperglycemia and glycosuria is rarely found in studies of animals in which increased total caloric intake is used as the variable. Even studies that focus on overingestion of specific nutrients, such as simple sugars, can often be criticized for failing to include pair-fed controls or for feeding the nutrient at levels unlikely to be encountered by humans or animals.

The metabolic responses associated with increased total caloric intake usually appear only after a long period of overeating. Thus, in addition to the associated adiposity, findings in many animal models of diet-induced diabetes are further confounded by the effects of aging inherent in most long-term feeding studies. In most cases, weight reduction and restoration of a more normal body composition reverse the effects of increased caloric intake on insulin resistance. Thus, it becomes exceedingly difficult to identify any specific effect of calories, independent of the effects on overall adiposity, on the development of diabetes.

There are several genetic models of both NIDDM and IDDM, for example, the female Yucatan miniature swine (Phillips et al., 1982), a strain of spiny mouse (*Acomy cahirihup*) (Obell, 1974), the desert sand rat (Kalderon et al., 1986; Rice and Robertson, 1980), and the Wistar fatty rat (WDF/Ta-*fa/fa*) (see Chapter 24 and Salans and Graham, 1982, for further details). Although there is some evidence that overingestion of specific nutrients may enhance (Kava et al., 1989) or provoke (Ikeda et al., 1981) the incipient diabetic condition and exacerbate specific pathologies, there is little evidence that the condition depends upon hyperphagia. One exception to this general statement is the development of diabetes in the sand rat. This strain of rat normally remains lean and nondiabetic in the wild, but when housed under laboratory conditions, it becomes hyperphagic and diabetic (Salans and Graham, 1982).

Cancer

Epidemiologic Studies

As reviewed in detail by the National Research Council's Committee on Diet, Nutrition, and Cancer (NRC, 1982), few investigators have specifically studied the association of total caloric intake with cancer risk. Different results were obtained in three case-control studies of colorectal cancer—one in Canada (Jain et al., 1980), one in Australia (Potter and McMichael, 1986), and one in Belgium (Tuyns et al., 1987). A higher caloric intake by cancer patients than by controls was reported in the Canadian and Australian studies,

but the opposite was found in the Belgian study. A recent reanalysis of the Canadian data (Howe et al., 1986) very clearly indicates that the risk in this study was associated with total fat and saturated fat intake for both males and females and that the relative risks associated with caloric intake were very close to unity.

In earlier studies, Gregor et al. (1969) concluded that as the per-capita food intake for gross national products increases, the mortality rates for gastric cancers fall and those for intestinal cancer rise. Lew and Garfinkel (1979) examined the relationship between mortality from cancer and other diseases and variations in weight among 750,000 men and women selected from the general population. Cancer mortality was significantly elevated in both sexes only among those 40% or more overweight. (See NRC for a detailed analysis of this and other studies up to 1981.)

Animal Studies

The early studies of Tannenbaum (1947, 1959) on diet and cancer were concerned mainly with effects of caloric restriction on carcinogenesis. His experiments and those in other laboratories showed that a variety of murine tumors, including skin tumors, mammary tumors, hepatomas, lung adenomas, sarcomas, and leukemia, are inhibited by reducing caloric intake (Carroll, 1975). In those experiments, food intake was usually restricted to between one-half and two-thirds of normal, in some cases by underfeeding and thus reducing the intake of all nutrients and in other cases by reducing either carbohydrates or fats alone. The inhibitory effect seemed to be exerted at later stages of tumor development rather than at initiation and was evidently not due to inanition, since the restricted animals were generally active and healthy and tended to live longer than animals fed ad libitum. Since many different types of tumors are inhibited by caloric restriction, the effect may be due simply to lack of energy intake or the metabolites required for tumor development, but other more specific factors such as pituitary hypofunction (Mulinos and Pomerantz, 1940), adrenal hyperfunction, lower insulin levels, and levels of a variety of growth factors may also be involved (Boutwell et al., 1948; Pariza, 1987).

Over the past few years, there has been a revival of interest in experiments in animals to study the influence of caloric intake on carcinogenesis (Kritchevsky, 1986; Kritchevsky and Klurfeld, 1987; Pariza, 1987). From the results of these experiments, it is clear that caloric restriction markedly inhibits tumors of the mammary gland and colon in rats, even when the diet is high in fat (Boissonneault et al., 1986; Klurfeld et al., 1987; Kritchevsky et al., 1984, 1986; Thompson et al., 1985). In most of these studies, dietary intake was restricted by 25% or more, and the body weights of restricted animals were substantially lower than those fed ad libitum. In one experiment, a 10% caloric restriction had no effect on mammary tumor incidence but reduced the tumor weights (Kritchevsky, 1986).

The effect of overfeeding on tumorigenesis is more difficult to investigate experimentally. However, animal species fed high-fat diets tend to gain more weight than those fed low-fat diets, even when the caloric intake is similar. This may be because less energy is required to store dietary fats as body fat than to convert dietary carbohydrates or protein to fat for storage (Pariza, 1987). The promoting effect of dietary fats may thus be due in part to increased caloric intake or to more efficient utilization of dietary calories (Carroll, 1986; Reddy, 1986). There is some evidence that cancer develops more readily in obese animals (Carroll, 1975).

EVIDENCE ASSOCIATING ENERGY EXPENDITURE WITH HEALTH AND CHRONIC DISEASES

Atherosclerotic Cardiovascular Diseases

Epidemiologic Studies

In reasonably homogeneous populations, people with jobs requiring high levels of physical activity have a lower incidence of CHD than those in sedentary occupations. Paffenbarger and Hale (1975) reported lower mortality rates from all causes and from CHD in longshoremen, who do physically demanding work, compared to those who engage in moderate or light activity. Morris et al. (1980) reported that British civil servants with high levels of physical activity during leisure experienced fewer coronary events and had fewer abnormalities in their electrocardiograms compared to those who exercised less. They emphasized the importance of bursts of increased physical activity, which at times exceeded 7.5 kcal/min (31 kJ/min or 5 METs/min). Paffenbarger et al. (1986) related leisure-time physical activity to the first heart attack in a follow-up of a large cohort of Harvard University alumni. For the entire range of energy expenditure, the risk of a first heart attack seemed to be lower in those who regularly participated in strenuous sports than in those with more casual activities. Siscovick et al. (1984) used a case-control technique to examine the relationship between habitual leisure-time activity and sudden death among people without a history of heart disease. The overall risk of primary cardiac arrest was increased among those who were habitually less active, compared to people who were more vigorous.

Sobolski et al. (1987) examined the relationship of physical fitness and physical activity to the development of CHD in approximately 1,734 men given a test to measure work capacity and followed for more than 5 years. They observed no association between physical activity on the job or at leisure and the development of CHD; however, there was an inverse relationship between work capacity (to produce a heart rate of 150) divided by body weight (in kilograms) to the risk of systemic heart disease. This variable, as well as HDL cholesterol and smoking, remained significant mediators of heart disease in multivariate analyses. The authors noted that physical fitness and personal estimates of physical activity may be poorly correlated.

The epidemiologic data presented here clearly suggest that there is an inverse association between the level of habitual, vigorous physical activity and the overall risk of CHD. Furthermore, the data indicate that the benefit results from exercise and that there are few who would not benefit from increased physical activity.

Clinical Studies

Clinical studies of people during physical training reveal a variety of physiologic changes relevant to cardiovascular diseases. Aerobic physical training improves cardiovascular function manifested by increased maximal oxygen uptake and a reduced heart rate. In many studies, physical training is associated with increased lean body mass as well as a reduction in body fat stores (Wilmore, 1983); the latter are related to the degree of negative energy balance during physical training. Physical training is also associated with a reduction in insulin levels and improved glucose tolerance.

Animal Studies

There is a substantial literature on the effects of physical fitness on cardiovascular function in animals. Similar to studies in humans, studies in animals have shown that cardiovascular fitness can be enhanced by regular exercise (Brooks and

White, 1978; Gleeson and Baldwin, 1981; Mazzeo et al., 1984; Starnes et al., 1983). It is also known that food intake by animals may increase to maintain energy balance over a wide range of energy expenditures.

Dynamic exercise lowers heart rate response (Frick et al., 1967; Ordway et al., 1982; Tipton, 1965) and may diminish maximal heart rate. These effects may be mediated through regulation of β-adrenergic receptor number or through modulation of the sympathetic nervous system input into cardiovascular dynamics (Hammond et al., 1987). Since the sympathetic nervous system may play an important role in the regulation of energy expenditure during physical activity as well as during rest, it may be that total energy expenditure and fitness over time are reflected in predictable changes in cardiovascular diseases, but the committee could identify no specific long-term studies in animals that specifically supported this hypothesis.

Diabetes Mellitus

Epidemiologic Studies

Jarrett et al. (1986) examined the relationship of physical activity levels to the risk of developing NIDDM in the Whitehall study. They found no association between blood glucose level and a physical activity score ascertained through questionnaires. There was also no evident relationship in this study between glucose tolerance or NIDDM and the time reportedly spent in leisure-time physical activity, or between glucose tolerance and energy expenditure. In the Tecumseh Study, physical activity was divided into three categories based on time spent in leisure and occupation-related physical activity (Montoye et al., 1977). As in the Whitehall study, there was no correlation between glucose tolerance and physical activity among 1,300 men ages 16 to 64 years.

Clinical Studies

In contrast to the epidemiologic studies, there is clear evidence from clinical studies that increasing physical activity can improve glucose tolerance and that physical inactivity can worsen it. Björntorp and colleagues (1973) placed overweight subjects in an extended physical training program under careful supervison and demonstrated that glucose tolerance, especially the secretion of insulin following an oral glucose tolerance test, is substantially improved by physical training. In contrast, after a few days of bed rest, glucose tolerance deteriorated in healthy subjects.

Animal Studies

Some studies in humans suggest that diet-induced thermogenesis is impaired in subjects with NIDDM. The few good animal models for NIDDM include the diabetic mouse, the Wistar fatty rat, and the sand rat. Studies of obese monkeys and dogs have not provided sufficient data to determine whether a reduction in diet-induced thermogenesis enhances the risk of adiposity and thus increases the incidence of diabetes. In a comparison of two diabetic mouse strains, Coleman (1979) concluded that the impairment in thermogenesis attributable to the mutant strains could not account for most of the observed metabolic efficiency. It is possible that increased adiposity contributes to the insulin resistance associated with diabetes. It is uncertain whether decreased thermogenesis contributes to the adiposity.

The effects of exercise on diabetic animals seem to be related primarily to effects on body weight and composition. Exercise training of obese, glucose-intolerant rodents leads to substantial reduction in plasma insulin (Walberg et al., 1982) and glucose. Exercise of sufficient intensity and endurance to affect muscle mass nevertheless affects glucose disposal rates and improves overall glucose tolerance (Ivy and Holloszy, 1981; Wardzala et al., 1982). Thus, it appears that increased energy expenditure may lessen the effects of incipient diabetes, but the data regarding prevention of initiation are inconclusive.

Cancers

Epidemiologic Studies

There are no reports of epidemiologic studies based on precise measurements of energy expenditure to determine if there is an association with cancer risk. In studies of college alumni, Frisch et al. (1985) found that formerly athletic women had a lower risk of cancers of the breast and reproductive organs than did nonathletes, and Paffenbarger et al. (1987) reported that people most active in college were subsequently at lower risk of rectal cancer but at a somewhat higher risk of prostate cancer. After college, leisure-time activity level was slightly positively associated in a dose-dependent manner with risk of colon and rectal cancers.

Paffenbarger et al. (1987) in their study of longshoremen found no association between estimated levels of energy expenditure and cancer risk. In a second group of dock workers, however, they found somewhat higher risks for colorectal cancer and lower risks for lung and prostate cancer in men engaged in heavy work as compared to men engaged in lighter work.

In two case-control studies of large bowel cancer (Garabrant et al., 1984; Vena et al., 1985), people with sedentary jobs or light workloads had a higher risk of colon cancer but not of rectal cancer compared to people who held more active jobs. A similar inverse relationship with job activity was found by Gerhardsson et al. (1986) in a retrospective cohort analysis.

The findings of these studies are inconsistent and permit no clear conclusion about the association of physical activity and cancer risk. Future studies based on better estimates of energy output are needed to clarify the relationship of energy expenditure to the risks of different types of cancer.

Animal Studies

A relationship between caloric restriction and reduced tumorigenesis has been observed in some rodent strains with specific types of tumors, as mentioned earlier. Reductions in tumor growth or burden have not been associated only with caloric restriction, however. They have also been noted under various conditions of energy store depletion, e.g., during physical activity. Only a few experiments directly examined the effects of energy expenditure on carcinogenesis, and these have provided limited data. For example, rats injected with dimethylbenzanthracene were subjected to food restriction or exercise or were pair-gained (i.e., weight gain of one animal was limited to the same level as that of the second animal in a pair) to the exercise group; however, all groups of rats lost weight and did not have the expected tumor growth (Moore and Tittle, 1973). Consequently, it was not possible to attribute the probable effect to either physical activity or caloric restriction per se.

In an experiment by Hoffman et al. (1962), Walker 256 tumors were transplanted by injection into Wistar rats who were either strenuously exercised or confined to small cages. The exercised group had smaller tumors than controls, but no pair-fed or pair-gained controls were included, which makes it difficult to attribute the decreased tumor load directly to exercise. In several more recent but preliminary reports (e.g., Bennink et al., 1986; Cohen, 1987; Thompson et al., 1988), comparisons of exercise and food restriction suggest that exercise interacts with either total caloric intake or dietary fats to determine the outcome (Yedinak et al., 1987). Cohen et al. (1988) recently reported that voluntary exercise inhibits

mammary carcinogenesis in rats. They have also reviewed earlier studies on forced exercise, but found the results to be inconsistent. The authors concluded that the promoting effects of high-fat diets fed ad libitum and the antipromoting effects of energy restriction and exercise are not due to alterations in energy homeostasis per se, but may be mediated indirectly, and perhaps independently, by endocrine, paracrine, or neurohormonal pathways. To date, the nature of this association or interaction remains to be elucidated. Therefore, the role of energy expenditure in the prevention or promotion of tumorigenesis remain unclear.

SUMMARY

Clinical and animal data indicate that increased energy intake leads to an increase in body energy stores and that reduced caloric intake lowers energy stores. In cross-sectional population studies, however, total caloric intake has no direct correlation with body weight and generally shows an inverse correlation with body weight. Thus, body fat acquired during adult life cannot be solely attributed to increased caloric intake, but probably also results from reduced energy expenditure. The association between total energy intake and energy expenditure and the risk of other chronic diseases, including diabetes and cancers, is unclear. For example, the results of epidemiologic studies regarding measurements of energy expenditure and risk of cancer are inconsistent. Animal studies have also yielded inconsistent results. No correlation has been reported between glucose tolerance and physical activity in epidemiologic studies; however, results of clinical studies suggest that increasing physical activity can improve glucose tolerance. Animal studies also suggest that increased energy expenditure may lessen the effects of incipient diabetes.

Total energy intake is influenced by age, sex, body weight, and ambient temperature. The highest caloric intake estimated for males and females occurs during the second decade of life and declines thereafter in both sexes. Total energy expenditure is influenced by age, sex, hormonal, and nutritional status and is related directly to body weight. RMR most likely has a familial component. Energy expenditure is directly associated with total energy intake in normal-weight subjects, but not necessarily in obese subjects. Increased energy expenditure resulting from increased physical activity has been associated with an overall decreased risk of CHD.

DIRECTIONS FOR RESEARCH

• The genetic basis for RMR, metabolic efficiency, and other components of energy balance is unknown and deserves further research.

• More information is needed about the relationship of physical activity to food intake. Increased physical activity may increase energy intake in lean subjects but not necessarily in overweight people. There is no current explanation for this phenomenon.

• The increased energy needed for fetal growth and development may not always stimulate a corresponding increase in food intake, suggesting recruitment of mechanisms for enhancing metabolic efficiency. The basis for this efficiency is unknown and should be studied.

• The proportion of fats in the diet may be a factor in the development of positive energy balance, but the validity of this claim and the possible mechanisms of action require elucidation.

• Lean body mass declines with age in most people. The relationship between energy expenditure, RMR, and lean body mass in the elderly warrants further investigation.

• The mechanism of the effects of exercise on carbohydrate tolerance and on HDL cholesterol levels is not adequately understood and requires further study.

REFERENCES

Arky, R.A. 1976. Environmental factors influencing the development of the diabetic state. Pp. 89–105 in S.S. Fajans, ed. Diabetes Mellitus. DHEW Publ. No. (NIH) 76–854, National Institutes of Health, Public Health Service, U.S. Department of Health, Education, and Welfare, Bethesda, Md.

Ashley, F.W., Jr., and W.B. Kannel. 1974. Relation of weight change to changes in atherogenic traits: the Framingham Study. J. Chronic Dis. 27:103–114.

Baecke, J.A., W.A. van Staveren, and J. Burema. 1983. Food consumption, habitual physical activity, and body fatness in young Dutch adults. Am. J. Clin. Nutr. 37:278–286.

Beaton, G.H., J. Milner, P. Corey, V. McGuire, M. Cousins, E. Stewart, M. de Ramos, D. Hewitt, P.V. Grambsch, N. Kassim, and J.A. Little. 1979. Sources of variance in 24-hour dietary recall data: implications for nutrition study design and interpretation. Am. J. Clin. Nutr. 32:2546–2559.

Beaudoin, R., and J. Mayer. 1953. Food intakes of obese and non-obese women. J. Am. Diet. Assoc. 29:29–33.

Bennink, M.R., H.J. Palmer, and M.J. Messina. 1986. Exercise and caloric restriction modify rat mammary carcinogenesis. Fed. Proc. 45:1087.

Björntorp, P., K. de Jounge, M. Krotkiewski, L. Sullivan, L. Sjöström, and J. Stenberg. 1973. Physical training in human obesity. 3. Effects of long-term physical training on body composition. Metabolism 22:1467–1475.

Bogardus, C., S. Lillioja, E. Ravussin, W. Abbott, J.K. Zawadzk, A. Young, W.C. Knowler, R. Jacobowitz, and P.P. Moll. 1986. Familial dependence of the resting metabolic rate. N. Engl. J. Med. 315:96–100.

Boissonneault, G.A., C.E. Elson, and M.W. Pariza. 1986. Net energy effects of dietary fat on chemically induced mammary carcinogenesis in F344 rats. J. Natl. Cancer Inst. 76:335–338.

Bouchard, C., R. Lesage, G. Lortie, J.A. Simoneau, P. Hamel, M.R. Boulay, L. Perusse, G. Theriault, and C. Leblanc. 1986. Aerobic performance in brothers, dizygotic and monozygotic twins. Med. Sci. Sports Exercise 18:639–646.

Boutwell, R.K., M.K. Brush, and H.P. Rusch. 1948. Some physiological effects associated with chronic caloric restriction. Am. J. Physiol. 154:517–524.

Boyle, P.C., L.H. Storlein, and R.E. Keesey. 1978. Increased efficiency of food utilization following weight loss. Physiol. Behav. 21:261–264.

Braitman, L.E., E.V. Adlin, and J.L. Stanton, Jr. 1985. Obesity and caloric intake: the National Health and Nutrition Examination Survey of 1971–1975 (NHANES I). J. Chronic Dis. 38:727–732.

Bray, G.A. 1976. The obese patient. Pp. 1–450 in Major Problems in Internal Medicine, Vol. 9. W.B. Saunders, Philadelphia.

Bray, G.A. 1983. The energetics of obesity. Med. Sci. Sports Exercise 15:32–40.

Bray, G.A., and D.S. Gray. 1988. Obesity. Part I—Pathogenesis. West. J. Med. 149:429–441.

Bray, G.A., F.L. Greenway, M. Molitch, W.T. Dahms, R.L. Atkinson, and K. Hamilton. 1978. Use of anthropometric measures to assess weight loss. Am. J. Clin. Nutr. 31:769–773.

Brooks, G.A., and T.P. White. 1978. Determination of metabolic and heart rate responses of rats to treadmill exercises. J. Appl. Physiol. 45:1009–1015.

Brownell, K.D., A.J. Stunkard, and J.M. Albaum. 1980. Evaluation and modification of exercise patterns in the natural environment. Am. J. Psychiatry 137:1540–1545.

Brownell, K.D., P.S. Bachorik, and R.S. Ayerle. 1982. Changes in plasma lipid and lipoprotein levels in men and women after a program of moderate exercise. Circulation 65:477–484.

Bullen, B.A., R.B. Reed, and J. Mayer. 1964. Physical activity of obese and nonobese adolescent girls appraised by motion picture sampling. Am. J. Clin. Nutr. 14:211–223.

Carroll, K.K. 1975. Experimental evidence of dietary factors and hormone-dependent cancers. Cancer Res. 35:3374–3383.

Carroll, K.K. 1986. Dietary fat and cancer: specific action or caloric effect? J. Nutr. 116:1130–1132.

Carroll, M.D., S. Abraham, and C.M. Dresser. 1983. Dietary Intake Source Data: United States, 1976–1980. Vital and Health Statistics, Series 11, No. 231. DHHS Publ. No. (PHS) 83-1681. National Center for Health Statistics, Public Health Service, U.S. Department of Health and Human Services, Hyattsville, Md. 483 pp.

Cleary, M.P., J.R. Vasselli, and M.R. Greenwood. 1980. Development of obesity in the Zucker obese (fafa) rat in absence of hyperphagia. Am. J. Physiol. 238:E284–E292.

Cohen, L.A. 1987. Fat and endocrine-responsive cancer in animals. Prev. Med. 16:468–474.

Cohen, L.A., K.W. Choi, and C.X. Wang. 1988. Influence of

dietary fat, caloric restriction, and voluntary exercise on N-nitrosomethylurea-induced mammary tumorigenesis in rats. Cancer Res. 48:4276–4283.

Coleman, D.L. 1979. Obesity genes: beneficial effects in heterozygous mice. Science 203:663–665.

Cox, J.E., and T.L. Powley. 1977. Development of obesity in diabetic mice pair-fed with lean siblings. J. Comp. Physiol. Psychol. 91:347–358.

de Boer, J.O., A.J. van Es, J.M. van Raaij, and J.G. Hautvast. 1987. Energy requirements and energy expenditure of lean and overweight women, measured by indirect calorimetry. Am. J. Clin. Nutr. 46:13–21.

Donato, K., and D.M. Hegsted. 1985. Efficiency of utilization of various sources of energy for growth. Proc. Natl. Acad. Sci. U.S.A. 82:4866–4870.

Drenick, E.J., A.S. Brickman, and E.M. Gold. 1972. Dissociation of the obesity–hyperinsulinism relationship following dietary restriction and hyperalimentation. Am. J. Clin. Nutr. 25:746–755.

Durnin, J.V.G.A. 1986. Energy requirements of pregnancy. An integration of the longitudinal data from the 5-country study. Pp. 147–154 in Nestlé Foundation for the Study of the Problems of Nutrition in the World, Annual Report 1986. Nestlé Foundation, Lausanne, Switzerland.

Edholm, O.G., J.M. Adam, M.J. Healy, H.S. Wolff, R. Goldsmith, and T.W. Best. 1970. Food intake and energy expenditure of army recruits. Br. J. Nutr. 24:1091–1107.

Fontaine, E., R. Savard, A. Tremblay, J.P. Despres, E. Poehlman, and C. Bouchard. 1985. Resting metabolic rate in monozygotic and dizygotic twins. Acta Genet. Med. Gemellol. 34:41–47.

Forbes, G.B. 1987. Lean body mass–body fat interrelationships in humans. Nutr. Rev. 45:225–231.

Frick, M.H., R.O. Elovainio, and T. Somer. 1967. The mechanism of bradycardia evoked by physical training. Cardiologia 51:46–54.

Frisch, R.E., G. Wyshak, N.L. Albright, T.E. Albright, I. Schiff, K.P. Jones, J. Witschi, E. Shiang, E. Koff, and M. Marguglio. 1985. Lower prevalence of breast cancer and cancers of the reproductive system among former college athletes compared to non-athletes. Br. J. Cancer 52:885–891.

Garabrant, D.H., J.M. Peters, T.M. Mack, and L. Bernstein. 1984. Job activity and colon cancer risk. Am. J. Epidemiol. 119:1005–1014.

Garrow, J.S. 1978. Energy Balance and Obesity in Man, 2nd ed. Elsevier/North-Holland, Amsterdam. 243 pp.

Geissler, C.A., D.S. Miller, and M. Shah. 1987. The daily metabolic rate of the post-obese and the lean. Am. J. Clin. Nutr. 45:914–920.

George, V., A. Tremblay, J.P. Després, C. Leblanc, L. Pérusse, and C. Bouchard. In press. Evidence for the existence of small eaters and large eaters of similar fat-free mass and activity level. Int. J. Obes.

Gerhardsson, M., S.E. Norell, H. Kiviranta, N.L. Pedersen, and A. Ahlbom. 1986. Sedentary jobs and colon cancer. Am. J. Epidemiol. 123:775–780.

Gleeson, T.T., and K.M. Baldwin. 1981. Cardiovascular response to treadmill exercise in untrained rats. J. Appl. Physiol. 50:1206–1211.

Glinsmann, W.H., H. Irausquin, and Y.K. Park. 1986. Evaluation of health aspects of sugars contained in carbohydrate sweeteners: report of Sugars Task Force, 1986. J. Nutr. 116:S1–S216.

Goor, R., J.D. Hosking, B.H. Dennis, K.L. Graves, G.T. Waldman, and S.G. Haynes. 1985. Nutrient intakes among selected North American populations in the Lipid Research Clinics Prevalence Study: composition of fat intake. Am. J. Clin. Nutr. 41:299–311.

Gordon, T., A. Kagan, M. Garcia-Palmieri, W.B. Kannel, W.J. Zukel, J. Tillotson, P. Sorlie, and M. Hjortland. 1981. Diet and its relation to coronary heart disease and death in three populations. Circulation 63:500–515.

Goto, Y., Y. Nakayama, and T. Yagi. 1958. Influence of the World War II food shortage on the incidence of diabetes mellitus in Japan. Diabetes 7:133–135.

Greenwood, M.R.C., M.P. Cleary, L. Steingrimsdottir, and J.R. Vasselli. 1981. Adipose tissue metabolism and genetic obesity: the LPL hypothesis. Recent Adv. Obesity Res. III: 75–79.

Gregor, O., R. Toman, and F. Prusova. 1969. Gastrointestinal cancer and nutrition. Gut 10:1031–1034.

Hammond, H.K., F.C. White, L.L. Brunton, and J.C. Longhurst. 1987. Association of decreased myocardial β-receptors and chronotropic response to isoproterenol and exercise in pigs following chronic dynamic exercise. Circ. Res. 60: 720–726.

Henry, R.R., T.A. Wiest-Kent, L. Scheaffer, O.G. Kolterman, and J.M. Olefsky. 1986. Metabolic consequences of very-low-calorie diet therapy in obese non-insulin-dependent diabetic and nondiabetic subjects. Diabetes 35: 155–164.

Himms-Hagen, J. 1985. Brown adipose tissue metabolism and thermogenesis. Annu. Rev. Nutr. 5:69–94.

Himsworth, H.P. 1935. Diet and incidence of diabetes mellitus. Clin. Sci. 2:117–148.

Hoffman, S.A., K.E. Paschkis, D.A. Debias, A. Cantarow, and T.L. Williams. 1962. The influence of exercise on the growth of transplanted rat tumors. Cancer Res. 22:597–599.

Horwitz, B.A., T. Inokuchi, B.J. Moore, and J.S. Stern. 1985. The effect of brown fat removal on the development of obesity in Zucker and Osborne-Mendel rats. Int. J. Obesity 2 suppl. 9:43–48.

Howe, G.R., A.B. Miller, and M. Jain. 1986. Re: "Total energy intake: implications for epidemiologic analyses." Am. J. Epidemiol. 124:157–159.

Hytten, F.E., and I. Leitch. 1971. The Physiology of Human Pregnancy, 2nd ed. Blackwell, Oxford. 599 pp.

Ikeda, H., A. Shino, T. Matsuo, H. Iwatsuka, and Z. Suzuoki. 1981. A new genetically obese-hyperglycemic rat (Wistar fatty). Diabetes 30:1045–1050.

Ivy, J.L., and J.O. Holloszy. 1981. Persistent increase in glucose uptake by rat skeletal muscle following exercise. Am. J. Physiol. 241:C200–C203.

Jain, M., G.M. Cook, F.G. Davis, M.G. Grace, G.R. Howe, and A.B. Miller. 1980. A case-control study of diet and colo-rectal cancer. Int. J. Cancer 26:757–768.

James, W.P. 1983. Energy requirements and obesity. Lancet 2: 386–389.

Jarrett, R.J., M.J. Shipley, and R. Hunt. 1986. Physical activity, glucose tolerance, and diabetes mellitus: the Whitehall Study. Diabetic Med. 3:549–551.

Jen, K.L., M.R.C. Greenwood, and S.A. Brasel. 1981. Sex differences in the effects of high-fat feeding on behavior and carcass composition. Physiol. Behav. 27:161–166.

Jequier, E. 1984. Energy expenditure in obesity. Clin. Endocrinol. Metab. 13:563–580.

Kalderon, B., A. Gutman, E. Levy, E. Shafrir, and J.H.

Adler. 1986. Characterization of stages in development of obesity–diabetes syndrome in sand rat (*Psammomys obesus*). Diabetes 35:717–724.

Kava, R.A., D.B. West, V.A. Lukasik, and M.R.C. Greenwood. 1989. Sexual dimorphism of hyperglycemia and glucose tolerance in Wistar fatty rat. Diabetes 38:159–163.

Kawate, R., M. Yamakido, Y. Nishimoto, P.H. Bennett, R.F. Hamman, and W.C. Knowler. 1979. Diabetes mellitus and its vascular complications in Japanese migrants on the island of Hawaii. Diabetes Care 2:161–170.

Keen, H., B.J. Thomas, R.J. Jarrett, and J.H. Fuller. 1979. Nutrient intake, adiposity, and diabetes. Br. Med. J. 1:655–658.

Keesey, R.E. 1980. Set point analysis of the regulation of body weight. Pp. 144–165 in A.J. Stunkard, ed. Obesity. W.B. Saunders, Philadelphia.

Keesey, R.E., and T.L. Powley. 1986. The regulation of body weight. Annu. Rev. Psychol. 37:109–133.

Kleiber, M. 1947. Body size and metabolic rate. Physiol. Rev. 15:511–541.

Klurfeld, D.M., M.M. Weber, and D. Kritchevsky. 1987. Inhibition of chemically induced mammary and colon tumor promotion by caloric restriction in rats fed increased dietary fat. Cancer Res. 47:2759–2762.

Kritchevsky, D. 1986. Fat, calories and fiber. Pp. 495–515 in C. Ip, D.F. Birt, A.E. Roges, and C. Mettlin, eds. Progress in Clinical and Biological Research, Vol. 222. Dietary Fat and Cancer. Alan R. Liss, New York.

Kritchevsky, D., and D.M. Klurfeld. 1987. Caloric effects in experimental mammary tumorigenesis. Am. J. Clin. Nutr. 45:236–242.

Kritchevsky, D., M.M. Weber, and D.M. Klurfeld. 1984. Dietary fat versus caloric content in initiation and promotion of 7,12-dimethylbenzanthracene-induced mammary tumorigenesis in rats. Cancer Res. 44:3174–3177.

Kritchevsky, D., M.M. Weber, C.L. Buck, and D.M. Klurfeld. 1986. Calories, fat and cancer. Lipids 21:272–274.

Kromhout, D. 1983a. Changes in energy and macronutrients in 871 middle-aged men during 10 years of follow-up (the Zutphen Study). Am. J. Clin. Nutr. 37:287–294.

Kromhout, D. 1983b. Energy and macronutrient intake in lean and obese middle-aged men (the Zutphen Study). Am. J. Clin. Nutr. 37:295–299.

Krotkiewski, M., L. Sjöström, P. Björntorp, G. Carlgren, G. Garellick, and U. Smith. 1977. Adipose tissue cellularity in relation to prognosis for weight reduction. Int. J. Obes. 1:395–416.

Lapidus, L., H. Andersson, C. Bengtsson, and I. Bosaeus. 1986. Dietary habits in relation to incidence of cardiovascular disease and death in women: a 12-year follow-up of participants in the population study of women in Gothenburg, Sweden. Am. J. Clin. Nutr. 44:444–448.

Leibel, R.L., and J. Hirsch. 1984. Diminished energy requirements in reduced-obese patients. Metabolism 33:164–170.

Lew, E.A., and L. Garfinkel. 1979. Variations in mortality by weight among 750,000 men and women. J. Chronic Dis. 32:563–576.

Lifson, N. 1966. Theory of use of the turnover rates of body water for measuring energy and material balance. J. Theor. Biol. 12:46–74.

Lincoln, J.E. 1972. Calorie intake, obesity, and physical activity. Am. J. Clin. Nutr. 25:390–394.

LRC (Lipid Research Clinic). 1980. Lipid Research Clinics Population Studies Data Book, Vol. I: The Prevalence Study. NIH Publ. No. 80-1527. National Institutes of Health, Public Health Service, U.S. Department of Health and Human Services, Bethesda, Md. 136 pp.

Mazzeo, R.S., G.A. Brooks, and S.M. Horvath. 1984. Effects of age on metabolic responses to endurance training in rats. J. Appl. Physiol. 57:1369–1374.

McGandy, R.B., C.H. Barrows, Jr., A. Spanias, A. Meredith, J.L. Stove, and A.H. Norris. 1966. Nutrient intakes and energy expenditure in men of different ages. J. Gerontol. 21:581–587.

McLean, J.A., and G. Tobin. 1988. Animal and Human Calorimetry. Cambridge University Press, New York. 352 pp.

Medalie, J.H., C.M. Papier, U. Goldbourt, and J.D. Herman. 1975. Major factors in the development of diabetes mellitus in 10,000 men. Arch. Intern. Med. 135:811–817.

Miller, W.H., Jr., and I.M. Faust. 1982. Alterations in rat adipose tissue morphology induced by a low-temperature environment. Am. J. Physiol. 242:E93–E96.

Montoye, H.J., W.D. Block, H. Metzner, and J.B. Keller. 1977. Habitual physical activity and glucose tolerance. Males age 16–64 in a total community. Diabetes 26:172–176.

Moore, C., and P.W. Tittle. 1973. Muscle activity, body fat, and induced rat mammary tumors. Surgery 73:329–332.

Morris, J.N., M.G. Everitt, R. Pollard, S.P. Chave, and A.M. Semmence. 1980. Vigorous exercise in leisure-time: protection against coronary heart disease. Lancet 2:1207–1210.

Mulinos, M.G., and L. Pomerantz. 1940. Pseudo-hypophysectomy; condition resembling hypophysectomy produced by malnutrition. J. Nutr. 19:493–504.

Noppa, H. 1980. Body weight change in relation to incidence of ischemic heart disease and change in risk factors for ischemic heart disease. Am. J. Epidemiol. 111:693–704.

NRC (National Research Council). 1980. Recommended Dietary Allowances, 9th ed. Report of the Food and Nutrition Board, Assembly of Life Sciences. National Academy Press, Washington, D.C. 185 pp.

NRC (National Research Council). 1982. Diet, Nutrition, and Cancer. Report of the Committee on Diet, Nutrition, and Cancer, Assembly of Life Sciences. National Academy Press, Washington, D.C. 478 pp.

Obell, A.E. 1974. Recent advances in mechanisms of causation of diabetes mellitus in man and *Acomy cahirinus*. East Afr. Med. J. 51:425–428.

Ordway, G.A., J.B. Charles, D.C. Randall, G.E. Billman, and D.R. Wekstein. 1982. Heart rate adaptation to exercise training in cardiac denervated dogs. J. Appl. Physiol. 52:1586–1590.

Owen, O.E., E. Kavle, R.S. Owen, M. Polansky, S. Caprio, M.A. Mozzoli, Z.V. Kendrick, M.C. Bushman, and G. Boden. 1986. A reappraisal of caloric requirements in healthy women. Am. J. Clin. Nutr. 44:1–19.

Owen, O.E., J.L. Holup, D.A. D'Alessio, E.S. Craig, M. Polansky, K.J. Smalley, E.C. Kavle, M.C. Bushman, L.R. Owen, M.A. Mozzoli, Z.V. Kendrick, and G.H. Boden. 1987. A reappraisal of the caloric requirements of men. Am. J. Clin. Nutr. 46:875–885.

Paffenbarger, R.S., and W.E. Hale. 1975. Work activity and coronary heart mortality. N. Engl. J. Med. 292:545–550.

Paffenbarger, R.S., Jr., R.T. Hyde, A.L. Wing, and C.C. Hsieh. 1986. Physical activity, all-cause mortality, and longevity of college alumni. N. Engl. J. Med. 314:605–613.

Paffenbarger, R.S., Jr., R.T. Hyde, and A.L. Wing. 1987.

Physical activity and incidence of cancer in diverse populations: a preliminary report. Am. J. Clin. Nutr. 45:312–317.

Pariza, M.W. 1987. Fat, calories, and mammary carcinogenesis: net energy effects. Am. J. Clin. Nutr. 45:261–263.

Phillips, R.W., N. Westmoreland, L. Panepinto, and G.L. Case. 1982. Dietary effects on metabolism of Yucatan miniature swine selected for low and high glucose utilization. J. Nutr. 112:104–111.

Potter, J.D., and A.J. McMichael. 1986. Diet and cancer of the colon and rectum: a case-control study. J. Natl. Cancer Inst. 76:557–569.

Ravussin, E., S. Lillioja, W.C. Knowler, L. Christin, D. Freymond, W.G. Abbott, V. Boyce, B.V. Howard, and C. Bogardus. 1988. Reduced rate of energy expenditure as a risk factor for body-weight gain. N. Engl. J. Med. 318:467–472.

Reddy, B.S. 1986. Dietary fat and cancer: specific action or caloric effect. J. Nutr. 116:1132–1135.

Rice, M.G., and R.P. Robertson. 1980. Reevaluation of the sand rat as a model for diabetes mellitus. Am. J. Physiol. 239:340E–345E.

Roberts, S.B., J. Savage, W.A. Coward, B. Chew, and A. Lucas. 1988. Energy expenditure and intake in infants born to lean and overweight mothers. N. Engl. J. Med. 318:461–466.

Romieu, I., W.C. Willett, M.J. Stampfer, G.A. Colditz, L. Sampson, B. Rosner, C.H. Hennekens, and F.E. Speizer. 1988. Energy intake and other determinants of relative weight. Am. J. Clin. Nutr. 47:406–412.

Salans, L., and B. Graham, eds. 1982. Proceedings of a task force on animals appropriate for studying diabetes mellitus and its complications. Diabetes 31 suppl. 1:1–102.

Schoeller D.A., E. Ravussin, Y. Schutz, K.J. Acheson, P. Baertschi, and E. Jequier. 1986. Energy expenditure by doubly labeled water: validation in humans and proposed calculation. Am. J. Physiol. 250:R823–R830.

Segal, K.R., M. Van Loan, P.I. Fitzgerald, J.A. Hodgdon, and T.B. Van Itallie. 1988. Lean body mass estimation by bioelectrical impedance analysis: a four-site cross-validation study. Am. J. Clin. Nutr. 47:7–14.

Sims, E.A., E. Danforth, Jr., E.S. Horton, G.A. Bray, J.A. Glennon, and L.B. Salans. 1973. Endocrine and metabolic effects of experimental obesity in man. Recent Prog. Horm. Res. 29:457–496.

Siscovick, D.S., N.S. Weiss, R.H. Fletcher, V.J. Schoenbach, and E.H. Wagner. 1984. Habitual vigorous exercise and primary cardiac arrest: effect of other risk factors on the relationship. J. Chronic Dis. 37:625–631.

Sjöström, L., H. Kvist, Å. Cederblad, and U. Tylén. 1986. Determination of total adipose tissue and body fat in women by computed tomography, ⁴⁰K, and tritium. Am. J. Physiol. 250:E736–E745.

Sobolski, J., M. Kornitzer, G. De Backer, M. Dramaix, M. Abramowicz, S. Degre, and H. Denolin. 1987. Protection against ischemic heart disease in the Belgian Physical Fitness Study: physical fitness rather than physical activity? Am. J. Epidemiol. 125:601–610.

Starnes, J.W., R.E. Beyer, and D.W. Edington. 1983. Myocardial adaptations to endurance exercise in aged rats. Am. J. Physiol. 245:H560–H566.

Stefanik, P.A., F.P. Heald, Jr., and J. Mayer. 1959. Caloric intake in relation to energy output of obese and non-obese adolescent boys. Am. J. Clin. Nutr. 7:55–62.

Stern, J.S., P.R. Johnson, B.R. Batchelor, L.M. Zucker, and J. Hirsch. 1975. Pancreatic insulin release and peripheral tissue resistance in Zucker obese rats fed high- and low-carbohydrate diets. Am. J. Physiol. 228:543–548.

Stock, M.J., and N.J. Rothwell. 1981. Sympathetic control of brown adipose tissue in the regulation of body weight. Biochem. Soc. Trans. 9:525–527.

Susini, C., and M. Lavau. 1978. *In-vitro* and *in-vivo* responsiveness of muscle and adipose tissue to insulin in rats rendered obese by a high-fat diet. Diabetes 27:114–120.

Tannenbaum, A. 1947. The role of nutrition in the origin and growth of tumors. Pp. 96–127 in F.R. Moulton, ed. Approaches to Tumor Chemotherapy. American Association for the Advancement of Science, Washington, D.C.

Tannenbaum, A. 1959. Nutrition and cancer. Pp. 517–562 in F.F. Homburger, ed. The Physiopathology of Cancer, 2nd ed. Hoeber-Harper, New York.

Thompson, H.J., L.D. Meeker, A.R. Tagliaferro, and J.S. Roberts. 1985. Effect of energy intake on the promotion of mammary carcinogenesis by dietary fat. Nutr. Cancer 7:37–41.

Thompson, H.J., A.M. Ronan, K.A. Ritacco, A.R. Tagliaferro, and L.D. Meeker. 1988. Effect of exercise on the induction of mammary carcinogenesis. Cancer Res. 48:2720–2723.

Tipton, C.M. 1965. Training and bradycardia in rats. Am. J. Physiol. 209:1089–1094.

Tryon, W.W. 1987. Activity as a function of body weight. Am. J. Clin. Nutr. 46:451–455.

Tuyns, A.J., M. Haelterman, and R. Kaaks. 1987. Colorectal cancer and the intake of nutrients: oligosaccharides are a risk factor, fats are not. A case control study in Belgium. Nutr. Cancer 10:181–196.

USDA (U.S. Department of Agriculture). 1980. Nationwide Food Consumption Survey 1977–78. Food and Nutrient Intakes of Individuals in 1 Day in the United States, Spring 1977. Preliminary Report No. 2. Consumer Nutrition Center, Human Nutrition, Science and Education Administration. Hyattsville, Md. 121 pp.

USDA (U.S. Department of Agriculture). 1984. Nationwide Food Consumption Survey. Nutrient Intakes: Individuals in 48 States, Year 1977–78. Report No. I-2. Consumer Nutrition Division, Human Nutrition Information Service, Hyattsville, Md. 439 pp.

USDA (U.S. Department of Agriculture). 1987. Nationwide Food Consumption Survey. Continuing Survey of Food Intakes of Individuals. Women 19–50 Years and Their Children 1–5 Years, 1 Day, 1986. Report No. 86-1. Nutrition Monitoring Division, Human Nutrition Information Service, Hyattsville, Md. 98 pp.

Vena, J.E., S. Graham, M. Zielezny, M.K. Swanson, R.E. Barnes, and J. Nolan. 1985. Lifetime occupational exercise and colon cancer. Am. J. Epidemiol. 122:357–365.

Walberg, J.L., P.A. Mole, and J.S. Stern. 1982. Effect of swim training on development of obesity in the genetically obese rat. Am. J. Physiol. 242:R204–R211.

Wardzala, L.J., M. Crettaz, E.D. Horton, B. Jeanrenaud, and E.S. Horton. 1982. Physical training of lean and genetically obese Zucker rats: effect on fat cell metabolism. Am. J. Physiol. 243:E418–E426.

Waxman, M., and A.J. Stunkard. 1980. Caloric intake and expenditure of obese boys. J. Pediatr. 96:187–193.

West, K.M., and J.M. Kalbfleisch. 1971. Influence of nutritional factors on prevalence of diabetes. Diabetes 20:99–108.

Wilkinson, P.W., J.M. Parkin, G. Pearlson, M. Strong, and

P. Sykes. 1977. Energy intake and physical activity in obese children. Br. Med. J. 1:756.

Willett, W., and M.J. Stampfer. 1986. Total energy intake: implications for epidemiologic analyses. Am. J. Epidemiol. 124:17–27.

Wilmore, J.H. 1983. Body composition in sport and exercise: directions for future research. Med. Sci. Sports Exercise 15: 21–31.

Woo, R., R. Daniels-Kush, and E.S. Horton. 1985. Regulation of energy balance. Annu. Rev. Nutr. 5:411–433.

Yedinak, R.A., D.K. Layman, and J.A. Milner. 1987. Influences of dietary fat and exercise on DMBA-induced mammary tumors. Fed. Proc. 46:436.

Young, J.B., and L. Landsberg. 1977. Stimulation of the sympathetic nervous system during sucrose feeding. Nature 269:615–617.

7

Fats and Other Lipids

Lipids are compounds that are insoluble in water but are soluble in organic solvents such as ether and chloroform. Lipids that are important to our discussion include fats and oils (triglycerides or triacyglycerols), fatty acids, phospholipids, and cholesterol.

Fats and oils are esters of glycerol and three fatty acids. They are important in the diet as energy sources and as sources of essential fatty acids and fat-soluble vitamins, which tend to associate with fats. They also contribute satiety, flavor, and palatability to the diet.

Fatty acids generally consist of a straight alkyl chain, terminating with a carboxyl group. The number of carbons in the chain varies, and the compound may be saturated (containing no double bonds) or unsaturated (containing one or more double bonds). Short- and medium-chain saturated fatty acids (SFAs) (4 to 12 carbons in length) are found in milk fat, palm oil, and coconut oil. Other animal and vegetable fats contain predominantly longer-chain SFAs (more than 14 carbons in length) and are found chiefly in meats, butterfat, and some vegetable oils. Monounsaturated fatty acids (MUFAs), such as oleic acid, contain one double bond per molecule, whereas polyunsaturated fatty acids (PUFAs), such as linoleic acid, contain more than one. Linoleic acid is classified as an essential nutrient, since the body requires it but cannot synthesize it. Arachidonic acid is also

required by the body but can be synthesized from linoleic acid, which is abundant in oils from corn, soybeans, and safflower seeds.

Linoleic acid (18 carbons with 2 double bonds) and arachidonic acid (20 carbons with 4 double bonds) belong to the omega(ω)-6 group of fatty acids, since the first double bond, counting from the methyl end of the molecule, occurs at carbon number 6. Since linoleic acid has 18 carbon atoms and 2 double bonds, it is usually represented in shorthand as C18:2, ω-6. Under this classification system, oleic acid (C18:1, ω-9) belongs to the ω-9 group, and the PUFAs in fish oils currently receiving much attention belong to the ω-3 group. Chief among these ω-3 fatty acids are eicosapentaenoic acid (EPA), which has 20 carbons and 5 double bonds (C20:5, ω-3), and docosahexaenoic acid (DHA), which has 22 carbons and 6 double bonds (C22:6, ω-3).

A growing body of evidence from studies in animals, including nonhuman primates, indicates that α-linolenic acid, or its longer-chain derivates EPA and DHA, are essential in the diet. These fatty acids appear to play distinctive roles in the structure and function of biologic membranes in the retina and central nervous system (Neuringer and Connor, 1986).

Unsaturated fatty acids form geometric isomers, i.e., the carbon chains are on the same side of the double bond in a *cis* isomer and on opposite sides of the bond in a *trans* isomer. Naturally occurring geometric isomers in food are mainly *cis* isomers, but hydrogenation of oils in the manufacture of margarine and shortening results in formation of some *trans* isomers. This latter process occurs naturally in the rumen of ruminants.

Phospholipids contain glycerol, fatty acids, phosphate, and, with such exceptions as phosphatidylglycerol and phosphatidylinositol, a nitrogenous component. Lecithin, for example, is made up of glycerol, two fatty acids (one saturated, usually), phosphate, and choline. Phospholipids are important structural components of brain and nervous tissue, of membranes throughout body tissues, and of lipoproteins—the carriers of cholesterol and fats in the blood.

Cholesterol and plant sterols, such as sitosterol, are high-molecular-weight alcohols with a characteristic cyclic nucleus and are unrelated to the structure of fats or phospholipids. Cholesterol frequently exists in foods and body tissues esterified to one fatty acid per molecule. It is a component of membranes in body cells and is required for normal development of the brain and nervous tissue. Furthermore, it is the precursor to bile acids, steroid hormones, and 7-dehydrocholesterol in the skin, which in turn is the precursor to vitamin D.

Cholesterol occurs naturally only in foods of animal origin. The highest concentrations are found in liver and egg yolk, but red meats, poultry (especially the skin), whole milk, and cheese make significant contributions to the diet.

TRENDS IN THE FOOD SUPPLY

Trends in the quantities of lipids present in the food supply have been recorded by the U.S. Department of Agriculture (USDA) since 1909. These data represent amounts of lipids that "disappear" into wholesale and retail markets. No account is taken of amounts wasted, and no effort is made to measure intakes by individuals. Thus, food supply data do not represent amounts of lipids actually consumed and are referred to here as amounts *available* for consumption (see Chapters 2 and 3). Total amounts available are divided by the U.S. population to obtain amounts per capita. The following data on time trends were obtained from Marston and Raper (1987).

Fat available in the food supply increased from an average of 124 g/day per capita in 1909 to 172 g/day in 1985. Although the chief sources of fat during that time have been fats and oils; meat, poultry, and fish; and dairy products, great changes

within each of these groups have occurred. The proportion of animal fat declined from 83 to 58% as butter and lard use declined, whereas the proportion of vegetable fat (in margarines and in salad and cooking oils) rose from 17 to 42%. Pork and beef have been major sources of fat in the food supply since 1909, but supplies of beef have declined somewhat recently from 90.7 lb/year per capita in 1975 to 79 lb/year in 1985. The supply of poultry has increased spectacularly since 1940 and continues to increase. In 1985, 70 lb per capita were available compared with 46 lb per capita from 1967 to 1969. The per-capita availability of whole milk dropped from 232 lb during 1967–1969 to 122 lb in 1985, whereas skim and low-fat milks increased from 44 to 112 lb (see Chapter 3).

Fatty acids available in the food supply have all increased since 1909, but the relative contributions of specific fatty acids have changed. The percentage of calories contributed by linoleic acid to total fat intake increased from 7% during 1909–1913 to about 16% in 1985, whereas the corresponding percentage from SFAs declined from approximately 42 to 34% (Figure 3–5). In 1985, linoleic acid was available at 7% of total calories, SFAs at 15%, and oleic acid at 17%.

Cholesterol availability reached its lowest levels of 464 mg/day per capita in 1917 and 1935, and its highest level of 596 mg/day in 1945. The supply declined to 480 mg/day per capita during 1977–1979, when it plateaued; the decline was due to diminished use of whole milk, butter, eggs, and lard. Food sources of cholesterol have changed somewhat over the century. In 1909, meat, poultry, and fish furnished 28% of the cholesterol in the food supply; in 1985, they supplied 40%. Fats and oils supplied 12% of the total cholesterol in 1909, but only 5% in 1985. Egg use has declined, but in 1985 still supplied 40% of the cholesterol in the food supply (see Chapter 3).

LIPID INTAKE: NATIONAL SURVEYS

Actual intakes of various lipids have been estimated in national surveys, but the different surveys fail to agree on trends in actual consumption of *fat*. Data from the USDA's Nationwide Food Consumption Surveys (NFCS) of 1955, 1965, and 1977–1978 show little change in fat levels used by *households*, but mean *individual* intakes were lower during 1977–1978 than in 1965 (USDA, 1984). Furthermore, compared with 1977–1978, a decline in fat intake was indicated in the 1985 and 1986 USDA Continuing Survey of Food Intakes of

Individuals (CSFII) (USDA 1986, 1987). On the other hand, data from the National Health and Nutrition Examination Surveys (NHANES) do not support a decline in fat intake. For example, data from the first and second NHANES (1971–1974 and 1976–1980, respectively) indicate that for women 19 to 50 years of age, mean fat intakes remained stable during the 1970s and early 1980s (see Table 3–4). Systematic biases due to methods used in the surveys appear to explain these differences in estimates of fat intake. For example, in the 1985 and 1986 CSFIIs, interviewers tried to determine whether or not fat was trimmed from meat and the skin removed from poultry before these foods were consumed, but this was not done in the 1977–1978 CSFII.

The 1985 and 1986 CSFIIs indicated that fat provided an average of 36 to 37% of total calories for men and women and 34% for children. The 1977–1978 NFCS reported an average of 41% of total calories as fat for women in this age group, but as noted above, the results of this survey were higher than those of other surveys.

On the basis of 4 nonconsecutive days of intake by women and their children, and on 1 day of intake by men, men and women 19 to 50 years of age consumed a mean of 13% of total calories from SFAs, 14% from MUFAs, and 7% from PUFAs. Children 1 to 5 years old consumed a mean of 14% of calories as SFAs, 13% as MUFAs, and 6% as PUFAs (USDA, 1986, 1987).

The daily intake of cholesterol averaged 280 mg for women 19 to 50 years old (187 mg/1,000 kcal) and 223 mg for children 1 to 5 years old (156 mg/1,000 kcal) (USDA, 1987). Intakes for men 19 to 50 years old averaged 439 mg/day (180 mg/1,000 kcal) (USDA, 1986). Cholesterol intake was higher in low-income groups than in high-income groups; black women had higher intakes than white women, but white men had higher intakes than other men.

In the 1977–1978 NFCS, people from infancy to 75 years of age and older averaged 385 mg of cholesterol per day (USDA, 1984). Dietary cholesterol levels, in absolute amounts and in mg/1,000 kcal, were higher for blacks, for those below the poverty level, for those living in the South and West, and for those living in inner cities.

In the 1985 CSFII, dietary cholesterol came chiefly from meat (48% for men and 45% for women). Eggs provided 18% of the cholesterol intake for men and 15% for women, and grain products furnished 17% of the cholesterol intake for women and 14% for men, but these figures are somewhat misleading in that grain products furnished cholesterol only because they contained milk, butter, and eggs. The milk group provided 14% of the cholesterol intake for men and 16% for women.

EVIDENCE ASSOCIATING DIETARY FATS AND OTHER LIPIDS WITH CHRONIC DISEASES

Atherosclerosis and Cardiovascular Disease

Arterial lesions characterized by intimal thickening, lipid accumulation, and calcification in humans were identified and described at least as early as the seventeenth century. The lesions were named *arteriosclerosis* in 1829, and the distinctive form associated with lipid deposition was named *atherosclerosis* in 1904. However, atherosclerosis was not considered a common cause of death until decades after Herrick (1912) linked coronary atherosclerosis to thrombosis and myocardial infarction. Coronary heart disease (CHD) reached epidemic proportions in the United States before dietary fats were seriously suspected of being causative agents around 1950.

The first recorded evidence that diet had any association with atherosclerosis was the observation by Ignatovski (1908) that rabbits fed meat, milk, and eggs developed arterial lesions resembling atherosclerosis in humans. Anitschkow and Chalatow (1913) then identified cholesterol as the dietary component responsible for hypercholesterolemia and atherosclerosis in rabbits. In subsequent years, investigators demonstrated that many animal species were susceptible to dietary cholesterol, but this phenomenon was considered a laboratory curiosity that had no relevance to human nutrition nor to the rising incidence of CHD and related diseases in the Western world during the first half of the twentieth century.

De Langen, a Dutch physician working in Java, reported in 1916 that native Indonesians had lower levels of plasma cholesterol than did colonists from the Netherlands and associated this observation with a much lower frequency of CHD in the natives. He also observed that Javanese stewards on Dutch passenger ships who ate typical Dutch food had high plasma cholesterol levels and precocious CHD. These observations, published in Dutch in an obscure journal (De Langen, 1916, 1922), lay unnoticed for more than 40 years. In 1934, Rosenthal noted that the distribution of atherosclerosis and atherosclerotic diseases in many parts of the world corresponded to the consumption of fats and cholesterol (Rosenthal, 1934a,b,c).

The next published association of dietary fats with atherosclerosis and cardiovascular disease was the comment by Snapper (1941), based on his experience at Peking Union Medical College, that the high unsaturated fatty acid and low cholesterol content of the Chinese diet might be responsible for the remarkable scarcity of arteriosclerosis in China. This observation also lay unnoticed until after World War II, when reports that deaths from cardiovascular disease, especially those due to arteriosclerosis, declined dramatically in Scandinavia during the war when meat, eggs, and dairy products were scarce (Biörk, 1956; Malmros, 1950; Strøm and Jensen, 1951; Vartiainen, 1946; Vartiainen and Kanerva, 1947).

During the same period, a number of case-control studies of patients with myocardial infarction showed that affected people had higher serum cholesterol levels than did controls (Davis et al., 1937; Gertler et al., 1950b; Lerman and White, 1946; Morrison et al., 1948; Poindexter and Bruger, 1938; Steiner, 1948). The association of serum cholesterol concentrations with atherosclerosis and myocardial infarction was widely recognized by 1946 (Dock, 1946). The predictive value of serum cholesterol concentration for CHD was firmly established by the Framingham Study in 1957 (Dawber et al., 1957) and was confirmed by many similar longitudinal studies in the 1950s and 1960s (Pooling Project Research Group, 1978).

Nevertheless, appreciation of the relationship of diet to serum cholesterol levels, and thereby to CHD, developed more slowly. Although there had been an accumulation of epidemiologic evidence (mainly ecological correlations) supporting the concept that diet, especially dietary fat, was associated with elevated serum cholesterol concentrations and with CHD (Keys, 1957; Keys and Anderson, 1954), there also was much skepticism, as illustrated by the comments of Yudkin (1957), Yerushalmy and Hilleboe (1957), and Mann (1957).

Early in the 1950s, the serum-cholesterol-lowering effects of PUFAs were discovered, and epidemiologic and human experimental studies were focused on this issue. The role of dietary cholesterol remained uncertain until the 1960s, when several careful experiments in humans showed that it had a modest but definite effect. The early development of these concepts, along with the controversies, are found in reviews of the topic by Keys (1957, 1975) and Ahrens (1957). Subsequent sections of this chapter review in detail the epidemiologic and experimental evidence on the relationship between serum cholesterol and CHD, between diet and serum cholesterol, and between diet and CHD.

Plasma Lipids and Lipoproteins

Functions and Transport Mechanisms

Lipids are insoluble in water and circulate in plasma in association with certain specific proteins called apolipoproteins. The lipoproteins are large, macromolecular complexes of apolipoproteins and lipids in varying proportions. The four classes of specific lipoproteins that circulate in plasma are called chylomicrons, very-low-density lipoproteins (VLDL), low-density lipoproteins (LDL), and high-density lipoproteins (HDL).

The primary function of plasma lipoproteins is lipid transport. The major lipid transported in lipoproteins—triglyceride—is only slightly soluble in water, yet up to several hundred grams must be transported through the blood daily. Hence, transport mechanisms have evolved to permit the packaging of thousands of triglyceride molecules in individual lipoprotein particles, which deliver the transported lipid to specific cells. Fatty acids esterified to glycerol constitute approximately 90% of the mass and about 95% of the potential energy of the triglyceride molecule. Free fatty acids are transported in noncovalent linkage as albumin–fatty acid complexes. This latter mode of transport does not permit the high degree of selective targeting of fatty acids to specific sites that is permitted by transport in lipoproteins, but these two modes of fatty acid transport together provide a more versatile system for bulk movement of a major substrate for energy metabolism.

Cholesterol is the other major lipid transported in lipoproteins. It is not used for energy; it is the precursor of steroid hormones and bile acids and is a structural component of cellular membranes. In higher animals, including all mammals, it is transported mainly in the form of cholesteryl esters, which are synthesized in cells or in the plasma compartment itself. As with triglycerides, the transport of cholesteryl esters in lipoproteins permits specific targeting of cholesterol to tissues that require it for structural purposes or for making its metabolic products.

Two of the lipoprotein classes, chylomicrons and VLDL, are composed primarily of triglyceride.

Chylomicrons transport exogenous (dietary) triglyceride, and VLDLs transport endogenous triglyceride. Chylomicrons are not normally present in postabsorptive plasma after an overnight fast. The VLDLs normally contain 10 to 15% of the plasma total cholesterol. LDLs contain cholesterol as their major component and normally contain most (60 to 70%) of the plasma cholesterol. HDLs are approximately half protein and half lipid and usually contain 20 to 30% of the total plasma cholesterol. Lipoproteins are lighter than the other plasma proteins because of their high lipid content. This characteristic permits both the operational classification and the ultracentrifugal separation of the different classes of lipoproteins.

Each lipoprotein class is heterogeneous in its protein constituents. Nine distinct apolipoproteins have been separated and described. Most investigators group the apolipoproteins into five families (designated apo A, apo B, apo C, apo D, and apo E) on the basis of their chemical, immunologic, and metabolic characteristics. Apo A refers to the apolipoproteins (apo A-I and apo A-II) that are primarily, but not exclusively, found in HDL. A third member of the apo A family, apo A-IV, is a minor component of chylomicrons. Apo B is the major apoprotein of LDL but also comprises about 35% of VLDL protein. There are two forms of apo B: a large form called apo B-100 and found in LDL and a smaller form called apo B-48 and produced mainly in the intestine. Apo C represents a group of apoproteins (apo C-I, apo C-II, apo C-III) that were originally described as major components of VLDL but that are also present as minor components in HDL. Apo D is a minor component of HDL. Apo E is a major component of VLDL and a minor one of HDL. The apolipoproteins serve both structural and functional roles. Some apoproteins are ligands for specific cell surface receptors, e.g., apo B-100 and apo E for the LDL (or apo B/E) receptor (Brown and Goldstein, 1986); others are cofactors for enzymes, e.g., apo C-II is a necessary activating cofactor for lipoprotein lipase. For reviews of lipoprotein structure and metabolism, see Havel (1987) and Stanbury et al. (1983).

Relationship of Plasma Lipid and Lipoprotein Levels to Atherosclerotic Cardiovascular Diseases

Epidemiologic Evidence for CHD

Most major epidemiologic studies have focused on white men, but a few have provided information about women and nonwhites of both sexes.

TOTAL CHOLESTEROL (TC) TC is used in this chapter as an abbreviation for the total cholesterol in either serum or plasma. TC concentration is usually expressed as milligrams of cholesterol per 100 ml of serum or plasma (mg/dl). TC concentrations in serum are about 2% higher than those measured in corresponding plasma (Folsom et al., 1983). Although this difference should be considered in comparing the results of studies with one another when numbers of subjects are large and small systematic biases might affect the comparison, it does not affect the major results or conclusions of studies discussed in this report in which serum or plasma is used in analyses of cholesterol. Thus, TC is used interchangeably for both serum and plasma total cholesterol.

Until the past decade, TC, rather than lipoprotein cholesterol, was measured in most epidemiologic studies because reliable methods for measuring lipoprotein cholesterol in large numbers of people were not available. Therefore, most data on disease risk are based on TC level.

Variation in Mean TC Among Populations Mean levels of TC vary widely among populations. In the Seven Countries Study, investigators studied 16 populations of middle-aged men residing in seven countries: Finland, the Netherlands, Italy, Yugoslavia, Greece, the United States, and Japan (Keys, 1970, 1980b). Examination methods, laboratory procedures, and quality control procedures were standardized. Mean TC for men ages 50 to 54 years varied from 157 mg/dl in a Japanese population to 262 mg/dl in eastern Finland (Keys, 1980b). In the Ni-Hon-San Study, three population-based samples of men of Japanese ancestry were compared. Mean TC levels for men ages 50 to 54 were 182, 219, and 228 mg/dl in Japan, Hawaii, and California, respectively (Nichaman et al., 1975). In the Israel Ischemic Heart Disease Study, the age-adjusted mean TC level in male civil servants age 40 and older varied from 195 mg/dl for those born in Africa to 219 mg/dl for those born in Central Europe (Kahn et al., 1969). Similar differences were found some 15 years later for male and female adolescents and adults in the Jerusalem Lipid Research Clinics Prevalence Study (Halfon et al., 1982a,b).

Other differences among populations have been observed for men in Puerto Rico, Hawaii, and Framingham, Massachusetts (Gordon et al., 1974), and for men and women in London, Naples, Uppsala, and Geneva (Lewis et al., 1978). Some of this evidence is reviewed in the report of a Conference on Health Effects of Blood Lipoproteins (1979). The results of these various studies, particularly the studies of migrants, indicate that the differences in mean TC levels among populations are due largely to environmental factors, principally diet, rather than to constitutional factors.

Large population differences in mean TC levels have also been observed among children and adolescents; the pattern of variation in these means closely parallels that of the adult values, but at lower absolute values (Conference on Blood Lipids in Children, 1983).

Variation in CHD Rates Among Populations   Large differences also exist among populations in the incidence of and mortality from CHD and in the prevalence and severity of atherosclerosis. For example, in the Seven Countries Study, age-standardized, 10-year incidence of first major CHD events (myocardial infarction and coronary death) among men free of CHD at entry varied from 3 in 1,000 on Crete to 107 in 1,000 in eastern Finland (Keys, 1980b). Corresponding figures for 10-year CHD mortality were 0 and 68 in 1,000, respectively. In the Ni-Hon-San Study, relative risks of first major CHD event were 0.46, 1.00, and 1.54 for the cohorts in Japan, Hawaii, and California, respectively (Kagan et al., 1981; Marmot et al., 1975; Robertson et al., 1977). Incidence of first major CHD events among middle-aged men in Framingham was twice that in Puerto Rico and Hawaii (Gordon et al., 1974).

Variation in Atherosclerosis Among Populations   In the International Atherosclerosis Project, the extent of atherosclerosis in the coronary arteries and aortas was measured in 23,207 autopsied people from 19 populations in 14 countries (McGill, 1968b). The mean percentage of intimal surface with raised lesions varied from 6% in Durban Bantu to 18% in New Orleans whites. Differences among populations were noticeable at ages 15 to 24 and marked at ages 25 to 34. With few exceptions, ranking the populations according to extent of raised lesions corresponded closely to ranking them by CHD mortality rate.

Correlations Between Mean TC and CHD Rates Among Populations   Variation in mean TC levels among populations is highly correlated with variation in CHD incidence and extent of atherosclerosis. The correlation coefficient for median level of TC with age-standardized, 10-year CHD death

rates for 16 cohorts in the Seven Countries Study was .82 (Keys, 1980b). The correlations between median TC and national CHD death rates for these seven countries at 0, 5, 10, and 15 years after TC was measured were .86, .90, .93, and .96, respectively (Rose, 1982). In the International Atherosclerosis Project, there was a correlation of .76 between the extent of atherosclerosis and mean TC concentration in 19 populations (Scrimshaw and Guzman, 1968). Populations with mean TC levels less than 180 mg/dl are largely free of atherosclerosis and CHD, whereas those with mean TC levels above 220 mg/dl are characterized by high rates of CHD (Conference on Health Effects of Blood Lipoproteins, 1979). These results support the conclusion that variation in CHD rates among populations is determined predominantly by differences in levels of TC.

CHD Incidence and Mortality Among Individuals Within Populations   In prospective studies of middle-aged men, TC levels above 200–220 mg/dl are positively associated with risk of CHD in the United States (Pooling Project Research Group, 1978; Stamler et al., 1986) as well as in Norway (Holme et al., 1981), France (Ducimetiere et al., 1980), Japan (Johnson et al., 1968), Israel (Goldbourt et al., 1985), England (Rose and Shipley, 1980), Italy (Italian National Research Council, 1982), Finland, the Netherlands, Greece, and Serbia (Keys, 1980b). The association may be weak or absent in some populations with low mean levels of TC and low absolute risk of CHD, e.g., in rural areas of Bosnia and Croatia (Keys, 1980b; Kozarevic et al., 1976, 1981).

Results have been less consistent regarding the association of TC levels below 200 mg/dl with the risk of CHD. In fact, questions have been raised as to whether the association of serum TC with CHD risk is continuous or whether there is some level of serum TC below which it is not related to risk of CHD (e.g., Goldbourt, 1987). In four of the eight studies in the U.S. Pooling Project, age-standardized incidence of CHD for men ages 40 to 64 years was lower in the second quintile of serum TC (194 to 218 mg/dl) than in the first quintile (<194 mg/dl) (Pooling Project Research Group, 1978). In the Israel Ischemic Heart Disease Study of 9,902 male civil servants 40 or more years old, age-standardized 15-year CHD mortality rates according to quintile of serum TC (<176, 176 to 197, 198 to 216, 217 to 241, and >241 mg/dl) were 4.5, 4.9, 4.4, 6.7, and 10.2 per 100, respectively (Goldbourt et al., 1985). In the same study, however, the corresponding 7-year CHD mortality rates previously showed a steadily increasing pattern: 10, 12, 16, 17, and 30 per 1,000, respectively (Yaari et al., 1981). Also, in that study, the 5-year incidence rates for myocardial infarction were 29, 39, and 60 per 1,000 for men in the serum TC tertiles of 77 to 189, 190 to 219, and 220 to 500 mg/dl, respectively (Medalie et al., 1973).

Many other large prospective studies have also shown a clear monotonic association of CHD with TC levels below 200 mg/dl. In the Hiroshima Adult Health Study of 4,256 men age 40 and older, 6-year age-standardized CHD morbidity ratios associated with three levels of TC (<180, 180 to 219, and >220 mg/dl) were 72, 162, and 333, respectively (100 representing risk for the whole group) (Johnson et al., 1968). Ten-year CHD mortality rates among 17,718 British civil servants ages 40 to 64 according to quintile of TC (<159, 159 to 183, 184 to 203, 204 to 233, and >233) were 28, 34, 36, 44, and 54 per 1,000, respectively (Rose and Shipley, 1980). In the Framingham Study, the 20-year CHD incidence for men ages 33 to 49 according to level of TC (114 to 193, 194 to 213, 214 to 230, 231 to 255, and 256 to 514 mg/ dl) was 86, 153, 220, 268, and 306 per 1,000, respectively (Kannel and Gordon, 1982). Among 356,222 men ages 35 to 57 who were initially screened in the Multiple Risk Factor Intervention Trial, age-standardized 6-year CHD mortality increased steadily according to decile of TC from 3 per 1,000 for TC <168 mg/dl to 13 per 1,000 for TC >263 mg/dl (Stamler et al., 1986). The data for that trial are shown in Figure 7–1.

In that trial the 6-year mortality rate doubled between 153 and 226 mg/dl (3.16 to 6.94 per 1,000) and doubled again between 226 and 290 mg/dl (6.94 to 13.05 per 1,000). The weight of evidence supports the idea that TC level, at least from 150 mg/dl upward, is positively associated in a continuous fashion with CHD risk. Because the incidence of CHD is low at TC levels under 200 mg/dl, occasional exceptions to this rule are more likely due to statistical artifact than to biologic diversity. Results from the observations of screenees in the Multiple Risk Factor Intervention Trial also indicated that the association between TC and 5-year risk of CHD death for 23,490 black men was similar to that for 325,384 white men (Neaton et al., 1984).

The association between TC and the *relative risk* of CHD declines with age. In the pooled results of five U.S. studies, the relative risk of CHD in the highest quintile of TC (>256 mg/dl) compared to

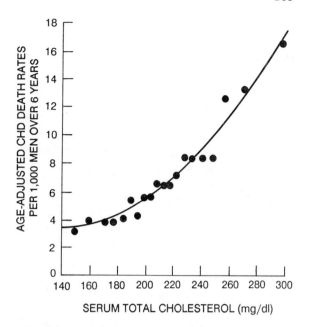

FIGURE 7–1 Relationship of serum cholesterol to CHD death in 361,662 men ages 35 to 57 during an average followup of 6 years. From Martin et al. (1986). Each point represents the median value for 5% of the population.

the lowest quintile (<194 mg/dl) (defined as the ratio of the risks in these two groups) was 3.6, 1.9, 1.8, and 1.5 for men ages 45 to 49, 50 to 54, 55 to 59, and 60 to 64, respectively (Pooling Project Research Group, 1978). This observation has sometimes been misinterpreted to mean that the level of TC is relatively unimportant in elderly people. The committee believes that this misinterpretation may arise from failure to distinguish between the concepts of *relative risk* (the ratio between two risks) and *attributable risk* (the difference between two risks). The former is commonly used to evaluate the magnitude of an epidemiologic association; the latter is commonly used to evaluate its public health importance. In fact, in the set of studies cited above, the attributable risk (calculated as the difference in risk between the highest and lowest quintiles) did not vary consistently with age. Thus, the corresponding attributable risks were 46, 28, 40, and 42 per 1,000 in 8 years for men ages 45 to 49, 50 to 54, 55 to 59, and 60 to 64, respectively.

Atherosclerosis at Autopsy TC measured by standardized procedures in apparently healthy men was strongly associated with extent of atherosclerosis at autopsy in the Hiroshima Adult Health Study (Rickert et al., 1968), Honolulu Heart Program (Reed et al., 1987; Rhoads et al., 1978), the Framingham Study (Feinleib et al., 1979), the Oslo Study (Holme et al., 1981), and the Puerto Rico Heart Study (Sorlie et al., 1981). There are few data on women.

In the Framingham Study, the extent of coronary atherosclerosis in men was positively correlated with TC measured 1, 5, and 9 years before death; in women, only TC measured 9 years before death but not TC measured 5 and 1 years before death correlated significantly (Feinleib et al., 1979). In the Bogalusa Heart Study, TC measured at 3 to 18 years of age was correlated ($R = .67$) with percentage of aortic intimal surface involved with fatty streaks as measured during the autopsies of 35 people who died between 7 and 24 years of age (Newman et al., 1986; Strong et al., 1986). Correlations with raised lesions and with lesions in the coronary arteries could not be reliably determined in this series because only 6 people had fibrous plaques and the extent of coronary intimal surface involved in fatty streaks was small, varying only from 0 to 6% (mean, 1%). In a follow-up of the initial report, Freedman et al. (1988) increased the number of cases to 44 and examined the relationship within races. As anticipated, blacks had more extensive fatty streaks than did whites, but there also was a strong positive association between the extent of aortic fatty streaks and the LDL cholesterol concentration within each race group.

In summary, epidemiologic findings among populations and for individuals within populations consistently indicate a strong, continuous, and positive relationship between TC levels and the prevalence and incidence of, as well as mortality from, atherosclerotic CHD. This relationship has been confirmed in autopsy studies.

LDL AND HDL CHOLESTEROL   There is less epidemiologic evidence on lipoprotein cholesterol than on TC. Few early studies included measurements of lipoprotein cholesterol because of technical difficulties and cost.

Differences Among Populations   Lipoprotein cholesterol was not measured in the Seven Countries Study; thus, variation among populations is less well characterized for LDL cholesterol (LDL-C) and HDL cholesterol (HDL-C) than for TC. Apparently, average values of LDL-C vary widely among populations, but the evidence is less clear for HDL-C. In the Four European Communities Study, mean LDL-C varied from 116 to 168 mg/dl for men and from 114 to 146 mg/dl for women; in

contrast, mean HDL-C varied only from 52 to 55 mg/dl for men and from 60 to 64 mg/dl for women (Lewis et al., 1978). In the 1950s, studies of three groups of sedentary Japanese men matched for fatness showed that mean β-lipoprotein cholesterol (LDL-C) was 120, 183, and 213 mg/dl for those residing in Shime, Honolulu, and Los Angeles, respectively; corresponding mean values for α-lipoprotein cholesterol (HDL-C) were 40, 40, and 35 mg/dl (Keys et al., 1958b). Results from the Jerusalem Lipid Research Clinic Study showed that differences in mean TC according to place of birth (Asia, North Africa, Europe, and Israel) were due mainly to differences in LDL-C (Harlap et al., 1982). On the other hand, a preliminary report of a survey of men in 13 countries indicated that mean HDL-C varied from 27 mg/dl in an African population to 58 mg/dl in eastern Finland (Knuiman and West, 1981). In a study of schoolboys 6 to 7 years old selected from 26 rural and urban populations in 16 countries (Knuiman et al., 1980), mean HDL-C varied from 31 mg/dl in rural Nigeria to 65 mg/dl in rural Finland and correlated (.90) with mean TC. The basis for these different results is not clear.

There is no firm evidence regarding the ecological association of mean HDL-C to risk of CHD. In one study, a correlation of $-.57$ was found between mean HDL-C and CHD mortality for 19 countries (Simons, 1986), but these results were based on nonstandardized measurements of undefined samples of people. Knuiman and West (1981) obtained standardized measurements of HDL-C in a survey of small samples of men in 13 countries and found a correlation of .57 with national CHD mortality in those countries. One of the lowest population mean values for HDL-C was found in Mexico in Tarahumara Indians, who also had very low values of LDL-C and TC (Connor et al., 1978). Thus, the extent to which variation among populations in CHD rates may be affected by (associated with) variations in mean HDL-C levels is uncertain. Clearly, the association is substantially less than that between population CHD rates and mean LDL-C levels.

Differences Among Individuals   Baseline levels of LDL-C were positively associated with risk of CHD in men and women ages 50 to 79 years in the Framingham Study (Gordon et al., 1977), in Israeli male civil servants age 40 and older (Medalie et al., 1973), and in men ages 35 to 57, black and white, separately identified, who were assigned to the Usual-Care Group in the Multiple Risk

Factor Intervention Trial (Watkins et al., 1986). Change in LDL-C level has also been related directly to change in CHD risk; among hypercholesterolemic men treated with cholestyramine, reduction of 11% in LDL-C was associated with a decrease of 19% in risk of CHD (Lipid Research Clinics Program, 1984b).

In the Framingham Study, HDL-C was inversely related to incidence of CHD in men and women ages 49 to 82 years (Castelli et al., 1986; Gordon et al., 1977); an increment in HDL-C of 25 mg/dl was associated with nearly a 50% decrement in risk of CHD for men and women after adjustment for age, body mass index (see Chapter 21 for definition), cigarette smoking, systolic blood pressure, and TC (Castelli et al., 1986). Among the hypercholesterolemic men treated with cholestyramine in the Lipid Research Clinics Coronary Primary Prevention Trial, 1 mg/dl increments in HDL-C at baseline and afterward were associated with decrements of 5.5 and 4.4% in risk of CHD, respectively (Gordon et al., 1986). Baseline level of HDL-C was inversely associated with risk of CHD among men assigned to the Usual-Care Group in the Multiple Risk Factor Intervention Trial (Watkins et al., 1986), but the association was weaker than that observed in the Framingham Study or the Lipid Research Clinics Program. These findings of an inverse relationship between HDL-C and CHD have been supported by observations in the Israel Ischemic Heart Disease Study (Goldbourt et al., 1985; Medalie et al., 1973) and in prospective case-comparison studies of frozen serum samples in Oslo (Enger et al., 1979) and in Tromsö, Norway (Miller et al., 1977).

HDL-C was not significantly associated with the 24-year CHD death rate in a cohort of 526 Finnish men ages 36 to 61 (Keys et al., 1984) and was only weakly associated with CHD death rate in a cohort of 284 Minneapolis business and professional men ages 45 to 55 at entry into the study (Keys, 1980a; Keys et al., 1963). HDL-C was weakly and not significantly (inversely) associated with the incidence of CHD after adjustment for age, body mass index, blood pressure, cigarette smoking, and non-HDL cholesterol in the British Regional Heart Study (Pocock et al., 1986). A study of men in the USSR also failed to find an inverse association between HDL-C and CHD (Levy and Klimov, 1987).

In the Oslo Study of men ages 40 to 49 years at entry in 1972 and 1973, antemortem measurements of plasma lipids and other characteristics were available for 129 men for whom there were also postmortem measurements of the extent of atherosclerosis. The percentage of the coronary intimal surface involved with raised lesions was positively correlated with TC (.32) and negatively correlated with HDL-C (−.25) (Holme et al., 1981).

Although changes in HDL-C are related to changes in CHD risk in most populations, the benefit that can be expected from raising HDL as a preventive strategy in itself is not entirely clear. Added benefit, over that derived from lowering LDL, is suggested, however, by the long-term results of the Coronary Drug Project (Canner et al., 1986), by the results of the Cholesterol Lowering Atherosclerosis Study (Blankenhorn et al., 1987), and by those of the Helsinki Heart Study (Frick et al., 1987; Manninen at al., 1988), in which HDL-C was raised and TC, LDL-C, and VLDL-C were lowered.

Among people ages 50 to 79 years in the Framingham Study, the ratio of TC to HDL-C was strongly associated with risk of CHD in men and women. The strength of the association was not significantly improved by adding TC or HDL-C to the equation containing this ratio (Castelli et al., 1983). A similar result was obtained with the ratio of LDL-C to HDL-C for women, but information about the level of LDL-C did add to the strength of the association in men. The authors concluded that ratios can be useful predictors of risk, but warned that they may not always be as informative as the joint use of the two individual figures used to calculate the ratio. It seems reasonable to expect that increasing knowledge about the various classes and subclasses of lipoproteins will lead to improved ability to predict risk of atherosclerotic diseases. Whether these prediction formulas will take the form of ratios or more detailed specifications of lipoprotein levels is uncertain.

Although the ratio of TC or LDL-C to HDL-C may be a very good predictor of CHD risk in the U.S. population, it is probably not the best target for clinical management or therapy. The recent report of the National Cholesterol Education Program (1988) identified the absolute level of LDL-C as the key index for clinical decision-making about cholesterol-lowering therapy and as the specific target for therapy. The authors of the report stated, "Reliance on a ratio of either total or LDL-cholesterol to HDL-cholesterol as a key factor in decisions regarding treatment is not a practice recommended in this report. Blood pressure and smoking are not combined into a single number because the clinician needs to know both facts separately in order to recommend an intervention. Similarly, HDL-cholesterol and LDL-cholesterol are independent risk factors with different determinants, and combining them into a single number conceals information that may be useful to the clinician" (National Cholesterol Education Program, 1988).

In summary, of the lipoprotein fractions, LDL has the strongest and most consistent relationship to individual and population risk of CHD. HDL has generally been found to be inversely associated with risk of CHD in individuals within a population, but in at least three long-term population studies, this inverse association was not seen (Keys et al., 1984; Levy and Klimov, 1987; Pocock et al., 1986). Population rates of CHD are much more strongly related to average TC and LDL-C values than to HDL-C.

These findings (together with the results of animal experiments and clinical research reviewed later in this chapter) strongly support the conclusions that LDL-C is centrally and causally important in the pathogenic chain leading to atherosclerosis and CHD. Variation in LDL-C levels explains a large part of individual risk within high-risk cultures and explains almost all the differences in CHD rates among populations. HDL-C is associated inversely with individual susceptibility to CHD within populations where there is widespread elevation of LDL-C and TC. Data are inadequate to characterize ratios of LDL to HDL as a major determinant of the atherosclerotic disease burden among populations; however, the ratio provides improved individual prediction, again within high-risk, high-LDL cultures.

APOLIPOPROTEINS Apolipoproteins play key roles in both the structure and function of plasma lipoproteins. Research on the molecular structure, genetic variability, and metabolism of plasma apolipoproteins has progressed rapidly in recent years, particularly with the application of the new techniques of molecular biology. Knowledge about apolipoproteins has added greatly to our understanding of lipoprotein metabolism and how it is related to atherosclerosis. In a number of instances, genetically controlled variations in apolipoproteins affect lipoprotein structure, composition, and metabolism. For example, polymorphic forms of apolipoprotein E (apo E) interact with dietary fats to influence plasma lipoprotein concentrations, and assessment of apo E phenotypes is an essential procedure in the diagnosis of familial dysbetalipoproteinemia. However, the evidence

currently available does not clearly show that plasma apolipoprotein levels are better predictors of CHD than are the plasma levels of cholesterol in the major lipoprotein classes.

Apo E Polymorphism and Hyperlipidemia In 1977, Utermann et al. (1977, 1979) demonstrated that genetic polymorphisms in apo E were associated with different plasma cholesterol, LDL-C, and β-VLDL concentrations. The apo E phenotypes were shown to be due to segregation of three alleles at a single locus (Zannis and Breslow, 1981) and the major isoforms to be determined by substitution of the amino acid cysteine for arginine (Weisgraber et al., 1981). The three major isoforms are called apo E2, E3, and E4. If the most common phenotype, designated E3/3, is considered to be normal, women who are heterozygous, with phenotype E3/2, have more than 40% higher plasma VLDL-C and intermediate-density-lipoprotein (IDL)-C levels, and 12% lower LDL-C levels (Robertson and Cumming, 1985). Men with the E3/2 phenotype have an approximately 15% increase in plasma VLDL-C and IDL-C concentrations and 20% lower LDL-C concentrations. The E2/2 phenotype is uncommon but is associated with extreme variations in plasma lipoprotein levels. Patients with familial dysbetalipoproteinemia (type 3 hyperlipoproteinemia) generally have the E2/2 phenotype. Most people with this phenotype do not have familial dysbetalipoproteinemia, however, and in fact have lower plasma cholesterol levels than the general population (see Davignon et al., 1988). In contrast, the presence of the E4 allele (and the E4/3 or 4/4 phenotype) appears to be associated with an increased level of LDL and an increase in coronary risk. Thus, a single amino acid substitution in one apolipoprotein can have a substantial effect on plasma cholesterol concentrations and on the plasma lipoprotein profile. This topic has been reviewed thoroughly by Davignon et al. (1988).

The Apolipoproteins and Atherosclerosis In the 1980s, the availability of better methods for fractionating lipoproteins, for measuring serum apolipoproteins, and for detecting apolipoprotein variants made possible a new series of studies that sought relationships among lipoproteins, apolipoproteins, and atherosclerosis. This topic was reviewed by Brunzell et al. (1984) and by Wallace and Anderson (1987).

Ishikawa et al. (1978) were among the first to examine the relationship of plasma apolipoprotein concentrations to CHD. In the Tromsö Heart

Study, apo A-I levels were associated inversely with CHD, but were less powerful predictors than HDL-C levels. A number of investigators subsequently compared CHD patients with controls and generally found apo B levels higher and apo A-I and apo A-II levels lower in diseased subjects (DeBacker et al., 1982; Fager et al., 1980, 1981; Franceschini et al., 1982; Maciejko et al., 1983; Naito, 1985; Onitiri and Jover, 1980; Riesin et al., 1980; Sniderman et al., 1980; Whayne et al., 1981). However, these investigators were not in agreement about whether apolipoprotein levels or lipoprotein cholesterol levels were better indicators of CHD. Pilger et al. (1983) used stepwise discriminant analysis to determine which measures best differentiated subjects with and without peripheral vascular disease. The best model included 14 variables, among which, in addition to HDL-C and LDL-C, were apo B, apo A-I, and apo A-II concentrations.

Menzel et al. (1983) examined the relationship of six different apo E phenotypes to coronary lesions assessed by angiography in 1,000 patients. Heterozygotes (E3/2) were more frequent in patients with little or no coronary atherosclerosis, but E2/2 homozygosity, despite the presence of β-VLDL in the plasma, was not associated with more severe coronary lesions.

Wallace and Anderson (1987) concluded their review by stating that apolipoprotein levels appeared promising as predictors of CHD, but that large cohort studies would be required to determine whether they are better predictors of atherosclerotic disease than plasma lipoprotein lipid levels and whether they are useful clinically.

Lp(a) and Human Atherosclerosis The role of lipoprotein(a) [Lp(a)] in atherosclerosis and atherosclerotic heart disease has been controversial ever since Lp(a) was discovered by Berg (1963). The apoprotein of Lp(a) has been shown to consist of two peptides—apo(a) and apo B—linked by one or more disulfide bonds (Gaubatz et al., 1983). The recent sequencing of a cloned apo(a) complementary DNA (cDNA) showed that apo(a) is very similar to plasminogen (McLean et al., 1987).

Several studies have shown a relationship between serum Lp(a) levels and CHD (Berg et al., 1974; Dahlén et al., 1975). High scores for coronary arteriosclerosis on angiography were correlated with serum Lp(a) levels (Dahlén et al., 1976). Walton et al. (1974) demonstrated Lp(a) in arterial lesions by immunofluorescence. Overall, the evidence concerning the association of Lp(a) with atherosclerosis is rather scanty, but highly suggestive. Lp(a) levels in plasma are generally believed not to be affected by diet.

Lipoproteins and Apolipoproteins in Atherosclerotic Lesions Kao and Wissler (1965) demonstrated the presence of LDL in human lesions by immunofluorescence with rabbit antisera to LDL. Hoff and associates have demonstrated the presence of apo B, apo A-I, and apo C in the arteries of humans and several animal species (Hoff and Gaubatz, 1975; Hoff et al., 1974, 1975a,b,c; Yomantas et al., 1984).

The same investigators quantified apo B in lesions (Hoff et al., 1977a,b, 1978, 1979b; reviewed by Hoff and Morton, 1985) and showed that LDL in lesions differed from plasma LDL (Hoff and Gaubatz, 1982; Hoff et al., 1979a). LDL in lesions stimulated the production of cholesteryl esters by macrophages (Clevidence et al., 1984; Goldstein et al., 1981). Apo A-I-containing lipoprotein extracted from arteries also differed in composition from plasma HDL (Heideman and Hoff, 1982).

These studies clearly show that apo B-containing lipoproteins accumulated in atherosclerotic lesions. LDL from atherosclerotic lesions contained particles larger than those found in plasma LDL, was more electronegative, and stimulated cholesterol esterification in mouse peritoneal macrophages. The extent to which these alterations in LDL occurred in the arterial intima, after the LDL had entered the vessel wall, is not clear. This combined evidence implicates apo B-containing lipoproteins in the pathogenesis of atherosclerosis.

Apolipoproteins and Dietary Responsiveness In view of the critical roles of apolipoproteins in lipoprotein metabolism, genetic variants in addition to those of apo E probably influence the lipemic responses of individuals to dietary fats and thereby affect the risk of CHD. This research area is quite active, and new findings are likely to be available in the near future.

Summary Apolipoproteins show promise of helping us to understand the mechanisms linking diet to atherosclerosis and cardiovascular disease, but as yet they have not provided predictive power for atherosclerotic diseases beyond that provided by plasma lipid and lipoprotein cholesterol concentrations. They are not now useful in assessing the relationship of dietary fats to atherogenesis or atherosclerotic cardiovascular diseases on a population-wide basis.

VLDL CHOLESTEROL (VLDL-C) AND TRIGLYCERIDES

Differences Among Populations Fasting plasma triglyceride or VLDL-C levels have not been systematically ascertained in standardized, population-based surveys designed to compare cultures. Nonfasting triglyceride levels were measured in the Framingham, Honolulu, and Puerto Rico studies. Results indicated that relatively high mean nonfasting triglyceride levels are compatible with low-population CHD rates when the mean TC is also low (Gordon et al., 1974). However, in most populations found to have low average TC levels, triglyceride levels are also low (Conference on Health Effects of Blood Lipoproteins, 1979). The correlation was small ($R = .26$) and not statistically significant between 1980 CHD death rates in 19 countries and mean triglyceride levels measured in undefined population samples in those countries during the 1970s (Simons, 1986).

Differences Among Individuals A fairly large number of epidemiologic studies have explored relationships between plasma triglyceride levels and the risk of CHD. The studies conducted before 1980 were reviewed in full by Hulley et al. (1980). In almost all reported studies, a significant positive association between triglyceride levels and CHD was found upon univariate analysis. However, triglyceride has not held up as an independent risk factor in most of the studies that have provided multivariate adjustment for a full set of major risk variables. It is well established that a reciprocal relationship generally exists, both within populations and within individuals, between plasma triglyceride (and, therefore, VLDL) and HDL levels. Thus, individuals with high triglyceride levels tend to have lower HDL levels, and an increase or decrease in triglyceride level in a patient is generally accompanied by an opposite change in HDL-C level. On the other hand, our understanding of the association of VLDL and VLDL remnants to atherosclerosis is still incomplete, and there is some evidence that the latter particles may have an important role in atherogenesis. Hence, the answer to the question of whether or not elevated triglyceride (and VLDL) levels are causally linked to atherosclerotic disease in some patients, or groups of people, is not clear. What is clear is that, as a group, people with high triglyceride levels have elevated coronary risk. Overall, however, the potential atherogenicity of the triglyceride-rich

lipoproteins has not been determined. (For reviews and reports of recent studies, see Aberg et al., 1985; Carlson and Bottiger, 1981; Hulley et al., 1980; NIH, 1984; Wallace and Anderson, 1987.)

In the Framingham Heart Study, the plasma triglyceride level was found to be an independent predictor of CHD in women (Castelli, 1986). Several studies have observed that triglycerides (and VLDL) may have independent predictive power for CHD in women and a greater association with peripheral arterial disease than with CHD, but none of the associations found was strong (Aberg et al., 1985; Gordon et al., 1977, 1981b).

The National Institutes of Health (NIH) Consensus Conference on Treatment of Hypertriglyceridemia concluded, "Careful evaluation of existing data indicates that in the presence of normal cholesterol levels mild elevations of plasma triglycerides do not necessarily increase the risk of CVD. When triglycerides are below 250 mg/dl, risk generally does not exceed that of other Americans, and changes in lifestyle are unnecessary beyond those recommended for the general public. The same can be said for many normocholesterolemic individuals with borderline hypertriglyceridemia (defined as triglyceride levels ranging from 250 to 500 mg/dl) who have no risk factors or family history for cardiovascular disease. However, triglyceride levels in the range of 250 to 500 mg/dl can be a marker for secondary disorders or for a subset of patients with genetic forms of hyperlipoproteinemia who are at increased risk and who need specific therapy. Dietary intervention is the primary approach to therapy in these patients, but drugs have a role in selected individuals not responding to dietary management. Finally, the danger of pancreatitis is present in frank hypertriglyceridemia (triglycerides >500 mg/dl), and triglyceride lowering by diet and, if necessary, by drugs is indicated" (NIH, 1984). The Committee on Diet and Health endorses these conclusions.

Summary The relationship between plasma triglyceride levels and cardiovascular diseases is somewhat controversial and unclear. In most within-population studies, plasma triglyceride levels were positively associated with increased risk for cardiovascular diseases but they were not independently predictive for CHD after statistical adjustment for closely associated attributes such as TC, HDL-C, hypertension, cigarette smoking, and obesity. As indicated above, however, in the Framingham Heart Study the plasma triglyceride level was found to be an independent predictor of

CHD in women. Even so, the plasma total triglyceride level, rather than being a direct cause of atherosclerotic disease, probably reflects the presence of certain atherogenic lipoproteins. It is well known that VLDLs are highly heterogeneous; a number of different kinds of lipoprotein particles are contained within this density class. Many disease entities that elevate triglyceride levels, such as diabetes mellitus, nephrotic syndrome, chronic renal disease, and certain primary hyperlipidemias, carry an increased risk of CHD. In these situations, the high triglyceride level may be a clue to the presence of other lipoprotein abnormalities that are more directly associated with CHD, such as low HDL-C, elevated apo B or LDL-C, or atherogenic remnant triglyceride-rich lipoprotein particles that have not been well defined. Thus, whether or not VLDL and triglycerides are directly involved in the atherogenic process, elevated levels can be helpful in identifying people at increased risk of cardiovascular diseases.

Clinical-Genetic Evidence of CHD

A number of genetic disorders of lipoprotein metabolism have been identified and characterized (Brown and Ginsberg, 1987; Stanbury et al., 1983). The study of these disorders has provided many insights into the structure, metabolism, and regulation of the plasma lipoproteins and apolipoproteins. Several of these disorders are characterized by severe hypercholesterolemia and premature atherosclerosis and CHD. Such disorders include familial hypercholesterolemia (FH), familial combined hyperlipidemia, and familial dysbetalipoproteinemia (type 3 hyperlipoproteinemia).

FH provides strong evidence that a high LDL level per se is a cause of accelerated atherosclerosis and premature CHD. FH is caused by a defect in the gene encoding for the LDL receptor—the cell surface receptor that normally removes LDL from the circulation (Brown and Goldstein, 1986). The defective gene results in the receptor being either absent or nonfunctional. One gene for the LDL receptor normally is inherited from each parent. In the heterozygous form of FH, the patient has one normal and one abnormal gene for LDL receptors, and LDL-C levels are approximately doubled to levels exceeding 200 mg/dl.

Heterozygous FH occurs in the general population at a frequency of about 1 in 500, making FH one of the most common single-gene-determined diseases in humans. FH heterozygotes have TC levels that usually exceed 300 mg/dl and frequently have tendon xanthomas, corneal arcus, premature

CHD, and a strong family history of hypercholesterolemia. Approximately 5% of patients with myocardial infarction before age 60 will have heterozygous FH. Affected men often develop CHD in their 30s and 40s; in women with FH, CHD often occurs in their 50s and 60s.

Rarely, about once per million people, individuals inherit two abnormal genes for LDL receptors and hence are homozygous for FH. Homozygous FH patients have TC levels that range from 600 to 1,000 mg/dl, and they usually have planar and tuberous xanthomas as well as tendon xanthomas. Severe and often fatal coronary disease frequently develops while these people are in their teens. One homozygote had an acute myocardial infarction as early as 18 months of age; another died of an acute myocardial infarction at 3 years of age. Very few FH homozygotes survive past age 30 (Goldstein and Brown, 1983).

An animal counterpart of FH has been identified in a strain of rabbits called the Watanabe heritable hyperlipidemic (WHHL) rabbit (Goldstein et al., 1983). These rabbits have very high TC and LDL-C levels and develop severe atherosclerosis that is similar to that seen in humans. This genetic animal model provides further strong evidence of the causal relationship between high LDL-C levels and atherosclerosis. Elevated LDL-C levels due to a defect in the LDL receptor have also been observed in a rhesus monkey family by Scanu et al. (1988).

The research on FH and on the LDL receptor has provided insights into the mechanisms that might be involved in the more common problem of the mild to moderately elevated blood cholesterol levels that are seen in the general population. Potential relationships between LDL receptors, diet, and atherosclerosis have been discussed by Brown and Goldstein (1986). It is likely that the dietary components that raise plasma TC and LDL-C levels (specifically, dietary SFAs and cholesterol, as discussed in detail later in this chapter) act, at least in part, by suppressing hepatic LDL receptor activity. Recent studies (Spady and Dietschy, 1988) in hamsters powerfully demonstrate the role of dietary saturated triglycerides in augmenting the effect of dietary cholesterol in suppressing hepatic LDL receptor activity and elevating plasma LDL-C levels.

Clinical Trials of CHD

SMALL-SCALE TRIALS (ANGIOGRAPHIC END POINTS) Evidence has been accumulating and a number of studies are under way to determine the effect of lowering TC by diet, drugs, or ileal bypass surgery on the progression or regression of atherosclerotic lesions of coronary and large peripheral arteries as determined by angiography and ultrasound. As shown angiographically, in the earliest reported randomized controlled trial, patients with intermittent claudication had less angiographic progression and more regression of plaques in the diet- and drug-treated group than did a control group over a 19-month period. This was directly related to change in plasma LDL-C concentration (Duffield et al., 1983). In a recently completed randomized controlled trial in which angiographic techniques were used, patients treated with diet and several TC-lowering drugs had less progression and more actual regression of plaques in natural and bypass graft coronary vessels compared to controls over a 2-year period (Blankenhorn et al., 1987). These results and those of other systematic studies cited below are generally consistent with the conclusion that reducing LDL-C in hyperlipidemic patients reduces the rate of progression (and can induce regression) of atherosclerosis according to the degree of blood lipid reduction (Arntzenius et al., 1985; Brensike et al., 1984; Cohn et al., 1975; Kuo et al., 1979; Nash et al., 1982; Nikkila et al., 1984).

LARGE-SCALE PREVENTIVE TRIALS (CHD END POINTS) Nine randomized controlled trials on the primary prevention of CHD have been conducted. Key elements of their designs are summarized in Table 7–1. In five trials, various methods were used to change the plasma lipid concentrations as the only intervention; in two, diet was used; and in three, drugs. The other four studies, in which diet was also used, were multifactorial trials in which effects of change in plasma lipids were confounded with effects of change in cigarette smoking and blood pressure. Only one of the six trials involving change in diet—the Los Angeles Veterans Administration Domiciliary Study—was conducted under double-blind conditions (Dayton et al., 1968). In two studies—the World Health Organization Multifactor Trial (WHO European Collaborative Group, 1983) and the Finnish Mental Hospital Study (Hjermann et al., 1981)—groups of participants were randomized. In the others, individuals were randomized. The number of participants in these studies varied from approximately 800 to nearly 50,000.

Results of the trials summarized in Table 7–2 have been listed according to the percentage difference in mean serum cholesterol that was created between the treatment and comparison groups—

from 0% in the Göteborg Multifactor Trial (Wilhelmsen et al., 1986) to −15% in the Finnish Mental Hospital Study (Hjermann et al., 1981; Miettinen et al., 1972). (A negative sign here indicates that the experimental group had a lower mean level than the control group.) These results indicate that the magnitude of the difference in risk of CHD varied directly with the magnitude of the difference in mean TC. Studies that achieved little or no difference in mean TC had little or no difference in rate of CHD, whereas studies that achieved larger difference in mean TC experienced larger differences in CHD rates.

As indicated in Table 7–2, differences in CHD rates were statistically significant in five of the seven studies that achieved a difference of 8% or more in mean TC. The number of cardiac events in the other two studies—in the entire cohort of men in the Los Angeles Veterans Administration Domiciliary Study and in the sample of women in the Finnish Mental Hospital Study—were relatively small, and the percentage differences in CHD rates, although comparable in magnitude to those that were statistically significant, did not reach the 5% criterion for statistical significance.

Combined with the evidence from epidemiologic, clinical, and laboratory animal studies, this body of evidence establishes unequivocally that lowering serum TC, particularly LDL-C, reduces the incidence of CHD in middle-aged, hypercholesterolemic men. High-risk populations were used in most of these studies for quite practical reasons; the cost and problems of conducting such a trial in the general population would be very large and the results might well be inconclusive. However, in light of the total body of evidence, it seems reasonable to extend this conclusion to the general population of men and women with serum TC of 200 mg/dl or higher. Results of the Los Angeles Veterans Administration Domiciliary Trial support the inference that the conclusion may extend to people over 65 years of age as well, perhaps with a somewhat smaller effect, but the evidence bearing on this important question is still weak.

Most of the trials listed in Tables 7–1 and 7–2 showed an excess of non-CHD deaths in the intervention group as compared to the comparison group. How much of this can be attributed to chance and whether any of it reflects adverse effects of intervention are complex questions that may never be completely resolved. An analysis of 20 randomized controlled clinical trials that involved change in serum TC as the only systematic intervention indicates no statistically significant

TABLE 7–1 Design of Randomized Controlled Trials on Primary Prevention of Coronary Heart Disease[a]

Study	Study Population	Double Blind	Interventions and Targets of Interventions
Göteborg Multifactor Trial[b]	20,015 men ages 47 to 55	No	Diet, cigarette smoking, high blood pressure
WHO Multifactor Trial[c]	66 employed groups totaling 49,781 men ages 40 to 59	No	Diet, cigarette smoking, high blood pressure
Multiple Risk Factor Intervention Trial[d]	12,886 high-risk men ages 35 to 57	No	Diet, cigarette smoking, high blood pressure
Lipid Research Clinics Coronary Primary Prevention Trial[e]	3,806 hypercholesterolemic men ages 35 to 59	Yes	Cholestyramine
WHO Clofibrate Trial[f]	11,627 hypercholesterolemic men ages 30 to 59	Yes	Clofibrate
Helsinki Heart Study[g]	4,081 hypercholesterolemic men ages 40 to 55	Yes	Gemfibrozil
Los Angeles Veterans Administration Domiciliary Study[h]	846 men ages 55 to 89	Yes	Diet only
Oslo Study[i]	1,232 hypercholesterolemic normotensive men ages 40 to 49	No	Diet, cigarette smoking
Finnish Mental Hospital Study[j]	2 mental hospitals totaling 4,178 male patients and 6,434 female patients ages 15 and older	No	Diet only

[a]Unpublished table compiled by R. Peto, University of Oxford, 1988. Not included in this table are data from a paper by the WHO European Collaborative Group (1983), which included populations in Warsaw, because it did not present results on percentage reduction in serum cholesterol, and a paper on the Finnish Mental Hospital Study (Turpeinen et al., 1979), because it lacked results for total mortality and for women.
[b]Wilhelmsen et al. (1986).
[c]WHO European Collaborative Group (1983).
[d]MRFIT (1982).
[e]Lipid Research Clinics Program (1984a).
[f]Committee of Principal Investigators (1978).
[g]Frick et al. (1987).
[h]Dayton et al. (1968). This study was not focused strictly on primary prevention; 20.1% of participants had evidence of old myocardial infarction at entry.
[i]Hjermann et al. (1981).
[j]Miettinen et al. (1972).

effect on risk of non-CHD death (Richard Peto, University of Oxford, personal communication, 1987). In the trials shown in Table 7–2, none of the percentage differences in risk of non-CHD death or total mortality was statistically significant except for the WHO Clofibrate Trial. In the final mortality follow-up, however, the Committee of Principal Investigators (1978) of that study found that the excess mortality in the clofibrate-treated group did not continue after the end of treatment, and they could not find a reasonable explanation for the excess mortality that did occur during the period of active treatment. The excess deaths were

due to a variety of non-CHD causes and had no apparent association either with the extent of reduction in TC or with duration of treatment with clofibrate. These results do not rule out the possibility of a toxic effect, but seem more consistent with the hypothesis that the excess of deaths in the treated group was the result of random sampling variation.

The possible adverse effects of the drugs used in these trials are not strictly relevant to a report on diet and health and are not discussed further. The safety of dietary changes to lower serum TC is discussed in Chapter 28 of this report. There is no

TABLE 7–2 Results of Randomized Controlled Trials on Primary Prevention of Coronary Heart Disease[a]

Study[b]	Serum Cholesterol at Entry (mg/dl)	Percentage Differences Between Treated and Control Groups[c]	
		Serum Cholesterol	CHD[d]
Göteborg Multifactor Trial	250	0	0
WHO Multifactor Trial	216	−1	−7
Multiple Risk Factor Intervention Trial	254	−2	−7
Lipid Research Clinics Coronary Primary Prevention Trial	292	−8	−19[e]
WHO Clofibrate Trial	242	−9	−20[e]
Helsinki Heart Study	270	−9	−34[e]
Finnish Mental Hospital Study (women)	275	−12	−34
Los Angeles Veterans Administration Domiciliary Study	233	−13	−24
Oslo Study	329	−13	−47[e]
Finnish Mental Hospital Study (men)	267	−15	−53[e]

[a]From R. Peto, University of Oxford, unpublished data, 1988.

[b]See footnotes to Table 7–1 for references.

[c]At the end of the trial.

[d]CHD death was the end point in the WHO Multifactor Trial, the Multiple Risk Factor Intervention Trial, and the Finnish Mental Hospital Study. CHD death and nonfatal myocardial infarction were end points in the other studies. The studies varied in their technical definitions of these events; the original reports should be consulted for these matters.

[e]$p < .05$.

firm evidence to indicate that any of the dietary interventions used in the trials described above increased the risk of non-CHD deaths. In the Los Angeles Veterans Administration Domiciliary Trial, an excess of cancer deaths was observed in the experimental group that ate a diet high in PUFAs (on average, 15% of calories as PUFAs), but the difference was larger in the subgroup that adhered poorly to the prescribed diets than in the subgroup that adhered well (Pearce and Dayton, 1971). Also, results from other clinical trials did not indicate an excess of cancer deaths in groups assigned to a high-PUFA diet (Ederer et al., 1971). These considerations support the conclusion that the excess of cancer deaths observed in the Los Angeles study did not result from the high-PUFA diet.

Rose et al. (1974) analyzed the pooled data from six prospective studies of CHD and found that the mean serum TC of men who subsequently developed colon cancer was significantly lower than expected. The extensive literature that has since developed on this topic has been reviewed by McMichael et al. (1984). In some studies, an inverse association was found over a protracted period; in others, an inverse association was ob-

served during the first few years of follow-up but disappeared during continued follow-up; in yet others, no association was observed between initial serum TC level and subsequent risk of cancer. Some of the results may have reflected a preclinical effect of cancer on serum TC and some may have been due to metabolic characteristics (e.g., increased secretion of bile) of people who maintain low serum TC despite a diet high in SFAs and cholesterol. There is no evidence from studies in humans that low consumption of SFAs and cholesterol are positively correlated with rates of mortality from colon cancer (Liu et al., 1979). This evidence is discussed in more detail later in this chapter and in Chapter 28.

Richard Peto (Oxford University, personal communication, 1987) contends that the primary information to be obtained from the randomized clinical trials is the time required for changes in TC to have an effect on CHD rates. He has obtained information on 18 published and 2 unpublished randomized trials that involved changes in TC as the only systematic intervention, regardless of the mode of intervention (diet or drugs) and regardless of whether they were trials of disease prevention or disease treatment. Analysis of all data from these trials indicates that a 10% reduction in TC was associated with an average reduction of 16% in CHD risk (95% confidence interval of 10.6 to 20.4%) in trials lasting 4 years. Peto also noted that the reduction in risk varied according to the duration of treatment: 11% ($\pm$5%) in 13 shorter trials and 21% ($\pm$4%) in 7 longer trials, for a 10% reduction in TC. There have been no trials lasting a decade or longer, but results from the observational studies suggest that a reduction of 10% in TC over decades would be associated with a 33% reduction in rate of fatal CHD.

Other Atherosclerotic Cardiovascular Diseases

PERIPHERAL VASCULAR DISEASES (PVD)   There are few systematic data on the relationship of blood lipids and lipoproteins to the prevalence or risk of PVD or large-vessel peripheral arterial disease (PAD). In the Framingham Study, the 26-year cumulative incidence of intermittent claudication showed a concentration of cases in the upper part of the distribution for TC values in men but not in women (i.e., 11.6% in the upper quintile versus 5.3% in the lower) (Kannel and McGee, 1985). The results are, however, inconsistent among studies. For example, serum cholesterol was strongly related in some studies (Bothig et al., 1976; Reunanen et al., 1982) but only weakly or not related in others (Cavallo-Perin et al., 1984; Davignon et al., 1977; Greenhalgh et al., 1971; Hughson et al., 1978; Isacsson, 1972; Sirtori et al., 1974).

Triglycerides (and VLDL) may be more highly related to PAD than either HDL or LDL. In a British in-patient case-control study, there was a suggestion that prebetalipoprotein (i.e., VLDL) and serum triglyceride levels were disproportionately elevated in PVD patients, leading the authors to speculate about differences in the time course or severity of atherosclerosis with this blood lipid pattern, compared to that in coronary disease (Greenhalgh et al., 1971). At any rate, the overlap was considerable, in that a third of their PVD patients also had CHD. Clustering of intermittent claudication with other atherosclerotic diseases was also very strong in the Framingham Study. Overt coronary disease, cerebrovascular disease, or congestive heart failure were found in one out of three cases of intermittent claudication at the time of diagnosis, indicating the strong likelihood of common risk characteristics (Kannel and McGee, 1985).

The linkage in the basic processes leading to manifestations of PVD and CHD is further suggested by the finding of a strong curvilinear relationship between a Framingham risk index involving multiple risk characteristics for coronary disease and the incidence over time of manifest intermittent claudication, primarily due to an excess risk of intermittent claudication in the upper quintile of the coronary index (Kannel and McGee, 1985). A similar predominance of hypertriglyceridemia was observed in older men and in women among a series of Swedish patients with PVD (Leren and Haabrekke, 1971).

Because the underlying pathogenesis of PVD and CHD is atherothrombotic disease, it is likely, but not established, that the same evidence outlined for the relationship of diet to CHD holds for PVD as well. This is also suggested by the epidemiologic evidence about PVD, i.e., the positive relationship of intermittent claudication to the coronary disease risk index in the Framingham population. Finally, although the pathogenesis of atherosclerosis is similar in the different arterial beds, the relative importance of different risk factors in causing the disease process clearly differs among different anatomic sites. This issue is discussed further in Chapter 19.

STROKE   There are few systematic data relating blood lipids and lipoproteins to stroke incidence. A U-shaped relationship between lipids and stroke was suggested in the Chicago Stroke Study, in which a lower stroke risk was found in the central part of the TC distribution (Ostfeld et al., 1974). This was more striking in the 20-year Framingham follow-up of the older population, ages 65 to 74, in which the highest risk of stroke and acute brain infarction was observed at TC levels below 190 and above 295 mg/dl. This U-shaped relationship was stronger for acute brain infarction than for all strokes. In the same series, there was a negative relationship between LDL-C and overall stroke as well as for HDL-C and overall stroke (Kannel and Wolf, 1983). A similar U-shaped relationship was also observed in the Honolulu Heart Program, both for TC and for LDL-C, whereas HDL-C was negatively related and VLDL was positively but not significantly related to stroke risk (D. Reed et al., 1986). The left side of the U-shaped relationship to stroke in the Honolulu Study was due primarily to the inverse relationship between TC and hemorrhagic stroke (Kagan et al., 1980).

In later studies involving improved ability to discriminate between intracerebral hemorrhage and thrombosis by the use of computed tomography (CT) scanning, a clearer epidemiologic picture emerges. For example, in recent data from the Multiple Risk Factor Intervention Trial on more than 360,000 screenees observed for 10 years, there is a clear, positive, monotonic, linear relationship between TC level and death ascribed to cerebral thrombosis (Iso et al., 1988). This explains the right side of the U-shaped distribution of TC to overall stroke risk. A strong linear negative relationship was found between TC level and deaths coded to cerebral hemorrhage, the major explanation for the left side of the U-shaped TC–stroke risk curve. However, the negative relationship between TC and cerebral hemorrhage was limited to people with TC levels under 160 mg/dl *and* diastolic pressures greater than 90 mm Hg (Iso et al., 1988).

Animal Studies of Atherosclerosis

Hypercholesterolemia has been the common denominator of experimental atherosclerosis in a variety of animal species since shortly after the turn of the century (reviewed by Anitschkow, 1967; Duff, 1935; Jokinen et al., 1985; Katz and Stamler, 1953; Roberts and Straus, 1965; Strong, 1976; Wissler and Vesselinovitch, 1987a,b). In most species, hypercholesterolemia is induced by a diet enriched in cholesterol, SFAs, or both. Some animal species, such as the rat and the dog, are resistant to diet-induced hypercholesterolemia and develop atherosclerotic lesions when hormonal or other manipulations are used in conjunction with diet to induce hypercholesterolemia. When hypercholesterolemia is prolonged over several years, these animals develop all the complications seen in advanced atherosclerosis in humans and, eventually, myocardial infarction and other clinical manifestations of atherosclerosis in humans (Taylor et al., 1963).

Not only has hypercholesterolemia been the sine qua non of experimental atherosclerosis, but the relationship of the specific plasma lipoproteins to atherosclerosis in animals is similar to that in humans. For example, in humans and nonhuman primates, LDL is positively, and HDL is negatively, associated with atherosclerosis. In multiple regression analyses, plasma LDL and HDL concentrations account for as much as 50% of the variance in the extent of atherosclerosis (McGill et al., 1981a, 1985; Rudel, 1980). In some experiments, physical characteristics of LDL, such as molecular size, are also associated with atherosclerosis (Rudel et al., 1985). When diet-induced hypercholesterolemia is combined with other conditions known to augment atherosclerosis in hu-

mans, such as hypertension, the experimental lesions also are increased in extent and severity (McGill et al., 1985). Thus, the association of altered plasma lipoprotein concentrations in laboratory animals is not only strong and consistent, but the pattern of the association is similar to that in humans.

Furthermore, many studies have demonstrated that reduction of plasma cholesterol concentrations by withdrawal of cholesterol or fat, or both, from the diet, or by administration of drugs, leads to regression of experimental atherosclerosis (reviewed by Malinow, 1983). These regression studies, which were conducted in nonhuman primates, gave considerable support to the concept that the progression of atherosclerosis in humans can be retarded and possibly that lesions can be reversed by treating hyperlipidemia with diet and drugs.

In Vitro Studies of Atherogenesis

The strong relationship between high levels of plasma LDL and atherosclerosis has provided an important background for in vitro studies dealing with the cellular and molecular mechanisms of atherogenesis. These in vitro studies have sought to determine how LDL and other atherogenic lipoproteins could lead to the formation of cholesteryl ester-filled macrophages (foam cells) and other elements of the atherosclerotic lesion. The results of such studies have, in turn, supported data on humans and animals that suggest a primary etiologic role for LDL and related lipoproteins in the development of atherosclerosis.

A prominent and early feature of atherosclerotic lesions is the foam cell. In order to understand the mechanisms of foam cell formation, investigators have studied the interaction of plasma lipoproteins with various types of cultured macrophages. Native LDL does not lead to the accumulation of cholesteryl ester in many types of macrophages (reviewed in Brown and Goldstein, 1983). This lack of native LDL-induced cholesteryl ester accumulation is due, at least in part, to down-regulation of the LDL receptor on these cells by small amounts of excess cellular cholesterol, thus preventing a large influx of LDL-C. However, modified forms of LDL, such as acetyl-LDL, oxidized LDL, and malondialdehyde-LDL, do lead to massive accumulations of cholesteryl ester in cultured macrophages. These modified forms of LDL enter the cell by a receptor (called the scavenger receptor) that is distinct from the LDL receptor and that is not subject to down-regulation (Brown and Goldstein, 1983, 1986). Thus, cellular influx of these modified forms of LDL continues at a high rate, leading to significant accumulation of cholesteryl ester.

These in vitro observations have spawned a widespread search for evidence of LDL modification in vivo. Several recent studies have shed light on this topic. Pitas et al. (1983) demonstrated that foam cell macrophages from explants of rabbit aorta atheroma have scavenger receptors capable of binding modified LDL. Kita et al. (1987) and Carew et al. (1987) took advantage of the in vitro finding that the drug probucol, which is an antioxidant transported in LDL, prevents oxidative modification of LDL. These investigators demonstrated that probucol treatment of LDL receptor-deficient WHHL rabbits decreased LDL uptake in foam cell lesions and reduced the rate of development of these lesions independently of plasma cholesterol levels. These results are consistent with the hypothesis that oxidative modification of LDL may be important in the development of foam cell lesions.

Haberland et al. (1988) found immunochemical evidence for the existence of malondialdehyde-LDL in atherosclerotic aortas. Malondialdehyde is a by-product of arachidonic acid metabolism, which is an active process in the arterial wall. Whether malondialdehyde-LDL is involved in foam cell formation in vivo has yet to be determined.

A potential role for native LDL in foam cell formation has recently been suggested by findings that another cultured macrophage, the J774 macrophage, accumulates large amounts of cholesteryl ester in the presence of native LDL (Tabas et al., 1985). In this case, the LDL receptor is poorly down-regulated by LDL-C because of intracellular shunting of cholesterol away from the regulatory pathway into a hyperactive cholesterol esterification pathway. Since LDL receptors are abundant on foam cells in vivo (see below), indicative of poor LDL receptor down-regulation, this mechanism of foam cell formation may help explain the atherogenic effects of native LDL.

Foam cell formation has also been demonstrated in vitro by lipoproteins other than native and modified forms of LDL. One such lipoprotein, β-VLDL, is a cholesterol-enriched lipoprotein in the plasma of cholesterol-fed animals and in the plasma of humans with the genetic disease familial dysbetalipoproteinemia. β-VLDL causes massive deposition of cholesteryl ester in macrophages in vitro (Brown and Goldstein, 1983; Koo et al., 1986) and enters the macrophage by binding to the same receptor as does native LDL, and this receptor demonstrates poor down-regulation (Koo et al., 1986). Receptors for β-VLDL (and thus for native

LDL) are located on foam cells from rabbit aorta atheroma (Pitas et al., 1983). These observations, together with the strong correlation between β-VLDL plasma levels and atherosclerosis in cholesterol-fed animals and dysbetalipoproteinemic humans, indicate that β-VLDL is atherogenic.

β-VLDL has been found only in humans with familial dysbetalipoproteinemia. However, chylomicron remnants, which occur commonly in humans, interact with macrophages as does β-VLDL and cause the accumulation of cholesteryl ester as well as a large amount of triglyceride (Van Lentern et al., 1985). These and other findings have led some investigators to speculate that postprandial lipoproteins, particularly cholesterol-enriched particles such as chylomicron remnants, may be atherogenic in humans.

Foam cell research is an active area of in vitro investigation exploring the relationship between LDL and atherogenesis. However, other areas of study have also focused on this relationship (reviewed in Steinberg, 1983). For instance, LDL, either native or oxidized, causes endothelial cell injury in vitro. Endothelial injury, in turn, has been hypothesized to initiate atherogenesis by causing platelet adherence to the vessel wall and release of growth factors. In addition, LDL has been reported to directly augment platelet aggregation and to stimulate the growth of smooth muscle cells—two important features of the atherosclerotic lesion. It is clear, moreover, that other components of cells and vessel walls, not yet well defined, are also important factors in atherogenesis. The potential roles of growth factors, endothelial injury, and the different cells in arterial walls in the pathogenesis of atherosclerosis have been reviewed by Ross (1986).

In summary, numerous in vitro studies have demonstrated the ability of LDL and related lipoproteins to cause the formation of foam cells and other elements of atherosclerosis. Although there may be other important metabolic, cellular, and vessel wall factors in atherogenesis, in vitro evidence strongly suggests an important causative role for LDL and related lipoproteins.

Summary

There are large interpopulation differences in mean plasma lipid and lipoprotein levels and CHD rates. Average population TC levels also differ between adults and children; levels in children parallel those in adults at lower absolute values. Population correlations between CHD risk and mean TC level are strong but are weak for VLDL, triglyceride, and HDL-C. TC means and CHD rates among migrants change toward those of the adopted country, whether higher or lower than the country of origin.

Individual correlations of TC and LDL-C levels with CHD risk within populations are strong, positive, and continuous. Individual HDL-C level is inversely related to CHD risk in studies in the United States, Norway, and Israel, but not in Finland and the USSR. HDL-C population means are weakly correlated, if at all, with population TC levels and CHD rates.

Randomized clinical trials show a consistent relationship between decreases in TC and LDL-C levels resulting from altered diets and drugs and decreases in CHD incidence; the magnitude of the difference in risk varies directly with the magnitude of the difference in mean TC between the experimental and control groups. Differences in CHD rates between the experimental and control groups were statistically significant in five of the seven trials that achieved a difference of 8% or more in mean TC. The magnitude of the benefit that can be expected from lowering TC and LDL levels can be estimated from observational epidemiologic studies and from clinical trials. The estimates from these different kinds of studies are consistent in projecting that for individuals with TC levels initially in the 250- to 300-mg/dl range, each 1% reduction in TC level reduces CHD rates by approximately 2%. Thus, observational studies and clinical trials indicate that relatively small differences or changes in average TC level have a relatively large population effect or public health impact on disease. In addition, the trials indicate that risk can be reduced in individuals at moderate to high risk and that much of the effect of a lower TC on risk is seen after only a very few years.

Effects of Dietary Fats on Plasma Lipids and Lipoproteins

Evidence concerning the effects of dietary fats on plasma lipid and lipoprotein levels is reviewed in this section. Evidence specifically about the effects of dietary sterols is reviewed later in the section on the Relationship Between Dietary Sterols and Cardiovascular Disease. However, it is often difficult to separate clearly the effects of SFAs from those of dietary cholesterol, especially in observational studies. Therefore, terms such as "SFAs and cholesterol" are sometimes used in order to avoid giving the impression that a statement applies only to the fatty acid intake.

In many early studies, only serum TC was measured. When reviewing that body of evidence, variation in TC has been interpreted as a surrogate for variation in LDL-C. Some of the early studies assessed only the percentage of calories from total fat and did not assess the fatty acid composition of the diets. Where it seemed appropriate, differences in percentage of calories from total fat have been interpreted as reflecting differences in percentage of calories from SFAs.

Epidemiologic Evidence

STUDIES OF POPULATIONS Before World War II, reports from many parts of the world indicated that the prevalence of atherosclerotic cardiovascular diseases varied according to intake of fat and cholesterol (Rosenthal, 1934a,b,c). In the decade following World War II, further studies provided evidence that populations with low mean intakes of SFAs and cholesterol had low mean levels of serum TC in comparison to populations with diets high in SFAs and cholesterol (Bronte-Stewart et al., 1955; Keys and Anderson, 1954; Scrimshaw et al., 1957). [Only representative publications have been cited here. This large body of literature was reviewed by Katz et al. (1958) and by Keys (1963).] Although consistent with the hypothesis that dietary factors play an important role in determining the distribution of TC in populations, these studies often suffered from inadequate sampling and lack of standardized procedures.

In the Seven Countries Study (Keys, 1970, 1980b), standardized procedures (including 7-day weighed food records, a central laboratory, and chemical analysis of duplicate meals) were used. Median TC levels varied from 156 to 264 mg/dl. The mean percentage of calories from fat varied from 9 to 40% of total calories, with 3 to 22% from SFAs, 3 to 29% from MUFAs, and 3 to 7% from PUFAs. The mean concentration of TC correlated with mean percentages of calories from total fats ($R = .67$) and from SFAs ($R = .87$), and with estimated mean serum TC ($R = .90$) calculated from the formula, $164 + 1.35 (2S - P)$, where S and P represent the percentage of calories from SFAs and PUFAs, respectively (Keys, 1980b). Neither mean intake of PUFAs nor mean relative body weight was significantly correlated with mean serum TC. Dietary cholesterol was not measured in this study, but mean intake of SFAs probably had a strong correlation with mean intake of cholesterol, and results for SFAs probably apply to cholesterol as well.

The strong correlation between mean serum TC and mean percentage of calories from SFAs has been observed in other studies in which groups have formed the unit of analysis. As noted by Keys (1980b), the correlation coefficient was .94 for participants in the Israeli Ischemic Heart Disease Study (Kahn et al., 1969) when categorized according to region of birth: Israel, Asia, Africa, and eastern, central, and southern Europe. Stallones (1983) reviewed a large array of data from population surveys and found that the correlations between mean percentage calories from fats and mean serum TC was .86 for 76 groups of men and .79 for 27 groups of women. Stallones found the magnitude of these correlations to be remarkable since the studies were conducted with different procedures at different times; measurements of diet and of serum TC were not always on the same people; dietary data were not always presented separately by gender; and serum TC and fat intake were subject to appreciable errors of measurement and are surrogates for the variables of real interest—serum LDL-C, dietary SFAs, and cholesterol.

These observations indicate that 60 to 80% of the variance among populations in mean serum TC can be accounted for on a statistical basis by variation in mean percentage of calories from SFAs. (Dietary cholesterol probably contributes to this result as well, but the evidence from cross-population studies on dietary cholesterol is much less than the evidence on SFAs). Many feeding experiments (reviewed below) have established that isocaloric changes in the lipid composition of the diet—i.e., in the percentage of calories from SFAs with 12 to 16 carbon atoms, the percentage of calories from PUFAs, and the amount of dietary cholesterol—affects the concentration of serum TC. However, these studies focused on the assessment of short-term effects; they did not attempt to determine whether long-term changes in the lipid composition of the diet would change the mean serum TC of populations characterized by a high incidence of CHD to levels (<200 mg/dl) commonly seen in populations with a low incidence of CHD. Evidence relating to this important question must come from a variety of sources, e.g., surveys of migrants, comparisons of socioeconomic classes that differ in access to meat and dairy products, analyses of secular trends, and feeding experiments. Some of this literature is reviewed below. Other reviews of this extensive literature have been done by Katz and Stamler (1953), Katz et al. (1958), Keys (1963), and Stamler (1967, 1979).

South Africa In a survey of employed, middle-aged men in Cape Town, South Africa, mean serum TC and mean consumption of fats were found to be lowest in Bantus, intermediate in "Cape Coloureds," and highest in "European Whites" (Bronte-Stewart et al., 1955). Mean TC levels were 166, 204, and 234 mg/dl, respectively; means for β-lipoprotein cholesterol were 122, 160, and 194 mg/dl; and means for fat intake were approximately 42, 62, and 88 g/day. (Given the differences among these groups in the sources of fats, it seems reasonable to infer that the groups differed substantially in intake of SFAs and cholesterol.) When each racial group was stratified according to income, differences in mean serum TC were closely paralleled by corresponding differences in mean consumption of fats, and racial groups similar in economic status also had similar intakes of fat and mean serum TC. The authors interpreted this evidence as supporting the hypothesis that the observed differences in serum TC could be accounted for by the observed differences in diet and that invoking genetic factors was unnecessary. This interpretation was supported by the results of feeding experiments in humans (Antonis and Bersohn, 1962b; Bronte-Stewart et al., 1955).

Southern Italy In the early 1950s, working-class inhabitants of Naples consumed 20% of their calories from fats (Keys et al., 1955). The great bulk of their diet consisted of bread and pasta. Cheese and meat were consumed in small amounts, olive oil was used sparingly, and butter was not used at all. Mean serum TC was 172 mg/dl in a sample of 230 clinically healthy male steel workers, firemen, and clerks 35 to 60 years of age (Keys et al., 1955).

In Boston, a survey was conducted on 189 clinically healthy male factory workers ages 20 to 50 who had lived all their adult lives in the United States but whose parents had been born near Naples. Investigators found that 43% of their calories came from fats (approximately 32% from animal fats) and that their mean serum TC was 239 mg/dl (Miller et al., 1958). It seems unlikely that the difference in mean serum TC between Naples and Boston was due to differences in body fatness; when the Boston sample was stratified according to relative weight, mean serum TC was 223, 243, and 232 mg/dl for men with relative weights less than 100, between 100 and 119, and 120% of standard or greater.

Ferro-Luzzi et al. (1984) partially substituted butter and other foods rich in SFAs and cholesterol for the customary olive oil in the diets of healthy middle-aged men and women who resided in a rural area south of Naples and who habitually consumed the traditional diet. Mean serum TC changed from 214 to 245 mg/dl in men and from 179 to 203 mg/dl in women. These differences were due almost entirely to changes in LDL-C, which were 148 to 182 mg/dl for men and 119 to 142 mg/dl for women.

The Japanese A survey of Japanese men in Japan, Hawaii, and Los Angeles indicated that mean serum TC was directly correlated with mean percentage of calories from fats, and that the mean serum TC of Japanese men in Los Angeles (about 240 mg/dl) was similar to that of American men generally (Keys et al., 1958b). A feeding experiment conducted in Japanese men indicated that the change in mean serum TC associated with change in lipid composition of the diet was comparable in magnitude to that of white subjects in Minnesota (Keys et al., 1957b).

In the Ni-Hon-San Study, standardized methods were used beginning in 1965 to investigate the three cohorts of middle-aged men of Japanese ancestry in Hiroshima and Nagasaki, in Honolulu, and in San Francisco (Kagan et al., 1974; Kato et al., 1973; Tillotson et al., 1973). In the latter two areas, more than 85% of the participants were Nisei who had been born in the United States to parents who had emigrated from Japan; the remainder were Issei who had migrated to the United States before the Exclusion Act of 1924. Sources of migration for more than 70% of the Issei and Nisei were the areas around Hiroshima and Nagasaki in the southwestern region of Japan. All three cohorts had similar distributions of the A, B, and O blood groups.

Data on diet were obtained by a 24-hour diet recall interview and a self-administered dietary acculturation questionnaire designed to ascertain adherence to a traditional Japanese diet (Tillotson et al., 1973). Information on fatty acid composition of foods in Japan was not available, and a food grouping system was used in order to categorize fats as primarily saturated or primarily unsaturated.

Mean values for serum TC for all cohorts in Japan, Honolulu, and San Francisco were 181, 218, and 228 mg/dl, respectively. Corresponding mean values for total energy intake were 2,164, 2,275, and 2,262 kcal/day; for percentage of calories from fats, 15, 33, and 38; for percentage of calories from saturated fats, 7, 23, and 26; for intake of cholesterol, 464, 545, and 533 mg/day; and for subscapular skinfold thickness, 10, 16, and 16 mm.

Although data on fatty acid composition of the diet were not available for the cohort in Japan, such data have been published for the cohorts in Hawaii and California (Tillotson et al., 1973). These data indicate that SFAs accounted for 54% of saturated fats in both Hawaii and California and that PUFAs accounted for 58% of unsaturated fats in Hawaii and 52% in California. The mean percentages of calories from SFAs and PUFAs in Japan were estimated, based on the assumption that the proportions were the same as those in Hawaii. The age-adjusted data for men ages 45 to 59 in Japan, Hawaii, and California are as follows: mean percentage of calories from SFAs was 3.5, 12.4, and 14.1% and from PUFAS, 5.3, 6.1, and 6.1%; mean intake of cholesterol was 217, 237, and 243 mg/1,000 kcal; and serum TC was 175.9, 219.2, and 226.1 mg/dl, respectively.

The effect of the differences in lipid composition of these diets on mean serum TC can be estimated by applying the equations of Keys et al. (1965c) and of Hegsted et al. (1965) (discussed in the next section of this chapter)—and subsequently modified by Hegsted (1986) for diets with 0 to 400 mg of dietary cholesterol per 1,000 kcal of intake. For men ages 45 to 59, the Keys equation accounts for more than 50% of the observed differences between the three groups. The Hegsted equation yields slightly lower values: 47% of the difference between Hawaii and Japan, 54% of the difference between California and Japan, and 57% of the difference between California and Hawaii. The predictive equations were based on short-term feeding experiments lasting for several weeks, and it is reasonable to expect that effects of long-term exposure to different diets would be greater. Therefore, these results support the concept that the major portion of the differences in mean serum TC between the cohorts in Japan, Hawaii, and California can be accounted for by differences in lipid composition of the diet.

The Yemenite Jews Toor et al. (1960) studied three groups of people who migrated from Yemen to Israel and had lived in Israel for approximately 5 years, 9 to 10 years, and more than 20 years, respectively. The economic status of the most recent migrants was very poor during 1953 and 1954. A survey showed that their diet was low in calories (mean, 1,750 kcal/day) and contained 12 g of animal protein and 30 g of total fat per day—almost all from vegetable sources. The economic status of the earliest migrants was better. Their mean intakes were: energy, 2,500 kcal/day;

animal protein, 29 g/day; and total fat, 65 g/day (28% from animal sources). For men ages 45 to 54, mean values for serum TC from the most recent to the earliest migrants were 158, 180, and 197 mg/dl, respectively. Corresponding values for women of the same age group were 172, 189, and 206 mg/dl. These differences in mean serum TC were due primarily to differences in β-lipoprotein (LDL) cholesterol; differences in the α-lipoprotein (HDL) fraction were small and not statistically significant. Mean weight-to-height ratios [weight in kg × 100/(height in cm − 100)] were 92, 98, and 96 for men and 95, 94, and 108 for women.

The Irish Results from the Ireland–Boston Diet–Heart Study (Kushi et al., 1985) indicate that migration without substantial change in lipid composition of the diet is not associated with substantial change in mean serum TC. Comparison of middle-aged Irishmen living in Ireland with their brothers and a sample of unrelated Irishmen living in Boston showed that the age-adjusted means for serum TC were similar—216, 218, and 215 mg/dl, respectively. Corresponding mean values for energy intake were 4,033, 3,099, and 2,946 kcal/day. The proportions of calories from SFAs were 18, 17, and 16% and from PUFAs, 2, 3, and 3%; the intakes of cholesterol were 233, 273, and 240 mg/1,000 kcal. Mean values for a diet score intended to estimate the effect of dietary lipids on serum TC were 60, 59, and 54 when calculated according to the equation of Keys et al. (1965c) and 89, 96, and 84 when calculated according to a modification of the equation of Hegsted et al. (1965). Mean relative weights were 100, 107, and 106% of standard.

These results indicate that the mean serum TC level of populations is strongly correlated with mean intake of SFAs (and probably of cholesterol as well, although data on this point are not adequate). Correlations of TC level are weaker with mean intake of PUFAs and mean relative weight. In short-term feeding experiments in small groups of people, mean TC changes predictably when intakes of SFAs, PUFAs, and cholesterol are changed under controlled conditions. Most of the differences among populations in mean TC can be accounted for by these short-term effects, and it seems reasonable to believe that long-term effects would be greater. Although populations differ in genetic factors, in body fatness, and in other factors affecting TC, it is not necessary to invoke such differences in order to account for the major portion of the differences among populations in mean TC levels. In view of the evidence, it seems reasonable to infer that variation among populations in the lipid composition of the diet, principally in mean intake of SFAs (and cholesterol), is an important factor, perhaps the major factor, in determining differences in mean serum TC.

STUDIES OF INDIVIDUALS Cross-sectional studies of individuals within populations have generally shown little or no association between the fatty acid composition of the diet and serum TC. [See reviews of the extensive literature by Stallones (1983) and Stamler (1979).] Initially, this observation was difficult to reconcile with the clear experimental evidence for groups of people that changes in the lipid composition of the diet predictably affect mean LDL-C and TC in the blood and with the evidence from observational studies that mean SFA intake is strongly correlated with mean TC across populations. However, subsequent investigations have shown that these results are not inconsistent and, in fact, are expected.

Levels of LDL-C (and consequently of TC) are determined by a variety of intrinsic and extrinsic factors—the lipid composition of the diet being a key extrinsic factor (Hegsted et al., 1965; Keys et al., 1965a). However, people differ substantially in their TC levels, even when maintained on the same diet under controlled conditions. Jacobs et al. (1979) showed that weak cross-sectional correlations between the individual intake of SFAs and level of TC are a consequence of the large variation in intrinsic TC levels among individuals. Moreover, random error in determining the usual intake of nutrients by individuals biases these already weak correlations further toward zero (Beaton et al., 1979; Keys, 1965; Liu et al., 1978; Rush and Kristal, 1982). Knowledge of hypercholesterolemia can lead people to change their diets, thereby producing a negative cross-sectional correlation between SFA intake and level of TC (Shekelle et al., 1981b). Although the correlations were weak, after adjustment for intraindividual variability Shekelle et al. (1981b) showed that the magnitude of the regression of TC on lipid composition of the diet was consistent with the effect demonstrated in controlled feeding experiments.

In summary, the epidemiologic evidence obtained between and within populations indicates that increased SFA intake is associated with increased plasma TC and that SFA intake is a major extrinsic determinant of TC levels.

Clinical and Metabolic Studies

EFFECTS OF SATURATION OF DIETARY FATTY ACIDS ON PLASMA CHOLESTEROL AND LIPOPROTEIN CONCENTRA-TIONS In 1952, Kinsell et al. (1952) studied the effects of formula diets on the responses of patients to various hormones and found that diets high in vegetable fat dramatically lowered TC concentrations. In the same year, Groen et al. (1952) observed that a diet rich in vegetable fat fed to volunteers resulted in much lower TC levels than a diet containing an equal amount of animal fat, regardless of cholesterol intake. Despite the skepticism typical of new findings, these initial observations were soon confirmed (Ahrens et al., 1954, 1957; Beveridge et al., 1955, 1957; Bronte-Stewart et al., 1955; Keys et al., 1957a,b; Kinsell et al., 1953; Malmros and Wigand, 1957). It was established that the serum cholesterol concentration was more responsive to the saturation of dietary fatty acids than to the total amount of fats or to the amount of dietary cholesterol. After many comparisons of different fats and oils, several investigators (Ahrens et al., 1957; Malmros and Wigand, 1957; Keys et al., 1957a) proposed that the presence of PUFAs in vegetable oils was responsible for the hypocholesterolemic effect. The effect was observed principally or exclusively on LDL-C.

Using the results of a series of experiments, Keys et al. (1957b, 1959) developed a formula predicting the change in serum cholesterol concentration from the change in the amounts of SFAs and PUFAs in the diet:

$$\Delta Chol = 2.74\ S - 1.31\ P,$$

where $\Delta Chol$ is the change in serum cholesterol in mg/dl and S and P are the changes in the percentage of calories derived from saturated (S) and polyunsaturated (P) fatty acids. At that time, the prevailing opinion was that dietary cholesterol did not affect the serum cholesterol concentration. Therefore, it was not part of the equation.

After additional experiments with dietary fats and cholesterol, Keys et al. (1965c) modified the equation and incorporated the effect of dietary cholesterol as follows:

$$\Delta Chol = 1.35\ (2\ S - P) + 1.5\ Z,$$

where Z is the difference between the square root of the initial intake of cholesterol and the square root of the subsequent intake of cholesterol, both expressed as mg per 1,000 kcal.

Hegsted et al. (1965) conducted a comprehensive experiment in which they examined the effects of different types of fats (safflower, olive, and coconut oils), amounts of fat (22 or 40% of calories), and amounts of cholesterol. The amounts of dietary fats within these limits did not influence serum cholesterol concentration; the proportion of saturated and unsaturated fatty acids was a major determinant. Dietary cholesterol produced a small but statistically significant effect independently of the amount or type of fat. These investigators also developed regression equations that predicted the responses of plasma cholesterol concentrations to changes in dietary fats. The most practical equation was the following:

$$\Delta Chol = 2.16\ S - 1.65\ P + 6.77\ C - 0.53,$$

where C is a change of 100 mg dietary cholesterol per day (or 100 mg per 2,600 kcal, or approximately 38 mg per 1,000 kcal) and S and P have the same meaning as above. This formula was subsequently modified by Hegsted (1986) to:

$$\Delta Chol = 2.16\ S - 1.65\ P + 0.097\ C,$$

where C is the difference in cholesterol intake between the two diets in mg/1,000 kcal. In these studies, the SFAs alone accounted for 72% of the variation in serum cholesterol concentrations.

Keys and Parlin (1966) compared the predictive power of the equation of Hegsted et al. (1965) with those he and his associates had proposed previously (Keys et al., 1957b, 1959, 1965c) and found them to be quite similar. The principal difference resided in the computation of the dietary cholesterol effect; the Keys equation treated it as a square-root function, whereas the Hegsted equation treated it as a linear function. Both equations predicted approximately 90% of the effect of the dietary fat changes on the observed serum cholesterol concentrations.

Equations of the type developed by Keys, Hegsted, and their associates in the publications cited above, and similar ones devised by other investigators, were intended to indicate an average effect of dietary modifications on plasma cholesterol concentrations in a group of individuals—not to represent precise physiological or metabolic mathematical models. The equations were useful in subsequent studies to compare the results of experiments that varied in proportions of dietary fatty acids and cholesterol. Most such experiments have confirmed the validity of these equations as predictors of group averages of responses to dietary manipulations, but at the same time many investigators have commented on the large individual variability in responses (Keys et al., 1959, 1965b). This individual variability was more prominent in experiments involving dietary cholesterol, but it also appeared in experiments involving types of dietary fats. For example, Grundy and Vega (1988) reviewed the results of four experiments on 46 subjects to determine the effects of PUFAs and SFAs on plasma cholesterol and LDL-C. Six (about 13%) of the 46 subjects did not respond to a change in dietary fatty acid saturation with any substantial change in plasma cholesterol concentration.

Katan et al. (1988) characterized the responsiveness of people to dietary cholesterol by subjecting them to repeated dietary challenges and then compared the responses of these same people to high-SFA and high-PUFA diets. Average egg eaters (who consumed an average of approximately 500 mg of cholesterol per day) showed a high degree of congruence between responsiveness to dietary cholesterol and responsiveness to dietary SFAs ($R = .62$, $p < .01$), whereas eaters of large amounts of eggs (approximately 1,130 mg of cholesterol per day) showed a low degree of congruence ($R = .15$, not significant). There was no ready explanation for the difference between the two groups. It will be important in future research to determine the extent to which the responsiveness to dietary fatty acids is a genetically determined characteristic, whether it is influenced by previous diets, whether it is dependent on an interaction between genetics and diet, and whether it involves the same metabolic processes as does responsiveness to dietary cholesterol.

One of the most convincing demonstrations of the effects of dietary fatty acid saturation was the Lipid Research Clinics Coronary Primary Prevention Trial, in which more than 6,000 hypercholesterolemic men were instructed to adopt a diet lower in cholesterol and higher in the relative proportion of PUFAs to SFAs. The change in dietary SFAs was correlated directly, and the change in PUFA intake was correlated inversely, with lowered plasma cholesterol concentration—mainly LDL-C (Gordon et al., 1982).

Within a few years of the initial observations, the weight of the evidence led to the clear conclusion that the effect was real and consistent, and research efforts thereafter were directed toward identifying the specific fatty acids responsible for the effect, the mechanisms of the effect, and the role of SFAs relative to that of cholesterol in causing hypercholesterolemia in humans. These topics have been reviewed by Ahrens (1957), Goodnight et al. (1982), Grundy (1979, 1987), Jackson et al. (1978), McNamara (1987), and Nestel (1987).

Saturated Fatty Acids   In early experiments concerned with the effects of fatty acid saturation on serum cholesterol concentrations, cocoa butter, which is approximately 35% stearic acid (C18:0), did not elevate serum cholesterol as did most other natural foods rich in SFAs (Ahrens et al., 1957; Erickson et al., 1964). Keys et al. (1965c) found that the predictive equations were more accurate when stearic acid was eliminated from the computation of the percentage of calories derived from SFAs. The SFAs with chain lengths shorter than 12 carbon atoms likewise appeared not to influence serum cholesterol levels, and the equations were more predictive when they were eliminated from consideration. Grande et al. (1970) demonstrated that stearic acid did not affect serum cholesterol concentrations. This finding was reconfirmed by Reiser et al. (1985), who compared the effects of beef fat, which is about 20% stearic acid, with those of coconut oil and safflower oil on serum cholesterol concentrations, and more recently by Bonanome and Grundy (1988), who compared the effects of formula diets high in palmitic, stearic, and oleic acids.

In early experiments, butter and coconut oil were strongly hypercholesterolemic. Because these fats have a high proportion of saturated medium- and short-chain fatty acids (C6 to C12), it was suspected that their effects might be due to these fatty acids. Beveridge et al. (1959) and Hashim et al. (1960) demonstrated that medium-chain triglycerides, which were 99% SFAs with chain lengths from C6 to C12, produced little or no elevations in serum cholesterol concentrations over those produced by corn oil diets. Keys et al. (1965c) found that SFAs with fewer than 12 carbon atoms did not contribute to the predictive accuracy of their equation for estimating serum cholesterol changes due to fatty acid intake, but included lauric acid (C12) in their equation. Hegsted et al. (1965) found that C10 and C12 SFAs did not contribute significantly to the predictive accuracy of their equation for estimating the cholesterol-raising effects of dietary fats. There has been little or no investigation of the metabolic effects of these fatty acids since 1965, and the role of lauric acid (C12) remains uncertain.

The average effects of the various fatty acids commonly encountered in human diets are summarized graphically in Figure 7–2 (Grundy, 1981). This figure compares the predictions of the Keys and Hegsted equations for serum cholesterol concentration changes when the fatty acid content of the diet is changed.

In conclusion, palmitic (C16) and myristic (C14) acids are the SFAs most effective in elevating serum cholesterol concentrations. Stearic acid (C18:0) and SFAs with chain lengths of 10 or less have no effect. Lauric acid (C12) also raises the serum cholesterol level but the quantitative extent of its effects, compared to those of C14 and C16 acids, requires further investigation.

Monounsaturated Fatty Acids   Early investigators noted that olive oil, which is rich in oleic acid (C18:1), lowered serum cholesterol concentrations when substituted for SFAs, as did the PUFAs (Ahrens et al., 1957; Bronte-Stewart et al., 1955; Keys 1957, 1958a). Keys et al. (1958a) found that substituting oleic acid for carbohydrates in isocaloric quantities did not affect the serum cholesterol level. Both Keys et al. (1965a) and Hegsted et al. (1965) reported that including MUFAs in regression equations did not increase the predictive value of the equation.

The effects of dietary MUFAs on serum lipoprotein levels were reexamined by Baggio et al. (1988), Becker et al. (1983), Grundy (1986), Grundy et al. (1986, 1988), Mattson and Grundy (1985), and Mensink and Katan (1987), all of whom confirmed that MUFAs did not elevate serum cholesterol concentrations as did SFAs. Furthermore, they found that high-MUFA diets did not lower HDL-C concentrations as did replacement of SFAs by carbohydrates.

The effects of MUFAs on serum lipoprotein levels are important, because olive oil or other oils rich in these fatty acids could be used, along with or as an alternative to carbohydrates, as replacement for SFAs in diets designed to lower serum cholesterol and, particularly, LDL-C levels. If the early and recent findings regarding the effects of MUFAs on LDL-C and HDL-C levels are consistently confirmed, the use of oils rich in these fatty acids makes possible the design of diets that would lower LDL-C levels, maintain HDL-C levels, and be more palatable than very-low-fat diets.

For patients with high serum cholesterol levels, it remains to be determined whether attempts to minimize HDL-C lowering (in the course of dietary treatment to lower LDL-C) by partial substitution

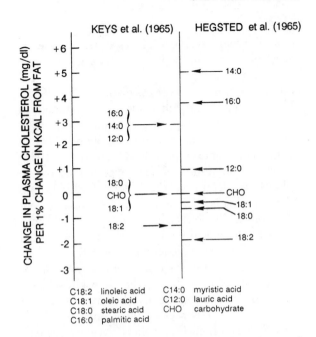

C18:2	linoleic acid	C14:0	myristic acid
C18:1	oleic acid	C12:0	lauric acid
C18:0	stearic acid	CHO	carbohydrate
C16:0	palmitic acid		

FIGURE 7–2   Responses to changes in dietary fatty acids predicted from the studies of Keys et al. (1965c) and Hegsted et al. (1965). Figure adapted from Grundy (1981).

of SFAs with MUFAs might be more beneficial than substitution with carbohydrates.

ω-6 PUFAs   The major dietary PUFA with the double bond in the ω-6 position is linoleic acid (C18:2). The proportion of linoleic acid in plant oils, expressed as percent of all fatty acids, ranges from 1 to 2% in coconut and palm kernel oils to 50 to 60% in corn, cottonseed, and soybean oils and to about 75% in safflower oil. Corn oil, cottonseed oil, and safflower oil are the natural sources most frequently used in the dietary experiments in humans cited in this report. The other important PUFA found in plants is linolenic acid (C18:3), which has a double bond in the ω-3 position.

Keys et al. (1957b, 1965a) and Hegsted et al. (1965) showed that isocaloric exchange of PUFAs for carbohydrates or MUFAs lowered the serum cholesterol concentration in men consuming mixed-food diets that provided 10 to 40% of calories from fat. Predictive equations developed by linear regression analysis of data from those experiments, described in the previous section, indicated that the isocaloric exchange of PUFAs for 10% of calories derived from MUFAs or from carbohydrates decreased serum cholesterol by 13 mg/dl (Keys et al., 1965c) or by 16.5 mg/dl (Hegsted et al., 1965) when other factors were held constant. This effect was observed directly in experiments in which PUFAs were exchanged for carbohydrates or for MUFAs with little change in intake of other nutrients.

Although Keys et al. (1957b, 1965a, 1965c) and Hegsted et al. (1965) published results only for serum cholesterol, both measured β-lipoprotein (the term then used for LDL) and stated that the changes observed in that fraction paralleled the changes in serum cholesterol. The observed differences in serum cholesterol were larger than would be accounted for by changes in HDL-C. These results suggested that PUFAs had a specific serum-cholesterol- (particularly, an LDL-C-) lowering effect when substituted isocalorically for carbohydrates as well as when substituted for SFAs.

Between 1959 and 1986, several studies in humans addressed the effects of PUFAs substituted for carbohydrates and suggested that dietary PUFAs did not lower serum TC or LDL-C levels when substituted for carbohydrates (Brussaard et al., 1980, 1982; Grundy et al., 1986; Horlick, 1959, 1960; Kuusi et al., 1985). Some of these experiments involved women, who may not have responded as did men, and the observations were not controlled for possible effects of the menstrual cycle on serum lipids and lipoproteins (Oliver and Boyd, 1953); some involved small numbers of subjects and had limited power; some were confounded by variation in other dietary components, particularly cholesterol; and in one, formula diets were used. These reports have, however, raised the question of whether there is a specific LDL-C-lowering effect of PUFAs when substituted for carbohydrates.

There have been no recent reports of experiments designed to test this question directly and rigorously in people eating mixed-food diets. The early experiments conducted by Keys, Hegsted, and their associates (described above) indicated that there was such an effect in men consuming mixed-food diets. Furthermore, the analysis of effects of dietary changes in the Lipid Research Clinics Coronary Primary Prevention Trial showed an association of increased intake of PUFAs with decreased serum cholesterol concentration (mainly in LDL-C). This association was independent of changes in body weight and intake of SFAs and cholesterol (Gordon et al., 1982).

This issue is not important in the design of practical diets for lowering serum cholesterol levels, because for other reasons, diets containing more than approximately 7% of calories as PUFAs are not recommended. The issue is of interest as part of the overall question of the mechanism by which dietary PUFAs lower LDL-C concentra-

tions. The evidence bearing on this mechanism is discussed below.

A consistent finding in all comparisons of isocaloric diets in which fats of any type were substituted for carbohydrates is that serum triglyceride levels were lowered. These studies have been of short duration. The effect may well be temporary, since populations that habitually consume a low-fat, high-carbohydrate diet are not characterized by a high prevalence of hypertriglyceridemia. The comparative effects of carbohydrates versus fats in both short- and long-term studies are discussed in more detail in Chapter 9.

ω-3 PUFAs Soon after the hypocholesterolemic effects of PUFAs were discovered in 1952, some investigators found that oils derived from fish and marine mammals were as effective as vegetable oils in lowering serum cholesterol levels in humans (Ahrens et al., 1959; Bronte-Stewart et al., 1955; Keys et al., 1957a). This observation received little attention for nearly 25 years until interest was stimulated by fragmented and poorly documented reports of low rates of CHD among fish-eating Greenland Eskimos. The recent literature on the effects of fish oils on plasma lipids, plasma lipoproteins, and lipoprotein metabolism has been reviewed by Carroll (1986a), Goodnight et al. (1982), Herold and Kinsella (1986), Klasing and Pilch (1986), Leaf and Weber (1988), Nestel (1987), von Schacky (1987), and Carroll and Woodward (1989).

Fish oils consistently reduce serum triglyceride concentrations, particularly in hypertriglyceridemic subjects (Harris et al., 1983, 1984; Illingworth et al., 1984; Nestel et al., 1984; Phillipson et al., 1985; Sanders et al., 1985; Sullivan et al., 1986). This effect appears to result from their inhibition of the synthesis of VLDL-triglycerides, leading to a reduced total secretion of VLDL-triglycerides (Connor, 1986; Nestel et al., 1984). Substitution of ω-3 PUFAs for SFAs in the diet results in a lowering of LDL-C. This response appears to be the result of removing SFAs from the diet. Thus, supplementation of the diet with ω-3 PUFAs without altering SFA intake has been reported not to cause a lowering of LDL-C levels (Rogers et al., 1986). In hypertriglyceridemic patients who are treated with ω-3 PUFAs, the lowering of plasma triglycerides is often associated with an increase in LDL-C levels (Connor, 1986). This response is typical of other triglyceride-lowering agents as well.

Fish oils also affect the hemostatic system (described below in the section on Effects of Dietary Fats and Other Lipids on Hemostasis and Eicosanoid Metabolism and reviewed in depth by Herold and Kinsella, 1986). The effects of the ω-3 PUFAs are currently being investigated intensively, and a considerable amount of new information regarding their effects on lipoprotein metabolism may be anticipated in the near future.

Hydrogenated Fatty Acids The hydrogenation of vegetable oils with high proportions of unsaturated fatty acids was developed as a process to make the oils more palatable and useful as substitutes for animal fats. This process not only reduces the degree of unsaturation of the oils, but also generates geometric isomers—the *trans* fatty acids (see section on *Trans* Fatty Acids below for a discussion of the effects of these isomers). In early experiments shortly after the discovery of the serum-cholesterol-lowering effects of the PUFAs, hydrogenation was found to raise serum cholesterol levels. Malmros and Wigand (1957) found that hydrogenated coconut oil elevated serum cholesterol more than other plant oils rich in PUFAs, but they did not test the effects of hydrogenation alone.

Anderson et al. (1961) reported that hydrogenated corn and safflower oils, compared to their native (naturally occurring) forms, consistently raised serum cholesterol concentrations, but the elevation was less than that predicted by the equations developed by Keys et al. (1957b). They attributed the less-than-predicted effect to the presence of *trans* fatty acids, which they tested in another experiment. Horlick (1960) observed that hydrogenated corn oil, as compared to a low-fat diet, elevated serum cholesterol in four subjects but not to the same degree as did butter. McOsker et al. (1962) found that the effects of hydrogenated cottonseed and soybean oils did not differ from effects of the native oils on serum cholesterol concentrations.

There is a widespread belief that hydrogenated vegetable oils, as consumed in margarines, shortenings, and salad oils, elevate serum cholesterol levels because of a reduction in the number of double bonds, but no controlled experiments have been conducted since 1962 to test this. The experiments with hydrogenated oils have focused on the *trans* fatty acids produced in the hydrogenation process and have attempted to eliminate saturation of fatty acids as a variable by using fat blends as controls.

Hydrogenated coconut oil was frequently used in the early experiments cited above. This oil was already rich in the cholesterol-raising SFAs (C12 to C16) and thus may not have been representative of the other vegetable oils. When oils rich in oleic and linoleic acids are hydrogenated, stearic and oleic acids, both of which do not elevate serum cholesterol, are produced; almost no myristic or palmitic acids (the main fatty acids responsible for raising serum cholesterol) are produced because the oils contain very few C14 or C16 unsaturated fatty acids. Furthermore, some PUFAs may remain. For example, analyses of more than 80 different margarines prepared by hydrogenation of vegetable oils showed that the palmitic acid content ranged from 8.5 to 13.2% of all fatty acids, with a mean of approximately 10% (Slover et al., 1985). Palmitic acid constituted 24% of one margarine made from lard. In the vegetable oil-based margarines, the linoleic acid content ranged from 6 to 46% (average, about 27%), and the linolenic acid content ranged from 0.2 to 3.6% (average, about 2%). Each hydrogenated oil preparation must be examined with regard to the spectrum of fatty acids it contains, and hydrogenated fats cannot be classified in general as cholesterol raising. This conclusion, based principally on the application of the predictive equations described above, needs verification by experimentation in humans.

The formation of *trans* fatty acids during hydrogenation is another matter that confounded many of the experiments with hydrogenated oils. This issue is discussed in the following section.

Trans Fatty Acids The *trans* fatty acids are geometric isomers of the unsaturated fatty acids (mostly oleic, linoleic, and linolenic acids) occurring naturally in the fats of ruminants and formed in vegetable oils during hydrogenation. From 2 to 7% of beef fat and butterfat, and from 10 to 30% of margarines, shortenings, and salad oils, are *trans* fatty acids. Between 1965 and 1983, the daily per-capita consumption was about 8 g/day or 6% of the total fat consumed in the United States. The estimates of daily consumption have been confirmed by analyses of *trans* fatty acids in the adipose tissue of humans (reviewed by Senti, 1985). The biologic properties of the *trans* fatty acids have been studied extensively, and the original reports have been reviewed by Applewhite (1981), Beare-Rogers (1983), Emken (1984), Hunter and Applewhite (1986), Kinsella et al. (1981), and Senti (1985). A recent survey of more than 80 samples of commercial margarines produced and sold in the United States showed that *trans*-unsaturated octadecanoic acids ranged from 10.7 to 30.1% of all fatty acids and that small amounts of *trans,trans, trans,cis,* and *cis,trans* isomers of linoleate were present (Slover et al., 1985).

Anderson et al. (1961) compared the effects of native and hydrogenated oils similar in their proportions of SFAs, MUFAS, and PUFAS, but varying in their proportions of *trans* isomers. The oils with high proportions of *trans* isomers produced higher serum levels of cholesterol and triglycerides than did the native oils. However, the hydrogenated corn oil contained half as much of the essential fatty acids as did the native corn oil. Beveridge and Connell (1962) compared the effects of margarines, corn oil, and butter in formula diets and found that margarines produced higher serum TC levels than did corn oil diets, but not as high as did butter. Grasso et al. (1962) found that the *trans* fatty acid composition of a hydrogenated oil lowered serum cholesterol levels as did an oil with the same distribution of SFAs, MUFAs, and PUFAs.

McOsker et al. (1962) reported no difference in serum cholesterol concentrations in six subjects fed hydrogenated oils containing 15 to 20% *trans* fatty acids. Erickson et al. (1964) compared the effects of partially hydrogenated oils with blends of native oils having a similar distribution of SFAs, MUFAs, and PUFAs, but up to 10% *trans* isomers, and found no difference in serum cholesterol levels and no interaction with dietary cholesterol. After a series of experiments, de Iongh et al. (1965) also concluded that *trans* fatty acid isomers had no effect on serum cholesterol concentrations; the levels attained followed the predictive equation of Keys et al. (1965c) and were not influenced by the *trans* fatty acid content. Mishkel and Spritz (1969) tested the effects of high levels of *trans* isomers of linoleic acid in six patients and found elevations of serum triglycerides but inconsistent changes in serum cholesterol concentrations.

Mattson et al. (1975) conducted the most thorough and controlled test of *trans* fatty acid effects in 33 men who consumed formula diets containing similar distributions of SFAs, MUFAs, and PUFAs, but differing to an extreme in *trans* fatty acid isomers. More than 60% of the MUFAs and approximately 50% of the PUFAs in the contrasting diet were in the *trans* configuration. There were no differences in serum cholesterol or triglyceride levels after 4 weeks on the diets.

In conclusion, some effects of the *trans* fatty acid isomers on lipid or lipoprotein metabolism may remain undetected. However, most evidence indicates that these isomers, in the quantities usually consumed in the U.S. diet, do not influence serum cholesterol concentrations. There may be other effects unrelated to lipid and lipoprotein metabolism. These possibilities deserve careful attention and additional investigation.

Peanut Oil Peanut oil, which is rich in MUFAs and PUFAs, was found to be unusually atherogenic in some experiments in animals (see following section on Animal Studies). Very few tests of the effects of peanut oil on serum lipoproteins have been conducted in humans. In a few experiments in humans (Ahrens et al., 1957; Baudet et al., 1984; Bronte-Stewart et al., 1955), peanut oil resulted in serum cholesterol and VLDL-C, LDL-C, and HDL-C concentrations similar to those produced by other unsaturated vegetable oils.

Fatty Acid Effects on Plasma Lipoproteins There have been many attempts to determine the mechanisms of action of the SFAs in raising serum cholesterol concentrations or of the PUFAs in lowering them. The unsaturated dietary fatty acids were incorporated into the lipoprotein lipids within 14 days (Spritz and Mishkel, 1969). In studies of humans fed high-PUFA diets, Shepherd et al. (1980a) found decreases in the cholesterol-to-protein ratio in LDL, and Pownall et al. (1980) observed a number of differences in the thermal properties of plasma LDL related to the fatty acid composition of the diet. Kuksis et al. (1982) found many changes in lipoprotein composition and decreased numbers of LDL particles, but no changes in the sizes of the particles, in people consuming a high-PUFA diet. Zanni et al. (1987) also found decreased numbers of LDL and HDL particles related to PUFA intake.

PUFA increased the fractional catabolic rate of LDL apo B (Shepherd et al., 1980a) and in some studies decreased the production of LDL (Cortese et al., 1983; Turner et al., 1981). However, these changes were small and did not occur consistently.

As yet, the only evidence regarding the type of effects exerted by fats on LDL receptor activity are the result of experiments in animals. Spady and Dietschy (1985) found that receptor-mediated uptake of LDL in hamsters was suppressed about 30% by dietary cholesterol when the animals were consuming PUFAs (safflower oil) and was suppressed about 90% when they were consuming SFAs (coconut oil). In more recent studies in hamsters, Spady and Dietschy (1988) observed that dietary cholesterol suppressed hepatic LDL receptor activity and raised plasma LDL levels in a dose-dependent manner. At each level of cholesterol intake, polyunsaturated triglycerides diminished and saturated triglycerides accentuated the effects of dietary cholesterol. In baboons, hepatic LDL receptor messenger RNA (mRNA) was decreased when the animals were fed SFAs with cholesterol as compared to those fed either MUFAs or PUFAs (Fox et al., 1987). In all these studies, the effects on LDL receptor activity were consistent with the observed fat-induced changes in plasma lipoprotein concentrations.

Plasma triglyceride levels, representing VLDL and other triglyceride-rich lipoproteins, were lower in humans on PUFA diets than on SFA diets. The difference was usually proportionally greater than for plasma cholesterol (Chait et al., 1974).

Initially, plasma HDL levels were believed to be insensitive to dietary factors (Keys et al., 1959). Between 1958 and 1980, 6 of 15 observational studies and experiments suggested an inverse relationship between HDL-C concentration and intake of PUFAs (reviewed by McGill et al., 1981c). PUFAs also decreased the synthesis of apo A-I but did not change its fractional catabolic rate (Shepherd et al., 1978).

Since 1981, a number of experiments in humans have been conducted to examine the effects of PUFAs on HDL. Brussaard et al. (1982), Ehnholm et al. (1984), Jackson et al. (1984), Kuusi et al. (1985), Mattson and Grundy (1985), Schonfeld et al. (1982), Shepherd et al. (1980b), and Vega et al. (1982) found that dietary PUFAs decreased HDL-C, but Baudet et al. (1984), Becker et al. (1983), Kraemer et al. (1982), McNamara et al. (1987), Oh and Miller (1985), and Weisweiler et al. (1985, 1986) reported no change in HDL-C in subjects on similar diets. Both Brussaard et al. (1982) and Kuusi et al. (1985) observed that the decrease in HDL was due primarily to a drop in HDL_2-C, whereas HDL_3-C was unchanged (HDL_2 and HDL_3 are the two major subfractions of HDL). Jones et al. (1987b) found that the reduction in HDL-C associated with an increased intake of PUFAs occurred only when total fat intake was low (20% of calories).

In conclusion, dietary PUFAs probably lower plasma HDL-C concentrations, particularly HDL_2 levels, to some degree, but individual variability in the response probably leads to varying results among experiments involving small numbers of subjects.

Effects of Fat on Cholesterol Absorption, Synthesis, and Excretion   There is little evidence that dietary fat saturation influences cholesterol absorption in humans (Grundy and Ahrens, 1970; Nestel et al., 1975). However, there are several reports of enhanced cholesterol absorption by PUFAs in squirrel monkeys (Tanaka and Portman, 1977). Measurements by sterol balance methods in humans (Grundy and Ahrens, 1970) and by in vitro methods in rat liver (Wilson and Siperstein, 1959) indicated that cholesterol synthesis was not influenced by saturation of dietary fat.

Although there is little support for the concept that fatty acid saturation influences cholesterol absorption or synthesis in humans, some results have shown a transient enhanced sterol excretion when PUFAs were substituted for SFAs in the diet (Connor et al., 1969; Moore et al., 1968; Nestel et al., 1973, 1975; Wood et al., 1966). The initial increase in sterol excretion may account for the reduction in plasma cholesterol resulting from dietary PUFAs. However, if cholesterol absorption and synthesis were not increased, increased sterol excretion would not be expected upon attainment of a new steady state. This may explain the failure to detect consistently enhanced sterol excretion in humans fed PUFAs as reported by Avigan and Steinberg (1965), Shepherd et al. (1980a), and Spritz et al. (1965) and in patients with hypertriglyceridemia (Grundy, 1975) or hypercholesterolemia (Grundy and Ahrens, 1970).

Grundy and Ahrens (1970) suggested that PUFAs cause a shift in cholesterol from plasma to liver. Hepatic cholesterol accumulation upon PUFA feeding has been reported in several animal experiments (Avigan and Steinberg, 1958; Bloomfield, 1964; Tidwell et al., 1962). However, in a group of 12 hypercholesterolemic patients, polyunsaturated fats, compared to saturated fats, decreased the liver cholesterol content (Frantz and Carey, 1961).

In summary, transient increased sterol excretion may explain the decrement in plasma cholesterol among normolipidemic subjects, but not among those with hypercholesterolemia. A plausible, but not firmly established, mechanism is that PUFAs accelerate the transport of lipoprotein cholesterol to the liver and promote higher sterol excretion until a new steady state is achieved. Precisely how PUFAs mediate the decrease in LDL production and LDL plasma concentration is not known. However, effects on LDL receptor activity in the liver are likely to play an important role in the mechanism of the effects of dietary SFAs and PUFAs. SFA intake may decrease LDL receptor activity, thereby leading to an increase in LDL and TC levels.

Summary Some dietary SFAs (palmitic, myristic, and lauric acids) elevate serum LDL-C and HDL-C concentrations. ω-6 PUFAs lower serum TC and LDL-C levels when substituted for SFAs and are also likely to do so to a small extent when isocalorically exchanged for MUFAs or carbohydrates in mixed-food diets that provide 10 to 40% of calories from fats. ω-6 PUFAs also lower HDL-C levels. MUFAs do not affect serum TC or LDL-C levels when isocalorically substituted for carbohydrates in mixed-food diets, but they do lower serum TC and LDL-C levels, without lowering HDL-C, when substituted for SFAs. The average effect on TC levels brought about by variations in the proportions of the various dietary fatty acids can be predicted largely from equations based on experimental observations. However, the mechanism of the effect is not clearly defined, despite many proposed hypothetical mechanisms. Recent results from experiments in animals suggest that the effects of dietary SFAs and PUFAs on hepatic LDL receptor activity play a role in this phenomenon. There is considerable interindividual variability in response of plasma lipoproteins to dietary fatty acid saturation. This is probably controlled genetically but has not been studied as intensively as has the response to dietary cholesterol.

Animal Studies

After the initial discovery that dietary cholesterol produced hypercholesterolemia and atherosclerosis in rabbits, a variety of species were found also to be sensitive to dietary cholesterol. Fat in the experimental diet was considered simply as a vehicle for the added cholesterol until the effects of SFAs and PUFAs on serum cholesterol levels were discovered in humans in 1952. Most studies of the effects of various types of fats on plasma lipid and lipoprotein levels and on lipoprotein metabolism have been conducted in humans, but a few investigators have examined these effects in animal models.

SFAS COMPARED TO PUFAS In 1954, Kritchevsky et al. (1954) demonstrated that dietary cholesterol elevated serum cholesterol to a greater extent when fed to rabbits with hydrogenated vegetable oil than when fed with corn oil. This effect was associated with saturation of dietary fatty acids (Kritchevsky et al., 1956).

Similar observations were made in nonhuman primates. SFAs usually produced higher serum cholesterol levels than did PUFAs when fed with low or moderate levels of dietary cholesterol to squirrel monkeys (Corey et al., 1974; Lofland et al., 1970; Robison et al., 1971), cebus monkeys (Corey et al., 1974; Portman and Andrus, 1965; Wissler et al., 1962), vervet monkeys (Mendelsohn et al., 1980), and rhesus monkeys, but not when fed to baboons (Strong and McGill, 1967). In some experiments, two or more types of fats differing in origin and in fatty acid chain length were compared. For example, in cebus monkeys (Wissler et al., 1962), coconut oil produced higher serum cholesterol levels than did butterfat. However, only a few such experiments were conducted, and it is difficult to reach a firm conclusion other than the generalization that SFAs elevate serum cholesterol and cause more severe atherosclerosis in most nonhuman primates than do PUFAs.

More recent experiments have been conducted to examine the effects of various types of fatty acids on the major serum lipoprotein classes. In baboons, for example, SFAs, as compared to unsaturated fatty acids, elevated serum LDL-C and HDL-C concentrations to approximately the same extent. (McGill et al., 1981b; Mott et al., 1982).

In rhesus monkeys, coconut oil, unlike corn oil, elevated plasma LDL-C proportionately more than it did HDL-C in a short-term experiment (Chong et al., 1987), but coconut oil elevated LDL-C only when fed with cholesterol in a long-term experiment (Ershow et al., 1981). Coconut oil also elevated serum cholesterol in cebus and squirrel monkeys (Corey et al., 1974). Although there are some variations among the results in nonhuman primates, the preponderance of evidence indicates that these animals respond to saturated and unsaturated fatty acids as do humans, i.e., with an elevation in the plasma concentrations of both LDL-C and HDL-C in response to SFAs.

A number of studies in animals have been conducted in an attempt to identify the mechanisms responsible for these effects of saturated and unsaturated fatty acids on plasma lipoproteins (Chong et al., 1987; Ershow et al., 1981; Johnson et al., 1985; Parks and Rudel, 1982; Rudel et al., 1981, 1983, 1986; Spady and Dietschy, 1985). The observation promising the most insight into the process (and discussed above) is that dietary SFAs fed with cholesterol suppress LDL receptor activity in the hamster liver to a much greater extent than does dietary cholesterol alone (Spady and Dietschy, 1985, 1988)—a change that would be expected to elevate plasma LDL-C levels.

Effects of Dietary Fats and Other Lipids on Hemostasis and Eicosanoid Metabolism

There is no conclusive evidence that hemostatic variables such as platelet function and blood coagulation as measured in vitro are influenced by dietary intake of SFAs, MUFAs, or ω-6 PUFAs, such as linoleic, dihomogamma linolenic, or arachidonic acids (von Schacky, 1987). However, some reports have suggested that long-term differences in the intake of SFAs or of ω-6 PUFAs may influence platelet function or thrombogenesis (Renaud et al., 1970, 1985). Additional definitive studies would be useful in this area.

More definite evidence about such effects is available for the ω-3 PUFAs, such as eicosapentaenoic acid (EPA, C20:5, ω-3) and docosahexaenoic acid (DHA; C22:6, ω-3). These ω-3 PUFAs appear to have inhibitory effects on platelet function and prolong bleeding time—phenomena somewhat similar to those elicited by aspirin (Knapp et al., 1986; Leaf and Weber, 1988). However, no studies have as yet determined whether ω-3 PUFAs reduce morbidity or mortality in cardiovascular disease (for full reviews and references, see Leaf and Weber, 1988, and von Schacky, 1987).

Shortened coagulation times measurable in hyperlipemic plasma were originally believed to represent hypercoagulability, but this was later shown to be an artifact induced by platelets trapped in the lipemic plasma (Marcus, 1966). With the possible exception of ω-3 PUFAs, dietary lipids do not influence eicosanoid metabolism as presently understood (Mahadevappa and Holub, 1987).

Of greatest interest concerning effects of dietary fats and other lipids on hemostasis and eicosanoid metabolism are the ω-3 PUFAs of marine origin (von Schacky et al., 1985b). Some investigators have reported that Eskimo populations in Greenland appear to have reduced mortality from occlusive vascular disease, putatively related to consumption of fish and fish oils containing ω-3 fatty acids (Bang and Dyerberg, 1980). However, the epidemiologic evidence on this assertion is quite incomplete. Furthermore, there is no evidence that dietary supplementation with ω-3 fish oils will reduce the risk of cardiovascular disease (Carroll, 1986a).

ω-3 POLYUNSATURATED FATTY ACIDS The ω-3 group of PUFAs includes not only EPA and DHA, but also α-linolenic acid (C18:3, ω-3). These PUFAs are cyclooxygenated and lipoxygenated in a manner similar to ω-6 fatty acids, but the end products may differ functionally from those of the ω-6 group.

The ω-6 PUFAs include linoleic acid (C18:2, ω-6), dihomogamma linolenic acid (C20:3, ω-6), and arachidonic acid (C20:4, ω-6). Arachidonic acid is cyclooxygenated to prostaglandins E_2, D_2, $F_{2\alpha}$, prostacyclin (PGI_2, measured as 6-keto-$PGF_{1\alpha}$), thromboxane (TX) A_2, HHT, and malondialdehyde (Marcus, 1978, 1984), whereas EPA is metabolized to PGE_3, $PGF_{3\alpha}$, PGI_3, and TXA_3. EPA is also lipoxygenated in stimulated leukocytes to the leukotrienes LTB_5, LTC_5, LTD_5, and LTE_5 and to 5-hydroxyeicosapentaenoic acid (5-HEPE). This is in contrast to leukocyte arachidonate, which is lipoxygenated to LTB_4, LTC_4, LTD_4, LTE_4, and 5-hydroxyeicosatetraenoic acid (5-HETE). In activated platelets, arachidonate is lipoxygenated to 12-HETE, and EPA to 12-HEPE (von Schacky, 1987).

Some studies indicate that TXA_3 does not possess the same proaggregatory or vasoconstrictory properties as TXA_2, whereas PGI_3 is reported to retain the vasodilatory and platelet inhibitory properties of PGI_2. More definitive studies are necessary to confirm and examine further the spectrum of biologic properties of PGI_3 and TXA_3.

TERMINOLOGY The widespread interdisciplinary interest in dietary lipids as possible modulators of hemostasis, eicosanoid metabolism, and cardiovascular disease has led to the inadvertent conceptualization of these different processes as synonymous events (Marcus, 1988b). Thrombogenesis, atherosclerosis, hypercoagulability, and platelet hyperreactivity are frequently referred to as phenomena occurring in parallel. Atherosclerosis, however, is not clearly related to blood coagulation or to platelet function, until it reaches the advanced occlusive stages in which thrombosis occurs.

Patients with clinically manifest coronary artery disease may have circulating hyperactive platelets, but these could result from increasing cell-to-cell encounters between platelets and atherosclerotic plaques. Platelet hyperreactivity may represent a secondary event such as a response to injury (Marcus, 1988a).

A direct relationship between diet and hemostasis or eicosanoid metabolism has not been established. The only possible exception may be an association with ω-3 PUFAs (Mahadevappa and Holub, 1987).

EFFECTS OF ω-3 FATTY ACIDS ON PLATELET FUNCTION   Studies have been conducted in volunteers and patients with vascular disease who have ingested cold water marine fish such as mackerel or salmon or fish oils per se. Cod liver oil, which contains 10% EPA and 15% DHA, has been administered in doses ranging from 10 to 40 ml daily for varying periods as has the commercial preparation known as MaxEPA—a blend of fish body oil containing 20% EPA and 10% DHA. Purified EPA and DHA also have been administered separately in a short-term study. Bleeding time, a major indicator of platelet function, was prolonged to some degree in almost all study participants (von Schacky, 1987). In Greenland Eskimos, bleeding time averaged 8 minutes; in a Danish control population, it was 5 minutes. Bleeding time in patients with atherosclerosis extended from a control of 3.3 minutes to 5.6 minutes during the third week in which their diet was supplemented with MaxEPA. Although these findings are suggestive, it is difficult to know with certainty whether such lengthening of the bleeding time indeed signifies protection against vascular disease. Nevertheless, the prolongation is consistent and is comparable to changes in bleeding time observed following the ingestion of aspirin (Knapp et al., 1986).

In addition to lengthening bleeding time, the ingestion of cod liver oil reduces ex vivo platelet aggregation in response to adenosine diphosphate (ADP) and collagen. Responsiveness to agonists would be more adequately interpretable if each stimulus were studied over a concentration curve, because high doses of agonists such as thrombin and collagen may mask mild inhibitory effects of fish oils.

When EPA and DHA were administered separately for 6 days at 6 g/day, EPA reduced platelet responsiveness to collagen. In contrast, DHA reduced platelet aggregation to both ADP and collagen. Thus, DHA may be an important antithrombotic agent in its own right (von Schacky et al., 1985b).

A COMPARISON OF ARACHIDONATE AND EPA METABOLISM IN HUMANS   Early in vitro studies on human or animal platelets demonstrated that added EPA was incorporated into all phospholipid subclasses whether or not arachidonate was also present. In contrast, EPA ingested by volunteers was incorporated mainly into platelet phosphatidylcholine and phosphatidylethanolamine, but *not* phosphatidylinositol or phosphatidylserine. Upon stimulation of washed platelets obtained from these volunteers, EPA was released by way of the phospholipase A_2 mechanism, acting on phosphatidylcholine and phosphatidylethanolamine. Moreover, the dietary EPA released was demonstrably converted to TXA_3 (von Schacky et al., 1985a).

When arachidonic acid is added to platelets in vitro, it is rapidly metabolized to TXA_2, HHT, and 12-HETE, and platelet aggregation ensues via release of ADP (Marcus, 1987). In contrast, the addition of EPA does not induce platelet aggregation. EPA will compete with free arachidonate for platelet cyclooxygenase; however, compared to arachidonate, EPA is a poor platelet agonist. More detailed research on the biologic action of TXA_3 in vitro is desirable (von Schacky et al., 1985b).

DHA is incorporated into platelets in vivo in a manner similar to EPA. At high concentrations (150 μM in vitro), DHA appears to inhibit platelet aggregation, but at low concentrations (2 to 10 μM) platelet aggregation is not inhibited. Following dietary supplementation, DHA is not released from stimulated human platelets or neutrophils. In contrast, dietary DHA is partially retroconverted to EPA (C20:5, ω-3). Further studies on the effects of DHA on platelets ex vivo should be of great interest (Mori et al., 1987; von Schacky et al., 1985b).

During ω-3 PUFA dietary supplementation of healthy volunteers or patients with atherosclerosis, the quantity of TXA_2 formed by stimulated platelets ex vivo is reduced. This could be due to preferential incorporation and may lead to less arachidonate being available for cyclooxygenation. There may also be competition for cyclooxygenase between arachidonate and EPA (which is oxygenated less efficiently than arachidonate), resulting in less TXA_2 formation. This may represent part of the suggested protective action of dietary ω-3 PUFAs.

METABOLISM OF EPA IN ENDOTHELIAL CELLS   EPA added to endothelial cells of human umbilical cord origin in the presence of arachidonate results in formation of PGI_3, whose biologic activity has been reported to be similar to that of PGI_2. During dietary supplementation with EPA, the urinary metabolite of PGI_3 is detectable. Metabolism of ω-3 PUFAs acids in various types of cultured cells should be a fruitful subject for future investigation. Results obtained thus far suggest that dietary lipid modification or supplementation may benefit blood vessel function (von Schacky, 1987).

SUMMARY There are many compelling reasons for pursuing basic and applied research on the effects of dietary ω-3 PUFAs in vascular, inflammatory, and allergy diseases. Among these are the broad spectrum of possible beneficial effects of two natural compounds (EPA and DHA), avoidance of pharmacologic intervention with its inherent side effects and problems of compliance, and the long-term economic advantages of successful prophylaxis in coronary artery disease and cerebrovascular disease. The effects of these ω-3 PUFAs can include reductions in platelet responsiveness, as well as favorable changes in blood lipids, blood pressure, blood rheology, and eicosanoid biosynthesis. More detailed information on the effects of ω-3 PUFAs on platelet function, coagulation, and eicosanoid metabolism is desirable. In studies of each disease entity possibly amenable to improvement by the ingestion of ω-3 PUFAs, problems of patient selection, precise dosages, criteria for evaluation of results, and definition of end points remain to be resolved.

Consumption of ω-3 PUFAs should be differentiated from that of fish. Epidemiologic data suggest that consumption of fish is associated with a reduced risk of CHD (Kromhout et al., 1985; Shekelle et al., 1981a). In contrast, it has not been established that intake of ω-3 fish oils per se will reduce the risk of CHD. Furthermore, it is not known whether long-term ingestion of these PUFAs will lead to undesirable side effects. The information available does not support a recommendation to use fish oil supplements to reduce the risk of CHD.

Associations of Dietary Fats and Fatty Acids with Cardiovascular Disease

Epidemiologic Evidence

Self-reported survey data from longitudinal population studies indicate that specific dietary fatty acids are related to CHD risk. Data from national sources on food consumption and vital statistics on causes of death also suggest an association.

STUDIES OF DIFFERENCES AMONG POPULATIONS In the Seven Countries Study, correlations between mean intake of SFAs and 10-year CHD mortality and incidence were .84 and .73, respectively (Keys, 1980b). CHD was not significantly associated with mean intake of PUFAs, which varied little among the cohorts. Another salient finding from these comparisons was the observation on Crete that a high intake of total fat (40% of daily calories) was compatible with very low risk of CHD, along with a very low total death rate, when the mean intake of SFA was low (8% of daily calories, while monounsaturates accounted for 29%).

Data from national food balance sheets and vital statistics show positive correlations of CHD deaths with eggs, meat, milk, sugar, and coffee, and negative correlations for flour (Armstrong et al., 1975; Stamler, 1979). However, such data have severe limitations, and the results should be interpreted with great caution, even when appropriate adjustments have been made for changes in the International Classification of Diseases and when data are used only from countries having the more reliable mortality statistics. These correlations require assumptions about lag time between measurement of diet and manifestation of disease. Moreover, confounders cannot usually be measured or accounted for in analysis. The diet and disease data bases are usually different, and the dietary data may not be representative for the populations of interest (e.g., middle-aged men). Nevertheless, these data suggest that more systematically acquired data, as from the Seven Countries Study, can be generalized.

Greenland Eskimos have been cited as an example of a population with a high intake of fats and oils from marine sources and very low rates of CHD (Bang and Dyerberg, 1980), but the epidemiologic data are insufficient to confirm this assertion. In fact, the risk of CHD is unknown in this small population, whose members live under harsh conditions and usually die before middle age.

The ecological associations between composition of the diet and CHD rates, based on systematic and standardized survey comparisons, indicate that low CHD rates may indeed occur in the presence of moderately high total (and monounsaturated) fatty acid intake—when intake of dietary SFAs and cholesterol is low. A low SFA intake, i.e., <10% of daily energy intake, along with a low intake of cholesterol, is common to all populations found to have truly low CHD rates.

STUDIES OF INDIVIDUALS WITHIN POPULATIONS Studies in which intake of nutrients was not adjusted for energy intake and dietary information was not obtained at the initial examination (when participants were unaware of their CHD risk status) have not been considered here. The committee considers their results to be uninterpretable with regard to associations between diet and CHD risk (Shekelle et al., 1981b; Willett and Stampfer, 1986).

Even studies that met these conditions have produced inconsistent results. For instance, the percentage of calories from SFAs was positively associated with risk of CHD in the rural sample of the Puerto Rico Study (Garcia-Palmieri et al., 1980), the Honolulu Heart Program (McGee et al., 1984), and the Ireland–Boston Diet–Heart Study (Kushi et al., 1985), but was not significantly associated in the Israel Ischemic Heart Disease Study (Medalie et al., 1973), the urban sample in Puerto Rico (Garcia-Palmieri et al., 1980), the Western Electric Study (Shekelle et al., 1981a), or the Zutphen Study (Kromhout and de Lezenne Coulander, 1984). The percentage of calories from PUFAs was inversely associated with risk of CHD in the Western Electric Study (Shekelle et al., 1981a), but not in the other studies; in fact, it was positively associated with CHD in the urban sample in Puerto Rico (Garcia-Palmieri et al., 1980). The ratio of PUFAs to SFAs (the P:S ratio) was inversely associated with risk of CHD in the small cohort of British men studied by Morris et al. (1977), but not in Israeli civil servants (Medalie et al., 1973).

In two studies, the Western Electric Study and the Ireland–Boston Diet–Heart Study, the lipid composition of the diet was characterized by scores based on the formulas developed by Keys et al. (1965c) and by Hegsted et al. (1965) to summarize the effect of change in dietary SFAs, PUFAs, and cholesterol on change in TC. In both studies, the scores were significantly associated with risk of CHD.

Animal foods in general were related to CHD risk and total deaths in Seventh-Day Adventists (Phillips et al., 1978). Fish-eating habits of men in the Zutphen Study and in the Western Electric Study were related to subsequent individual CHD risk. In these studies, men who rarely or never ate fish had a higher risk of CHD in comparison to men who usually consumed fish one or more times per week (Kromhout et al., 1985; Shekelle et al., 1985). In other population studies, however, fish intake was not significantly related to risk of death from CHD (Curb and Reed, 1985; Snowdon, 1981; Vollset et al., 1985).

The results of studies of individuals within populations have in general been somewhat inconsistent and inconclusive. Investigation of the basis for these inconsistencies has led to greater awareness of the problems inherent in using cohort and case-comparison studies to investigate a diet–disease hypothesis. These problems include the limited variation in characteristic intake of dietary lipids among individuals within populations; the

large misclassification of persons according to characteristic intake of dietary lipids; and the substantial misclassification of individuals according to severity of coronary atherosclerosis (the dependent variable of real interest) when classification is based on signs and symptoms of CHD. These factors will produce weak and inconsistent associations in case-comparison and cohort studies of dietary lipids and CHD, even when important causal associations exist. When combined with results from metabolic ward studies, data from carefully conducted ecological studies, such as the Seven Countries Study (Keys, 1980b), provide a more accurate estimate of the role of dietary lipids in producing widespread atherosclerosis and CHD.

TRANS FATTY ACIDS Thomas et al. (1981, 1983a,b) compared the *trans* fatty acid content of adipose tissues from men dying of CHD and from other causes. CHD subjects had a higher proportion of shorter chain *trans* fatty acids than did non-CHD subjects. The investigators concluded that the CHD subjects had consumed more hydrogenated fats than had the controls; however, they did not adjust their findings for other risk factors. In contrast, Heckers et al. (1977) found no differences in tissue *trans* fatty acids related to atherosclerosis in a few cases. No other systematic epidemiologic data regarding the possible association of *trans* fatty acid consumption and atherosclerotic disease are available.

ATHEROSCLEROSIS AT AUTOPSY In an autopsy study of 253 men in New Orleans (Moore et al., 1976), data on diet were obtained retrospectively from surviving spouses. The extent of raised lesions in the coronary arteries was positively associated with reported intake (expressed as percentage of total calories) of fat and animal protein and was inversely associated with intake of vegetable protein and starch. In contrast, however, antemortem data on diet in the prospective Honolulu Heart Program (Reed et al., 1987) were not significantly associated with the extent of coronary atherosclerosis. Results from the prospective Puerto Rico Heart Health Program (Sorlie et al., 1981) showed small negative correlations between extent of coronary atherosclerosis and reported intake of calories, starch, and fat, but the results are difficult to interpret because the data on intake of nutrients were not adjusted for intake of calories.

DIET AND OTHER CARDIOVASCULAR DISEASE MANIFESTATIONS Even though data may be collected systematically, they are insufficient for comparing habitual diet and rates of brain infarction and peripheral vascular disease among populations. This is partly because of the difficulty of obtaining accurate diagnoses and because rates of stroke and peripheral vascular disease rates are much lower than those for CHD, thus giving less power for analysis.

Animal fat, saturated fat, and total fat have been positively related to the risk of thrombotic brain infarction (D. Reed et al., 1986). However, where hemorrhage accounts for most cases of stroke, as in Japan, animal protein and saturated fat are inversely related to cerebral hemorrhage and overall incidence (Kagan et al., 1980, 1985; Kato et al., 1973; Takeya et al., 1984). The components of diets consumed by omnivorous Seventh-Day Adventists, including meat, eggs, milk, and cheese, were shown to be unrelated to risk of stroke (Snowden, 1988).

In studies of Japanese populations, investigators have hypothesized that a Western-type diet (i.e., with a fat content higher than the usual Japanese diet), which is associated with higher TC levels, is protective against stroke in Japan (Komachi 1977). This idea arose not only from the findings of the negative association of TC level to cerebral hemorrhage, but also from the decline in overall stroke rates in Japan with acculturation to Western ways in the last 20 years (Shimamoto et al., 1989). This hypothesis has been supported in Western countries by the negative association of TC with cerebral hemorrhage deaths among hypertensives in the Multiple Risk Factor Intervention Trial screening population and by the positive association of TC with cerebral thrombotic deaths cited above. However, it is still questionable whether the Western diet with its higher saturated and total fat intake and resultant higher TC levels is *causally* related to *decreased* risk of cerebral hemorrhage, because obvious confounders, such as the traditional Japanese diet of high salt and relatively low fat and protein intake, have not been sufficiently considered. Another potential confounder, alcohol and alcohol-related bleeding diseases, has also not been excluded.

Randomized Trials of Diet and Coronary Heart Disease

The randomized controlled trials on primary prevention of CHD are summarized above in Tables 7-1 and 7-2. Results indicated that the percentage difference in risk of CHD between the experimental and control groups varied directly

with the percentage difference in mean serum TC: the larger the difference in mean TC, the larger the difference in risk of CHD.

Only two small studies included changes in diet as the only intervention. The double-blind Los Angeles Veterans Administration Domiciliary Study (Dayton et al., 1968) of 846 men ages 55 to 89 years was not strictly focused on primary prevention, since 20% of the participants had evidence of old myocardial infarction at entry. In this study, investigators compared the effects of two diets, each providing approximately 40% of calories as fat, but with a much higher proportion of PUFAs and a lower proportion of SFAs in the experimental diet than in the control diet. The experimental diet (which contained linoleic and oleic acid each at 35 to 40% of total fatty acids) induced a prompt and sustained difference in mean TC level between the experimental and control groups, amounting to 12.7% of the starting level. Incidence of the primary end point, sudden death and definite myocardial infarction, was 24% lower in the experimental group than in the control group (54 compared to 71 cases, respectively), but the difference was not statistically significant. However, when these end points were pooled with cerebral infarction and other secondary end points, the totals were 66 in the experimental group and 96 in the control group (31% reduction; $p = .01$). Fatal atherosclerotic events numbered 48 in the experimental group and 70 in the control group (31% reduction; $p < .05$).

Initially, there was some concern that the experimental diet might have increased the risk of cancer, since 31 of 174 deaths in the experimental group were due to cancer as compared to 17 of 178 deaths in the control group ($p = .06$) (Pearce and Dayton, 1971). However, analysis of results from four other clinical trials in which high-PUFA diets were used to lower serum TC (Ederer et al., 1971) showed that the incidence of and mortality from all cancers were lower in the experimental group than in the control group; the relative risks were .75 for incidence and .62 for death. None of the relative risks were significantly different from unity, and the combined results from all five studies were consistent with the conclusion that the cholesterol-lowering diets did not influence risk of cancer. However, these studies could not rule out the possibility of small effects in either direction (increasing or decreasing the risk of cancer).

Further examination of the results of the Los Angeles Veterans Administration Domiciliary

Study showed an association between the experimental diet and cholelithiasis (Sturdevant et al., 1973). Autopsied men who had eaten more than 33% of the experimental meals served from entry into the trial to death were more likely to have gallstones than were control subjects; the prevalence rates were 34 and 14%, respectively ($p <$ .01). The prevalence of gallstones at autopsy was positively correlated with number of trial meals eaten by men in the experimental group ($p < .05$) but not by men in the control group.

High-PUFA diets (i.e., more than 10% of total calories from PUFAs) are no longer recommended in the United States for lowering serum TC, in part because of concerns about the long-term safety of such diets.

In the Finnish Mental Hospital Study (Turpenien et al., 1979), participants were 450 men ages 34 to 64 who were hospitalized in one of two mental hospitals near Helsinki. At the beginning of the study, one hospital received a diet low in SFA and cholesterol and relatively high in PUFA, while the other hospital continued with the usual hospital diet. Six years later, the diets were reversed, and the study was continued for another 6 years. In both hospitals, the special (high PUFA) diet was associated with markedly lower mean TC. The difference in one hospital was −50.9 mg/dl (−19%) and in the other, −32.0 mg/dl (−12%). The mean difference between the special-diet and usual-diet periods in the two hospitals was −41.4 mg/dl (−15%). The incidence of coronary events in the special-diet and usual-diet periods for both hospitals combined was 2.3 and 4.3 per 1,000 person-years, respectively, for coronary death ($p = .10$); 4.2 and 12.7 per 1,000 person-years for coronary death plus major electrocardiogram (ECG) change ($p = .001$); and 13.5 and 24.3 per 1,000 person-years for coronary death plus intermediate or major ECG changes ($p = .008$).

A large-scale trial on primary prevention of CHD with change in diet as the only intervention was never conducted because of concerns about feasibility (NHLBI, 1971). Thus, the remaining diet–heart trials are either 2-factor or 3-factor trials in which any effect of dietary change was confounded with effects of changes in the other factors. Three of those trials (the Göteborg Multifactor Trial, the WHO Multifactor Trial, and Multiple Risk Factor Intervention Trial) achieved differences in mean TC between the intervention and comparison groups of 0, −1, and −2%, respectively; the differences in coronary rates were

correspondingly small (0, −4, and −7%, respectively).

The Oslo Study (Hjermann et al., 1981), which began with 1,232 hypercholesterolemic men ages 40 to 49, achieved a 13% reduction in mean TC levels in the experimental group as compared to the control group. At the end of the follow-up period, 7.5 years later, the incidence of myocardial infarction (fatal and nonfatal) plus sudden death was 47% lower in the experimental group than in the control group ($p = .028$). Total mortality in the experimental and control groups was 26/1,000 and 38/1,000, respectively ($p = .25$). From their own analysis of the data in this study, the authors concluded that changes in cigarette smoking accounted for at most approximately one-fourth of the observed difference in risk of CHD and that most of the difference in CHD was apparently due to diet-induced changes in serum cholesterol. Although this quantitative conclusion is subject to some question, it is clear that the diet-induced lowering of TC played a major role in the observed significant reduction in CHD.

SUMMARY   Epidemiologic evidence shows that serum TC levels are positively associated with risk of CHD, experimental studies in animals and clinical research have elucidated in large part the mechanisms for this association, and results of clinical trials strongly support the concept that lowering TC levels reduces incidence of CHD. Experimental studies in humans have demonstrated that intake of dietary SFAs, PUFAs, and cholesterol affects the level of serum TC. The mechanisms of these effects are now being elucidated. Epidemiologic studies support the concept that variation among populations in mean intake of SFAs (and probably cholesterol) is a major factor accounting for variation in mean TC levels. Results of dietary intervention clinical trials are consistent with the conclusion that changing the lipid composition of the diet in ways expected to lower the TC levels (i.e., decreasing SFA and cholesterol intake, and increasing PUFA intake) in fact does lower mean levels of serum TC and reduces incidence of CHD.

Animal Studies

SFAS AND PUFAS   The relationship of dietary fatty acid saturation to experimental atherosclerosis parallels closely the fatty acid effects on levels of serum cholesterol, particularly LDL-C. Cholesterol fed with hydrogenated vegetable oil (source unspecified) produced more severe atherosclerosis in rabbits than cholesterol fed with corn oil (Kritchevsky et al., 1954). Subsequently, SFAs were found to be more atherogenic than unsaturated fatty acids in several species of monkeys (Lofland et al., 1970; Mendelsohn et al., 1980; Robison et al., 1971; Wissler et al., 1962).

EFFECTS OF DIETARY FATS WITH NO CHOLESTEROL Hypercholesterolemia and atherosclerosis were produced in rabbits by feeding them semisynthetic diets enriched with hydrogenated coconut oil, butterfat, or margarines and no added cholesterol (Carroll, 1971; Funch et al., 1960, 1962; Lambert et al., 1958; Malmros and Wigand, 1959; Wigand, 1959). It was later shown, however, that these diets were deficient in essential fatty acids, and a small amount of PUFAs prevented hypercholesterolemia (Diller et al., 1961). Finally, an improved semisynthetic diet eliminated the essential fatty acid deficiency, and it was shown that hypercholesterolemia and atherosclerosis were related to fatty acid saturation when fed with a low dose of cholesterol (Wilson et al., 1973). These results were confirmed by other investigators (Kritchevsky and Tepper, 1965a,b; McMillan et al., 1960). Cholesterol-free semisynthetic diets also produced hypercholesterolemia and atherosclerosis in vervet monkeys and in baboons (Kritchevsky et al., 1974a,b).

PEANUT OIL Gresham and Howard (1960) reported that peanut oil, which has a high proportion of PUFAs, had the unanticipated effect of being more atherogenic than other fats when fed with cholesterol to rats. This finding was confirmed in rats (Scott et al., 1964) and extended to rabbits (Imai et al., 1966; Kritchevsky et al., 1971) and rhesus monkeys (Scott et al., 1967a,b; Vesselinovitch et al., 1974, 1980). Later experiments suggest that the unusual atherogenicity may be related to triglyceride structure (Kritchevsky et al., 1973, 1981; Myher et al., 1977), but there are no studies that explain this effect in terms of an effect on lipoprotein metabolism.

In cynomolgus monkeys, peanut oil fed with a concentration of dietary cholesterol equivalent to that consumed by humans affected serum lipoproteins and atherosclerosis as did other unsaturated vegetable oils (Alderson et al., 1986).

The contradictory results have not been explained. Kritchevsky (1988) suggested that because positional randomization of the triglyceride fatty acids of peanut oil reduced its atherogenicity, the unusual effect might be due to its triglyceride

structure or that a lectin in peanut oil might be responsible. Further investigation is needed to resolve these discrepant results.

TRANS FATTY ACIDS Effects of *trans* fatty acid isomers have been studied in laboratory animals (reviewed by Kritchevsky, 1982; Senti, 1985). These isomers are not metabolized in the same way as the *cis* isomers. However, at dietary intakes similar to those consumed by humans, and with a small proportion of linoleic acid in the diets, the *trans* fatty acid isomers appear to have no deleterious health effects (Jackson et al., 1977; Kritchevsky, 1983; Royce et al., 1984).

SUMMARY AND CONCLUSIONS In most animal species, SFA intake is associated with more severe atherosclerosis than that achieved with similar diets without (or with little) SFA. Some types of SFAs, especially coconut oil, are more atherogenic than indicated by their effects on plasma lipoproteins alone. The observations in animals support the putative role of SFAs in causing hypercholesterolemia and atherosclerosis in humans.

Relationship Between Dietary Sterols and Cardiovascular Disease

The first evidence that dietary cholesterol may be involved in the etiology of atherosclerosis and its sequelae (CHD, stroke, or peripheral vascular disease) came from the demonstration by Anitschkow and Chalatow in 1913 that cholesterol fed to rabbits produced arterial lesions similar to those of human atherosclerosis (Anitschkow, 1967; Anitschkow and Chalatow, 1913). Over the next 50 years, it was shown that almost all animal species were to some degree susceptible to dietary cholesterol-induced hyperlipidemia and experimentally induced atherosclerosis.

In the late 1940s, interest in the possible dietary etiology of atherosclerosis in humans was stimulated by the observations on CHD in Europe during World War II. A large number of epidemiologic, clinical, and animal studies were conducted from 1950 to the present to examine the roles of dietary fats, including cholesterol, in causing hyperlipidemia, atherosclerosis, and clinical atherosclerotic disease. Dietary SFAs became the major focus, because their effects on serum cholesterol levels in humans were more consistent and their associations with atherosclerotic diseases were stronger than those of cholesterol. Despite the high susceptibility of many test animals to dietary cholesterol, evidence regarding dietary cholesterol in humans was for many years variable and often conflicting. In the past decade, a number of studies have shed light on this difference in findings by indicating that there is considerable variability in the plasma lipid responses to dietary cholesterol among individuals and that a substantial proportion of the population is highly susceptible to the cholesterol-raising effects of dietary cholesterol. This variability probably accounts for much of the initial uncertainty about the role of dietary cholesterol and for many of the apparently conflicting results (reviewed by McGill, 1979).

Epidemiologic Studies

STUDIES OF POPULATIONS Stamler et al. (1970, 1972) examined the relationship of mean per-capita consumption of dietary cholesterol to arteriosclerotic disease mortality rates in 20 developed countries. The correlation coefficient for daily cholesterol intake and mortality from CHD in 1964 was .617 ($p < .01$) for 45- to 54-year-old men and .685 ($p < .01$) for 55- to 64-year-old men. These mortality rates were also correlated with national per-capita income, cigarette smoking, total protein consumption, total fat consumption, and other environmental variables.

Armstrong et al. (1975) compared the consumption of various commodities with mortality from ischemic heart disease in nine regions of the United Kingdom and in 30 countries. They found strong correlations between egg consumption and ischemic heart disease. These results are consistent with the hypothesis that dietary cholesterol is causally associated with incidence of CHD, but evidence from other types of studies must be considered in order to assess alternative hypotheses and to reach a conclusion.

STUDIES OF INDIVIDUALS

The Effect of Dietary Cholesterol on Plasma Lipids With one exception (Connor et al., 1978), cross-sectional studies of individuals within populations have shown little or no association between dietary cholesterol and concentration of serum TC (Frank et al., 1978; Garcia-Palmieri et al., 1977; Harlan et al., 1983; Kahn et al., 1969; Nichols et al., 1976; Shekelle et al., 1981a; U.S.–U.S.S.R. Steering Committee, 1984; Yano et al., 1986). Jacobs et al. (1979) reported that correlations close to zero are a necessary result of cross-sectional studies because of the large differences in intrinsic TC levels among individuals. They concluded that cross-sectional studies are inappropri-

ate for studying the effects of dietary cholesterol on serum TC.

In contrast, longitudinal observational studies have generally shown a positive association between changes in dietary cholesterol and changes in TC concentrations. For example, in the Lipid Research Clinics Coronary Primary Prevention Trial, 6,000 hypercholesterolemic men were advised to lower their intake of cholesterol and SFAs (Gordon et al., 1982). Multiple regression analysis showed that the reduction in dietary cholesterol was independently associated with reduction in serum TC concentrations. The reduction in TC was due primarily to a reduction in LDL-C. A similar association of changes in dietary cholesterol with changes in serum TC was found in the Zutphen Study (Kromhout, 1983) and in the Western Electric Study (Shekelle et al., 1981a). The magnitude of the association found in observational studies has been less than that found in experimental studies due to the well-known effects of day-to-day intraindividual variation in intake of nutrients and in serum TC levels (Beaton et al., 1979; Keys, 1965; Liu et al., 1978).

Dietary Cholesterol and Coronary Heart Disease Before 1981, epidemiologic studies of individuals within populations showed little or no association between dietary cholesterol and risk of CHD (Garcia-Palmieri et al., 1980; Gertler et al., 1950a; Gordon et al., 1981a; Paul et al., 1963; Yano et al., 1978). However, in these studies, investigators did not adequately consider one or more of three important methodological issues: adjustment for the confounding effect of caloric intake (Willett and Stampfer, 1986); limitations in the reliability of dietary measurements (Beaton et al., 1979; Keys, 1965; Liu et al., 1978); and bias resulting from systematic dietary changes made by hypercholesterolemic persons after learning of their condition (Shekelle et al., 1981b). Since then, four long-term cohort studies—the Western Electric Study (Shekelle et al., 1981a), the Zutphen Study (Kromhout and de Lezenne Coulander, 1984; Kromhout et al., 1985), the Ireland–Boston Diet–Heart Study (Kushi et al., 1985), and the Honolulu Heart Program (McGee et al., 1984)—have shown that dietary cholesterol, assessed reliably at entry and expressed as mg/1,000 kcal, was positively associated with risk of CHD after adjustment for age, blood pressure, cigarette smoking, and serum cholesterol level. Combining the results of these studies, Stamler and Shekelle (1988) calculated that a dietary cholesterol increment of 200 mg/1,000 kcal daily was associated with a 30% greater risk of CHD.

Considering the difficulties in measuring cholesterol intake, the many etiologic factors involved in CHD, the long natural history of the underlying atherosclerosis, and the variability among individuals in response to diet, the committee interprets these observations as supporting an etiologic role of dietary cholesterol in CHD. Since the association between dietary cholesterol and CHD persisted after adjustment for serum TC, the results suggest that dietary cholesterol may affect atherogenesis and CHD by other mechanisms in addition to its effect on LDL-C concentration (Zilversmit, 1979). The possible contribution of dietary cholesterol to cerebral vascular disease and peripheral vascular disease was not addressed in these studies.

Clinical and Metabolic Studies

RESPONSE OF SERUM TOTAL CHOLESTEROL   Many experiments have been conducted to measure the response of serum or lipoprotein cholesterol concentrations in humans to different amounts of dietary cholesterol. Cholesterol intake was usually modulated by adding or removing eggs from the diet. These experiments have varied widely in the degree of control of dietary intake among the subjects. They range from experiments in which the subjects were confined to a metabolic ward and fed laboratory-prepared formula diets to those in which noninstitutionalized subjects were advised to add eggs to or remove eggs from their habitual diets.

Examples of rigorously controlled experiments include those reported by Connor et al. (1961a,b, 1964). In each of three experiments, six men were placed on cholesterol-free and high-cholesterol diets that were either formula diets or carefully selected natural foods. Cholesterol was added as egg yolk. In all three experiments, substantial increases in serum TC resulted from the addition of egg yolk to the diet.

Beveridge et al. (1960) fed formula diets containing varying amounts of added crystalline cholesterol for 8 days to 67 noninstitutionalized university students. There was a linear increase in serum TC with increases in daily intake up to about 600 mg. A similar study was conducted by Mattson et al. (1972) in 56 healthy prison inmates who consumed formula diets with varying amounts of added egg yolk. There was an approximately linear relationship between cholesterol intake and elevation of serum TC levels.

An unusual opportunity to examine the effects of changes in habitual diet on plasma lipoprotein cholesterol levels was provided by the Lipid Research Clinics Coronary Primary Prevention Trial (Gordon et al., 1982). As in other cross-sectional studies, there was no association of any dietary component with either LDL-C or HDL-C before subjects were instructed to change their diets. However, the *change* in cholesterol intake (of about 27 mg/1,000 kcal per day) was associated with a *change* in plasma cholesterol concentration in a multiple regression model. The association was independent of the effects of changes in saturated and unsaturated fat and of weight loss, and there was no interaction between the type of fat and cholesterol intake. The change in plasma cholesterol was almost entirely due to a change in LDL-C.

In a follow-up analysis of data from the same trial after it was terminated, serum TC and LDL-C levels were less strongly and less consistently correlated with decreases in cholesterol intake up to 7 years after the initial dietary instruction period (Glueck et al., 1986). The partial regression coefficients were statistically significant at 4 years, but not at 0.8 and 7 years. In contrast, the coefficients for SFA intake were significant at all times.

In another cross-sectional dietary study, the investigators focused on subfractions of the lower-density lipoproteins measured by analytic ultracentrifugation (Williams et al., 1986). Daily cholesterol intake averaged 190 mg/1,000 kcal. Dietary cholesterol was not significantly correlated with serum TC or LDL-C, but was significantly correlated with the mass of small LDL in the $S_f 0$–7 range ($Rs = .30$, $p < .01$). Although there is considerable interest in the relative atherogenicity of lipoprotein subclasses, we do not know whether $S_f 0$–7 LDL has any special significance.

PREDICTIVE EQUATIONS RELATING DIETARY CHOLESTEROL TO SERUM CHOLESTEROL   The first report of an equation to describe the effect of dietary cholesterol or serum cholesterol was made by Grande et al. (1965) in 1965. Keys (1984) reviewed this equation in light of 39 subsequent reports and concluded that the same equation, shown below, remained the best description:

$$\Delta Chol = 1.5 \, (C_2^{1/2} - C_1^{1/2}),$$

where $\Delta Chol$ is the change in serum TC concentration in mg/dl, C_2 is the new intake of cholesterol in mg/1,000 kcal per day, and C_1 is the initial intake.

Hegsted (1986) reviewed the same 39 reports plus several others and concluded that the association was essentially linear from 0 to 400 mg per 1,000 kcal and could be described by the following equation:

$$\Delta Chol = 0.0974\ C,$$

where $\Delta Chol$ is the change in serum cholesterol in mg/dl and C is the difference in cholesterol intake between the two diets in mg/1,000 kcal.

VARIABILITY IN RESPONSE TO DIETARY CHOLESTEROL   Most reports of experiments on dietary cholesterol in humans mention the high variability of responses of serum cholesterol and LDL-C among individuals. Some people do not respond at all; many have small responses; and a few have large responses. Indeed, as discussed above, the variability among individuals is so great that it obscures correlations in cross-sectional studies.

Reports after 1980 began to focus more attention on this variability. A group of investigators in the Netherlands conducted an intensive study of individual variability in responsiveness to dietary cholesterol. Katan et al. (1986) tested 94 people on diets providing 121 and 625 mg of cholesterol per day in egg yolk. The highest quartile and the lowest quintile of responders were challenged 1 month and again 7 months after the initial challenge. The high and low responders were significantly different from one another in the repeated challenges. Standardized correlation coefficients of the responses to the three challenges, taken in pairs, ranged from .34 to .53 (all $p < .05$). The mean of each subject's responses during the three challenges, taken as the best estimate of the response, showed a normal unimodal distribution from -12 to $+46$ mg/dl. Approximately 90% of the change in serum TC was accounted for by changes in LDL-C. McNamara et al. (1987) found that people who responded to dietary cholesterol with an increase in TC were also those in whom endogenous cholesterol synthesis was not suppressed.

There now appears to be convincing evidence that consistent differences in responsiveness of serum cholesterol to dietary cholesterol do exist in humans. When these responses are measured in terms of specific lipoprotein classes, the differences among individuals become even more prominent. No simple marker for sensitivity is available. A test for responsiveness involves feeding a controlled diet for 6 weeks or longer and analyzing several blood samples. The procedure is laborious and cannot be performed on large numbers of people. The definition of a responder, or a high responder, is arbitrary, but is the basis for determining the proportion affected, since the distribution of responses is continuous. However, the results indicate that approximately 20% of adults are likely to have a response more than 10% higher than that predicted by the Hegsted (1986) or Keys (1984) equations.

EFFECTS OF DIETARY CHOLESTEROL ON LIPOPROTEIN METABOLISM   In most studies up to about 1980, the effects of dietary cholesterol were measured only as changes in serum TC. As new analytical methods became available, investigators began to measure the effects of dietary cholesterol on the major lipoprotein classes or the apolipoproteins or on variables such as lipoprotein secretion or degradation. Only in the late 1970s did reliable techniques become available for measuring cholesterol in major lipoprotein fractions and apolipoproteins in a large number of plasma samples. Many cholesterol feeding experiments were repeated to take advantage of these new techniques. For example, Applebaum-Bowden et al. (1979) found that elevations in serum cholesterol were due principally to an elevation of LDL-C and that plasma apolipoprotein B concentrations were also increased. Similar results were obtained by Mistry et al. (1981), Packard et al. (1983), and Schonfeld et al. (1982).

Beynen and Katan (1985) and Schonfeld et al. (1982) reported that most of the change in serum cholesterol was accounted for by a change in LDL-C. Zanni et al. (1987) demonstrated that dietary cholesterol affected HDL-C and found considerable heterogeneity in response among individuals. Applebaum-Bowden et al. (1984) observed that LDL receptor activity in mononuclear cells, as measured by ability to degrade LDL, was decreased by dietary cholesterol proportionally to the increase in serum LDL-C levels. Lin and Connor (1980) found that the percentage of dietary cholesterol absorbed in two subjects did not change within the range of intake from 45 mg to 1,000 mg per day. Ginsberg et al. (1981) reported no change in the rates of production or clearance of VLDL or LDL with changes in dietary cholesterol in five subjects. In all the studies in which the characteristics of the elevated serum LDL were examined, the LDL particles were essentially normal in size and other characteristics; there were simply more particles.

Katan and Beynen (1987) looked for differences in metabolic characteristics between high and low responders and found that only habitual cholesterol intake and HDL$_2$ cholesterol levels were associated with responsiveness. McNamara et al. (1987) observed that two-thirds of a group of 75 men responded to a 600 mg/day increase in dietary cholesterol with no change in plasma cholesterol level, whereas approximately one-third of the subjects responded with an increase greater than 5%. The nonresponders suppressed cholesterol biosynthesis in blood mononuclear cells, but endogenous biosynthesis was not decreased in the responders.

Zilversmit (1979) suggested that absorbed dietary cholesterol is concentrated in the postprandial lipoproteins, which are thereby made more atherogenic. Investigation of the postprandial lipoproteins on a larger scale has been hampered by limitations in the methods for separating and quantitating these lipoproteins. Therefore, this mechanism remains an attractive but speculative possibility.

In summary, the effect of dietary cholesterol on serum lipoprotein concentrations is principally an increase in the concentration of normal serum LDL particles. There may be other effects on the characteristics of VLDL or HDL that are related to the increased LDL, but these have not been clearly identified and linked to the change in LDL.

INTERACTIONS OF DIETARY CHOLESTEROL WITH OTHER NUTRIENTS   Many investigators have looked for an interaction between dietary cholesterol and type of fat with regard to their effects on serum lipoproteins. A positive interaction with SFAs was found by the National Diet–Heart Study Research Group in the Faribault Study (1968). Bronsgeest-Schoute et al. (1979a) observed no significant interaction in one experiment, but did find one in a later experiment (1979b). Neither Chenoweth et al. (1981) nor Oh and Monaco (1985) reported an interaction with any type of fat.

In summary, despite the widespread belief that there is a positive interaction between dietary cholesterol and SFAs in their effects on serum lipid or lipoprotein concentrations, the evidence from studies in humans is inconsistent, perhaps due to varying proportions of responders and nonresponders in the different studies. Further research is needed to resolve this question.

Animal Studies

Since the initial demonstration of dietary cholesterol-induced atherosclerosis in rabbits in 1913 (Anitschkow, 1967; Anitschkow and Chalatow,

1913), a variety of animal species have been shown to be sensitive to cholesterol. Guinea pigs (Bailey, 1916), mice (Löwenthal, 1925), goats (Chalatow, 1929), swine (Bragdon et al., 1957), chickens (Dauber and Katz, 1942), and most species of nonhuman primates (Clarkson et al., 1976a,b) are quite sensitive; dogs (Steiner and Kendall, 1946) and rats (Wissler et al., 1954) are relatively resistant. Among the nonhuman primates, rhesus, cynomolgus, squirrel, and vervet monkeys are moderately sensitive, whereas baboons are only slightly sensitive (Corey et al., 1974; Eggen, 1974; McGill et al., 1976; Portman and Andrus, 1965; Srinivasan et al., 1976). In each species, as in humans, there is considerable interindividual variability, and it has been shown in several species that much of this variability is under genetic control (Clarkson et al., 1971, 1985; Flow et al., 1981). The metabolic basis of the genetic variability has not been identified.

In animal models, as in humans, the elevated serum cholesterol resulting from dietary cholesterol is carried primarily in LDL (McGill et al., 1981b). Effects on HDL vary considerably from one species to another. In some, dietary cholesterol increases HDL; in others, it decreases HDL.

The increases in serum lipids and lipoproteins caused by dietary cholesterol (usually accompanied by a high level of dietary SFAs) result in arterial lesions similar to those found in humans with atherosclerosis. A few experiments with prolonged feeding of a cholesterol-supplemented diet showed that arterial lesions in animals can undergo complications typical of those seen in advanced atherosclerosis in humans and occasionally result in thrombotic occlusion of the coronary artery and myocardial infarction or occlusion of the iliac or femoral arteries and peripheral vascular disease (Taylor et al., 1963).

In summary, dietary cholesterol is the dominant feature of experimental hyperlipidemia and atherosclerosis in animal models. Humans resemble the more resistant species of nonhuman primates in their sensitivity to dietary cholesterol. The results of studies in which cholesterol is fed to laboratory animals are of particular value in examining physiological mechanisms. The role of dietary cholesterol as an etiologic agent in atherosclerosis in humans should be interpreted with caution, because the relative amount of cholesterol fed to animals usually is much greater than that consumed by human populations. Experimental diets often contain 1,000 to 2,000 mg of cholesterol per 1,000 kcal, whereas a high intake for humans is

300 to 500 mg per 1,000 kcal. These very high cholesterol diets are used to produce high serum cholesterol levels and atherosclerotic lesions within a limited time. Lower dietary intakes, well within the range of human intakes, fed over longer periods to susceptible species have produced atherosclerotic lesions. Thus, the observations in laboratory animals are consistent with the causative role of dietary cholesterol in human disease.

Cholesterol Autoxidation Products

There has been much speculation about the possible toxicity of cholesterol derivatives. Several reports, all from one laboratory (Imai et al., 1976, 1980; Janakidevi et al., 1984; K.T. Lee et al., 1985; Murray et al., 1981; Peng et al., 1978, 1979; Taylor et al., 1979) indicate that 25-hydroxycholesterol and cholestane triol cause necrosis of arterial smooth muscle cells and influence the growth of these cells in culture. None of these effects has been confirmed by other investigators. There is no epidemiologic or clinical evidence suggesting that these derivatives cause hyperlipidemia or atherosclerosis in humans.

Plant Sterols

The intake of plant sterol by humans ranges from 150 to 400 mg/day—about the same daily intake as cholesterol. Most plant sterols are poorly absorbed by the intestinal tract, and those that are absorbed are rapidly excreted. Sitosterol is the most abundant plant sterol; others include stigmasterol, campesterol, brassicasterol, and 24-methylene cholesterol. The amounts that are absorbed are inversely proportional to the molecular weight of the sterols.

Long ago, plant sterols (β-sitosterol and related compounds) were found to prevent the absorption of dietary cholesterol (Best et al., 1955; Farquhar and Sokolow, 1958; Farquhar et al., 1956; Lees et al., 1977; Peterson et al., 1959), apparently by blocking absorption of cholesterol in the intestine (Davis, 1955; Grundy and Mok, 1977; Jandacek et al., 1977; Mattson et al., 1977). More recent reports indicate that these compounds may be more effective in small doses than previously believed (Mattson et al., 1982). No deleterious side effects have been identified, but β-sitosterol has not been widely used in a lipid-lowering diet.

A rare genetic disorder causes people to absorb a large proportion of dietary plant sterols (Bhattacharyya and Connor, 1974; Lin et al., 1983; McArthur et al., 1986; Miettinen, 1980; Shulman et al., 1976; Tilvis and Miettinen, 1986). In this condition, known as phytosterolemia, the affected subjects have high plasma levels of plant sterols and xanthomas. The patients appear to be at an increased risk for atherosclerotic cardiovascular disease and should therefore greatly limit their intake of plant sterols.

Summary

Dietary cholesterol causes hypercholesterolemia and atherosclerosis in a variety of animal species. In humans, within the usual range of intakes (300 to 600 mg/day, or about 150 to 300 mg/1,000 kcal), dietary cholesterol influences the plasma cholesterol concentration, primarily LDL-C. On average, 100 mg of dietary cholesterol per 1,000 kcal elevates LDL-C by 8 to 10 mg/dl. Individual responses vary considerably on both sides of this average response in a continuous distribution. Some people are resistant to the cholesterol-raising effects of dietary cholesterol; others are quite sensitive. For those in the upper range of this distribution—at least one-third of the population—dietary cholesterol is a substantial contributor to serum TC and LDL-C concentration and thus to the progression of atherosclerosis and to the risk of clinically manifest atherosclerotic disease. The only way to identify a susceptible person is by repeated dietary challenges—a procedure that is not feasible on a large scale. For the overall population, the evidence indicates that dietary cholesterol contributes to the development of atherosclerosis and the risk of CHD.

Dietary Lipids/Fats and Hypertension
Human Studies

Epidemiologic studies suggest that people who subsist on complete vegetarian diets have lower mean blood pressure levels than those consuming omnivorous diets (Sacks et al., 1974) (see Chapters 8 and 10). The specific dietary components involved have not been identified, but they probably do not include sodium since salt intake is similar in many vegetarian and omnivorous groups (Armstrong et al., 1974). The fact that complete vegetarians tend to eat more PUFAs and less total fat, SFAs, and cholesterol (Rouse et al., 1981) has led researchers to design a number of observational, clinical, and community intervention studies to examine the relationship of dietary fatty acids to blood pressure (Weinsier and Norris, 1985).

In general, observational studies of blood pressure and of indirect indices of high blood pressure such as stroke in noninstitutionalized populations offer little support for an effect of total fat, but suggest a modest and more consistent effect for specific fatty acids. Tuomilhehto et al. (1984) compared random samples of the Finnish population, ages 30 to 59, living in two counties in eastern Finland in 1972, 1977, and 1982, and reported that intake of total fat was positively associated with blood pressure in each study period and with change in blood pressure over the three study periods. In two other studies, no association with total fat was found. McCarron et al. (1983) used cross-sectional data from the 1971–1974 NHANES I to evaluate representative subgroups of the U.S. population for whom intake of 17 nutrients was determined and a single blood pressure measurment was taken. They found no difference in total fat intake between hypertensive (>160/95 mm Hg) and normotensive (<160/95 mm Hg) individuals. The lack of association was found in both men and women and across the three age categories examined: 20 to 34, 35 to 54, and 55 to 74 years. Thulin et al. (1980) compared the nutrient intakes of 36 untreated hypertensive women to that of an equal number of normotensive age-matched women and found no difference in total fat intake between the two groups. The authors did not, however, control for other dietary variables.

A lack of association of hypertension with total fat has also been observed in studies using stroke as a surrogate end point. In a 10-year follow-up study of 7,895 men of Japanese ancestry ages 45 to 68 living in Hawaii with no history of stroke at baseline, Kagan et al. (1985) observed an inverse association of total dietary fat with incidence of thromboembolic stroke and total stroke in univariate analysis. This association disappeared when the investigators controlled other factors associated with stroke (e.g., age, blood pressure, serum glucose, and cigarette smoking). No association of total fat with hemorrhagic stroke was seen in either univariate or multivariate analyses.

In a pilot cross-sectional study comparing blood pressure level to dietary variables in a small number of people living in rural Finland, Italy, and the United States, no association with total dietary fat was found (Carvalho et al., 1981; Iacono et al., 1982). The authors did report, however, that the Finnish sample, which had the highest mean blood pressures of all three groups, also had a higher intake of SFAs and a lower intake of PUFAs than did the two other national samples. Groen et al. (1962) compared dietary intakes by Benedictine and Trappist monks who had a prevalence of hypertension (diastolic blood pressure >95 mm Hg) of 51 and 12%, respectively, and found no difference in total fat consumption between the two groups. Trappist monks, however, consumed a greater percentage of their fat as vegetable fat.

The types and amounts of dietary lipids and their relationships to blood pressure have been examined in clinical studies of both normotensive and hypertensive people but have produced inconsistent results. In a study at the USDA Lipid Nutrition Laboratory, Judd et al. (1981) compared blood pressures among four groups of normal and mildly hypertensive male subjects fed natural diets of either high fat (43% of calories from fat) or low fat (25% of calories from fat) with a high P:S ratio (1.0) or low P:S ratio (0.3) for 6 weeks. Salt intake was slightly decreased (from 8.6 to 8.1 g/day) and potassium intake was slightly increased (from ≃4.1 to ≃5.1 g/day) in the groups consuming low compared to high fat. Body weights changed only slightly. On average, systolic and diastolic blood pressures were lower in persons on the high P:S diets than in those on the low P:S diets, regardless of total fat intake, although the magnitude of the difference between the groups (<4 mm Hg for both diastolic and systolic blood pressure) was modest (Iacono et al., 1982).

Vergroesen et al. (1978) assessed blood pressure changes in eight normotensive people (five men and three women) who were fed a diet with a moderately increased level of linoleic acid and no other dietary changes. A decrease in diastolic but not systolic blood pressure was noted after approximately 4 weeks on the diet. The diastolic pressure returned to baseline values after the subjects resumed their normal dietary regimen. In a similar but larger study, Fleischman et al. (1979) reported decreases in both systolic and diastolic blood pressures in 28 mildly hypertensive subjects fed a diet substituting linoleic-rich lipids for SFAs. Further evidence for an effect of linoleic acid was provided by Rao et al. (1981), who randomized 24 hypertensive Indians into one of three treatment groups receiving capsules containing groundnut oil (21% PUFA), safflower oil (12% PUFA), or starch. The authors calculated that the groundnut and safflower oil supplements increased linoleic acid intake by 7 to 10%. All three groups received a standard diet containing 2,000 kcal and 15 to 18% energy from fat. After 1 month of treatment, diastolic blood pressure decreased approximately 6.5 and 9.0% in the groups consuming supplements of groundnut and safflower oil, respectively;

no change was observed in the group consuming starch.

Not all clinical studies have demonstrated that a change in dietary fatty acids affects blood pressure. Sacks et al. (1984) reduced SFAs from 21 g/day to 10 g/day (maintaining a constant level of PUFA, carbohydrate, and total fiber) in the diets of 19 normotensive volunteers and observed no change in blood pressure. Margetts et al. (1984), in a randomized double-blind study of 54 normotensive volunteers, reported no change in blood pressure in people allocated to either a low or high P:S ratio diet. In a subsequent randomized, double-blind crossover study, 21 mildly hypertensive subjects were fed dietary supplements of cream, safflower oil, and carbohydrate for 6 weeks in random sequence (Sacks et al., 1987). The investigators noted no difference in blood pressure among the three study groups.

Three metabolic epidemiologic studies comparing blood pressure levels to fatty acid concentrations in tissue and erythrocytes in noninstitutionalized populations offer conflicting data. Oster et al. (1979) studied 650 German males and observed a small inverse correlation ($R = -.16$ to $-.12$) between the concentration of linoleic acid in adipose tissue and both systolic and diastolic blood pressure. These small correlations were reduced even further when the investigators controlled for age and body weight. Berry and Hirsch (1986) found no association between linoleic acid concentration in adipose tissue and blood pressure in 399 males in the United States, but they reported that there was an inverse association between linolenic acid concentrations in adipose tissue and systolic and diastolic blood pressure, both of which decreased approximately 5 mm Hg for every 1% increase in adipose linolenic acid content. The authors concluded that the level of dietary linolenic acid has a disproportionate effect on blood pressure since it constituted only one-eighth as much of the fatty acid content of the adipose tissue as did linoleic acid. Ciocca et al. (1987) compared the fatty acid composition of erythrocytes to arterial blood pressure in a large population of urban Italian females and noted no differences in the relative amounts of SFAs, MUFAs, and PUFAs or in the mean P:S ratio and linoleic:oleic acid ratio in erythrocytes across quartiles of systolic and diastolic blood pressure.

Several population intervention studies on dietary lipids and blood pressure have been conducted. In Finland and Italy, 30 normotensive couples were given an experimental diet in which total fat was decreased and the P:S ratio and vegetable intake were increased. The authors observed a reduction in blood pressure that was reversed when the couples resumed their usual diets (Ehnholm et al., 1982; Puska et al., 1982).

Using a different approach, Strazzullo et al. (1986) investigated whether or not adding SFAs to the typical Mediterranean diet of rural southern Italians would raise blood pressure. Fifty-seven normotensive people (29 males and 28 females) ages 30 to 50 were followed for 2 weeks on their customary diet (P:S ratio of 0.44), then switched to a 6-week isocaloric diet with a 70% increase in SFAs and a corresponding decrease in carbohydrate and MUFAs (P:S ratio of 0.23). By the end of 6 weeks, systolic blood pressure had increased by 2.6 mm Hg in men and 4.8 mm Hg in women; no change in diastolic blood pressure was observed in either sex.

In an intervention study on 57 adult normotensive spouse pairs (diastolic blood pressure <90 mm Hg) and untreated hypertensive people (diastolic blood pressure >90 mm Hg) living in two communities in North Karelia, Finland, Puska et al. (1983) randomly allocated couples to one of three study groups: Group 1 followed a low-fat diet (23% of energy intake) with a high P:S ratio (1.0); Group II reduced daily salt intake from 192 mmol to 77 mmol; and Group III continued their usual diet. After a 6-week intervention period, systolic blood pressure in Group I declined from 138.4 to 129.5 mm Hg, while diastolic pressure decreased from 88.9 to 81.3 mm Hg. The mean decrease in blood pressure was greater in hypertensive than in normotensive subjects. Both diastolic and systolic blood pressures returned to baseline values once couples in Group I resumed their usual diets. No blood pressure differences were observed over the course of the study in Groups II or III.

In a subsequent study of 84 middle-aged people from the same population, Puska et al. (1985) randomly allocated subjects to one of two study groups. Total fat intake was reduced from 38 to 24% in both groups. The dietary P:S ratio was increased from 0.2 to 0.9 in Group I and from 0.2 to 0.4 in Group II. During the 12-week intervention period, systolic and diastolic blood pressure in Group I decreased 4 mm Hg and 5 mm Hg, respectively. The corresponding decrease in Group II was 3 mm Hg and 4 mm Hg, respectively. Again, blood pressure reduction was reversed when subjects assumed their usual diets. The findings suggest that in people on a low fat diet, a moderate increase in the dietary P:S ratio is as effective in lowering blood pressure as is a greater increase.

In a study in 36 children ages 8 to 18 in the same two communities in North Karelia, Vartiainen et al. (1986) assessed the effect of total fat reduction (from 35 to 24% of total energy) and an increase in P:S ratio (from 0.18 to 0.61) on blood pressure. Neither systolic nor diastolic blood pressure changed significantly over the 12-week study period.

A few reports indicate that MUFAs, like PUFAs, may reduce blood pressure. In a cross-sectional survey of 76 middle-aged persons, Williams et al. (1987) found a strong inverse correlation between MUFA intake and both systolic and diastolic blood pressures that persisted after controlling for other potentially confounding variables, including age, cigarette smoking, stress, Quetelet Index, percentage of body fat, and waist-to-hip ratio. Rao et al. (1981) reported an inverse association between supplemental dietary MUFAs and blood pressure in hypertensive Indians on a traditional low-fat diet. Further studies, especially controlled clinical studies, are needed to replicate these findings.

In summary, studies of dietary lipids and blood pressure in humans suggest that a diet with a high P:S ratio and low total fat can produce modest reductions in blood pressure in normotensive and hypertensive people. Reduced total fat intake by itself appears to have little influence on blood pressure.

The inconsistency among study findings may reflect, in part, the inadequacy of the P:S ratio as a measure of the fatty acid composition of the diet, imprecise measurements of the dietary PUFAs and SFAs consumed by study participants, and inadequate control of other dietary and nondietary variables that may confound the association between dietary lipids and blood pressure.

Animal Studies

Studies in animals provide additional evidence for an association between intake of specific fatty acids (e.g., PUFAs) and blood pressure. In many animal studies, however, hypertension is induced by extremely high levels of dietary salt, which can confound interpretation of results. The following section distinguishes such studies from those restricting dietary salt or providing basal salt levels.

LIPID STUDIES ON HYPERTENSION NOT INDUCED BY SALT Smith-Barbaro et al. (1981) investigated the relative effects of diets high in PUFAs (20%

corn oil), high in SFAs (5% corn oil and 15% coconut oil), and low in total fat (5% corn oil) in Sprague Dawley rats. Salt was maintained at normal levels in all three diets. After 9 weeks, blood pressure was highest in animals fed the high SFA diets, intermediate in animals fed the high PUFA diets, and lowest in animals fed the low-fat diet.

Dusing et al. (1983) reported that the addition of even small amounts (5%) of linoleic acid to the diets of rats was sufficient to blunt the increase in blood pressure associated with diets deficient in linoleic acid. The moderating effect was evident even when animals were fed varying amounts of SFAs. The authors concluded that reduced linoleic acid intake was a more important factor in elevating blood pressure than increased SFAs. MacDonald et al. (1981) noted that the effect of linoleic acid intake on blood pressure is not continuous but, rather, exhibits a threshold (between 4.2 and 9.4% of total calories) above which little effect on blood pressure is observed.

Total dietary fat appears to modify the effect of dietary linoleate on blood pressure. Moritz et al. (1985) reported that low dietary fat (15% of energy from fat) can moderate the development of hypertension in susceptible rats and that high PUFA diets (15% sunflower or linseed oil by weight) can lower blood pressure in both hypertensive and normotensive animals.

Like studies in humans, studies in animals have not produced consistent results. Murray et al. (1986) reported higher blood pressures in Wistar-Kyoto spontaneously hypertensive rats (SHRs) fed high fat (40% of energy from fat) maize-oil diets compared to SHRs fed high-fat coconut-oil diets. Wexler (1981) observed that the onset of hypertension was blocked in Okamoto-Aoki SHRs fed a high SFA (20% suet) diet but not a low-fat (4% fat) diet.

In one study in rabbits (Bursztyn and King, 1986) and one in the SHR and normotensive Wistar-Kyoto and Wistar-Schonwalde rat strains (Singer et al., 1986), no effect on blood pressure was observed from specific fatty acids with diets that differed in their proportions of linoleic, γ-linolenic, α-linolenic, and eicosapentaenoic acids.

LIPID STUDIES ON SALT-INDUCED HYPERTENSION Studies on salt-induced hypertension in sodium-sensitive Wistar (Ten Hoor and Van de Graaf, 1978) and Dahl rats (Tobian et al., 1985) indicate that the addition of linoleic acid can blunt the hypertensive response of dietary salt and result in lower blood pressures. Hoffman et al. (1978) compared blood pressures in Wistar rats fed low saturated fat (7% hydrogenated palm kernel oil) or unsaturated fat (7% sunflower seed oil) diets with 1.5% added salt. They concluded that when chain length is similar, degree of unsaturation is inversely associated with systolic blood pressure.

Smith-Barbaro et al. (1981) compared blood pressure responses in Sprague Dawley rats on low total fat (5% corn oil), high PUFA (20% corn oil), and high SFA (5% corn oil and 15% coconut oil) diets who were also randomized to two levels of salt intake (8 and 15% sodium chloride). The authors reported that high salt intake produced hypertension when consumed with the low-fat diet. However, substitution of a high-SFA diet appeared to minimize the hypertensive effect of salt.

Codde and colleagues (1987a,b) conducted two studies comparing the effects of ω-3 PUFA (fish oil), ω-6 PUFA (safflower oil), and SFAs on blood pressure in rats challenged with desoxycorticosterone and salt. In the first study (Codde et al., 1987a), blood pressure in all three groups increased markedly by the end of the study (8 weeks), but rats fed the ω-3 and ω-6 PUFA diets had significantly lower blood pressures than those fed the SFA diet. In the second study (Codde et al., 1987b), SHRs and normotensive Wistar-Kyoto rats fed either an ω-3-rich diet of fish oil or an SFA-rich diet exhibited no differences in blood pressure before the addition of 1.5% saline to the diet. With salt loading, however, the blood pressure of SHRs on the SFA diet increased 21 mm Hg over that of the SHRs given the fish oil diets. No change was seen in the Wistar-Kyoto group.

The effect of dietary lipids on blood pressure has also been investigated by Kennedy et al. (1978), who reported that blood pressure in New Zealand white rabbits fed palm oil diets (high in SFAs) increased more than in rabbits fed safflower oil diets high in ω-6 PUFAs. Elevations in blood pressure have also been observed in rabbits fed a high SFA diet of coconut oil (Gardey et al., 1978).

In summary, animal studies indicate that diets deficient in linoleic acid increase blood pressure, and they provide weaker and less consistent evidence that diets with high levels of PUFAs lower blood pressure whereas those high in SFAs increase blood pressure. A few studies suggest that the hypertensive effect of high salt intake is moderated by high-fat diets.

The mechanism by which unsaturated fatty acids, especially linoleic acid, influence blood pressure has not been identified. Postulated mechanisms include alterations in prostaglandin production or effects on the renin–angiotensin system (Comberg et al., 1978; Frohlich, 1977; Weinsier and Norris, 1985).

Summary

Observational, clinical, and community intervention studies in humans suggest that although reduction of total dietary fat alone has little to no effect on reducing blood pressure in normotensive and mildly hypertensive individuals, increasing the dietary P:S ratio, with or without decreasing total intake of fat, results in a modest decrease in the blood pressure of hypertensives. The inconsistency of findings in humans, however, may reflect the inadequacy of the P:S ratio as an accurate measure of the dietary composition of fatty acids, as well as inadequate control of other dietary factors (e.g., total calories, salt, potassium, calcium, and alcohol) that might confound the association between lipids and blood pressure.

Findings in animal studies support an association of dietary lipids with blood pressure. The strongest and most consistent evidence links linoleic acid restriction to elevated blood pressure. Weaker evidence suggests that increasing the proportion of MUFAs or PUFAs relative to SFAs reduces blood pressure but that increasing dietary SFAs alone increases blood pressure. The exact nature of the response of blood pressure to graded increases in the intake of linoleic acid beyond the amounts necessary to prevent deficiency is unclear.

Cancer

The National Research Council's Committee on Diet, Nutrition, and Cancer (NRC, 1982) concluded "that of all the dietary components it studied, the combined epidemiological and experimental evidence is most suggestive for a causal relationship between fat intake and the occurrence of cancer. Both epidemiological studies and experiments in animals provide convincing evidence that increasing the intake of total fat increases the incidence of cancer at certain sites, particularly the breast and colon, and, conversely, that the risk is lower with lower intakes of fat. Data from studies in animals suggest that when fat intake is low, polyunsaturated fats are more effective than saturated fats in enhancing tumorigenesis, whereas the data on humans do not permit a clear distinction to be made between the effects of different components of fat. In general, however, the evidence from epidemiological and laboratory studies is consistent."

The committee further concluded that "the relationship between dietary cholesterol and cancer is not clear. Many studies of serum cholesterol levels and cancer mortality in human populations have demonstrated an inverse correlation with colon cancer among men, but the evidence is not conclusive. Data on cholesterol and cancer risk from studies in animals are too limited to permit any inferences to be drawn" (NRC, 1982, pp. 1–4 and 1–5).

The conclusion on fat was based largely on the consistency between epidemiologic and animal evidence. International correlation studies show direct associations between per-capita availability of dietary fat and the incidence of mortality from cancer at such sites as the breast, prostate, and gastrointestinal tract. Further evidence is provided by observational epidemiologic studies and by experimental results showing that animals fed high-fat diets develop cancers of the mammary gland, pancreas, and intestinal tract more readily than do animals on low-fat diets (NRC, 1982).

Rather than repeat discussions of the evidence on dietary fat, cholesterol, and cancer reviewed by the Committee on Diet, Nutrition, and Cancer (NRC, 1982), this section is concerned primarily with data that have accumulated since that time. Much work continues to be focused on breast cancer and colon cancer. Other studies have focused on the effects of dietary fat on pancreatic cancer and on the development of better models of prostate cancer that can be used to study effects of dietary fat. Interest has been concentrated primarily on effects of different levels and types of dietary fat. The mechanisms by which dietary fat may influence carcinogenesis have also been the subject of much speculation and some studies.

Epidemiologic data from different countries show that cancer incidence and mortality correlate more positively with total dietary fat than with any one type of dietary fat. On the other hand, results of experiments in animals demonstrate that vegetable oils containing ω-6 PUFAs promote carcinogenesis more effectively than SFAs, whereas fish oils containing ω-3 PUFAs tend to inhibit carcinogenesis. These findings are not necessarily in conflict with the epidemiologic data, since the studies were conducted primarily with individual fats and oils with fatty acid compositions that are quite different from those of the mixtures of fats and oils present in the diets of humans.

Recent studies on dietary fat and carcinogenesis

are summarized in books, conference proceedings, and review articles (e.g., ACS, 1983, 1986; Carroll, 1985; CAST, 1982; ECP/IUNS, 1986; Finley and Schwass, 1985; Hayashi et al., 1986; Holman et al., 1986; Hopkins and Carroll, 1985; ILSI/NF, 1987; Ip et al., 1986; Joosens et al., 1985; Knudsen, 1986; Milner and Perkins, 1984; Perkins and Wisek, 1983; Poirier et al., 1987; Reddy and Cohen, 1986a,b; Roe, 1983; Stich, 1982; Walker, 1986; Wynder et al., 1983).

Epidemiologic Evidence

The National Research Council's report *Diet, Nutrition, and Cancer* (NRC, 1982) indicated that fat has probably been studied more thoroughly and has been associated with various cancers more frequently than any other dietary factor. Since that report was published, studies have focused on the relationship between dietary fat and risk of colorectal, breast, and some other cancers, including cancers of the prostate and ovary. In this section, the committee considers the evidence first on dietary fat and then on dietary and serum cholesterol.

Dietary Fat

The evidence from epidemiologic studies has been based in part on geographical comparisons correlating differences in incidence of and mortality from various cancers with estimated fat intake by populations. Strong associations were found for cancer of the breast, colorectum, endometrium, and prostate, and, to a lesser extent, kidney and testicles (Armstrong and Doll, 1975; Carroll, 1975; Hems, 1980; Knox, 1977). In studies based on data from personal interviews in Hawaii, Kolonel et al. (1981) found significant associations of total fat, animal fat, and saturated and unsaturated fat intakes with ethnic patterns of breast, prostate, and corpus uteri cancer incidence but not of colon cancer.

Other studies have suggested an association of dietary fat with breast cancer (Lubin et al., 1981; Miller et al., 1978; Nomura et al., 1978; Phillips, 1975), prostate cancer (Hirayama, 1977; Rotkin, 1977; Schuman et al., 1982), and colorectal cancer (Dales et al., 1979; Jain et al., 1980; Martinez et al. 1979; Phillips, 1975). Negative studies were also reported, especially for colorectal cancer (Bjelke, 1978; Graham et al., 1978; Haenzel et al., 1980). As noted by the Committee on Diet, Nutrition, and Cancer (NRC, 1982), however, some of these studies were conducted on groups of relatively homogeneous populations, and some were not specifically designed to test the hypothesis that fat consumption is associated with colorectal cancer. The studies specifically designed to test the dietary fat hypothesis (e.g., Dales et al., 1979; Jain et al., 1980) tend to show the most striking direct associations.

The remainder of this section presents the evidence by cancer site, the way most of it is reported.

BREAST CANCER Since the 1982 report of the Committee on Diet, Nutrition, and Cancer (NRC, 1982), data from an earlier case-control study in Canada (Miller et al., 1978) have been reanalyzed with more modern methods and in light of the contribution made by different dietary factors (Howe, 1985). As a result of this analysis, the strongest association was found for SFA intake, and the dose–response relationship was particularly significant in premenopausal women. In this group, the risk for those in the highest SFA consumption tertile (>35.4 g of SFAs per day) relative to the lowest (<23.4 g of SFAs per day) was 5.9. Hirohata et al. (1987) studied 183 case-control sets of Japanese and 161 case-control sets of Caucasian subjects in Hawaii. Each case was matched to one hospital and one neighborhood control, and all were between the ages of 45 and 74. No statistically significant differences were found between cases and controls in their mean intake of total fat, SFAs, oleic acid, linoleic acid, animal protein, and cholesterol. However, there was a suggestion that cases consumed more SFAs and oleic acid than did neighborhood controls. As the authors noted, one difficulty with this investigation may have been the use of a relatively limited dietary questionnaire, which was designed to collect information on a selected list of 43 food items believed to represent the major sources of total and saturated fat, cholesterol, and animal protein.

Lubin et al. (1986) reported the findings of a large case-control study in Israel in which neighborhood controls were also used. When consumption levels were considered in quartiles, an increased risk of breast cancer was found among high fat, high animal protein, and low fiber consumers compared to those with the lowest consumption of fat and animal protein and highest consumption of fiber. For women under the age of 50, the relative risk was 1.6; for women age 50 or more, it was 2.0. A significant trend (p <.02) was found for the latter group.

In British Columbia, Canada, Hislop et al. (1986) administered a food frequency questionnaire on current diet and dietary practices in childhood. Although unable to determine nutrient intake, they found positive associations of breast cancer with current intake of fat-associated foods, especially whole milk and beef, and an increased risk among those who consumed visible fat on meat, both recently and in childhood. In northern Italy, risk estimates for indices of fat intake based on selected food items with a high fat content were found to be moderately elevated (Talamini et al., 1984). In a large case-control study in France involving 1,010 breast cancer cases and 1,950 controls with nonmalignant diseases, increased risk was found for consumption of dairy products but not for butter or yogurt; for the latter, there was a suggestion of a protective effect (Lê et al., 1986). For daily cheese consumption relative to never, the risk was 1.5, and for full cream milk consumption relative to none, the risk was 1.8.

At least three recent studies, however, were negative. In a case-control study in Greece involving 120 patients with breast cancer and 120 controls from an orthopedic hospital, Katsouyanni et al. (1986) found no association with consumption of fats and oils, but a protective effect for the consumption of vegetables. However, the authors pointed out that animal fat consumption in Greece is less than one-third of that in the United States or Canada and all study subjects may have therefore been at low risk of breast cancer, whereas vegetable consumption in Greece is twice as high. In a case-control study in Australia involving 451 cases and 451 controls, Rohan et al. (1988) found no association between dietary fat, protein, or caloric intake, but a protective effect of β-carotene.

A cohort study of nurses who completed a self-administered questionnaire also showed no association between dietary fat and risk of breast cancer (Willett et al., 1987). Among the possible reasons for discrepancies between this large cohort study (89,538 nurses ages 34 to 59 who had 601 breast cancers during 4 years' follow-up) and most case-control studies are recall bias in the case-control studies, and in the cohort study, less than complete estimates of fat intake in the self-administered questionnaire compared to a detailed dietary history (Jain et al., 1982), a short follow-up period (4 years), a narrow range of fat intakes in the study sample, and measurement error combined with a weak association. Another cohort study based on NHANES I data showed an inverse association between dietary fat and breast cancer occurrence that was no longer significant when adjusted for total energy intake. However, the findings may have been influenced by methodologic problems with the dietary assessment; indeed, the design of the NHANES study has been considered unsuitable for analyses based on individual intakes (Jones et al., 1987a) (see Chapter 2).

In addition to the limitations noted above, part of the inconsistencies in the epidemiologic studies could be that fat intake early in life may have a greater influence on breast cancer risk than intake later in life. This could account for the slow change in breast cancer rates in some migrant groups and could be reflected in the failure to observe reduced breast cancer incidence in population groups who as adults have made major dietary changes resulting in lower total fat intake. This applies to groups of nuns who adopted a low-fat diet in adult life (Kinlen, 1982). Furthermore, measurement errors in dietary recall in case-control and cohort studies can account for weak or absent associations of dietary fat with breast cancer, even if the relationship is real (Freudenheim and Marshall, 1988; Prentice et al., 1988).

In summary, the overall evidence is inconsistent. Nevertheless, it tends to support a weak association between dietary fat and breast cancer risk in humans.

COLORECTAL CANCER   Miller et al. (1983) compared the intake of food groups and various nutrients, particularly SFAs, in relation to risk of colorectal cancer. This was a further analysis of the case-control study first reported by Jain et al. (1980). The risk associated with a higher consumption of SFAs relative to lower consumption, considered in tertiles, for colon and rectal cancer cases combined relative to the combined neighborhood and surgical control series was 2.4 for males and 2.6 for females. In females, increased intake of SFAs consistently increased risk for colon cancer and also had an important independent effect over and above an apparent effect of some meats in increasing risk of rectal cancers. In males, different meat products appeared to increase risk and intake of SFAs did not appear to have an independent effect. Nevertheless, it seems possible that imprecision in consumption estimates, particularly for men, may have contributed to this result.

Willett and Stampfer (1986), in a commentary on differences in total energy intake in dietary studies, recalculated nutrient densities for SFA intake (SFAs divided by total calories) from the study of Jain et al. (1980) and found that the association with colorectal cancer largely disap-

peared. They noted, however, that inverse associations (as observed for crude fiber intake) can be produced by this process even when such nutrients are not independently associated with disease. This caused Howe et al. (1986) to reanalyze the data from the Jain et al. (1980) study once more, constructing logistic regression models that included variables representing the effect of SFAs and calories from sources other than SFAs. In this approach, the risk for highest, relative to low, consumption levels for SFAs was found to be 2.0 for males and 2.3 for females. No effects were found for calories or for fiber.

Manousos et al. (1983) in a case-control study conducted in Greece based on a food frequency questionnaire observed a positive association between intake of beef and lamb and colorectal cancer risk and a negative association with intake of cabbage, lettuce, spinach, and beets.

Stemmermann et al. (1984) reported the results of a 14- to 17-year follow-up of 8,006 men of Japanese ancestry whose intake of total fat was assessed by a 24-hour recall administered at baseline. The estimated mean intake of fat by the 99 cases was 69 g/day. For the 378 controls, it was 77 g/day. Thus this study did not support the dietary fat hypothesis.

In the Marseilles region of southern France, 399 cases and a corresponding number of surgical controls were studied by Macquart-Moulin et al. (1986), who used a food frequency dietary questionaire and estimated consumption of fat. There was no evidence of any difference in the consumption of total fat between cases and controls. Indeed, a reduced risk appeared to be associated with increasing consumption of oil, largely monounsaturated oil. Vegetables, particularly vegetables with low fiber content, appeared to be protective in this study.

In Belgium, a study conducted with a similar questionnaire showed no effect of fat intake, but there was a clear dose–response effect for intake of mono- and disaccharides. A protection effect was found for linoleic acid and dietary fiber (Tuyns et al., 1987).

In a case-control study conducted in Adelaide, Australia, Potter and McMichael (1986) found evidence of increasing risk with increasing consumption of a number of nutrients and a pattern of food intake involving high dietary fat and possibly SFAs. Although risk associated with SFAs and various components of fat was increased, it was the impression of the authors that the major contribution to increased risk came from dietary protein.

A case-control study of colorectal cancer in Melbourne, Australia, included 715 cases and 727 age- and sex-matched community controls. Fat intake was found to be a risk factor for both males and females (Kune et al., 1987); however, the relative risk associated with high fat intake was not large (1.4) and became apparent only after adjustment for meat and vegetable intake. The effect was similar, however, for colon and rectal cancer.

In summary, the weight of the evidence points to an association between colorectal cancer and a pattern of food intake involving high dietary fat. The negative outcome of some studies may be partly attributable to methodological difficulties, but it is possible that different cultures differ in the extent to which factors operate either in increasing risk or in providing protection against colorectal cancer.

PROSTATE CANCER   Results from at least four case-control studies have been published since the 1982 report *Diet, Nutrition, and Cancer* (NRC, 1982). Heshmat et al. (1985) reported a case-control study of 181 blacks with histologically confirmed prostate cancer and 181 controls from Washington, D.C. Risk enhancement was associated with increased intake of proteins, total fat, SFAs, and oleic acid. These items were related to intake by people ages 30 to 49 years, but not for those age 50 or more.

Graham et al. (1983) compared 262 patients from Buffalo, New York, with two different control series. Risk of prostate cancer increased with increasing ingestion of animal fats. Risk ratios of approximately 2.0 were found for fat consumption greater than 2,100 g/month relative to fat consumption of less than 1,200 g/month.

In a study of 452 prostate cancer cases and 899 age-matched population controls in Hawaii, Kolonel et al. (1988) found a dose–response gradient in risk of prostate cancer associated with intake of SFAs among men 70 years of age and older. The risk ratio was 1.7 for the highest relative to the lowest quartile of SFA intake.

In a follow-up study of 6,763 Seventh-Day Adventists who completed a dietary questionnaire in 1960, Snowdon et al. (1984) found positive associations between fatal prostate cancer and the consumption of milk, cheese, eggs, and meat. There was a graded dose–response between each of the four animal products and risk. The predicted relative risk of fatal prostate cancer was 3.6 for those who consumed all four animal products heavily. Although the dietary instrument used

could not provide an estimate of fat consumption, it does seem possible that dietary fat at least contributed to the increased risk of fatal prostate cancer in this study.

In summary, though not entirely consistent, there is evidence of an association of dietary fat, especially from animal sources, with prostate cancer. In one study, there was an association with incidence of prostate cancer, particularly in younger men, and in another, with fatal prostate cancer.

OVARIAN CANCER   Two case-control studies on dietary fat and risk of ovarian cancer have produced contradictory results. In one, based on data collected between 1957 and 1965, 274 white women ages 30 to 79 with epithelial carcinoma of the ovary were compared with 1,034 hospital controls (Byers et al., 1983). The investigators found no risk associated with consumption of fat at any age. However, Cramer et al. (1984), who studied 215 white women with epithelial ovarian cancer and 215 control women matched by age, race, and residence, found that the women with ovarian cancer favored, and consumed greater amounts of, foods high in animal fats and significantly less vegetable fat compared with control subjects. There was a significant trend toward an increased risk of ovarian cancer with increasing animal fat consumption. The risk controlling for Quetelet's Index for those with a high intake of animal fat (intake score of 225 or more) was 1.83 compared to those with a low intake (intake score of less than 125).

Details of the methods of dietary assessment used by Cramer et al. (1984) were not given. It is known that in the method used by Byers et al. (1983), relatively limited information was collected on food items contributing to dietary fat.

The geographic correlations for dietary fat and ovarian cancer are somewhat lower than those found for breast, colorectal, and prostate cancer (Armstrong and Doll, 1975). The positive results of Cramer et al. (1984) suggest that further study of this reported association is warranted.

CONCLUSIONS   In summary, evidence suggests that the risk of breast cancer and, to a possibly greater extent, of colon, prostate, and ovarian cancers, is associated with dietary fat. Although studies on diet and endometrial cancer have not been reported since 1982, the incidence of endometrial cancer has also been associated geographically with high total fat intake and with the incidence of these other cancers. The data suggest that the endocrine-related cancers of the breast, prostate, ovary, and endometrium, and also colorectal cancer, which itself has some features of an endocrine-related disease, are all associated with diet and possibly with total fat or SFA intake. This evidence supports the evidence from animals in studies reviewed below in the section on Animal Studies.

Dietary Cholesterol

Cholesterol intake was greater in premenopausal cases than in controls in a case-control study of diet and breast cancer (Miller et al., 1978). However, this association was not statistically significant and was quantitatively weaker than an association with dietary fat. In a reanalysis of the same data, dietary cholesterol did not have an effect independent of SFA intake (Howe, 1985). Cholesterol intake by cases was greater than that by controls in a case-control study of colorectal cancer, but the risk ratios were lower than for SFA intake (Jain et al., 1980). Risk ratios were also elevated for dietary cholesterol and colon cancer in a second case-control study, but they were lower for rectal cancer where risk was more strongly associated with dietary protein (Potter and McMichael, 1986). In a study comparing cholesterol intake by Seventh-Day Adventist lacto-ovovegetarians and nonvegetarians, differences were not "striking" (Turjman et al., 1984b). However, Liu et al. (1979), using food disappearance data from 20 countries, found that when they controlled for dietary cholesterol, the associations of dietary fat and fiber with colon cancer mortality that they previously observed were no longer significant.

Dietary cholesterol was associated with an increased risk of lung cancer in a case-control study by Hinds et al. (1983). The association was found in cigarette smokers and in males but not in females. Dietary cholesterol has also been associated with an increased risk of bladder cancer in a case-control study by Risch et al. (1988). In these studies, however, relatively restricted dietary questionnaires were used and it was not possible to determine whether the association with dietary cholesterol was due to other dietary factors associated with cholesterol intake.

No significant association was found between dietary cholesterol and cancer mortality in a 10-year follow-up of the Honolulu Heart Program (McGee et al., 1985), but data for individual cancer sites were not reported. In a cohort study of 89,538 U.S. nurses, no association between dietary cholesterol and breast cancer was found (Willett et al., 1987).

Serum Cholesterol

Some studies suggest that low serum TC is associated with an increased risk of cancer. These are discussed in the following paragraphs. The topic of competing risks is discussed further in Chapter 28.

Data on TC and cancer collected up to 1983 were reviewed by McMichael et al. (1984), who concluded that observational studies provide substantial evidence that preclinical cancer causes a lowering of TC and that limited but biologically plausible evidence suggests that males with low TC despite a diet high in SFAs and cholesterol are at increased risk of colon cancer. Since the studies reviewed by McMichael and colleagues (i.e., from 1983 on), there have been reports of seven studies primarily related to follow-up of cohorts established for the study of cardiovascular disease. In a study of 4,035 residents of California ages 40 to 89, Wingard et al. (1984) found no association between serum TC and cancer morbidity or mortality over a 7-year period for either men or women for any cancer site.

In a 5-year follow-up of 10,940 participants in the Hypertension Detection and Follow-up Program, a small but statistically significant inverse relationship was found between baseline TC and cancer incidence (Morris et al., 1983). When cases diagnosed during the first 2 years were excluded, the association was similar in magnitude but no longer statistically significant. The number of cases did not permit analysis by cancer site. In up to 6 years of follow-up (mean, 3 years) of 10,000 middle-aged men in the Malmo Prevention Program (Peterson and Trell, 1983), TC was inversely related to cancer mortality (44 deaths)—a relationship also observed for the 25 cancer deaths that occurred more than 2.5 years after screening. Serum urate levels at screening in this study were correlated with early but not late (more than 2.5 years after screening) cancer mortality (Peterson and Trell, 1983). As urate levels might indicate proliferation of cancer cells, the association of elevated TC with the late deaths may be due to a factor other than cancer operating at the time of screening.

In the Busselton Community Study in western Australia, 1,564 subjects ages 40 to 74 were followed for 13 years (Cullen et al., 1983). In men ages 60 to 74, but not in men ages 40 to 59 or in women, a negative association was found between serum TC and cancer mortality. In this study, however, it was not indicated whether the association persisted if early cancer deaths were excluded. In New Zealand, 630 Maoris ages 25 to 74 were followed for more than 17 years (Salmond et al., 1985). A significant inverse relationship between cancer mortality and TC was found for men and women considered together. The relative risk derived by comparing cancer mortality in men and women in the 10th and 90th percentiles of TC concentration decreased from 3.0 to 2.4 after excluding deaths during the first 5 years.

In the Seven Countries Study, 11,325 healthy men ages 40 to 59 were followed for 15 years (Keys et al., 1985). Among 477 cancer deaths 5 or more years after TC measurement, there was a significant excess of deaths from lung cancer in the lowest 20% of the TC distribution. Nevertheless, regional comparisons of cancer mortality showed that the highest cancer rates occurred in northern Europe where the TC levels were highest. In contrast, in a cohort study of 92,000 subjects less than 75 years old examined during 1963–1965 and followed by linkage to the Swedish Cancer Registry to 1975, there was a positive association between TC levels and risk of rectal cancer in men (Tornberg et al., 1986). The risk for men with elevated levels of both serum TC ($\geq$250 mg per deciliter) and β-lipoprotein ($\geq$2.2 g/liter), relative to those with lower levels of both, was 1.62 for colon cancer (95% confidence interval [CI], 1.18–2.22) and 1.70 for rectal cancer (95% CI, 1.18–2.44).

Cancer incidence was determined in 160,135 men and women who were members of a prepaid health plan and whose TC was determined as part of a multiphasic health examination (Hiatt and Fireman, 1986). These subjects were followed from 8 to 16 years. No consistent association of low TC with cancer incidence was found, but cancer incidence was highest among those in the lowest quintile of TC in the first 2 years after the measurement. In the largest study so far reported, a follow-up of the 361,662 men screened for the MRFIT study, there was a significant excess of cancer in those in the lowest decile of TC (<168 mg/dl), which attenuated over time (Sherwin et al., 1987).

Serum TC was assessed in five case-control studies. In one, elevated levels of TC were found in 37 cases of primary brain tumors compared to 74 controls (Abramson and Kark, 1985). The difference was not reduced by controlling for potential confounders (including weight). In another case-control study, TC was measured in 244 patients with adenomatous polyps of the colon, 182 patients with Dukes' A or B colon cancer, and 688 hospital controls (Neugat et al., 1986). The mean

TC levels were lower in the cancer cases than in the controls, the Dukes' B cases accounting for most of the difference. There was no difference between the mean levels for those with adenomatous polyps and the controls. After adjustment for nutritional status based on serum albumin level, however, there were no differences among any of the groups. In a nested case-control study within a cohort of members of a prepaid health care plan, 245 newly diagnosed cases of large bowel cancer and 5 matched controls for each case were compared on the basis of TC levels measured during a multiphasic health examination before diagnosis of the cases (Sidney et al., 1986). No direct or inverse relationship between TC and large bowel cancer was found. A fourth case-control study was based on a cohort of 18,995 people examined at a health center between 1970 and 1973 (Gerhardsson et al., 1986). The investigators found medical records for 100 of 176 cancer cases who died by 1979, for 393 of 900 controls still alive in 1979, and for 69 of 153 people who died of cardiovascular disease by 1979. Serum TC levels in the cancer cases were significantly lower than those of controls only in the 2-year period before death.

In a fifth study, a positive association was found between TC levels and the prevalence of adenomatous polyps found during colonoscopies of 842 patients (Mannes et al., 1986). For large bowel adenoma, the odds ratio between the highest and lowest quintiles of serum cholesterol was 1.9 (95% CI, 1.1–3.5) after adjustment for age and was 2.0 (95% CI, 1.1–3.6) after adjustment for body mass index. In a study by Tartter et al. (1984), serum TC was assessed in relation to disease-free survival of 279 colon cancer patients. There was an 11% but nonsignificant lower cumulative disease-free survival at 5 years in those whose TC levels were below the median than in those with levels above the median. In another study, a family history of cancer was found to be positively associated with TC levels in young adults (T. Reed et al., 1986).

Thus, although some epidemiologic studies of cohorts assembled to study cardiovascular disease risk show associations of low serum TC with cancer incidence and mortality, the studies designed specifically to assess the relationship have not in general found an association. When site-specific data are available, they are not consistent.

Clinical and Metabolic Studies

Metabolic studies have explored variables possibly related to the question of whether or not diet plays a role in the etiology of colon cancer. Several studies of fecal steroids have been undertaken in a number of different populations. Antonis and Bersohn (1962a) found that an increase in calories from dietary fat from 15 to 40% of the diet consumed by 43 white and Bantu prisoners resulted in an increased fecal excretion of neutral sterols and bile acids. The effect was greater for unsaturated fat. Cummings et al. (1978) observed that healthy volunteers placed on controlled diets containing first high and then low levels of animal fat had significant increases in fecal steroid excretion when on the high-fat diet. In a similar study, Reddy et al. (1980a) observed an increase in the enzymic activity of fecal microflora in addition to increases in excretion of fecal steroids.

Studies in various populations have shown an association of fecal excretion of steroids and cholesterol metabolites with the incidence of colorectal cancer in volunteers from England, Scotland, the United States, Uganda, Japan, India, and Hong Kong (Crowther et al. 1976; Hill et al., 1971). Finegold et al. (1974, 1975) were unable to confirm the findings reported by the previous investigators. Hill (1981) pointed out the limitations of traditional bacteriological techniques to investigate the microflora of the colonic lumen.

Reddy et al. (1978) found that volunteers in the United States and from rural Kuopio in Finland excreted the same amount of secondary bile acids daily, but the concentration of fecal bile acids in the U.S. subjects was 2.5 times greater than that of the Finns due to the greater stool output of the Finns. Similar studies conducted in New York and Sweden produced comparable results (Reddy et al., 1983). In another international study, dietary intake and fecal characteristics of random population samples from Kuopio, Finland, and Copenhagen, Denmark, were compared (Maclennan and Jensen, 1977). This study failed to confirm the correlation between the incidence of large bowel cancer and fecal steroid output or concentration. No difference was found in fat intake, but there were higher intakes of dietary fiber and milk in low-incidence Kuopio.

Another study conducted by the same group included areas with intermediate colon cancer risks in Finland and Denmark (Jensen et al., 1982). Daily fecal loss of bile acids was found to be identical among high-, medium-, and low-risk groups, but fecal bile acid concentrations among these groups were positively correlated with large bowel cancer risk, a finding probably related to the negative association between fecal bulk—which increases with increased fiber intake—and fecal bile acid concentration. Comparisons between Japanese living in Hawaii and those in Japan showed rather similar findings (Nomura et al., 1983).

Turjman et al. (1984a) found different concentrations of total bile acids among pure vegetarians, lacto-ovovegetarians, nonvegetarian Seventh-Day Adventists, and a demographically comparable group from the general population—groups that have different risks for colon cancer. Fecal cholesterol and its metabolites were lower among vegetarians; the ratio of secondary to primary bile acids also differed among the groups, suggesting a positive correlation between the formation of secondary bile acids and risk for developing colon cancer (Nair et al., 1984).

Several investigators have studied the excretion of bile acids in patients with colon cancer and in controls (Hill et al., 1977; Murray et al., 1980; Reddy and Wynder, 1977). These studies have generally produced inconsistent findings, possibly because of sampling limitations and the difficulties in sorting out causal factors from metabolic side effects of the disease or its treatment.

A completely different line of investigation has been followed by some investigators who studied the relationship between fecal mutagens and potential colon cancer. Ehrich et al. (1979) compared three South African populations with different colon cancer risks and observed that 19% of the fecal samples from urban white South Africans who are at higher risk of colon cancer were mutagenic compared to only 2% for urban blacks and 0% for rural blacks who are at lower risk. Reddy et al. (1980b) studied fecal mutagen activity among omnivorous volunteers and vegetarian Seventh-Day Adventists from New York, and rural Finns from Kuopio. A significantly higher percentage of omnivorous volunteers had fecal mutagenic activity compared to subjects in Finland. None of the samples from Seventh-Day Adventists had mutagenic activity. Similar results were obtained by Kuhnlein et al. (1981), but two small case-control studies failed to show a significant association of fecal mutagens with adenomatous polyps in autopsy specimens (Correa et al., 1981) or with colon cancer in newly diagnosed patients (Bruce and Dion, 1980). Bruce and Dion (1980) also found no differences in fecal mutagenic activity among people with different fat intakes.

In summary, clinical and metabolic studies focusing on colon cancer have explored three postulated intermediate mechanisms in colonic carcinogenesis, involving fecal bacteria, steroids and bile acids, and mutagens. Some consistency in research findings has been attained only for fecal steroids and bile acids, possibly because of the complexity of metabolic pathways and, in some instances, inadequate attention to appropriate sampling procedures. These findings have suggested that it is the concentrations of fecal steroids and bile acids that may enhance carcinogenesis rather than the total amounts excreted.

Animal Studies

Recent studies on dietary fat and carcinogenesis in laboratory animals have generally confirmed earlier evidence that animals fed high-fat diets develop tumors of the mammary gland, intestinal tract, and pancreas more readily that those fed low-fat diets ad libitum (NRC, 1982). The results can be modified, however, by the type of dietary fat.

Dietary fats increase the yield of mammary tumors only when they contain adequate amounts of ω-6 PUFAs, which are normally present as linoleate in fats derived from plants and land animals. This probably explains why fats such as butter, coconut oil, and beef tallow have little effect on mammary carcinogenesis (Carroll et al., 1981). The requirements for ω-6 PUFAs in mammary tumor promotion have been explored systematically by Ip et al. (1985), who reported 4 to 5% of total calories as the threshold at which the yield of mammary tumors increased. Increasing the amount of linoleate above this level appeared to have little additional effect on tumor promotion (Ip, 1987).

The amount of linoleate required to promote pancreatic tumors in rats appears to be somewhat higher (up to 8% of calories) (Birt and Roebuck, 1986; Roebuck et al., 1985). Much smaller amounts are evidently required for colon cancer (Bull et al., 1988), but in general, PUFAs appear to promote tumorigenesis more effectively than SFAs or MUFAs (Reddy, 1986a; Reddy and Maeura, 1984). However, some investigators have failed to observe the promotion of colon cancer by either SFAs or PUFAs (Nauss et al., 1987; Newberne and Nauss, 1986).

There is some evidence that tumor initiation can be influenced by the type of dietary fat. For example, lard has been observed to increase the yield of mammary tumors (Rogers and Lee, 1986; Rogers et al., 1986; Sylvester et al., 1986a) and colon tumors (Reddy, 1986a) when fed before or during the initiation.

The effects of dietary PUFAs on tumor metastasis have been investigated in two animal studies. Katz and Boylan (1987) found that a high-fat diet containing 23% corn oil stimulated metastasis of a mammary adenocarcinoma in retired female breeder rats compared to a diet containing 5% corn oil. Hubbard and Erickson (1987) reported that metastasis from transplanted mammary tumors in mice was enhanced by diets containing 8 to 12% linoleic acid as compared to diets with lower levels of linoleic acid.

In contrast to fats containing ω-6 PUFAs, fish oils, which contain mainly ω-3 PUFAs, fail to promote tumorigenesis when fed at high levels in the diet and may even have an inhibitory effect. This has been observed for tumors of the mammary gland (Braden and Carroll, 1986; Jurkowski and Cave, 1985; Karmali et al., 1984), intestine (Reddy, 1986a), and pancreas (O'Connor et al., 1985).

Diets used in these experiments may have been deficient in ω-6 PUFAs, because fish oils contain only small amounts of these PUFAs and because ω-3 PUFAs act as competitive inhibitors of reactions involving ω-6 PUFAs. This may have affected the results of the experiments on tumorigenesis (Karmali, 1987). In more recent studies, vegetable oils have been added to fish oil diets to provide a source of ω-6 PUFAs. In one such study, Kort et al. (1987a) reported that dietary menhaden oil inhibited the growth of transplantable mammary adenocarcinomas in rats but had no effect on metastases. In another, the tumor growth inhibition was not observed when the fish oil diet was fed only after transplantation of the tumor (Kort et al., 1987b). Other studies on experimental models of mammary cancer (Cave and Jurkowski, 1987), colon cancer (Reddy, 1987), and pancreatic cancer (O'Connor et al., 1987) indicate that a relatively high ratio of dietary fish oil to polyunsaturated vegetable oil is required to counteract the promoting effects of the vegetable oil.

Studies on animal models of mammary cancer and colon cancer indicate that *trans* fatty acids behave like SFAs with respect to their effects on tumorigenesis and do not promote tumors to a greater extent than do the *cis* isomers (Ip et al., 1986; Reddy et al., 1985; Selenskas et al., 1984). The evidence regarding dietary MUFAs, such as that derived from studies with olive oil, whose principal MUFA is oleic acid, is somewhat variable. In some experiments, olive oil promoted tumorigenesis about as well as PUFAs containing a high proportion of linoleic acid (Carroll and Khor,

1971), but more recent reports suggest that olive oil is not a good promoter (L.A. Cohen et al., 1986; Reddy, 1986a). The amount of linoleic acid in olive oil is insufficient for maximum promoting activity (Ip et al., 1985), and variations in linoleic acid content may account for some of the difference among results.

Although experiments in animals indicate that the promoting effect of dietary fat is influenced by its fatty acid composition, cancer mortality in human populations seems to correlate with total dietary fat about as well as with animal fat, and there is little or no correlation with vegetable fat or PUFAs (Carroll, 1983; Carroll et al., 1986). This does not necessarily conflict with the results of animal studies that show a tumor-promoting effect of PUFAs. In fact, the experiments in animals suggest a twofold requirement in promotion of carcinogenesis by dietary fat (Carroll, 1986b). The dietary fat must provide a certain amount of ω-6 PUFA. When this requirement is satisfied, the promoting effect of additional dietary fat appears to be unrelated to the type of fat (Ip, 1987). This promotion related to total fat intake may correspond to the positive correlations between total dietary fat and cancer incidence and mortality seen in epidemiologic data.

Dietary cholesterol has been studied primarily with respect to intestinal cancer. Although the data are inconsistent, Broitman (1986) in his review of the literature concluded that most evidence points to a possible relationship between dietary cholesterol and colon tumor development.

Mechanism of Action of Dietary Fat

In animals treated with a single dose of a chemical carcinogen to induce mammary tumors, the predominant effect of dietary fat is exerted after exposure to the carcinogen, is positively correlated with the duration of feeding the high-fat diet, and is inversely related to the time between exposure to carcinogen and introduction of the high-fat diet (Dao and Chan, 1983; Rogers and Lee, 1986). This indicates that dietary fat is acting primarily as a promoter (Carroll and Khor, 1975).

As indicated above, some dietary fats, e.g., lard and beef tallow (Rogers et al., 1986; Sylvester et al., 1986a), enhance mammary tumorigenesis when fed only at or before exposure to a carcinogen (Cohen, 1986; Rogers and Lee, 1986; Welsch, 1986). The mechanism of action for this is not known (Rogers and Lee, 1986) but could involve alteration of the rates of formation and inactivation of carcinogens or an influence on their binding to DNA (Hopkins and West, 1976; Wade and Dhardwadkar, 1986).

Many of the hypotheses advanced to account for the promoting action of dietary fat have been concerned specifically with mammary cancer (Carroll, 1986a; Cohen, 1986; Kidwell, 1986; Rogers et al., 1986; Welsch, 1986; Welsch and Aylsworth, 1983). One of the first and most intensively studied hypotheses is that dietary fat perturbs the endocrine system, especially prolactin (Cohen, 1986). After reviewing this literature, Welsch (1986) concluded that there is no consistent support for the concept that dietary fat enhances mammary tumorigenesis by increasing blood levels of pituitary or ovarian hormones. This concept is also weakened by evidence that high-fat diets promote the development of tumors that both are and are not dependent on hormones (Sylvester et al., 1986b: Welsch, 1986). Other studies have shown little difference between target tissue receptor levels and responsiveness to estrogen and prolactin in animals fed moderate and high levels of fat. Animals fed low levels of fat have reduced hormone receptor levels, which may be related to essential fatty acid deficiency (Welsch, 1986).

Other proposed mechanisms are related to the observation that dietary PUFAs promote mammary carcinogenesis in animals more effectively than SFAs (Carroll et al., 1986). As indicated above, this difference appears to be related to a requirement for ω-6 PUFAs, which are precursors of a variety of biologically active eicosanoids, including prostaglandins, thromboxanes, and leucotrienes. Evidence that the promoting effect of dietary fat can be prevented by inhibitors of prostaglandin synthesis (Carter et al., 1983; Hillyard and Abraham, 1979) suggests that the effect of fat may be mediated by eicosanoids. Further support for this idea is provided by the failure of dietary fish oils to promote mammary carcinogenesis (see the section on Breast Cancer). The ω-3 PUFAs in fish oils competitively inhibit the formation of eicosanoids from ω-6 PUFAs, and eicosanoids formed from ω-3 PUFAs differ in structure and biologic properties from those derived from ω-6 PUFAs. However, the prostaglandin synthesis inhibitor carprofen marginally enhanced the induction of mammary tumors induced by dimethylbenzanthracene in rats fed diets containing 5 or 20% corn oil, although the average weight of tumors was reduced significantly (Carter et al., 1987).

Although this is an attractive hypothesis, it is based mainly on speculation. The highly unsaturated fatty acids in fish oils are very susceptible to oxidation. Furthermore, while products of lipoxidation may initiate or promote carcinogenesis (Carroll, 1986a), there is also the alternative possibility that such compounds may inhibit carcinogenesis by exerting a toxic effect on tumor cells.

PUFAs of the ω-6 and ω-3 families can be incorporated into cellular membrane lipids. Since these fatty acids cannot be synthesized by animals, the amounts in tissues are influenced by the dietary supply (Holman, 1986). A model in which dietary unsaturated fatty acids are first taken up by adipose tissue and then transferred to epithelial tissue of the mammary gland has been described by Kidwell (1986).

The effects of dietary fat on the composition and properties of cellular membranes could influence carcinogenesis in a number of different ways. One possibility is an alteration in immune responses, which are known to be affected by PUFAs. These effects may be mediated by alterations in structure and function of cellular membranes or by modulation of prostaglandin biosynthesis (Erickson, 1986). Alterations in membrane structure may affect gap junction-mediated intercellular communication and thus serve as a mechanism by which dietary fat may promote carcinogenesis (Aylsworth, 1986).

These and other studies have led to an interest in diglyceride and protein kinase C as potential mediators of the effects of dietary fat on carcinogenesis. Protein kinase C is activated by diglyceride and also by phorbol ester—a known tumor promoter. Activation of protein kinase C has in turn been associated with cellular proliferation. Since unsaturated diglycerides activate protein kinase C more effectively than saturated diglycerides, it is possible that these compounds could mediate effects of dietary fat on carcinogenesis (Welsch, 1986).

Most proposed mechanisms involve the possible effects of dietary fat on cellular proliferation. Evidence presented by Hillyard and Abraham (1979) suggests, however, that dietary PUFAs may enhance tumor growth by prolonging the life of tumor cells and thus altering the balance between accretion and loss of cells by the tumor.

In epidemiologic studies, total dietary fat shows the strongest correlation with breast cancer incidence and mortality, whereas dietary PUFAs show little or no correlation (Carroll et al., 1986). This has been explained on the basis that human diets normally contain enough PUFAs to satisfy the threshold requirement for tumor promotion observed in animal studies. The positive correlations observed in epidemiologic studies are consistent

with the promotional effect of dietary fat observed in animal models (Carroll, 1986a). Therefore, mechanisms by which high-fat diets per se may promote carcinogenesis should be considered.

There is a strong positive correlation between caloric intake and level of dietary fat (Carroll and Khor, 1975), and it is well known that carcinogenesis can be inhibited in animals by caloric restriction (Beth et al., 1987; Cohen et al., 1988; Klurfeld et al., 1987; Kritchevsky, 1986; Reddy et al., 1987; Sylvester, 1986; Tannenbaum, 1959). It is therefore possible that promotion of tumorigenesis by high-fat diets is due to excess caloric intake, but this has not been demonstrated experimentally. The metabolism of animals on high-fat diets is substantially different from that of animals on low-fat diets (Clarke, 1986); some of these differences may favor carcinogenesis.

The mechanisms by which dietary fat affects mammary carcinogenesis are not necessarily the same as those by which it affects other sites. In colon cancer, excretion of secondary bile acids has been positively correlated with the promotion of colon cancer by different types of dietary fat (Reddy, 1986a,b). No specific mechanisms have yet been proposed for effects of dietary fat on pancreatic cancer (Birt and Roebuck, 1986).

Summary

Together, the epidemologic and animal data generally support an association between dietary fat and risk of several cancers. The data are most consistent for colorectal cancer and less so for prostate and breast cancer. Overall, the association with total fat is the strongest and most consistent. However, some evidence obtained in studies on humans suggests that high SFA intake is associated with an increased risk of and mortality from cancers of the colon, prostate, and breast. In animals, ω-6 PUFAs increase risk to the greatest extent, but high SFA intake also increases risk, provided that the minimum requirement for ω-6 PUFAs is satisfied. There is some evidence from animal experiments that diets with a high content of ω-3 PUFAs may decrease risk of cancers of the mammary gland, intestine, and pancreas. In some studies, MUFAs have been shown either to have no effect on cancer risk or to be protective. Dietary cholesterol is highly correlated with SFA intake in humans. There is no consistent evidence that low levels of serum cholesterol increase the risk of cancer in any site, including the colon and rectum.

Dietary Phospholipids

Phospholipids are major constituents of biologic membranes and as such are normal constituents of the diet. Phosphatidylcholine (PtdCho), also called lecithin, makes up approximately 40 to 70% of mammalian membrane phospholipids. It is also added to foods as an emulsifying agent. Lipid emulsions used for parenteral nutrition contain about 1% PtdCho. In the United States, the intake of PtdCho from natural sources is 3 to 6 g per day (Wurtman, 1979; Zeisel et al., 1980). Some people also take nutritional supplements containing PtdCho.

Two phospholipids, PtdCho and phosphatidyl-serine, are undergoing testing for their use as drugs for treatment or prophylaxis for various diseases. This section focuses mainly on PtdCho and on the nutritional aspects of dietary phospholipids.

Choline as an Essential Nutrient

Phospholipids and their constituents can be synthesized in the body and are thus not normally required in the diet. Choline, a constituent of PtdCho, may, however, be an essential dietary ingredient under certain circumstances (Zeisel, 1981).

Chronic ingestion of a diet deficient in choline has been associated with memory impairment and with hepatic, renal, and growth disorders. In the rat, hamster, pig, dog, chicken, and baboon, choline deficiency resulted in fatty infiltration of the liver (Zeisel, 1981), probably by disturbing the synthesis of PtdCho needed to secrete triglycerides as part of the lipoproteins. Renal function was also compromised. Infertility, growth impairment, bony abnormalities, decreased hematopoiesis, and hypertension have also been associated with consumption of diets low in choline (Zeisel, 1981). Deficiency of choline and methionine produces a high incidence of liver tumors in rats in the absence of any known carcinogen (Ghoshal and Farber, 1984; Mikol et al., 1983; Newberne and Rogers, 1986). A relatively short exposure to severe methyl group deficiency also enhanced development of carcinogen-induced liver tumors (Hoover et al., 1984). In mice, choline deficiency was associated with memory impairment (Bartus et al., 1980).

Decreased serum choline concentrations have been observed in humans fed by total parenteral nutrition with commercial solutions low in choline. Liver disease associated with parenteral nutrition may be related to choline deficiency

(Sheard et al., 1986). Marked depressions of plasma choline levels were noted among trained athletes running the Boston Marathon, and this might have affected performance (Conlay et al., 1986).

Despite this evidence of pathology associated with choline-deficient diets, it is not possible to state definitely that humans require dietary choline, because there is uncertainty about the extent to which methionine and other labile methyl donors can be substituted for choline. In rats, biosynthesis of PtdCho by methylation is decreased by dietary deficiencies of methionine and vitamin B_{12} (Akesson et al., 1978; Hoffman et al., 1980).

PtdCho and Other Choline-Containing Compounds in the Treatment of Human Diseases

Diseases of the Nervous System

Administration of choline or PtdCho can benefit patients with tardive dyskinesia (Gelenberg et al., 1979; Zeisel, 1981). This disorder is a side effect of virtually all antipsychotic drugs marketed in the United States and presumably results from an imbalance between dopaminergic and cholinergic neurotransmission.

Cholinergic neurons are essential for memory and other cognitive functions in rats and humans. An age-related diminution of memory in mice was exacerbated by a diet low in choline and was alleviated by a choline-rich diet (Bartus et al., 1980). Administration of choline reportedly improved memory in serial-learning and selective-reminding tasks among humans who were poor initial learners (Sitaram et al., 1978; Zeisel, 1981).

Supplemental choline (usually as PtdCho) has also been tested in the prophylaxis or treatment of memory disorders associated with Alzheimer's disease in which central cholinergic neurotransmission is known to be deficient (Zeisel, 1981). Preliminary nonblinded studies in Alzheimer's patients yielded positive findings, but most well-controlled, double-blind studies have failed to show clear-cut improvement (Corkin et al., 1982). In a single long-term, double-blind study, approximately 20 g of highly purified PtdCho or placebo given daily for 6 months led to a significant improvement in the oldest third of 50 patients (Little et al., 1985).

Supplemental choline has also been used to treat mania, which may reflect excessive activation of adrenergic receptors in the brain. When PtdCho was given to manic patients with lithium, the improvement in behavior was marked but temporary (Cohen et al., 1980).

PtdCho produced mild improvement in a few patients with Friedreich's ataxia, but no improvement in patients with another ataxic disorder, spinocerebellar degeneration (Barbeau, 1978). Administration of choline only occasionally resulted in reproducible improvement in other ataxic disorders (Lawrence et al., 1980). Some improvement was observed in one patient with the myasthenic syndrome (Kranz et al., 1980). Supplemental choline does not appear to be beneficial in myasthenia gravis, but this difference has not been explored extensively.

The Cardiovascular System

Choline increases release of acetylcholine by the heart in vitro (Loffelholz et al., 1979) but has not been found to affect cardiac function in healthy humans. Rats exposed to transient periods of choline deficiency develop irreversible hypertension (Kratzing and Perry, 1971; Michael et al., 1975). This may be related to renal as well as cardiovascular function.

Lipid Transport

In a study on rabbits fed an atherogenic diet, soya lecithin (1 or 5 g daily) was found to decrease serum cholesterol and atherosclerosis (Kesten and Silbowitz, 1942). Other investigators reported reductions in serum cholesterol in hypercholesterolemic patients treated with soya lecithin (Morrison, 1958; Steiner and Domanski, 1944), but subsequent studies had less encouraging results (Cobb et al., 1980; Davies and Murdoch, 1959; ter Welle et al., 1974). Childs et al. (1981) observed small but significant reductions in LDL-C and an increase in HDL-C in normolipidemic and familial hypercholesterolemic subjects given 36 g of an oral soya lecithin daily. Since soy lecithin preparations used for such studies generally contained less than 30% PtdCho, observed effects could have been due to other components.

High-PUFA PtdCho has been given in some studies. Svanberg et al. (1974) reported a decrease in serum triglycerides and VLDL-C and an increase in HDL-C in hypertriglyceridemic subjects treated with lecithin high in linoleate. Greten et al. (1980) observed no change in serum lipid or lipoprotein concentrations in patients with familial hypercholesterolemia or normal controls treated with lecithin with high linoleate content, but fecal stool excretion was increased. PtdCho

has been found to interfere with intestinal absorption of cholesterol both in humans and in laboratory animals (Beil and Grudy, 1980; Rampone and Machida, 1981). In some of these studies, care was taken to distinguish between effects of PtdCho and its constituent PUFAs. Disaturated PtdChos adsorb to surfaces more readily than those with unsaturated fatty acids. Elevated levels of disaturated PtdChos have been observed in some patients with atherosclerotic heart disease and may constitute a risk factor (Gershfeld, 1979).

Inositol and Phosphoinositides

Although phosphoinositides are minor components of the lipids of cellular membranes, they have recently attracted much attention as precursors of second messenger molecules (Majerus et al., 1986). In this capacity, they can exert profound effects on cellular function and metabolism.

Like most other phospholipids, phosphoinositides and their component parts can normally be synthesized in adequate amounts in the body. There are reports, however, of deficiency symptoms associated with inositol-deficient diets in animals (Holub, 1982, 1986). Liver triglycerides accumulate in inositol-deficient animals, possibly because of inadequate release of lipoproteins (Hoover et al., 1978) or increased mobilization of fatty acids from adipose depots to the liver due to activation of hormone-sensitive lipase in adipose tissue (Hayashi et al., 1978). Further research on the role of inositol in cardiovascular disease may therefore be warranted.

Gallbladder Disease

Pathophysiology of Gallbladder Disease

Gallstones are the major cause of gallbladder disease in the United States, affecting approximately 10% of the adult population. Cholecystectomy for gallstones is one of the most common surgical procedures. Gallstones are composed primarily of cholesterol and bilirubin. The pathogenesis of cholesterol gallstones has been reviewed by Admirand and Small (1968), Bennion and Grundy (1978a,b), Carey and Small (1978), Grundy (1979), Schoenfield (1980), and Small (1976).

Cholesterol, bile acids, and phospholipids are secreted by the liver in varying proportions. Cholesterol is solubilized in bile by the detergent properties of the bile salts and phospholipids. When cholesterol exceeds a certain level relative to the concentrations of other lipids, the bile becomes supersaturated, increasing the probability that cholesterol crystals will precipitate and begin to form stones. Thus, supersaturated bile predisposes to cholesterol gallstones, and conditions that increase the proportion of cholesterol in bile relative to that of bile salts are considered to be possible etiologic factors. Gallstones are frequently asymptomatic, but they predispose to cholecystitis and obstruction of the biliary duct—complications requiring surgical intervention.

Epidemiology of Gallstones

As with most chronic diseases, the wide geographic and ethnic variations in the frequency of cholesterol and pigment gallstones (Brett and Barker, 1976; reviewed by Heaton, 1973; Yamase and McNamara, 1972) suggest that both environmental and genetic factors are involved in their causation. Cholesterol gallstones are much more common among American Indians (Comess et al., 1967; Sampliner et al., 1970) and Hispanics (Arevalo et al., 1987; Weiss et al., 1984) than among black or white Americans. They are the predominant type of gallstones in North and South America and in Europe, but are rare in the Orient (Sutor and Wooley, 1971; Trotman and Soloway, 1975). Pigment gallstones are most frequent in the Orient, but cholesterol stones are becoming more frequent in Japan (Nagase et al., 1978).

Within the U.S. white population, the major conditions associated with a greater probability of developing cholesterol gallstones are obesity, female sex, number of pregnancies, and age (Friedman et al., 1966). Despite widespread suspicion in the medical community and the general population that diet contributes to cholesterol gallstone formation, no convincing epidemiologic evidence except for that pertaining to obesity supports this concept (see review by Low-Beer, 1985).

Clinical and Metabolic Studies

The major body of evidence linking dietary fats and sterols to cholesterol gallstones and thereby to chronic gallbladder disease derives from many observational and experimental studies of humans indicating that dietary cholesterol and PUFAs may increase the cholesterol saturation of bile, thereby increasing the probability of stone formation.

Dietary Cholesterol

Case-control studies have shown no association between cholelithiasis and consumption of eggs (Sarles et al., 1969) or cholesterol (Scragg et al.,

1984). In a cohort study, cholesterol intake did not predict the occurrence of cholelithiasis (Friedman et al., 1966). The lithogenicity of bile (bile saturation index) was increased modestly by large intakes of cholesterol as egg yolk in one experiment (DenBesten et al., 1973) and was increased substantially in another experiment (D.W. Lee et al., 1985), especially in patients who already had gallstones. However, dietary cholesterol did not increase the bile saturation index in three other experiments (Andersen and Hellstrom, 1979; Dam et al., 1971; Sarles et al., 1970). Thus, despite the obvious logic relating cholesterol intake to cholesterol gallstones, little evidence from studies in humans supports the relationship. The variability in results from different experiments, each involving small numbers of subjects, suggests that a few persons may be sensitive to the lithogenic effects of dietary cholesterol but that most persons are not.

Polyunsaturated Fats

A number of experiments in humans between 1958 and 1967 showed no effect of dietary PUFAs on the lithogenicity of bile (Dam et al., 1967; Hellstrom and Lindstedt, 1966; Lewis, 1958; Lindstedt et al., 1965; Sodhi et al., 1967; Watanabe et al., 1962). In 1973, attention was redirected to this issue by an observation from a dietary trial to prevent coronary heart disease. The prevalence of cholelithiasis (as detected at autopsy) was about twice as high in men who had consumed a low-cholesterol, high-PUFA diet as in men who had consumed a high-cholesterol, high-SFA diet (Sturdevant et al., 1973). However, no difference related to PUFAs was observed in another, similar dietary trial (Miettinen et al., 1976).

Grundy (1975) identified 4 of 11 patients with hypertriglyceridemia in whom bile cholesterol saturation was increased by PUFA feeding. However, this difference could not be distinguished from random or individual variability, and it could not be extrapolated to the general population because the subjects were highly selected. More recently, Kohlmeier et al. (1985) found extreme variability in the response of bile cholesterol saturation to a high-PUFA, low-cholesterol diet fed to 12 women, 2 of whom developed much higher cholesterol saturation indices, while the rest experienced no significant change.

In summary, the evidence suggests that a few people may be susceptible to the lithogenic effects of PUFAs when the cholesterol saturation index of bile is increased, but that most humans do not seem to be susceptible. It would be important to identify such subjects if they exist.

Caloric Intake

Numerous epidemiologic studies have shown that gallstones are more frequent among obese persons than among persons of appropriate weight for height (for example, Friedman et al., 1966; Scragg et al., 1984). Obese people have higher bile saturation indices than do nonobese persons, and the condition is reversible (Bennion and Grundy, 1975). This is caused by increased hepatic secretion of cholesterol into the bile (Leijd, 1980) (see also Chapter 21, Obesity and Digestive Diseases). A high-calorie diet also increases the bile cholesterol saturation index (Sarles et al., 1971; Scragg et al., 1984).

Obesity is at least one factor involved in the predisposition of Pima Indians to gallstones (Howard, 1986). Thus, it is well established that obesity possibly resulting from high caloric intake is associated with increased risk of cholelithiasis through greater secretion of cholesterol by the liver and higher bile cholesterol saturation.

Other Factors in Cholelithiasis

Recent research indicates that the lithogenicity of bile may be much more complex than the interrelationships among cholesterol, bile salts, and phospholipids (reviewed by Somjen and Gilat, 1986). Vesicles composed mainly of phospholipids and cholesterol have been observed in the bile of humans, and some proteins may be involved in the processes that influence stone formation. Thus, the cholesterol saturation index, which does not take into account other carriers and other mechanisms stabilizing cholesterol in bile, may be limited in its ability to detect the conditions that favor the formation of gallstones. There is no information concerning the effects of dietary cholesterol, fat, or other nutrients on these newly identified properties of bile that are likely to influence gallstone formation. Such information should lead to new insights into the genetic–environmetal interactions involved in cholelithiasis.

Animal Studies

Early Observations

Scattered reports between 1912 and 1950 describe gallstones induced in rabbits by feeding them excess cholesterol, but the results were inconsistent and many cholesterol-fed rabbits did not develop gallstones (reviewed by Freston and Bouchier, 1968). Interest in animal models was stimulated by the discovery of diet-induced gallstones in hamsters in 1952. Subsequently, cholesterol gallstones were observed in mice, prairie dogs, and several species of monkeys. These animal models appear to involve different mechanisms. Dam (1971), Freston and Bouchier (1968), Gurll and DenBesten (1978), and Holzbach (1984) reviewed animal models of gallstones.

Hamster

While examining the relationship of nutrition to muscular dystrophy in hamsters, Dam and Christensen (1952) found that a high-carbohydrate, low-fat diet produced gallstones. These investigators carried out a number of experiments (reviewed by Dam, 1971) concerned with the etiology and pathogenesis of this phenomenon. It was eventually determined that the nutritional factor was an essential fatty acid deficiency that did not alter the secretion of bile salts but did increase biliary cholesterol secretion severalfold (Robins and Fasulo, 1973). The enhanced biliary cholesterol secretion was not accompanied by increased tissue cholesterol levels. The addition of cholesterol to the diet yielded varying results, but most investigators have found that increased lithogenicity of bile was associated with dietary cholesterol, e.g., as reported by Singhal et al. (1983). The hamster, which appears to be genetically more susceptible than other rodents to the lithogenic effects of dietary cholesterol (Ho, 1976), continues to be the subject of studies to investigate the pathogenesis and prevention of lithogenic bile and gallstones, but this animal model is of little help in identifying nutritional factors contributing to gallstones in humans.

Prairie Dog

A high-cholesterol (1.2% by weight, derived from egg yolk), high-fat (41% of calories from egg yolk) diet for 6 months invariably produced cholesterol gallstones in prairie dogs (Cynomys ludovicianus) (Brenneman et al., 1972). The bile became lithogenic primarily through the increased secretion of cholesterol. The mechanism was interpreted as a massive overloading of the hepatic system for metabolism of cholesterol, apparently because the prairie dog absorbed cholesterol efficiently from the intestine. The overload occurred quite rapidly after beginning the diet, since bile cholesterol was increased within 36 hours, cholesterol crystals were found in the gallbladder within 5 days, and most animals had gallstones within 14 days (DenBesteen et al., 1974). A semisynthetic diet with cholesterol was even more effective in inducing gallstones (B.I. Cohen et al., 1986). Susceptibility was not due to lack of responsiveness of 7α-hydroxylase in the liver (Howell et al., 1983). Thus, this animal model also may be useful in studying the pathogenesis of gallstones.

Ground Squirrel

MacPherson et al. (1987) produced cholesterol gallstones rapidly in ground squirrels (*Spermphilus richardsonii*) by giving them a cholesterol-enriched (2%) rat chow diet. The features of this model appear to be similar to those of the cholesterol-fed prairie dog.

Mouse

Tepperman et al. (1964) produced cholesterol gallstones in mice by feeding them a diet containing 1% cholesterol, 0.5% cholic acid, and 31% lard. There has been no subsequent exploration of this phenomenon in inbred strains of mice.

Nonhuman Primates

Osuga and Portman (1971, 1972) and Osuga et al. (1974) produced lithogenic bile and cholesterol gallstones in squirrel monkeys (*Saimiri sciureus*) with a diet containing 0.9 mg of cholesterol per kcal and 45% of total calories from butter. They concluded that dietary cholesterol was the major factor in the production of these effects (Osuga et al., 1976). Armstrong et al. (1982) found that dietary cholesterol increased the cholesterol bile saturation index of squirrel monkeys, whereas dietary fat saturation (corn vs. coconut oil) had no independent effect. The effect of cholesterol was greater when it was fed with PUFAs (Melchior et al., 1978; Tanaka et al., 1976). African green monkeys (*Cercopithecus aethiops*) also developed a more lithogenic bile when fed cholesterol with PUFAs (St. Clair et al., 1980). In contrast, the bile of *Cebus* monkeys, which do not develop gallstones from dietary cholesterol, was much less influenced by diet.

Baboons (*Papio* sp.) occasionally develop cholesterol gallstones spontaneously (Glenn and Mc-Sherry, 1970), and their bile is frequently supersaturated with cholesterol (McSherry et al., 1971a). The bile of these animals has a cyclic variation that reflects the enterohepatic circulation of bile salts (McSherry et al., 1971b).

Summary

The animal models of cholelithiasis present a mixed picture. Several species of rodents (but not the rat) are susceptible to the lithogenic effects of dietary cholesterol, but they require large doses of cholesterol and are accompanied by high levels of serum cholesterol. The common denominator of these rodent models is enhanced secretion of cholesterol into the bile, as in humans with cholelithiasis, but the underlying genetically determined metabolic characteristic that makes them susceptible to dietary cholesterol is not known. Among nonhuman primates, the squirrel monkey is similar to humans in its sensitivity to dietary cholesterol. The baboon appears to simulate more closely the human pathophysiology. The extreme susceptibility of some species to dietary cholesterol does not seem to have any parallel in humans with cholelithiasis.

Summary

Cholesterol gallstones are the major cause of chronic gallbladder disease in the United States and are responsible for substantial morbidity (see Chapter 5). Excessive secretion of cholesterol into the bile relative to the secretion of bile salts and phospholipids is the common denominator in both human and test animals with cholelithiasis. The only nutritional factor clearly identified in humans is obesity possibly due to excessive caloric intake. The major nutritional factor identified from animal models is dietary cholesterol, although other conditions, such as essential fatty acid deficiency, also may produce gallstones. Remarkably few intensive epidemiologic studies have been undertaken to determine whether dietary fats and sterols are causative agents in cholelithiasis. And despite the evidence from studies in animals, no conclusive statements about their role in the development of cholelithiasis in humans can be made. It seems likely that, as with hyperlipidemia and atherosclerosis, lithogenic bile and cholelithiasis result from an interaction between dietary factors (such as dietary fats and sterols) and unidentified, genetically programmed metabolic characteristics. Research to identify both dietary and metabolic factors responsible for cholelithiasis, following the pattern of investigation used in hyperlipidemia and atherosclerosis, might lead to dietary recommendations to prevent cholelithiasis and chronic gallbladder disease in susceptible persons.

Dietary Fat and Obesity

Epidemiologic Studies

As noted in Chapter 6, epidemiologic studies indicate that average caloric intake has been decreasing while mean body weight and body mass index have increased. There is no epidemiologic evidence indicating that total fat intake per se, independent of total caloric intake, is associated with increased adiposity in the overall population. Although some diseases commonly associated with obesity (e.g., cardiovascular disease and some cancers) are associated either with an increase in type of fat in the diet or with the percentage of fat in the diet (see earlier sections in this chapter), no clear association of either *percentage* or *type* of fat (independent of total caloric intake) has been associated with human obesity in epidemiologic studies. Thus, although the type or amount of dietary fat may be associated with diseases common in obese individuals, obesity itself has not been found to be associated with dietary fat in either between- or within-population studies.

Clinical Studies

Most knowledge of the effect of dietary fat on obesity in humans comes from studies in which diets differing in percent or type of fat have been fed to individuals for short periods. This was most frequently done through isocaloric substitution of fat for carbohydrate in isonitrogenous diets. In the typical study design, weight gain on a high-fat diet can be compared to gains on a low-fat or high-carbohydrate diet. Thus, the evidence does not permit an effective analysis of changes in weight or adiposity over a *range* of dietary fat intakes. In some studies, weight gain on a high-fat diet, or weight loss on a low-fat diet, have been been observed (e.g., Duncan et al., 1983). However, when dietary fat was replaced with sucrose polyester (Glueck et al., 1982) or carbohydrate (Porikos et al., 1977), the subjects compensated partially or completely for the calories deleted from the diet as fat.

In one study (Lissner et al., 1987), caloric compensation was studied in 24 women who consumed in sequence three 2-week diets with low (15–20%), medium (30–35%), and high (40–45%) fat contents, similar in appearance and apparent palatability. Subjects on the low-fat diet spontaneously consumed 11.3% fewer calories, and those on the high-fat diet consumed 15.4% more calories than did those on the medium-fat diet. Thus these diets, differing in fat content and consumed spontaneously, resulted in significant short-term changes in body weight due to changes in caloric intake.

Some data suggest that obese people and formerly obese people prefer high-fat stimuli

(Drewnowski et al., 1985) and may overconsume high-fat foods (Gates et al., 1975). A few studies suggest that a high SFA intake may be associated with obesity. For example, Berry et al. (1986) reported a positive association between body mass index and SFAs as a marker of animal fat intake. In addition, an analysis of the Nurses' Health Study (Romieu et al., 1988) suggests that obese women report higher intakes of both total fat and SFAs. Some people spontaneously reduce total caloric consumption when regularly given a low-fat diet; others spontaneously increase caloric intake when a high-fat diet is easily available.

Hence, the short-term clinical studies suggest that low-fat diets may be beneficial to obese people or those at risk for obesity. Nonetheless, it is difficult to implicate excess dietary fat ingestion per se (independent of total caloric intake) as a mechanism for the cause of obesity and the development of obesity. It is more likely that a combination of increased total caloric intake and decreased physical activity are the variables directly associated with the onset of human obesity.

Animal Studies

Studies in animals have provided evidence that both the type and the amount of dietary fat are significant in the production of obesity in rodents and other animal species. Several spontaneously obese rodent models show preferences for dietary fat at least under some experimental conditions (Maggio et al., 1983). When rats are allowed to spontaneously select macronutrient diets, they will consume approximately 30% of their calories as fat (Kanarek et al., 1981) and sometimes higher percentages during weight cycling (i.e., repeated episodes of weight loss and regain) (Reed, 1988). When medium-chain triglycerides are substituted isocalorically for long-chain triglycerides, both obese and lean rats gain less weight (Turkenkopf, 1982).

Some effects of high-fat intake have been attributed to the fact that the energy cost of converting dietary fat to stored triglycerides is lower than the cost of converting dietary carbohydrates to stored triglyceride (Donato and Hegsted, 1985). Furthermore, early exposure to a high-fat diet may predispose to future weight gain on high-fat diets (Peckham et al., 1962).

There is considerable genetic heterogeneity in animal populations, even among inbred strains of normally lean rats. Some rats, normally lean when fed standard chow, will gain body fat and develop hyperphagia when fed isonitrogenous diets containing increasingly higher percentages of fat (Schemmel et al., 1982).

Responses to high-fat diets are different between the sexes. Female rats spontaneously overingest high-fat diets compared to male rats and become fatter than males when fed isocaloric high-fat and high-carbohydrate diets (Hoyenga and Hoyenga, 1982; Sclafani and Gorman, 1977).

Summary

Animal data suggest that dietary fat, independent of total caloric intake, may contribute to obesity, possibly through more efficient metabolism of this nutrient relative to other nutrients. This effect is particularly prominent in female rats of some inbred strains (e.g., Wistar and Sprague Dawley rats) and certain genetic backgrounds (e.g., Osborne-Mendel). Unfortunately, there are no equivalent data on humans. Short-term studies in humans, primarily clinical studies, indicate that reduced fat content may be accompanied by weight loss. Reductions in caloric intake were noted in some of these reports and although not always specifically noted, may have occurred in others. This in itself is significant and may indicate that substantial reductions in the percentages of fat in the diet of humans may result in beneficial total caloric reductions as well, perhaps because diets with reduced dietary fat are generally regarded as less palatable. From a public health perspective, this phenomenon may be important, regardless of whether obesity is decreased by reduced percentages of dietary fat per se or is secondary only to concomitant reductions in caloric intake.

EFFECTS OF DIETARY FATS AND OTHER LIPIDS ON HEALTH AND DISEASE IN CHILDREN

Cardiovascular Diseases

The Origin of Atherosclerosis in Childhood

Childhood Atherosclerotic Lesions

Atherosclerosis and its clinical sequelae are found primarily in adults. In rare cases (about 1 in a million), however, children with homozygous familial hypercholesterolemia develop severe atherosclerosis and clinical CHD. Holman—a pioneer in the exploration of atherosclerosis in childhood (Holman et al., 1958)—in 1959 presented a paper posing the question, "Atherosclerosis—a pediatric nutrition problem?" at the Ninth International Congress of Pediatrics (Holman, 1961). At that time, the question could not be answered with certainty, because there was no evidence supporting the relationship in children between diet and subsequent atherosclerosis, in contrast to the considerable amount of data supporting such an association in adults. Abnormal lipid deposits (fatty streaks), believed by many to be the precursors of raised atherosclerotic lesions, were found in the aortas of all children by 3 years of age in all populations around the world, regardless of dietary fat and cholesterol intake (Strong et al., 1958; Tejada et al., 1968). Furthermore, these simple lipid deposits had not been firmly linked to the fibrous plaques that lead directly to arterial occlusion (see Chapter 19).

Progression of Fatty Streaks to Fibrous Plaques

Long before there was any concern about hyperlipidemia or atherosclerosis in children, Enos et al. (1953) described advanced coronary artery lesions in young American adults in a landmark study of Korean battlefield casualties. In this study, 77% of men averaging 22 years of age had grossly detectable coronary artery lesions, and 15% had coronary artery lesions that obstructed the lumen by 50% or more. This remarkable prevalence of coronary atherosclerosis in young men was confirmed in other studies of young people who died from accidental causes in the United States (Strong and McGill, 1962).

Subsequent intensive examination of large numbers of children and young adults showed that a continuous progression of lesions could be traced from fatty streaks to fibrous plaques (Geer et al., 1968; McGill, 1984; Robertson et al., 1963; Stary, 1987a,b; Strong and McGill, 1969; reviewed by McGill et al., 1963, 1980). These observations and many more left little doubt that many fatty streaks in the coronary arteries and some fatty streaks in the aortas of children are converted to fibrous plaques in adolescents and young adults.

Effects of Dietary Fats and Cholesterol in Infants

Immediate Effects

Preweaning (suckling) infants are quite sensitive to the plasma cholesterol-raising (or lowering) effects of dietary fat and cholesterol. Approximately 50% of the calories in human breast milk is supplied by fat, half of which is SFA (Lo, 1985; reviewed by Jensen et al., 1978). Its cholesterol content averages 11 mg/dl (range, 3 to 29 mg/dl)

(Picciano et al., 1978; reviewed by Jensen et al., 1978). In comparison to human milk, cow's milk has more SFA (65.6 versus 48.2% of total fatty acids), less MUFA (30.3 versus 39.8%), and much less PUFA (4.1 versus 12.0%) (Lo, 1985). In contrast, commercially prepared infant formulas are made with soy, corn, safflower, and coconut oils. Although these formulas provide the same proportion of calories as fat as does breast milk, they contain a higher proportion of PUFAs (up to 50% as linoleic acid) and virtually no cholesterol (Benson, 1981; Jensen et al., 1978). In several studies, as might be anticipated from their higher intake of cholesterol and SFAs, breast-fed infants had higher serum cholesterol concentrations than did formula-fed infants (Carlson et al., 1982; Pomeranze, 1961; reviewed by Wissler and McGill, 1983).

In a study of the nutrient composition of diets given to infants over the age of 6 months, Montaldo and coworkers (1985) compared solid food diets supplemented with whole milk from cows or with formula. Using data from NHANES II, they found that infants fed the cow's milk received less iron and linoleic acid. Manipulation of the fat and cholesterol content of infant formulas showed the anticipated effects (Sweeney et al., 1961). Similar observations have been made in animals, particularly nonhuman primates, whose breast milk is similar in composition to that of humans (Mott et al., 1978). The effect of plasma cholesterol concentrations in the suckling child on the subsequent development of atherosclerosis is totally unknown. It has generally been believed not to be significant because of the limited duration of exposure and the overriding importance of other nutritional considerations during the first year of life.

Deferred Effects

In 1972, Reiser proposed that a high cholesterol intake before weaning, such as that provided by breast milk, would induce a higher level of tolerance for dietary cholesterol in adulthood and presented results from studies in swine and rats to support this hypothesis (Reiser and Sidelman, 1972; Reiser et al., 1979). Tests of this hypothesis in other animal species, including nonhuman primates, have generally been negative (Mott et al., 1982; reviewed by Innis, 1985). However, Mott et al. (1982) found that breast-fed infant baboons had lower plasma HDL-C and apo AI concentrations when they reached adolescence than did formula-fed baboons, regardless of the cholesterol content of the formula. In another experiment,

Lewis et al. (1988) also found that breast-fed baboon infants reared on an atherogenic diet had lower HDL-C levels and more extensive atherosclerosis at age 5 than baboons fed a formula as infants and reared on an identical diet. No similar effects have been detected in humans.

Summary

Plasma lipid and lipoprotein concentrations in infants and children under 2 years of age are quite sensitive to dietary fat and cholesterol, but there is no evidence that elevated plasma lipoproteins in this age group are factors in the etiology of atherosclerosis. Other nutritional considerations are more important during this period. Results from experiments in animals indicate that breast feeding, as compared to formula feeding, exerts a long-term deferred effect on lipoprotein metabolism that continues into adulthood, but no such effect has yet been detected in humans. Therefore, the remaining concerns regarding dietary fat and cholesterol during childhood are focused on children over the age of 2 years.

Relationship of Childhood Lesions to Plasma Lipids and Lipoproteins

It has been difficult to obtain information relating the arterial lesions observed in children and young adults to plasma lipid and lipoprotein levels. Many early observations seemed to indicate that there was no relationship when population means were compared (McGill, 1968; Tejada et al., 1968).

Fatty streaks were found to be ubiquitous among children throughout the world. Little or no excess was observed in populations such as that of the United States where TC levels were high. Indeed, aortic fatty streaks were equally prevalent in poorly nourished children in post-World War I Europe (Zinserling, 1925). Holman et al. (1959) observed that children dying from cystic fibrosis had difficulty in absorbing fat, had very low TC concentrations, and had one-fourth the fatty streaks as did the children without the disease.

An unusual opportunity to study the relationship of childhood lesions to plasma lipid or lipoprotein concentrations was provided by examinations of the arteries of young accidental death victims (average age, 18 years) whose plasma lipids and lipoproteins had been measured in the Bogalusa Heart Study (Berenson, 1980). In this study, both aortic and coronary fatty streaks were correlated strongly with antemortem LDL-C levels (Newman et al., 1986). The relationship continued to be strong, even when the confounding effect of race was taken into account in a larger number of cases (Freedman et al., 1988). These findings from a small number of cases are the only observations that relate atherosclerotic lesions directly to plasma lipid or lipoprotein concentrations in children.

Plasma Lipids and Lipoproteins in Children

Age and Sex Distributions

Until about 1970, descriptive studies of the distribution of serum cholesterol and lipoprotein cholesterol concentrations focused on adults. In the early 1970s, several research groups began to survey these variables in U.S. children (Berenson et al., 1979; Frerichs et al., 1976, 1978a,b; Friedman and Goldberg, 1973; Lauer et al., 1975; Morrison et al., 1979a,b; NHLBI, 1978; Wilmore and McNamara, 1974). Results of these studies indicate that TC concentrations at birth were approximately 70 mg/dl (half of it as HDL-C) and rose rapidly to approximately double that value at 1 year and increased slowly thereafter to about 160 mg/dl (roughly two-thirds LDL-C and one-third HDL-C) at 10 years of age. Between 12 and 18 years of age, TC in boys declined slightly to about 150 mg/dl. The 10 mg/dl decrease was accounted for primarily by HDL-C and was associated with an increase in plasma testosterone levels (Kirkland et al., 1987). Serum TC concentrations and lipoprotein cholesterol distributions in girls remained at about the same level. At any age, the frequency distribution of TC levels was skewed to the high end similar to that of the adult population. In the 10- to 14-year age group, the fifth percentile levels were approximately 120 mg/dl, and the 95th percentile levels were about 200 mg/dl (Lipid Research Clinics Population Studies Data Book, 1980).

Dietary Intakes by Children

In the Bogalusa Heart Study, which periodically screens a pediatric population of approximately 5,000 children from a semirural community, Berenson et al. (1988) found that the schoolchildren's daily diet contained an average of 38% fat and 300 mg of cholesterol; the P:S ratio was 0.4. These data are similar to the findings of the National Health Survey (Carroll et al., 1983).

Emmons (1986) studied the nutritional adequacy of diets consumed by low-income people participating in the Special Supplemental Food Program for Women, Infants, and Children (WIC Program) and found that both white and black children consumed approximately 35% of their calories as fat. However, black children consumed more animal fat than vegetable fat and thus had a diet with a lower P:S ratio than that of white children. On average, therefore, it appears that children in the United States, especially those in lower socioeconomic groups, consume diets that tend to increase their LDL-C.

The H.J. Heinz Company of Canada conducted a longitudinal survey of the eating habits of infants and children (Leung et al., 1984). The food intake of more than 400 4-year-old children was obtained from data collected from a 4-day dietary record. This study documented that preschool Canadian children obtained 34% of their calories as fat. Their snacks, unlike typical processed food snacks in the United States, had the lowest caloric density of any of the meals, suggesting that they were composed mainly of carbohydrates. These Canadian data contrast strongly with the diet of U.S. children (Carroll et al., 1983).

The Lipid Research Clinics Program Prevalence Study presented the dietary data for white American males and females between the ages of 6 and 25 years. Enrolled within that study were more than 1,100 schoolchildren. The percentage of calories as fat was 39% for the boys and 38% for the girls. The P:S ratio was 0.4 for both sexes (Beaglehole et al., 1980).

Ecological and Familial Associations

Serum cholesterol levels in U.S. children were considerably higher than those in children of other regional groups or countries where CHD was much less frequent (Knuiman et al., 1980; Savage et al., 1976; Sullivan et al., 1987). The families of children with high TC levels had a greater incidence of deaths from CHD than did the families of children with low TC levels (Schrott et al., 1979). Families of children with low HDL-C levels also had an excess of deaths from CHD (Bodurtha et al., 1987). Conversely, approximately one-third of the children selected because their parents had precocious CHD had serum TC or triglyceride levels in the upper percentiles for their age (Chase et al., 1974; Glueck et al., 1974; Tamir et al., 1972).

Tracking

Of importance in studies of childhood serum lipid levels is tracking, that is, whether children maintain similar levels (relative to one another) of serum total and lipoprotein cholesterol as they grow. Tracking is important in determining whether a child in a high percentile of serum cholesterol concentration would remain in the same high percentile several years later when he or she entered adulthood and therefore would be at high risk of CHD. Most studies have demonstrated that serum TC concentrations track to a moderate degree during childhood (Clarke et al., 1978; Frerichs et al., 1979; Laskarzewski et al., 1979; Webber et al., 1983, 1986) and from childhood into young adulthood (Orchard et al., 1983). For example, in the study by Orchard and colleagues, 49% of children with a TC level in the top quintile at 12 years of age were in the top quintile when 21 years old, and the correlation coefficient between the 12- and 21-year values was .52. Children who were obese had both higher TC and blood pressure and increased left ventricular mass (Frerichs et al., 1978a; Schieken et al., 1981).

Walter and Hofman (1987) studied the differences in the distribution of risk factors in children stratified by race and socioeconomic status in the "Know Your Body" program. They found that white children in the lower socioeconomic strata had the highest level of risk as defined by blood pressure, physical conditioning, and serum lipoprotein levels. These children also reportedly consumed the most atherogenic diets of the groups in the study. Thus, the evidence indicates that children with high TC values will be likely to become adults with high serum cholesterol values.

Effects of Diet on Serum Lipids and Lipoproteins in Children

Observational Studies

Observational cross-sectional studies of diet and serum lipids in children have yielded results similar to those obtained from adults—correlations that are either zero or weak (Frank et al., 1978; McGandy, 1971; Morrison et al., 1980; Rasanen et al., 1978; Vartiainen et al., 1982). For example, Frank et al. (1978) studied 185 10-year-old children and found a positive but statistically insignificant association of TC concentration with total fat and SFA intake and no association with dietary cholesterol. Some statistically significant correlations emerged from other surveys, but they were low in magnitude (Frank et al., 1986).

Experimental Results

Like studies in adults, early experiments on the effects of dietary cholesterol on serum TC levels in children were negative (Heymann and Rack, 1943). In later studies, positive results were obtained. In one study conducted in a boys' boarding school, meals were modified to reduce total fat intake from 38 to 33% of calories, SFAs from 16 to 10% of calories, and cholesterol from 720 mg/day to 380 mg/day; PUFA intake was increased from 3 to 13% of calories (Ford et al., 1972; McGandy et al., 1972). The average TC concentration of the 63 13- to 18-year-old boys fell from approximately 190 mg/dl, equivalent to that of other age-matched boys in similar schools (McGandy et al., 1972), to about 170 mg/dl—a reduction of 15%. The boys with the highest TC levels experienced the greatest decreases. Several other dietary interventions in children subsequently showed a similar responsiveness of TC concentrations to reductions in dietary SFAs and cholesterol (Nestel et al., 1979; Puska et al., 1985; Stein et al., 1982; Vartiainen et al., 1986). Thus, adolescent children are as responsive to dietary fat modification as are adults.

Safety of Fat-Modified Diets for Children

When it was first recommended in 1970 that the diets of children as well as those of adults be reduced in fat and cholesterol content, the question of safety was immediately raised. This concern stemmed from the natural conservatism of physicians combined with the great improvements in growth and health of children in the United States associated with the conventional diets they consumed. Many major childhood infectious diseases and conditions related to nutritional deficiency, e.g., rheumatic fever, tuberculosis, rickets, scurvy, and others, had virtually disappeared, and their disappearance was attributed in large part to improved nutrition. Therefore, physicians were reluctant to tamper with success.

Cholesterol as an Essential Nutrient

Since cholesterol is an essential component of mammalian tissues, and since it is a precursor of steroid hormones, dietary cholesterol has been hypothesized to be necessary for optimum growth and development, particularly of the central nervous system. However, there is no experimental or observational evidence to support the concept that cholesterol is an essential nutrient.

The well-known capacity of mammalian cells to synthesize cholesterol suggests that dietary cholesterol is not required for normal growth. However, there have been no experiments testing the effects of cholesterol deprivation on children or on growing animals, probably because the hypothesis is considered to be very unlikely. As in other situations, proving the lack of a requirement is more difficult than proving that a requirement exists.

Total Fat Requirements of Children

Evidence indicates that there is no need for a fat intake of more than 10% of calories, provided the diet contains an adequate amount of essential fatty acids. The requirement for essential fatty acids in infants is met if they ingest 3% of their total calories as linoleic acid. This requirement drops to between 1 and 2% of total calories as linoleic acid in adults (NRC, 1980)—an amount well below the usually recommended 30% of calories from fat or even the 20% of calories from fat sometimes recommended. Energy requirements can readily be met by an increased intake of carbohydrate.

Observational Studies

Friedman and Goldberg (1976) found no differences associated with a low-fat, low-cholesterol diet for a number of developmental and biochemical variables of children. Dwyer (1980) discussed the preparation of diets for children that would fulfill the recommendations for lowering fat and cholesterol intake, but would also meet the Recommended Dietary Allowances for other nutrients. If care is not taken, she pointed out, deficiencies in the intakes of some vitamins and minerals might result. These and other aspects of safety have been reviewed by Kwiterovich (1980, 1986) and by Voller and Strong (1981). It is clear that caloric intake needs to be monitored to ensure its adequacy, if fat intake is decreased, in order to maintain optimal growth and development.

Recommendations of Other Expert Groups Regarding Dietary Modifications for Children

The American Heart Association recommended in 1983 that all children over 2 years of age should reduce total fat intake to no more than 30% of calories, 10% or less being provided by SFAs and not more than 10% by PUFAs, and should reduce cholesterol intake to 100 mg/1,000 kcal (Weidman et al., 1983). That report did not discuss safety concerns, which had been the basis for earlier reluctance to extend to children recommendations made for adults. About the same time, the Committee on Nutrition of the American Academy of Pediatrics stated, "Current dietary trends in the United States toward a reduced consumption of saturated fats, cholesterol, and salt and an in-

creased intake of polyunsaturated fats should be followed with caution. Diets that avoid extremes are safe for children" (AAP, 1983). However, the committee did not recommend specific targets.

The recommendations of these two committees are rather similar. Dietary fat and cholesterol intakes of children have declined along with those of adults, and continued reductions would bring actual intakes very close to those recommended by the American Heart Association. Thus, the only real difference between the two recommendations is the absence of quantitative targets in the statement issued by the American Academy of Pediatrics.

The most recent recommendation regarding fat-modified diets for children was made by the National Institutes of Health Consensus Conference on Cholesterol (NIH, 1985). This recommendation corresponds closely to that of the American Heart Association for children over 2 years of age. Subsequent published comments have both supported and opposed these recommendations. In a detailed and comprehensive review, Kwiterovich (1986) concluded that the recommendation by the American Heart Association was safe and beneficial. Barness (1986) approved the recommendations to limit total fat to 30% of calories, but believed that PUFA intake should be less than 10% of calories and saw no reason to limit cholesterol intake.

Conclusions and Recommendations of the Committee on Diet and Health

After reviewing the evidence, the Committee on Diet and Health concluded that recommendations concerning dietary fats and other lipids for children over 2 years of age should be generally similar to those for adults. In general, children over 2 years of age should eat a diet that includes a total fat intake of no more than 30% of calories, with less than 10% of calories from SFAs, and PUFAs at approximately current levels—6 to 8% of calories and not to exceed 10% of calories in any individual and a cholesterol intake of 100 mg or less per 1,000 calories—not to exceed 300 mg per day. A diet supplying macronutrients from the major food groups, with an increase in fruits and vegetables rather than refined sugar, should provide ample amounts of essential fatty acids, protein for growth, and an abundance of trace minerals and vitamins.

Between the ages of 2 and 4, children are often fed diets rather different from those consumed by older members of their family. Thus, it would not be unreasonable to gradually phase in the recommended diet by slowly limiting the intake of fat and cholesterol, so that by age 5 the child is eating the recommended diet (similar to the rest of the family).

Diets similar to this recommended diet are consumed by children in Mediterranean countries where the prevalence of CHD is much lower than in the United States. No abnormalities of growth and development have been observed in these children. The evidence indicates that the recommended diet is both safe and hygienically advisable.

OVERALL SUMMARY

A substantial body of evidence supports the conclusion that there is a direct relationship between dietary fat and the risk of both CHD and certain kinds of cancer, and possibly also obesity. The evidence is extremely powerful for CHD and is somewhat more limited for cancer. Fortunately, the major public health conclusions and recommendations that flow from the evidence, namely, that Americans should eat less total fat, especially less SFAs, are congruent with respect to both CHD and cancer, and possibly obesity.

Cardiovascular Disease

Many lines of evidence—from epidemiologic, clinical, genetic, and laboratory animal studies—indicate that high plasma levels of total and LDL cholesterol are causally related to atherosclerosis and increased risk of CHD. The epidemiologic evidence includes comparisons among various populations and prospective studies of individuals within populations. The predictive association between serum TC levels and the future occurrence of CHD is a continuous one throughout the range of values seen in the U.S. population and meets all the criteria for an etiological relationship. Clinically, premature CHD can result from high LDL-C levels, even in the absence of any other contributing risk factors. This is most clearly demonstrated in patients with familial hypercholesterolemia.

Many animal species (including monkeys and baboons) develop atherosclerosis when fed diets that raise their TC levels. Severe atherosclerotic lesions in monkeys regress when the TC is lowered substantially for an extended period by diet or by drugs.

Clinical trials have shown that lowering TC and LDL-C levels by diet or drugs decreases the subsequent incidence of CHD. The direct evidence

from such trials is strongest in middle-aged men with highest initial cholesterol levels. However, the complete set of evidence, including that from epidemiologic studies and experiments in animals, strongly suggests that reducing TC and LDL-C levels is also likely to decrease CHD incidence in younger and older men, in women, and in individuals with more moderate levels of TC. Moreover, the epidemiologic studies and clinical trials are remarkably consistent in their quantitative conclusions. The data suggest that for people with TC levels in the upper range, each 1% of reduction in serum TC levels leads to an approximately 2% reduction in CHD rates after 5 to 7 years and an even greater reduction in CHD rates after decades.

Consumption of specific fatty acids strongly influences plasma levels of TC and LDL-C in individuals and in populations. Many kinds of studies of relationships between diet, serum cholesterol, and CHD, including clinical–metabolic, epidemiologic, and animal studies, have implicated both the amount and nature of dietary fats as important determinants of serum cholesterol levels and CHD risk.

Clinical and controlled metabolic ward studies have clearly shown that increased intakes of some SFAs (palmitic, myristic, and lauric acids) raises TC and LDL-C levels in humans and, conversely, that reduced intake of these SFAs has the opposite effect. Although there is much interindividual variability in quantitative response to changes in SFA intake, the average response in the population can be quantitatively described by formulas developed in the laboratories of Keys and of Hegsted.

There are two kinds of PUFAs: ω-6 and ω-3. In general, ω-6 PUFAs lower TC, including reductions in both LDL-C and HDL-C levels. Substitution of linoleic acid for dietary SFAs results in a significant drop in TC levels. Although high intakes of linoleic acid were once advocated as a means of lowering TC, lack of information about the consequences of long-term ingestion of large amounts of linoleic acid, including concern about effects on cancer risk (see below), has led most public health authorities to recommend a ceiling of 10% or less of total calories from such fatty acids.

The major sources of ω-3 PUFAs are fish oils. Whether ω-3 PUFAs are useful in the prevention of CHD has not been determined. They have been found to lower serum triglyceride levels when given in relatively high doses; however, there is little evidence that they lead to reductions in concentrations of LDL-C beyond those obtained by removal of SFAs from the diet. It is not known whether long-term ingestion of these oils will lead to undesirable side effects, but there is no evidence that such side effects occur when intake of fish oils is through ingestion of fresh fish.

MUFAs have long been considered to be neutral in their effects on serum TC levels. However, recent evidence indicates that replacing SFAs with oleic acid may lead to a significant decrease in LDL-C levels without the concomitant decrease in HDL-C observed when linoleic acid is substituted for SFAs in the diet.

A variety of epidemiologic studies have focused on the relationships between dietary fat (both the amount and kind), serum cholesterol levels, and CHD. Several types of international and population studies have explored population (group) differences in diet, TC distributions in the population, and CHD rates. These studies have included comparisons of populations in different countries, of migrant groups from a single origin, and of special population groups within a country. These studies have generally demonstrated that mean intake of SFAs is strongly correlated with mean TC and LDL-C levels and with CHD rates in populations.

In contrast to the strong correlations observed between dietary fat and serum TC between populations, only weak (albeit significant) associations have been found between diet and TC in cross-sectional studies of individuals within a given population. There are methodological difficulties, however, suggesting that this might be a false-negative result. Thus, a number of factors identified would make it difficult to demonstrate such relationships in individuals within a fairly homogeneous population.

Studies in animals have shown that SFAs increase TC levels in a variety of species. In most species, SFA intake also is associated with severe atherosclerosis. These observations further support the conclusion that SFAs are important contributors to high TC levels and to atherosclerosis in humans.

Many studies have explored relationships between dietary cholesterol intake, serum cholesterol, and CHD. The evidence includes results from epidemiologic, clinical–metabolic, and experimental animal studies. Epidemiologic studies have shown high correlations between populations (both within and between countries) with respect to average dietary cholesterol intake, average TC levels, and CHD rates. In contrast to these high ecological correlations, however, individual correlations of dietary cholesterol with TC levels and CHD rates within a population have generally been found to be weak. These two methods of assessing correlations measure different kinds of correlations, and several factors could weaken the ability to demonstrate individual correlations within a given group. Moreover, since 1980, a small but definite power of dietary cholesterol to predict subsequent CHD within given populations has emerged from several longitudinal epidemiologic studies.

Dietary cholesterol causes hypercholesterolemia and atherosclerosis in a variety of animal species, including nonhuman primates. In clinical and controlled metabolic ward studies in humans, variable effects of dietary cholesterol (from large to negligibly small) have been reported. In general, however, within the range of intakes ordinarily consumed (200 to 600 mg/day, or approximately 150 to 400 mg/1,000 kcal), dietary cholesterol influences serum TC concentration, primarily LDL-C. On the average, in a large group of people, 100 mg of dietary cholesterol per 1,000 kcal elevates LDL-C by approximately 8 mg/dl. There is, however, much individual variability in the response to dietary cholesterol. Some people are resistant to the TC-elevating effect of dietary cholesterol, and others are quite sensitive. For the one-third or more of the population in the upper range of the distribution of response, dietary cholesterol is a meaningful contributor to TC and LDL-C concentrations and thereby to CHD risk. Dietary cholesterol may also have an effect on atherogenesis independent of its effect on fasting plasma lipid concentrations. Thus, for the overall population, it is clear that dietary cholesterol definitely contributes to the development of atherosclerosis and risk of CHD, although there is extensive interindividual variability in response.

Cancer

The National Research Council's Committee on Diet, Nutrition, and Cancer (NRC, 1982) concluded "that of all the dietary components [it] studied, the combined epidemiological and experimental evidence is most suggestive for a causal relationship between fat intake and the occurrence of cancer." This conclusion was based largely on the consistency between the epidemiologic and experimental evidence.

Epidemiologic and laboratory animal evidence obtained since 1981 bears on the possible relationship between dietary fat and the risk of certain kinds of cancer. The epidemiologic evidence includes comparisons of populations in different geographical areas as well as case-control studies of cancer of the colon and rectum, prostate, ovary, and breast. In general, these studies support conclusions from the earlier studies, namely, that there are significant associations between dietary fat and risk of these cancers; however, such associations have not been found in all studies.

In the epidemiologic studies, cancer incidence and mortality have generally had a stronger positive correlation with total dietary fat than with any particular type of dietary fat. Some studies of breast and prostate cancer have shown especially strong associations of cancer risk with the intake of SFAs and with dietary fat from animal sources, much of which is saturated. Overall, however, cancer mortality in human populations seems to correlate with total dietary fat about as well as with animal fat, and there is little or no correlation with vegetable fat or PUFAs.

Recent studies in animals have generally confirmed earlier evidence that animals fed high-fat diets develop tumors of the mammary gland, intestinal tract, and pancreas more readily than those fed low-fat diets. Dietary fat has its greatest effect during the promotion phase of carcinogenesis, but a lesser effect on initiation has been observed in some studies. The effect of dietary fat differs according to the type of fat. Vegetable oils containing ω-6 PUFAs promote carcinogenesis in animals more effectively than SFAs. Fish oils containing ω-3 PUFAs tend to have an inhibitory effect on carcinogenesis in animals. These findings are not necessarily in conflict with the epidemiologic data on humans that show the greatest effects from total and SFA intake, since the animals are usually fed large amounts of specific fats and oils, representing extremes of intake not found in the diets of human.

Epidemiologic studies have focused on potential relationships between low levels of serum cholesterol and cancer risk. In some studies of cohorts assembled to study cardiovascular disease risk, low serum cholesterol levels have been associated with increased cancer incidence and mortality. Such associations have not been found in some other studies and have been found inconsistently in subgroups within a given study population. The site-specific cancer data that are available are not consistent. In general, studies designed specifically to assess the relationship do not confirm the association. Thus, the complete set of evidence does not support the existence of a causally linked association between low levels of serum cholesterol and cancer risk.

Obesity and Gallbladder Disease

High-fat intake is associated with the development of obesity in animals and possibly in humans. In short-term clinical studies, a marked reduction in the percentage of calories derived from dietary fat has been associated with weight loss.

Obesity is the only nutritional factor clearly identified with cholesterol gallstones (gallbladder disease) in humans. In several animal models, increased dietary cholesterol causes cholelithiasis. However, few epidemiologic studies have been conducted to examine relationships between dietary fats and sterols and cholelithiasis. No conclusive evidence exists about the possible roles of dietary fat and cholesterol in the development of cholelithiasis.

Conclusions

The evidence concerning cardiovascular disease, summarized above, clearly indicates that dietary changes to lower the plasma levels of TC and LDL-C in North America would be desirable from a public health perspective. Two approaches can be used to accomplish this. First is a population (public health) strategy to shift the distribution of cholesterol levels in the entire population to a lower range. Second is a high-risk, patient-based approach that seeks to identify individuals at high risk and bring them into medical intervention. These two approaches are complementary and together represent a coordinated strategy to reduce cholesterol levels and coronary risk. Both approaches merit pursuit.

Although the evidence relating dietary fat to cancer is weaker than that relating dietary fat to CHD, the conclusions for both of these major chronic diseases are entirely congruent. Thus, recommendations to reduce the dietary intake of total fat and of SFAs will lead to reductions in coronary risk and perhaps in cancer risk.

DIRECTIONS FOR RESEARCH

More information is needed on many issues concerning relationships between dietary fats and other lipids and health and disease. Thus, the committee believes that future research directed at the following issues would be of value.

Cardiovascular Disease

• The role of postprandial lipoproteins and their remnants in atherogenesis and in coronary risk;

relationships between intake of specific fats and lipids and postprandial and remnant lipoproteins.

• The nature and regulation (including the dietary regulation) of heterogeneity within each major class of lipoproteins and the roles of different lipoprotein subclasses in atherosclerosis and CHD.

• The major dietary determinants of plasma HDL and the role and mechanism of HDL as protective against CHD.

• Characterization of the extent of interindividual variability in response to SFA intake. Are there human hyper- and hyporesponders to SFA intake? Can markers of such responsiveness be identified?

• Further characterization of the effects of MUFAs and stearic acid on serum lipid and lipoprotein profiles and levels.

• More systematic study of the effects of *trans* fatty acids on health.

• Is there a threshold for the unusually atherogenic effects of peanut oil observed in animals? Does peanut oil, consumed above a certain level, increase the risk of atherosclerotic disease in humans?

• Further characterization of the long-term consequences of the ingestion of different levels of ω-6 PUFA vegetable oils (i.e., on lipoproteins, atherosclerosis, cancer, and gallstones). What is the desirable level of intake of ω-6 PUFAs?

• The effects of ω-3 PUFAs (fish oils) on serum lipids and lipoproteins and on other parameters (including platelet function, coagulation, and eicosanoid metabolism). What are the long-term effects of ω-3 PUFA ingestion (e.g., potential benefits, untoward effects, possible regression of atherosclerosis)? More information is needed on the biologic actions of thromboxane A3.

• Characterization of the basis, particularly the genetic basis, of the variability in response to dietary cholesterol. Can we define human hyper- and hyporesponders?

• Effects of dietary cholesterol and dietary fats, and their interactions, on receptor-mediated clearance of IDL and LDL.

• Is there a minimum level of dietary cholesterol that affects plasma LDL level? Does dietary cholesterol lead to the formation of particularly atherogenic postprandial remnant lipoproteins?

• The associations of diet, and the levels and profiles of serum lipoproteins, with peripheral vascular and cerebrovascular diseases.

• Mechanisms and extent to which genetic factors control responses to dietary fats and other lipids, their interaction, and impact on specific chronic diseases, especially cardiovascular diseases, cancer, and gallbladder disease.

• The influence of dietary factors other than fats on serum lipids, the atherosclerotic process, and cardiovascular disease.

Cancer

• Further characterization of the association of dietary fat and caloric intake with increased risk of breast, colorectal, prostate, endometrial, and ovarian cancer.

• Further exploration of the possible mechanisms through which the amount and type of dietary fat (e.g., SFAs, ω-6 and ω-3 PUFAs) may influence different stages of carcinogenesis.

• Clarification of the relationship between dietary fat and other macronutrients (e.g., protein, carbohydrate) in colorectal cancer.

• Evaluation of the possible reciprocal relationship of dietary fat and dietary fiber intake to risk of colorectal cancer.

• Further assessment of the relationship between specific types of dietary fat (SFAs, MUFAs, ω-6 and ω-3 PUFAs) and risk of breast, colorectal, and prostate cancer.

• Evaluation of the possible relationship of dietary fat and elevated cholesterol intake to risk of lung and bladder cancer.

• Exploration of the quantitative relationship between reduced fat intake and decreased cancer rates, and thus the optimal range of intake of dietary fat and its component types.

• Consideration of the feasibility of intervention studies, preferably on defined populations, to determine the effects of reduced fat intake on the incidence of common cancers, especially colorectal and perhaps breast cancer. Large sample sizes and long-term follow-up will be required for such studies.

Obesity

• The proportion of fats in the diet may be a factor in the development of positive energy balance and possibly obesity, but the validity of this claim and the possible mechanisms of action require elucidation.

Gallstones

• Further exploration of the epidemiology of cholesterol gallstones. Identification of dietary and metabolic factors, and their interplay, in the etiology of cholelithiasis.

• Dietary studies in humans to relate defined dietary components to changes in the lithogenicity of bile.

REFERENCES

AAP (American Academy of Pediatrics). 1983. Committee on Nutrition: toward a prudent diet for children. Pediatrics 71: 78–80.

Aberg, H., H. Lithell, I. Selinus, and H. Hedstrand. 1985. Serum triglycerides are a risk factor for myocardial infarction but not for angina pectoris. Results from a 10-year followup of Uppsala Primary Preventive Study. Atherosclerosis 54:89–97.

Abramson, Z.H., and J.D. Kark. 1985. Serum cholesterol and primary brain tumours: a case-control study. Br. J. Cancer 52:93–98.

ACS (American Cancer Society). 1983. Workshop conference on nutrition in cancer causation and prevention. Fort Lauderdale, Florida, October 18–20, 1982. Cancer Res. 43: 2398S–2519S.

ACS (American Cancer Society). 1986. Second National Conference on Diet, Nutrition and Cancer. Houston, Texas, September 5–7, 1985. Cancer 58:1791–1962.

Admirand, W.H., and D.M. Small. 1968. The physicochemical basis of cholesterol gallstone formation in man. J. Clin. Invest. 47:1043–1052.

Ahrens, E.H., Jr. 1957. Nutritional factors and serum lipid levels. Am. J. Med. 23:928–952.

Ahrens, E.H., Jr., D.H. Blankenhorn, and T.T. Tsaltas. 1954. Effect on human serum lipids of substituting plant for animal fat in diet. Proc. Soc. Exp. Biol. Med. 86:872–878.

Ahrens, E.H., Jr., J. Hirsch, W. Insull, Jr., T.T. Tsaltas, R. Blomstrand, and M.L. Peterson. 1957. The influence of dietary fats on serum-lipid levels in man. Lancet 1:943–953.

Ahrens, E.H., Jr., W. Insull, Jr., J. Hirsch, W. Stoffel, M.L. Peterson, J.W. Farquher, T. Miller, and H.J. Thomasson. 1959. The effect on human serum-lipids of a dietary fat, highly unsaturated, but poor in essential fatty acids. Lancet 1:115–119.

Akesson, B., C. Fehling, and M. Jagerstad. 1978. Effect of vitamin B deficiency on phosphatidylethanolamine methylation in rat liver. Br. J. Nutr. 40:521–527.

Alderson, L.M., K.C. Hayes, and R.J. Nicholosi. 1986. Peanut oil reduces diet-induced atherosclerosis in cynomolgus monkeys. Arteriosclerosis 6:465–474.

American Health Foundation. 1979. Conference on the health effects of blood lipids: optimal distributions for populations. Prev. Med. 8:580–759.

Andersen, E., and K. Hellstrom. 1979. The effect of cholesterol feeding on bile acid kinetics and biliary lipids in normolipidemic and hypertriglyceridemic subjects. J. Lipid Res. 20:1020–1027.

Anderson, J.T., F. Grande, and A. Keys. 1961. Hydrogenated fats in the diet and lipids in the serum of man. J. Nutr. 75: 388–394.

Anitschkow, N.N. 1967. A history of experimentation on arterial atherosclerosis in animals. Pp. 21–44 in H.T. Blumenthal, ed. Cowdry's Arteriosclerosis: A Survey of the Problem, 2nd ed. C.C. Thomas, Springfield, Ill.

Anitschkow, N., and S. Chalatow. 1913. Ueber Experimentelle Cholesterinsteatose und ihre Bedeutung für die Entstehung einiger pathologischer Prozesse. Zentralbl. Allg. Pathol. Pathol. Anat. 24:1–9.

Antonis, A., and I. Bersohn. 1962a. The influence of diet on fecal lipids in South African White and Bantu prisoners. Am. J. Clin. Nutr. 11:142–155.

Antonis, A., and I. Bersohn. 1962b. The influence of diet on serum lipids in South African White and Bantu prisoners. Am. J. Clin. Nutr. 10:484–499.

Applebaum-Bowden, D., W.R. Hazzard, J. Cain, M.C. Cheung, R.S. Kushwaha, and J.J. Albers. 1979. Short-term egg yolk feeding in humans. Increase in apolipoprotein B and low density lipoprotein cholesterol. Atherosclerosis 33:385–396.

Applebaum-Bowden, D., S.M. Haffner, E. Hartsook, K.H. Luk, J.J. Albers, and W.R. Hazzard. 1984. Down-regulation of the low-density lipoprotein receptor by dietary cholesterol. Am. J. Clin. Nutr. 39:360–367.

Applewhite, T.H. 1981. Nutritional effects of hydrogenated soya oil. J. Am. Oil Chem. Soc. 58:260–269.

Arevalo, J.A., A.O. Wollitzer, M.B. Corporon, M. Larios, D. Huante, and M.T. Ortiz. 1987. Ethnic variability in cholelithiasis—an autopsy study. West. J. Med. 147:44–47.

Armstrong, B., and R. Doll. 1975. Environmental factors and cancer incidence and mortality in different countries, with special reference to dietary practices. Int. J. Cancer 15:617–631.

Armstrong, B.K., J.I. Mann, A.M. Adelstein, and F. Eskin. 1975. Commodity consumption and ischemic heart disease mortality, with special reference to dietary practices. J. Chronic Dis. 28:455–469.

Armstrong, M.J., Z. Stephan, and K.C. Hayes. 1982. Biliary lipids in New World monkeys: dietary cholesterol, fat, and species interactions. Am. J. Clin. Nutr. 36:592–601.

Arntzenius, A.C., D. Kromhout, J.D. Barth, J.H. Reiber, A.V. Bruschke, B. Buis, C.M. van Gent, N. Kempen-Voogd, S. Strikwerda, and E.A. van der Bruschke. 1985. Diet, lipoproteins, and the progression of coronary atherosclerosis: the Leiden Intervention Trial. N. Engl. J. Med. 312:805–811.

Avigan, J., and D. Steinberg. 1958. Effects of saturated and unsaturated fat on cholesterol metabolism in the rat. Proc. Soc. Exp. Biol. Med. 97:814–816.

Avigan, J., and D. Steinberg. 1965. Sterol and bile acid excretion in man and the effects of dietary fat. J. Clin. Invest. 44:1845–1856.

Aylsworth, C.F. 1986. Effects of lipids on gap junctionally-mediated intercellular communication: possible role of the promotion of tumorigenesis by dietary fat. Prog. Clin. Biol. Res. 222:607–622.

Baggio, G., A. Pagnan, M. Muraca, S. Martini, A. Opportuno, A. Bonanome, G.B. Ambrosio, S. Ferrari, P. Guarini, D. Piccolo, E. Manzato, R. Corrocher, and G. Crepaldi. 1988. Olive-oil-enriched diet: effect on serum lipoprotein levels and biliary cholesterol saturation. Am. J. Clin. Nutr. 47:960–964.

Bailey, C.H. 1916. Observations on cholesterol-fed guinea pigs. Proc. Soc. Exp. Biol. Med. 13:60–62.

Bang, H.O., and J. Dyerberg. 1980. Lipid metabolism and ischemic heart disease in Greenland Eskimos. Pp. 1–22 in H.H. Draper, ed. Advances in Nutritional Research, Vol. 3. Plenum Press, New York.

Barbeau, A. 1978. Lecithin in neurologic disorders. N. Engl. J. Med. 299:200–201.

Barness, L.A. 1986. Cholesterol and children. J. Am. Med. Assoc. 256:2871.

Bartus, R.T., R.L. Dean, J.A. Goas, and A.S. Lippa. 1980.

Age-related changes in passive avoidance retention: modulation with dietary choline. Science 209:301–303.

Baudet, M.F., C. Dachet, M. Lasserre, O. Esteva, and B. Jacotot. 1984. Modification in the composition and metabolic properties of human low density and high density lipoproteins by different dietary fats. J. Lipid. Res. 25:456–468.

Beaglehole, R., D.C. Trost, I. Tamir, P. Kwiterovich, C.J. Glueck, W. Insull, and B. Christensen. 1980. Plasma high-density lipoprotein cholesterol in children and young adults. The Lipid Research Clinics Program Prevalence Study. Circulation 62:IV83–IV92.

Beare-Rogers, J.L. 1983. Trans- and positional isomers of common fatty acids. Adv. Nutr. Res. 5:171–200.

Beaton, G.H., J. Milner, P. Corey, V. McGuire, M. Cousins, E. Stewart, M. de Ramos, D. Hewitt, P.V. Grambsch, N. Kassim, and J.A. Little. 1979. Sources of variance in 24-hour dietary recall data: implications for nutrition study design and interpretation. Am. J. Clin. Nutr 32:2546–2549.

Becker, N., D.R. Illingworth, P. Alaupovic, W.E. Connor, and E.E. Sundberg. 1983. Effects of saturated, monounsaturated, and omega-6 polyunsaturated fatty acids on plasma lipids, lipoproteins, and apoproteins in humans. Am. J. Clin. Nutr. 37:355–360.

Beil, F.U., and S.M. Grundy. 1980. Studies on plasma lipoproteins during absorption of exogenous lecithin in man. J. Lipid Res. 21:525–536.

Bennion, L.J., and S.M. Grundy. 1975. Effects of obesity and caloric intake on biliary lipid metabolism in man. J. Clin. Invest. 56:996–1011.

Bennion, L.J., and S.M. Grundy. 1978a. Risk factors for the development of cholelithiasis in man (first of two parts). N. Engl. J. Med. 299:1161–1167.

Bennion, L.J., and S.M. Grundy. 1978b. Risk factors for the development of cholelithiasis in man (second of two parts). N. Engl. J. Med. 299:1221–1227.

Benson, J. 1981. Fats of human milk and infant formulas. Pp. 553–560 in E. Lebenthal, ed. Textbook of Gastroenterology and Nutrition in Infancy, Vol. 1. Gastrointestinal Development in Perinatal Nutrtion. Raven Press, New York.

Berenson, G.A. 1980. Cardiovascular Risk Factors in Children: The Early Natural History of Atherosclerosis and Essential Hypertension. Oxford University Press, New York. 453 pp.

Berenson, G.S., and F.H. Epstein. 1983. Conference on blood lipids in children: optimal levels for early prevention of coronary artery disease. Workshop report: epidemiological section. April 18 and 19, 1983, American Health Foundation. Prev. Med. 12:741–797.

Berenson, G.S., S.R. Srinivasan, R.R. Frerichs, and L.S. Webber. 1979. Serum high density lipoprotein and its relationship to cardiovascular disease risk factor variables in children—the Bogalusa Heart Study. Lipids 14:91–98.

Berenson, G.S., S.R. Srinivasan, T.A. Nicklas, and L.S. Webber. 1988. Cardiovascular risk factors in children and early prevention of heart disease. Clin. Chem. 34:B115–B122.

Berg, K. 1963. A new serum type system in man—the Lp system. Acta Pathol. Microbiol. Scand. 59:369–382.

Berg, K., G. Dahlen, and M.H. Frick. 1974. Lp(a) lipoprotein and pre-β_1-lipoprotein in patients with coronary heart disease. Clin. Genet. 6:230–235.

Berry, E.M., and J. Hirsch. 1986. Does dietary linoleic acid influence blood pressure? Am. J. Clin. Nutr. 44:336–340.

Berry, E.M., J. Hirsch, J. Most, D.J. McNamara, and J. Thorton. 1986. The relationship of dietary fat to plasma lipid levels as studied by factor analysis of adipose tissue fatty acid composition in a free living population of middle aged American men. Am. J. Clin. Nutr. 44:220–231.

Best, M.M., C.H. Duncan, E.J. Van Loon, and J.D. Wathen. 1955. The effects of sitosterol on serum lipids. Am. J. Med. 19:61–70.

Beth, M., M.R. Berger, M. Aksoy, and D. Schmahl. 1987. Comparison between the effects of dietary fat level and of calorie intake on methylnitrosourea-induced mammary carcinogenesis in female SD rats. Int. J. Cancer 39:737–744.

Beveridge, J.M.R., and W.F. Connell. 1962. The effect of commercial margarines on plasma cholesterol levels in man. Am. J. Clin. Nutr. 10:391–397.

Beveridge, J.M.R., W.F. Connell, G.A. Mayer, J.B. Firstbrook, and M.S. DeWolfe. 1955. The effects of certain vegetable and animal fats on the plasma lipids of humans. J. Nutr. 56:311–320.

Beveridge, J.M.R., W.F. Connell, and G.A. Mayer. 1957. The nature of the substances in dietary fat affecting the level of plasma cholesterol in humans. Can. J. Biochem. Physiol. 35:257–270.

Beveridge, J.M.R., W.F. Connell, H.L. Haust, and G.A. Mayer. 1959. Dietary cholesterol and plasma cholesterol levels in man. Can. J. Biochem. Physiol. 37:575–582.

Beveridge, J.M.R., W.F. Connell, G.A. Mayer, and H.L. Haust. 1960. The response of man to dietary cholesterol. J. Nutr. 71:61–65.

Beynen, A.C., and M.B. Katan. 1985. Effect of egg yolk feeding on the concentration and composition of serum lipoprotein in man. Atherosclerosis 54:157–166.

Bhattacharyya, A.K., and W.E. Connor. 1974. Beta-sitosterolemia and xanthomatosis. A newly described lipid storage disease in two sisters. J. Clin. Invest. 53:1033–1043.

Biörck, G. 1956. Wartime lessons on arteriosclerotic heart disease from northern Europe. Pp. 8–21 in A. Keys and P.D. White, eds. Cardiovascular Epidemiology. Second World Congress of Cardiology and Twenty-Seventh Annual Scientific Sessions of the American Heart Association. Hoeber-Haper, New York.

Birt, D.F., and B.D. Roebuck. 1986. Enhancement of pancreatic carcinogenesis by dietary fat in the hamster and rat models. Prog. Clin. Biol. Res. 222:331–335.

Bjelke, E. 1978. Dietary factors and the epidemiology of cancer of the stomach and large bowel. Aktuel. Ernaehrungsmed. Klin. Prax. Suppl. 2:10–17.

Blankenhorn, D.H., S.A. Nessim, R.L. Johnson, M.E. Sanmarko, S.P. Azen, and L. Cashin-Hemphill. 1987. Beneficial effects of combined colestipol-niacin therapy on coronary atherosclerosis and coronary venous bypass grafts. J. Am. Med. Assoc. 257:3233–3240.

Bloomfield, D.K. 1964. Cholesterol metabolism. III. Enhancement of cholesterol absorption and accumulation in safflower oil-fed rats. J. Lab. Clin. Med. 64:613–623.

Bodurtha, J.N., R.M. Schieken, J. Segrest, and W.E. Nance. 1987. High-density lipoprotein-cholesterol subfractions in adolescent twins. Pediatrics 79:181–189.

Bonanome, A., and S.M. Grundy. 1988. Effect of dietary stearic acid on plasma cholesterol and lipoprotein levels. N. Engl. J. Med. 318:1244–1248.

Bothig, S., V.I. Metelitsa, W. Barth, A.A. Aleksandrov, I. Schneider, T.P. Ostrovskaya, E.V. Kokurina, I.I. Saposhinkov, I.P. Iliushina, and L.S. Gurevich. 1976. Prevalence of ischaemic heart disease, arterial hypertension and intermittent claudication, and distribution of risk factors among middle-aged men in Moscow and Berlin. Cor Vasa 18:104–118.

Braden, L.M., and K.K. Carroll. 1986. Dietary polyunsaturated fat in relation to mammary carcinogenesis in rats. Lipids 21:285–288.

Bragdon, J.H., J.H. Zeller, and J.W. Stevenson. 1957. Swine and experimental atherosclerosis. Proc. Soc. Exp. Biol. Med. 95:282–284.

Brenneman, D.E., W.E. Connor, E.L. Forker, and L. DenBesten. 1972. The formation of abnormal bile and cholesterol gallstones from dietary cholesterol in the prairie dog. J. Clin. Invest. 51:1495–1503.

Brensike, J.F., R.I. Levy, S.F. Kelsey, E.R. Passamani, J.M. Richardson, I.K. Loh, N.J. Stone, R.F. Aldrich, J.W. Battaglini, D.J. Moriarity, M.R. Fisher, L. Friedman, W. Friedewald, K.M. Detre, and S.E. Epstein. 1984. Effects of therapy with cholestyramine on progression of coronary arteriosclerosis: results of the NHLBI Type II Coronary Intervention Study. Circulation 69:313–324.

Brett, M., and D.J. Barker. 1976. The world distribution of gallstones. Int. J. Epidemiol. 5:355–341.

Broitman, S.A. 1986. Cholesterol conundrums: the relationship between dietary and serum cholesterol in colon cancer. Prog. Clin. Biol. Res. 222:435–459.

Bronsgeest-Schoute, D.C., J.G. Hautvast, and R.J. Hermus. 1979a. Dependence of the effects of dietary cholesterol and experimental conditions on serum lipids in man. I. Effects of dietary cholesterol in a linoleic acid-rich diet. Am. J. Clin. Nutr. 32:2183–2187.

Bronsgeest-Schoute, D.C., R.J. Hermus, G.M. Dallinga-Thie, and J.G. Hautvast. 1979b. Dependence of the effects of dietary cholesterol and experimental conditions on serum lipids in man. II. Effects of dietary cholesterol in a linoleic acid-poor diet. Am. J. Clin. Nutr. 32:2188–2192.

Bronte-Stewart, B., A. Keys, J.F. Brock, A.D. Moodie, M.H. Keys, and A. Antonis. 1955. Serum-cholesterol, diet, and coronary heart-disease: an inter-racial survey in the Cape Peninsula. Lancet 269:1103–1108.

Brown, M.S., and J.L. Goldstein. 1983. Lipoprotein metabolism in the macrophage: implications for cholesterol deposition in atherosclerosis. Annu. Rev. Biochem. 52:223–261.

Brown, M.S., and J.L. Goldstein. 1986. A receptor-mediated pathway for cholesterol homeostasis. Science 232:34–47.

Brown, W.V., and H. Ginsberg. 1987. Classification and diagnosis of the hyperlipidemias. Pp. 143–168 in D. Steinberg and J.M. Olefsky, eds. Hypercholesterolemia and Atherosclerosis: Pathogenesis and Prevention. Churchill Livingstone, New York.

Bruce, W.R., and P.W. Dion. 1980. Studies relative to a fecal mutagen. Am. J. Clin. Nutr. 33:2511–2512.

Brunzell, J.D., A.D. Sniderman, J.J. Albers, and P.O. Kwiterovich, Jr. 1984. Apoproteins B and A-I and coronary artery disease in humans. Arteriosclerosis 4:79–83.

Brussaard, J.H., F. Dallinga-Thie, P.H. Groot, and M.B. Katan. 1980. Effects of amount and type of dietary fat on serum lipids, lipoproteins and apolipoproteins in man. A controlled 8-week trial. Atherosclerosis 36:515–527.

Brussaard, J.H., M.B. Katan, P.H. Groot, L.M. Havekes, and J.G. Hautvast. 1982. Serum lipoproteins of healthy persons fed a low-fat diet or a polyunsaturated fat diet for three months. A comparison of two cholesterol-lowering diets. Atherosclerosis 42:205–219.

Bull, A.W., J.C. Bronstein, and N.D. Nigro. 1988. Role of essential fatty acids in azoxymethane-induced colon carcinogenesis. Proc. Am. Assoc. Cancer Res. 29:149.

Bursztyn, P.G., and M.H. King. 1986. Fat-induced hypertension in rabbits: the effects of dietary linoleic and linolenic acid. J. Hypertens. 4:699–702.

Byers, T., J. Marshall, S. Graham, C. Mettlin, and M. Swanson. 1983. A case-control study of dietary and nondietary factors in ovarian cancer. J. Natl. Cancer Inst. 71: 681–686.

Canner, P.L., K.G. Berge, N.K. Wenger, J. Stamler, L. Friedman, R.J. Prineas, and W. Friedewald. 1986. Fifteen year mortality in Coronary Drug Project patients: long-term benefit with niacin. J. Am. Coll. Cardiol. 8:1245–1255.

Carew, T.E., D.C. Schwenke, and D. Steinberg. 1987. Antiatherogenic effect of probucol unrelated to its hypocholesterolemic effect: evidence that antioxidants in vivo can selectively inhibit low density lipoprotein degradation in macrophage-rich fatty streaks and slow the progression of atherosclerosis in the Watanabe heritable hyperlipidemic rabbit. Proc. Natl. Acad. Sci. U.S.A. 84:7725–7729.

Carey, M.C., and D.M. Small. 1978. The physical chemistry of cholesterol solubility in bile. Relationship to gallstone formation and dissolution in man. J. Clin. Invest. 61: 998–1026.

Carlson, L.A., and L.E. Bottiger. 1981. Serum triglycerides, to be or not to be a risk factor for ischaemic heart disease? Atherosclerosis 39:287–291.

Carlson, S.E., P.W. DeVoe, and L.A. Barness. 1982. Effect of infant diets with different polyunsaturated to saturated fat ratios on circulating high-density lipoproteins. J. Pediatr. Gastroenterol. Nutr. 1:303–309.

Carroll, K.K. 1971. Plasma cholesterol levels and liver cholesterol biosynthesis in rabbits fed commercial or semisynthetic diets with and without added fats or oils. Atherosclerosis 13:67–76.

Carroll, K.K. 1975. Experimental evidence of dietary factors and hormone-dependent cancers. Cancer Res. 35:3374–3383.

Carroll, K.K. 1983. Diet and carcinogenesis. Pp. 223–227 in F.G. Schettler, A.M. Gotto, G. Middelhoff, A.J.R. Habenicht, and K.R. Jurutka, eds. Atherosclerosis: Proceedings of the Sixth International Symposium. Springer-Verlag, Berlin.

Carroll, K.K. 1985. Dietary fat and breast cancer. Pp. 29–47 in J. Weininger, ed. Nutrition Update, Vol. 2. Wiley, New York.

Carroll, K.K. 1986a. Biological effects of fish oils in relation to chronic diseases. Lipids 21:731–732.

Carroll, K.K. 1986b. Experimental studies on dietary fat and cancer in relation to epidemiological data. Prog. Clin. Biol. Res. 222:231–248.

Carroll, K.K., and H.T. Khor. 1971. Effects of level and type of dietary fat on incidence of mammary tumors induced in female Sprague-Dawley rats by 7,12-dimethylbenz(a)anthracene. Lipids 6:415–420.

Carroll, K.K., and H.T. Khor. 1975. Dietary fat in relation to tumorigenesis. Prog. Biochem. Pharmacol. 10:308–353.

Carroll, K.K., and C.J.H. Woodward. 1989. Nutrition and human health aspects of marine oils and lipids. Pp. 435–456 in R.G. Ackman, ed. Marine Biogenic Lipids, Fats, and Oils, Vol. 2. CRC Press, Boca Raton, Fla.

Carroll, K.K., G.J. Hopkins, T.G. Kennedy, and M.B. Davidson. 1981. Essential fatty acids in relation to mammary carcinogenesis. Prog. Lipid. Res. 20:685–690.

Carroll, K.K., L.M. Braden, J.A. Bell, and R. Kalameghan. 1986. Fat and cancer. Cancer 58:1818–1825.

Carroll, M.D., S. Abraham, and C.M. Dresser. 1983. Dietary Intake Source Data: United States, 1976–80. Vital and Health Statistics, Ser. 11, No. 231. DHHS Publ. No. (PHS) 83-1681. National Center for Health Statistics, Public Health Service, U.S. Department of Health and Human Services, Hyattsville, Md. 483 pp.

Carter, C.A., R.J. Milholland, W. Shea, and M.M. Ip. 1983. Effect of the prostaglandin synthetase inhibitor indomethacin on 7,12-dimethylbenz(a)anthracene-induced mammary tumorigenesis in rats fed different levels of fat. Cancer Res. 43:3559–3562.

Carter, C.A., M.M. Ip, and C. Ip. 1987. Response of mammary carcinogenesis to dietary linoleate and fat levels and its modulation by prostaglandin synthesis inhibitors. Pp. 253–260 in W.E.M. Lands, ed. Proceedings of the AOCS Short Course on Polyunsaturated Fatty Acids and Eicosanoids. American Oil Chemists' Society, Champaign, Ill.

Carvalho, A.C.A., C. Galli, R. Paoletti, J.M. Iacono, and A. Keys. 1981. Platelets, thrombosis and dietary fats. International pilot epidemiological study in thrombosis. Pp. 125–142 in N.G. Basán, R. Paoletti, and J.M. Iacono, eds. New Trends in Nutrition, Lipid Research, and Cardiovascular Diseases. Current Topics in Nutrition and Disease, Vol. 5. Alan R. Liss, New York.

CAST (Council for Agricultural Science and Technology). 1982. Diet, Nutrition, and Cancer: A Critique. Report of the Task Force on Diet, Nutrition, and Cancer. Special Publ. No. 13. CAST, Ames, Iowa. 80 pp.

Castelli, W.P. 1986. The triglyceride issue: a view from Framingham. Am. Heart J. 112:432–437.

Castelli, W.P., R.D. Abbott, P.M. McNamara. 1983. Summary estimates of cholesterol used to predict coronary heart disease. Circulation 67:730–734.

Castelli, W.P., R.J. Garrison, P.W. Wilson, R.D. Abbott, S. Kalousdian, and W.B. Kannel. 1986. Incidence of coronary heart disease and lipoprotein cholesterol levels. The Framingham Study. J. Am. Med. Assoc. 256:2835–2838.

Cavallo-Perin, P., C. Barile, A. Ozzello, M. La Rosa, G. Pagano, and G. Lenti. 1984. Peripheral vascular disease and risk factors of atherosclerosis: an epidemiologic study. Panminerva Med. 26:139–143.

Cave, W.T., Jr., and J.J. Jurkowski. 1987. Comparative effects of omega-3 and omega-6 dietary lipids on rat mammary tumor development. Pp. 261–266 in W.E.M. Lands, ed. Proceedings of the AOCS Short Course on Polyunsaturated Fatty Acids and Eicosanoids. American Oil Chemists' Society, Champaign, Ill.

Chait, A., A. Onitiri, A. Nicoll, E. Rabaya, J. Davies, and B. Lewis. 1974. Reduction of serum triglyceride levels by polyunsaturated fat. Studies on the mode of action and on very low density lipoprotein composition. Atherosclerosis 20:347–364.

Chalatow, S.S. 1929. Bemerkungen zu den Arbeiten über die sogenannte. Experimentelle Cholesterinsteatose oder Experimentelle Cholesterinkrankheit des Kaninchens und anderer Tiere. Virchows. Arch. f. Pathol. Anat. 272:691–708.

Chase, H.P., R.J. O'Quin, and D. O'Brien. 1974. Screening for hyperlipidemia in childhood. J. Am. Med. Assoc. 230: 1535–1537.

Chenoweth, W., M. Ullmann, R. Simpson, and G. Leveille.

1981. Influence of dietary cholesterol and fat on serum lipids in men. J. Nutr. 111:2069–2080.

Childs, M.T., J.A. Bowlin, J.T. Ogilvie, W.R. Hazzard, and J.J. Albers. 1981. The contrasting effects of a dietary soya lecithin product and corn oil on lipoprotein lipids in normolipidemic and familial hypercholesterolemic subjects. Atherosclerosis 38:217–228.

Chong, K.S., R.J. Nicolosi, R.F. Rodger, D.A. Arrigo, R.W. Yuan, J.J. MacKey, S. Georas, and P.N. Herbert. 1987. Effect of dietary fat saturation on plasma lipoproteins and high density lipoprotein metabolism of the rhesus monkey. J. Clin. Invest. 79:675–683.

Ciocca, S., M. Arca, A. Montali, S. Fazio, A. Bucci, and F. Angelico. 1987. Lack of association between arterial blood pressure and erythrocyte fatty acid composition in an Italian population sample. Scand. J. Clin. Lab. Invest. 47:105–110.

Clarke, S.D. 1986. Metabolic adaptations to dietary fats. Prog. Clin. Biol. Res. 222:531–553.

Clarke, W.R., H.G. Schrott, P.E. Leaverton, W.E. Connor, and R.M. Lauer. 1978. Tracking of blood lipids and blood pressures in school age children: the Muscatine Study. Circulation 58:626–634.

Clarkson, T.B., H.B. Lofland, Jr., B.C. Bullock, and H.O. Goodman. 1971. Genetic control of plasma cholesterol. Studies on squirrel monkeys. Arch. Pathol. 92:37–45.

Clarkson, T.B., N.D. Lehner, B.C. Bullock, H.B. Lofland, and W.D. Wagner. 1976a. Atherosclerosis in new world monkeys. Primates Med. 9:90–144.

Clarkson, T.B., T.E. Hamm, B.C. Bullock, and N.D. Lehner. 1976b. Atherosclerosis in old world monkeys. Primates Med. 9:66–89.

Clarkson, T.B., J.R. Kaplan, and M.R. Adams. 1985. The role of individual differences in lipoprotein, artery wall, gender, and behavioral responses in the development of atherosclerosis. Ann. N.Y. Acad. Sci. 454:28–45.

Clevidence, B.A., R.E. Morton, G. West, D.M. Dusek, and H.F. Hoff. 1984. Cholesterol esterification in macrophages. Stimulation by lipoproteins containing apo B isolated from human aortas. Arteriosclerosis 4:196–207.

Cobb, M., P. Turkki, W. Linscheer, and K. Raheja. 1980. Lechithin supplementation in healthy volunteers: effect on cholesterol esterification and plasma, and bile lipids. Nutr. Metab. 24:228–237.

Codde, J.P., K.D. Croft, and L.J. Beilin. 1987a. Dietary suppression of prostaglandin synthesis does not accelerate DOCA/salt hypertension in rats. Clin. Exp. Pharmacol. Physiol. 14:513–523.

Codde, J.P., L.J. Beilin, K.D. Croft, and R. Vandongen. 1987b. The effect of dietary fish oil and salt on blood pressure and eicosanoid metabolism of spontaneously hypertensive rats. J. Hypertens. 5:137–142.

Cohen, B.I., E.H. Mosbach, C.K. McSherry, R.J. Stenger, S. Kuroki, and B. Rzigalinski. 1986. Gallstone prevention in prairie dogs: comparison of chow vs semisynthetic diets. Hepatology 6:874–880.

Cohen, B.M., A.L. Miller, J.F. Lipinski, and H.G. Pope. 1980. Lecithin in mania: a preliminary report. Am. J. Psychiatry 137:242–243.

Cohen, L.A. 1986. Dietary fat and mammary cancer. Pp. 77–100 in B.S. Reddy and L.A. Cohen, eds. Diet, Nutrition and Cancer: A Critical Evaluation, Vol. 1. Macronutrients and Cancer. CRC Press, Boca Raton, Fla.

Cohen, L.A., D.O. Thompson, V. Maeura, K. Choi, M.E.

Blank, and D.P. Rose. 1986. Dietary fat and mammary cancer. 1. Promoting effects of different dietary fats on N-nitrosomethylurea-induced rat mammary tumorigenesis. J. Natl. Cancer Inst. 77:33–42.

Cohen, L.A., K.W. Choi, and C.X. Wang. 1988. Influence of dietary fat, caloric restriction, and voluntary exercise on N-nitrosomethylurea-induced mammary tumorigenesis in rats. Cancer Res. 48:4276–4283.

Cohn, K., F.J. Sakai, and M.F. Langston, Jr. 1975. Effect of clofibrate on progression of coronary disease: a prospective angiographic study in man. Am. Heart J. 89:591–598.

Comberg, H.U., S. Heyden, C.G. Hames, A.J. Vergroesen, and A.I. Fleischman. 1978. Hypotensive effect of dietary prostaglandin precursor in hypertensive man. Prostaglandins 15:193–197.

Comess, L.J., P.H. Bennett, and T.A. Burch. 1967. Clinical gallbladder disease in Pima Indians. Its high prevalence in contrast to Framington, Massachusetts. N. Engl. J. Med. 277:894–898.

Committee of Principal Investigators. 1978. A co-operative trial in the primary prevention of ischaemic heart disease using clofibrate. Br. Heart J. 40:1069–1118.

Conlay, L.A., R.J. Wurtman, K. Blusztajn, I.L. Coviella, T.J. Maher, and G.E. Evoniuk. 1986. Decreased plasma choline concentrations in marathon runners. N. Engl. J. Med. 315:892.

Connor, W.E. 1986. Hypolipidemic effects of dietary omega-3 fatty acids in normal and hyperlipidemic humans: effectiveness and mechanisms. Pp. 173–210 in A.P. Simopoulos, R.R. Kifer, and R.E. Martin, eds. Health Effects of Polyunsaturated Fatty Acids in Seafoods. Academic Press, New York.

Connor, W.E., R.E. Hodges, and R.E. Bleiler. 1961a. Effect of dietary cholesterol upon serum lipids in man. J. Lab. Clin. Med. 57:331–342.

Connor, W.E., R.E. Hodges, and R.E. Bleiler. 1961b. The serum lipids in men receiving high cholesterol and cholesterol-free diets. J. Clin. Invest. 40:894–901.

Connor, W.E., D.B. Stone, and R.E. Hodges. 1964. The interrelated effects of dietary cholesterol and fat upon human serum lipid levels. J. Clin. Invest. 43:1691–1696.

Connor, W.E., D.T. Witiak, D.B. Stone, and M.L. Armstrong. 1969. Cholesterol balance and fecal neutral steroid and bile acid excretion in normal men fed dietary fats of different fatty acid composition. J. Clin. Invest. 48:1363–1375.

Connor, W.E., M.T. Cerqueira, R.W. Connor, R.B. Wallace, M.R. Malinow, and H.R. Casdorph. 1978. The plasma lipids, lipoproteins, and diet of the Tarahumara Indians of Mexico. Am. J. Clin. Nutr. 31:1131–1142.

Corey, J.E., K.C. Hayes, B. Dorr, and D.M. Hegsted. 1974. Comparative lipid response of four primate species to dietary changes in fat and carbohydrate. Atherosclerosis 19:119–134.

Corkin, S., K.L. Davis, J.H. Growdon, E. Usdin, and R.J. Wurtman, eds. 1982. Aging, Vol. 19. Alzheimer's Diseases: A Report of Progress in Research. Raven Press, New York. 525 pp.

Correa, P., J. Paschal, P. Pizzolato, W. Pelon, and D.E. Lesley. 1981. Fecal mutagens and colorectal polyps: preliminary report of an autopsy study. Pp. 119–127 in W.R. Bruce, P. Correa, M. Lipkin, S.R. Tannenbaum, and T.D. Wilkins, eds. Banbury Report 7. Gastrointestinal Cancer: Endogenous Factors. Cold Spring Harbor Laboratory, New York.

Cortese, C., Y. Levy, E.D. Janus, P.R. Turner, S.N. Rao, N.E. Miller, and B. Lewis. 1983. Modes of action of lipid-lowering diets in man: studies of apolipoprotein B kinetics in relation to fat consumption and dietary fatty acid composition. Eur. J. Clin. Invest. 13:79–85.

Cramer, D.W., W.R. Welch, G.B. Hutchinson, W. Willett, and R.E. Scully. 1984. Dietary animal fat in relation to ovarian cancer risk. Obstet. Gynecol. 63:833–838.

Crowther, J.S., B.S. Drasar, M.J. Hill, B. Maclennen, D. Magnin, S. Peach, and C.H. Teoh-Chan. 1976. Faecal steroids and bacteria and large bowel cancer in Hong Kong by socio-economic groups. Br. J. Cancer 34:191–198.

Cullen, K., N.S. Stenhouse, K.L. Wearne, and T.A. Welborn. 1983. Multiple regression analysis of risk factors for cardiovascular disease and cancer mortality in Busselton, Western Australia—13-year study. J. Chronic Dis. 36:371–377.

Cummings, J.H., H.S. Wiggins, D.J. Jenkins, H. Houston, T. Jivraj, B.S. Drasar, and M.J. Hill. 1978. Influence of diets high and low in animal fat on bowel habit, gastrointestinal transit time, fecal microflora, bile acid, and fat excretion. J. Clin. Invest. 61:953–963.

Curb, J.D., and D.M. Reed. 1985. Fish consumption and mortality from coronary heart disease. N. Engl. J. Med. 313:821.

Dahlén, G., K. Berg, T. Gillnäs, and C. Ericson. 1975. Lp(a) lipoprotein/pre-β_1-lipoprotein in Swedish middle-aged males and in patients with coronary heart disease. Clin. Genet. 7:334–341.

Dahlén, G., K. Berg, and M.H. Frick. 1976. Lp(a) lipoprotein/pre-beta$_1$-lipoprotein, serum lipids and atherosclerotic disease. Clin. Genet. 9:558–566.

Dales, L.G., G.D. Friedman, H.K. Ury, S. Grossman, and S.R. Williams. 1979. A case-control study of relationships of diet and other traits to colorectal cancer in American blacks. Am. J. Epidemiol. 109:132–144.

Dam, H. 1971. Determinants of cholesterol cholelithiasis in man and animals. Am. J. Med. 51:596–613.

Dam, H., and F. Christensen. 1952. Alimentary production of gallstones in hamsters. Acta Path. Microbiol. Scand. 30:236–242.

Dam, H., I. Kruse, M.K. Jensen, and H.E. Kallehauge. 1967. Studies on human bile. II. Influence of two different fats on the composition of human bile. Scand. J. Clin. Lab. Invest. 19:367–378.

Dam, H., I. Prange, M.K. Hensen, H.E. Kallehauge, and H.J. Fenger. 1971. Studies on human bile. IV. Influence of ingestion of cholesterol in the form of eggs on the composition of bile in healthy subjects. Z. Ernaehrungswiss. 10:178–187.

Dao, T.L., and P.C. Chan. 1983. Effect of duration of high fat intake on enhancement of mammary carcinogenesis in rats. J. Natl. Cancer Inst. 71:201–205.

Dauber, D.V., and L.N. Katz. 1942. Experimental cholesterol atheromatosis in an omnivorous animal, the chick. Arch. Pathol. 34:937–950.

Davies, L.G.G., and L. Murdoch. 1959. "Lipostabil": A pilot study. Br. Med. J. 2:619–620.

Davignon, J., S. Lussier-Cacan, M. Ortin-George, M. Lelievre, D. Bertagna, A. Gattereau, and A. Fontaine. 1977. Plasma lipids and lipoprotein patterns in angiographically graded atherosclerosis of the legs and in coronary heart disease. Can. Med. Assoc. J. 116:1245–1250.

Davignon, J., R.E. Gregg, and C.F. Sing. 1988. Apolipoprotein E polymorphism and atherosclerosis. Arteriosclerosis 8:1–21.

Davis, D., B. Stern, and G. Lesnick. 1937. The lipid and cholesterol content of blood of patients with angina pectoris and arteriosclerosis. Ann. Int. Med. 11:354–369.

Davis, W.W., III. 1955. Symposium on sitosterol. III. The physical chemistry of cholesterol and β-sitosterol related to the intestinal absorption of cholesterol. Trans. N.Y. Acad. Sci. 18:123–128.

Dawber, T.R., F.E. Moore, and G.V. Mann. 1957. Coronary heart disease in the Framingham Study. Am. J. Public Health 47 Suppl. April:4–24.

Dayton, S., M.L. Pearce, H. Goldman, A. Harnish, D. Plotkin, M. Schickman, M. Winfield, A. Zager, and W. Dixon. 1968. Controlled trial of a diet high in unsaturated fat for prevention of atherosclerotic complications. Lancet 2:1060–1062.

DeBacker, G., M. Rosseneu, and J.P. Deslypere. 1982. Discriminative value of lipids and apoproteins in coronary heart diease. Atherosclerosis 42:197–203.

de Iongh, H., R.K. Beerthuis, C. den Hartog, L.M. Dalderup, and P.A. van der Spek. 1965. The influence of some dietary fats on serum lipids in man. Bibl. Nutr. Dieta. 7:137–152.

de Langen, C.D. 1916. Cholesterine-Stofwisseling en Rassenpathologie. Geneeskd. Tijdschr. Ned. Indie 56:1–34.

de Langen, C.D. 1922. Het cholesterinegehalte van het bloed in Indie. Geneeskd. Tijdschr. Ned. Indie 62:1–4.

DenBesten, L., W.E. Connor, and S. Bell. 1973. The effect of dietary cholesterol on the composition of human bile. Surgery 73:266–273.

DenBesten, L., S. Safaie-Shirazi, W.E. Connor, and S. Bell. 1974. Early changes in bile composition and gallstone formation induced by a high cholesterol diet in prairie dogs. Gastroenterology 66:1036–1045.

Diller, E.R., M. Korzenovsky, and O.A. Harvey. 1961. Endogenous hypercholesterosis in rabbits fed a fat-free purified diet and the effect of unsaturated lipid. J. Nutr. 73:14–16.

Dock, W. 1946. The predilection of atherosclerosis for the coronary arteries. J. Am. Med. Assoc. 131:875–878.

Donato, K., and D.M. Hegsted. 1985. Efficiency of utilization of various sources of energy for growth. Proc. Natl. Acad. Sci. U.S.A. 82:4866–4870.

Drewnowski, A., J.D. Brunzell, K. Sande, P.H. Iverius, and M.R. Greenwood. 1985. Sweet tooth reconsidered: taste responsiveness in human obesity. Physiol. Behav. 35:617–622.

Ducimetiere, P., J.L. Richard, F. Cambien, R. Rakotovao, and J.R. Claude. 1980. Coronary heart disease in middle-aged Frenchmen: comparisons between Paris Prospective Study, Seven Countries Study, and Pooling Project. Lancet 1:1346–1350.

Duff, G.L. 1935. Experimental cholesterol arteriosclerosis and its relationship to human arteriosclerosis. Arch. Pathol. 20:81–124, 259–304.

Duffield, R.G., B. Lewis, N.E. Miller, C.W. Jamieson, J.N. Brunt, and A.C. Colchester. 1983. Treatment of hyperlipidemia retards progression of symptomatic femoral atherosclerosis. A randomized control trial. Lancet 2:639–642.

Duncan, K.H., J.A. Bacon, and R.L. Weinsier. 1983. The effects of high and low energy density diets on satiety, energy intake, and eating time of obese and nonobese subjects. Am. J. Clin. Nutr. 37:763–767.

Dusing, R., R. Scherhag, K. Glanzer, U. Budde, and H.J. Kramer. 1983. Dietary linoleic acid deprivation: effects on blood pressure and PGI2 synthesis. Am. J. Physiol. 244:H228–H233.

Dwyer, J. 1980. Diets for children and adolescents that meet the dietary goals. Am. J. Dis. Child. 134:1073–1080.

ECP/IUNS (European Organization for Cooperation on Cancer Prevention Studies/International Union for Nutritional Sciences). 1986. Proceedings of a joint ECP-IUNS workshop on diet and human carcinogenesis (Århus, Denmark; June 1985). Nutr. Cancer 8:1–40.

Ederer, F., P. Leren, O. Turpeinen, and I.D. Frantz, Jr. 1971. Cancer among men on cholesterol-lowering diets. Experience from five clinical trials. Lancet 2:203–206.

Eggen, D.A. 1974. Cholesterol metabolism in rhesus monkey, squirrel monkey, and baboon. J. Lipid Res. 15:139–145.

Ehnholm, C., J. Huttunen, P. Pietinen, U. Leino, M. Mutanen, E. Kostiainen, J Pikkarainen, R. Dougherty, J.M. Iacono, and P. Puska. 1982. Effect of diet on serum lipoproteins in a population with a high risk of coronary heart disease. N. Engl. J. Med. 307:850–855.

Ehnholm, C., J.K. Huttunen, P. Pietinen, U. Leino, M. Mutanen, E. Kostiainen, J.M. Iacono, R. Dougherty, and P. Puska. 1984. Effect of a diet low in saturated fatty acids on plasma lipids, lipoproteins, and HDL subfractions. Arteriosclerosis 4:265–269.

Ehrich, M., J.E. Aswell, R.L. Van Tassell, T.D. Wilkins, A.R. Walker, and N.J. Richardson. 1979. Mutagens in the feces of 3 South-African populations at different levels of risk for colon cancer. Mutagen. Res. 64:231–240.

Emken, E.A. 1984. Nutrition and biochemistry of trans and positional fatty acid isomers in hydrogenated oils. Annu. Rev. Nutr. 4:339–376.

Emmons, L. 1986. Food procurement and the nutritional adequacy of diets in low-income families. J. Am. Diet. Assoc. 86:1684–1693.

Enger, S.C., I. Hjermann, O.P. Foss, A. Helgeland, I. Holme, P. Leren, and K.R. Norum. 1979. High density lipoprotein cholesterol and myocardial infarction or sudden coronary death: a prospective case-control study in middle-aged men of the Oslo Study. Artery 5:170–181.

Enos, W.F., R.H. Holmes, and J. Beyer. 1953. Coronary disease among United States soldiers killed in action in Korea. J. Am. Med. Assoc. 152:1090–1093.

Erickson, B.A., R.H. Coots, F.H. Mattson, and A.M. Kligman. 1964. The effect of partial hydrogenation of dietary fats, of the ratio of polyunsaturated to saturated fatty acids, and of dietary cholesterol upon plasma lipids in man. J. Clin. Invest. 43:2017–2025.

Erickson, K.L. 1986. Mechanisms of dietary fat modulation of tumorigenesis: changes in immune response. Prog. Clin. Biol. Res. 222:555–586.

Ershow, A.G., R.J. Nocolosi, and K.C. Hayes. 1981. Separation of the dietary fat and cholesterol influences on plasma lipoproteins of rhesus monkeys. Am. J. Clin. Nutr. 34:830–840.

Fager, G., O. Wiklund, S.O. Olofsson, C. Wihelmsson, and G. Bondjers. 1980. Serum apolipoprotein levels in relation to acute myocardial infarction and its risk factors. Apolipoprotein A-I levels in male survivors of myocardial infarction. Atherosclerosis 36:67–74.

Fager, G., O. Wiklund, S.O. Olofsson, L. Wilhelmsen, and G. Bondjers. 1981. Multivariate analyses of serum apolipoproteins and risk factors in relation to acute myocardial infarction. Arteriosclerosis 1:273–279.

Farquhar, J.W., and M. Sokolow. 1958. Response of serum lipids and lipoproteins of man to beta-sitosterol and safflower oil: a long-term study. Circulation 17:890–899.

Farquhar, J.W., R.E. Smith, and M.E. Dempsey. 1956. The effect of beta-sitosterol on the serum lipids of young men with arteriosclerotic heart disease. Circulation 14:77–82.

Feinleib, M., W.B. Kannel, C.G. Tedeschi, T.K. Landau, and R.J. Garrison. 1979. The relation of antemortem characteristics to cardiovascular findings at necropsy—The Framingham Study. Atherosclerosis 34:145–157.

Ferro-Luzzi, A., P. Strazzullo, C. Scaccini, A. Siani, S. Sette, M.A. Mariani, P. Mastranzo, R.M. Dougherty, J.M. Iacono, and M. Mancini. 1984. Changing the Mediterranean diet: effects on blood lipids. Am. J. Clin. Nutr. 40:1027–1037.

Finegold, S.M., H.R. Attebery, and V.L. Sutter. 1974. Effect of diet on human fecal flora: comparison of Japanese and American diets. Am. J. Clin. Nutr. 27:1456–1469.

Finegold, S.M., D.J. Flora, H.R. Attebery, and V.L. Sutter. 1975. Fecal bacteriology of colonic polyp patients and control patients. Cancer Res. 35:3407–3417.

Finley, J.W., and D.E. Schwass. 1985. Xenobiotic Metabolism: Nutritional Effects. American Chemical Society Symposium Series 277. American Chemical Society, Washington, D.C. 382 pp.

Fleischman, A.T., M.L. Bierenbaum, A. Stier, H. Somol, P. Watson, and A.M. Naso. 1979. Hypotensive effect of increased dietary linoleic acid in mildly hypertensive humans. J. Med. Soc. N.J. 76:181–183.

Flow, B.L., T.C. Cartwright, T.J. Keuhl, G.E. Mott, D.C. Kraemer, A.W. Kruski, J.D. Williams, and H.C. McGill, Jr. 1981. Genetic effects on serum cholesterol concentrations in baboons. J. Hered. 72:97–103.

Folsom, A.R., K. Kuba, R.V. Leupker, D.R. Jacobs, and I.D. Frantz, Jr. 1983. Lipid concentrations in serum and EDTA-treated plasma from fasting and nonfasting normal persons, with particular regard to high-density lipoprotein cholesterol. Clin. Chem. 29:505–508.

Ford, C.H., R.B. McGandy, and F.J. Stare. 1972. An institutional approach to the dietary regulation of blood cholesterol in adolescent males. Prev. Med. 1:426–445.

Fox, J.C., H.C. McGill, Jr., K.D. Carey, and G.S. Getz. 1987. In vivo regulation of hepatic LDL receptor mRNA in the baboon. J. Biol. Chem. 262:7014–7020.

Franceschini, G., A. Bondioli, M. Mantero, M. Sirtori, G. Tattoni, G. Biasi, and C.R. Sirtori. 1982. Increased apoprotein B in very low density lipoproteins of patients with peripheral vascular disease. Arteriosclerosis 2:74–80.

Frank, G.C., G.S. Berenson, and L.S. Webber. 1978. Dietary studies and the relationship of diet to cardiovascular disease risk factor variables in 10-year-old children—The Bogalusa Heart Study. Am. J. Clin. Nutr. 31:328–340.

Frank, G.C., R.P. Farris, J.L. Cresanta, and T.A. Nicklas. 1986. Dietary intake as a determinant of cardiovascular risk factor variables. Part A: observations in a pediatric population. Pp. 254–291 in G.S. Berenson, ed. Causation of Cardiovascular Risk Factors in Children: Perspectives on Cardiovascular Risk in Early Life. Raven Press, New York.

Frantz, I.D., Jr., and J.B. Carey, Jr. 1961. Cholesterol content of human liver after feeding of corn oil and hydrogenated coconut oil. Proc. Soc. Exp. Biol. Med. 106:800–801.

Freedman, D.S., W.P. Newman III, R.E. Tracy, A.E. Voors, S.R. Srinivasan, L.S. Webber, C. Restrepo, J.P. Strong, and G.S. Berenson. 1988. Black-white differences in aortic fatty streaks in adolescence and early adulthood: the Bogalusa Heart Study. Circulation 77:856–864.

Frerichs, R.R., S.R. Srinivasan, L.S. Webber, and G.S. Berenson. 1976. Serum cholesterol and triglyceride levels in 3,446 children from a biracial community: the Bogalusa Heart Study. Circulation 54:302–309.

Frerichs, R.R., L.S. Webber, S.R. Srinivasan, and G.S. Berenson. 1978a. Relation of serum lipids and lipoproteins to obesity and sexual maturity in white and black children. Am. J. Epidemiol. 108:486–496.

Frerichs, R.R., S.R. Srinivasan, L.S. Webber, M.C. Rieth, and G.S. Berenson. 1978b. Serum lipids and lipoproteins at birth in a biracial population: the Bogalusa Heart Study. Pediatr. Res. 12:858–863.

Frerichs, R.R., L.S. Webber, A.W. Voors, S.R. Srinivasan, and G.S. Berenson. 1979. Cardiovascular disease risk factor variables in children at two successive years—the Bogalusa Heart Study. J. Chronic Dis. 32:251–262.

Freston, J.W., and I.A. Bouchier. 1968. Experimental cholelithiasis. Gut 9:2–4.

Freudenheim, J.L., and J.R. Marshall. 1988. The problem of profound mismeasurement and the power of epidemiological studies of diet and cancer. Nutr. Cancer 11:243–250.

Frick, M.H., O. Elo, K. Haapa, O.P. Heinonen, P. Heinsalmi, P. Helo, J.K. Huttunen, P. Kaitaniemi, P. Koskinen, V. Manninen, H. Maenpaa, M. Malkonen, M. Manttari, S. Norola, A. Pasternack, J. Pikkarainen, M. Romo, T. Sjoblom, and E.A. Nikkila. 1987. Helsinki Heart Study: primary-prevention trial with gemfibrozil in middle-aged men with dyslipidemia. Safety of treatment, changes in risk factors, and incidence of coronary heart disease. N. Engl. J. Med. 317:1237–1245.

Friedman, G., and S.J. Goldberg. 1973. Normal serum cholesterol values. Percentile ranking in a middle-class pediatric population. J. Am. Med. Assoc. 225:610–612.

Friedman, G., and S.J. Goldberg. 1976. An evaluation of the safety of a low-saturated-fat, low-cholesterol diet beginning in infancy. Pediatrics 58:655–657.

Friedman, G.D., W.B. Kannel, and T.R. Dawber. 1966. The epidemiology of gallbladder disease: observations in the Framingham Study. J. Chronic Dis. 19:273–292.

Frohlich, E.D. 1977. Hemodynamics of hypertension. Pp. 15–49 in J. Genest, E. Koiw, and O. Kuchel, eds. Hypertension: Physiopathology and Treatment. McGraw-Hill, New York.

Funch, J.P., B. Krogh, and H. Dam. 1960. Effects of butter, some margarines and arachis oil in purified diets on serum lipids and atherosclerosis in rabbits. Br. J. Nutr. 14:355–360.

Funch, J.P., G. Kristensen, and H. Dam. 1962. Effects of various dietary fats on serum cholesterol, liver lipids and tissue pathology in rabbits. Br. J. Nutr. 16:497–506.

Garcia-Palmieri, M.R., J. Tillotson, E. Cordero, R. Costas, Jr., P. Sorlie, T. Gordon, W.B. Kannel, and A.A. Colon. 1977. Nutrient intake and serum lipids in urban and rural Puerto Rican men. Am. J. Clin. Nutr. 30:2092–2100.

Garcia-Palmieri, M.R., P. Sorlie, J. Tillotson, R. Costas, Jr., E. Cordero, and M. Rodriguez. 1980. Relationship of dietary intake to subsequent coronary heart disease incidence: the Puerto Rico Heart Health Program. Am. J. Clin. Nutr. 33:1818–1827.

Gardey, T., P.G. Burstyn, and T.G. Taylor. 1978. Fat induced hypertension in rabbits. I. The effects of fibre on the blood pressure increase induced by coconut oil. Proc. Nutr. Soc. 37:97A.

Gates, J.C., R.L. Huenemann, and R.J. Brand. 1975. Food

choices of obese and non-obese persons. J. Am. Diet. Assoc. 67:339–343.

Gaubatz, J.W., C. Heideman, A.M. Gotto, Jr., J.D. Morrisett, and G.H. Dahlen. 1983. Human plasma lipoprotein [a]. Structural properties. J. Biol. Chem. 258:4582–4589.

Geer, J.C., H.C. McGill, Jr., W.B. Robertson, and J.P. Strong. 1968. Histologic characteristics of coronary artery fatty streaks. Lab. Invest. 18:565–570.

Gelenberg, A.J., J.D. Wojcik, and J.H. Growdon. 1979. Lecithin for the treatment of tardive dyskinesia. Pp. 285–303 in A. Barbeau, J.H. Growdon, and R.J. Wurtman, eds. Nutrition and the Brain, Vol. 5. Choline and Lecithin in Brain Disorders. Raven Press, New York.

Gerhardsson, M., U. Rosenqvist, A. Ahlbom, and L.A. Carlson. 1986. Serum cholesterol and cancer—a retrospective case-control study. Int. J. Epidemiol. 15:155–159.

Gershfeld, N.L. 1979. Selective phospholipid adsorption and atherosclerosis. Science 204:506–508.

Gertler, M.M., S.M. Garn, and P.D. White. 1950a. Diet, serum cholesterol and coronary artery disease. Circulation 2: 696–704.

Gertler, M.M., S.M. Garn, and J. Lerman. 1950b. The interrelationships of serum cholesterol, cholesterol esters and phospholipids in health and in coronary artery disease. Circulation 2:205–214.

Ghoshal, A.K., and E. Farber. 1984. The induction of liver cancer by dietary deficiency of choline and methionine without added carcinogens. Carcinogenesis 5:1367–1370.

Ginsberg, J., N.A. Le, C. Mays, J. Gibson, and W.V. Brown. 1981. Lipoprotein metabolism in nonresponders to increased dietary cholesterol. Arteriosclerosis 1:463–470.

Glenn, F., and C.K. McSherry. 1970. The baboon and experimental cholelithiasis. Arch. Surg. 100:105–108.

Glueck, C.J., R.W. Fallat, R. Tsang, and C.R. Buncher. 1974. Hyperlipidemia in progeny of parents with myocardial infarction before age 50. Am. J. Dis. Child. 127:70–75.

Glueck, C.J., M.M. Hastings, C. Allen, E. Hogg, L. Baehler, P.S. Gartside, D. Phillips, M. Jones, E.J. Hollenbach, B. Braun, and J.B. Anastasia. 1982. Sucrose polyester and covert caloric dilution. Am. J. Clin. Nutr. 35:1352–1359.

Glueck, C.J., D.J. Gordon, J.J. Nelson, C.E. Davis, and H.A. Tyroler. 1986. Dietary and other correlates of changes in total and low density lipoprotein cholesterol in hypercholesterolemic men: the Lipid Research Clinics Coronary Primary Prevention Trial. Am. J. Clin. Nutr. 44:489–500.

Goldbourt, U. 1987. High risk versus public health strategies in primary prevention of coronary heart disease. Am. J. Clin. Nutr. 45 Suppl. 5:1185–1192.

Goldbourt, U., E. Holtzman, and H.N. Neufeld. 1985. Total and high density lipoprotein cholesterol in the serum and risk of mortality: evidence of a threshold effect. Br. Med. J. 290:1239–1243.

Goldstein, J.L., and M.S. Brown. 1983. Familial hypercholesterolemia. Pp. 672–712 in J.B. Stanbury, J.B. Wyngaarden, D.S. Fredrickson, J.L. Goldstein, and M.S. Brown, eds. The Metabolic Basis of Inherited Disease, 5th ed. McGraw-Hill, New York.

Goldstein, J.L., H.F. Hoff, Y.K. Ho, S.K. Basu, and M.S. Brown. 1981. Stimulation of cholesteryl ester synthesis in macrophages by extracts of atherosclerotic human aortas and complexes of albumin/cholesteryl esters. Arteriosclerosis 1: 210–226.

Goldstein, J.L., T. Kita, and M.S. Brown. 1983. Defective lipoprotein receptors and atherosclerosis. Lessons from an animal counterpart of familial hypercholesterolemia. N. Engl. J. Med. 309:288–296.

Goodnight, S.H., Jr., W.S. Harris, W.E. Connor, and D.R. Illingworth. 1982. Polyunsaturated fatty acids, hyperlipidemia, and thrombosis. Arteriosclerosis 2:87–113.

Gordon, D.J., K.M. Salz, K.J. Roggenkamp, and F.A. Franklin, Jr. 1982. Dietary determinants of plasma cholesterol change in the recruitment phase of the Lipid Research Clinics Coronary Primary Prevention Trial. Arteriosclerosis 2:537–548.

Gordon, D.J., J. Knoke, J.L. Probstfield, R. Superko, and H.A. Tyroler. 1986. High-density lipoprotein cholesterol and coronary heart disease in hypercholesterolemic men: the Lipid Research Clinics Coronary Primary Prevention Trial. Circulation 74:1217–1225.

Gordon, T., M.R. Garcia-Palmieri, A. Kagan, W.B. Kannel, and J. Schiffman. 1974. Differences in coronary heart disease mortality in Framingham, Honolulu and Puerto Rico. J. Chronic Dis. 27:329–344.

Gordon, T., W.P. Castelli, M.C. Hjortland, W.B. Kannel, and T.R. Dawber. 1977. High density lipoprotein as a protective factor against coronary heart disease. The Framingham Study. Am. J. Med. 62:707–714.

Gordon, T., A. Kagan, M. Garcia-Palmieri, W.B. Kannel, W.J. Zukel, J. Tillotson, P. Sorlie, and M. Hjortland. 1981a. Diet and its relation to coronary heart disease and death in three populations. Circulation 63:500–515.

Gordon, T., W.B. Kannel, W.P. Castelli, and T.R. Dawber. 1981b. Lipoproteins, cardiovascular disease, and death: the Framingham Study. Arch. Intern. Med. 141:1128–1131.

Graham, S., H. Dayal, M. Swanson, A. Mittelman, and G. Wilkinson. 1978. Diet in the epidemiology of cancer of the colon and rectum. J. Natl. Cancer Inst. 61:709–714.

Graham, S., B. Humphey, J. Marshall, R. Priore, T. Byers, T. Rzepka, C. Mettlin, and J.E. Pontes. 1983. Diet in the epidemiology of carcinoma of the prostate gland. J. Natl. Cancer Inst. 70:687–692.

Grande, F., J.T. Anderson, C. Chlouverakis, M. Proja, and A. Keys. 1965. Effect of dietary cholesterol on man's serum lipids. J. Nutr. 87:52–62.

Grande, F., J.T. Anderson, and A. Keys. 1970. Comparison of effects of palmitic and stearic acids in the diet on serum cholesterol in man. Am. J. Clin. Nutr. 23:1184–1193.

Grasso, S., B. Gunning, K. Imaichi, G. Michaels, and L. Kinsell. 1962. Effects of natural and hydrogenated fats of approximately equal dienoic acid content upon plasma lipids. Metabolism 11:920–924.

Greenhalgh, R.M., D.S. Rosengarten, I. Mervart, J.S. Calnan, B. Lewis, and P. Martin. 1971. Serum lipids and lipoproteins in peripheral vascular disease. Lancet 2:947–950.

Gresham, G.A., and A.N. Howard. 1960. The independent production of atherosclerosis and thrombosis in the rat. Br. J. Exp. Pathol. 41:395–402.

Greten, H., H. Raetzer, A. Stiehl, and G. Schettler. 1980. The effect of polyunsaturated phosphatidylcholine on plasma lipids and fecal sterol excretion. Atherosclerosis 36: 81–88.

Groen, J., B.K. Tjiong, C.E. Kamminga, and A.F. Willebrands. 1952. The influence of nutrition, individuality and some other factors, including various forms of stress, on the serum cholesterol; an experiment of nine months' duration in 60 normal human volunteers. Voeding 13:556–587.

Groen, J.J., K.B. Tijong, M. Koster, A.F. Willebrands, G. Verdonck, and M. Pierloot. 1962. The influence of nutrition and ways of life on blood cholesterol and the prevalence of hypertension and coronary heart disease among Trappist and Benedictine Monks. Am. J. Clin. Nutr. 10:456–470.

Grundy, S.M. 1975. Effects of polyunsaturated fats on lipid metabolism in patients with hypertriglyceridemia. J. Clin. Invest. 55:269–282.

Grundy, S.M. 1979. Dietary fats and sterols. Pp. 89–118 in R.I. Levy, B.M. Rifkind, B.H. Dennis, and N. Ernst, eds. Nutrition, Lipids, and Coronary Heart Disease: A Global View. Nutrition in Health and Disease, Vol. 1. Raven Press, New York.

Grundy, S.M. 1981. Saturated fats and coronary heart disease. Pp. 57–78 in M. Winick, ed. Nutrition and the Killer Diseases. Wiley, New York.

Grundy, S.M. 1986. Comparison of monounsaturated fatty acids and carbohydrates for lowering plasma cholesterol. N. Engl. J. Med. 314:745–748.

Grundy, S.M. 1987. Monounsaturated fatty acids, plasma cholesterol, and coronary heart disease. Am. J. Clin. Nutr. 45:1168–1175.

Grundy, S.M., and E.H. Ahrens, Jr. 1970. The effects of unsaturated dietary fats on absorption, excretion, synthesis, and distribution of cholesterol in man. J. Clin. Invest. 49:1135–1152.

Grundy, S.M., and H.Y. Mok. 1977. Determination of cholesterol absorption in man by intestinal perfusion. J. Lipid Res. 18:263–271.

Grundy, S.M., and G.L. Vega. 1988. Plasma cholesterol responsiveness to saturated fatty acids. Am. J. Clin. Nutr. 47:822–824.

Grundy, S.M., D. Nix, M.F. Whelan, and L. Franklin. 1986. Comparison of three cholesterol-lowering diets in normolipidemic men. J. Am. Med. Assoc. 256:2351–2355.

Grundy, S.M., L. Florentin, D. Nix, and M.F. Whelan. 1988. Comparison of monounsaturated fatty acids and carbohydrates for reducing raised levels of plasma cholesterol in man. Am. J. Clin. Nutr. 47:965–969.

Gurll, N., and L. DenBesten. 1978. Animal models of human cholesterol gallstone disease: a review. Lab. Animal Sci. 28:428–432.

Haberland, M.E., D. Fong, and L. Cheng. 1988. Malondialdehyde-altered protein occurs in atheroma of Watanabe heritable hyperlipidemic rabbits. Science 241:215–218.

Haenzel, W., F.B. Locke, and M. Segi. 1980. A case-control study of large bowel cancer in Japan. J. Natl. Cancer Inst. 64:17–22.

Halfon, S.T., S. Eisenberg, M. Baras, A.M. Davies, G. Halperin, and Y. Stein. 1982a. Plasma cholesterol, triglyceride and high-density lipoprotein-cholesterol levels in 17-year-old Jerusalem offspring of Jews from 19 countries of birth. Isr. J. Med. Sci. 18:1121–1130.

Halfon, S.T., B.M. Rifkind, S. Harlap, N.A. Kaufmann, M. Baras, P.E. Slater, G. Halperin, S. Eisenberg, A.M. Davies, and Y. Stein. 1982b. Plasma lipids and lipoproteins in adult Jews of different origin: the Jerusalem Lipid Research Clinic prevalence study. Isr. J. Med. Sci. 18:1113–1120.

Harlan, W.R., A.L. Hull, R.P. Schmouder, F.E. Thompson, F.A. Larkin, and J.R. Landis. 1983. Dietary Intake and Cardiovascular Risk Factors, Part II. Serum Urate, Serum Cholesterol, and Correlates. Vital and Health Statistics, Ser. 11, No. 227. DHHS Publ. No. (PHS) 83-1677. National Center for Health Statistics, Public Health Service, U.S. Department of Health and Human Services, Hyattsville, Md. 94 pp.

Harlap, S., M. Baras, Y. Friedlander, N.A. Kaufmann, S. Eisenberg, A.M. Davies, and Y. Stein. 1982. Contributions of different lipoprotein fractions to variations in total cholesterol between Israeli origin groups and social classes. Isr. J. Med. Sci. 18:1131–1136.

Harris, W.S., W.E. Connon, and M.P. McMurry. 1983. The comparative reductions of the plasma lipids and lipoproteins by dietary polyunsaturated fats: salmon oil versus vegetable oils. Metabolism 32:179–184.

Harris, W.S., W.E. Connor, S.B. Inkeles, and D.R. Illingworth. 1984. Dietary omega-3 fatty acids prevent carbohydrate-induced hypertriglyceridemia. Metabolism 33:1016–1019.

Hashim, S.A., A. Argeaga, and T.B. Van Itallie. 1960. Effect of a saturated medium-chain triglyceride on serum-lipids in man. Lancet 1:1105–1108.

Havel, R.J. 1987. Origin, metabolic fate, and metabolic function of plasma lipoproteins. Pp. 117–141 in D. Steinberg and J.M. Olefsky, eds. Hypercholesterolemia and Atherosclerosis: Pathogenesis and Prevention. Churchill Livingstone, New York.

Hayashi, E., T. Maeda, R. Hasegawa, and T. Tomita. 1978. The effect of myo-inositol deficiency on lipid metabolism in rats. III. The mechanism of an enhancement in lipolysis due to myo-inositol deficiency in rats. Biochem. Biophys. Acta 531:197–205.

Hayashi, Y., M. Nagao, T. Sugimura, S. Takayama, L. Tomatis, L.W. Wattenberg, and G.N. Wogan. 1986. Proceedings of the 16th International Symposium of the Princess Takamatsu Cancer Research Fund, Tokyo, 1985. Diet, Nutrition and Cancer. Japan Scientific Society Press, Tokyo. 345 pp.

Heaton, K.W. 1973. The epidemiology of gallstones and suggested aetiology. Clin. Gastroenterol. 2:67–83.

Heckers, H., M. Korner, T.W.L. Tuschen, and F.M. Melcher. 1977. Occurrence of individual trans-isomeric fatty acids in human myocardium, jejunum and aorta in relation to different degrees of atherosclerosis. Atherosclerosis 28:389–398.

Hegsted, D.M. 1986. Serum-cholesterol reponse to dietary cholesterol: a re-evaluation. Am. J. Clin. Nutr. 44:299–305.

Hegsted, D.M., R.B. McGandy, M.L. Myers, and F.J. Stare. 1965. Quantitative effects of dietary fat on serum cholesterol in man. Am. J. Clin. Nutr. 17:281–295.

Heideman, C.L., and H.F. Hoff. 1982. Lipoproteins containing apolipoprotein A-I extracted from human aortas. Biochem. Biophys. Acta 711:431–444.

Hellstrom, K., and S. Lindstedt. 1966. Studies on the formation of cholic acid in subjects given standardized diet with butter or corn oil as dietary fat. Am. J. Clin. Nutr. 18:46–59.

Hems, G. 1980. Associations between breast-cancer and mortality rates, childbearing and diet in the United Kingdom. Br. J. Cancer 41:429–437.

Herold, P.M., and J.E. Kinsella. 1986. Fish oil consumption and decreased risk of cardiovascular disease: a comparison of findings from animal and human feeding trials. Am. J. Clin. Nutr. 43:566–598.

Herrick, J.B. 1912. Clinical features of sudden obstruction of the coronary arteries. J. Am. Med. Assoc. 59:2015–2020.

Heshmat, M.Y., L. Kaul, J. Kovi, M.A. Jackson, A.G. Jackson, G.W. Jones, M. Edson, J.P. Enterline, R.G. Worrell, and S.L. Perry. 1985. Nutrition and prostate cancer: a case-control study. Prostate 6:7–17.

Heymann, W., and F. Rack. 1943. Independence of serum cholesterol from exogenous cholesterol in infants and in children. Am. J. Dis. Child. 65:235–246.

Hiatt, R.A., and B.H. Fireman. 1986. Serum cholesterol and the incidence of cancer in a large cohort. J. Chronic Dis. 39: 861–870.

Hill, M.J. 1981. Diet and the human intestinal flora. Cancer Res. 41:3778–3780.

Hill, M.J., B.S. Drasar, G. Hawksworth, V. Aries, J.S. Crowther, and R.E. Williams. 1971. Bacteria and aetiology of cancer of the large bowel. Lancet 1:95–100.

Hill, M.J., B.S. Drasar, R.E. Williams, T.W. Meade, A.G. Cox, J.E. Simpson, and B.C. Morson. 1977. Faecal bile-acids and clostridia in patients with cancer of the large bowel. Lancet 1:535–539.

Hillyard, L.A., and S. Abraham. 1979. Effect of dietary polyunsaturated fatty acids on growth of mammary adeno-carcinomas in mice and rats. Cancer Res. 39:4430–4437.

Hinds, M.W., L.N. Kolonel, J.H. Hankin, and J. Lee. 1983. Dietary cholesterol and lung cancer risk in a multiethnic population in Hawaii. Int. J. Cancer 32:727–732.

Hirayama, T. 1977. Changing patterns of cancer in Japan with special reference to the decrease in stomach cancer mortality. Pp. 55–75 in H.H. Hiatt, J.D. Watson, and J.A. Winston, eds. Origins of Human Cancer, Book A. Incidence of Cancer in Humans. Cold Spring Harbor Laboratory, New York.

Hirohata, T., A.G. Nomura, J.H. Hankin, L.N.Kolonel, and J. Lee. 1987. An epidemiologic study on the association between diet and breast cancer. J. Natl. Cancer Inst. 78: 595–600.

Hislop, T.G., A.J. Coldman, J.M. Elwood, G. Brauer, and L. Kan. 1986. Childhood and recent eating patterns and risk of breast cancer. Cancer Detect. Prev. 9:47–58.

Hjermann, I., K. Velve Byre, I. Holme, and P. Leren. 1981. Effect of diet and smoking intervention on the incidence of coronary heart disease. Report from the Oslo Study Group of a randomised trial in healthy men. Lancet 2:1303–1310.

Ho, K.J. 1976. Comparative studies on the effect of cholesterol feeding on biliary composition. Am. J. Clin. Nutr. 29:698–704.

Hoff, H.F., and J.W. Gaubatz. 1975. Ultrastructural localization of plasma lipoproteins in human intracranial arteries. Virchows Arch. 369:111–121.

Hoff, H.F., and J.W. Gaubatz. 1982. Isolation, purification, and characterization of a lipoprotein containing Apo B from the human aorta. Atherosclerosis 42:273–297.

Hoff, H.F., and R.E. Morton. 1985. Lipoproteins containing apo B extracted from human aortas. Structure and function. Ann. N.Y. Acad. Sci. 454:183–194.

Hoff, H.F., R.L. Jackson, S.J. Mao, and A.M. Gotto, Jr. 1974. Localization of low-density lipoproteins in atherosclerotic lesions from human normolipemics employing a purified fluorescent-labeled antibody. Biochem. Biophys. Acta 351:407–415.

Hoff, H.F., J.L. Titus, R.J. Bajardo, R.L. Jackson, A.M. Gotto, M.E. DeBakey, and J.T. Lie. 1975a. Lipoproteins in atherosclerotic lesions. Localization by immunofluorescence of apo-low-density lipoproteins in human atherosclerotic arteries from normal and hyperlipoproteinemics. Arch. Pathol. 99:253–258.

Hoff, H.F., C.L. Heideman, G.P. Noon, and J.S. Meyer. 1975b. Localization of apo-lipoproteins in human carotid artery plaques. Stroke 6:531–534.

Hoff, H.F., C.L. Heideman, R.L. Jackson, R.J. Bayardo, H.S. Kim, and A.M. Gotto, Jr. 1975c. Localization patterns of plasma apolipoproteins in human atherosclerotic lesions. Circ. Res. 37:72–79.

Hoff, H.F., C.L. Heideman, A.M. Gotto, Jr., and J.W. Gaubatz. 1977a. Apolipoprotein B retention in the grossly normal and atherosclerotic human aorta. Circ. Res. 41:684–690.

Hoff, H.F., C.L. Heideman, J.W. Gaubatz, A.M. Gotto, Jr., E.E. Erickson, and R.L. Jackson. 1977b. Quantification of apolipoprotein B in grossly normal human aorta. Circ. Res. 40:56–64.

Hoff, H.F., J.W. Gaubatz, and A.M. Gotto, Jr. 1978. Apo B concentration in the normal human aorta. Biochem. Biophys. Res. Commun. 85:1424–1430.

Hoff, H.F., W.A. Bradley, C.L. Heideman, J.W. Gaubatz, M.D. Karagas, and A.M. Gotto, Jr. 1979a. Characterization of low density lipoprotein-like particle in the human aorta from grossly normal and atherosclerotic regions. Biochem. Biophys. Acta 573:361–374.

Hoff, H.F., M. Karagas, C.L. Heideman, J.W. Gaubatz, and A.M. Gotto, Jr. 1979b. Correlation in the human aorta of apo B fractions with tissue cholesterol and collagen content. Atherosclerosis 32:259–268.

Hoffman, D.R., E.O. Uthus, and W.E. Cornatzer. 1980. Effect of diet on choline phosphotransferase, phosphatidyl-ethanolamine methyltransferase and phosphatidyldimethyl-ethanolamine methyltransferase in liver microsomes. Lipids 15:439–446.

Hoffmann, P., C. Taube, K. Pönicke, W. Forster, L. Somova, V. Orbetova, and F. Davidova. 1978. Influence of linoleic acid content on arterial blood pressure of salt loaded rats. I. Effects on prostaglandin metabolism and sympathetic nervous system. Acta Bio. Med. Ger. 37:863–867.

Holman, R.L. 1961. Atherosclerosis—a pediatric nutrition problem? Am. J. Clin. Nutr. 9:565–569.

Holman, R.L., H.C. McGill, Jr., J.P. Strong, and J.C. Geer. 1958. The natural history of atherosclerosis. The early aortic lesions as seen in New Orleans in the middle of the 20th century. Am. J. Pathol. 34:209–235.

Holman, R.L., W.A. Blanc, and D. Andersen. 1959. Decreased aortic atherosclerosis in cystic fibrosis of the pancreas. Pediatrics 24:34–39.

Holman, R.T. 1986. Nutrition and functional requirements for essential fatty acids. Prog. Clin. Biol. Res. 222:211–228.

Holman, R.T., W.W. Christie, H. Sprecher, M. Crawford, B. Lewis, K.K. Carroll, and K.K. Wahle, eds. 1986. Dietary fats and cancer. Pp. 527–553 in Progress in Lipid Research, Vol. 25. Essential Fatty Acids, Prostaglandins and Leukotrienes. Pergamon Press, Oxford.

Holme, I., S.C. Enger, A. Helgeland, I. Hjermann, P. Leren, P.G. Lund-Larsen, L.A. Solberg, and J.P. Strong. 1981. Risk factors and raised atherosclerotic lesions in coronary and cerebral arteries. Statistical analysis from the Oslo study. Arteriosclerosis 1:250–256.

Holub, B.J. 1982. The nutritional significance, metabolism, and function of myo-inositol and phosphatidylinositol in health and disease. Adv. Nutr. Res. 4:107–141.

Holub, B.J. 1986. Metabolism and function of myo-inositol and inositol phospholipids. Annu. Rev. Nutr. 6:563–597.

Holzbach, R.T. 1984. Animal models of cholesterol gallstone disease. Hepatology 4:191S–198S.

Hoover, G.A., R.J. Nocolosi, J.E. Corey, M. el Lozy, and K.C. Hayes. 1978. Inositol deficiency in the gerbil: altered hepatic lipid metabolism and triglyceride secretion. J. Nutr. 108:1588–1594.

Hoover, K.L., P.H. Lynch, and L.A. Poirier. 1984. Profound postinitiation enhancement by short-term severe methionine, choline, vitamin B12 and folate deficiency of hepatocarcinogenesis in F344 rats given a single low-dose diethylnitrosamine injection. J. Natl. Cancer Inst. 73:1327–1336.

Hopkins, G.J., and K.K. Carroll. 1985. Role of diet in cancer prevention. J. Environ. Pathol. Toxicol. Oncol. 5:279–298.

Hopkins, G.J., and C.E. West. 1976. Possible roles of dietary fats in carcinogenesis. Life Sci. 19:1103–1116.

Horlick, L. 1959. Studies on the regulation of serum-cholesterol levels in man; the effects of corn oil, ethyl stearate, hydrogenated soybean oil, and nicotinic acid when added to a very low-fat basal diet. Lab. Invest. 8:723–735.

Horlick, L. 1960. The effect of artificial modification of food on the serum cholesterol level. Can. Med. Assoc. J. 83: 1186–1192.

Howard, B.V. 1986. Obesity, cholelithiasis, and lipoprotein metabolism in man. Atherosclerosis Rev. 15:169–186.

Howe, G.R. 1985. The use of polytomous dual response data to increase power in case-control studies: an application to the association between dietary fat and breast cancer. J. Chronic Dis. 38:663–670.

Howe, G.R., A.B. Miller, and M. Jain. 1986. Re: "Total energy intake": implications for epidemiologic analyses. Am. J. Epidemiol. 124:157–159.

Howell, J.H., M.E. Marsh, E.S. Thiel, and R.T. Holzbach. 1983. Hepatic microsomal activities of cholesterol 7 alpha-hydroxylase and 3-hydroxy-3-methylglutaryl-CoA reductase in the prairie dog. An animal model for cholesterol gallstone disease. Biochim. Biophys. Acta 753:32–39.

Hoyenga, K.B., and K.T. Hoyenga. 1982. Gender and energy balance: sex differences in adaptations for feast and famine. Physiol. Behav. 28:545–563.

Hubbard, N.E., and K.L. Erickson. 1987. Enhancement of metastasis from a transplantable mouse mammary tumor by dietary linoleic acid. Cancer Res. 47:6171–6175.

Hughson, W.G., J.I. Mann, and A. Garrod. 1978. Intermittent claudication: prevalence and risk factors. Br. Med. J. 1: 1379–1381.

Hulley, S.B., R.H. Rosenman, R.D. Bawol, and R.J. Brand. 1980. Epidemiology as a guide to clinical decisions. The association between triglycerides and coronary heart disease. N. Engl. J. Med. 302:1383–1389.

Hunter, J.E., and T.H. Applewhite. 1986. Isometric fatty acids in the U.S. diet: levels and health perspectives. Am. J. Clin. Nutr. 44:707–717.

Iacono, J.M., R.M. Dougherty, and P. Puska. 1982. Reduction of blood pressure associated with dietary polyunsaturated fat. Hypertension 4:III34–III42.

Ignatovski, A.I. 1908. Influence of animal food on the organism of rabbits. Izv. Imp. Voyenno-Med. Akad. Peter. 16:154–176.

Illingworth, D.R., W.S. Harris, and W.E. Connor. 1984. Inhibition of low density lipoprotein synthesis by dietary omega-3 fatty acids in humans. Arteriosclerosis 4:270–275.

ILSI/NF (International Life Sciences Institute/Nutrition Foundation). 1987. Calories and energy expenditure in carcinogenesis. Proceedings of a symposium, Washington, D.C., February 24 and 25, 1986. Am. J. Clin. Nutr. 45:149–372.

Imai, H., K.T. Lee, S. Pastori, E. Panlilio, R. Florentin, and W.A. Thomas. 1966. Arteriosclerosis in rabbits. Architectural and subcellular alterations of smooth muscle cells of aortas in response to hyperlipemia. Exp. Mol. Pathol. 5: 273–310.

Imai, H., N.T. Werthessen, C.B. Taylor, and K.T. Lee. 1976. Angiotoxicity and atherosclerosis due to contaminants to USP-grade cholesterol. Arch. Pathol. Lab. Med. 100:565–572.

Imai, H., N.T. Werthessen, V. Subramanyam, P.W. LeQuesne, A.H. Soloway, and M. Kanisawa. 1980. Angiotoxicity of oxygenated sterols and possible precursors. Science 207:651–653.

Innis, S.M. 1985. The role of diet during development on the regulation of adult cholesterol homeostasis. Can. J. Physiol. Pharmacol. 63:557–564.

Ip, C. 1987. Fat and essential fatty acid in mammary carcinogenesis. Am. J. Clin. Nutr. 45:218–224.

Ip, C., C.A. Carter, and M.M. Ip. 1985. Requirement of essential fatty acid for mammary tumorigenesis in the rat. Cancer Res. 45:1997–2001.

Ip, C., M.M. Ip, and P. Sylvester. 1986. Relevance of trans fatty acids and fish oil on animal tumorigenesis studies. Prog. Clin. Biol. Res. 222:283–294.

Isacsson, S.O. 1972. Venous occlusion plethysmography in 55-year old men. A population study in Malmo, Sweden. Acta Med. Scand., Suppl. 537:1–62.

Ishikawa, T., N. Fidge, D.S. Thelle, O.H. Forde, and N.E. Miller. 1978. The Tromso Heart Study: serum apolipoprotein AI concentration in relation to future coronary heart disease. Eur. J. Clin. Invest. 8:179–182.

Iso, H., D.R. Jacobs, Jr., D. Wentworth, J.D. Neaton, and J. Cohen. 1988. Relationship of serum cholesterol to risk of different types of stroke: 28th conference on cardiovascular disease epidemiology. CVD Epidemiol. Newsletter (AHA) 43:40.

Italian National Research Council. 1982. Incidence and prediction of coronary heart disease in two Italian rural population samples followed-up for 20 years. Acta Cardiol. 37: 129–145.

Jackson, R.L., J.D. Morrisett, H.J. Pownall, A.M. Gotto, Jr., A. Kamio, H. Imai, R. Tracy, and F.A. Kummerow. 1977. Influence of dietary trans-fatty acids on swine lipoprotein composition and structure. J. Lipid Res. 18:182–190.

Jackson, R.L., O.D. Taunton, J.D. Morrisett, and A.M. Gotto, Jr. 1978. The role of dietary polyunsaturated fat in lowering blood cholesterol in man. Circ. Res. 42:447–453.

Jackson, R.L., M.L. Kashyap, R.L. Barnhart, C. Allen, E. Hogg, and C.J. Glueck. 1984. Influence of polyunsaturated and saturated fats on plasma lipids and lipoproteins in man. Am. J. Clin. Nutr. 39:589–597.

Jacobs, D.R., Jr., J.T. Anderson, and H. Blackburn. 1979. Diet and serum cholesterol: do zero correlations negate the relationship? Am. J. Epidemiol. 110:77–87.

Jain, M., G.M. Cook, F.G. Davis, M.G. Grace, G.H. Howe, and A.B. Miller. 1980. A case-control study of diet and colo-rectal cancer. Int. J. Cancer 26:757–768.

Jain, M.G., L. Harrison, G.R. Howe, and A.B. Miller. 1982. Evaluation of a self-administered dietary questionnaire for use in a cohort study. Am. J. Clin. Nutr. 36:931–935.

Janakidevi, K., K.T. Lee, M. Kroms, H. Imai, and W.A. Thomas. 1984. Mosaicism in female hybrid hares heterozygous for glucose-6-phospate dehydrogenase. VI. Production of monotypism in the aortas of 4 of 10 mosaic hares fed cholesterol oxidation products. Exp. Mol. Pathol. 41:354–362.

Jandacek, R.J., M.R. Webb, and F.H. Mattson. 1977. Effect

of an aqueous phase on the solubility of cholesterol in an oil phase. J. Lipid Res. 18:203–210.

Jensen, O.M., R. MacLennan, and J. Wahrendorf. 1982. Diet, bowel function, fecal characteristics, and large bowel cancer in Denmark and Finland. Nutr. Cancer 4:5–19.

Jensen, R.G., M.M. Hagerty, and K.E. McMahon. 1978. Lipids of human milk and infant formulas: a review. Am. J. Clin. Nutr. 31:990–1016.

Johnson, F.L., R.W. St. Clair, and L.L. Rudel. 1985. Effects of the degree of saturation of dietary fat on the hepatic production of lipoproteins in the African green monkey. J. Lipid Res. 26:403–417.

Johnson, K.G., K. Yano, and H. Kato. 1968. Coronary heart disease in Hiroshima, Japan: a report of a six-year period of surveillance, 1958–1964. Am. J. Public Health 58:1355–1367.

Jokinen, M.P., T.B. Clarkson, and R.W. Prichard. 1985. Animal models in atherosclerosis research. Exp. Mol. Pathol. 42:1–28.

Jones, D.Y., A. Schatzkin, S.B. Green, G. Block, L.A. Brinton, R.G. Ziegler, R. Hoover, and P.R. Taylor. 1987a. Dietary fat and breast cancer in the National Health and Nutrition Examination Survey. I. Epidemiological Follow-up Study. J. Natl. Cancer Inst. 79:465–471.

Jones, D.Y., J.T. Judd, P.R. Taylor, W.S. Campbell, and P.P. Nair. 1987b. Influence of caloric contribution and saturation of dietary fat on plasma lipids in premenopausal women. Am. J. Clin. Nutr. 45:1451–1456.

Joossens, J.V., M.J. Hill, and J. Geboers, eds. 1985. Diet and Human Carcinogenesis: Proceeding of the 3rd Annual Symposium of the European Organization for Cooperation in Cancer Prevention Studies (ECP). International Congress Series No. 685. Excerpta Medica, Amsterdam. 343 pp.

Judd, J.T., M.W. Marshall, and J.J. Canary. 1981. Changes in blood pressure and blood lipids of adult men consuming modified fat diets. Pp. 129–141 in G.R. Beecher, ed. Beltsville Symposia in Agricultural Research, IV. Human Nutrition Research. Allanheld, Osmun, & Co., Totowa, N.J.

Jurkowski, J.J., and W.T. Cave, Jr. 1985. Dietary effects of menhaden oil on the growth and membrane lipid composition of rat mammary tumors. J. Natl. Cancer Inst. 74:1145–1150.

Kagan, A., B.R. Harris, W. Winkerstein, Jr., K.G. Johnson, H. Kato, S.L. Syme, G.G. Rhoads, M.L. Gay, M.Z. Nichaman, H.B. Hamilton, and J. Tillotson. 1974. Epidemiologic studies of coronary heart disease and stroke in Japanese men living in Japan, Hawaii and California: Demographic, physical, dietary and biochemical characteristics. J. Chronic Dis. 27:345–364.

Kagan, A.K, J.S. Popper, and G.G. Rhoads. 1980. Factors related to stroke incidence in Hawaii Japanese men. The Honolulu Heart Study. Stroke 11:14–21.

Kagan, A., D.L. McGee, K. Yano, G.G. Rhoads, and A. Nomura. 1981. Serum cholesterol and mortality in a Japanese-American population: the Honolulu Heart Program. Am. J. Epidemiol. 114:11–20.

Kagan, A., J.S. Popper, G.G. Rhoads, and K. Yano. 1985. Dietary and other risk factors for stroke in Hawaiian Japanese men. Stroke 16:390–396.

Kahn, H.A., J.H. Medalie, H.N. Neufeld, E. Riss, M. Balogh, and J.J. Groen. 1969. Serum cholesterol: its distribution and association with dietary and other variables in a survey of 10,000 men. Isr. J. Med. Sci. 5:1117–1127.

Kanarek, R.B., T.G. Feldman, and C. Hanes. 1981. Patterns of dietary self selection in VMH lesioned rats. Physiol. Behav. 29:337–343.

Kannel, W.B., and T. Gordon. 1982. The search for an optimum serum cholesterol. Lancet 2:374–375.

Kannel, W.B., and D.L. McGee. 1985. Update on some epidemiologic features of intermittent claudication: the Framingham Study. J. Am. Geriatr. Soc. 33:13–18.

Kannel, W.B., and P.A. Wolf. 1983. Epidemiology of cerebrovascular disease. Pp. 1–24 in R.W.R. Russel, ed. Vascular Disease of the Central Nervous System, 2nd ed. Churchill Livingstone, Edinburgh.

Kao, V.C., and R.W. Wissler. 1965. A study of the immunohistochemical localization of serum lipoproteins and other plasma proteins in human atherosclerotic lesions. Exp. Mol. Pathol. 4:465–479.

Karmali, R.A. 1987. Omega-3 fatty acids and cancer: a review. Pp. 222–232 in W.E.M. Lands, ed. Proceedings of the AOCS Short Course on Polyunsaturated Fatty Acids and Eicosanoids. American Oil Chemists' Society, Champaign, Ill.

Karmali, R.A., J. Marsh, and C. Fuchs. 1984. Effect of omega-3 fatty acids on growth of a rat tumor. J. Natl. Cancer Inst. 73:457–461.

Katan, M.B., and A.C. Beynen. 1987. Characteristics of human hypo- and hyperresponders to dietary cholesterol. Am. J. Epidemiol. 125:387–399.

Katan, M.B., A.C. Beynen, J.H. de Vries, and A. Nobels. 1986. Existence of consistent hypo- and hyperresponders to dietary cholesterol in man. Am. J. Epidemiol. 123:221–234.

Katan, M.B., M.A. Berns, J.F. Glatz, J.T. Knuiman, A. Nobels, and J.H. de Vries. 1988. Congruence of individual responsiveness to dietary cholesterol and to saturated fat in humans. J. Lipid Res. 29:883–892.

Kato, H., J. Tillotson, M.Z. Nichaman, G.G. Rhoads, and H.B. Hamilton. 1973. Epidemiologic studies of coronary heart disease and stroke in Japanese men living in Japan, Hawaii and California. Serum lipids and diet. Am. J. Epidemiol. 97:372–385.

Katsouyanni, K., D. Trichopoulos, P. Boyle, E. Xirouchaki, A. Trichopoula, B. Lisseos, S. Vasilaros, and B. MacMahon. 1986. Diet and breast cancer: a case-control study in Greece. Int. J. Cancer 38:815–820.

Katz, E.B., and E.S. Boylan. 1987. Stimulating effect of high polyunsaturated fat diet on lung metastasis from the 13762 mammary adenocarcinoma in female retired breeder rats. J. Natl. Cancer Inst. 79:351–358.

Katz, L.N., and J. Stamler. 1953. Experimental atherosclerosis. Pp. 120–290 in Experimental Atherosclerosis. C.C. Thomas, Springfield, Ill.

Katz, L.N., J. Stamler, and R. Pick. 1958. Nutrition and Atherosclerosis. Lea & Febiger, Philadelphia. 146 pp.

Kennedy, M., P.G. Burstyn, and D.R. Husbands. 1978. Fat induced hypertension in rabbits. 2. The effect of feeding diets containing high concentrations of safflower oil and palm oil. Proc. Nutr. Soc. 37:98A.

Kesten, A.D., and R. Silbowitz. 1942. Experimental atherosclerosis and soya lecithin. Proc. Soc. Exp. Biol. Med. 49:71–73.

Keys, A. 1957. Diet and the epidemiology of coronary heart disease. J. Am. Med. Assoc. 164:1912–1919.

Keys, A. 1963. The role of the diet in human atherosclerosis and its complications. Pp. 263–299 in M. Sandler and G.H. Bourne, eds. Atherosclerosis and Its Origin. Academic Press, New York.

Keys, A. 1965. Dietary survey methods in studies on cardiovascular epidemiology. Voeding 26:464–483.

Keys, A. 1970. Coronary heart disease in seven countries. Circulation Suppl. 41:I1–I211.

Keys, A. 1975. Coronary heart disease—the global picture. Atherosclerosis 22:149–192.

Keys, A. 1980a. Alpha lipoprotein (HDL) cholesterol in the serum and the risk of coronary heart disease and death. Lancet 2:603–606.

Keys, A. 1980b. Seven Countries: A Multivariate Analysis of Death and Coronary Heart Disease. Harvard University Press, Cambridge, Mass. 381 pp.

Keys, A. 1984. Serum cholesterol response to dietary cholesterol. Am. J. Clin. Nutr. 40:351–359.

Keys, A., and J.T. Anderson. 1954. The relationship of the diet to the development of atherosclerosis in man. Pp. 181–197 in Symposium on Atherosclerosis. Publ. No. 338. National Research Council, National Academy of Sciences, Washington, D.C.

Keys, A., and R.W. Parlin. 1966. Serum cholesterol response to changes in dietary lipids. Am. J. Clin. Nutr. 19:175–181.

Keys, A., F. Fidanza, and M.H. Keys. 1955. Further studies on serum cholesterol of clinically healthy men in Italy. Voeding 16:492–498.

Keys, A., J.T. Anderson, and F. Grande. 1957a. "Essential" fatty acids, degree of unsaturation, and effect of corn (maize) oil on the serum-cholesterol level in man. Lancet 1:66–68.

Keys, A., J.T. Anderson, and F. Grande. 1957b. Prediction of serum-cholesterol responses of man to changes in fats in the diet. Lancet 2:959–966.

Keys, A., J.T. Anderson, and F. Grande. 1958a. Effect on serum cholesterol in man of mono-ene fatty acid (oleic acid) in the diet. Proc. Soc. Exp. Biol. Med. 98:387–391.

Keys, A., N. Kimura, A. Kusukawa, B. Bronte-Stewart, N. Larsen, and M.H. Keys. 1958b. Lessons from serum cholesterol studies in Japan, Hawaii and Los Angeles. Ann. Intern. Med. 48:83–94.

Keys, A., J.T. Anderson, and F. Grande. 1959. Serum cholesterol in man: diet fat and intrinsic responsiveness. Circulation 19:201–214.

Keys, A., H.L. Taylor, H. Blackburn, J. Brozek, J.T. Anderson, and E. Simonson. 1963. Coronary heart disease among Minnesota business and professional men followed fifteen years. Circulation 28:381–395.

Keys, A., J.T. Anderson, and F. Grande. 1965a. Serum cholesterol response to changes in the diet. I. Iodine value of dietary fat versus 2S-P. Metabolism 14:747–758.

Keys, A., J.T. Anderson, and F. Grande. 1965b. Serum cholesterol response to changes in the diet. III. Differences among individuals. Metabolism 14:766–775.

Keys, A., J.T. Anderson, and F. Grande. 1965c. Serum cholesterol response to changes in the diet. IV. Particular saturated fatty acids in the diet. Metabolism 14:776–787.

Keys, A., M.J. Karvonen, S. Punsar, A. Menotti, F. Fidanza, and G. Farchi. 1984. HDL serum cholesterol and 24-year mortality of men in Finland. Int. J. Epidemiol. 13:428–435.

Keys, A., C. Aravanis, H. Blackburn, R. Buzina, A.S. Dontas, F. Fidanza, M.J. Karvonen, A. Menotti, S. Nedeljkovic, S. Punsar, and H. Toshima. 1985. Serum cholesterol and cancer mortality in the Seven Countries Study. Am. J. Epidemiol. 121:870–883.

Kidwell, W.R. 1986. Fatty acid growth requirements of normal and neoplastic mammary epithelium. Prog. Clin. Biol. Res. 222:699–706.

Kinlen, L.J. 1982. Meat and fat consumption and cancer mortality: a study of strict religious orders in Britain. Lancet 1:946–949.

Kinsell, L.W., J. Partridge, L. Boling, S. Margen, and G. Michaels. 1952. Dietary modification of serum cholesterol and phospholipid levels. J. Clin. Endocrinol. 12:909–913.

Kinsell, L.W., G.D. Michaels, J.W. Partridge, L.A. Boling, H.E. Balch, and G.C. Cochrane. 1953. Effect upon serum cholesterol and phospholipids of diets containing large amounts of vegetable fat. J. Clin. Nutr. 1:224–231.

Kinsella, J.E., G. Bruckner, J. Mai, and J. Shimp. 1981. Metabolism of trans fatty acids with emphasis on the effects of trans, trans-octadecadienoate on lipid composition, essential fatty acid, and prostaglandins: an overview. Am. J. Clin. Nutr. 34:2307–2318.

Kirkland, R.T., B.S. Keenan, J.L. Probstfield, W. Patsch, T.L. Lin, G.W. Clayton, and W. Insull, Jr. 1987. Decrease in plasma high-density lipoprotein cholesterol levels at puberty in boys with delayed adolescence. Correlation with plasma testosterone levels. J. Am. Med. Assoc. 257:502–507.

Kita, T., Y. Nagano, M. Yokode, K. Ishii, N. Kume, A. Ooshima, H. Yoshida, and C. Kawai. 1987. Proc. Natl. Acad. Sci. U.S.A. 84:5928–5931.

Klasing, S.A., and S.M. Pilch. 1986. Review of Epidemiological and Clinical Evidence on the Role of Omega-3 Fatty Acids in Health and Disease. Quick Response Report #3. Life Sciences Research Office, Federation of American Societies for Experimental Biology, Bethesda, Md. 66 pp.

Klurfeld, D.M., M.M. Weber, and D. Kritchevsky. 1987. Inhibition of chemically induced mammary and colon tumor promotion by caloric restriction in rats fed increased dietary fat. Cancer Res. 47:2759–2762.

Knapp, H.R., I.A. Reilly, P. Alessandrini, and G.A. FitzGerald. 1986. In vivo indexes of platelet and vascular function during fish-oil administration in patients with atherosclerosis. N. Engl. J. Med. 314:937–942.

Knox, E.G. 1977. Foods and diseases. Br. J. Prev. Soc. Med. 31:71–80.

Knudsen, I., ed. 1986. Genetic Toxicology of the Diet. Progress in Clinical and Biological Research, Vol. 206. Alan R. Liss, New York. 351 pp.

Knuiman, J.T., and C.E. West. 1981. HDL-cholesterol in men from thirteen countries. Lancet 2:367–368.

Knuiman, J.T., R.J. Hermus, and J.G. Hautvast. 1980. Serum total and high density lipoprotein (HDL) cholesterol concentrations in rural and urban boys from 16 countries. Atherosclerosis 36:529–537.

Kohlmeier, M., G. Stricker, and G. Schlierf. 1985. Influences of "normal" and "prudent" diets on biliary and serum lipids in healthy women. Am. J. Clin. Nutr. 42:1201–1205.

Kolonel, L.N., J.H. Hankin, J. Lee, S.Y. Chu, A.M. Nomura, and M.W. Hinds. 1981. Nutrient intakes in relation to cancer incidence in Hawaii. Br. J. Cancer 44:332–339.

Kolonel, L.N., C.N. Yoshizawa, and J.H. Hankin. 1988. Diet and prostatic cancer: a case-control study in Hawaii. Am. J. Epidemiol. 127:999–1012.

Komachi, Y. 1977. Recent problems in cerebrovascular accidents: characteristics of stroke in Japan. Nippon Ronen Igakkai Zasshi 14:359–364.

Koo, C., M.E. Wernette-Hammond, and T.L. Innerarity. 1986. Uptake of canine beta-very low density lipoproteins by mouse peritoneal macrophages is mediated by a low density lipoprotein receptor. J. Biol. Chem. 261:11194–11201.

Kort, W.J., I.M. Weijma, A.J. Vergroesen, and D.L. Westbroek. 1987a. Conversion of diets at tumor induction shows the pattern of tumor growth and metastasis of the first given diet. Carcinogenesis 8:611–614.

Kort, W.J., I.M. Weijma, A.M. Bijma, W.P. van Schalkwijk, A.J. Vergroesen, and D.L. Westbroek. 1987b. Omega-3 fatty acids inhibiting the growth of a transplantable rat mammary adenocarcinoma. J. Natl. Cancer Inst. 79:593–599.

Kozarevic, D., B. Pirc, Z. Racic, T.R. Dawber, T. Gordon, and W.J. Zukel. 1976. The Yugoslavia cardiovascular disease study. II. Factors in the incidence of coronary heart disease. Am. J. Epidemiol. 104:133–140.

Kozarevic, D., D. McGee, N. Vojvodic, T. Gordon, Z. Racic, W. Zukel, and T. Dawber. 1981. Serum cholesterol and mortality: the Yugoslavia Cardiovascular Disease Study. Am. J. Epidemiol. 114:21–28.

Kraemer, F.B., M. Greenfield, T.A. Tobey, and G.M. Reaven. 1982. Effects of moderate increases in dietary polyunsaturated:saturated fat on plasma triglyceride and cholesterol levels in man. Br. J. Nutr. 47:259–266.

Kranz, H., D.J. Caddy, A.M. Williams, and W. Gay. 1980. Myasthenic syndrome: effect of choline, plasmapheresis and tests for circulating factor. J. Neurol. Neurosurg. Psychiatry 43:483–488.

Kratzing, C.C., and J.J. Perry. 1971. Hypertension in young rats following choline deficiency in maternal diets. J. Nutr. 101:1657–1661.

Kritchevsky, D. 1982. Trans fatty acid effects in experimental atherosclerosis. Fed. Proc. 41:2813–2817.

Kritchevsky, D. 1983. Influence of trans unsaturated fat on experimental atherosclerosis. Pp. 403–413 in E.G. Perkins and W.J. Visek, eds. Dietary Fats and Health. American Oil Chemists' Society, Champaign, Ill.

Kritchevsky, D. 1986. Fat, calories and fiber. Prog. Clin. Biol. Res. 222:495–515.

Kritchevsky, D. 1988. Cholesterol vehicle in experimental atherosclerosis. A brief review with special reference to peanut oil. Arch. Pathol. Lab. Med. 112:1041–1044.

Kritchevsky, D., and S.A. Tepper. 1965a. Cholesterol vehicle in experimental atherosclerosis. VII. Influence of naturally occurring saturated fats. Med. Pharmacol. Exp. 12:315–320.

Kritchevsky, D., and S.A. Tepper. 1965b. Cholesterol vehicle in experimental atherosclerosis. 8. Effect of a medium chain triglyceride (MCT). Exp. Mol. Pathol. 4:489–499.

Kritchevsky, D., A.W. Moyer, W.C. Tesar, J.B. Logan, R.A. Brown, M.C. Davies, and H.R. Cox. 1954. Effect of cholesterol vehicle in experimental atherosclerosis. Am. J. Physiol. 178:30–32.

Kritchevsky, D., A.W. Moyer, W.C. Tesar, R.F.J. McCandless, J.B. Logan, R.A Brown, and M.E. Englert. 1956. Cholesterol vehicle in experimental atherosclerosis. II. Influence of unsaturation. Am. J. Physiol. 185:279–280.

Kritchevsky, D., S.A. Tepper, D. Vesselinovitch, and R.W. Wissler. 1971. Cholesterol vehicle in experimental atherosclerosis. 11. Peanut oil. Atherosclerosis 14:53–64.

Kritchevsky, D., S.A. Tepper, D. Vesselinovitch, and R.W. Wissler. 1973. Cholesterol vehicle in experimental atherosclerosis. 13. Randomized peanut oil. Atherosclerosis 17:225–243.

Kritchevsky, D., L.M. Davidson, J.J. van der Watt, P.A. Winter, and I. Bersohn. 1974a. Hypercholesterolaemia and atherosclerosis induced in vervet monkeys by cholesterol-free, semisynthetic diets. S. Afr. Med. J. 48:2413–2414.

Kritchevsky, D., L.M. Davidson, I.L. Shapiro, H.K. Kim, M. Kitagawa, S. Malhotra, P.P. Nair, T.B. Clarkson, I. Bersohn, and P.A. Winter. 1974b. Lipid metabolism and experimental atherosclerosis in baboons: influence of cholesterol-free, semi-synthetic diets. Am. J. Clin. Nutr. 27:29–50.

Kritchevsky, D., S.A. Tepper, D.A. Scott, D.M. Klurfeld, D. Vesselinovitch, and R.W. Wissler. 1981. Cholesterol vehicle in experimental atherosclerosis. 18. Comparison of North American, African and South American peanut oils. Atherosclerosis 38:291–299.

Kromhout, D. 1983. Body weight, diet, and serum cholesterol in 871 middle-aged men during 10 years of follow-up (the Zutphen Study). Am. J. Clin. Nutr. 38:591–598.

Kromhout, D., and C. de Lezenne Coulander. 1984. Diet, prevalence and 10-year mortality from coronary heart disease in 871 middle-aged men. The Zutphen Study. Am. J. Epidemiol. 119:733–741.

Kromhout, D., E.B. Bosschieter, and C. de Lezenne Coulander. 1985. The inverse relation between fish consumption and 20-year mortality from coronary heart disease. N. Engl. J. Med. 312:1205–1209.

Kuhnlein, U., D. Bergstrom, and H. Kuhnlein. 1981. Mutagens in feces from vegetarians and non-vegetarians. Mutat. Res. 85:1–12.

Kuksis, A., J.J. Myher, K. Geher, G.J. Jones, J. Shepherd, C.J. Packard, J.D. Morrisett, O.D. Taunton, and A.M. Gotto. 1982. Effect of saturated and unsaturated fat diets on lipid profiles of plasma lipoproteins. Atherosclerosis 41:221–240.

Kune, S., G.A. Kune, and L.F. Watson. 1987. Case-control study of dietary etiological factors: the Melbourne Colorectal Cancer Study. Nutr. Cancer 9:21–42.

Kuo, P.T., K. Hayase, J.B. Kostis, and A.E. Moreyra. 1979. Use of combined diet and colestipol in long-term (7–7½ years) treatment of patients with type II hyperlipoproteinemia. Circulation 59:199–211.

Kushi, L.H., R.A. Lew, F.J. Stare, C.R. Ellison, M. el Lozy, G. Bourke, L. Daly, I. Graham, N. Hickey, R. Mulcahy, and J. Kevaney. 1985. Diet and 20-year mortality from coronary heart disease. The Ireland–Boston Diet–Heart Study. N. Engl. J. Med. 312:811–818.

Kuusi, T., C. Ehnholm, J.K. Huttunen, E. Kostiainen, P. Pietinen, U. Leino, U. Uusitalo, T. Nikkari, J.M. Iacono, and P. Puska. 1985. Concentration and composition of serum lipoproteins during a low-fat diet at two levels of polyunsaturated fat. J. Lipid. Res. 26:360–367.

Kwiterovich, P.O., Jr. 1980. Can an effective fat-modified diet be safely recommended after weaning for infants and children in general? a. Some theoretical and practical considerations of the use of a low-fat diet in childhood. Pp. 375–382 in R.M. Lauer and R.B. Shekelle, eds. Childhood Prevention of Atherosclerosis and Hypertension. Raven Press, New York.

Kwiterovich, P.O., Jr. 1986. Biochemical, clinical, epidemiologic, genetic, and pathologic data in the pediatric age group relevant to the cholesterol hypothesis. Pediatrics 78:349–362.

Lambert, G.F., J.P. Miller, R.T. Olsen, and D.V. Frost. 1958. Hypercholesterolemia and atherosclerosis induced in rabbits by purified high fat rations devoid of cholesterol. Proc. Soc. Exp. Biol. 97:544–549.

Laskarzewski, P., J.A. Morrison, I. deGroot, K.A. Kelly, M.J. Mellies, P. Khoury, and C.J. Glueck. 1979. Lipid and lipoprotein tracking in 108 children over a four-year period. Pediatrics 64:584–591.

Lauer, R.M., W.E. Connor, P.E. Leaverton, M.A. Reiter, and W.R. Clarke. 1975. Coronary heart disease risk factors in school children: the Muscatine Study. J. Pediatr. 86:697–706.

Lawrence, C.M., P. Millac, G.S. Stout, and J.W. Ward. 1980. The use of choline chloride in ataxic disorders. J. Neurol. Neurosurg. Psychiatry 43:452–454.

Lê, M.G., L.H. Moulton, C. Hill, and A. Kramer. 1986. Consumption of dairy produce and alcohol in a case-control study of breast cancer. J. Natl. Cancer Inst. 77:633–636.

Leaf, A., and P.C. Weber. 1988. Cardiovascular effects of n-3 fatty acids. N. Engl. J. Med 318:549–557.

Lee, D.W., C.J. Gilmore, G. Bonorris, H. Cohen, J.W. Marks, M. Cho-Sue, M.S. Meiselman, and L.J. Schoenfield. 1985. Effect of dietary cholesterol on biliary lipids in patients with gallstones and normal subjects. Am. J. Clin. Nutr. 42:414–420.

Lee, K.T., K. Janakidevi, M. Kroms, J. Schmee, and W.A. Thomas. 1985. Mosaicism in female hybrid hares heterozygous for glucose-6-phosphate dehydrogenase. VII. Evidence for selective advantage of one phenotype over the other in ditypic samples from aortas of hares fed cholesterol oxidation products. Exp. Mol. Pathol. 42:71–77.

Lees, A.M., H.Y. Mok, R.S. Lees, M.A. McCluskey, and S.M. Grundy. 1977. Plant sterols as cholesterol-lowering agents: clinical trials in patients with hypercholesterolemia and studies of sterol balance. Atherosclerosis 28:325–338.

Leijd, B. 1980. Cholesterol and bile acid metabolism in obesity. Clin. Sci. 59:203–206.

Leren, P., and O. Haabrekke. 1971. Blood lipids in patients with atherosclerosis obliterans of the lower limbs. Acta Med. Scand. 189:511–513.

Lerman, J., and P.D. White. 1946. Metabolic changes in young people with coronary heart disease. J. Clin. Invest. 25:914.

Leung, M., D.L. Yeung, M.D. Pennell, and J. Hall. 1984. Dietary intakes of preschoolers. J. Am. Diet. Assoc. 84:551–554.

Levy, R.I., and A.N. Klimov. 1987. High density lipoprotein cholesterol (HDL-C) and mortality in U.S.S.R. and U.S. middle-aged men: Collaborative U.S.–U.S.S.R. Mortality Follow-up Study. Arteriosclerosis 7:508a.

Lewis, B. 1958. Effect of certain dietary oils on bile-acid secretion and serum-cholesterol. Lancet 1:1090–1092.

Lewis, B., A. Chait, and G. Sigurdsson. 1978. Serum lipoproteins in four European communities: a quantitative comparison. Eur. J. Clin. Invest. 8:165–173.

Lewis, D.S., G.E. Mott, C.A. McMahan, E.J. Masoro, K.D. Carey, and H.C. McGill, Jr. 1988. Deferred effects of preweaning diet on atherosclerosis in adolescent baboons. Arteriosclerosis 8:274–280.

Lin, D.S., and W.E. Connor. 1980. The long term effects of dietary cholesterol upon the plasma lipids, lipoproteins, cholesterol absorption, and the sterol balance in man: the demonstration of feedback inhibition of cholesterol biosynthesis and increased bile acid excretion. J. Lipid. Res. 21:1042–1052.

Lin, H.J., C. Wang, G. Salen, K.C. Lam, and T.K. Chan. 1983. Sitosterol and cholesterol metabolism in a patient with coexisting phytosterolemia and cholestanolemia. Metabolism 32:126–133.

Lindstedt, S., J. Avigan, D.S. Goodman, J. Sjovall, and D. Steinberg. 1965. The effect of dietary fat on the turnover of cholic acid and on the composition of the biliary bile acids in man. J. Clin. Invest. 44:1754–1765.

Lipid Research Clinics Program. 1984a. The Lipid Research Clinics Coronary Primary Prevention Trial results. I. Reduction in incidence of coronary heart disease. J. Am. Med. Assoc. 251:351–364.

Lipid Research Clinics Program. 1984b. The Lipid Research Clinics Coronary Primary Prevention Trial results. II. The relationship of reduction in incidence of coronary heart disease to cholesterol lowering. J. Am. Med. Assoc. 251:365–374.

Lissner, L., D.A. Levitsky, B.J. Strupp, H.J. Kalkwarf, and D.A. Roe. 1987. Dietary fat and the regulation of energy intake in human subjects. Am. J. Clin. Nutr. 46:886–892.

Little, A., R. Levy, P. Chuaqui-Kidd, and D. Hand. 1985. A double-blind, placebo controlled trial of high-dose lecithin in Alzheimer's disease. J. Neurol. Neurosurg. Psychiatry 48:736–742.

Liu, K., J. Stamler, A. Dyer, J. McKeever, and P. McKeever. 1978. Statistical methods to assess and minimize the role of intra-individual variability in obscuring the relationship between dietary lipids and serum cholesterol. J. Chronic Dis. 31:399–418.

Liu, K., J. Stamler, D. Moss, D. Garside, V. Persky, and I. Soltero. 1979. Dietary cholesterol, fat, and fibre, and colon-cancer mortality. An analysis of international data. Lancet 2:782–785.

Lo, C.W. 1985. Human milk: nutritional properties. Pp. 797–818 in W.A. Walker and J.B. Watkins, eds. Nutrition in Pediatrics: Basic Science and Clinical Application. Little, Brown and Co., Boston.

Löffelholz, K., R. Lindmar, and W. Weide. 1979. The relationship between choline and acetylcholine release in the autonomic nervous system. Pp. 233–241 in A. Barbeau, J.H. Growdon, and R.J. Wurtman, eds. Nutrition and the Brain, Vol. 5. Choline and Lecithin in Brain Disorders. Raven Press, New York.

Lofland, H.B., Jr., T.B. Clarkson, and B.C. Bullock. 1970. Whole body sterol metabolism in squirrel monkeys (*Saimiri sciureus*). Exp. Mol. Pathol. 13:1–11.

Low-Beer, T.S. 1985. Nutrition and cholesterol gallstones. Proc. Nutr. Soc. 44:127–134.

Löwenthal, K. 1925. Cholesterinfütterung bei der Maus. Verh. Dtsch. Pathol. Ges. 20:137–139.

Lubin, F., Y. Wax, and B. Modan. 1986. Role of fat, animal protein, and dietary fiber in breast cancer etiology: a case-control study. J. Natl. Cancer Inst. 77:605–612.

Lubin, J.H., P.E. Burns, W.J. Blot, R.G. Ziegler, A.W. Lees, and J.F. Fraumeni, Jr. 1981. Dietary factors and breast cancer risk. Int. J. Cancer 28:685–689.

MacDonald, M.C., R.L. Kline, and G.J. Mogenson. 1981. Dietary linoleic acid and salt-induced hypertension. Can. J. Physiol. Pharmacol. 59:872–875.

Maciejko, J.J., D.R. Holmes, B.A. Kottke, A.R. Zinsmeister, D.M. Dinh, and S.J. Mao. 1983. Apolipoprotein A-I as a marker of angiographically assessed coronary-artery disease. N. Engl. J. Med. 309:385–389.

Maclennan, R., and O.M. Jensen. 1977. Dietary fibre, transit-time, faecal bacteria, steroids and colon cancer in two Scandinavian populations. Report from the International Agency for Research on Cancer Intestinal Microecology Group. Lancet 2:207–211.

MacPherson, B.R., R.S. Pemsingh, and G.W. Scott. 1987. Experimental cholelithiasis in the ground squirrel. Lab. Invest. 56:138–145.

Macquart-Moulin, G., E. Riboli, J. Cornee, B. Charnay, P. Berthezene, and N. Day. 1986. Case-control study on colorectal cancer and diet in Marseilles. Int. J. Cancer. 38:183–191.

Maggio, C.A., M.R.C. Greenwood, and J.R. Visselli. 1983. The satiety effects of intragastric macronutrient infusions in fatty and lean Zucker rats. Physiol. Behav. 31:367–372.

Mahadevappa, V.G., and B.J. Holub. 1987. Quantitative loss of individual eicosapentaenoyl-relative to arachidonoyl-containing phospholipids in thrombin-stimulated human platelets. J. Lipid Res. 28:1275–1280.

Majerus, P.W., T.M. Connolly, H. Deckmyn, T.S. Ross, T.E. Bross, H. Ishii, V.S. Bansal, and D.B. Wilson. 1986. The metabolism of phosphoinositide-derived messenger molecules. Science 234:1519–1526.

Malinow, M.R. 1983. Experimental models of atherosclerosis regression. Atherosclerosis 48:105–118.

Malmros, H. 1950. The relation of nutrition to health: a statistical study of the effect of the war-time on arteriosclerosis, cardiosclerosis, tuberculosis and diabetes. Acta Med. Scand. Suppl. 246:137–153.

Malmros, H., and G. Wigand. 1957. The effect on serum-cholesterol of diets containing different fats. Lancet 2:1–7.

Malmros, H., and G. Wigand. 1959. Atherosclerosis and deficiency of essential fatty acids. Lancet 2:749–751.

Mann, G.V. 1957. The epidemiology of coronary heart disease. Am. J. Med. 23:463–480.

Mannes, G.A., A. Maier, C. Thieme, B. Wiebecke, and G. Paumgartner. 1986. Relation between the frequency of colorectal adenoma and the serum cholesterol level. N. Engl. J. Med. 315:1634–1638.

Manninen V., M.O. Elo, M.H. Frick, K. Haapa, O.P. Heinonen, P. Heinsalmi, P Helo, J.K. Huttunen, P. Kaitaniemi, P. Koskinen, H. Mäenpää, M. Mälkönen, M. Mänttäri, S. Norola, A. Pasternack, J. Pikkarainen, M. Romo, T. Sjöblom, and E.A. Nikkilä. 1988. Lipid alterations and decline in the incidence of coronary heart disease in the Helsinki Heart Study. J. Am. Med. Assoc. 260:641–651.

Manousos, O., N.E. Day, D. Trichopoulos, F. Gerovassilis, A. Tzonou, and A. Polychronopoulou. 1983. Diet and colorectal cancer: a case-control study in Greece. Int. J. Cancer. 32:1–5.

Marcus, A.J. 1966. The role of lipids in blood coagulation. Adv. Lipid Res. 4:1–37.

Marcus, A.J. 1978. The role of lipids in platelet function: with particular reference to the arachidonic acid pathway. J. Lipid Res. 19:793–826.

Marcus, A.J. 1984. The eicosanoids in biology and medicine. J. Lipid Res. 25:1511–1516.

Marcus, A.J. 1987. Platelet eicosanoid metabolism. Pp. 676–688 in R.W. Coleman, J. Hirsch, V.J. Marder, and E.W. Salzman, eds. Hemostasis and Thrombosis: Basic Principles and Clinical Practice, 2nd ed. J.B. Lippincott, Philadelphia.

Marcus, A.J. 1988a. Eicosanoids: transcellular metabolism. Pp. 129–137 in J.I. Gallin, I.M. Goldstein, and R. Snyderman, eds. Inflammation: Basic Principles and Clinical Correlates. Raven Press, New York.

Marcus, A.J. 1988b. Hemorrhagic disorders: abnormalities of platelet and vascular function. Pp. 1042–1060 in J.B. Wyngaarden and L.H. Smith, Jr., eds. Cecil Textbook of Medicine, 18th ed., Vol. 1. Saunders, Philadelphia.

Margetts, B.M., L.J. Beilin, B.K. Armstrong, R. Vandongen, and K.D. Croft. 1984. Dietary fat intake and blood pressure: a double blind controlled trial of changing polyunsaturated to saturated fat ratio. J. Hypertens. 2:S201–S203.

Marmot, S.G., S.L. Syme, A. Kagan, H. Kato, J.B. Cohen, and J. Belsky. 1975. Epidemiologic studies of coronary heart disease and stroke in Japanese men living in Japan, Hawaii and California: prevalence of coronary and hypertensive heart disease and associated risk factors. Am. J. Epidemiol. 102:514–525.

Marston R., and N. Raper. 1987. Nutrient content of the U.S. food supply. National Food Review (Winter-Spring) 36:18–23.

Martin, M.J., S.B. Hulley, W.S. Browner, L.H. Kuller, and D. Wentworth. 1986. Serum cholesterol, blood pressure, and mortality: implications from a cohort of 361,662 men. Lancet 2:933–936.

Martinez, I., R. Torres, Z. Frias, J.R. Colón, and M. Fernàndez. 1979. Factors associated with adenocarcinomas of the large bowel in Puerto Rico. Pp. 45–52 in J.M. Birch, ed. Advances in Medical Oncology, Research and Education, Vol. III. Epidemiology. Pergamon Press, Oxford.

Mattson, F.H., and S.M. Grundy. 1985. Comparison of effects of dietary saturated, monounsaturated, and polyunsaturated fatty acids on plasma lipids and lipoproteins in man. J. Lipid Res. 26:194–202.

Mattson, F.H., B.A. Erickson, and A.M. Kligman. 1972. Effect of dietary cholesterol on serum cholesterol in man. Am. J. Clin. Nutr. 25:589–594.

Mattson, F.H., E.J. Hollenbach, and A.M. Kligman. 1975. Effect of hydrogenated fat on the plasma cholesterol and triglyceride levels of man. Am. J. Clin. Nutr. 28:726–731.

Mattson, F.H., R.A. Volpenhein, and B.A. Erikson. 1977. Effect of plant sterol esters on the absorption of dietary cholesterol. J. Nutr. 107:1139–1146.

Mattson, F.H., S.M. Grundy, and J.R. Crouse. 1982. Optimizing the effect of plant sterols on cholesterol absorption in man. Am. J. Clin. Nutr. 35:697–700.

McArthur, R.G., D.A. Roncari, J.A. Little, A. Kuksis, J.J. Myher, and L. Marai. 1986. Phytosterolemia and hypercholesterolemia in childhood. J. Pediatr. 108:254–256.

McCarron, D.A., J. Stanton, H. Henry, and C. Morris. 1983. Assessment of nutritional correlates of blood pressure. Ann. Intern. Med. 98:715–719.

McGandy, R.B. 1971. Adolescence and the onset of atherosclerosis. Bull. N.Y. Acad. Med. 47:590–600.

McGandy, R.B., B. Hall, C. Ford, and F.J. Stare. 1972. Dietary regulation of blood cholesterol in adolescent males: a pilot study. Am. J. Clin. Nutr. 25:61–66.

McGee, D.L., D.M. Reed, K. Yano, A. Kagan, and J. Tillotson. 1984. Ten-year incidence of coronary heart disease in the Honolulu Heart Program. Relationship to nutrient intake. Am. J. Epidemiol. 119:667–676.

McGee, D., D. Reed, G. Stemmerman, G. Rhoads, K. Yano, and M. Feinleib. 1985. The relationship of dietary fat and cholesterol to mortality in 10 years: the Honolulu Heart Program. Int. J. Epidemiol. 14:97–105.

McGill, H.C., Jr. 1968a. Fatty streaks in the coronary arteries and aorta. Lab. Invest. 18:560–564.

McGill, H.C., Jr., ed. 1968b. The Geographic Pathology of Atherosclerosis. Williams & Wilkins, Baltimore. 193 pp.

McGill, H.C., Jr. 1979. The relationship of dietary cholesterol to serum cholesterol concentration and to atherosclerosis in man. Am. J. Clin. Nutr. 32:2664–2702.

McGill, H.C., Jr. 1980. Morphologic development of the atherosclerotic plaque. Pp. 41–49 in R.M. Lauer and R.B. Shekelle, eds. Childhood Prevention of Atherosclerosis and Hypertension. Raven Press, New York.

McGill, H.C., Jr. 1984. George Lyman Duff memorial lecture. Persistent problems in the pathogenesis of atherosclerosis. Arteriosclerosis 4:443–451.

McGill, H.C., Jr., J.C. Geer, and J.P. Strong. 1963. Natural history of human atherosclerotic lesions. Pp. 39–65 in M. Sandler and G.H. Bourne, eds. Atherosclerosis and Its Origin. Academic Press, New York.

McGill, H.C., Jr., G.E. Mott, and C.A. Bramblett. 1976. Experimental atherosclerosis in the baboon. Primates Med. 9:41–65.

McGill, H.C., Jr., C.A. McMahan, A.W. Kruski, and G.E. Mott. 1981a. Relationship of lipoprotein cholesterol concentrations to experimental atherosclerosis in baboons. Arteriosclerosis 1:3–12.

McGill, H.C., Jr., C.A. McMahan, A.W. Kruski, J.L. Kelley, and G.E. Mott. 1981b. Responses of serum lipoproteins to dietary cholesterol and type of fat in the baboon. Arteriosclerosis 5:337–344.

McGill, H.C., Jr., C.A. McMahan, and J.D. Wene. 1981c. Unresolved problems in the diet–heart issue. Arteriosclerosis 1:164–176.

McGill, H.C., Jr., K.D. Carey, C.A. McMahan, Y.N. Marinez, T.E. Cooper, G.E. Mott, and C.J. Schwartz. 1985. Effects of two forms of hypertension on atherosclerosis in the hyperlipidemic baboon. Arteriosclerosis 5:481–493.

McLean, J.W., J.E. Tomlinson, W.J. Kuang, D.L. Eaton, E.Y. Chen, G.M. Fless, A.M. Scanu, and R.M. Lawn. 1987. cDNA sequence of human apolipoprotein(a) is homologous to plasminogen. Nature 330:132–137.

McMichael, A.J., O.M. Jensen, D.M. Parkin, and D.G. Zaridze. 1984. Dietary and endogenous cholesterol and human cancer. Epidemiol. Rev. 6:192–216.

McMillan, G.C., B.I. Weigensberg, and A.C. Ritchie. 1960. Effects of dietary fats in rabbits fed cholesterol. Arch. Pathol. 70:220–225.

McNamara, D.J. 1987. Effects of fat-modified diets on cholesterol and lipoprotein metabolism. Annu. Rev. Nutr. 7:273–290.

McNamara, D.J., R. Kolb, T.S. Parker, H. Batwin, P. Samuel, C.D. Brown, and E.H. Ahrens, Jr. 1987. Heterogeneity of cholesterol homeostasis in man. Response to changes in dietary fat quality and cholesterol quantity. J. Clin. Invest. 79:1729–1739.

McOsker, D.E., F.H. Mattson, H.B. Sweringen, and A.M. Kligman. 1962. The influence of partially hydrogenated dietary fats on serum cholesterol levels. J. Am. Med. Assoc. 180:380–385.

McSherry, C.K., N.B. Javitt, J.M. De Carvalho, and F. Glenn. 1971a. Cholesterol gallstones and the chemical composition of bile in baboons. Ann. Surg. 173:569–577.

McSherry, C.K., F. Glenn, and N.B. Javitt. 1971b. Composition of basal and stimulated hepatic bile in baboons, and the formation of cholesterol gallstones. Proc. Natl. Acad. Sci. U.S.A. 68:1564–1568.

Medalie, J.H., H.A. Kahn, H.N. Neufeld, E. Riss, and U. Goldbourt. 1973. Five-year myocardial infarction incidence. II. Association of single variables to age and birthplace. J. Chronic Dis. 26:325–349.

Melchior, G.W., H.B. Lofland, and R.W. St. Clair. 1978. The effect of polyunsaturated fats on bile acid metabolism and cholelithiasis in squirrel monkeys. Metabolism 27:1471–1484.

Mendelsohn, D., L. Mendelsohn, and D.G. Hamilton. 1980. Effect of polyunsaturated fat on atheroma formation in the non-human primate. S. Afr. J. Sci. 76:225–228.

Mensink, R.P., and M.B. Katan. 1987. Effect of monounsaturated fatty acids versus complex carbohydrates on high-density lipoproteins in healthy men and women. Lancet 1:122–125.

Menzel, H.J., R.G. Kladetzky, and G. Assmann. 1983. Apolipoprotein E polymorphism and coronary artery disease. Arteriosclerosis 3:310–315.

Michael, U.F., S.L. Cookson, R. Chavez, and V. Pardo. 1975. Renal function in the choline deficient rat. Proc. Soc. Exp. Biol. Med. 150:672–676.

Miettinen, M., O. Turpeinen, M.J. Karvanon, R. Elosuo, and E. Paavilainen. 1972. Effect of cholesterol-lowering diet on mortality from coronary heart-disease and other causes. A twelve-year clinical trial in men and women. Lancet 2:835–838.

Miettinen, M., O. Turpeinen, M.J. Karvonen, E. Paavilainen, and R. Elosuo. 1976. Prevalence of cholelithiasis in men and women ingesting a serum-cholesterol-lowering diet. Ann. Clin. Res. 8:111–116.

Miettinen, T.A. 1980. Phytosterolaemia, xanthomatosis and premature atherosclerotic arterial disease: a case with high plant sterol absorption, impaired sterol elimination and low cholesterol synthesis. Eur. J. Clin. Invest. 10:27–35.

Mikol, Y.B., K.L. Hoover, D. Creasia, and L.A. Poirier. 1983. Hepatocarcinogenesis in rats fed methyl-deficient, amino acid-defined diets. Carcinogenesis 4:1619–1629.

Miller, A.B., A. Kelly, N.W. Choi, V. Matthews, R.W. Morgan, L. Munan, J.D. Burch, J. Feather, G.R. Howe, and M. Jain. 1978. A study of diet and breast cancer. Am. J. Epidemiol. 107:499–509.

Miller, A.B., G.R. Howe, M. Jain, K.J. Craib, and L. Harrison. 1983. Food items and food groups as risk factors in a case-control study of diet and colo-rectal cancer. Int. J. Cancer 32:155–161.

Miller, D.C., M.F. Trulson, M.B. McCann, P.D. White, and F.J. Stare. 1958. Diet, blood lipids and health of Italian men in Boston. Ann. Intern. Med. 49:1178–1200.

Miller, N.E., D.S. Thelle, O.H. Forde, and O.D. Mjos. 1977. The Tromso Heart-Study. High-density lipoprotein and coronary heart-disease: a prospective case-control study. Lancet 1:965–968.

Milner, J.A., and E.G. Perkins, chairmen. 1984. Papers from the symposium on cancer—a molecular event. J. Am. Oil. Chem. Soc. 61:1881–1918.

Mishkel, M.A., and N. Spritz. 1969. The effects of trans isomerized trilinolein on plasma lipids of man. Pp. 355–364 in W.L. Holmes, L.A. Carlson, and R. Paoletti, eds. Drugs Affecting Lipid Metabolism. Advances in Experimental Medicine and Biology, Vol. 4. Plenum Press, New York.

Mistry, P., N.E. Miller, M. Laker, W.R. Hazzard, and B. Lewis. 1981. Individual variation in the effects of dietary cholesterol on plasma lipoproteins and cellular cholesterol homeostasis in man. Studies of low density lipoprotein receptor activity and 3-hydroxy-3-methylglutaryl coenzyme A reductase activity in blood mononuclear cells. J. Clin. Invest. 67:493–502.

Montaldo, M.B., J.D. Benson, and G.A. Martinez. 1985. Nutrient intakes of formula-fed infants and infants fed cow's milk. Pediatrics 75:343–351.

Moore, M.C., M.A. Guzman, P.E. Schilling, and J.P. Strong. 1976. Dietary-atherosclerosis study on deceased persons. Relation of selected dietary components to raised coronary lesions. J. Am. Diet. Assoc. 68:216–223.

Moore, R.B., J.T. Anderson, H.L. Taylor, A. Keys, and I.D. Frantz, Jr. 1968. Effect of dietary fat on the fecal excretion of cholesterol and its degradation products in man. J. Clin. Invest. 47:1517–1534.

Mori, T.A., J.P. Codde, R. Vandongen, and L.J. Beilin. 1987. New findings in the fatty acid composition of individual platelet phospholipids in man after dietary fish oil supplementation. Lipids 22:744–750.

Moritz, V., P. Singer, D. Forster, I. Bergen, and S. Massow. 1985. Changes of blood pressure in spontaneously hypertensive rats dependent on the quantity and quality of fat intake. Biomed. Biochim. Acta 44:1491–1505.

Morris, D.L., N.O. Borhani, E. Fitzsimmons, R.J. Hardy, C.M. Hawkins, J.F. Kraus, D.R. Labarthe, L. Mastbaum, and G.H. Payne. 1983. Serum cholesterol and cancer in the Hypertension Detection and Follow-up Program. Cancer 52:1754–1759.

Morris, J.N., J.W. Marr, and D.G. Clayton. 1977. Diet and heart: a postscript. Br. Med. J. 2:1307–1314.

Morrison, J.A., I. deGroot, K.A. Kelly, B.K. Edwards, M.J. Mellies, S. Tillett, P. Khoury, and C.J. Glueck. 1979a. High and low density lipoprotein cholesterol levels in hypercholesterolemic school children. Lipids 14:99–104.

Morrison, J.A., P.M. Laskarzewski, J.L. Rauh, R. Brookman, M. Mellies, M. Frazer, P. Khoury, I. deGroot, K. Kelly, and C.J. Glueck. 1979b. Lipids, lipoproteins, and sexual maturation during adolescence: the Princeton maturation study. Metabolism 28:641–649.

Morrison, J.A., R. Larsen, L. Glatfelter, D. Boggs, K. Burton, C. Smith, K. Kelly, M.J. Mellies, P. Khoury, and C.J. Glueck. 1980. Interrelationships between nutrient intake and plasma lipids and lipoproteins in schoolchildren aged 6 to 19: the Princeton School District Study. Pediatrics 65:727–734.

Morrison, L.M. 1958. Serum cholesterol reduction with lecithin. Geriatrics 13:12–19.

Morrison, L.M., L. Hall, and A.L. Chaney. 1948. Cholesterol metabolism: blood serum cholesterol and ester levels in 200 cases of acute coronary thrombosis. Am. J. Med. Sci. 216:32–38.

Mott, G.E., C.A. McMahan, and H.C. McGill, Jr. 1978. Diet and sire effects on serum cholesterol and cholesterol absorption in infant baboons (Papio cynocephalus). Circ. Res. 43:364–371.

Mott, G.E., C.A. McMahan, J.L. Kelly, C.M. Farley, and H.C. McGill, Jr. 1982. Influence of infant and juvenile diets on serum cholesterol, lipoprotein cholesterol, and apolipoprotein concentrations in juvenile baboons (Papio sp.). Atherosclerosis 45:191–202.

MRFIT (Multiple Risk Factor Intervention Trial) Research Group. 1982. Multiple Risk Factor Intervention Trial: risk factor changes and mortality results. J. Am. Med. Assoc. 248:1465–1477.

Murray, C.D., K.T. Lee, W.A. Thomas, J.M. Reiner, and K. Janakidevi. 1981. Mosaicism in female hybrid hares heterozygous for glucose-6-phosphate dehydrogenase (G-6-PD). III. Changes in the ratios of G-6-PD types in skin fibroblast cultures exposed to 25-hydroxycholesterol. Exp. Mol. Pathol. 34:209–215.

Murray, G.E., R. Nair, and J. Patrick. 1986. The effect of dietary polyunsaturated fat on cation transport and hypertension in the rat. Br. J. Nutr. 56:587–593.

Murray, W.R., A. Backwood, J.M. Trotter, K.C. Calman, and C. MacKay. 1980. Faecal bile acids and clostridia in the aetiology of colorectal cancer. Br. J. Cancer 41:923–928.

Myher, J.J., L. Marai, and A. Kuksis. 1977. Acylglycerol structure of peanut oils of different atherogenic potential. Lipids 12:775–785.

Nagase, M., H. Tanimura, M. Setoyama, and Y. Hikasa. 1978. Present features of gallstones in Japan. A collective review of 2,144 cases. Am. J. Surg. 135:788–790.

Nair, P.P., N. Turjman, G.T. Goodman, C. Guidry, and B.M. Calkins. 1984. Diet, nutrition intake, and metabolism in populations at high and low risk for colon cancer. Metabolism of neutral sterols. Am. J. Clin. Nutr. 40:931–936.

Naito, H.K. 1985. The association of serum lipids, lipoproteins, and apolipoproteins with coronary artery disease assessed by coronary arteriography. Ann. N.Y. Acad. Sci. 454:230–238.

Nash, D.T., G. Gensini, and P. Esente. 1982. Effect of lipid-lowering therapy on the progression of coronary atherosclerosis assessed by scheduled repetitive coronary arteriography. Int. J. Cardiol. 2:43–55.

National Cholesterol Education Program. 1988. Report of the National Cholesterol Education Program Expert Panel on Detection, Evaluation, and Treatment of High Blood Cholesterol in Adults. 1988. Arch. Intern. Med. 148:36–69.

National Diet–Heart Study Research Group. 1968. The National Diet–Heart Study Final Report. Chapter XVII: Faribault Second Study. Circulation 37:I260–I274.

Nauss, K.M., L.R. Jacobs, and P.M. Newberne. 1987. Dietary fat and fiber: relationship to caloric intake, body growth, and colon tumorigenesis. Am. J. Clin. Nutr. 45:243–251.

Neaton, J.D., L.H. Kuller, D. Wentworth, and N.O. Borhani. 1984. Total and cardiovascular mortality in relation to cigarette smoking, serum cholesterol concentration, and diastolic blood pressure among black and white males followed up for five years. Am. Heart J. 108:759–769.

Nestel, P.J. 1987. Polyunsaturated fatty acids (n-3, n-6). Am. J. Clin. Nutr. 45:1161–1167.

Nestel, P.J., N. Havenstein, H.M. Whyte, T.J. Scott, and L.J. Cook. 1973. Lowering of plasma cholesterol and enhanced sterol excretion with the consumption of polyunsaturated ruminant fats. N. Engl. J. Med. 288:379–382.

Nestel, P.J., N. Havenstein, Y. Homma, T.W. Scott, and L.J. Cook. 1975. Increased sterol excretion with polyunsaturated-fat high-cholesterol diets. Metabolism 24:189–198.

Nestel, P.J., A. Poyser, and T.J. Boulton. 1979. Changes in cholesterol metabolism in infants in response to dietary cholesterol and fat. Am. J. Clin. Nutr. 32:2177–2182.

Nestel, P.J., W.E. Connor, M.F. Reardon, S. Connor, S. Wong, and R. Boston. 1984. Suppression by diets rich in fish oil of very low density lipoprotein production in man. J. Clin. Invest. 74:82–89.

Neugat, A.I., C.M. Johnsen, and D.J. Fink. 1986. Serum cholesterol levels in adenomatous polyps and cancer of the colon. A case-control study. J. Am. Med. Assoc. 255:365–367.

Neuringer, M., and W.E. Connor. 1986. N-3 fatty acids in the brain and retina: evidence for essentiality. Nutr. Rev. 44:285–294.

Newberne, P.M., and K.M. Nauss. 1986. Dietary fat and colon cancer: variable results in animal models. Prog. Clin. Biol. Res. 222:311–330.

Newberne, P.M., and A.E. Rogers. 1986. Labile methyl groups and the promotion of cancer. Annu. Rev. Nutr. 6: 407–432.

Newman, W.P., III, D.S. Freedman, A.W. Voors, P.D. Gard, S.R. Srinivasan, J.L. Cresanta, G.D. Williamson, L.S. Webber, and G.S. Berenson. 1986. Relation of serum lipoprotein levels and systolic blood pressure to early atherosclerosis. The Bogalusa Heart Study. N. Engl. J. Med. 314: 138–144.

NHLBI (National Heart, Lung, and Blood Institute). 1971. Arteriosclerosis: A Report by the National, Heart, Lung and Blood Task Force on Arteriosclerosis, Vol. 1. DHEW Publ. No. (NIH) 72-219. National Institutes of Health, Public Health Service, U.S. Department of Health, Education, and Welfare, Bethesda, Md. 365 pp.

NHLBI (National Heart, Lung, and Blood Institute). 1978. Cardiovascular Profile of 15,000 Children of School Age in Three Communities 1971–1975. DHEW Publ. No. (NIH) 78-1472. National Institutes of Health, Public Health Service, U.S. Department of Health, Education, and Welfare, Bethesda, Md. 806 pp.

NHLBI (National Heart, Lung, and Blood Institute). 1980. The Lipid Research Clinics Population Studies Data Book, Vol. I. The Prevalence Study: Aggregate Distributions of Lipids, Lipoproteins and Selected Variables in 11 North American Populations. NIH Publ. No. 80-1527. National Institutes of Health, Public Health Service, U.S. Department of Health and Human Services, Bethesda, Md. 136 pp.

Nichaman, M.Z., H.B. Hamilton, A. Kagan, T. Grier, T. Sacks, and S.L. Syme. 1975. Epidemiologic studies of coronary heart disease and stroke in Japanese men living in Japan, Hawaii and California: distribution of biochemical risk factors. Am. J. Epidemiol. 102:491–501.

Nichols, A.B., C. Ravenscroft, D.E. Lamphiear, and L.D. Ostrander, Jr. 1976. Daily nutritional intake and serum lipid levels. The Tecumseh Study. Am. J. Clin. Nutr. 29:1384–1392.

NIH (National Institutes of Health). 1984. Treatment of hypertriglyceridemia: consensus conference. J. Am. Med. Assoc. 251:1196–1200.

NIH (National Institutes of Health). 1985. Lowering blood cholesterol to prevent heart disease: consensus conference. J. Am. Med. Assoc. 253:2080–2086.

Nikkila, E.A., P. Viikinkoski, M. Valle, and M.H. Frick. 1984. Prevention of progression of coronary atherosclerosis by treatment of hyperlipidaemia: a seven year prospective angiographic study. Br. Med. J. 289:220–223.

Nomura, A., B.E. Henderson, and J. Lee. 1978. Breast cancer and diet among the Japanese in Hawaii. Am. J. Clin. Nutr. 31:2020–2025.

Nomura, A.M., T.D. Wilkins, S. Kamiyama, L.K. Heilbrun, A. Shimada, G.N. Stemmerman, and H.F. Mower. 1983. Fecal neutral steroids in two Japanese populations with different colon cancer risks. Cancer Res. 43:1910–1913.

NRC (National Research Council). 1980. Recommended Dietary Allowances, 9th ed. Report of the Committee on Dietary Allowances, Food and Nutrition Board, Division of Biological Sciences, Assembly of Life Sciences. National Academy Press, Washington, D.C. 185 pp.

NRC (National Research Council). 1982. Diet, Nutrition, and Cancer. Report of the Committee on Diet, Nutrition, and Cancer, Assembly of Life Sciences. National Academy Press, Washington, D.C. 478 pp.

O'Connor, T.P., B.D. Roebuck, F. Peterson, and T.C. Campbell. 1985. Effect of dietary intake of fish oil and fish protein on the development of L-azaserine-induced preneoplastic lesions in the rat pancreas. J. Natl. Cancer Inst. 75: 959–962.

O'Connor, T.P., B.D. Roebuck, and T.C. Campbell. 1987. Effect of varying dietary omega-3:omega-6 fatty acid ratio on L-azaserine induced preneoplastic development in rat pancreas. Pp. 238–240 in W.E.M. Lands, ed. Proceedings of the AOCS Short Course on Polyunsaturated Fatty Acids and Eicosanoids. American Oil Chemists' Society, Champaign, Ill.

Oh, S.Y., and L.T. Miller. 1985. Effect of dietary egg on variability of plasma cholesterol levels and lipoprotein cholesterol. Am. J. Clin. Nutr. 42:421–431.

Oh, S.Y., and P.A. Monaco. 1985. Effect of dietary cholesterol and degree of fat unsaturation on plasma lipid levels, lipoprotein composition, and fecal steroid excretion in normal young adult men. Am. J. Clin. Nutr. 42:399–413.

Oliver, M.F., and G.S. Boyd. 1953. Changes in the plasma lipids during the menstrual cycle. Clin. Sci. 12:217–222.

Onitiri, A.C., and E. Jover. 1980. Comparative serum apolipoprotein studies in ischaemic heart disease and control subjects. Clin. Chim. Acta 108:25–30.

Orchard, T.J., R.P. Donahue, L.H. Kuller, P.N. Hodge, and A.L. Drash. 1983. Cholesterol screening in childhood: does it predict adult hypercholesterolemia? The Beaver County experience. J. Pediatr. 103:687–691.

Oster, P., L. Arab, B. Schellenberg, C.C. Hueck, R. Mordasini, and G. Schlierf. 1979. Blood pressure and adipose tissue linoleic acid. Res. Exp. Med. 175:287–291.

Ostfeld, A.M., R.B. Shekelle, H. Klawans, and H.M. Tufo. 1974. Epidemiology of stroke in an elderly welfare population. Am. J. Public Health 64:450–458.

Osuga, T., and O.W. Portman. 1971. Experimental formation of gallstones in the squirrel monkey. Proc. Soc. Exp. Biol. Med. 136:722–726.

Osuga, T., and O.W. Portman. 1972. Relationship between bile composition and gallstone formation in squirrel monkeys. Gastroenterology 63:122–133.

Osuga, T., O.W. Portman, K. Matamura, and M. Alexander. 1974. A morphologic study of gallstone development in the squirrel monkey. Lab. Invest. 30:486–493.

Osuga, T., O.W. Portman, N. Tanaka, M. Alexander, and A.J. Ochsner III. 1976. The effect of diet on hepatic bile formation and bile acid metabolism in squirrel monkeys with and without cholesterol gallstones. J. Lab. Clin. Med. 88: 649–661.

Packard, C.J., L. McKinney, K. Carr, and J. Shepherd. 1983. Cholesterol feeding increases low density lipoprotein synthesis. J. Clin. Invest. 72:45–51.

Parks, J.S., and L.L. Rudel. 1982. Different kinetic fates of apolipoproteins A-I and A-II from lymph chylomicra of nonhuman primates. Effect of saturated versus polyunsaturated dietary fat. J. Lipid Res. 23:410–421.

Paul, O., M.H. Lepper, W.H. Phelan, G.W. Dupertuis, A. MacMillan, H. McKean, and H. Park. 1963. A longitudinal study of coronary heart disease. Circulation 28:20–31.

Pearce, M.L., and S. Dayton. 1971. Incidence of cancer in men on a diet high in polyunsaturated fat. Lancet 1:464–467.

Peckham, S.C., C. Entenman, and H.W. Carroll. 1962. The influence of a hypercaloric diet on gross body and adipose tissue composition in the rat. J. Nutr. 77:187–197.

Peng, S.K., C.B. Taylor, P. Tham, N.T. Werthessen, and B. Mikkelson. 1978. Effect of auto-oxidation products from cholesterol on aortic smooth muscle cells: an in vitro study. Arch. Pathol. Lab. Med. 102:57–61.

Peng, S.K., P. Tham, C.B. Taylor, and B. Mikkelson. 1979. Cytotoxicity of oxidation derivatives of cholesterol on cultured aortic smooth muscle cells and their effect on cholesterol biosynthesis. Am. J. Clin. Nutr. 32:1033–1042.

Perkins, E.G., and W.J. Wisek, eds. 1983. Dietary Fats and Health. American Oil Chemists' Society, Champaign, Ill. 978 pp.

Peterson, B., and E. Trell. 1983. Premature mortality in middle-aged men: Serum cholesterol as risk factor. Klin. Wochenschr. 61:795–801.

Peterson, D.W., C.W. Nichols, Jr., N.F. Peek, and I.L. Chaikoff. 1959. Depression of plasma cholesterol in human subjects consuming butter containing soy sterols. Fed. Proc. 15:569.

Petersson, B., and E. Trell. 1983. Raised serum urate concentration as risk factor for premature mortality in middle-aged men: relation to death from cancer. Br. Med. J. 287:7–9.

Phillips, R.L. 1975. Role of life-style and dietary habits in risk of cancer among Seventh-Day Adventists. Cancer. Res. 35: 3513–3522.

Phillips, R.L., F.R. Lemon, W.L. Beeson, and J.W. Kuzma. 1978. Coronary heart disease mortality among Seventh-Day Adventists with differing dietary habits: a preliminary report. Am. J. Clin. Nutr. 31:S191–S198.

Phillipson, B.E., D.W. Rothrock, W.E. Connor, W.S. Harris, and D.R. Illingworth. 1985. Reduction of plasma lipoproteins, and apoproteins by dietary fish oils in patients with hypertriglyceridemia. N. Engl. J. Med. 312:1210–1216.

Picciano, M.F., H.A. Guthrie, and D.M. Sheehe. 1978. The cholesterol content of human milk. A variable constituent among women and within the same woman. Clin. Pediatr. 17:359–362.

Pilger, E., H. Pristautz, K.P. Pfeiffer, and G. Kostner. 1983. Risk factors for peripheral atherosclerosis. Retrospective evaluation by stepwise discriminant analysis. Arteriosclerosis 3:57–63.

Pitas, R.E., T.L. Innerarity, and R.W. Mahley. 1983. Foam cells in explants of atherosclerotic rabbit aortas have receptors for beta-very low density lipoproteins and modified low density lipoproteins. Arteriosclerosis 3:2–12.

Pocock, S.J., A.G. Shaper, A.N. Phillips, M. Walker, and T.P. Whitehead. 1986. HDL cholesterol is not a major risk factor for ischaemic heart disease in British men. Br. Med. J. 292:515–519.

Poindexter, C.A., and M. Bruger. 1938. Cholesterol content of the blood in heart disease. Arch. Intern. Med. 61:714–719.

Poirier, L.A., P.M. Newberne, and M.W. Pariza. 1987. Essential Nutrients in Carcinogenesis. Advances in Experimental Medicine and Biology, Vol. 206. Plenum Publishing Company, New York. 562 pp.

Pomeranze, J. 1961. Serum cholesterol studies in infants. A comparison of infants fed breast milk, evaporated milk and prepared milk formulas. Am. J. Clin. Nutr. 9:570–572.

Pooling Project Research Group. 1978. Relationship of blood pressure, serum cholesterol, smoking habit, relative weight and ECG abnormalities to incidence of major coronary events: final report of the Pooling Project. J. Chronic Dis. 31:201–306.

Porikos, K.P., G. Booth, and T.B. Van Itallie. 1977. Effect of covert nutritive dilution on the spontaneous food intake of obese individuals: a pilot study. Am. J. Clin. Nutr. 30: 1638–1644.

Portman, O.W., and S.B. Andrus. 1965. Comparative evaluation of three species of new world monkeys for studies of dietary factors, tissue lipids, and atherogenesis. J. Nutr. 87: 429–438.

Potter, J.D., and A.J. McMichael. 1986. Diet and cancer of the colon and rectum: a case-control study. J. Natl. Cancer Inst. 76:557–569.

Pownall, H.J., J. Shepherd, W.W. Mantulin, L.A. Sklar, and A.M. Gotto, Jr. 1980. Effect of saturated and polyunsaturated fat diets on the composition and structure of human low density lipoproteins. Atherosclerosis 36:299–314.

Prentice, R.L., F. Kakar, S. Hursting, L. Sheppard, R. Klein, and L.H. Kushi. 1988. Aspects of the rationale for the women's health trial. J. Natl. Cancer Inst. 80:802–814.

Puska, P., E. Vartiainen, U. Pallonen, J.T. Salonen, P. Poyhia, K. Koskela, and A. McAlister. 1982. The North Karelia Youth Project: evaluation of two years of intervention on health behavior and CVD risk factors among 13- to 15-year old children. Prev. Med. 11:550–570.

Puska, P., J.M. Iacono, A. Nissinen, H.J. Korhonen, E. Vartianinen, P. Pietinen, R. Dougherty, U. Leino, M. Mutanen, S. Moisio, and J. Huttunen. 1983. Controlled, randomized trial of the effect of dietary fat on blood pressure. Lancet 1:1–5.

Puska, P., J.M. Iacono, A. Nissinen, E. Vartiainen, R. Dougherty, P. Pietinen, U. Leino, U. Uusitalo, T. Kuusi, E. Kostiainen, T. Nikkari, E. Seppälä, H. Vapaatalo, and J.K. Huttunen. 1985. Dietary fat and blood pressure: an intervention study on the effects of a low-fat diet with two levels of polyunsaturated fat. Prev. Med. 14:573–584.

Rampone, A.J., and C.M. Machida. 1981. Mode of action of lecithin in suppressing cholesterol absorption. J. Lipid Res. 22:744–752.

Rao, R.H., U.B. Rao, and S.G. Srikantia. 1981. Effect of polyunsaturate-rich vegetable oils on blood pressure in essential hypertension. Clin. Exper. Hypertens. 3:27–38.

Rasanen, L., M. Wilska, R.L. Kantero, V. Nanto, A. Ahlstrom, and N. Hallman. 1978. Nutrition survey of Finnish rural children. IV. Serum cholesterol values in relation to dietary variables. Am. J. Clin. Nutr. 31:1050–1056.

Reddy, B.S. 1986a. Amount and type of dietary fat and colon cancer: animal model studies. Prog. Clin. Biol. Res. 222: 295–309.

Reddy, B.S. 1986b. Diet and colon cancer: evidence from human and animal model studies. Pp. 47–65 in B.S. Reddy and L.A. Cohen, eds. Diet, Nutrition, and Cancer: A Critical Evaluation, Vol. I. Macronutrients and Cancer. CRC Press, Boca Raton, Fla.

Reddy, B.S. 1987. Dietary fat and colon cancer: effect of fish oil. Pp. 233–237 in W.E.M. Lands, ed. Proceedings of the AOCS Short Course on Polyunsaturated Fatty Acids and Eicosanoids. American Oil Chemists' Society. Champaign, Ill.

Reddy, B.S., and L.A. Cohen, eds. 1986a. Diet, Nutrition, and Cancer: A Critical Evaluation, Vol. I. Macronutrients and Cancer. CRC Press, Boca Raton, Fla. 175 pp.

Reddy, B.S., and L.A. Cohen, eds. 1986b. Diet, Nutrition, and Cancer: A Critical Evaluation, Vol. II. Micronutrients, Nonnutritive Dietary Factors, and Cancer. CRC Press, Boca Raton, Fla. 181 pp.

Reddy, B.S., and Y. Maeura. 1984. Tumor promotion by

dietary fat in azoxymethane-induced colon carcinogenesis in female F344 rats: influence of amount and source of dietary fat. J. Natl. Cancer Inst. 72:745–750.

Reddy, B.S., and E.L. Wynder. 1977. Metabolic epidemiology of colon cancer. Fecal bile acids and neutral sterols in colon cancer patients and patients with adenomatous polyps. Cancer 39:2533–2539.

Reddy, B.S., A.R. Hedges, K. Laakso, and E.L. Wynder. 1978. Metabolic epidemiology of large bowel cancer: fecal bulk and constituents of high-risk North American and low-risk Finnish population. Cancer 42:2832–2838.

Reddy, B.S., B. Hanson, S. Mangat, L. Mathews, M. Sbaschnig, C. Sharma, and B. Simi. 1980a. Effect of high-fat, high-beef diet and of mode of cooking of beef in the diet on fecal bacterial enzymes and fecal bile acids and neutral sterols. J. Nutr. 110:1880–1887.

Reddy, B.S., C. Sharma, L. Darby, K. Laakso, and E.L. Wynder. 1980b. Metabolic epidemiology of large bowel cancer. Fecal mutagens in high- and low-risk population for colon cancer. A preliminary report. Mutat. Res. 72:511–522.

Reddy, B.S., G. Ekelund, M. Bohe, A. Engle, and L. Domellof. 1983. Metabolic epidemiology of colon cancer: dietary pattern and fecal sterol concentrations of three populations. Nutr. Cancer 5:34–40.

Reddy, B.S., T. Tanaka, and B. Simi. 1985. Effect of different levels of dietary *trans* fat or corn oil on azoxymethane-induced colon carcinogenesis in F344 rats. J. Natl. Cancer Inst. 75:791–798.

Reddy, B.S., C.X. Wang, and H. Maruyama. 1987. Effect of restricted caloric intake on azoxymethane-induced colon tumor incidence in male F344 rats. Cancer Res. 47:1226–1228.

Reed, D., K. Yano, and A. Kagan. 1986. Lipids and lipoproteins as predictors of coronary heart disease, stroke, and cancer in the Honolulu Heart Program. Am. J. Med. 80:871–878.

Reed, D.M., C.J. MacLean, and T. Hayashi. 1987. Predictors of atherosclerosis in the Honolulu Heart Program. I. Biologic, dietary, and lifestyle characteristics. Am. J. Epidemiol. 126:214–225.

Reed, D., R.J. Contreras, C. Maggio, M.R.C. Greenwood, and J. Rodin. 1988. Weight cycling in female rats increases dietary fat selection and adiposity. Physiol. Behav. 42:389–395.

Reed, T., D.K. Wagner, R.P. Donahue, and L.H. Kuller. 1986. Family history of cancer related to cholesterol level in young adults. Genet. Epidemiol. 3:63–71.

Reisen, W.F., R. Mordasini, C. Salzmann, A. Theler, and H.P. Gurtner. 1980. Apoproteins and lipids as discriminators of severity of coronary heart disease. Atherosclerosis 37:157–162.

Reiser, R., and Z. Sidelman. 1972. Control of serum cholesterol homeostasis by cholesterol in the milk of the suckling rat. J. Nutr. 102:1009–1016.

Reiser, R., B.C. O'Brien, G.R. Henderson, and R.W. Moore. 1979. Studies on a possible function for cholesterol in milk. Nutr. Rep. Int. 19:835–849.

Reiser, R., J.L. Probstfield, A. Silvers, L.W. Scott, M.L. Shorney, R.D. Wood, B.C. O'Brien, A.M. Gotto, Jr., and W. Insull, Jr. 1985. Plasma lipid and lipoprotein response of humans to beef fat, coconut oil and safflower oil. Am. J. Clin. Nutr. 42:190–197.

Renaud, S., K. Kuba, C. Goulet, Y. Lemire, and C. Allard. 1970. Relationship between fatty acid composition of platelets and platelet aggregation in the rat and man. Relation to thrombosis. Circ. Res. 26:553–561.

Renaud, S., R. Morazain, F. Godsey, C. Thevenon, J. Martin, and F. Mendy. 1986. Nutrients, platelet function and composition in nine groups of French and British farmers. Atherosclerosis 60:37–48.

Reunanen, A., H. Takkunen, and A. Aromaa. 1982. Prevalence of intermittent claudication and its effect on mortality. Acta Med. Scand. 211:249–256.

Rhoads, G.G., W.C. Blackwelder, G.N. Stemmerman, T. Hayashi, and A. Kagan. 1978. Coronary risk factors and autopsy findings in Japanese-American men. Lab. Invest. 38:304–311.

Rickert, R.R., K.G. Johnson, H. Kato, T. Yamamoto, and K. Yano. 1968. Atherosclerosis in a defined Japanese population: a clinicopathologic appraisal. Am. J. Clin. Pathol. 49:371–386.

Risch, H.A., J.D. Burch, A.B. Miller, G.B. Hill, R. Steele, and G.R. Howe. 1988. Dietary factors and the incidence of cancer of the urinary bladder. Am. J. Epidemiol. 127:1179–1191.

Roberts, J.C., Jr., and R. Straus, eds. 1965. Comparative Atherosclerosis; the Morphology of Spontaneous and Induced Atherosclerotic Lesions in Animals and Its Relation to Human Disease, by 56 Authors. Harper & Row, New York. 426 pp.

Robertson, F.W., and A.M. Cumming. 1985. Effects of apoprotein E polymorphism on serum lipoprotein concentration. Arteriosclerosis 5:283–292.

Robertson, T.L., H. Kato, G.G. Rhoads, A. Kagan, M. Marmot, S.L. Syme, T. Gordon, R.M. Worth, J.L. Belsky, D.S. Dock, M. Miyanishi, and S. Kawamoto. 1977. Epidemiologic studies of coronary heart disease and stroke in Japanese men living in Japan, Hawaii and California. Am. J. Cardiol. 39:239–243.

Robertson, W.B., J.C. Geer, J.P. Strong, and H.C. McGill, Jr. 1963. The fate of the fatty streak. Exp. Mol. Pathol. 2 Suppl. 1:28–39.

Robins, S.J., and J. Fasulo. 1973. Mechanism of lithogenic bile production: studies in the hamster fed an essential fatty acid-deficient diet. Gastroenterology 65:104–114.

Robison, R.L., K.C. Hayes, H.L. McCombs, and T.P. Faherty. 1971. Effect of dietary fat and cholesterol on circulating lipids and aortic ultrastructure of squirrel monkeys. Exp. Mol. Pathol. 15:281–303.

Roe, D.A., ed. 1983. Diet, Nutrition, and Cancer: From Basic Research to Policy Implications. Current Topics in Nutrition and Disease, Vol. 9. Alan R. Liss, New York. 294 pp.

Roebuck, B.D., D.S. Longnecker, K.J. Baumgartner, and C.D. Thron. 1985. Carcinogen-induced lesions in the rat pancreas: effects of varying levels of essential fatty acid. Cancer Res. 45:5252–5256.

Rogers, A.E., and S.Y. Lee. 1986. Chemically-induced mammary gland tumors in rats: modulation by dietary fat. Prog. Clin. Biol. Res. 222:255–282.

Rogers, A.E., B. Connor, C. Boulanger, and S. Lee. 1986. Mammary tumorigenesis in rats fed diets high in lard. Lipids 21:275–280.

Rohan, T.E., A.J. McMichael, and P.A. Baghurst. 1988. A population-based case-control study of diet and breast cancer in Australia. Am. J. Epidemiol. 128:478–489.

Romieu, I., W.C. Willett, M.J. Stampfer, G.A. Colditz, L. Sampson, B. Rosner, C.H. Hennekens, and F.E. Speizer.

1988. Energy intake and other determinants of relative weight. Am. J. Clin. Nutr. 47:406–412.

Rose, G. 1982. Incubation period of coronary heart disease. Br. Med. J. 284:1600–1601.

Rose, G., and M.J. Shipley. 1980. Plasma lipids and mortality: a source of error. Lancet 1:523–526.

Rose, G., H. Blackburn, A. Keys, H.L. Taylor, W.B. Kannel, O. Paul, D.D. Reid, and J. Stamler. 1974. Colon cancer and blood-cholesterol. Lancet 1:181–183.

Rosenthal, S.R. 1934a. Studies in atherosclerosis: chemical, experimental and morphologic. I and II. Roles of cholesterol metabolism, blood pressure and structure of the aorta; the fat angle of the aorta (f.a.a.), and the infiltration-expression theory of lipoid deposit. Arch. Pathol. 18:473–506.

Rosenthal, S.R. 1934b. Studies in atherosclerosis: chemical, experimental and morphologic. III and IV. Roles of cholesterol metabolism, blood pressure and structure of the aorta; the fat angle of the aorta (f.a.a.), and the infiltration-expression theory of lipoid deposit. Arch. Pathol. 18:660–698.

Rosenthal, S.R. 1934c. Studies in atherosclerosis: chemical, experimental and morphologic. V. Possible dangers of iodine therapy in atherosclerosis of aorta seen from an experimental standpoint. Arch. Pathol. 18:827–842.

Ross, R. 1986. The pathogenesis of atherosclerosis—an update. N. Engl. J. Med. 314:488–500.

Rotkin, I.D. 1977. Studies in the epidemiology of prostatic cancers: expanded sampling. Cancer Treat. Rep. 61:173–180.

Rouse, I.L., B.K. Armstrong, B.M. Margetts, and L.J. Beilin. 1981. The dietary habits and nutrient intakes of Seventh-Day Adventists vegetarians and Mormon omnivores. Proc. Nutr. Soc. Aust. 6:117.

Royce, S.M., R.P. Holmes, T. Takagi, and F.A. Kummerow. 1984. The influence of dietary isomeric and saturated fatty acids on atherosclerosis and eicosanoid synthesis in swine. Am. J. Clin. Nutr. 39:215–222.

Rudel, L.L. 1980. Plasma lipoproteins in atherogenesis in nonhuman primates. Pp. 37–57 in S.S. Kalter, ed. The Use of Nonhuman Primates in Cardiovascular Diseases. University of Texas Press, Austin, Tex.

Rudel, L.L., J.A. Reynolds, and B.C. Bullock. 1981. Nutritional effects on blood lipid and HDL cholesterol concentrations in two subspecies of African green monkeys (Cercopithecus aethiops). J. Lipid Res. 22:278–286.

Rudel, L.L., J.S. Parks, and R.M. Carroll. 1983. Effects of polyunsaturated versus saturated dietary fat on nonhuman primate HDL. Pp. 649–666 in E.G. Perkins and W.J. Visek, eds. Dietary Fats and Health. American Oil Chemists' Society, Champaign, Ill.

Rudel, L.L., M.G. Bond, and B.C. Bullock. 1985. LDL heterogeneity and atherosclerosis in nonhuman primates. Ann. N.Y. Acad. Sci. 454:248–253.

Rudel, L.L., J.S. Parks, and M.G. Bond. 1986. Dietary polyunsaturated fat effects on atherosclerosis and plasma lipoproteins in African green monkeys. Pp. 501–523 in D.G. Scarpelli and G. Migaki, eds. Nutritional Diseases: Research Directions in Comparative Pathobiology. Current Topics in Nutrition and Disease, Vol. 15. Alan R. Liss, New York.

Rush, D., and A.R. Kristal. 1982. Methodologic studies during pregnancy: the reliability of the 24-hour dietary recall. Am. J. Clin. Nutr. 35:1259–1268.

Sacks, F.M., B. Rosner, and E.H. Kass. 1974. Blood pressure in vegetarians. Am. J. Epidemiol. 100:390–398.

Sacks, F.M., G.E. Marais, G. Handysides, J. Salazar, L. Miller, J.M. Foster, B. Rosner, and E.H. Kass. 1984. Lack of an effect of dietary saturated fat and cholesterol on blood pressure in normotensives. Hypertension 6:193–198.

Sacks, F.M., I.L. Rouse, M.J. Stampfer, L.M. Bishop, C.F. Lenherr, and R.J. Walther. 1987. Effect of dietary fats and carbohydrate on blood pressure of mildly hypertensive patients. Hypertension 10:452–460.

Salmond, C.E., R. Beaglehole, and I.A.M. Prior. 1985. Are low cholesterol values associated with excess mortality? Br. Med. J. 290:422–424.

Sampliner, R.E., P.H. Bennett, L.J. Comess, F.A. Rose, and T.A. Burch. 1970. Gallbladder disease in Pima Indians. Demonstration of high prevalence and early onset by cholecystography. N. Engl. J. Med. 283:1358–1364.

Sanders, T.A., D.R. Sullivan, J. Reeve, and G.R. Thompson. 1985. Triglyceride-lowering effect of marine polyunsaturates in patients with hypertriglyceridemia. Arteriosclerosis 5: 459–465.

Sarles, H., C. Chabert, Y. Pommeau, E. Save, H. Mouret, and A. Gerolami. 1969. Diet and cholesterol gallstones. A study of 101 patients with cholelithiasis compared to 101 matched controls. Am. J. Dig. Dis. 14:531–537.

Sarles, H., J. Hauton, N.E. Planche, H. Lafont, and A. Gerolami. 1970. Diet, cholesterol gallstones, and composition of the bile. Am. J. Dig. Dis. 15:251–260.

Sarles, H., C. Crotte, A. Gerolami, A. Mule, N. Domingo, and J. Hauton. 1971. The influence of calorie intake and of dietary protein on the bile lipids. Scand. J. Gastroenterol. 6: 189–191.

Savage, P.J., R.F. Hamman, G. Bartha, S.E. Dippe, M. Miller, and P.H. Bennett. 1976. Serum cholesterol levels in American (Pima) Indian children and adolescents. Pediatrics 58:274–282.

Scanu, A.M., A. Khalil, L. Neven, M. Tidore, G. Dawson, D. Pfaffinger, E. Jackson, K.D. Carey, H.C. McGill, and G.M. Fless. 1988. Genetically determined hypercholesterolemia in a rhesus monkey family due to a deficiency of the LDL receptor. J. Lipid Res. 29:1671–1681.

Schemmel, R., O. Mickelsen, and K. Motawi. 1982. Conversion of dietary to body energy in rats as affected by strain, sex and ration. J. Nutr. 102:1187–1197.

Schieken, R.M., W.R. Clarke, and R.M. Lauer. 1981. Left ventricular hypertrophy in children with blood pressures in the upper quintile of the distribution. The Muscatine Study. Hypertension 3:669–675.

Schoenfield, L.J. 1980. Diseases of the gallbladder and bile ducts. Pp. 1489–1498 in K.J. Isselbacher, R.D. Adams, E. Braunwald, R.G. Petersdorf, and J.D. Wilson, eds. Harrison's Principles of Internal Medicine, 9th ed., Vol. 2. McGraw-Hill, New York.

Schonfeld, G., W. Patsch, L.L. Rudel, C. Nelson, M. Epstein, and R.E. Olson. 1982. Effects of dietary cholesterol and fatty acids on plasma lipoproteins. J. Clin. Invest. 69: 1072–1080.

Schrott, H.G., W.R. Clarke, D.A. Wiebe, W.E. Connor, and R.M. Lauer. 1979. Increased coronary mortality in relatives of hypercholesterolemic school children: the Muscatine Study. Circulation 59:320–326.

Schuman, L.M., J.S. Mandel, A. Radke, U. Seal, and F. Halberg. 1982. Some selected features of the epidemiology of prostatic cancer: Minneapolis-St. Paul, Minnesota Case-Control Study, 1976–1979. Pp. 345–354 in K. Magnus, ed.

Trends in Cancer Incidence: Causes and Practical Implications. Hemisphere Publishing Corp., Washington, D.C.

Sclafani, A., and A.N. Gorman. 1977. Effects of age, sex, and prior body weight on the development of dietary obesity in adult rats. Physiol. Behav. 18:1021–1026.

Scott, R.F., E.S. Morrison, W.A. Thomas, R. Jones, and S.C. Nam. 1964. Short-term feeding of unsaturated versus saturated fat in the production of atherosclerosis in the rat. Exp. Mol. Pathol. 3:421–443.

Scott, R.F., E.S. Morrison, J. Jarmolych, S.C. Nam, M. Kroms, and F. Coulston. 1967a. Experimental atherosclerosis in rhesus monkeys. I. Gross and light microscopy features and lipid values in serum and aorta. Exp. Mol. Pathol. 7:11–33.

Scott, R.F., R. Jones, A.S. Daoud, O. Zumbo, F. Coulston, and W.A. Thomas. 1967b. Experimental atherosclerosis in rhesus monkeys. II. Cellular elements of proliferative lesions and possible role of cytoplasmic degeneration in pathogenesis as studied by electron microscopy. Exp. Mol. Pathol. 7: 34–57.

Scragg, R.K.R, A.J. McMichael, and P.A. Baghurst. 1984. Diet, alcohol, and relative weight in gall stone disease: a case-control study. Br. Med. J. 288:1113–1119.

Scrimshaw, N.S., and M.A. Guzman. 1968. Diet and atherosclerosis. Lab. Invest. 18:623–628.

Scrimshaw, N.S., M. Trulson, C. Tejada, D.M. Hegsted, F.J. Stare. 1957. Serum lipoprotein and cholesterol concentrations; comparison of rural Costa Rican, Guatemalan, and United States populations. Circulation 15:805–813.

Selenskas, S.L., M.M. Ip, and C. Ip. 1984. Similarity between trans fat and saturated fat in the modification of rat mammary carcinogenesis. Cancer Res. 44:1321–1326.

Senti, F.R., ed. 1985. Health Aspects of Dietary trans Fatty Acids. Federation of American Societies for Experimental Biology, Bethesda, Md. 148 pp.

Sheard, N.F., J.A. Tayek, B.R. Bistrian, G.L. Blackburn, and S.H. Zeisel. 1986. Plasma choline concentration in humans fed parenterally. Am. J. Clin. Nutr. 43:219–224.

Shekelle, R.B., A.M. Shryock, O. Paul, M. Lepper, J. Stamler, S. Liu, and W.J. Raynor, Jr. 1981a. Diet, serum cholesterol, and death from coronary heart disease. The Western Electric Study. N. Engl. J. Med. 304:65–70.

Shekelle, R.B., J. Stamler, O. Paul, A.M. Shryock, S. Liu, and M. Lepper. 1981b. Dietary lipids and serum cholesterol level: change in diet confounds the cross-sectional association. Am. J. Epidemiol. 115:506–514.

Shekelle, R.B., L. Missell, O. Paul, A.M. Shryock, and J. Stamler. 1985. Fish consumption and mortality from coronary heart disease. N. Engl. J. Med. 313:820.

Shepherd, J., C.J. Packard, J.R. Patsch, A.M. Gotto, Jr., and O.D. Taunton. 1978. Effects of dietary polyunsaturated and saturated fat on the properties of high density lipoproteins and the metabolism of apolipoprotein A-I. J. Clin. Invest. 61:1582–1592.

Shepherd, J., C.J. Packard, S.M. Grundy, D. Yeshurun, A.M. Gotto, Jr., and O.D. Taunton. 1980a. Effects of saturated and polyunsaturated fat diets on the chemical composition and metabolism of low density lipoproteins in man. J. Lipid Res. 21:91–99.

Shepherd, J., J.M. Stewart, J.G. Clark, and K. Carr. 1980b. Sequential changes in plasma lipoproteins and body fat composition during polyunsaturated fat feeding in man. Br. J. Nutr. 44:265–271.

Sherwin, R.W., D.N. Wentworth, J.A. Cutler, S.B. Hulley, L.H. Kuller, and J. Stamler. 1987. Serum cholesterol levels and cancer mortality in 361,662 men screened for the Multiple Risk Factor Intervention Trial. J. Am. Med. Assoc. 257:943–948.

Shimamoto, T., Y. Komachi, H. Inada, M. Doi, H. Iso, S. Sato, A. Kitamura, M. Iida, M. Konishi, N. Nakanishi, A. Terao, Y. Naito, and S. Kojima. 1989. Trends for coronary heart disease and stroke and their risk factors in Japan. Circulation 79:503–516.

Shulman, R.S., A.K. Bhattacharyya, W.E. Connor, and D.S. Fredrickson. 1976. Beta-sitosterolemia and xanthomatosis. N. Engl. J. Med 294:482–483.

Sidney, S., G.D. Friedman, and R.A. Hiatt. 1986. Serum cholesterol and large bowel cancer. A case-control study. Am. J. Epidemiol. 124:33–38.

Simons, L.A. 1986. Interrelations of lipids and lipoproteins with coronary artery disease mortality in 19 countries. Am. J. Cardiol. 57:5G–10G.

Singer, P., U. Gerhard, V. Moritz, D. Förster, I. Berger, and H. Heine. 1986. Different changes of N-6 and N-3 fatty acids in adipose tissue from spontaneously hypertensive (SHR) and normotensive rats after diets supplemented with linolenic or eicosapentaenoic acids. Prost. Leuk. Med. 24: 163–172.

Singhal, A.K., J. Finver-Sadowsky, C.K. McSherry, and E.H. Mosbach. 1983. Effect of cholesterol and bile acids on the regulation of cholesterol metabolism in hamster. Biochim. Biophys. Acta 752:214–222.

Sirtori, C.R., G. Biasi, G. Vercellio, E. Agradi, and E. Malan. 1974. Diet, lipids and lipoproteins in patients with peripheral vascular disease. Am. J. Med. Sci. 268:325–332.

Sitaram, N., H. Weingartner, E.D. Caine, and J.C. Gillin. 1978. Choline: selective enhancement of serial learning and encoding of low imagery words in man. Life Sci. 22:1555–1560.

Slover, H.T., R.H. Thompson, Jr., C.S. Davis, and G.V. Merola. 1985. Lipids in margarines and margarine-like foods. J. Am. Oil Chem. Soc. 62:775–786.

Small, D.M. 1976. Part I. The etiology and pathogenesis of gallstones. Adv. Surg. 10:63–85.

Smith-Barbaro, P., M.R. Quinn, H. Fisher, and D.M. Hegstead. 1981. The effect of dietary fat and salt on blood pressure, renal and aortic prostaglandins. Nutr. Res. 1:277–287.

Snapper, I. 1941. Chinese Lessons to Western Medicine. Interscience Publishers, New York. 380 pp.

Sniderman, A., S. Shapiro, D. Marpole, B. Skinner, B. Teng, and P.O. Kwiterovich, Jr. 1980. Association of coronary atherosclerosis with hyperapobetalipoproteinemia [increased protein but normal cholesterol levels in human plasma low density (beta) lipoproteins]. Proc. Natl. Acad. Sci. U.S.A. 77:604–608.

Snowdon, D.A. 1981. Alcohol Use and Mortality from Cancer and Heart Disease Among Members of the Lutheran Brotherhood Cohort. University Microfilms, Ann Arbor, Mich.

Snowdon, D.A. 1988. Animal product consumption and mortality because of all causes combined, coronary heart disease, stroke, diabetes, and cancer in Seventh-Day Adventists. Am. J. Clin. Nutr. 48:739–748.

Snowdon, D.A., R.L. Phillips, and W. Choi. 1984. Diet, obesity, and risk of fatal prostate cancer. Am. J. Epidemiol. 120:244–250.

Sodhi, H.S., P.D. Wood, G. Schlierf, and L.W. Kinsell.

1967. Plasma, bile and fecal sterols in relation to diet. Metabolism 16:334–344.

Somjen, G.J., and T. Gilat. 1986. Changing concepts of cholesterol solubility in bile. Gastroenterology 91:772–775.

Sorlie, P.D., M.R. Garcia-Palmieri, M.I. Castillo-Stabb, R. Costas, Jr., M.C. Oalmann, and R. Havlik. 1981. The relation of antemortem factors to atherosclerosis at autopsy. The Puerto Rico Heart Health Study. Am. J. Pathol. 103: 345–352.

Spady, D.K., and J.M. Dietschy. 1985. Dietary saturated triacylglycerols suppress hepatic low density lipoprotein receptor activity in the hamster. Proc. Natl. Acad. Sci. U.S.A. 82:4526–4530.

Spady, D.K., and J.M. Dietschy. 1988. Interaction of dietary cholesterol and triglycerides in the regulation of hepatic low density lipoprotein transport in the hamster. J. Clin. Invest. 81:300–309.

Spritz, N., and M.A. Mishkel. 1969. Effects of dietary fats on plasma lipids and lipoproteins: an hypothesis for the lipid-lowering effect of unsaturated fatty acids. J. Clin. Invest. 48: 78–86.

Spritz, N., E.H. Ahrens, Jr., and S. Grundy. 1965. Sterol balance in man as plasma cholesterol concentrations are altered by exchanges of dietary fats. J. Clin. Invest. 44: 1482–1493.

Srinivasan, S.R., B. Radhakrishnamurthy, C.C. Smith, R.H. Wolf, and G.S. Berenson. 1976. Serum lipid and lipoprotein responses of six nonhuman primate species to dietary changes in cholesterol levels. J. Nutr. 106:1757–1767.

St. Clair, R.W., G.R. Henderson, V. Heaster, W.D. Wagner, M.G. Bond, and M.R. McMahan. 1980. Influence of dietary fats and oral contraceptive on plasma lipids, high density lipoproteins, gallstones, and atherosclerosis in African green monkeys. Atherosclerosis 37:103–121.

Stallones, R.A. 1983. Ischemic heart disease and lipids in blood and diet. Annu. Rev. Nutr. 3:155–185.

Stamler, J. 1967. Lectures on Preventive Cardiology. Grune & Stratton, New York. 434 pp.

Stamler, J. 1979. Population studies. Pp. 25–88 in R.I. Levy, B.M. Rifkind, B.H. Dennis, and N. Ernst, eds. Nutrition, Lipids, and Coronary Heart Disease: A Global View. Nutrition in Health and Disease, Vol. 1. Raven Press, New York.

Stamler, J., and R. Shekelle. 1988. Dietary cholesterol and human coronary heart disease: the epidemiologic evidence. Arch. Pathol. Lab. Med. 112:1032–1040.

Stamler, J., R. Stamler, and R.B. Shekelle. 1970. Regional differences in prevalence, incidence and mortality from atherosclerotic coronary heart disease. Pp. 84–127 in J.H. de Haas, H.C. Hemker, and H.A. Snellen, eds. Ischaemic Heart Disease. Leiden University Press, Leiden, The Netherlands.

Stamler, J., D.M. Berkson, and H.A. Lindberg. 1972. Risk factors: their role in the etiology and pathogenesis of the atherosclerotic diseases. Pp. 41–119 in R.W. Wissler, J.C. Geer, and N. Kaufman, eds. The Pathogenesis of Atherosclerosis. Williams & Wilkins, Baltimore.

Stamler, J., D. Wentworth, and J.D. Neaton. 1986. Is the relationship between serum cholesterol and risk of premature death from coronary heart disease continuous and graded? Findings in 356,222 primary screenees of the Multiple Risk Factor Intervention Trial (MRFIT). J. Am. Med. Assoc. 256:2823–2828.

Stanbury, J.B., J.B. Wyngaarden, D.S. Fredrickson, J.L.

Goldstein, and M.S. Brown, eds. 1983. The Metabolic Basis of Inherited Disease, 5th ed., Part 4. McGraw-Hill, New York. 2032 pp.

Stary, H.C. 1987a. Evolution and progression of atherosclerosis in the coronary arteries of children and adults. Pp. 20–36 in S.R. Bates and E.C. Gangloff, eds. Atherogenesis and Aging. Springer-Verlag, New York.

Stary, H.C. 1987b. Macrophages, macrophage foam cells, and eccentric intimal thickening in the coronary arteries of young children. Atherosclerosis 64:91–108.

Stein, E.A., J. Shapero, C. McNerney, C.J. Glueck, T. Tracy, and P. Gartside. 1982. Changes in plasma lipid and lipoprotein fractions after alteration in dietary cholesterol, polyunsaturated, saturated, and total fat in free-living normal and hypercholesterolemic children. Am. J. Clin. Nutr. 35:1375–1390.

Steinberg, D. 1983. Lipoproteins and atherosclerosis. A look back and a look ahead. Arteriosclerosis 3:283–301.

Steiner, A. 1948. Significance of cholesterol in coronary arteriosclerosis. N.Y. State J. Med. 48:1814–1818.

Steiner, A., and B. Domanski. 1944. Effect of feeding of "soya lecithin" on serum cholesterol level of man. Proc. Soc. Exp. Biol. Med. 55:236–238.

Steiner, A., and F.E. Kendall. 1946. Atherosclerosis and arteriosclerosis in dogs following ingestion of cholesterol and thiouracil. Arch. Pathol. 42:433–444.

Stemmerman, G.N., A.M. Nomura, and L.K. Heilbrun. 1984. Dietary fat and the risk of colorectal cancer. Cancer Res. 44:4633–4637.

Stich, H.F., ed. 1982. Carcinogens and Mutagens in the Environment, Vol. I. Food Products. CRC Press, Boca Raton, Fla. 310 pp.

Strazzullo, P., A. Ferro-Luzzi, A. Siani, C. Scaccini, S. Sette, G. Catasta, and M. Mancini. 1986. Changing the Mediterranean diet: effects on blood pressure. J. Hypertens. 4:407–412.

Strøm, A., and R.A. Jensen. 1951. Mortality from circulatory diseases in Norway 1940–1945. Lancet 1:126–129.

Strong, J.P. 1976. Atherosclerosis in primates. Introduction and overview. Primates Med. 9:1–15.

Strong, J.P., and H.C. McGill, Jr. 1962. The natural history of coronary atherosclerosis. Am. J. Pathol. 40:37–49.

Strong, J.P., and H.C. McGill, Jr. 1967. Diet and experimental atherosclerosis in baboons. Am. J. Pathol. 50:669–690.

Strong, J.P., and H.C. McGill, Jr. 1969. The pediatric aspects of atherosclerosis. J. Atheroscler. Res. 9:251–265.

Strong, J.P., H.C. McGill, Jr., C. Tejada, and R.L. Holman. 1958. The natural history of atherosclerosis. Comparison of the early aortic lesions in New Orleans, Guatemala, and Costa Rica. Am. J. Pathol. 34:731–744.

Strong, J.P., W.P. Newman III, D.S. Freedman, P.D. Gard, R.E. Tracy, and L.A. Solberg. 1986. Atherosclerotic disease in children and young adults: relationship to cardiovascular risk factors. Pp. 27–41 in G.S. Berenson, ed. Causation of Cardiovascular Risk Factors in Children. Perspectives on Cardiovascular Risk in Early Life. Raven Press, New York.

Sturdevant, R.A., M.L. Pearce, and S. Dayton. 1973. Increased prevalence of cholelithiasis in men ingesting a serum-cholesterol-lowering diet. N. Engl. J. Med. 288:24–27.

Sullivan, D.R., T.A. Sanders, I.M. Trayner, and G.R. Thompson. 1986. Paradoxical elevation of LDL apoprotein B levels in hypertriglyceridaemic patients and normal subjects ingesting fish oil. Atherosclerosis 61:129–134.

Sullivan, D.R., C.E. West, M.B. Katan, I. Halferkamps, and H. van der Torre. 1987. Atherogenic and protective lipoproteins in boys from ten countries differing in dietary carbohydrate intake. Pp. 73–81 in B.S. Hetzel and G.S. Berenson, eds. Cardiovascular Risk Factors in Childhood: Epidemiology and Prevention. Elsevier, Amsterdam.

Sutor, D.J., and S.E. Wooley. 1971. A statistical survey of the composition of gallstones in eight countries. Gut 12:55–64.

Svanberg, U., A. Gustafson, and R. Ohlson. 1974. Polyunsaturated fatty acids in hyperlipoproteinemia. II. Administration of essential phospholipids in hypertriglyceridemia. Nutr. Metab. 17:338–346.

Sweeney, M.J., J.N. Etteldorf, W.T. Dobbins, B. Somervil, R. Fischer, and C. Ferrell. 1961. Dietary fat and concentrations of lipid in the serum during the first six to eight weeks of life. Pediatrics 27:765–771.

Sylvester, P.W. 1986. Role of acute caloric-restriction in murine tumorigenesis. Prog. Clin. Biol. Res. 222:517–528.

Sylvester, P.W., M. Russell, M.M. Ip., and C. Ip. 1986a. Comparative effects of different animal and vegetable fats fed before and during carcinogen administration on mammary tumorigenesis, sexual maturation, and endocrine function in rats. Cancer Res. 46:757–762.

Sylvester, P.W., C. Ip., and M.M. Ip. 1986b. Effects of high dietary fat on the growth and development of ovarian-independent carcinogen-induced mammary tumors in rats. Cancer Res. 46:763–769.

Tabas, I., D.A. Weiland, and A.R. Tall. 1985. Unmodified low density lipoprotein causes cholesteryl ester accumulation in J774 macrophages. Proc. Natl. Acad. Sci. U.S.A. 82:416–420.

Takeya, Y., J.S. Popper, Y. Shimizu, H. Kato, G.G. Rhoads, and A. Kagan. 1984. Epidemiologic studies of coronary heart disease and stroke in Japanese men living in Japan, Hawaii and California: incidence of stroke in Japan and Hawaii. Stroke 15:15–23.

Talamini, R., C. La Veccia, A. Decarli, S. Franceschi, E. Grattoni, E. Grigoletto, A. Liberati, and G. Tognoni. 1984. Social factors, diet and breast cancer in a northern Italian population. Br. J. Cancer 49:723–729.

Tamir, I., Y. Bojanower, O. Levtow, D. Heldenberg, Z. Dickerman, and B. Werbin. 1972. Serum lipids and lipoproteins in children from families with early coronary heart disease. Arch. Dis. Child. 47:808–810.

Tanaka, N., and O.W. Portman. 1977. Effect of type of dietary fat and cholesterol on cholesterol absorption rate in squirrel monkeys. J. Nutr. 107:814–821.

Tanaka, N., O.W. Portman, and T. Osuga. 1976. Effect of type of dietary fat, cholesterol and chenodeoxycholic acid on gallstone formation, bile acid kinetics and plasma lipids in squirrel monkeys. J. Nutr. 106:1123–1134.

Tannenbaum, A. 1959. Nutrition and cancer. Pp. 517–562 in F. Homburger, ed. The Physiopathology of Cancer by 32 Authors, 2nd ed. Hoeber-Harper, New York.

Tartter, P.I., G. Slater, A.E. Paptestas, and A.H. Aufses, Jr. 1984. Cholesterol, weight, height, Quetelet's index, and colon cancer recurrence. J. Surg. Oncol. 27:232–235.

Taylor, C.B., D.E. Patton, and G.E. Cox. 1963. Atherosclerosis in rhesus monkeys. VI. Fatal myocardial infarction in a monkey fed fat and cholesterol. Arch. Pathol. 76:404–423.

Taylor, C.B., S.K. Peng, N.T. Werthessen, P. Tham, and K.T. Lee. 1979. Spontaneously occurring angiotoxic derivatives of cholesterol. Am. J. Clin. Nutr. 32:40–57.

Tejada, C., J.P. Strong, M.R. Montenegro, C. Restrepo, and L.A. Solberg. 1968. Distribution of coronary and aortic atherosclerosis by geographic location, race, and sex. Lab. Invest. 18:509–526.

ten Hoor, F., and H.M. van de Graaf. 1978. The influence of a linoleic acid-rich diet and of acetyl salicylic acid on NaCl induced hypertension, Na+—and H$_2$O-balance and urinary prostaglandin excretion in rats. Acta Biol. Med. Ger. 37:875–877.

Tepperman, J., F.T. Caldwell, and H.M. Tepperman. 1964. Induction of gallstones in mice by feeding a cholesterol-cholic acid containing diet. Am. J. Physiol. 206:628–634.

ter Welle, H.F., C.M. van Gent, W. Dekker, and A.F. Willebrands. 1974. The effect of soya lecithin on serum lipid values in type II hyperlipoproteinemia. Acta Med. Scand. 195:267–271.

Thomas, L.H., P.R. Jones, J.A. Winter, and H. Smith. 1981. Hydrogenated oils and fats: the presence of chemically-modified fatty acids in human adipose tissue. Am. J. Clin. Nutr. 34:877–886.

Thomas, L.H., J.A. Winter, and R.G. Scott. 1983a. Concentration of transunsaturated fatty acids in the adipose body tissue of decedents dying of ischaemic heart disease compared with controls. J. Epidemiol. Community Health 37:22–24.

Thomas, L.H., J.A. Winter, and R.G. Scott. 1983b. Concentration of 18:1 and 16:1 transunsaturated fatty acids in the adipose body tissue of decedents dying of ischaemic heart disease compared with controls: analysis by gas liquid chromatography. J. Epidemiol. Community Health 37:16–21.

Thulin, T., M. Abdulla, I. Denker, M. Jagerstad, A. Melander, A. Norden, B. Schersten, and B. Akesson. 1980. Comparison of energy and nutrient intakes in women with high and low blood pressure levels. Acta Med. Scand. 208:367–373.

Tidwell, H.C., J.C. McPherson, and W.W. Burr, Jr. 1962. Effect of the saturation of fats upon the disposition of ingested cholesterol. Am. J. Clin. Nutr. 11:108–114.

Tillotson, J.L., H. Kato, M.Z. Nichaman, D.C. Miller, M.L. Gay, K.G. Johnson, and G.G. Rhoads. 1973. Epidemiology of coronary heart disease and stroke in Japanese men living in Japan, Hawaii, and California: methodology for comparison of diet. Am. J. Clin. Nutr. 26:177–184.

Tilvis, R.S., and T.A. Miettinen. 1986. Serum plant sterols and their relation to cholesterol absorption. Am. J. Clin. Nutr. 43:92–97.

Tobian, L., M. Ganguli, M.A. Johnson, and J. Iwai. 1985. The influence of renal prostaglandins and dietary linoleate on hypertension of Dahl salt-sensitive rats. Pp. 349–359 in M.J. Horan, M. Blaustein, J.B. Dunbar, W. Kachadorian, N.M. Kaplan, and A.P. Simopoulos, eds. NIH Workshop on Nutrition and Hypertension: Proceedings from a Symposium. Biochemical Information Corp., New York.

Toor, M., A. Katchalsky, J. Agmon, and D. Allalouf. 1960. Atherosclerosis and related factors in immigrants to Israel. Circulation 22:265–279.

Tornberg, S.A., L.E. Holm, J.M. Carstensen, and G.A. Eklund. 1986. Risks of cancer of the colon and rectum in relation to serum cholesterol and beta-lipoprotein. N. Engl. J. Med. 315:1629–1633.

Trotman, B.W., and R.D. Soloway. 1975. Pigment vs cholesterol cholelithiasis: clinical and epidemiological aspects. Am. J. Dig. Dis. 20:735–740.

Tuomilehto, J., P. Puska, A. Nissinen, J. Salonen, A.

Tanskanen, P. Pietinen, and E. Wolf. 1984. Community-based prevention of hypertension in North Karelia, Finland. Ann. Clin. Res. 16 Suppl. 43:18–27.

Turjman, N., G.T. Goodman, B. Jaeger, and P.P. Nair. 1984a. Diet, nutrition intake, and metabolism in populations at high and low risk for colon cancer. Metabolism of bile acids. Am. J. Clin. Nutr. 40:937–941.

Turjman, N., B. Calkins, R. Phillips, G.T. Goodman, and P.P. Nair. 1984b. Dietary intake of plant sterols and cholesterol among population groups at different risks for colon cancer. Fed. Proc. 43:855.

Turkenkopf, I.J., C.A. Maggio, and M.R. Greenwood. 1982. Effect of high fat weaning diets containing either medium-chain triglycerides or long-chain triglycerides on the development of obesity in the Zucker rat. J. Nutr. 112:1254–1263.

Turner, J.D., N.A. Le, and W.V. Brown. 1981. Effect of changing dietary fat saturation on low-density lipoprotein metabolism in man. Am. J. Physiol. 241:E57–E63.

Turpeinen, O., M.J. Karvonen, M. Pekkarinen, M. Miettinen, R. Elosuo, and E. Paavilainen. 1979. Dietary prevention of coronary heart disease: the Finnish Mental Hospital Study. Int. J. Epidemiol. 8:99–118.

Tuyns, A.J., M. Haelterman, and R. Kaaks. 1987. Colorectal cancer and the intake of nutrients: oligosaccharides are a risk factor, fats are not. A case-control study in Belgium. Nutr. Cancer 10:181–196.

USDA (U.S. Department of Agriculture). 1984. Nationwide Food Consumption Survey. Nutrient Intakes: Individuals in 48 States, Year 1977–78. Report No. I-2. Consumer Nutrition Division, Human Nutrition Information Service, Hyattsville, Md. 439 pp.

USDA (U.S. Department of Agriculture). 1986. Nationwide Food Consumption Survey. Continuing Survey of Food Intakes of Individuals. Men 19–50 Years, 1 Day, 1985. Report No. 85-3. Nutrition Monitoring Division, Human Nutrition Information Service, Hyattsville, Md. 94 pp.

USDA (U.S. Department of Agriculture). 1987. Nationwide Food Consumption Survey. Continuing Survey of Food Intakes of Individuals. Women 19–50 Years and Their Children 1–5 Years, 4 Days, 1985. Report No. 85-4. Nutrition Monitoring Division, Human Nutrition Information Service, Hyattsville, Md. 182 pp.

U.S.-U.S.S.R. Steering Committee. 1984. Nutrient intake and its association with high-density lipoprotein and low-density lipoprotein cholesterol in selected U.S. and U.S.S.R. subpopulations. The U.S.-U.S.S.R. Steering Committee for Problem Area I: the pathogenesis of atherosclerosis. Am. J. Clin. Nutr. 39:942–952.

Utermann, G., M. Hees, and A. Steinmetz. 1977. Polymorphism of apolipoprotein E and occurrence of dysbetalipoproteinaemia in man. Nature 269:604–607.

Utermann, G., N. Pruin, and A. Steinmetz. 1979. Polymorphism of apolipoprotein E. III. Effect of a single polymorphic gene locus on plasma lipid levels in man. Clin. Genet. 15:63–72.

Van Lenten, B.J., A.M. Fogelman, R.L. Jackson, S. Shapiro, M.E. Haberland, and P.A. Edwards. 1985. Receptor-mediated uptake of remnant lipoproteins by cholesterol-loaded human monocyte-macrophages. J. Biol. Chem. 260:8783–8788.

Vartiainen, E., P. Puska, and J.T. Salonen. 1982. Serum total cholesterol, HDL cholesterol and blood pressure levels in 13-year-old children in Eastern Finland. The North Karelia Youth Project. Acta Med. Scand. 211:95–103.

Vartiainen, E., P. Puska, P. Pietinen, A. Nissinen, U. Leino, and U. Uusitalo. 1986. Effects of dietary fat modifications on serum lipids and blood pressure in children. Acta Pediatr. Scand. 75:396–401.

Vartiainen, I. 1946. War-time and mortality in certain diseases in Finland. Ann. Med. Int. Fenn. 35:234–240.

Vartiainen, I., and K. Kanerva. 1947. Arteriosclerosis and war-time. Ann. Med. Int. Fenn. 36:748–758.

Vega, G.L., E. Groszek, R. Wolf, and S.M. Grundy. 1982. Influence of polyunsaturated fats on composition of plasma lipoproteins and apolipoproteins. J. Lipid Res. 23:811–822.

Vergroesen, A.J., A.I. Fleischman, H.U. Comberg, S. Heyden, and C.G. Hames. 1978. The influence of dietary linoleate on essential hypertension in man. Acta Biol. Med. Ger. 37:879–883.

Vesselinovitch, D., G.S. Getz, R.H. Hughes, and R.W. Wissler. 1974. Atherosclerosis in the rhesus monkey fed three food fats. Atherosclerosis 20:303–321.

Vesselinovitch, D., R.W. Wissler, T.J. Schaffner, and J. Borensztajn. 1980. The effect of various diets on atherogenesis in rhesus monkeys. Atherosclerosis 35:189–207.

Voller, R.D., Jr., and W.B. Strong. 1981. Pediatric aspects of atherosclerosis. Am. Heart J. 101:815–836.

Vollset, S.E., I. Heuch, and E. Bjelke. 1985. Fish consumption and mortality from coronary heart disease. N. Engl. J. Med. 313:820–821.

von Schacky, C. 1987. Prophylaxis of atherosclerosis with marine omega-3 fatty acids. A comprehensive strategy. Ann. Intern. Med. 107:890–899.

von Schacky, C., W. Siess, S. Fischer, and P.C. Weber. 1985a. A comparative study of eicosapentaenoic acid metabolism by human platelets in vivo and in vitro. J. Lipid Res. 26:457–464.

von Schacky, C., S. Fischer, and P.C. Weber. 1985b. Long-term effects of dietary marine omega-3 fatty acids upon plasma and cellular lipids, platelet function, and eicosanoid formation in humans. J. Clin. Invest. 76:1626–1631.

Wade, A.E., and S. Dhardwadkar. 1986. Metabolic activation of carcinogens. Prog. Clin. Biol. Res. 222:587–606.

Walker, B.L. (Memorial Symposium). 1986. Lipids and cancer. Papers from the Brian L. Walker Memorial Symposium presented at the 76th AOCS Annual Meeting in Philadelphia, Pennsylvania, May 1985. Lipids 21:271–307.

Wallace, R.B., and R.A. Anderson. 1987. Blood lipids, lipid-related measures, and the risk of atherosclerotic cardiovascular disease. Epidemiol. Rev. 9:95–119.

Walter, H.J., and A. Hofman. 1987. Socioeconomic status, ethnic origin, and risk factors for coronary heart disease in children. Am. Heart. J. 113:812–818.

Walton, K.W., J. Hitchens, H.N. Magnani, and M. Khan. 1974. A study of methods of identification and estimation of LP(a) lipoprotein and of its significance in health, hyperlipidaemia and atherosclerosis. Atherosclerosis 20:323–346.

Watanabe, N., N.S. Gimbel, and C.G. Johnston. 1962. Effect of polyunsaturated and saturated fatty acids on the cholesterol holding capacity of human bile. Arch. Surg. 85:136–141.

Watkins, L.O., J.D. Neaton, and L.H. Kuller. 1986. Racial differences in high-density lipoprotein cholesterol and coronary heart disease incidence in the usual-care group of the Multiple Risk Factor Intervention Trial. Am. J. Cardiol. 57:538–545.

Webber, L.S., J.L. Cresanta, A.W. Voors, and G.S. Berenson. 1983. Tracking of cardiovascular disease risk factor variables in school-age children. J. Chronic Dis. 36:647–660.

Webber, L.S., D.S. Freedman, and J.L. Cresanta. 1986. Tracking of cardiovascular disease risk factor variables in school-age children. Pp. 42–64 in G.S. Berenson, ed. Causation of Cardiovascular Risk Factors in Children. Perspectives on Cardiovascular Risk in Early Life. Raven Press, New York.

Weidman, W., P. Kwiterovich, Jr., M.J. Jesse, and E. Nugent. 1983. Diet in the healthy child. Task Force Committee of the Nutrition Committee and the Cardiovascular Disease in the Young Council of the American Heart Association. Circulation 67:1411A–1414A.

Weinsier, R.L., and D. Norris. 1985. Recent developments in the etiology and treatment of hypertension: dietary calcium, fat, and magnesium. Am. J. Clin. Nutr. 42:1331–1338.

Weisgraber, K.H., S.C. Rall, Jr., and R.W. Mahley. 1981. Human E apoprotein heterogeneity. Cysteine-arginine interchanges in the amino acid sequence of the apo-E isoforms. J. Biol. Chem. 256:9077–9083.

Weiss, K.M., R.E. Ferrell, C.L. Hanis, and P.N. Styne. 1984. Genetics and epidemiology of gallbladder disease in new world native peoples. Am. J. Hum. Genet. 36:1259–1278.

Weisweiler, P., P. Janetschek, and P. Schwandt. 1985. Influence of polyunsaturated fats and fat restriction on serum lipoproteins in humans. Metabolism 34:83–87.

Weisweiler, P., P. Janetschek, and P. Schwandt. 1986. Fat restriction alters the composition of apolipoprotein B-100 containing very low-density lipoproteins in humans. Am. J. Clin. Nutr. 43:903–909.

Welsch, C.W. 1986. Interrelationship between dietary fat and endocrine processes in mammary gland tumorigenesis. Prog. Clin. Biol. Res. 222:623–654.

Welsch, C.W., and C.F. Aylsworth. 1983. Enhancement of murine mammary tumorigenesis by feeding high levels of dietary fat: a hormonal mechanism? J. Natl. Cancer Inst. 70:215–221.

Wexler, B.C. 1981. Inhibition of the pathogenesis of spontaneous hypertension in spontaneously hypertensive rats by feeding a high fat diet. Endocrinology 108:981–989.

Whayne, T.F., P. Alaupovic, M.D. Curry, E.T. Lee, P.S. Anderson, and E. Schechter. 1981. Plasma apolipoprotein B and VLDL-, LDL-, and HDL-cholesterol as risk factors in the development of coronary artery disease in male patients examined by angiography. Atherosclerosis 39:411–424.

WHO (World Health Organization). 1982. Prevention of Coronary Heart Disease. Technical Report Series No. 678. World Health Organization, Geneva. 53 pp.

WHO (World Health Organization) European Collaborative Group. 1983. Multifactorial trial in the prevention of coronary heart disease: 3. Incidence and mortality results. Eur. Heart J. 4:141–147.

Wigand, G. 1959. Production of hypercholesterolemia and atherosclerosis in rabbits by feeding different fats without supplementary cholesterol. Acta Med. Scand. 166 suppl. 351:1–91.

Wilhelmsen, L., G. Berglund, D. Elmfeldt, G. Tibblin, H. Wedel, K. Pennert, A. Vedin, C. Wilhelmsson, and L. Werkö. 1986. The multifactor primary prevention trial in Göteborg, Sweden. Eur. Heart J. 7:279–288.

Willett, W., and M.J. Stampfer. 1986. Total energy intake: implications for epidemiologic analyses. Am. J. Epidemiol. 124:17–27.

Willett, W., M.J. Stampfer, G.A. Colditz, B.A. Rosner, C.H. Hennekens, and F.E. Speizer. 1987. Dietary fat and the risk of breast cancer. N. Engl. J. Med. 316:22–28.

Williams, P.T., R.M. Krauss, S. Kindel-Joyce, D.M. Dreon, K.M. Vranizan, and P.D. Wood. 1986. Relationship of dietary fat, protein, cholesterol, and fiber intake to atherogenic lipoproteins in men. Am. J. Clin. Med. 44:788–797.

Williams, P.T., S.P. Fortmann, R.B. Terry, S.C. Garay, K.M. Vranizan, N. Ellsworth, and P.D. Wood. 1987. Associations of dietary fats, regional adiposity, and blood pressure in men. J. Am. Med. Assoc. 257:3251–3256.

Wilmore, J.H., and J.J. McNamara. 1974. Prevalence of coronary heart disease risk factors in boys, 8 to 12 years of age. J. Pediatr. 84:527–533.

Wilson, J.D., and M.D. Siperstein. 1959. Effect of saturated and unsaturated fats on hepatic synthesis and biliary excretion of cholesterol by the rat. Am. J. Physiol. 196:599–602.

Wilson, R.B., P.M. Newberne, and M.W. Conner. 1973. An improved semisynthetic atherogenic diet for rabbits. Dietary fat–carbohydrate interaction in atherogenesis. Arch. Pathol. 96:355–359.

Wingard, D.L., M.H. Criqui, M.J. Holbrook, and E. Barrett-Connor. 1984. Plasma cholesterol and cancer morbidity and mortality in an adult community. J. Chronic Dis. 37:401–406.

Wissler, R.W., and H.C. McGill, Jr. 1983. Conference on blood lipids in children: optimal levels for early prevention of coronary artery disease. Workshop report: experimental section. American Health Foundation, April 18 and 19, 1983. Prev. Med. 12:868–902.

Wissler, R.W., and D. Vesselinovitch. 1987a. Animal models for hyperlipidemia-induced atherosclerosis. Pp. 111–116 in R. Paoletti, D. Kritchevsky, and W.L. Holmes, eds. Drugs Affecting Lipid Metabolism. Springer-Verlag, Berlin.

Wissler, R.W., and D. Vesselinovitch. 1987b. The development and use of animal models in atherosclerosis research. Pp. 337–357 in L.L. Gallo, ed. Cardiovascular Disease: Molecular and Cellular Mechanisms, Prevention and Treatment. Plenum Press, New York.

Wissler, R.W., M.L. Eilert, M.A. Schroeder, and L. Cohen. 1954. Production of lipomatous and atheromatous arterial lesions in the albino rat. Arch. Pathol. 57:333–351.

Wissler, R.W., L.E. Frazier, R.H. Hughes, and R.A. Rasmussen. 1962. Atherogenesis in the cebus monkey. I. A comparison of three food fats under controlled dietary conditions. Arch. Pathol. 74:312–322.

Wood, P.D.S., R. Shioda, and L.W. Kinsell. 1966. Dietary regulation of cholesterol metabolism. Lancet 2:604–607.

Wurtman, J.J. 1979. Sources of choline and lecithin in the diet. Pp. 73–81 in A. Barbeau, J.H. Growdon, and R.J. Wurtman, eds. Nutrition and the Brain, Vol. 5. Choline and Lecithin in Brain Disorders. Raven Press, New York.

Wynder, E.L., G.A. Leveille, J.H. Weisburger, and G.E. Livingston, eds. 1983. Environmental Aspects of Cancer: The Role of Macro and Micro Components of Foods. Proceedings of an International Conference Sponsored by the American Health Foundation, March 31–April 1, 1982, New York, New York. Food & Nutrition Press, Westport, Conn. 295 pp.

Yaari, S., U. Goldbourt, S. Even-Zohar, and H.N. Neufeld. 1981. Associations of serum high density lipoprotein and total cholesterol with total, cardiovascular, and cancer mortality in a 7-year prospective study of 10,000 men. Lancet 1:1011–1015.

Yamase, H., and J.J. McNamara. 1972. Geographic differences in the incidence of gallbladder disease. Influence of environment and ethnic background. Am. J. Surg. 123: 667–670.

Yano, K., G.G. Rhoads, A. Kagan, and J. Tillotson. 1978. Dietary intake and the risk of coronary heart disease in Japanese men living in Hawaii. Am. J. Clin. Nutr. 31: 1270–1279.

Yano, K., D.M. Reed, J.D. Curb., J.H. Hankin, and J.J. Albers. 1986. Biological and dietary correlates of plasma lipids and lipoproteins among elderly Japanese men in Hawaii. Arteriosclerosis 6:422–433.

Yerushalmy, J., and H.E. Hilleboe. 1957. Fat in the diet and mortality from heart disease: a methodologic note. N.Y. State J. Med. 57:2343–2354.

Yomantas, S., V.M. Elner, T. Schaffner, and R.W. Wissler. 1984. Immunohistochemical localization and apolipoprotein B in human atherosclerotic lesions. Arch. Pathol. Lab. Med. 108:374–378.

Yudkin, J. 1957. Diet and coronary thrombosis: hypothesis and fact. Lancet 2:155–162.

Zanni, E.E., Zannis, V.I., C.B. Blum, P.N. Herbert, and J.L. Breslow. 1987. Effect of egg cholesterol and dietary fats on plasma lipids, lipoproteins, and apoproteins of normal women consuming natural diets. J. Lipid Res. 28: 518–527.

Zannis, V.I., and J.L. Breslow. 1981. Human very low density lipoprotein apolipoprotein E isoprotein polymorphism is explained by genetic variation and posttranslational modification. Biochemistry 20:1033–1041.

Zeisel, S.H. 1981. Dietary choline: biochemistry, physiology, and pharmacology. Annu. Rev. Nutr. 1:95–121.

Zeisel, S.H., J.H. Growdon, R.J. Wurtman, S.G. Magil, and M. Logue. 1980. Normal plasma choline responses to ingested lecithin. Neurology 30:1226–1229.

Zilversmit, D.B. 1979. Atherogenesis: a postprandial phenomenon. Circulation 60:473–485.

Zinserling, W.D. 1925. Untersuchungen über Atherosklerose. I. Über die Aortaverfettung bei Kindern. Virchows Arch. f. Pathol. Anat. 255:677–705.

8

Protein

Proteins account for about three-fourths of the dry matter in most human tissues other than bone and adipose tissue. They are macromolecules with molecular weights ranging from a few thousand to many millions, and they are required for practically every essential function in the body. From the standpoint of nutrition, the human body does not require dietary protein per se. Rather, it requires the nine essential amino acids that are present in dietary proteins. Dietary sources of utilizable carbon, usually from carbohydrates, and nitrogen are required for the synthesis of nonessential amino acids.

The nine essential amino acids are histidine, isoleucine, leucine, lysine, methionine, phenylalanine, threonine, tryptophan, and valine. They are deemed essential because they cannot be synthesized by mammals, at least in the amounts needed, and are therefore essential constituents of an adequate diet for humans. The earlier classification of amino acids as either indispensable or dispensable (Rose and Wixom, 1955) now requires refinement, since in some conditions (e.g., premature births and liver damage) the so-called dispensable amino acids (e.g., cystine and tyrosine) may be important components of the diet and should be considered to be conditionally dispensable (Horowitz et al., 1981).

It has long been known that proteins differ in their growth-promoting ability. These differences in nutritional or biologic value are often expressed in terms of high-quality reference proteins (i.e.,

foods such as eggs, cow's milk, meat, and fish, which contain all the essential amino acids in relatively high concentrations). Because amino acid requirements change with growth and development (FAO/WHO/UNU, 1985), it is now accepted that the biologic or nutritional value is not an unchanging attribute of a protein but can vary with the age of the consumer. However, the degree to which the mixed proteins in typical diets differ in their nutritional value for younger children through adulthood seems rather small (FAO/WHO/UNU, 1985), especially when the usual diet contains a mixture of good protein sources (e.g., milk, eggs, meat, fish, legumes, and nuts) whose amino acid content complements that of such staple foods as cereals and potatoes (Bressani, 1977).

PATTERNS OF INTAKE IN THE U.S. DIET

Protein available in the U.S. food supply has amounted to about 100 g/person/day, or 11% of total energy, since 1909 when the U.S. Department of Agriculture (USDA) began to report food supply data (see Figure 3–3 and Table 3–3 in Chapter 3). A major change since 1909 has been a marked increase (from 52 to 68%) in the proportion of total protein from animal sources and a concomitant decrease in protein from plant sources. Food supply data indicate only the amount of protein available for consumption in wholesale and retail markets, however, and not the amounts actually consumed.

According to USDA's Nationwide Food Consumption Survey (NFCS) of 1977–1978, the mean protein intake for all respondents (infancy to over 75 years of age) was 74 g/day or 16.5% of total calories and exceeded the RDA for all 22 age–sex groups (USDA, 1984). In later USDA surveys, conducted in 1985 and 1986, protein intake averaged 15 to 16% of calories for children 1 to 5 years, 16% of calories for women 19 to 50 years, and 16.5% for men 19 to 50 years, regardless of income (USDA, 1986, 1987a,b). There was little variation in intake with race or urbanization. The 1977–1978 NFCS indicated that meats, poultry, and fish contributed approximately 49%, dairy products 18%, eggs 4%, legumes 3%, cereal products 18%, and fruits and vegetables 7 to 8% of the protein in the U.S. diet (USDA, 1983).

EVIDENCE ASSOCIATING PROTEIN WITH CHRONIC DISEASES

Several considerations must be borne in mind in reviewing studies on dietary protein and chronic diseases:

• Because intakes of animal protein and saturated fat tend to be highly correlated, it is not possible in most epidemiologic studies to separate their independent effects.

• Many epidemiologic studies rely on evidence from vegetarians (e.g., complete vegetarians and lacto-ovovegetarians) that should be evaluated carefully for several reasons: The total protein intake of vegetarians is not much lower than that of omnivores; however, the lifestyles of vegetarians are likely to differ from those of omnivores in many ways that may confound the association between vegetable or animal protein intake and health. In addition, there is a lack of consistency among and within some studies regarding the length of time that subjects have followed a vegetarian diet.

• Laboratory animal studies are often conducted with large, nonphysiologic doses of protein. Thus, the applicability of their findings to human populations may be severely limited.

Coronary Heart Disease

Epidemiologic Studies

The epidemiologic literature on the etiology of coronary heart disease (CHD) emphasizes the role of dietary fats, particularly saturated fat, rather than dietary protein (see Chapter 7). Because animal protein and saturated fat intake tend to be highly correlated, however, it is not surprising that animal protein intake is positively correlated with CHD mortality as are intakes of total and saturated fats. This is so whether one compares populations among different countries, within countries, or migrant populations, or whether one examines secular trends (Aravanis and Loannidis, 1984; Berkson and Stamler, 1981; Kritchevsky, 1976; Toshima et al., 1984).

Findings from the major cohort studies of heart disease have generally failed to demonstrate an independent effect for total dietary protein. For example, Keys et al. (1986) found no association between 15-year mortality from CHD and dietary protein intake (as a percentage of total calories) in an ecological correlation analysis of 15 male cohorts in seven countries. Similarly, Gordon et al. (1981) found no relationship between age-adjusted mean daily protein intake (based on 24-hour dietary recalls) and the occurrence of CHD over periods as long as 6 years in three prospective cohorts of men (in Framingham, Honolulu, and Puerto Rico). A more recent analysis of the Honolulu cohort confirmed the finding; however, because total caloric intake was lower for CHD cases than for the noncases (reflecting a lower intake of carbohydrates and alcohol), protein *as a percentage of total calories* was significantly higher for the CHD cases (McGee et al., 1984).

Clinical Studies

The importance of the source of the protein as a factor in CHD risk is supported indirectly by studies of the effects of different dietary proteins on serum cholesterol—a well-established risk factor for CHD (see Chapter 7). Soy protein-based diets have been shown to have a substantial serum cholesterol-lowering effect in hypercholesterolemic subjects, and the major decrease is in low-density liproprotein (LDL) cholesterol (Descovich et al., 1980; Gaddi et al., 1987; Goldberg et al., 1982; Sirtori et al., 1979, 1985; Verillo et al., 1985; Widhalm, 1986; Wolfe et al., 1981).

The effect of soy-based protein diets on people with normal serum cholesterol is less consistent. For example, Wolfe et al. (1986) and Carroll et al. (1978b) reported that the substitution of vegetable protein (primarily soy) for meat and dairy protein resulted in a substantial lowering of mean serum cholesterol in healthy adults of both sexes. Van Raaij et al. (1981) reported that substitution of

65% soy protein for casein in diets containing 13% of total calories from protein resulted in a marked decline in LDL cholesterol and a weaker but still significant increase in high-density liproprotein (HDL) cholesterol. In other studies, however, no cholesterol-lowering effect of different dietary proteins (e.g., soy protein) was found in subjects with normal serum cholesterol (Bodwell et al., 1980; Terpstra et al., 1983b; van Raaij et al., 1979). The variability in these findings for subjects with normal cholesterol may reflect such factors as interindividual differences in lipid metabolism, differences among studies in the preparation and type of protein sources, and the failure in some studies to exclude animal protein completely from the experimental diets.

Animal Studies

Early animal studies suggesting an effect of protein on atherosclerosis (Ignatovski, 1908) were largely discounted because the diets also contained cholesterol, which is known to be atherogenic. Subsequent studies (Meeker and Kesten, 1940, 1941), however, showed that rabbits fed a cholesterol-free casein diet developed hypercholesterolemia and atherosclerosis in contrast to rabbits fed a similar diet containing soy protein. Again, these findings were largely discounted for nearly two decades (Carroll, 1978; Kritchevsky et al., 1987).

In the late 1950s, workers in two different laboratories reported that rabbits became hypercholesterolemic and developed atherosclerosis when fed cholesterol-free, semipurified diets and that the effect persisted over time (Lambert et al., 1958; Malmros and Wigand, 1959). Subsequent experiments implicated casein as the causative agent (Carroll et al., 1979; Hamilton and Carroll, 1976). The effects of casein were found to be dose related (Huff et al., 1977; Terpstra et al., 1981) and appeared to be associated with enhanced intestinal absorption of cholesterol, decreased fecal excretion of cholesterol and bile acids, slower rate of turnover of plasma cholesterol, reduction in apolipoprotein B/E receptor activity in liver, and inhibition of hepatic cholesterol biosynthesis (Chao et al., 1982; Huff and Carroll, 1980a; Nagata et al., 1982; Sirtori et al., 1984).

Most animal proteins produce some degree of hypercholesterolemia independent of body weight, whereas plant proteins uniformly produce low levels of plasma cholesterol. The hypercholesterolemic effects of animal proteins vary according to the type of protein (e.g., mixtures or single animal proteins) and the animal model used (Beynen and

West, 1987; Hermus et al., 1983; Jacques et al., 1986; Kim et al., 1983; Kritchevsky et al., 1983; Van der Meer and Beynen, 1987), as well as to the type and amount of other dietary constituents. For example, high levels (20% of total calories) of certain polyunsaturated fats such as corn oil and sunflower oil (Lambert et al., 1958; Malmros and Wigand, 1959), fiber-rich foods such as alfalfa (Hamilton and Carroll, 1976; Kritchevsky et al., 1977), dietary carbohydrates such as potato starch (Carroll et al., 1978a; Hamilton and Carroll, 1976), and calcium and zinc (Samman and Roberts, 1987) have all been reported to attenuate the hypercholesterolemic effect of semipurified cholesterol-free diets.

The different effects of animal and plant proteins on serum cholesterol and lipoprotein levels in rabbits (Huff and Carroll, 1980b; Huff et al., 1977) and baboons (Wolfe and Grace, 1987) are largely due to their amino acid composition, although the specific amino acids, or combinations of amino acids, responsible for these observed effects are not known (Huff and Carroll, 1980b). The ratio of lysine to arginine (Kritchevsky, 1979; Kritchevsky et al., 1983, 1987) and the absolute amounts of methionine and glycine (Terpstra et al., 1983a) in the diet have been reported to influence serum cholesterol levels. These findings have not been uniformly replicated (Carroll, 1981), however, and their interpretation is complicated because such studies may not mimic the feeding of intact proteins, which are acted upon by the digestive process (Woodward and Carroll, 1985).

Hypertension

Epidemiologic Studies

Many of the data on the effect of protein on blood pressure are derived from studies of people with chronic protein malnutrition. Many chronically malnourished people have low blood pressure (Viart, 1977); however, the relative contribution of protein deficiency to this condition cannot be readily determined since many such people also suffer from caloric and other nutrient deficiencies as well as other illnesses.

Malhotra (1970) found no association of animal protein intake with blood pressure in a study of two omnivorous populations in India. In a large prospective study of omnivorous Japanese men in Hawaii with *threefold higher protein intakes*, Reed et al. (1983) found significant inverse associations between protein, calcium, potassium, and milk intake (determined from 24-hour diet recalls) and both systolic and diastolic blood pressure levels, although it was not possible to determine whether any of these dietary components had an independent effect on blood pressure. A similar inverse association between dietary protein intake and systolic blood pressure was found in a group of male college students in the United States (Pellum and Medeiros, 1983).

Most epidemiologic studies of protein and blood pressure involve comparisons of groups of vegetarians with other populations that include meat and fish in their diets. These studies consistently reported lower blood pressures among the vegetarians independent of age, weight, and pulse, but it was not possible to determine whether these findings resulted from decreased animal protein intake or from some other dietary components or nondietary factors that differed among the comparison groups (Armstrong et al., 1977; Donaldson, 1926; Ophir et al., 1983; Rouse and Beilin, 1984; Sacks et al., 1974). Nevertheless, these studies suggest that some component of animal products in the diet, possibly animal protein or fat, may influence blood pressure in well-nourished populations.

Clinical Studies

In a randomized trial of 59 omnivorous volunteers, Rouse et al. (1983) found a lowering of both systolic and diastolic blood pressures in those placed on a lacto-ovovegetarian diet as compared to controls on an omnivorous diet. The specific components of the lacto-ovovegetarian diet responsible for this effect were not determined. In a randomized trial of 69 normotensive subjects in Holland, Brussaard et al. (1981) found that blood pressure was not affected differently by the various types of protein in the diet (e.g., vegetable or animal).

Yamori et al. (1984) suggested that deficiencies of certain amino acids, specifically tyrosine and possibly tryptophan, may influence blood pressure in hypertensives either at the vascular level or through the neuronal control of the cardiovascular system. In contrast, Wurtman and Milner (1985) found no convincing evidence that plasma amino acids in general, or tyrosine or tryptophan specifically, are involved in the pathogenesis of human hypertension.

Animal Studies

Most studies of animals with experimentally induced hypertension suggest that dietary protein restriction alone does not lower blood pressure. In rats that have undergone extensive ablation of

renal tissue, protein restriction severe enough to limit body growth does not lower blood pressure (Madden and Zimmerman, 1983; Meyer et al., 1983), nor does protein restriction lower blood pressure in the uninephrectomized spontaneously hypertensive rat (Dworkin and Feiner, 1986). However, protein restriction coupled with alterations in other dietary factors (e.g., added dietary salt) accelerates the development of severe hypertension in the spontaneously hypertensive rat (Kimura, 1977; Yamori, 1980).

Different effects by type of protein have also been noted. For example, consumption of diets rich in milk protein (either casein or whey) limits the development of severe hypertension in stroke-prone spontaneously hypertensive rats (Ikeda et al., 1987).

Stroke

Epidemiologic Studies

There are few epidemiologic studies on dietary protein and stroke. Kagan et al. (1985) found weak evidence of a positive association between consumption of a low-fat, low animal-protein diet and the incidence of stroke in a cohort of Japanese men in Hawaii. The finding for animal protein persisted in a further analysis of these data (Lee et al., 1988) and was supported by the results of an autopsy study of cerebral atherosclerosis in the same study population (Reed et al., 1988). In intercountry comparisons, per capita intake of plant proteins (except those from cereals) was also inversely correlated with cerebrovascular mortality rates (Seely, 1982). However, these data are insufficient to reach any conclusion about the effect of dietary protein on the risk of stroke in humans.

Animal Studies

Very high-protein diets (≈50% of total calories) limit the development of severe hypertension and reduce the incidence of stroke in various strains of spontaneously hypertensive rats (Lovenberg and Yamori, 1984; Wang et al., 1984; Yamori et al., 1978, 1984), whereas diets with a moderately low protein content (approximately 10% protein but with 1% added saline) have the opposite effect (Wexler, 1983a). The type of protein may influence the outcome; for example, diets low in fish protein cause more rapid increases in blood pressure in stroke-prone, spontaneously hypertensive rats than do diets low in animal protein (Wexler, 1983b), and in the same animal model, diets rich in milk protein restrict the development of severe hypertension and extend lifespan (Ikeda et al., 1987).

Specific Cancer Sites

Epidemiogic Studies

A direct effect of dietary protein on cancer risk has been difficult to assess in epidemiologic studies because of the very high correlation between fat and protein intake in the Western diet (Armstrong and Doll, 1975; Carroll and Khor, 1975; Jain et al., 1980; Kolonel et al., 1981). Thus, the effects of these two macronutrients cannot easily be separated. Research has focused more on fat than on protein, and where both have been examined together, associations have generally been stronger for fat (NRC, 1982). Most of the evidence on protein pertains to cancers of the large bowel and the breast, but other sites have been implicated as well.

Large-bowel cancer

Ecological correlations of protein consumption with large-bowel cancer rates are not consistent. In international comparisons, large-bowel cancer incidence and mortality were positively correlated with per-capita total protein, and especially animal protein intake, particularly in developing countries (Armstrong and Doll, 1975; Gregor et al., 1969; Thind, 1986). In contrast, more rigorous dietary assessments in less extensive comparisons, e.g., between two Scandinavian populations or among regional populations in Britain, did not suggest any associations of large-bowel cancer with dietary protein intake (Bingham et al., 1979; IARC–IMG, 1977; Jensen et al., 1982).

In four recent case-control studies, investigators assessed protein intake in relation to risk for large-bowel cancer. In two of these (Jain et al., 1980; Potter and McMichael, 1986), protein consumption was associated with cancers of both the colon and the rectum in both sexes after adjustment for other risk factors. However, this association with protein could not be clearly separated from a similar association with dietary fat in the former study and with total energy intake in the latter. In the other two reports (Kune et al., 1987; Macquart-Moulin et al., 1986), no associations with protein were found in more detailed analyses of the data.

Two prospective cohort studies do not support an association between dietary protein and colon cancer risk. Neither Garland et al. (1985) nor Stemmermann et al. (1984) found any differences in intakes of animal or vegetable protein between colon cancer cases and noncases.

In several epidemiologic studies, both correlation and case-control, positive associations were found between meat consumption (an important source of protein and saturated fat in Western diets) and colon cancer risk, whereas no association was found in many other studies (Kolonel, 1987). Thus, taken together, these findings do not provide added support for a role of dietary protein in the etiology of colon cancer.

Breast cancer

Several studies demonstrate a strong ecological correlation between dietary protein, particularly animal protein, and breast cancer incidence or mortality (Armstrong and Doll, 1975; Carroll and Khor, 1975; Gaskill et al., 1979; Gray et al., 1979; Hems, 1978; Knox, 1977; Kolonel et al., 1981). In the study by Armstrong and Doll (1975) and in a further analysis by Hems (1980), the association of breast cancer with dietary fat was stronger than with protein. Furthermore, in the analysis by Gaskill et al. (1979), no association with protein was observed after controlling for age at first marriage.

Several case-control studies have looked at dietary protein in relation to breast cancer risk. In most of these studies (Hirohata et al., 1985, 1987; Miller et al., 1978; Phillips, 1975), no convincing evidence of an effect of protein was found. On the other hand, J. Lubin et al. (1981) found a positive association between breast cancer risk and level of consumption of animal protein (estimated from only eight food items on a questionnaire). F. Lubin et al. (1986) addressed the problem of intercorrelation among dietary variables (fat, animal protein, and fiber) by stratifying their study sample by four consumption levels in a conditional logistic regression analysis. They showed increased risks associated with animal protein, but not a clear dose-response trend, and concluded that the combination of a high-fat, high-animal-protein, low-fiber diet increased the risk for breast cancer in their population.

Meat consumption was positively associated with breast cancer mortality in a cohort of women in Japan (Hirayama, 1986), but not in a cohort of omnivorous Seventh-Day Adventists in the United States (Mills et al., 1986; Phillips and Snowdon, 1983).

Other cancers

Pancreatic cancer has been associated with dietary protein intake in several geographic correlation analyses (Armstrong and Doll, 1975; Böing et al., 1985; Lea, 1967). High frequency of meat consumption has also been associated with risk for this cancer in some analytic studies (Hirayama, 1981; Ishii et al., 1968; Mack et al., 1986) but not in others (Gold et al., 1985; Norell et al., 1986).

Prostate cancer was positively correlated with protein intake (animal as well as total) in several ecological analyses (Armstrong and Doll, 1975; Böing et al., 1985; Kolonel et al., 1981). In one case-control study, Heshmat et al. (1985) found a nonsignificant increase in protein intake by cases. In another, Graham et al. (1983) did not examine protein but found a statistically significant trend in risk associated with higher frequency of consumption of meats and fish in men 70 years or older.

The relationship of dietary protein to other cancer sites has received little attention. Positive associations with endometrial and stomach cancers (Jedrychowski et al., 1986; Kolonel et al., 1981), and a lack of association with renal and ovarian cancers (Armstrong et al., 1976; Byers et al., 1983), have been reported.

Animal Studies

The evidence associating protein intake with incidence of spontaneous tumors in rodents is inconsistent. Some studies have shown negative associations (Slonaker, 1931), others have been positive (Ross et al., 1970; White and Andervont, 1943; White and White, 1944), whereas still others have shown no association (Tannenbaum and Silverstone, 1949).

Studies have been conducted in rodents to investigate how proteins influence transplanted tumors and tumors induced by such chemicals as aflatoxins, N-acetyl-2-aminofluorene, dimethylbenz(a)anthracene (DMBA), methylcholanthrene, and dimethylhydrazine. Their results indicate that diets with protein at approximately 5% of calories (i.e., below the requirement for optimum growth) generally suppress the development of tumors as well as their subsequent growth and development (Clinton et al., 1984, 1986; Elson, 1958; Engel and Copeland, 1951; Madhavan and Gopalan, 1968; Morris et al., 1948; Temcharoen et al., 1978; Topping and Visek, 1976; Visek, 1985; Walters and Roe, 1964; Wells et al., 1976). The only apparent exception is the increase in DMBA-induced tumor yield in rats fed a low protein diet (Clinton et al., 1979; Elson, 1958; Miller et al., 1941; Silverstone, 1948).

Increasing dietary protein to 20 or 25% of total calories generally enhances tumorigenesis. Further increases have little effect or, in many cases, even inhibit tumorigenesis (Appleton and Campbell, 1982; Engel and Copeland, 1952; Ross and Bras, 1973; Ross et al., 1970; Saxton et al., 1948; Tannenbaum and Silverstone, 1949; Topping and Visek, 1976; Wells et al., 1976). It is not clear whether the general inhibition or the absence of effect on tumorigenesis at very high levels of dietary protein is due to a reduced intake of food and total calories, or whether it is due to other adverse effects, e.g., renal toxicity due to high levels of protein (NRC, 1982). However, tumor enhancement by dietary protein occurs only when there is amino acid balance, suggesting that the effect is not due to specific amino acids or to amino acid imbalance (NRC, 1982).

Osteoporosis

Epidemiologic and Clinical Studies

High dietary protein taken as a purified isolated nutrient increases urinary excretion of calcium (Allen et al., 1979; Anand and Linkswiler, 1974; Chu et al., 1975; Hegsted and Linkswiler, 1981; Hegsted et al., 1981; Johnson et al., 1970; Kim and Linkswiler, 1979; Margen et al., 1974; McCance and Widdowson, 1942; Schwartz et al., 1973; Walker and Linkswiler, 1972). There is little evidence, however, that natural diets high in protein increase osteoporosis risk.

In the U.S. Ten-State Nutrition Survey, a very low, nonsignificant correlation was found between average daily protein intake and metacarpal cortical bone area in elderly adults (Garn et al., 1981). However, these intakes were based on 24-hour dietary recalls, which are poor measures of intake for individuals (see Chapter 2). Furthermore, because bone mass at older ages is determined primarily by the mass achieved at maturity (Draper and Scythes, 1981; Matkovic et al., 1979), correlations of bone density with contemporaneous dietary intake in the elderly may be misleading.

Bone mineral mass appears to be lower in omnivorous women than in lacto-ovovegetarian women (Marsh et al., 1980; Sanchez et al., 1980) and lower in North Alaskan Eskimos consuming an extremely high animal-protein diet than in North American Caucasians (Mazess and Mather, 1974). It has not been shown, however, that either the type or the amount of protein in the diet is responsible for these differences.

In a 4-year clinical trial of postmenopausal women who did not take calcium supplements, Freudenheim et al. (1986) observed a positive correlation between protein intake and changes in bone mineral content of the radius. However, although such short-term studies in the elderly suggest that high-protein diets produce an increase in urinary calcium excretion and often a worsening in calcium balance (Licata et al., 1981; Lutz and Linkswiler, 1981), the long-term effects of such diets, particularly on bone mass, are unknown.

In addition, urinary calcium excretion increases with increased protein intake only if phosphorus intake is held constant (see Chapter 13). If phosphorus intake rises with protein intake as it does in typical U.S. diets, the effect of protein is minimized (Hegsted et al., 1981; Schuett and Linkswiler, 1982). Thus, although it has been suggested that a habitual high intake of protein may contribute to an increased risk of osteoporosis, this is not supported by current evidence.

Chronic Renal Disease

Epidemiologic and Clinical Studies

Brenner et al. (1982) hypothesized that glomerular capillary hypertension (which is associated with an increase in glomerular filtration rate and capillary blood flow) results from unrestricted intake of protein-rich foods and leads to glomerular sclerosis, thus accounting for the progressive decrease in renal function observed with age. However, although both glomerular filtration rate and capillary blood flow increase in response to a high protein intake (Bosch et al., 1983; Pullman et al., 1954), thus far there are no epidemiologic or clinical data to support this hypothesis.

Animal Studies

In animals, as in humans, glomerular sclerosis increases with age (Couser and Stilmant, 1975; Guttman and Andersen, 1968). In rats fed ad libitum standard chows containing about 20 to 25% protein, most glomeruli showed signs of sclerosis by 2 years of age (Coleman et al., 1977). However, development of glomerular sclerosis in rats can be delayed either by decreasing the amount of standard chow by one-half to two-thirds that consumed by animals fed ad libitum (Berg and Simms, 1960; Tucker et al., 1976; Yu et al., 1982) or by decreasing the amount of protein in the chow to 6% of total calories (Meyer et al., 1983). Conversely, increasing dietary animal protein to 31% or more of total calories has been shown to accelerate development of glomerular sclerosis (Newburgh and Curtis, 1928). These findings suggest that dietary protein influences renal blood flow, glomerular filtration rate, and, ultimately, progression of age-related glomerular sclerosis in the healthy animal.

SUMMARY

Animal proteins in the diet have not been linked specifically to CHD risk in humans, although high levels induce hypercholesterolemia and atherosclerosis in laboratory animals. Substitution of soybean protein for animal protein in the diet reduces the level of serum cholesterol in humans, particularly in hypercholesterolemic subjects, and there is evidence that groups eating vegetarian diets have lower average blood cholesterol levels than the general population. The data linking elevated intakes of animal protein to increased risk of hypertension are weak.

Some epidemiologic studies suggest that higher intakes of animal protein may be associated with increased risk of cancer at certain sites, although the data are not entirely consistent. However, because of the strong positive correlation between dietary protein and fat over the range of normal intakes in most Western populations, it is not clear whether dietary protein exerts an independent effect on cancer. In laboratory experiments, the relationship of dietary protein to carcinogenesis appears to depend upon protein level. Chemically induced carcinogenesis is enhanced as protein intake is increased up to 2 or 3 times the normal requirement. Higher levels produce no further enhancement and, in many cases, may inhibit tumorigenesis.

Although high dietary protein taken as a purified isolated nutrient increases urinary excretion of calcium, there is little evidence that natural diets high in protein increase osteoporosis risk. High intakes of animal protein are hypothesized to lead to progressive glomerular sclerosis and deterioration of renal function by promoting sustained increases in renal blood flow and glomerular filtration rates. Although both human and animal studies indicate that a high-protein intake can increase glomerular filtration rate and age-related progression of renal disease, the effect of high dietary protein on the risk of chronic renal disease in humans needs further investigation.

DIRECTIONS FOR RESEARCH

• The relative effects of different levels of total protein and different types of protein (animal or vegetable) in chronic disease etiology and their mechanisms of action (e.g., in CHD, hypertension, specific cancers, osteoporosis, chronic renal disease, and stroke).

- The long-term effects of protein intake above nutritional requirements on renal function in humans and the relationship of dietary protein to increased risk of end-stage renal disease.

- The role of specific amino acids or combinations of amino acids in augmenting chronic disease risk.

- The optimal range of protein intake (animal or vegetable) for reducing chronic disease risk.

- The effect of the kind and amount of protein upon various stages and mechanisms of neoplastic development.

REFERENCES

Allen, L.H., E.A. Oddoye, and S. Margen. 1979. Protein-induced hypercalciuria: a longer term study. Am. J. Clin. Nutr. 32:741–749.

Anand, C.H., and H.M. Linkswiler. 1974. Effect of protein intake on calcium balance of young men given 500 mg calcium daily. J. Nutr. 104:695–700.

Appleton, B.S., and T.C. Campbell. 1982. Inhibition of aflatoxin-initiated preneoplastic liver lesions by low dietary protein. Nutr. Cancer 3:200–206.

Aravanis, C., and P.J. Loannidis. 1984. Nutritional factors and cardiovascular diseases in the Greek Islands Heart Study. Pp. 125–135 in W. Lovenberg and Y. Yamori, eds. Nutritional Prevention of Cardiovascular Disease. Academic Press, Orlando, Fla.

Armstrong, B., and R. Doll. 1975. Environmental factors and cancer incidence and mortality in different countries, with specific reference to dietary practices. Int. J. Cancer 15:617–631.

Armstrong, B., A. Garrod, and R. Doll. 1976. A retrospective study of renal cancer with special reference to coffee and animal protein consumption. Br. J. Cancer 33:127–136.

Armstrong, B., A.J. Van Merwyk, and H. Coates. 1977. Blood pressure in Seventh-Day Adventist vegetarians. Am. J. Epidemiol. 105:444–449.

Berg, B.N., and H.S. Simms. 1960. Nutrition and longevity in the rat. II. Longevity and onset of disease with different levels of food intake. J. Nutr. 71:255–263.

Berkson, D.M., and J. Stamler. 1981. Epidemiology of the killer chronic diseases. Pp. 17–55 in M. Winick, ed. Nutrition and the Killer Diseases. Wiley, New York.

Beynen, A.C., and C.E. West. 1987. Cholesterol metabolism in swine fed diets containing either casein or soybean protein. J. Am. Oil Chem. Soc. 64:1178–1182.

Bingham, S., D.R.R. Williams, T.C. Cole, and W.P.T. James. 1979. Dietary fibre and regional large-bowel cancer mortality in Britain. Br. J. Cancer 40:456–463.

Bodwell, C.E., E.M. Schuster, P.S. Steele, J.T. Judd, and J.C. Smith. 1980. Effects of dietary soy protein on plasma lipid profiles of adult men. Fed. Proc. 39:1113.

Böing, H., L. Martinez, R. Frentzel-Beyme, and U. Oltersdorf. 1985. Regional nutritional pattern and cancer mortality in the Federal Republic of Germany. Nutr. Cancer 7:121–130.

Bosch, J.P., A. Saccaggi, A. Lauer, C. Ronco, M. Belledonne, and S. Glabman. 1983. Renal functional reserve in humans. Effect of protein intake on glomerular filtration rate. Am. J. Med. 75:943–950.

Brenner, B.M., T.W. Meyer, and T.H. Hostetter. 1982. Dietary protein intake and the progressive nature of kidney disease: the role of hemodynamically mediated glomerular injury in the pathogenesis of progressive glomerular sclerosis in aging, renal ablation, and intrinsic renal disease. N. Engl. J. Med. 307:652–659.

Bressani, R. 1977. Protein supplementation and complementation. Pp. 204–232 in C.E. Bodwell, ed. Evaluation of Proteins for Humans. AVI Publ. Co., Westport, Conn.

Brussaard, J.H., J.M. van Raaij, M. Stasse-Wolthuis, M.B. Katan, and J.G. Hautvast. 1981. Blood pressure and diet in normotensive volunteers: absence of an effect of dietary fiber, protein, or fat. Am. J. Clin. Nutr. 34:2023–2029.

Byers, T., J. Marshall, S. Graham, C. Mettlin, and M. Swanson. 1983. A case-control study of dietary and nondietary factors in ovarian cancer. J. Natl. Cancer Inst. 71:681–686.

Carroll, K.K. 1978. Dietary protein in relation to plasma cholesterol levels and atherosclerosis. Nutr. Rev. 36:1–5.

Carroll, K.K. 1981. Soya protein and atherosclerosis. J. Am. Oil Chem. Soc. 58:416–419.

Carroll, K.K., and H.T. Khor. 1975. Dietary fat in relation to tumorigenesis. Prog. Biochem. Pharmacol. 10:308–353.

Carroll, K.K., R.M. Hamilton, M.W. Huff, and A.D. Falconer. 1978a. Dietary fiber and cholesterol metabolism in rabbits and rats. Am. J. Clin. Nutr. 31:S203–S207.

Carroll, K.K., P.M. Giovannetti, M.W. Huff, O. Moase, D.C.K. Roberts, and B.M. Wolfe. 1978b. Hypocholesterolemic effect of substituting soybean protein for animal protein in the diet of healthy young women. Am. J. Clin. Nutr. 31:1312–1321.

Carroll, K.K., M.W. Huff, and D.C.K. Roberts. 1979. Vegetable protein and lipid metabolism. Pp. 261–280 in H.L. Wilcke, D.T. Hopkins, and D.H. Waggle, eds. Soy Protein and Human Nutrition. Academic Press, New York.

Chao, Y., T.T. Yamin, and A.W. Alberts. 1982. Effects of cholestyramine on low density lipoprotein binding sites on liver membranes from rabbits with endogenous hypercholesterolemia induced by a wheat starch-casein diet. J. Biol. Chem. 257:3623–3627.

Chu, J.Y., S. Margen, and F.M. Costa. 1975. Studies in calcium metabolism. II. Effects of low calcium and variable protein intake on human calcium metabolism. Am. J. Clin. Nutr. 28:1028–1035.

Clinton, S.K., C.R. Truex, and W.J. Visek. 1979. Dietary protein, aryl hydrocarbon hydroxylase and chemical carcinogenesis in rats. J. Nutr. 109:55–62.

Clinton, S.K., P.B. Imrey, J.M. Alster, J. Simon, C.R. Truex, and W.J. Visek. 1984. The combined effects of dietary protein and fat on 7,12-dimethylbenz(a)anthracene-induced breast cancer in rats. J. Nutr. 114:1213–1223.

Clinton, S.K., J.M. Alster, P.B. Imrey, S. Nandkumar, C.R. Truex, and W.J. Visek. 1986. Effects of dietary protein, fat and energy intake during an initiation phase study of 7,12-dimethylbenz(a)anthracene-induced breast cancer in rats. J. Nutr. 116:2290–2302.

Coleman, G.L., W. Barthold, G.W. Osbaldiston, S.J. Foster, and A.M. Jonas. 1977. Pathological changes during aging in barrier-reared Fischer 344 male rats. J. Gerontol. 32:258–278.

Couser, W.G., and M.M. Stilmant. 1975. Mesangial lesions and focal glomerular sclerosis in the aging rat. Lab. Invest. 33:491–501.

Descovich, G.C., A. Gaddi, G. Mannino, L. Cattin, U. Senin, C. Caruzzo, C. Fragiacomo, M. Sirtori, C. Ceredi,

M.S. Benassi, L. Colombo, G. Fontana, E. Mannarino, E. Bertelli, G. Noseda, and C.R. Sirtori. 1980. Multicentre study of soybean protein diet for outpatient hypercholesterolaemic patients. Lancet 2:709–712.

Donaldson, A.N. 1926. Relation of protein foods to hypertension. Calif. West. Med. 24:328–331.

Draper, H.H., and C.A. Scythes. 1981. Calcium, phosphorus, and osteoporosis. Fed. Proc. 40:2434–2438.

Dworkin, L.D., and H.D. Feiner. 1986. Glomerular injury in uninephrectomized spontaneously hypertensive rats. A consequence of glomerular capillary hypertension. J. Clin. Invest. 77:797–809.

Elson, L.A. 1958. Some dynamic aspects of chemical carcinogenesis. Br. Med. Bull. 14:161–164.

Engel, R.W., and D.H. Copeland. 1951. Influence of diet on the relative incidence of eye, mammary, ear-duct, and liver tumors in rats fed 2-acetylaminofluorene. Cancer Res. 11:180–183.

Engel, R.W., and D.H. Copeland. 1952. The influence of dietary casein level on tumor induction with 2-acetylaminofluorene. Cancer Res. 12:905–908.

FAO/WHO/UNU (Food and Agriculture Organization/World Health Organization/United Nations University). 1985. Energy and Protein Requirements. Report of a Joint FAO/WHO/UNU Expert Consultation. Technical Report Series No. 724. World Health Organization, Geneva. 206 pp.

Freudenheim, J.L., N.E. Johnson, and E.L. Smith. 1986. Relationships between usual nutrient intake and bone-mineral content of women 35–65 years of age: longitudinal and cross-sectional analysis. Am. J. Clin. Nutr. 44:863–876.

Gaddi, A., G.C. Descovich, G. Noseda, C. Fragiocomo, A. Nicolini, G. Montanari, G. Vanetti, M. Sirtori, E. Gatti, and C.R. Sirtori. 1987. Hypercholesterolaemia treated by soybean protein diet. Arch. Dis. Child. 62:274–278.

Garland, C., R.B. Shekelle, E. Barrett-Connor, M.H. Criqui, A.H. Rossof, and O. Paul. 1985. Dietary vitamin D and calcium and risk of colorectal cancer: a 19-year prospective study in men. Lancet 1:307–309.

Garn, S.M., M.A. Solomon, and J. Friedl. 1981. Calcium intake and bone quality in the elderly. Ecol. Food Nutr. 10:131–133.

Gaskill, S.P., W.L. McGuire, C.K. Osborne, and M.P. Stern. 1979. Breast cancer mortality and diet in the United States. Cancer Res. 39:3628–3637.

Gold, E.B., L. Gordis, M.D. Diener, R. Seltser, J.K. Boitnott, T.E. Bynum, and D.F. Hutcheon. 1985. Diet and other risk factors for cancer of the pancreas. Cancer 55:460–467.

Goldberg, A.P., A. Lim, J.B. Kolar, J.J. Grundhauser, F.H. Steinke, and G. Schonfeld. 1982. Soybean protein independently lowers plasma cholesterol levels in primary hypercholesterolemia. Atherosclerosis 43:355–368.

Gordon, T., A. Kagan, M. Garcia-Palmieri, W.B. Kannel, W.J. Zukel, J. Tillotson, P. Sorlie, and M. Hjortland. 1981. Diet and its relation to coronary heart disease and death in three populations. Circulation 63:500–515.

Graham, S., B. Haughey, J. Marshall, R. Priore, T. Byers, T. Rzepka, C. Mettlin, and J.E. Pontes. 1983. Diet in the epidemiology of carcinoma of the prostate gland. J. Natl. Cancer Inst. 70:687–692.

Gray, G.E., M.C. Pike, and B.E. Henderson. 1979. Breast-cancer incidence and mortality rates in different countries in relation to known risk factors and dietary practices. Br. J. Cancer 39:1–7.

Gregor, O., R. Toman, and F. Prusova. 1969. Gastrointestinal cancer and nutrition. Gut 10:1031–1034.

Guttman, P.H., and A.C. Andersen. 1968. Progressive intercapillary glomerulosclerosis in aging and irradiated beagles. Radiol. Res. 35:45–60.

Hamilton, R.M., and K.K. Carroll. 1976. Plasma cholesterol levels in rabbits fed low fat, low cholesterol diets: effects of dietary proteins, carbohydrates and fibre from different sources. Atherosclerosis 24:47–62.

Hegsted, M., and H.M. Linkswiler. 1981. Long-term effects of level of protein intake on calcium metabolism in young adult women. J. Nutr. 111:244–251.

Hegsted, M., S.A. Schuette, M.B. Zemel, and H.M. Linkswiler. 1981. Urinary calcium and calcium balance in young men as affected by level of protein and phosphorus intake. J. Nutr. 111:553–562.

Hems, G. 1978. The contributions of diet and childbearing to breast-cancer rates. Br. J. Cancer 37:974–982.

Hems, G. 1980. Associations between breast-cancer mortality rates, child bearing and diet in the United Kingdom. Br. J. Cancer 41:429–437.

Hermus, R.J.J., C.E. West, and E.J. van Weerden. 1983. Failure of dietary-casein-induced acidosis to explain the hypercholesterolemia of casein-fed rabbits. J. Nutr. 113:618–629.

Heshmat, M.Y., L. Kaul, J. Kovi, M.A. Jackson, A.G. Jackson, G.W. Jones, M. Edson, J.P. Enterline, R.G. Worrell, and S.L. Perry. 1985. Nutrition and prostate cancer: a case-control study. Prostate 6:7–17.

Hirayama, T. 1981. A large-scale cohort study on the relationship between diet and selected cancers of digestive organs. Pp. 409–429 in W.R. Bruce, P. Correa, M. Lipkin, S.R. Tannenbaum, and T.D. Wilkins, eds. Banbury Report 7—Gastrointestinal Cancer: Endogenous Factors. Cold Spring Harbor, New York.

Hirayama, T. 1986. A large scale cohort study on cancer risks by diet—with special reference to the risk reducing effects of green-yellow vegetable consumption. Pp. 41–53 in Y. Hayashi, M. Nagao, T. Sugimura, S. Takayama, L. Tomatis, L.W. Wattenberg, and G.N. Wogan, eds. Diet, Nutrition and Cancer. Japan Scientific Societies Press, Tokyo.

Hirohata, T., T. Shigematsu, A.M.Y. Nomura, Y. Nomura, A. Horie, and I. Hirohata. 1985. Occurrence of breast cancer in relation to diet and reproductive history: a case-control study in Fukuoka, Japan. Natl. Cancer Inst. Monogr. 69:187–190.

Hirohata, T., A.M.Y. Nomura, J.H. Hankin, L.N. Kolonel, and J. Lee. 1987. An epidemiologic study on the association between diet and breast cancer. J. Natl. Cancer Inst. 78:595–600.

Horowitz, J.H., E.B. Rypins, J.M. Henderson, S.B. Heymsfield, S.D. Moffitt, R.P. Bain, R.K. Chawla, J.C. Bleier, and D. Rudman. 1981. Evidence for impairment of transsulfuration pathway in cirrhosis. Gastroenterology 81:668–675.

Huff, M.W., and K.K. Carroll. 1980a. Effects of dietary protein on turnover, oxidation, and absorption of cholesterol, and on steroid excretion in rabbits. J. Lipid Res. 21:546–558.

Huff, M.W., and K.K. Carroll. 1980b. Effects of dietary proteins and amino acid mixtures on plasma cholesterol levels in rabbits. J. Nutr. 110:1676–1685.

Huff, M.W., R.M.G. Hamilton, and K.K. Carroll. 1977. Plasma cholesterol levels in rabbits fed low fat, cholesterol-free semipurified diets: effects of dietary proteins, protein hydrolysates and amino acid mixtures. Atherosclerosis 28: 187–195.

IARC–IMG (International Agency for Research on Cancer-Intestinal Microecology Group). 1977. Dietary fibre, transit-time, faecal bacteria, steroids, and colon cancer in two Scandinavian populations. Lancet 2:207–211.

Ignatovski, A.I. 1908. Influence of animal food on the organism of rabbits. Izv. Imp. Voyenno-Med. Akad. Peter. 16:154–176.

Ikeda, K., S. Mochizuki, Y. Nara, R. Horie, and Y. Yamori. 1987. Effect of milk protein and fat intake on blood pressure and the incidence of cerebrovascular diseases in stroke-prone spontaneously hypertensive rats (SHRSP). J. Nutr. Sci. Vitaminol. 33:31–36.

Ishii, K., K. Nakamura, H. Ozaki, N. Yamada, and T. Takeuchi. 1968. Epidemiological problems of pancreas cancer. Jpn. J. Clin. Med. 26:1839–1842.

Jacques, H., Y. Deshaies, and L. Savoie. 1986. Relationship between dietary proteins, their in vitro digestion products, and serum cholesterol in rats. Atherosclerosis 61:89–98.

Jain, M., G.M. Cook, F.G. Davis, M.G. Grace, G.R. Howe, and A.B. Miller. 1980. A case-control study of diet and colo-rectal cancer. Int. J. Cancer 26:757–768.

Jedrychowski, W., J. Wahrendorf, T. Popiela, and J. Rachtan. 1986. A case-control study of dietary factors and stomach cancer risk in Poland. Int. J. Cancer 37:837–842.

Jensen, O.M., R. MacLennan, and J. Wahrendorf. 1982. Diet, bowel function, fecal characteristics, and large bowel cancer in Denmark and Finland. Nutr. Cancer 4:5–19.

Johnson, N.E., E.N. Alcantara, and H. Linkswiler. 1970. Effect level of protein intake on urinary and fecal calcium and calcium retention of young adult males. J. Nutr. 100: 1425–1430.

Kagan, A., J.S. Popper, G.G. Rhoads, and K. Yano. 1985. Dietary and other risk factors for stroke in Hawaiian Japanese men. Stroke 16:390–396.

Keys, A., A. Menotti, M.J. Karvonen, C. Aravanis, H. Blackburn, R. Buzina, B.S. Djordjevic, A.S. Dontas, F. Fidanza, M.H. Keys, D. Kromhout, S. Nedeljkovic, S. Punsar, F. Seccareccia, and H. Toshima. 1986. The diet and 15-year death rate in the Seven Countries Study. Am. J. Epidemiol. 124:903–915.

Kim, D.N., K.T. Lee, J.M. Reiner, and W.A. Thomas. 1983. Effects of soy protein on cholesterol metabolism in swine. Pp. 101–110 in M.J. Gibney and D. Kritchevsky, eds. Current Topics in Nutrition and Disease, Vol. 8. Animal and Vegetable Proteins in Lipid Metabolism and Atherosclerosis. Alan R. Liss, New York.

Kim, Y., and H.M. Linkswiler. 1979. Effect of level of protein intake on calcium metabolism and on parathyroid and renal function in the adult human male. J. Nutr. 109:1399–1404.

Kimura, N. 1977. Atherosclerosis in Japan: epidemiology. Pp. 209–221 in R. Paoletti and A.M. Gotto, Jr., eds. Atherosclerosis Reviews, Vol. 2. Raven Press, New York.

Knox, E.G. 1977. Foods and diseases. Br. J. Prev. Soc. Med. 31:71–80.

Kolonel, L.N. 1987. Fat and colon cancer: how firm is the epidemiologic evidence? Am. J. Clin. Nutr. 45:336–341.

Kolonel, L.N., J.H. Hankin, J. Lee, S.Y. Chu, A.M.Y. Nomura, and M.W. Hinds. 1981. Nutrient intakes in relation to cancer incidence in Hawaii. Br. J. Cancer 44:332–339.

Kritchevsky, D. 1976. Diet and atherosclerosis. Am. J. Pathol. 84:615–632.

Kritchevsky, D. 1979. Vegetable protein and atherosclerosis. J. Am. Oil Chem. Soc. 56:135–140.

Kritchevsky, D., S.A. Tepper, D.E. Williams, and J.A. Story. 1977. Experimental atherosclerosis in rabbits fed cholesterol-free diets. 7. Interaction of animal or vegetable protein with fiber. Atherosclerosis 26:397–403.

Kritchevsky, D., S.A. Tepper, S. Czarnecki, D.M. Klurfeld, and J.A. Story. 1983. Effects of animal and vegetable protein in experimental atherosclerosis. Pp. 85–100 in M.J. Gibney and D. Kritchevsky, eds. Animal and Vegetable Proteins in Lipid Metabolism and Atherosclerosis. Alan R. Liss, New York.

Kritchevsky, D., S.A. Tepper, and D.M. Klurfeld. 1987. Dietary protein and atherosclerosis. J. Am. Oil Chem. Soc. 64:1167–1171.

Kune, S., G.A. Kune, and L.F. Watson. 1987. Case-control study of dietary etiological factors: The Melbourne Colorectal Cancer Study. Nutr. Cancer 9:21–42.

Lambert, G.F., J.P. Miller, R.T. Olsen, and D.V. Frost. 1958. Hypercholesteremia and atherosclerosis induced in rabbits by purified high fat rations devoid of cholesterol. Proc. Soc. Exp. Biol. Med. 97:544–549.

Lea, A.J. 1967. Neoplasms and environmental factors. Ann. R. Coll. Surg. Engl. 41:432–438.

Lee, C.N., D.M. Reed, C.J. MacLean, K. Yano, and D. Chiu. 1988. Dietary potassium and stroke. N. Engl. J. Med. 318: 995–996.

Licata, A.A., E. Bou, F.C. Bartter, and F. West. 1981. Acute effects of dietary protein on calcium metabolism in patients with osteoporosis. J. Gerontol. 36:14–19.

Lovenberg, W., and Y. Yamori. 1984. Nutritional factors and cardiovascular disease. Clin. Exp. Hypertens. A6:417–426.

Lubin, F., Y. Wax, and B. Modan. 1986. Role of fat, animal protein, and dietary fiber in breast cancer etiology: a case-control study. J. Natl. Cancer Inst. 77:605–612.

Lubin, J.H., W.J. Blot, and P.E. Burns. 1981. Breast cancer following high dietary fat and protein consumption. Am. J. Epidemiol. 114:422.

Lutz, J., and H.M. Linkswiler. 1981. Calcium metabolism in postmenopausal and osteoporotic women consuming two levels of dietary protein. Am. J. Clin. Nutr. 34:2178–2186.

Mack, T.M., M.C. Yu, R. Hanisch, and B.E. Henderson. 1986. Pancreas cancer and smoking, beverage consumption, and past medical history. J. Natl. Cancer Inst. 76:49–60.

Macquart-Moulin, G., E. Riboli, J. Cornée, B. Charnay, P. Berthezène, and N. Day. 1986. Case-control study on colorectal cancer and diet in Marseilles. Int. J. Cancer 38:183–191.

Madden, M.A., and S.W. Zimmerman. 1983. Protein restriction and renal function in the uremic rat. Kidney Int. 23: 217.

Madhavan, T.V., and C. Gopalan. 1968. The effect of dietary protein on carcinogenesis of aflatoxin. Arch. Pathol. 85: 133–137.

Malhotra, S.L. 1970. Dietary factors causing hypertension in India. Am. J. Clin. Nutr. 23:1353–1363.

Malmros, H., and G. Wigand. 1959. Atherosclerosis and deficiency of essential fatty acids. Lancet 2:749–751.

Margen, S., J.Y. Chu, N.A. Kaufmann, and D.H. Calloway. 1974. Studies in calcium metabolism. I. The calciuretic effect of dietary protein. Am. J. Clin. Nutr. 27:584–589.

Marsh, A.G., T.V. Sanchez, O. Midkelsen, J. Keiser, and G. Mayor. 1980. Cortical bone density of adult lacto-ovo-vegetarian and omnivorous women. J. Am. Diet. Assoc. 76: 148–151.

Matkovic, V., K. Kostial, I. Simonovic, R. Buzina, A. Brodarec, and B.E.C. Nordin. 1979. Bone status and fracture rates in two regions of Yugoslavia. Am. J. Clin. Nutr. 32:540–549.

Mazess, R.B., and W. Mather. 1974. Bone mineral content of North Alaskan Eskimos. Am. J. Clin. Nutr. 27:916–925.

McCance, R.A., and E.M. Widdowson. 1942. Mineral metabolism of healthy adults on white and brown bread dietaries. J. Physiol. 101:44–85.

McGee, D.L., D.M. Reed, K. Yano, A. Kagan, and J. Tillotson. 1984. Ten-year incidence of coronary heart disease in the Honolulu Heart Program: relationship to nutrient intake. Am. J. Epidemiol. 119:667–676.

Meeker, D.R., and H.D. Kesten. 1940. Experimental atherosclerosis and high protein diets. Proc. Soc. Exp. Biol. Med. 45:543–545.

Meeker, D.R., and H.D. Kesten. 1941. Effect of high protein diets on experimental atherosclerosis of rabbits. Arch. Pathol. 31:147–162.

Meyer, T.W., T.H. Hostetter, H.G. Rennke, J.L. Noddin, and B.M. Brenner. 1983. Preservation of renal structure and function by long term protein restriction in rats with reduced nephron mass. Kidney Int. 23:218.

Miller, A.B., A. Kelly, N.W. Choi, V. Matthews, R.W. Morgan, L. Munan, J.D. Burch, J. Feather, G.R. Howe, and M. Jain. 1978. A study of diet and breast cancer. Am. J. Epidemiol. 107:499–509.

Miller, J.A., D.L. Miner, H.P. Rusch, and C.A. Baumann. 1941. Diet and hepatic tumor formation. Cancer Res. 1:699–708.

Mills, P., J.F. Annegers, and R.L. Phillips. 1986. Dietary relationships to fatal breast cancer among Seventh-Day Adventists. Am. J. Epidemiol. 124:531.

Morris, H.P., B.B. Westfall, C.S. Dubnik, and T.B. Dunn. 1948. Some observations on carcinogenicity, distribution and metabolism of N-acetyl-2-aminofluorene in the rat. Cancer Res. 8:390.

Nagata, Y., N. Ishiwaki, and M. Sugano. 1982. Studies on the mechanism of antihypercholesterolemic action of soy protein and soy protein-type amino acid mixtures in relation to the casein counterparts in rats. J. Nutr. 112:1614–1625.

Newburgh, L.H., and A.C. Curtis. 1928. Production of renal injury in white rat by protein of diet; dependence of injury on duration of feeding, and on amount and kind of protein. Arch. Intern. Med. 42:801–821.

Norell, S.E., A. Ahlbom, R. Erwald, G. Jacobson, I. Lindberg-Navier, R. Olin, B. Törnberg, and K.L. Wiechel. 1986. Diet and pancreatic cancer: a case-control study. Am. J. Epidemiol. 124:894–902.

NRC (National Research Council). 1982. Diet, Nutrition, and Cancer. Report of the Committee on Diet, Nutrition, and Cancer, Assembly of Life Sciences. National Academy Press, Washington, D.C. 478 pp.

Ophir, O., G. Peer, J. Gilad, M. Blum, and A. Aviram. 1983. Low blood pressure in vegetarians: the possible role of potassium. Am. J. Clin. Nutr. 37:755–762.

Pellum, L.K., and D.M. Medeiros. 1983. Blood pressure in young adult normotensives: effect of protein, fat, and cholesterol intakes. Nutr. Rep. Int. 27:1277–1285.

Phillips, R.L. 1975. Role of life-style and dietary habits in risk of cancer among Seventh-Day Adventists. Cancer Res. 35:3513–3522.

Phillips, R.L., and D.A. Snowdon. 1983. Association of meat and coffee use with cancers of the large bowel, breast, and prostate among Seventh-Day Adventists: preliminary results. Cancer Res. 43:2403s-2408s.

Potter, J.D., and A.J. McMichael. 1986. Diet and cancer of the colon and rectum: a case-control study. J. Natl. Cancer Inst. 76:557–569.

Pullman, T.N., A.S. Alving, R.J. Dern, and M. Landowne. 1954. Influence of dietary protein intake on specific renal functions in normal man. J. Lab. Clin. Med. 44:320–332.

Reed, D., D. McGee, K. Yano, and J. Hankin. 1983. Diet, blood pressure and multicollinearity. Pp. 155–166 in W. Lovenberg and Y. Yamori, eds. Nutritional Prevention of Cardiovascular Disease. Academic Press, Orlando, Fla.

Reed, D.M., J.A. Resch, T. Hayashi, C. MacLean, and K. Yano. 1988. A prospective study of cerebral artery atherosclerosis. Stroke 19:820–825.

Rose, W.C., and R.L. Wixom. 1955. The amino acid requirements of man. XVI. The role of the nitrogen intake. J. Biol. Chem. 217:997–1004.

Ross, M.H., and G. Bras. 1973. Influence of protein under- and overnutrition on spontaneous tumor prevalence in the rat. J. Nutr. 103:944–963.

Ross, M.H., G. Bras, and M.S. Ragbeer. 1970. Influence of protein and caloric intake upon spontaneous tumor incidence of the anterior pituitary gland of the rat. J. Nutr. 100:177–189.

Rouse, I.L., and L.J. Beilin. 1984. Vegetarian diet and blood pressure. J. Hypertens. 2:231–240.

Rouse, I.L., L.J. Beilin, B.K. Armstrong, and R. Vandongen. 1983. Blood-pressure-lowering effect of a vegetarian diet: controlled trial in normotensive subjects. Lancet 1:5–10.

Sacks, F.M., B. Rosner, and E.H. Kass. 1974. Blood pressure in vegetarians. Am. J. Epidemiol. 100:390–398.

Samman, S., and D.C. Roberts. 1987. The importance of the non-protein components of the diet in the plasma cholesterol response of rabbits to casein: zinc and copper. Br. J. Nutr. 57:27–33.

Sanchez, T.V., O. Mickelsen, A.G. Marsh, S.M. Garn, and G.H. Mayor. 1980. Bone mineral in elderly vegetarian and omnivorous females. Pp. 94–98 in R.B. Mazess, ed. Proceedings: Fourth International Conference on Bone Measurement, Toronto, June 1978. NIH Publ. No. 80–1938. National Institute of Arthritis, Metabolism, and Digestive Diseases, National Institutes of Health, Public Health Service, U.S. Department of Health and Human Services. Bethesda, Md.

Saxton, J.A., Jr., G.A. Sperling, L.L. Barnes, and C.M. McCay. 1948. The influence of nutrition upon the incidence of spontaneous tumors of the albino rat. Acta Unio Int. Contra Cancrum 6:423–431.

Schuette, S.A., and H.M. Linkswiler. 1982. Effects on Ca and P metabolism in humans by adding meat, meat plus milk, or purified proteins plus Ca and P to allow protein diet. J. Nutr. 112:338–349.

Schwartz, R., N.A. Woodcock, J.D. Blakely, and I. MacKellar. 1973. Metabolic responses of adolescent boys to two levels of dietary magnesium and protein. II. Effect of magnesium and protein level on calcium balance. Am. J. Clin. Nutr. 26:519–523.

Seely, S. 1982. Diet and cerebrovascular disease: search for linkages. Med. Hypotheses 9:509–515.

Silverstone, H. 1948. The levels of carcinogenic azo dyes in the livers of rats fed various diets containing p-dimethylaminoazobenzene: relationship to the formation of hepatomas. Cancer Res. 8:301–308.

Sirtori, C.R., E. Gatti, O. Mantero, F. Conti, E. Agradi, E. Tremoli, M. Sirtori, L. Fraterrigo, L. Tavazzi, and D. Kritchevsky. 1979. Clinical experience with the soybean protein diet in the treatment of hypercholesterolemia. Am. J. Clin. Nutr. 32:1645–1658.

Sirtori, C.R., G. Galli, M.R. Lovati, P. Carrara, E. Bosisio, and M.G. Kienle. 1984. Effects of dietary proteins on the regulation of liver lipoprotein receptors in rats. J. Nutr. 114:1493–1500.

Sirtori, C.R., C. Zucchi-Dentone, M. Sirtori, E. Gatti, G.C. Descovich, A. Gaddi, L. Cattin, P.G. Da Col, U. Senin, E. Mannarino, G. Avellone, L. Colombo, C. Fragiacomo, G. Noseda, and S. Lenzi. 1985. Cholesterol-lowering and HDL-raising properties of lecithinated soy proteins in type II hyperlipidemic patients. Ann. Nutr. Metab. 29:348–357.

Slonaker, J.R. 1931. The effect of different percents of protein in the diet. VII. Life span and cause of death. Am. J. Physiol. 98:226–275.

Stemmermann, G.N., A.M.Y. Nomura, and L.K. Heilbrun. 1984. Dietary fat and the risk of colorectal cancer. Cancer Res. 44:4633–4637.

Tannenbaum, A., and H. Silverstone. 1949. The genesis and growth of tumors. IV. Effects of varying the proportion of protein (casein) in the diet. Cancer Res. 9:162–173.

Temcharoen, P., T. Anukarahanonta, and N. Bhamarapravati. 1978. Influence of dietary protein and vitamin B_{12} on the toxicity and carcinogenicity of aflatoxins in rat liver. Cancer Res. 38:2185–2190.

Terpstra, A.H.M., L. Harkes, and F.H. van der Veen. 1981. The effect of different proportions of casein in semipurified diets on the concentration of serum cholesterol and the lipoprotein composition in rabbits. Lipids 16:114–119.

Terpstra, A.H.M., R.J.J. Hermus, and C.E. West. 1983a. Dietary protein and cholesterol metabolism in rabbits and rats. Pp. 19–49 in M.J. Gibney and D. Kritchevsky, eds. Current Topics in Nutrition and Disease, Vol. 8. Animal and Vegetable Proteins in Lipid Metabolism and Atherosclerosis. Alan R. Liss, New York.

Terpstra, A.H.M., R.J.J. Hermus, and C.E. West. 1983b. The role of dietary protein in cholesterol metabolism. World Rev. Nutr. Diet. 42:1–55.

Thind, I.S. 1986. Diet and cancer—an international study. Int. J. Epidemiol. 15:160–163.

Topping, D.C., and W.J. Visek. 1976. Nitrogen intake and tumorigenesis in rats injected with 1,2-dimethylhydrazine. J. Nutr. 106:1583–1590.

Toshima, H., H. Tashiro, M. Sumie, Y. Koga, and N. Kimura. 1984. Changes in risk factors and cardiovascular mortality and morbidity within Tanushimaru 1958–1982. Pp. 203–210 in W. Lovenberg and Y. Yamori, eds. Nutritional Prevention of Cardiovascular Disease. Academic Press, Orlando, Fla.

Tucker, S.M., R.L. Mason, and R.E. Beauchene. 1976. Influence of diet and feed restriction on kidney function of aging male rats. J. Gerontol. 31:264–270.

USDA (U.S. Department of Agriculture). 1983. Nationwide Food Consumption Survey 1977–78. Food Intakes: Individuals in 48 States, Year 1977–78. Report No. I-1. Consumer Nutrition Division, Human Nutrition Information Service, Hyattsville, Md. 617 pp.

USDA (U.S. Department of Agriculture). 1984. Nationwide Food Consumption Survey. Nutrient Intakes: Individuals in 48 States, Year 1977–78. Report No. I-2. Consumer Nutrition Division, Human Nutrition Information Service, Hyattsville, Md. 439 pp.

USDA (U.S. Department of Agriculture). 1986. Nationwide Food Consumption Survey. Continuing Survey of Food Intakes of Individuals. Men 19–50 Years, 1 Day, 1985. Report No. 85–3. Nutrition Monitoring Division, Human Nutrition Information Service, Hyattsville, Md. 94 pp.

USDA (U.S. Department of Agriculture). 1987a. Nationwide Food Consumption Survey. Continuing Survey of Food Intakes of Individuals. Women 19–50 Years and Their Children 1–5 Years, 1 Day, 1986. Report No. 86–1. Nutrition Monitoring Division, Human Nutrition Information Service, Hyattsville, Md. 98 pp.

USDA (U.S. Department of Agriculture). 1987b. Nationwide Food Consumption Survey. Continuing Survey of Food Intakes of Individuals. Women 19–50 Years and Their Children 1–5 Years, 4 Days, 1985. Report No. 85–4. Nutrition Monitoring Division, Human Nutrition Information Service, Hyattsville, Md. 182 pp.

Van der Meer, R., and A.C. Beynen. 1987. Species-dependent responsiveness of serum cholesterol to dietary proteins. J. Am. Oil Chem. Soc. 64:1172–1177.

van Raaij, J.M.A., M.B. Katan, and J.G.A.J. Hautvast. 1979. Casein, soya protein, serum-cholesterol. Lancet 2:958.

van Raaij, J.M.A., M.B. Katan, J.G.A.J. Hautvast, and R.J.J. Hermus. 1981. Effects of casein versus soy protein diets on serum cholesterol and lipoproteins in young healthy volunteers. Am. J. Clin. Nutr. 34:1261–1271.

Verrillo, A., A. de Teresa, P.C. Giarrusso, and S. La Rocca. 1985. Soybean protein diets in the management of type II hyperlipoproteinaemia. Atherosclerosis 54:321–331.

Viart, P. 1977. Hemodynamic findings in severe protein-caloric malnutrition. Am. J. Clin. Nutr. 30:334–348.

Visek, W.J. 1985. Dietary protein and experimental carcinogenesis. Pp. 163–186 in L.A. Poirier, P.M. Newberne, and M.W. Pariza, eds. Advances in Experimental Medicine and Biology, Vol. 206: Essential Nutrients in Carcinogenesis. Plenum Press, New York.

Walker, R.M., and H.M. Linkswiler. 1972. Calcium retention in the adult human male as affected by protein intake. J. Nutr. 102:1297–1302.

Walters, M.A., and F.J.C. Roe. 1964. The effect of dietary casein on the induction of lung tumours by the injection of 9,10-dimethyl-1,2-benzanthracene (DMBA) into newborn mice. Br. J. Cancer 18:312–316.

Wang, H., K. Ikeda, M. Kihara, Y. Nara, R. Horie, and Y. Yamori. 1984. Effect of dietary urea on blood pressure in spontaneously hypertensive rats. Clin. Exp. Pharmacol. Physiol. 11:555–561.

Wells, P., L. Alftergood, and R.B. Alfin-Slater. 1976. Effect of varying levels of dietary protein on tumor development and lipid metabolism in rats exposed to aflatoxin. J. Am. Oil. Chem. Soc. 53:559–562.

Wexler, B.C. 1983a. Enovid-induced exacerbation of the propensity for stroke in low protein fish diet-fed stroke-prone/SHR. Stroke 14:995–1000.

Wexler, B.C. 1983b. Low protein fish vs low protein animal diet enhances the propensity for stroke in stroke-prone/SHR. Stroke 14:585–590.

White, F.R., and J. White. 1944. Effect of a low lysine diet on mammary-tumor formation in strain C3H mice. J. Natl. Cancer Inst. 5:41–42.

White, J., and H.B. Andervont. 1943. Effect of a diet relatively low in cystine on the production of spontaneous mammary-gland tumors in strain C3H female mice. J. Natl. Cancer Inst. 3:449–451.

Widhalm, K., 1986. Effect of diet on serum lipids and lipoprotein in hyperlipoproteinemic children. Pp. 133–140 in A.C. Beynen, ed. Nutritional Effects on Cholesterol Metabolism. Transmondial, Voorthuizen, The Netherlands.

Wolfe, B.M., and D.M. Grace. 1987. Substitution of mixed amino acids resembling soy protein for mixed amino acids resembling casein in the diet reduces plasma cholesterol in slowly, but not rapidly fed nor fasted baboons. Metabolism 36:223–229.

Wolfe, B.M., P.M. Giovannetti, D.C.H. Cheng, D.C.K. Roberts, and K.K. Carroll. 1981. Hypolipidemic effect of substituting soybean protein isolate for all meat and dairy protein in the diets of hypercholesterolemic men. Nutr. Rep. Int. 24:1187–1198.

Wolfe, B.M., E.H. Taves, and P.M. Giovannetti. 1986. Low protein diet decreases serum cholesterol in healthy human subjects. Clin. Invest. Med. 9:A43.

Woodward, C.J., and K.K. Carroll. 1985. Digestibilities of casein and soya-bean protein in relation to their effects on serum cholesterol in rabbits. Br. J. Nutr. 54:355–366.

Wurtman, R.J., and J.D. Milner. 1985. Dietary amino acids, the central nervous system, and hypertension. Pp. 231–240 in M.J. Horan, M. Blaustein, J.B. Dunbar, W. Kachadorian, N.M. Kaplan, and A.P. Simopoulos, eds. NIH Workshop on Nutrition and Hypertension: Proceedings from a Symposium. Biomedical Information Corp., New York.

Yamori, Y. 1980. Gene-environment interaction in the pathogenesis of hypertensive diseases. Pp. 263–269 in R.M. Lauer and R.B. Shekelle, eds. Childhood Prevention of Atherosclerosis and Hypertension. Raven Press, New York.

Yamori, Y., R. Horie, M. Ohtaka, Y. Nara, and K. Ikeda. 1978. Genetic and environmental modification of spontaneous hypertension. Jpn. Circ. J. 42:1151–1159.

Yamori, Y., R. Horie, H. Tanase, K. Fujiwara, Y. Nara, and W. Lovenberg. 1984. Possible role of nutritional factors in the incidence of cerebral lesions in stroke-prone spontaneously hypertensive rats. Hypertension 6:49–53.

Yu, B.P., E.J. Masoro, I. Murata, H.A. Bertrand, and F.T. Lynd. 1982. Life span study of SPF Fischer 344 male rats fed ad libitum or restricted diets: longevity, growth, lean body mass and disease. J. Gerontol. 37:130–141.

9

Carbohydrates

Carbohydrates are the most important source of calories for the world's population because of their relatively low cost and wide availability. This chapter discusses the role of digestible (simple and complex) carbohydrates in the etiology and prevention of chronic diseases. The indigestible carbohydrates (components of dietary fiber) are considered in Chapter 10.

Simple carbohydrates are sugars and include monosaccharides, which consist of one sugar (saccharide) unit per molecule, and disaccharides, which contain two sugar units per molecule. The monosaccharides glucose and fructose and the disaccharides sucrose, maltose, and lactose occur naturally. Glucose and fructose are found in honey and fruits, whereas sucrose (common table sugar) is found in molasses, maple syrup, and in small amounts in fruits. Sucrose is made up of 1 unit each of glucose and fructose per molecule, whereas lactose (milk sugar) consists of 1 glucose and 1 galactose unit per molecule. Maltose consists of two glucose molecules and is present in sprouting grains, malted milk, malted cereals, and some corn syrups.

Sugars added during food processing include sucrose, fructose, and syrups that contain glucose or fructose. Ordinary corn syrups are made by hydrolyzing corn starch and contain glucose, maltose, and higher polymers of glucose. High-fructose corn syrups (HFCSs), which are made by the isomerization of glucose-containing syrups, contain both fructose and glucose in varying amounts. The most commonly used HFCSs contain from 42 to 55% fructose on a dry weight basis (Glinsmann et al., 1986).

Complex carbohydrates, or *polysaccharides*, are large molecules consisting of many sugar units. Starches (polymers of glucose) are the most abundant polysaccharides in the diet and occur in many foods, including cereal grains, legumes, and potatoes. Glucose, fructose, and galactose are produced during the digestion of the carbohydrate mixture found in the usual diet. After absorbtion, fructose and galactose are converted in the liver to glucose, the blood sugar. Although liver and muscles can store excess glucose as glycogen (animal starch), small amounts of glycogen remain in muscle meats after slaughter. Consequently, practically all dietary carbohydrates come from plant sources, except for lactose, which comes from milk.

DIETARY INTAKE OF CARBOHYDRATES

Historical trends in the amounts of carbohydrates in the food supply since 1909 have been reported by the U.S. Department of Agriculture (Marston and Raper, 1987). These data do not represent the amount of carbohydrates actually consumed, however, because there are no estimates of losses or waste and no measurements of actual intake. Total carbohydrate availability has declined since 1909; per-capita amounts fell from 493 g/day during 1909–1913 to a low of 378 g/day during 1967–1969 and rose to 413 g/day in 1985 (Chapter 3, Table 3–3). The decline was due to decreased use of flour and cereal products.

From the early part of this century to the 1980s, there was a notable shift in the proportion of total carbohydrate derived from starch and sugars. During 1909–1913, 68% of total carbohydrates came from starch, in comparison to 47% in 1980. Conversely, the contribution of sugars increased from 32% during 1909–1913 to 53% in 1980 (Welsh and Marston, 1982).

Over the past 20 years, the relative contribution of sugars to the food supply has changed. In 1965, sucrose predominated, comprising 85% of total sugars; sugars in corn syrups comprised only 13%. There were no HFCS sweeteners at that time. By 1985, the use of all types of corn syrups had increased to 47% of total sugars but there was a concomitant decline in sucrose use. The marked increase in corn syrup use during the last decade was due chiefly to greater use of HFCS—a popular sweetener of soft drinks and other processed foods. In 1985, HFCS accounted for 30% of the total sugar supply (Glinsmann et al., 1986).

The 1977–1978 Nationwide Food Consumption Survey (NFCS) (USDA, 1984) indicated that carbohydrates furnished an average of 43% of calories, whereas the NFCS Continuing Survey of Food Intakes by Individuals (CSFII) (USDA, 1986, 1987, 1988) suggested that women and children derived closer to 47% of their calories from carbohydrates. Both surveys indicated that children had higher proportionate intakes of carbohydrates than did adults and that women had higher intakes of carbohydrates compared to men of the same age group. Because these surveys did not take into account the percentage of calories from alcohol, the reported percentages of calories from carbohydrates, fats, and proteins are inaccurate. Carbohydrate intake was not affected by region, urbanization, or season; however, it was higher for those below than above the poverty level (USDA 1984, 1987, 1988).

In 1986, the Food and Drug Administration (FDA) estimated that the average daily intake of all sugars by the U.S. population accounted for 21% of total calories—half coming from added sugars and half from naturally occurring sugars. On the average, approximately 4% of calories came from fructose, 9% from sucrose, and 5% from

sugars in corn syrups (see Chapter 3, Tables 3–6 and 3–7, and Glinsmann et al. 1986).

EVIDENCE ASSOCIATING CARBOHYDRATE INTAKE WITH CHRONIC DISEASES

Noninsulin-Dependent Diabetes Mellitus

Epidemiologic Evidence

Most epidemiologic studies were conducted at the time when distinction was still made between juvenile-onset and adult-onset diabetes rather than the most recently adopted more distinct classifications of Type I, or insulin-dependent diabetes mellitus (IDDM), and Type II, or noninsulin-dependent diabetes mellitus (NIDDM), respectively. Although the studies referenced here generally concern adult-onset diabetes, it seems reasonable to extend the results to all cases of diabetes.

Increased intake of sugars or total carbohydrates is not associated with increased risk of NIDDM. In a prospective study of 9,494 male Israeli government employees who were nondiabetic and 40 years of age or older at baseline, Medalie et al. (1974) found no association between calories from sugars or intake of total carbohydrates and incidence of diabetes mellitus over a 5-year follow-up. In a cross-sectional study of 3,454 employed people in England, Keen et al. (1979) observed that intake of carbohydrates, fats, and protein tended to be inversely correlated with concentration of blood sugar and indices of glucose tolerance; they inferred that the correlations probably were confounded by caloric expenditure. Baird (1972) reported an inverse association between sugar intake and prevalence of previously undetected diabetes among the siblings of diabetic propositi. West et al. (1976) found no association between sugar consumption and occurrence of diabetes in 286 Plains Indians, whose intake of refined sugar ranged from less than 70 g/day to more than 200 g/day.

In a study involving 22 countries, Yudkin (1964) reported a correlation of 0.73 between mean per-capita supply of sugars from 1934 to 1938 and risk of death due to diabetes from 1955 to 1956. West (1978) pointed out that this result was not consistently observed; in a sample of 44 countries, the correlation was only 0.18 for sugar intake in 1951 and diabetes mortality in 1971. Furthermore, sugar consumption is high in several countries where rates of diabetes are low (Walker, 1977). In a correlation analysis study of data obtained from 1894 to 1934 in several countries, Himsworth (1935–1936) observed an inverse association between rates of death from diabetes and the mean percentage of total calories obtained from carbohydrates in the diets of urban working-class families. West (1978) reported an inverse correlation between prevalence of diabetes and mean percentage of calories from carbohydrates in surveys of persons 35 years of age and older in seven countries. To the extent that such correlations do exist, it seems reasonable to infer that they do not reflect direct associations but, rather, that they reflect confounding by variables such as caloric expenditure and obesity.

Clinical Studies

No long-term prospective studies have attempted to alter the incidence of NIDDM by changing the carbohydrate content of the diet. On the other hand, shifts in the proportion of carbohydrates in the diet have been used in the clinical management of both types of diabetes and have had a controversial history (Bierman, 1979). High-carbohydrate diets have been recommended for the management of diabetes, because they appear to improve glucose tolerance and insulin sensitivity, and with a change to such a diet, there is a concomitant reduction in the proportion of calories as fat, which reduces risk of atherosclerosis—a major cause of death among diabetics (American Diabetes Association, 1987). There have been no prospective studies on the influence of diet on the complications of diabetes, and the role of diet in the increased prevalence and severity of atherosclerosis among diabetics has not been documented. In studies of high-carbohydrate, low-fat diets given to people with NIDDM, investigators have observed reduced incidence of hyperglycemia, hypercholesterolemia, and hypertriglyceridemia, and decreased treatment requirements (Anderson and Ward, 1979; Blanc et al., 1983; Kiehm et al., 1976; Simpson et al., 1979a,b; Stone and Connor, 1963; Story et al., 1985). An increase in insulin sensitivity observed in vivo after high-carbohydrate diets (Kolterman et al., 1979) is consistent with enhanced insulin action at the cellular level (Olefsky and Saekow, 1978).

A change from a diet of average composition to a very-high-carbohydrate, low-fat diet (more than 60% of calories as carbohydrates and moderate to large amounts of sucrose, i.e., up to 220 g/day) is associated with short-term (2- to 4-week) increases in fasting plasma very-low-density lipoprotein (VLDL) and triglyceride levels in NIDDM patients (Emanuele et al., 1986; Jellish et al., 1984; Reaven, 1986) similar to those seen in nondiabetics. A 5-week study in which a diet high in complex-carbohydrates (65% of total calories) was substituted for saturated fat in NIDDM patients with normal lipid levels failed to show an increase in fasting serum triglyceride levels (Abbott et al., 1989). In a study by Reiser et al. (1981a,b), graded amounts of sucrose (up to 33% of total calories) were fed for 6 weeks in a gorging pattern (most of the daily calories at dinner) to subjects preselected on the basis of exaggerated insulin responses to a sucrose load. Higher fasting glucose, insulin, and triglyceride levels were observed at higher sucrose intakes. In contrast to fasting levels, postprandial triglyceride levels have been shown to decrease in hypertriglyceridemic NIDDM patients on high-sucrose, high-carbohydrate diets (Emanuele et al., 1986). However, in part based on their short-term metabolic studies (15-day periods comparing 60% and 40% carbohydrate diets in nine subjects), Reaven and colleagues (Coulston et al., 1987; Reaven 1988) have cautioned against using this type of diet for long-term management of NIDDM on the basis of observed increases in postprandial glucose and insulin levels and in basal triglyceride levels. Recently, these studies were repeated with longer (6-week) dietary periods yielding similar findings (Coulston et al., 1989). These diets were already reduced in saturated fat and cholesterol.

Studies in which smaller amounts of mixed carbohydrate (de Bont et al., 1981; Weinsier et al., 1974) or sucrose (Peterson et al., 1986) were substituted for fat in diets tested on diabetics failed to show elevations of fasting triglyceride levels. This was confirmed in a recent metabolic ward study comparing a 60% mixed-carbohydrate diet with a 50% carbohydrate baseline diet in 10 subjects with NIDDM, but fasting triglyceride levels were increased in comparison to a high monounsaturated (50% fat, 33% monounsaturated) fat diet (Garg et al., 1988). Thus, evidence from some short-term metabolic studies suggests that normolipidemic diabetics whose diet is changed from one that is high in saturated fat to a diet containing very high carbohydrate levels and moderate to large amounts of sucrose respond with an increase in fasting triglyceride levels but do not consistently have increased postprandial triglyceride levels. Lesser degrees of substitution of carbohydrate for saturated fat usually do not increase fasting triglyceride levels. The increase in fasting triglyceride levels in hypertriglyceridemic diabetics is exaggerated; after 2 weeks, these levels tend to revert toward control levels. High-carbohydrate, low-saturated fat diets lower both low-density lipoprotein (LDL) and high-density lipoprotein (HDL) cholesterol levels (Abbott et al., 1989; Katan, 1984) and usually the degree of hyperglycemia as well.

Diabetic populations, such as those in Asia, that subsist on high-carbohydrate diets have lower levels of plasma cholesterol, LDL cholesterol, and plasma triglycerides and higher levels of HDL cholesterol and apolipoprotein A1 than do persons with diabetes in the United States (Pan et al., 1986). The relatively low frequency and severity of atherosclerotic disease among these diabetic populations compared to Western diabetics have long been known (West, 1978; WHO, 1985). Studies in migrant populations have shown that diabetic men adopting a higher-fat, lower-carbohydrate diet after moving from Japan to Hawaii have increased triglyceride and cholesterol levels and a higher incidence of cardiovascular diseases (Kawate et al., 1979). Nevertheless, although some diet-specific effects on the complications and severity of already diagnosed diabetes may continue to be suspected or remain controversial, there is little evidence to implicate dietary carbohydrates, either complex or simple, in the etiology of diabetes.

Animal Studies

Evaluation of the hypothesis that a high-carbohydrate diet is an independent risk factor in the development of glucose intolerance or diabetes is complicated by such factors as hyperphagia and meal patterns (ad libitum versus meal feeding), which can influence plasma insulin curves, body weight, and fat pad weight (Glinsmann et al., 1986). Data derived from studies in several animal species have been somewhat difficult to interpret and are frequently contradictory. For example, in a prediabetic line of female Yucatan miniature swine genetically selected for diminished glucose tolerance, a diet containing 42% of calories as sucrose or starch for 3 months appeared to improve glucose tolerance (Phillips et al., 1982). In contrast, a strain of the spiny mouse (Acomy cahirinus), a desert animal with pancreatic beta-cell hyperplasia and abnormal carbohydrate metabolism, developed decreased glucose tolerance, increased plasma triglycerides and cholesterol levels, and an increase in liver enzymes involved in lipid metabolism after consuming a diet containing 55% sucrose for 4 months (Obell, 1974).

In a study by Cohen (1978), genetically selected prediabetic rats (Hebrew University) were fed diets containing 72% (by weight) of sucrose, fructose, glucose, or starch for 8 months. Rats fed the high-sucrose and high-fructose diets had high glucose peaks, relatively higher tissue insulin resistance, and increased serum cholesterol, but those on the high-starch diet did not. The high-fructose diet also resulted in elevated triglyceride levels. None of these adverse effects was noticed in the normal rat strains used as controls. Prediabetic male rats developed proteinuria (nephropathy) and testicular atrophy and lost weight after eating these high-sucrose (72% by weight) diets (Rosenmann et al., 1974). In pregnant females, this diet caused an increase in fetal malformations (Ornoy and Cohen, 1980). Thus, although these studies suggest that glucose intolerance may be worsened or provoked in animals predisposed to that condition, their results have to be extrapolated with caution because of the very high levels of sugar used, which far exceed levels in the common U.S. diet, especially the usual diets of patients with diabetes.

The desert sand rat (Psammomys obesus) has been used as a laboratory model for both adult-onset diabetes and spontaneous obesity, since it overeats when given free access to food and becomes obese and hyperinsulinemic (Kalderon et al., 1986). In a study by Rice and Robertson (1980), sand rats fed a sucrose-rich (56%) diet for 18 months did not differ from sand rats fed a starch-rich (56%) diet in development of obesity and insulin resistance; diabetes was not reliably produced in either case.

A new rodent model of NIDDM was described by Ikeda et al. (1981). This Wistar rat (now designated WDF/Ta-fa/fa) was produced by transferring the mutant gene Fa (fatty) from the obese, hyperinsulinemic but normoglycemic Zucker fatty rat to a lean albino Wistar Kyoto background rat using a combination of inbreeding and backcrossing. Unlike the obese Zucker rat, which becomes insulin resistant and hyperinsulinemic but does not become hyperglycemic or glucosuric, the WDF/Ta-fa/fa male becomes frankly diabetic. If the obese male is fed a diet high in sucrose, it becomes diabetic earlier and the hyperglycemia is worsened in the already hyperglycemic animal (Greenwood et al., 1988). The female WDF/Ta-fa/fa rat does not respond to the high sucrose diet by developing hyperglycemia. Thus, this new strain provides a sexually dimorphic rodent model in which to examine the interaction of diet with sex-associated obesity and diabetic traits.

Genetically obese young male SHR/N-*cp/cp* (corpulent) rats fed diets containing 54% (by weight) sucrose or cornstarch for 9 weeks had increased body weight, hyperlipidemia, hyperinsulinemia, and abnormal glucose tolerance. Their lean litter mates (+/*cp*) had increased blood insulin levels but were normoglycemic (Michaelis et al., 1984). Thus, it seems that obesity may be the most important dietary factor in the development of diabetes in this and other animal models.

In a study by Stearns and Smith (1985), female WDF/Ta-*fa/fa* rats were fed diets containing 77% (by weight) sucrose or cornstarch for 60 days. The sucrose-fed rats had increased body weight, but exhibited no differences from cornstarch-fed rats in their plasma glucose, insulin, or triglyceride levels, triglyceride secretion rates, or pancreatic insulin content. That study shows that hyperglycemia, hypertriglyceridemia, and hyperinsulinemia do not necessarily accompany sucrose feeding of rats.

Insulin-Dependent Diabetes Mellitus

Epidemiologic Evidence

The role of carbohydrates has not been examined in epidemiologic studies, at least in recent years, because there is considerable consensus that the etiology of IDDM is not diet dependent.

Clinical Studies

Alterations in carbohydrate intake have been used as an adjunct to the management of IDDM patients with the goal of preventing chronic diseases, especially atherosclerosis. As with NIDDM, increasing the proportion of total calories from carbohydrates improves insulin sensitivity; lowers glucose, triglyceride, and cholesterol levels; and decreases insulin requirements (Simpson et al., 1979b; Stone and Connor, 1963). Also, as with NIDDM, very-long-term clinical studies have not been performed.

Some short-term metabolic studies on high-carbohydrate diets have shown transient increases in basal triglyceride levels (Bierman and Hamlin, 1961; Hollenbeck et al., 1985), but others have not (Riccardi et al., 1984). Female patients with IDDM who were fed a 65% carbohydrate, low-cholesterol diet for 6 weeks had slightly increased triglyceride levels, reduced cholesterol, apolipoprotein B, and apolipoprotein A1 levels but did not have altered glycemic control (Hollenbeck et al., 1985). These observations are similar to those described for NIDDM patients and nondiabetics.

Animal Studies

In a diabetic strain of mice (C57BL/KsJ-*db/db*), pancreatic islet destruction results in insulin insufficiency and glucose intolerance, but the relevance of this model to humans is not yet known. Diets containing 60% (by weight) simple sugars (e.g., sucrose, fructose, or glucose) caused additional obesity, hyperglycemia, atrophy of pancreatic islets, and early death in this strain, whereas dextrin or meals without carbohydrates did not. In normal littermates (+/*db*), no adverse effects were observed (Leiter et al., 1983).

Other animal models of IDDM are created by chemical destruction of insulin-producing cells with streptozotocin, which produces moderate diabetes (hyperglycemia with glycosuria). Sucrose-rich diets fed to such animals usually produce increased adiposity and variable deterioration of glucose tolerance, making it difficult to determine whether observed effects are due to differences in adiposity or to specific effects of sucrose on glucose homeostasis (Goda et al., 1982; Gray and Olefsky, 1982; Hallfrisch et al., 1979). It appears that in animals, as in humans, carbohydrate-rich diets given in the untreated diabetic state may lead to further deterioration of glucose homeostasis. In contrast to studies of humans, few dietary studies have been conducted in animal models of IDDM during treatment of hyperglycemia.

Carbohydrates have been implicated in the development of microvascular changes in diabetic rodents. Studies of eye changes showed that there were increases in sorbitol, fructose, and lactate levels in the retina when either sucrose or cornstarch at 68% of the diet was fed for 15 days to steptozotocin-diabetic Wistar rats (Heath and Hamlett, 1976; Heath et al., 1975). Six months of feeding the same high-sucrose diet to normal Wistar rats produced retinopathy similar in severity to retinal changes in diabetic rats on high-starch diets (Papachristodoulou et al., 1976). Fructose alone was found to cause comparable retinal changes in the same strain of diabetic rats (Boot-Hanford and Heath, 1981). Thornber and Eckhert (1984) suggest that retinopathy following high-sucrose diets may be due to dietary deficiencies, since supplementation of experimental diets containing 68% (by weight) of sucrose with chromium, selenium, and corn oil prevented capillary damage.

Increased kidney weight and glomerulosclerosis were observed in streptozotocin-diabetic Wistar rats on cornstarch diets and in normal rats consuming 68% of their diet as sucrose or fructose for

6 months (Boot-Hanford and Heath, 1981). Other authors also reported kidney changes in diabetic rats fed high levels of sucrose or cornstarch and in normal rats fed high levels of sucrose (Kang et al., 1982; Taylor et al., 1980).

Streptozotocin-diabetic Sprague-Dawley rats, but not normal rats, fed diets containing 66% (by weight) sucrose for 13 weeks had elevated HDL, VLDL, and total cholesterol (Bar-On et al., 1981). Sucrose fed at 66% of the diet for 21 days caused hypertriglyceridemia in diabetic male Sprague-Dawley rats, but not when the rats exercised daily (Dallaglio et al., 1983). The presence of 12% bran in a high-sucrose (32 or 72%) diet fed to Sprague-Dawley rats for 14 to 32 days reduced the plasma triglyceride levels to normal (Lin and Anderson, 1977).

The effects of high-sucrose diets on serum triglyceride and cholesterol levels seem to depend on the animal model used. For example, diabetic Wistar rats had increased lipid levels, whereas genetically diabetic mice had no change (Gonnermann et al., 1982).

Caution needs to be exercised in extrapolating the results of these animal studies to humans because very high levels of sugars were used, species appeared to differ in their responses, chronic effects on glycemia and metabolic changes often were not monitored, metabolic responses were not tested for reversibility, and some of the reported changes may have been due to nutrient deficiencies that also produce glucose intolerance (Glinsman et al., 1986).

Atherosclerotic Cardiovascular Diseases

Variations in the prevalence of coronary heart disease (CHD) among populations correlate directly with the proportion of calories derived from fats (Chapter 7) and, therefore, inversely with the proportion of calories derived from carbohydrates. Yudkin (1964) compared the per-capita sugar consumption in various countries with mortality from CHD and proposed that sugar contributes to the occurrence of heart disease. However, several subsequent studies have failed to substantiate this. Recent animal and epidemiologic data were reviewed in the 1986 report of the Sugars Task Force of the FDA, *Evaluation of Health Aspects of Sugars Contained in Carbohydrate Sweeteners* (Glinsmann et al., 1986). This task force stated, "There was no conclusive evidence that dietary sugars are an

independent risk factor for coronary artery disease in the general population."

A change from a Western-type diet to a very-high-carbohydrate, low-fat diet (60% or more of calories from any type of carbohydrate, e.g., simple sugars or starches) has been shown in short-term studies to cause a reduction of HDL (Gonen et al., 1981; Katan, 1984) and LDL (Abbott et al., 1989; Nestel et al., 1979) and a transient increase in fasting plasma triglyceride levels (Jellish et al., 1984; Reaven, 1986). Glucose, sucrose, fructose, and starch appear to have comparable effects on fasting triglyceride levels in short-term metabolic studies (Dunnigan et al., 1970; Mann and Truswell, 1970; McDonald, 1972; Nikkilä and Kekki, 1972; Porte et al., 1966; Turner et al., 1979). The increased basal triglyceride levels decline after several weeks to months on the high-carbohydrate diets, whereas reduced HDL levels persist (Katan, 1984). A high mixed carbohydrate diet (65% of calories) fed to normolipidemic subjects did not increase basal triglyceride levels after 4 to 6 weeks (Grundy et al., 1988). The transient increase in basal circulating triglycerides may be exaggerated in hypertriglyceridemic people (Ahrens, 1986; Liu et al., 1983) regardless of the type of carbohydrate and appears to be greater in men than in women (McDonald, 1985). High-carbohydrate diets lead to a short-term increase in overnight triglyceride levels, whereas postprandial triglyceride levels are actually lower in normal and hypertriglyceridemic subjects given high-carbohydrate diets than when fed high-fat diets (Barter et al., 1971; Schlierf and Dorow, 1973; Schlierf et al., 1971).

On the other hand, long-term feeding of diets high in carbohydrates and soluble fiber (e.g., oat bran) do not raise and may actually lower fasting triglyceride levels in hypertriglyceridemic people (Anderson and Tietyen-Clark, 1986). Such effects have not been observed in hypertriglyceridemic subjects consuming high levels of insoluble fiber (e.g., wheat bran). High-complex-carbohydrate diets (60% of total calories) fed to hypertriglyceridemic subjects for as long as 3 months have also been shown to reduce fasting triglyceride levels (Cominacini et al., 1988). Increased levels of cholesterol-rich and triglyceride-rich lipoproteins are not found in some populations, such as vegetarians or people living in parts of Asia, who have adapted to very-high-carbohydrate and low-fat intakes (Cerqueria et al., 1979) and who also have low levels of HDL, LDL, and VLDL as well as a low prevalence of CHD. The low HDL levels

(Connor et al., 1978; Katan, 1984; Knuiman et al., 1987) do not appear to adversely influence their low CHD prevalence rate.

A prospective study of the relationship of dietary intake to subsequent CHD was undertaken in Puerto Rico by Garcia-Palmieri et al. (1980). A 6-year follow-up of 10,000 men age 45 to 64 years in that study indicated that urban men who developed new CHD had significantly lower carbohydrate intakes. Similar results have been reported for populations in Framingham, Massachusetts (Gordon et al., 1981) and in Hawaii (Yano et al., 1978). In the Hawaii study, men who developed CHD during a 6-year follow-up consumed less total carbohydrates, starches, and sugars than did those without CHD. Thus the development of CHD does not appear to be associated with high-carbohydrate diets, and no differences among types of carbohydrate have been demonstrated.

Dental Caries

Epidemiologic Evidence

Experimental studies such as the classic 5-year cohort study of 436 institutionalized mental patients in Vipeholm, Sweden (Gustafsson et al., 1954), have established that sugars consumed in sticky form, particularly between meals, increases the risk of dental caries. Restricting the intake of sugars (Becks, 1950) or substituting a nonfermentable sugar alcohol (xylitol) for sucrose (Scheinin et al., 1975) decreases the incidence of caries.

Cross-sectional studies support the inference that consumption of sugars is an important determinant of the incidence of dental caries. In 47 countries from which data were available in the late 1960s and 1970s, Sreebny (1982) found a correlation of 0.72 between the prevalence of dental caries in 12-year-old children and the mean per-capita supply of sugars. For 6-year-olds in 23 countries, the correlation was 0.31. The prevalence of dental caries in Japanese children decreased precipitously during the 1940s in conjunction with the severe reduction in supply of sugars (Takeuchi, 1961). Similar changes were noted in Europe (Sognnaes, 1948; Toverud, 1957).

Clinical Studies

Many clinical studies of diet and its association with plaque formation and composition are confounded by such variations in oral hygiene as brushing of teeth (Glinsmann et al., 1986). The bulk of the evidence from clinical studies, however, is consistent, indicating that all dietary carbohydrates are potentially cariogenic (Brown, 1975).

Telemetry analysis of plaque in situ demonstrates that plaque pH is lowered not only after consumption of a sugar cube (Geddes et al., 1977) and after rinsing with sucrose solutions (Tenovuo et al., 1984) but also after ingestion of starch (Mormann and Muhlemann, 1981). Abelson and Pergola (1984) determined the effects of three sucrose concentrations (10, 40, and 70%) on in vivo plaque pH in caries-prone 18- to 26-year-old adults. Above a certain concentration, additional sucrose did not heighten the acidogenic response. Schachtele and Jensen (1983) inserted a pH electrode in teeth to measure oral pH after consumption of various foods and found that several foods high in starch produced a marked decline in oral pH. These foods (white bread, white rice, and cooked carrots) are notable in that they contain either none or only low levels of individual sugars such as sucrose, glucose, and fructose; most of their carbohydrate content is starch.

The preponderance of clinical evidence, however, indicates that dietary sugars are of major etiologic importance in caries formation. Sucrose in solution has been shown to stimulate plaque formation (Geddes et al., 1978) and to alter the composition of plaque and saliva to a form suggestive of increased mineral resorption from the teeth (Tenovuo et al., 1984). In five subjects, who frequently rinsed their mouths with a sucrose solution for 2 months, there were changes characteristic of early demineralization of tooth surfaces (Geddes et al., 1978). Slabs of bovine enamel mounted in the human mouth likewise underwent demineralization when frequently exposed to sucrose (Pearce and Gallagher, 1979; Tehrani et al., 1983).

Sucrose in foods has also been shown to be cariogenic. In one clinical trial (Scheinin et al., 1975), three groups consuming diets containing sucrose, frutose, or xylitol were followed for 2 years. By the study's end, the average number of decayed, missing, or filled teeth (DMFT) was higher in the sucrose group than in the fructose group. Subjects consuming only xylitol had virtually no DMFT. The authors attributed the low cariogenicity of xylitol to the fact that it is not metabolized by oral microbes (Scheinin, 1976; Scheinin et al., 1975). The inability of other studies to demonstrate a cariogenic effect of presweetened cereals in schoolchildren (Finn and Jamison, 1980; Glass and Fleisch, 1974) may reflect differences in the specific sugars added to the cereals (Glinsmann et al., 1986).

The form of dietary carbohydrates also appears to influence cariogenicity. Consumption of canned pears and apples, for example, lowers plaque pH to a greater degree than do sugars alone (Imfeld et al., 1978; Jensen and Schachtele, 1983). Edgar et al. (1975) found that there was a wide variation in the ability of different snack foods to increase plaque acid formation. However, the extent of plaque acid formation from foods does not necessarily indicate either the amount of enamel destruction that will occur or the number and severity of the related caries.

The sequence in which carbohydrate-containing foods and other foods are eaten also appears to influence caries formation. A sharp increase in oral hydrogen-ion concentration and in plaque scraped at regular intervals from the mouth has been noted after use of a sugar rinse; the concentration of hydrogen ions returns to baseline after approximately 30 minutes. If cheese is consumed 5 minutes after the sugar rinse, however, the sharp increase in hydrogen-ion concentration is diminished and the concentration returns quickly to baseline (Edgar, 1981; Edgar et al., 1982; Schachtele and Jensen, 1983). The frequency of carbohydrate consumption also appears to influence caries formation. In the Vipeholm study, caries activity in adult patients was monitored over several years while their diet and eating schedule were controlled. There were two important findings. First, the extent of caries activity appeared to be influenced more by the frequency of sucrose intake than by total amount consumed. Second, consumption of solid forms of sugar appeared to be more cariogenic than liquid forms (Gustafsson et al., 1954).

In summary, clinical evidence suggests that all carbohydrates are cariogenic to various degrees, but that the form of carbohydrate-containing foods, as well as their sequence and frequency of consumption, can substantially influence their cariogenicity. Beyond this observation, little is known about the cariogenic potential of specific carbohydrate-containing foods because of the complex and interactive role of diet in caries formation. Dental caries is a multifactorial bacterial disease; dietary factors, host resistance, fluoride exposure, and the nature of bacterial flora in the mouth all play important roles (Shaw, 1987). In addition, most clinical studies have involved adults whose teeth are much less caries-prone than those of children, which suggests caution in generalizing such findings.

Animal Studies

Rats exhibit a dose-dependent increase in caries formation as sucrose is added to the diet; a cariogenic effect is observed at dietary levels as low as 0.1% (by weight) of diet (Michalek et al., 1977). However, a saturation point on the dose–response curve has been noted at anywhere from 8% (Kreitzman and Klein, 1976) to 40% dietary sucrose (Hefti and Schmid, 1979); there is no increase in caries formation above these levels. The cariogenic potential of sucrose is greater than that of equivalent amounts of glucose, fructose, or invert sugars (mixture of dextrose and fructose obtained by hydrolyzing sucrose) (Birkhed et al., 1981; Horton et al., 1985).

Frequency, form, and composition of the diet appear to influence the cariogenicity of dietary carbohydrates in animals as in humans. For example, frequent consumption of carbohydrates markedly accelerates caries formation (Firestone et al., 1982; Skinner et al., 1982). Certain carbohydrate-containing foods, such as bananas, are much more cariogenic than sucrose alone or even frequently fed sucrose-topped chocolate (Shrestha and Kreutler, 1983). Consumption of an unsweetened cereal to which sucrose has been added has been shown to cause fewer caries than consumption of cereals presweetened with equal sucrose levels (McDonald and Stookey, 1977), and carbohydrates in the form of maize or wheat starch have virtually no cariogenic activity (Beighton and Hayday, 1984; Horton et al., 1985). With respect to dietary composition, addition of cheese to a cariogenic diet has been shown to be protective against buccal (cheek side) decay in some studies (Edgar et al., 1982; Harper et al., 1987) and against buccal as well as sulcal (toward the linear depression or valley in the occlusal surface of the tooth) caries in others (Rosen et al., 1984).

The rat is the most favored animal species in studies of dietary carbohydrates and dental caries. This is due to the rapidity with which it develops experimentally induced dental caries and to the similarity of its sulcal and smooth-surface carious lesions to those of humans (Glinsmann et al., 1986). Most findings in rats seem likely to be applicable to humans. Generalizations should still be made with caution, however, since feeding patterns and oral physiology differ. For example, microbial flora, oral pH, salivary composition, flow rate, and buffering capacity are known to differ between the two species (McDonald, 1985). Also, rats nibble throughout the day, and it is known that meal frequency correlates positively, and strongly, with caries formation in animals (Firestone et al., 1982; Skinner et al., 1982) and in humans (Gustafsson et al., 1954). Also, assessment of the cariogenicity of foods in animals is complicated by the fact that foods must be given in powdered form and not in the physical form usually consumed by humans (Krasse, 1985). Differences in oral physiology further complicate the issue. For example, most types of phosphates effectively reduce caries in rats when added to sucrose-containing diets, whereas phosphate supplemention of the human diet has been markedly unsuccessful in reducing caries incidence (Nizel and Harris, 1964). Although some caution is warranted in interpreting evidence obtained from the rat model, animal studies are essential to our understanding of the role of dietary carbohydrates in cariogenesis.

Interactions

The cariogenic action of dietary sucrose is influenced by other dietary constituents. For animals (Edgar et al., 1982; Harper et al., 1987) and humans (Edgar, 1981; Edgar et al., 1982; Schachtele and Jensen, 1983), cheese exerts a protective effect by blunting the short-term increase in hydrogen-ion concentration characteristically associated with a cariogenic diet. Cheese extracts administered after sucrose rinses have also been shown to inhibit demineralization of bovine enamel blocks fitted into the mouths of volunteers (Silva et al., 1987). Dietary substances inhibiting sucrose cariogenicity in animals include cheddar cheese (Rosen et al., 1984); mineral concentrates containing protein, calcium, and phosphate (Harper et al., 1987); cocoa (Paolino, 1982); lycasin, a hydrogenated corn syrup product (Leach et al., 1984); xylitol (Leach and Green, 1981; Shyu and Hsu, 1980); and saccharin (Linke, 1980). The mechanisms by which these substances inhibit sucrose cariogenicity are not fully understood; they may include enzyme inhibition in oral bacteria (Paolino, 1982), the stimulation of saliva, which maintains plaque pH in a neutral range (Krasse, 1985), and, for cheeses, the influences of texture and the casein or calcium-phosphate content (Harper et al., 1987).

Obesity

Epidemiologic and Clinical Studies

An inverse association between caloric intake and body fatness has been found in some epidemiologic studies (Baeke et al., 1983; Johnson et al., 1956; Keen et al., 1979; Keys et al., 1967; Kromhout, 1983a,b; Lincoln, 1972; Maxfield and Konishi, 1966; McCarthy, 1966; Stefanik et al., 1959; Wilkinson et al., 1977) but not in others (Morris et al., 1977). It is likely that variation in caloric intake along with variation in amount of physical activity are factors in the causation of obesity (Sopko et al., 1984). This issue is discussed in Chapter 6.

Studies in which the influence of calorie sources was assessed indicate that compared to lean people, fatter people generally have a lower mean intake of calories from all sources including carbohydrates (but excluding alcohol). Keen et al. (1979) found small inverse correlations (-0.01 to -0.31) of body mass index with intake of total energy, protein, fats, total carbohydrates, and sucrose in three samples of employed men and women in Great Britain. These results show that in the general population obese adults do not consume more sugars or more complex carbohydrates than lean people; in fact, they seem to consume less.

Psychophysical taste testing in obese and normal humans also consistently indicates that obese subjects do not have stronger preferences for sucrose or sweet solutions (Drewnowski et al., 1985; Grinker, 1978; Malcolm et al., 1980). Interpretation of the epidemiologic results is complicated, however, by the association of physical activity as well as total caloric intake with body fatness (see Chapter 6).

Animal Studies

In contrast to the clinical and epidemiologic data, studies in animals show that various types of high-carbohydrate diets can lead to obesity. For example, a diet containing sucrose produced greater weight gains in lean and corpulent (SHR/N-cp/cp) rats than did a diet containing cooked cornstarch (Michaelis et al., 1984). Although the sweet taste of sugar has been thought to encourage overeating in rats, Hill et al. (1980) found no differences in carbohydrate or caloric intake when adult male rats were offered either a sweet-tasting sucrose solution or a bland dextrin powder in addition to a chow diet, but the sucrose group gained more weight. In a similar experiment, Sclafani and Xenakis (1984) compared solutions of sucrose, Polycose (a bland-tasting polysaccharide), or Polycose sweetened with saccharin. They concluded that sweetness was not essential for production of carbohydrate-induced obesity, although it did increase the intake of polysaccharide.

Kanarek and Hirsch (1977) have described a method of producing obesity in rats by feeding them sucrose solutions. In later experiments, Kanarek and Orthen-Gambill (1982) observed that obesity could also be induced by supplementing the standard diet with solutions of glucose or fructose. Rattigan and Clark (1984) reported that the effect of a sucrose solution depends on the composition of the solid diet. Body weight and body fat increased without a significant increase in total caloric intake in rats given a low-fat, high-carbohydrate diets and the sucrose solution. Body weight, body fat, and total caloric intake were all decreased, however, in rats given high-fat, low-carbohydrate diets and the sugar solution.

Cancer

Epidemiologic and Clinical Studies

There is little epidemiologic evidence to support a role for carbohydrates per se in the etiology of cancer. No definitive conclusion is justified, however, because carbohydrates have often been reported in epidemiologic studies only as a component of total energy and not analyzed separately.

In several international correlation studies, investigators have evaluated the role of sugar and sometimes carbohydrates in the etiology of some cancers. Armstrong and Doll (1975) found that sugar intake was positively correlated with both the incidence of and mortality from cancer of the colon, rectum, breast, and ovary, and with the incidence of cancer of the corpus uteri. Similar positive correlations were found between sugar intake and the incidence of and mortality from cancer of the prostate, kidney, and nervous system and the incidence of cancer of the testes. Sugar intake was inversely correlated with liver cancer incidence, but positively correlated with mortality from pancreatic cancer in women. Armstrong and Doll (1975) also reported a weak association between liver cancer incidence and the intake of potatoes—a starch-rich vegetable. For most of the sites reported, however, particularly the colon, rectum, and breast, the positive correlations with fat intake were greater than for sugar intake. Other investigations have produced similar findings. For example, Hems (1978) and Carroll (1977) found a positive correlation between breast cancer and sugar intake. Subsequently, however, Carroll (1986) found that whereas breast cancer mortality is positively correlated with the percent of calories derived from dietary fat, it varies inversely with the percent of calories from carbohydrates. This mirrors an earlier finding by Hems and Stuart (1975), who also found

an inverse relationship between breast cancer incidence and starch consumption.

Hakama and Saxen (1967) reported a strong correlation between the per-capita intake of cereal used as flour and mortality from stomach cancer. The possible association of carbohydrate intake with gastric cancer was further evaluated by Modan et al. (1974), who found that high-starch foods were consumed more frequently by cases than by controls. Similarly, in a case-control study of diet and stomach cancer in Canada, Risch et al. (1985) found an increasing risk with total carbohydrate consumption but the relative risk for each 100-g/day increase in carbohydrates was only 1.53.

The effect of monosaccharides was evaluated in two studies of colorectal cancer. In a case-control study conducted in Marseilles (Macquart-Moulin et al., 1986), there appeared to be no evidence of increasing risk with increasing consumption of monosaccharides. However, in another case-control study conducted in Belgium (Tuyns et al., 1987), with essentially the same dietary survey technique, increasing monosaccharide and disaccharide intake was related to increasing risk of both colon and rectal cancer. The relative risks for the highest compared to the lowest consumption level was 1.7 for colon cancer and 2.4 for rectal cancer.

Animal Studies

In an extensive survey of the literature, the National Research Council's Committee on Diet, Nutrition, and Cancer (NRC, 1982) found relatively few animal studies dealing with the effects of dietary carbohydrates on carcinogenesis, and those studies provided little evidence of significant effects. Two research groups investigated the effects of diets containing different starches and sugars on mammary tumors induced by 7,12-dimethylbenz-(a)anthracene (Hoehn and Carroll, 1978; Klurfeld et al., 1984). The results provided some evidence that rats fed sucrose or dextrose developed tumors more readily than those fed lactose or starch. Gridley et al. (1983) found that mice had a much higher incidence of spontaneous mammary tumors when fed a diet containing sucrose than when given a diet with dextrin.

Two other studies focused on the effects of dietary carbohydrates on liver carcinogenesis. Hei and Sudilovsky (1985) used diethylnitrosamine to induce hepatocarcinogenesis and found more γ-glutamyltranspeptide-positive foci in rats fed a sucrose-containing diet compared to those on a diet containing glucose. In other experiments on liver carcinogenesis induced by 3'-methylamino-azobenzene in rats fed liquid or powdered diets, Sato et al. (1984) found that tumorigenesis was enhanced by reducing sugar intake.

Other Disorders

Hyperactivity

Several reports examined the effects on human behavior of reactive or postprandial hypoglycemia, which is defined by decreased blood glucose after eating coupled with a characteristic group of clinical symptoms. Hypoglycemia in children has been alleged to be associated with hyperkinesis, attention-deficit disorders, juvenile delinquency, and criminality (Harper and Gans, 1986; Kruesi and Rapoport, 1986; Milich, 1986). Furthermore, hypoglycemia has been specifically associated with the ingestion of sucrose. A review by Harper and Gans (1986) points to a lack of scientific experimentation or support of claims in this area.

There have been suggestions that dietary components, particularly sugars, cause changes in the behavior of children and adults. Some reports (e.g., Prinz et al., 1980) have linked sugar consumption to hyperactivity in children (hyperkinesis). This has some biologic plausibility, since experimental evidence in animals indicates that sugars as well as other dietary components may affect the level of brain neurotransmitters. Sugar consumption by humans, however, results in increased levels of serotonin (Crane and Ladene, 1983; Fernstrom and Wurtman, 1971), which should reduce activity levels.

Studies to determine whether there is a relationship between blood glucose levels and behavioral change failed to find any correlation (Behar et al., 1984; Brody and Wolinsky, 1983). The subjects of these studies included normal children as well as hyperactive children who, according to their parents, had behavioral deterioration following intake of sugars. Glucose and fructose were compared to a placebo (saccharin) by using standard tests for memory and attention as the dependent variables. There was no evidence for behavioral excitation and some weak evidence for a calming effect of sugars. These studies cast doubt on the hypothesized clinical significance of sugar intake in the etiology of behavioral disturbances (Prinz et al., 1980). A similar experimental design was used in a study by Wolraich et al. (1985) to test the effects of sucrose and aspartame on behavioral and cognitive parameters in 16 hyperactive boys. No differences were observed. Based on a review of the literature, several investigators (e.g., Kruesi and Rapoport, 1986; Milich, 1986) have concluded that there is no scientific basis for a relationship between sugar consumption and hyperactivity or other behavioral changes in children.

Criminality

Some people claim that juvenile delinquency as well as aggressive, antisocial, and even criminal behavior can result from reactive or postprandial hypoglycemia following the ingestion of sucrose and other carbohydrates (Gray, 1987; Harper and Gans, 1986; Schauss, 1980). Schoenthaler (1982) contends that a high proportion (up to 90%) of prison inmates are hypoglycemic and attributes that to a particularly high consumption of refined sugar. Studies undertaken to support this contention are characterized by inadequate diagnosis of hypoglycemia and lack of valid control groups (Gray, 1987). Another set of studies of violent adult male habitual offenders in Finland failed to support a relationship between violent behavior and hypoglycemia (Virkunen, 1982; Virkunen and Huttunen, 1982). Thus, the claims that high sugar intake can cause aggressive, antisocial behavior are based largely on conclusions drawn from anecdotal evidence and inadequately designed studies (Gray, 1987; Harper and Gans, 1986).

Documented reactive hypoglycemia based on accepted criteria (American Diabetes Association, 1982) is an uncommon condition (Cahill and Soeldner, 1974; Yager and Young, 1974) and occurs only in a very small percentage of people who commit crimes (Gray and Gray, 1983; Jukes, 1986). Apparently, no objective studies have been published to support the contention that aggressive or criminal behavior is influenced by sugar or carbohydrate intake. Despite the absence of any supporting data, however, some prison authorities have altered their institutional diets (Gray, 1987).

Lactose Intolerance

Primary lactose intolerance is the inability to digest the disaccharide lactose (the main carbohydrate in milk), breaking it down into glucose and galactose. This results from a progressive decrease, early in childhood, of the enzyme lactase, which is normally present at birth. As described in Chapter 4, some adults maintain lactase activity, which is controlled by a single gene. Lactose ingestion (milk drinking) will not induce lactase activity after its decrease nor will lactose restriction reduce enzyme activity if still present. Thus, the ingestion of lactose plays no role in the genetic expression of primary lactose intolerance. However, symptoms of lactose intolerance can be ameliorated by restriction of lactose-containing dairy products. Total elimination of lactose is rarely necessary, since most affected individuals can tolerate 1 to 2 glasses of milk daily (Gray, 1983).

Secondary lactose intolerance is associated with chronic gastrointestinal disease in people with persistent lactase activity. This condition will lessen as the disease is reversed. Also, chronic alcoholics without malnutrition have an increase in lactase deficiency, which is reversible with alcohol abstinence (Perlow et al., 1977).

Sucrose intolerance due to sucrase deficiency is a rarer genetic disorder. Its symptoms are indistinguishable from those of lactose intolerance, except that they are elicited by table sugar rather than by milk. Starch is usually well tolerated and digested. Dietary sucrose plays no role in the expression of this disorder, but its restriction will ameliorate symptoms (Gray, 1983).

SUMMARY

The role of sugar-containing foods in the etiology of a variety of disorders and disabilities in humans has generated considerable attention. Carbohydrates are still believed by some to be fattening beyond their contribution to total calories, and sugars themselves are sometimes regarded as contributors to diabetes and heart disease. Sugars have also been implicated in a variety of behavioral aberrations associated with hypoglycemia, but rarely confirmed by acceptable criteria as discussed earlier.

Epidemiologic studies have shown that populations eating high-carbohydrate diets usually have a lower prevalence of NIDDM and CHD compared to populations eating lower-carbohydrate and higher-fat diets. The role of carbohydrates has not been completely established, but it seems reasonable to infer that the correlations of NIDDM and CHD with carbohydrates do not reflect a direct association but, rather, are due to confounding by variables such as caloric expenditure and obesity. Paradoxically, obesity also is associated with lower caloric intake, including low carbohydrate intake, in population studies. Evidence supports the contention that consumption of sugars, in particular sucrose, is the major dietary factor associated with the incidence of dental caries. Population studies suggesting a link between carbohydrate intake and colorectal cancer have been inconclusive.

With the exception of dental caries, clinical studies of carbohydrate intake and chronic diseases have focused more on dietary management of chronic diseases than on the role of diet in causation. High-carbohydrate, low-fat diets have been recommended both for the management of diabetes mellitus and for lowering glucose and lipid levels and reducing insulin requirements. However, short-term metabolic studies suggest that for some individuals, such diets may raise glucose and triglyceride levels, thereby pointing to the need for further long-term population studies and for intervention trials.

The scientific data supporting beliefs that high-carbohydrate diets are associated with hypoglycemia, hyperactivity, or criminality are inadequate. Controlled clinical studies to test the carbohydrate–hypoglycemia–hyperactivity connection have been negative.

DIRECTIONS FOR RESEARCH

• Long-term prospective studies are needed to evaluate the effects of increasing the proportion of carbohydrate calories in the diet on morbidity and mortality from CHD among diabetics.

• Longer-term clinical studies are needed to characterize the metabolic adaptive changes in lipoproteins associated with switching from a low-carbohydrate to a high-carbohydrate diet from various dietary sources.

• Additional studies should be conducted to test for a possible link between intake of total or individual carbohydrates and the incidence of colorectal and other cancers.

• Research on the effect of fluoridation on dental caries among people with a wide spectrum of carbohydrate intakes would help elucidate whether the contributory role of carbohydrates in the pathogenesis of caries can be effectively offset by fluoride.

REFERENCES

Abbott, W.G.H., V.L. Boyce, S.M. Grundy, and B.V. Howard. 1989. Effects of replacing saturated fat with complex carbohydrate in diets of subjects with NIDDM. Diabetes Care 12:102–107.

Abelson, D.C., and G. Pergola. 1984. The effect of sucrose concentration on plaque pH in vivo. Clin. Prev. Dent. 6: 23–26.

Ahrens, E.H. 1986. Carbohydrates, plasma triglycerides and coronary heart disease. Nutr. Rev. 44:60–64.

American Diabetes Association. 1982. Statement on hypoglycemia. Diabetes Care 5:72–73.

American Diabetes Association. 1987. Nutritional recommendations and principles for individuals with diabetes mellitus: 1986. Diabetes Care 10:126–132.

Anderson, J.W., and J. Tietyen-Clark. 1986. Dietary fiber: hyperlipidemia, hypertension, and coronary heart disease. Am. J. Gastroenterol. 81:907–919.

Anderson, J.W., and K. Ward. 1979. High carbohydrate, high-fiber diets for insulin-treated men with diabetes mellitus. Am. J. Clin. Nutr. 32:2312–2321.

Armstrong, B.K., and R. Doll. 1975. Environmental factors and cancer incidence and mortality in different countries with special reference to dietary practices. Int. J. Cancer 15: 617–631.

Baeke, J.A.H., W.A. van Staveren, and J. Burema. 1983. Food consumption, habitual physical activity, and body fatness in young Dutch adults. Am. J. Clin. Nutr. 37:278–286.

Baird, J.D. 1972. Diet and development of clinical diabetes. Acta Diabetol. Lat. 9 suppl. 1:621–637.

Bar-On, H., Y.I. Chen, and G.M. Reaven. 1981. Evidence for a new cause of defective plasma removal of very low density lipoproteins in insulin-deficient rats. Diabetes 30: 496–499.

Barter, P.J., K.F. Carroll, and P. Nestel. 1971. Diurnal fluctuations in triglyceride, free fatty acids and insulin during sucrose consumption and insulin infusion in man. J. Clin. Invest. 50:583–591.

Becks, H. 1950. Carbohydrate restriction in the prevention of dental caries using the L.a. count as one index. J. Calif. State Dent. Assoc. 26:53–58.

Behar, D., J.L. Rapoport, A.J. Adams, C.J. Berg, and M. Cornblath. 1984. Sugar challenge testing with children considered behaviorally "sugar reactive." Nutr. Behav. 1: 277–288.

Beighton, D., and H. Hayday. 1984. The establishment of the bacterium *Streptococcus mutans* in dental plaque and the introduction of caries in macaque monkeys (*Macaca fascicularis*) fed a diet containing cooked wheat flour. Arch. Oral Biol. 29:369–372.

Bierman, E.L. 1979. Nutritional management of adult and juvenile diabetics. Pp. 107–117 in M. Winick, ed. Nutritional Management of Genetic Disorders. Wiley, New York.

Bierman, E.L., and J.T. Hamlin III. 1961. The hyperlipemic effect of a low-fat, high-carbohydrate diet in diabetic subjects. Diabetes 10:432–437.

Birkhed, D., V. Topitsoglou, S. Edwardsson, and G. Frostell. 1981. Cariogenicity of invert sugar in long-term experiments. Caries Res. 15:302–307.

Blanc, M.H., O.P. Ganda, R.E. Gleason, and J.S. Soeldner. 1983. Improvement of lipid status in diabetic boys: the 1971 and 1979 Joslin Camp lipid levels. Diabetes Care 6:64–66.

Boot-Hanford, R.P., and H. Heath. 1981. The effect of dietary fructose and diabetes on the rat kidney. Br. J. Exp. Pathol. 62:398–406.

Brody, S., and D.L. Wolinsky. 1983. Lack of mood changes following sucrose loading. Psychosomatics 24:155–162.

Brown, A.T. 1975. The role of dietary carbohydrates in plaque formation and oral disease. Nutr. Rev. 33:353–361.

Cahill, G.F., Jr., and J.S. Soeldner. 1974. A non-editorial on nonhypoglycemia. N. Engl. J. Med. 291:905–906.

Carroll, K.K. 1977. Dietary factors in hormone-dependent cancers. Pp. 25–40 in M. Winick, ed. Current Concepts in Nutrition, Vol. 6: Nutrition and Cancer. Wiley, New York.

Carroll, K.K. 1986. Experimental studies on dietary fat and cancer in relation to epidemiological data. Pp. 231–248 in C. Ip, D.F. Birt, A.E. Rogers, and C. Mettle, eds. Progress in Clinical and Biological Research, Vol. 222: Dietary Fat and Cancer. Alan R. Liss, Inc., New York.

Cerqueria, M.P., M. McMurry, and W.E. Connor. 1979. The food and nutrient intakes of the Tarahumara Indians of Mexico. Am. J. Clin. Nutr. 32:905–913.

Cohen, A.M. 1978. Genetically determined response to different ingested carbohydrates in the production of diabetes. Horm. Metab. Res. 10:86–92.

Cominacini, L., I. Zocce, U. Gorbin, A. Doviol, R. Compri, L. Brunetti, and O. Bosello. 1988. Long-term effect of a low-fat, high-carbohydrate diet on plasma lipids of patients affected by familial endogenous hypertriglyceridemia. Am. J. Clin. Nutr. 48:57–65.

Connor, W.E., M.P. Cerqueria, R.W. Connor, R.B. Wallace, M.R. Malinow, and H.R. Casdorph. 1978. The plasma lipids, lipoproteins and diet of the Tarahumara Indians of Mexico. Am. J. Clin. Nutr. 31:1131–1142.

Coulston, A.M., C.B. Hollenbeck, A.L.M. Swislocki, Y.D.I. Chen, and G.M. Reaven. 1987. Deleterious metabolic effect of high carbohydrate, sucrose-containing diets in patients with non-insulin-dependent diabetes mellitus. Am. J. Med. 82:213–220.

Coulston, A.M., C.B. Hollenbeck, A.L.M. Swislocki, and G.M. Reaven. 1989. Persistence of hypertriglyceridemic effect of high-carbohydrate low-fat diets in NIDDM patients. Diabetes Care 12:94–101.

Crane, S.C., and P.A. Ladene. 1983. Effects of sucrose, glucose and fructose on spontaneous activity and brain monamines in rat pups. Nutr. Rep. Int. 28:991–997.

Dallaglio, E., F. Chang, H. Chang, J. Stern, and G.M. Reaven. 1983. Effect of exercise and diet on triglyceride metabolism in rats with moderate insulin deficiency. Diabetes 32:46–50.

de Bont, A.J., I.A. Baker, A.S. St. Leger, P.M. Sweetnam, K.G. Wragg, S.M. Stephens, and T.M. Hayes. 1981. A randomised controlled trial of the effect of low fat diet advice on dietary response in insulin dependent diabetic young women. Diabetologia 21:529–533.

Drewnowski, A., J.B. Brunzell, K. Sande, P.H. Iverius, and M.R.C. Greenwood. 1985. Sweet tooth reconsidered: taste responsiveness in human obesity. Physiol. Behav. 35:617–622.

Dunnigan, M.G., T. Fyfe, M.T. McKiddie, and S.M. Crosbie. 1970. The effects of isocaloric exchange of dietary starch and sucrose on glucose tolerance, plasma insulin and serum lipids in man. Clin. Sci. 38:1–9.

Edgar, W.M. 1981. Effect of sequence in food intake on plaque pH. Pp. 279–287 in J.J. Hefferren and H.M. Koehler, eds. Foods, Nutrition and Dental Health, Vol. 1. Pathotox Publishing, Park Forest South, Ill.

Edgar, W.M., B.G. Bibby, S. Mundorff, and J. Rowley. 1975. Acid production in plaques after eating snacks: modifying factors in foods. J. Am. Dent. Assoc. 90:418–425.

Edgar, W.M., W.H. Bowen, S. Amsbaugh, E. Monell-Torrens, and J. Brunelle. 1982. Effects of different eating patterns on dental caries in the rat. Caries Res. 16:384–389.

Emanuele, M.A., C. Abraira, W.S. Jellish, and M. De Bartlo. 1986. A crossover trial of high and low sucrose carbohydrate diets in Type II diabetics with hypertriglyceridemia. J. Am. Coll. Nutr. 5:429–437.

Fernstrom, J.D., and R.J. Wurtman. 1971. Brain serotonin content: increase following ingestion of carbohydrate diet. Science 174:1023–1025.

Finn, S.B., and H.C. Jamison. 1980. The relative effects of three dietary supplements on dental caries. ASDC J. Dent. Child. 47:109–113.

Firestone, A.R., R. Schmid, and H.R. Muhlemann. 1982. Cariogenic effects of cooked wheat starch alone or with sucrose and frequency controlled feedings in rats. Arch. Oral Biol. 27:759–763.

Garcia-Palmieri, M.R., P. Sorlie, J. Tillotson, R. Costas, Jr., E. Cordero, and M. Rodriguez. 1980. Relationship of dietary intake to subsequent coronary heart disease incidence: the Puerto Rico Heart Health Program. Am. J. Clin. Nutr. 33:1818–1827.

Garg, A., A. Bonanome, S.M. Grundy, Z.J. Zhang, and R.H. Unger. 1988. Comparison of a high-carbohydrate diet with a high-monounsaturated-fat diet in patients with non-insulin-dependent diabetes mellitus. N. Engl. J. Med. 319:829–834.

Geddes, D.A.M., W.M. Edgar, G.N. Jenkins, and A.J. Rugg-Gunn. 1977. Apples, salted peanuts and plaque pH. Br. Dent. J. 142:317–319.

Geddes, D.A.M., J.A. Cooke, W.M. Edgar, and G.N. Jenkins. 1978. The effect of frequent sucrose mouthrinsing on the induction in vivo of caries-like changes in human dental enamel. Arch. Oral Biol. 23:663–665.

Glass, R.L., and S. Fleisch. 1974. Diet and dental caries: dental caries incidence and the consumption of ready-to-eat cereals. J. Am. Dent. Assoc. 88:807–813.

Glinsmann, W.H., H. Irausquin, and Y.K. Park. 1986. Evaluation of health aspects of sugars contained in carbohydrate sweeteners: report of Sugars Task Force, 1986. J. Nutr. 116:S1–S216.

Goda, T., K. Yamada, M. Sugiyama, S. Moriuchi, and N. Hosoya. 1982. Effect of sucrose and acarbose feeding on the development of streptozotocin-induced diabetes in the rat. J. Nutr. Sci. Vitaminol. 78:41–56.

Gonen, B., W. Patsch, I. Kvisk, and G. Schoenfeld. 1981. The effect of short-term feeding of a high carbohydrate diet on HDL subclasses in normal subjects. Metabolism 30:1125–1129.

Gonnermann, B., R. Schafer-Spiegel, H. Laube, and H. Schatz. 1982. The effect of a saccharose-rich diet on carbohydrate and lipid metabolism of streptozotocin-diabetic rats and genetically determined "diabetic" mice (gg-diab). Int. J. Obesity 6 suppl. 1:41–48.

Gordon, T., A. Kagan, M. Garcia-Palmieri, W.B. Kannel, W.J. Tukel, J. Tillotson, P. Sorlie, and M. Hjortland. 1981. Diet and its relation to coronary heart disease and death in three populations. Circulation 63:500–515.

Gray, G.E. 1987. Crime and diet: is there a relationship? World Rev. Nutr. Diet. 49:66–86.

Gray, G.E., and L.K. Gray. 1983. Diet and juvenile delinquency. Nutr. Today 18:14–22.

Gray, G.M. 1983. Intestinal disaccharidose deficiencies and glucose-galactose malabsorption. Pp. 1729–1742 in J.B. Stanbury, J.B. Wyngaarden, D.S. Fredrickson, J.L. Goldstein, and M.S. Brown, eds. The Metabolic Basis of Inherited Disease. McGraw-Hill, New York.

Gray, R.S., and J.M. Olefsky. 1982. Effect of a glucosidase inhibitor on the metabolic response of diabetic rats to a high carbohydrate diet, consisting of starch and sucrose, or glucose. Metabolism 31:88–92.

Greenwood, M.R.C., R. Kava, D.B. West, and V.A. Lukasik. 1988. Wistar fatty rat: a sexually dimorphic model of human noninsulin-dependent diabetes. Pp. 316–318 in E. Shafrir and A.E. Renold, eds. Frontiers in Diabetes Research: Lessons from Animal Diabetes II. John Libbey, London.

Gridley, D.S., J.D. Kettering, J.M. Slater, and R.L. Nutter. 1983. Modification of spontaneous mammary tumors in mice fed different sources of protein, fat and carbohydrate. Cancer Lett. 19:133–146.

Grinker, J.A. 1978. Obesity and sweet taste. Am. J. Clin. Nutr. 31:1078–1087.

Grundy, S.M., L. Florentin, D. Nix, and M.F. Whelan. 1988. Comparison of monounsaturated fatty acids and carbohydrates for reducing raised levels of plasma cholesterol in man. Am. J. Clin. Nutr. 47:965–969.

Gustafsson, B.E., C.E. Quensel, L.S. Lanke, C. Lundquist, H. Grahnen, B.E. Bonow, and B. Krasse. 1954. The Vipeholm Dental Caries Study. The effect of different levels of carbohydrate intake on caries activity in 436 individuals observed for five years. Acta Ondontol. Scand. 11:232–364.

Hakama, M., and E.A. Saxen. 1967. Cereal consumption and gastric cancer. Int. J. Cancer 2:265–268.

Hallfrisch, J., F. Lazar, and S. Reiser. 1979. Effect of feeding sucrose or starch to rats made diabetic with streptozotocin. J. Nutr. 109:1909–1915.

Harper, A.E., and D.A. Gans. 1986. Claims of antisocial behavior from consumption of sugar: an assessment. Food Technol. 40:142–149.

Harper, D.S., J.C. Osborn, R. Clayton, and J.J. Hefferren. 1987. Modification of food cariogenicity in rats by mineral-rich concentrates from milk. J. Dent. Res. 66:42–45.

Heath, H., and Y.C. Hamlett. 1976. The sorbitol pathway: effect of streptozotocin-induced diabetes and the feeding of a sucrose-rich diet on glucose, sorbitol and fructose in the retina, blood and liver of rats. Diabetes 12:43–46.

Heath, H., S.S. Kang, and D. Philippou. 1975. Glucose, glucose-6-phosphate, lactate and pyruvate content of the retina, blood and liver of streptozotocin-diabetic rats fed sucrose- or starch-rich diets. Diabetes 11:57–62.

Hefti, A., and R. Schmid. 1979. Effect on caries incidence in rats of increasing dietary sucrose levels. Caries Res. 13:298–300.

Hei, T.K., and O. Sudilovsky. 1985. Effects of a high-sucrose diet on the development of enzyme-altered foci in chemical hepatocarcinogenesis in rats. Cancer Res. 45:2700–2705.

Hems, G. 1978. The contributions of diet and childbearing breast-cancer rates. Br. J. Cancer 37:974–982.

Hems, G., and A. Stuart. 1975. Breast cancer rate in populations of single women. Br. J. Cancer 31:118–123.

Hill, W., T.W. Castonguary, and G.H. Collier. 1980. Taste or diet balancing? Physiol. Behav. 24:765–767.

Himsworth, H.P. 1935–1936. Diet and the incidence of diabetes mellitus. Clin. Sci. Mol. Med. 2:117–148.

Hoehn, S.K., and K.K. Carroll. 1978. Effects of dietary carbohydrate on the incidence of mammary tumors induced by rats by 7,12-dimethylbenz(a)anthracene. Nutr. Cancer 1:27–30.

Hollenbeck, C.B., W.E. Connor, U.C. Riddle, P. Alaupovic, and J.E. Leklem. 1985. The effects of a high-CHO, low-fat cholesterol-restricted diet on plasma lipid, lipoprotein, and apoprotein concentrations in insulin-dependent (Type I) diabetes mellitus. Metabolism 34:559–566.

Horton, W.A., A.E. Jacobs, R.M. Green, V.F. Hillier, and D.B. Drucker. 1985. The cariogenicity of sucrose, glucose, and maize starch in gnotobiotic rats mono-infected with strains of the bacteria Streptococcus mutans, Streptococcus salivarius, and Streptococcus milleri. Arch. Oral Biol. 30:777–780.

Ikeda, H., A. Shino, T. Matsuo, H. Iwatsuka, and Z. Suzuoki. 1981. A new genetically obese-hyperglycemic rat (Wistar fatty). Diabetes 30:1045–1050.

Imfeld, T., R.S. Hirsch, and H.R. Muhlemann. 1978. Telemetric recordings of interdental plaque pH during different meal patterns. Br. Dent. J. 144:40–45.

Jellish, W.S., M.A. Emanuele, and C. Abraira. 1984. High sucrose carbohydrate diets vs sucrose restricted diets in overt diabetics. Am. J. Med. 77:1015–1022.

Jensen, M.E., and C.F. Schachtele. 1983. The acidogenic potential of reference foods and snack at interproximal sites in the human dentition. J. Dent. Res. 62:889–892.

Johnson, M.L., B.S. Burke, and J. Mayer. 1956. Relative importance of inactivity and overeating in the energy balance of obese high school girls. Am. J. Clin. Nutr. 4:37–44.

Jukes, T.H. 1986. Sugar and Health. World Rev. Nutr. Diet. 48:137–194.

Kalderon, B., A. Gutman, E. Levy, E. Shafrir, and J. Adler. 1986. Characterization of stages in development of obesity-diabetes syndrome in sand rat (*Psammomys obesus*). Diabetes 35:717–724.

Kanarek, R.B., and E. Hirsch. 1977. Dietary-induced overeating in experimental animals. Fed. Proc. 36:154–158.

Kanarek, R.B., and N. Orthen-Gambill. 1982. Differential effects of sucrose, fructose and glucose on carbohydrate-induced obesity in rats. J. Nutr. 112:1546–1554.

Kang, S.S., R. Fears, S. Noirot, J.N. Mbanya, and J. Yudkin. 1982. Changes in metabolism of rat kidney and liver caused by experimental diabetes and by dietary sucrose. Diabetes 22:285–288.

Katan, M.J. 1984. Diet and HDL. Pp. 103–131 in N.E. Miller and G.J. Miller, eds. Metabolic Aspects of Cardiovascular Disease, Vol. 3. Clinical and Metabolic Aspects of HDL. Elsevier, Oxford.

Kawate, R., M. Yamakido, Y. Nishimoto, P.H. Bennett, R.F. Hamman, and W.C. Knowler. 1979. Diabetes mellitus and its vascular complications in Japanese migrants on the island of Hawaii. Diabetes Care 2:161–170.

Keen, J., B.J. Thomas, R.J. Jarrett, and J.H. Fuller. 1979. Nutrient intake, adiposity, and diabetes. Br. Med. J. 1:655–658.

Keys, A., C. Aravanis, H. Blackburn, F.S.P. Van Buchem, K. Buzina, B.S. Djordjevic, A.S. Dontas, F. Fidanz, M.J. Karvonen, N. Kimura, D. Lekos, M. Monti, V. Puddu, and H.L. Taylor. 1967. Epidemiologic studies related to coronary heart disease: characteristics of men aged 40–59 in seven countries. Acta Med. Scand., Suppl. 460:1–392.

Kiehm, G., J.W. Anderson, and K. Ward. 1976. Beneficial effects of a high carbohydrate, high fiber diet on hyperglycemic diabetic men. Am. J. Clin. Nutr. 29:895–899.

Klurfeld, D.M., M.M. Webber, and D. Kritchevsky. 1984. Comparison of dietary carbohydrates for promotion of DMBA-induced mammary tumorigenesis in rats. Carcinogenesis 5:423–425.

Knuiman, J.T., C.E. West, M.J. Katan, and J.G.A.J. Houtvast. 1987. Total cholesterol levels in populations differing in fat and carbohydrate intake. Arteriosclerosis 7:612–619.

Kolterman, O.G., M. Greenfield, G.M. Reaven, M. Saekow, and J.M. Olefsky. 1979. Effect of a high carbohydrate diet on insulin binding to adipocytes and on insulin action *in vivo* in man. Diabetes 28:731–736.

Krasse, B. 1985. The cariogenic potential of foods—a critical review of current methods. Int. Dent. J. 35:36–42.

Kreitzman, S.N., and R.M. Klein. 1976. Non-linear relationship between dietary sucrose and dental caries. J. Dent. Res. (sp. iss.) 55:B175.

Kromhout, D. 1983a. Changes in energy and macronutrients in 871 middle-aged men during 10 years of follow-up (the Zutphen Study). Am. J. Clin. Nutr. 37:287–294.

Kromhout, D. 1983b. Energy and macronutrient intake in lean and obese middle-aged men (the Zutphen Study). Am. J. Clin. Nutr. 37:295–299.

Kruesi, M.J.P., and J.L. Rapoport. 1986. Diet and human behavior: how much do they affect each other? Annu. Rev. Nutr. 6:113–130.

Leach, S.A., and R.M. Green. 1981. Reversal of fissure caries in the albino rat by sweetening agents. Caries Res. 15:508–511.

Leach, S.A., R. Connell, J.A. Speechley, and R.M. Green. 1984. Reversal of dental caries by the sugar substitute lycasin *in vivo*. J. Dent. Res. (sp. iss.) 63:334.

Leiter, E.H., D.L. Coleman, D.K. Ingram, and M.A. Reynolds. 1983. Influence of dietary carbohydrate on the induction of diabetes in C57BL/KsJ-*db/db* diabetes mice. J. Nutr. 113:184–195.

Lin, W.J., and J.W. Anderson. 1977. Effects of high sucrose or starch-bran diets on glucose and lipid metabolism of normal and diabetic rats. J. Nutr. 107:584–595.

Lincoln, J.E. 1972. Calorie intake, obesity, and physical activity. Am. J. Clin. Nutr. 25:390–394.

Linke, H.A.B. 1980. Inhibition of dental caries in the inbred hamster by saccharin. Ann. Dent. 39:71–74.

Liu, G.C., A.M. Coulston, and G.M. Reaven. 1983. Effects of high-carbohydrate low-fat diets on plasma glucose, insulin, and lipid responses in hypertriglyceridemic humans. Metabolism 32:750–753.

Macquart-Moulin, G., E. Riboli, J. Correa, B. Charnay, P. Berthezene, and N. Day. 1986. Case-control study on colorectal cancer and diet in Marseilles. Int. J. Cancer 38:183–191.

Malcolm, R., P.M. O'Neil, A.A. Hirsch, H.S. Currey, and G. Moskowitz. 1980. Taste hedonics and thresholds in obesity. Int. J. Obesity 4:203–212.

Mann, J.I., and A.S. Truswell. 1970. Effects of isocaloric exchange of dietary sucrose and starch of fasting serum lipids, post-prandial insulin secretion and alimentary lipaemia in human subjects. Br. J. Nutr. 27:295.

Marston, R., and N. Raper. 1987. Nutrient content of the U.S. food supply. National Food Review, Winter-Spring, NFR-36:18–23.

Maxfield, E., and F. Konishi. 1966. Patterns of food intake and physical activity in obesity. J. Am. Diet. Assoc. 49:406–408.

McCarthy, M.C. 1966. Dietary and activity patterns of obese women in Trinidad. J. Am. Diet. Assoc. 48:33–37.

McDonald, I. 1972. Relationship between dietary carbohydrates and fats in their influence on serum lipid concentrations. Clin. Sci. 43:265–274.

McDonald, J.L., Jr. 1985. Cariogenicity of foods. Pp. 320–345 in R.L. Pollack and E. Kravitz, eds. Nutrition in Oral Health and Disease. Lea & Febiger, Philadelphia.

McDonald, J.L., Jr., and J.K. Stookey. 1977. Animal studies concerning the cariogenicity of dry breakfast cereals. J. Dent. Res. 56:1001–1006.

Medalie, J.H., C. Papier, J.B. Herman, U. Goldbourt, S. Tamir, H.N. Neufeld, and E. Riss. 1974. Diabetes mellitus among 10,000 adult men. I. Five-year incidence and associated variables. Isr. J. Med. Sci. 10:681–697.

Michaelis, O.E., IV, K.C. Ellwood, J.M. Judge, N.W. Schoene, and C.T. Hansen. 1984. Effect of dietary sucrose on the SHR/N-corpulent rat: a new model for insulin-independent diabetes. Am. J. Clin. Nutr. 39:612–618.

Michalek, S.M., J.R. McGhee, T. Shiota, and D. Devenyns. 1977. Low sucrose levels promote extensive Streptococcus mutans-induced dental caries. Infect. Immun. 16:712–714.

Milich, R. 1986. Sugar and hyperactivity: a critical review of empirical findings. Clin. Psychol. Rev. 6:493–513.

Modan, B.W., V. Barrell, F. Lubin, R.A. Greenberg, M. Modan, and S. Graham. 1974. The role of starches in the etiology of gastric cancer. Cancer 34:2087–2092.

Mormann, J.E., and H.R. Muhlemann. 1981. Oral starch degradation and its influence on acid production in human dental plaque. Caries Res. 15:166–175.

Morris, J.N., J.W. Marr, and D.G. Clayton. 1977. Diet and heart: a post-script. Br. Med. J. 2:1307–1314.

Nestel, P.J., M. Reardon, and N.H. Fidge. 1979. Sucrose-induced changes in VLDL- and LDL-B apoprotein removal rates. Metabolism 28:531–535.

Nikkilä, W.A., and M. Kekki. 1972. Effects of dietary fructose and sucrose on plasma triglyceride metabolism in patients with endogenous hypertriglyceridemia. Acta Med. Scand., Suppl. 542:221–227.

Nizel, A.E., and R.S. Harris. 1964. The effects of phosphates on experimental dental caries: a literature review. J. Dent. Res. 43:1123–1136.

NRC (National Research Council). 1982. Diet, Nutrition, and Cancer. Report of the Committee on Diet, Nutrition, and Cancer, Assembly of Life Sciences. National Academy Press, Washington, D.C. 478 pp.

Obell, A.E. 1974. Recent advances in mechanism of causation of diabetes mellitus in man and Acomy cahirinus. East Afr. Med. J. 51:425–428.

Olefsky, J.M., and M. Saekow. 1978. The effects of dietary carbohydrate content on insulin binding and glucose metabolism by isolated rat adipocytes. Endocrinology 103:2252–2263.

Ornoy, A., and A.M. Cohen. 1980. Teratogenic effects of sucrose diet in diabetic and nondiabetic rats. Isr. J. Med. Sci. 16:789–791.

Pan, X.R., C.E. Walden, G.R. Warnick, S.X. Hue, J.J. Albers, M. Cheung, and E.L. Bierman. 1986. A comparison of plasma lipoproteins and apoproteins in Chinese and American non-insulin dependent diabetics and controls. Diabetes Care 9:395–400.

Paolino, V. 1982. Anti-plaque activity of cocoa. Pp. 43–58 in J.J. Hefferren and H.M. Koehler, eds. Foods, Nutrition and Dental Health, Vol. 2: Third Annual Conference. American Dental Association, Chicago.

Papachristodoulou, D., H. Heath, and S.S. Kang. 1976. The development of retinopathy in sucrose fed and streptozotocin-diabetic rats. Diabetes 12:367–374.

Pearce, E.I.F., and I.H.C. Gallagher. 1979. The behavior of sucrose and xylitol in an intra-oral caries test. N.Z. Dent. J. 75:8–14.

Perlow, W., E. Baraona, and C.S. Lieber. 1977. Symptomatic intestinal disaccharidase deficiency in alcoholics. Gastroenterology 72:680–684.

Peterson, D.B., J. Lambert, S. Geiring, P. Darling, R.D. Carter, R. Jelfs, and J.I. Mann. 1986. Sucrose in the diet of diabetic patients—just another carbohydrate? Diabetologia 29:216–220.

Phillips, R.W., N. Westmoreland, L. Panepinto, and G.L. Case. 1982. Dietary effects on metabolism of Yucatan miniature swine selected for low and high glucose utilization. J. Nutr. 112:104–111.

Porte, D., Jr., E.L. Bjerman, and J.D. Bagdade. 1966. Substitution of dietary starch for dextrose in hyperlipemic subjects. Proc. Soc. Exp. Biol. Med. 123:84–86.

Prinz, R.J., W.A. Roberts, and E. Hantman. 1980. Dietary correlates of hyperactive behavior in children. J. Consult. Clin. Psychol. 48:760–769.

Rattigan, S., and M.G. Clark. 1984. Effect of sucrose solution drinking option on the development of obesity in rats. J. Nutr. 114:1971–1977.

Reaven, G.R. 1986. Effect of dietary carbohydrate on the metabolism of patients with non-insulin dependent diabetes mellitus. Nutr. Rev. 44:65–73.

Reaven, G.R. 1988. Dietary therapy for non-insulin dependent diabetes mellitus. N. Engl. J. Med. 319:862–864.

Reiser, S., M.C. Bickard, J. Hallfrisch, O.E. Michaelis IV, and E.S. Prather. 1981a. Blood lipids and their distribution in lipoproteins in hyperinsulinemic subjects fed three different levels of sucrose. J. Nutr. 111:1045–1057.

Reiser, S., E. Bohn, J. Hallfrisch, O.E. Michaelis IV, M. Keeney, and E.S. Prather. 1981b. Serum insulin and glucose in hyperinsulinemic subjects fed three different levels of sucrose. Am. J. Clin. Nutr. 34:2348–2358.

Riccardi, G., A. Rivellese, D. Pocioni, S. Genovese, P. Mastranzo, and M. Mancini. 1984. Separate influence of dietary carbohydrate and fibre on the metabolic control in diabetes. Diabetologia 26:116–121.

Rice, M.G., and R.P. Robertson. 1980. Reevaluation of the sand rat as a model for diabetes mellitus. Am. J. Physiol. 239E:340–345.

Risch, H.A., M. Jain, N.W. Choi, J.G. Fodor, C.J. Pfeiffer, G.R. Howe, L.W. Harrison, K.J. Craib, and A.B. Miller. 1985. Dietary factors and the incidence of cancer of the stomach. Am. J. Epidemiol. 122:947–959.

Rosen, S., D.B. Min, D.S. Harper, W.J. Harper, W.X. Beck, and F.M. Beck. 1984. Effect of cheese, with and without sucrose, on dental caries and recovery of Streptococcus mutans in rats. J. Dent. Res. 63:894–896.

Rosenmann, E., Z. Palti, A. Teitelbaum, and A.M. Cohen. 1974. Testicular degeneration in genetically selected sucrose-fed diabetic rats. Metabolism 23:343–348.

Sato, A.T., Y. Nakagima, T. Koyama, T. Shirai, and N. Ito. 1984. Dietary carbohydrate level as a modifying factor on 3'-methyl-4-dimethylaminoazobenzene liver carcinogenesis in rats. Gann 75:665–671.

Schachtele, C.F., and M.E. Jensen. 1983. Can foods be ranked according to their cariogenic potential? Pp. 136–146 in B. Guggenheim, ed. Cariology Today. S. Karger, Basel.

Schauss, A.G. 1980. Diet, Crime and Delinquency. Parker House, Berkeley, Calif. 108 pp.

Scheinin, A. 1976. Caries control through the use of sugar substitutes. Int. Dent. J. 26:4–13.

Scheinin, A., K.K. Makinen, and K. Ylitalo. 1975. Turku sugar studies. I. An intermediate report on the effect of sucrose, fructose, and xylitol diets on the caries incidence in man. Acta Ondontol. Scand. 33 suppl. 70:5–34.

Schlierf, G., and E. Dorow. 1973. Diurnal patterns of triglycerides, free fatty acids, blood sugar, and insulin during carbohydrate-induction in man and their modification by nocturnal suppression of lipolysis. J. Clin. Invest. 42:732–746.

Schlierf, G., V. Stossberg, and W. Reinheimer. 1971. Diurnal patterns of plasma triglycerides and free fatty acids in normal subjects and in patients with endogenous (type IV) hyperlipoproteinemia. Nutr. Metabol. 13:80.

Schoenthaler, S.J. 1982. The effect of sugar on the treatment and control of antisocial behavior: a double-blind study of an incarcerated juvenile population. Int. J. Biosocial Res. 3:1–9.

Sclafani, A., and S. Xenakis. 1984. Sucrose and polysaccharide induced obesity in the rat. Physiol. Behav. 32:169–174.

Shaw, J.H. 1987. Causes and Control of Dental Caries. N. Engl. J. Med. 317:996–1004.

Shrestha, B.M., and P.A. Kreutler. 1983. A comparative rat caries study on cariogenicity of foods using the intubation and gel methods. J. Dent. Res. 62:685.

Shyu, K.W., and M.Y. Hsu. 1980. The cariogenicity of xylitol, mannitol, sorbitol, and sucrose. Proc. Natl. Sci. Council Rep. China 4:21–26.

Silva, M.F., R.C. Burgess, H.J. Sandham, and G.N. Jenkins. 1987. Effects of water-soluble components of cheese on experimental caries in humans. J. Dent. Res. 66:38–41.

Simpson, R.W., J.I. Mann, J. Eaton, R.D. Carter, and T.D.R. Hockaday. 1979a. High-carbohydrate diets and insulin-dependent diabetes. Br. Med. J. 2:523–525.

Simpson, R.W., J.I. Mann, J. Eaton, R.A. Moore, R. Carter, and T.D.R. Hockaday. 1979b. Improved glucose control in maturity-onset diabetes treated with high-carbohydrate-modified fat diet. Br. Med. J. 1:1753–1756.

Skinner, A., P. Connolly, and M.N. Naylor. 1982. Influence of the replacement of dietary sucrose by maltose in solid and in solution on rat caries. Caries Res. 16:443–452.

Sognnaes, R.F. 1948. Analysis of war time reduction of dental caries in European children. Am. J. Dis. Child. 75:792–821.

Sopko, G., D.R. Jacobs, Jr., and H.L. Taylor. 1984. Dietary measures of physical activity. Am. J. Epidemiol. 120:900–911.

Sreebny, L.M. 1982. Sugar availability, sugar consumption, and dental caries. Community Dent. Oral Epidemiol. 10:1–7.

Stearns, S.B., and P.H. Smith. 1985. Sucrose-feeding does not alter triglyceride secretion rates or insulin release in female rats. Nutr. Int. 1:26–29.

Stefanik, P.A., F.P. Heald, and J. Mayer. 1959. Caloric intake in relation to energy output of obese and non-obese adolescent boys. Am. J. Clin. Nutr. 7:55–62.

Stone, D.B., and W.E. Connor. 1963. The prolonged effects of a low cholesterol, high carbohydrate diet upon the serum lipids in diabetic patients. Diabetes 12:127–132.

Story, L., J.W. Anderson, W.J. Chen, D. Karounos, and B. Jefferson. 1985. Adherence to high-carbohydrate, high-fiber diets: long-term studies of non-obese diabetic men. J. Am. Diet. Assoc. 85:1105–1110.

Takeuchi, M. 1961. Epidemiological study on dental caries in Japanese children before, during, and after World War II. Int. Dent. J. 11:443–457.

Taylor, S.A., R.G. Price, S.S. Kang, and J. Yudkin. 1980. Modification of the glomerular basement membrane in sucrose-fed and streptozotocin-diabetic rats. Diabetes 19:364–378.

Tehrani, A., F. Brudevold, F. Attarzadeh, J. Van Houte, and J. Russo. 1983. Enamel demineralization by mouth rinses containing different concentrations of sucrose. J. Dent. Res. 62:1216–1217.

Tenovuo, J., K.K. Makinen, and K. Paunio. 1984. Effects on oral health of mouth rinses containing xylitol, sodium cyclamate, and sucrose sweeteners in the absence of oral hygiene. IV. Analysis of whole saliva. Proc. Finn. Dent. Soc. 80:28–34.

Thornber, J.M., and C.D. Eckhert. 1984. Protection against sucrose induced retinol capillary damage at the Wistar rat. J. Nutr. 114:1070–1075.

Toverud, G. 1957. The influence of war and post-war conditions on the teeth of Norwegian school children. III. Discussion of food supply and dental condition in Norway and other European countries. Milbank Mem. Fund Quart. 35:373–459.

Turner, J.L., E.L. Bierman, J.D. Brunzell, and A. Chait. 1979. Effect of dietary fructose on triglyceride transport and glucoregulatory hormones in hypertriglyceridemic man. Am. J. Clin. Nutr. 32:1043–1050.

Tuyns, A.J., M. Haelterman, and R. Kaaks. 1987. Colorectal cancer and the intake of nutrients: oligosaccharides are a risk factor, fats are not. A case control study in Belgium. Nutr. Cancer 10:181–196.

USDA (U.S. Department of Agriculture). 1984. Nationwide Food Consumption Survey. Nutrient Intakes: Individuals in 48 States, Year 1977–78. Report No. I-2. Consumer Nutrition Division, Human Nutrition Information Service, Hyattsville, Md. 439 pp.

USDA (U.S. Department of Agriculture). 1986. Nationwide Food Consumption Survey. Continuing Survey of Food Intakes by Individuals. Men 19–50 Years, 1 Day, 1985. Report No. 85-3. Nutrition Monitoring Division, Human Nutrition Information Service, Hyattsville, Md. 94 pp.

USDA (U.S. Department of Agriculture). 1987. Nationwide Food Consumption Survey. Continuing Survey of Food Intakes by Individuals. Women 19–50 Years and Their Children 1–5 Years, 4 Days, 1985. Report No. 85-4. Nutrition Monitoring Division, Human Nutrition Information Service, Hyattsville, Md. 182 pp.

USDA (U.S. Department of Agriculture). 1988. Nationwide Food Consumption Survey. Continuing Survey of Food Intakes by Individuals. Low-Income Women 19–50 Years and Their Children 1–5 Years, 4 Days, 1985. Report No. 85-5. Nutrition Monitoring Division, Human Nutrition Information Service, Hyattsville, Md. 220 pp.

Virkunen, M. 1982. Reactive hypoglycemic tendency among habitually violent offenders. Neuropsychobiology 8:35–40.

Virkunen, M., and M.O. Huttunen. 1982. Evidence for abnormal glucose tolerance test among violent offenders. Neuropsychobiology 8:30–34.

Walker, A.R.P. 1977. Sugar intake and diabetes mellitus. S. Afr. Med. J. 51:842–851.

Weinsier, R.L., A. Seeman, M.G. Herrera, J.P. Assal, J.S. Soeldner, and R.E. Gleason. 1974. High- and low-carbohydrate diets in diabetes mellitus. Ann. Intern. Med. 80:332–341.

Welsh, S.O., and R.M. Marston. 1982. Review of trends in food use in the United States, 1909 to 1980. J. Am. Diet. Assoc. 81:120–125.

West, K.M. 1978. Epidemiology of Diabetes and Its Vascular Lesions. Elsevier, New York. 579 pp.

West, K.M., M.E. Sanders, E.L. McCulloch, R.P. Robinson, and J.A. Stober. 1976. Does sugar consumption increase risk of diabetes and obesity? Diabetes 25 suppl. 1:342.

WHO (World Health Organization) Multinational Study of Vascular Disease in Diabetics. 1985. Prevalence of small vessel and large vessel disease in diabetic patients from 14 centres. Diabetologia 28:615–640.

Wilkinson, P.W., J.M. Parkin, G. Pearlson, M. Strong, and P. Sykes. 1977. Energy intake and physical activity in obese children. Br. Med. J. 1:756.

Wolraich, M., R. Milich, P. Stumbo, and F. Schultz. 1985. Effects of sucrose ingestion on the behavior of hyperactive boys. J. Pediatr. 106:675–682.

Yager, J., and R.T. Young. 1974. Non-hypoglycemia is an epidemic condition. N. Engl. J. Med. 291:907–908.

Yano, K., G.G. Rhoads, A. Kagan, and J. Tillotson. 1978. Dietary intake and risk of coronary heart disease in Japanese men living in Hawaii. Am. J. Clin. Nutr. 31: 1270–1279.

Yudkin, J. 1964. Dietary fat and dietary sugar in relation to ischemic heart disease and diabetes. Lancet 2:4–5.

10

Dietary Fiber

Dietary fiber is a complex material; its composition varies from one food to another. Trowell (1972) first defined dietary fiber as components of the plant cell wall that resist digestion by secretions of the human alimentary tract. These include cellulose, hemicelluloses, pectin, and lignin. Later, he extended the definition to include indigestible plant materials that are not cell-wall components. These materials include gums, such as guar and locust bean gums, algal polysaccharides, such as alginates and carrageenan, and mucilages (Trowell et al., 1976). This expanded definition recognizes that analytical methods failed to distinguish indigestible plant cell-wall components from indigestible storage polysaccharides that exist within plant cells. The term *edible fiber* has also been suggested and includes, in addition to the above-named components, chitins from fungi and crustaceans, indigestible fiberlike materials such as aminopolysaccharides from animals, and partially synthetic polysaccharides such as methyl cellulose (Trowell et al., 1978). Recently, the Life Sciences Research Office of the Federation of American Societies for Experimental Biology defined dietary fiber as "the endogenous components of plant materials in the diet which are resistant to digestion by enzymes produced by humans" (LSRO, 1987). This definition excludes such substances as cutin, saponins, phytates, lectins, proteins, waxes, nonenzymatic browning products, resistant starch, silicon, and other inorganic constituents, which are associated with the plant cell wall. A Canadian report on dietary fiber contained a similar definition, but it included some nonnutritive substances (e.g., phytates) associated with the plant cell wall (Health and Welfare Canada, 1985). The term *endogenous* in the 1987 LSRO definition of dietary fiber excludes indigestible substances (e.g., nonenzymatic browning products) formed during food processing.

Analytically, dietary fiber is defined as nonstarch polysaccharides and lignin from plants. Lignin is a complex polymer of phenylpropane residues; the remaining dietary fiber components are polysaccharides. These polysaccharides resist digestion because they are non-α-linked-glucan-polysaccharides, whereas the human digestive tract appears to secrete only α-glucosidases (Southgate, 1982). Any degradation of dietary fiber in the human gastrointestinal tract results from the action of enzymes secreted by the intestinal microflora.

Various fractionations of dietary fiber are shown in Figure 10–1. The nonstarch polysaccharides consist of cellulose, hemicelluloses, pectin, gums, and mucilages, whereas noncellulosic polysaccharides include all of these except cellulose.

It is difficult to analyze dietary fiber chemically and thus to understand its role in health. Problems in analyzing this complex substance are reviewed by Dintzis (1982), Lanza and Butrum (1986),

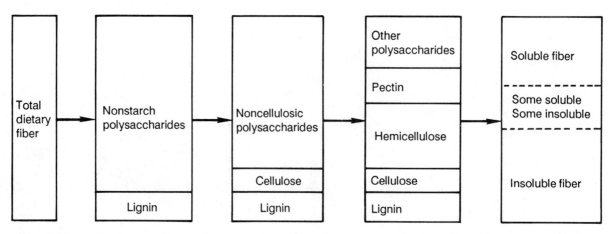

FIGURE 10–1. Total dietary fiber can be categorized as shown above. For example, total dietary fiber can be divided into nonstarch polysaccharides and lignin. Nonstarch polysaccharides can be further divided into noncellulosic polysaccharides and cellulose. Note: Cellulose, lignin, and most hemicelluloses are not soluble in water, whereas pectins and other polysaccharides (such as gums and mucilages) are water soluble. Adapted from Asp and Johansson (1984).

Selvendran and Du Pont (1984), Southgate et al. (1978), and Theander (1981).

Pectins, gums, and mucilages are soluble in water, as are some hemicelluloses, whereas lignins, cellulose, and most hemicelluloses are insoluble in water. Although the physical and chemical properties of different dietary fiber components, such as viscosity, water-holding capacity, ion-exchange capacity, and binding capacity, have been studied, these properties do not adequately predict the physiological properties of specific dietary fibers and of high-fiber whole foods.

PHYSIOLOGICAL EFFECTS OF DIETARY FIBER

Some physiological effects of dietary fiber are systemic, whereas others are localized in the gastrointestinal tract. Diets with a high fiber content are high-volume diets, requiring longer mastication and ingestion time (Heaton, 1980), and subjective assessments indicate that they may increase satiety (Bolton et al., 1981; Duncan et al., 1983; Kay and Stitt, 1978). Although guar gum and pectin, both viscous fibers, have been shown in some studies to delay gastric emptying (Holt et al., 1979; Tadesse, 1982; Wilmshurst and Crawley, 1980), other studies fail to confirm this (Rydning et al., 1985).

Some soluble dietary fiber components, such as oat bran, pectin, and guar gum, stimulate fecal excretion of bile acids. However, wheat bran has no such effect; it promotes a different composition of bile acids than does pectin (Hillman et al., 1986; Pomare and Heaton, 1973; Pomare et al.,

1976). Some soluble fibers also lower serum cholesterol (Judd and Truswell, 1985). In short-term studies (a single meal or a few days), soluble fiber fed to healthy subjects enhanced glucose tolerance and increased insulin sensitivity, but the results of longer studies are conflicting (LSRO, 1987).

Dietary fiber affects colonic function and activities of the microflora. High fiber intakes promote increased bacterial mass but do not alter the microflora composition (Baird et al., 1977; Drasar et al., 1976; Finegold and Sutter, 1978). Colonic bacteria attack fermentable fiber components and degrade at least a portion of them to short-chain fatty acids and gases. The role and importance of these short-chain fatty acids in the colon have not been determined.

Insoluble fibers such as wheat bran decrease intestinal transit time and increase stool weight and volume. Increased stool volume observed after high intakes of dietary fiber is due in part to indigestible remnants of plant cell walls and in part to increased bacterial mass, but certain dietary fibers may also result in increased fecal nitrogen excretion. Most studies have not assessed the source of the increased nitrogen excretion. Stephen and Cummings (1980b) concluded that most of it can be attributed to bacterial mass and to mucosal cell debris and intestinal secretions.

SOURCES OF DIETARY FIBER

Quantifying total dietary fiber as well as the different fiber components in foods has been extremely difficult, because the complex nature of dietary fiber demands complex analytical techniques. Until recently, food composition data bases quantified only crude fiber, which was obtained by extracting the fiber from plant foods with acid and alkali. This process resulted in the destruction of large and inconsistent portions of dietary fiber components. More recently, R.A. McCance and E.M. Widdowson developed a table containing the estimated composition of dietary fiber in different foods (Paul and Southgate, 1978), but the method used to obtain these data has been criticized because the removal of starch is incomplete (Selvendran and Du Pont, 1980) and the calorimetric methods used to measure sugars are nonspecific (Hudson and Bailey, 1980). The Association of Official Analytical Chemists approved a method for quantifying total dietary fiber (Prosky et al., 1985), but no data on dietary fiber in foods have been published with this method. At present, there are no satisfactory data bases on the individual components of dietary fiber in foods.

Lanza and Butrum (1986) compiled provisional dietary fiber tables based on published values derived from a variety of analytical methods. The magnitude of the error introduced by combining data in this way is unknown, but the variation among laboratories using the same analytical method is known to be large (Theander, 1981). In addition, most values in Lanza and Butrum's tables are based on analysis of only one or a few samples; genetic varieties and changes in fiber due to food processing could not be taken into account (Lanza and Butrum, 1986).

In general, foods with a high fiber content include whole-grain breads and cereals, fruits, vegetables, legumes, and nuts. Fruit skins, seeds, berries, and the bran layers of cereal grains contain higher concentrations of fiber than do the remainder of these foods (Lanza and Butrum, 1986).

Components of dietary fiber vary from food to food, as noted in a comprehensive review by Selvendran (1984). Plant species, stage of maturity, and parts of the plant consumed all influence the composition of dietary fiber. High levels of cellulose are found in root and leafy vegetables, legumes, and some fruits such as pears and apples. Lignin content is highest in fruits, particularly strawberries and peaches, whereas pectin levels are highest in citrus fruits and apples. Cereals and grains contain high levels of the insoluble fibers cellulose and hemicelluloses (Lanza and Butrum, 1986; Selvendran, 1984).

PATTERNS OF FIBER INTAKE IN THE UNITED STATES

The paucity of accurate population-based data on fiber intake, due largely to the lack of data on fiber in foods, hinders interpretation of epidemiologic studies of the relationship of dietary fiber to chronic diseases. In addition, many of these studies used only crude fiber data. Crude fiber in the U.S. food supply declined from 6.1 g/day per capita during 1909–1913 to 4.1 g/day in 1982. Using the dietary fiber data published by Paul and Southgate (1978), Bingham and Cummings (1980) estimated that the availability (not the actual consumption) of total dietary fiber fell from 40 g/day per capita during 1909–1913 to 26.7 g/day in 1980. Most of the decline resulted from decreased use of cereal grains and potatoes.

The Nationwide Food Consumption Survey (NFCS) of the U.S. Department of Agriculture (USDA) contained the first estimates of total fiber intake in its reports of the 1985 Continuing Survey of Food Intakes of Individuals (CSFII) (USDA 1985, 1986a,b, 1987a,b, 1988). Estimates of the amount of dietary fiber in foods were derived chiefly by the methods of Englyst et al. (1982) and, to a lesser extent, Prosky et al. (1985). The mean intake of women 19 to 50 years of age, based on four nonconsecutive days of intake, was 10.9 g/day (7.3 g/1,000 kcal); for children 1 to 5 years of age, mean intake was 9.8 g/day (6.9 g/1,000 kcal) (USDA, 1987a). Low-income women in the same age group averaged, on the one day surveyed, 10.1 g/day (6.7 g/1,000 kcal) in 1985 (USDA, 1986a) and 10.2 g/day (6.9 g/1,000 kcal) in 1986 (USDA, 1987b). Low-income children averaged 8.6 g/day (6.2 g/1,000 kcal) in 1985 (USDA, 1986a) and 9.3 g/day (6.2 g/1,000 kcal) in 1986 (USDA, 1987b). The 1-day fiber intakes of men 19 to 50 years of age surveyed in 1985 averaged 17.5 g/day (7.0 g/1,000 kcal) (USDA, 1986b).

The provisional dietary fiber table of Lanza and Butrum (1986) was used to calculate the fiber intake of adults in the Second National Health and Nutrition Examination Survey (NHANES II) (Lanza et al., 1987). Mean intakes for the total adult population, men as well as women, were 11.1 g/day, compared with 13.3 g/day using the table of Paul and Southgate (1978). Women in the NHANES II study consumed an average of 6.5 g/1,000 kcal, whereas men consumed 5.5 g/1,000 kcal.

The USDA and NHANES II surveys indicate that men have a higher absolute daily intake of dietary fiber than do women, but that women's intakes are higher per 1,000 kcal. Limited data suggest that dietary fiber intake per 1,000 kcal may be higher among the elderly than among young adults and that adolescents may have low intakes (LSRO, 1987).

A more definitive assessment of current fiber intake patterns must await improvement in the food composition data base, now in progress, and more accurate information about dietary practices.

METHODOLOGICAL PROBLEMS IN ASSESSING FIBER-DISEASE INTERRELATIONSHIPS

Several caveats must be borne in mind when reviewing studies on dietary fiber and chronic disease etiology. First, as noted above, the term *fiber* is used to define a complex mixture of dietary substances with differing chemical, physical, and physiological properties. Analyses of studies in terms of total dietary fiber content could be misleading if the effect of one component of fiber masks differing effects of the other components. This problem is compounded by the lack of complete data on the various components of dietary fiber in different foods and the imprecision of current methods for estimating fiber intake in epidemiologic studies.

Second, in some populations consuming Western diets, fiber intake is positively correlated with total caloric intake, which itself is highly correlated with fat intake. There may therefore be a positive correlation between fiber intake and fat intake. When the effect of caloric intake is controlled, however, fiber and fat intakes of individuals are usually negatively correlated (i.e., among people with the same caloric intake, those with a higher fat intake tend to have a lower fiber intake and vice versa). Thus, in assessing associations with fiber intake, it is necessary to consider caloric as well as fat intakes. Nevertheless, statistical analyses of fiber intake that specifically take caloric and fat intake into account simultaneously may be unstable due to multicollinearity.

Third, any fiber effect could be interactive (e.g., high fiber intake could be protective only in people with high fat intake). Such interactions can usually be detected only in much larger studies than those required to detect main effects.

Fourth, epidemiologic studies that rely on evidence from vegetarians (who as a rule consume more fiber than nonvegetarians) should be evaluated carefully, since most types of vegetarians (e.g., complete vegetarians, lacto-ovovegetarians, and others) differ from omnivores in many ways that may confound the association between fiber intake and health. In addition, there is a general lack of consistency among and within some studies regarding the length of time that subjects have followed a vegetarian diet.

Finally, many populations are fairly homogeneous in their fiber intake. Studies in such populations may fail to detect a true effect of fiber.

EVIDENCE ASSOCIATING DIETARY FIBER WITH CHRONIC DISEASES

Hyperlipidemia and Coronary Heart Disease

Epidemiologic Studies

The effects of dietary fiber on lipid metabolism in humans have been described in several comprehensive reviews (Judd and Truswell, 1985; Kay and Truswell, 1980; Story, 1980; Vahouny, 1982, 1985). Most epidemiologic data on fiber intake and levels of serum lipid, lipoprotein, and apolipoprotein come from comparisons of vegetarian and nonvegetarian populations. In a study of complete vegetarians, lacto-ovovegetarians, and nonvegetarians, Hardinge and colleagues observed that serum cholesterol levels were significantly lower in complete vegetarians (Hardinge and Stare, 1954; Hardinge et al., 1958). Intakes of fiber, presumably crude fiber, among complete vegetarians, lacto-ovovegetarians, and nonvegetarians were 7.9, 5.4, and 2.9 g/1,000 kcal, respectively, for males and 8.6, 5.2, and 3.1, respectively, for females. Subsequent studies (Burslem et al., 1978; Knuiman and West, 1982; Sacks et al., 1975) confirmed the lower serum lipid levels in complete vegetarians and also noted that vegetarians have higher ratios of high-density lipoprotein (HDL) cholesterol to total cholesterol and lower levels of apo-B and apo-AI lipoproteins than either lacto-ovovegetarians or nonvegetarians.

The epidemiologic evidence linking fiber intake to coronary heart disease (CHD) risk is less consistent than the data on serum lipids. Although the rate of CHD in 20 economically advanced countries varied inversely with estimated fiber intake (Liu et al., 1982), adjustment for fat intake removed the association. In the Ireland–Boston Diet–Heart Study—a 20-year cohort study of 1,001 middle-aged men—decreased fiber consumption was associated with increased risk of CHD, but the association was no longer significant when other risk factors were taken into account (Kushi et al., 1985). A 10-year follow-up study of diet and mortality in the Netherlands (Kromhout et al., 1982) showed no significant difference in fiber intake between people dying of CHD (9.5 g/1,000 kcal) and noncases (10.0 g/1,000 kcal). In a subsequent follow-up, Kromhout and de Lezenne Coulander (1984) found a negative association between fiber intake and risk of CHD, but the association disappeared after controlling for total caloric intake. Similarly, in a study of 200 males, Kay et al. (1980) showed that serum cholesterol levels were inversely associated with fiber intake, but this association no longer held when caloric intake was taken into account in the analysis. The significance of such observations is not clear, however, since people with CHD tend to have lower caloric intakes than those without the disease (see Chapter 7) and, thus, will inevitably tend to have lower fiber intakes.

Morris et al. (1977) reported a protective effect of dietary fiber from cereals on risk of CHD independent of caloric intake. Khaw and Barrett-Connor (1987) found that fiber intake was inversely associated with ischemic heart disease mortality in a 12-year follow-up study of 859 men and women aged 50 to 79 years. In this study, intake was measured by 24-hour dietary recall, which, as noted in Chapter 2, has limited applicability in the assessment of the usual dietary intake of individuals in the United States. Relative risks in those with a 24-hour fiber intake of 16 g or more compared with those with an intake less than 16 g were 0.33 for men and 0.37 for women. A 6 g increment in daily fiber intake was associated with a 25% reduction in ischemic heart disease mortality. This effect was independent of other dietary variables, including calories, fats, cholesterol, protein, carbohydrates, alcohol, calcium, and potassium. In England, 10,943 vegetarians were shown to be at lower risk of CHD, but their decreased risk could not be accounted for by increased fiber consumption alone (Burr, 1982).

Clinical and Metabolic Studies

Metabolic studies (Anderson et al., 1984; Challen et al., 1983; Kay et al., 1985; Schweizer et al., 1983) suggest that increasing consumption of fiber-rich foods can reduce serum cholesterol levels. For example, serum cholesterol concentrations have been lowered by diets providing 45 g of dietary fiber per day in fresh fruits, vegetables, and legumes (Grande et al., 1965; Jenkins et al., 1979b; Keys et al., 1960) and by isocaloric substi-

tution of either sugar or bread by a mixture of vegetables, providing 40 g/day, but not fruit, providing 20 g/day (Grande et al., 1974). Unlike vegetables, legumes, and possibly fruits, the addition of cereals to the diet has little effect on serum cholesterol levels.

Not all dietary fibers appear to influence serum lipid levels to the same degree or in the same manner. Soluble fibers such as guar gum, pectin, and oat gum have some hypocholesterolemic effect in hyperlipidemics. Guar supplements tend to lower low-density lipoprotein (LDL) cholesterol but not to influence HDL cholesterol, whereas oat bran has been shown in some studies to reduce triglycerides (LSRO, 1987). In contrast, supplements containing insoluble fibers have been shown to have little influence on serum lipid levels in hyperlipidemic people (Jenkins et al., 1986; LSRO, 1987; Schneeman and Lefevre, 1986).

Animal Studies

Studies on dietary fiber in relation to atherosclerosis in different animal models have been reviewed by Kritchevsky (1986a). Early studies in animals were undertaken to determine why natural-ingredient (chow) diets appear to be less atherogenic than semipurified diets, even when the latter contain no cholesterol (Kritchevsky, 1964). The casein used as the protein component of semipurified diets was subsequently found to be primarily responsible for the hypercholesterolemia and the atherogenic effects of the semipurified diets (Hamilton and Carroll, 1976), but experiments in which the fiber component was varied showed that fiber could also influence serum cholesterol levels and the development of atherosclerosis in animals (Kritchevsky, 1986a; Kritchevsky and Story, 1986).

The effects depend on the animal model used and the type of fiber added to the diet. For example, grain residues and wheat straw reduce the atherogenicity of a semipurified, high-fat, cholesterol-free diet in rabbits (Kritchevsky and Tepper, 1965; Kritchevsky et al., 1977) but have less effect in vervet monkeys than does cellulose (Kritchevsky, 1986a,b). Pectin inhibits atherogenesis in cholesterol-fed chickens (Fisher et al., 1966) but does not appear to affect cholesterolemia in vervet monkeys (Kritchevsky, 1986a,b). In general, the water-soluble, viscous, polysaccharide types of dietary fiber appear to be most effective in lowering plasma cholesterol and LDL cholesterol (Schneeman and Lefevre, 1986). Dietary fiber of this type has been shown to inhibit the intestinal absorption of cholesterol and other lipids in rats (Vahouny and Cassidy, 1986a,b).

Mechanisms of Action

Several mechanisms have been suggested to explain the hypocholesterolemic effect of certain dietary fibers. Since dietary fibers do not appear to be readily absorbable, it might be expected that their effects on serum cholesterol levels and atherosclerosis would be exerted in the gastrointestinal tract. This has led to studies on adsorption of bile acids by dietary fiber in relation to fecal steroid excretion. Story (1986) concluded, however, that the effects of dietary fiber on bile acid excretion were not consistent or large enough to account for observed changes in serum cholesterol levels. They suggested two other possible mechanisms: (1) The site at which lipids are absorbed from the intestine could be altered by dietary fiber, which could affect the composition of chylomicrons and influence cholesterol metabolism. (2) Absorbable products of the bacterial degradation of dietary fiber (e.g., short-chain fatty acids) in the colon may modify some aspect of cholesterol metabolism such as cholesterol synthesis (Story, 1986). Tocotrienols, which are effective inhibitors of cholesterol synthesis, have been found in some plant sources of dietary fiber (Qureshi et al., 1986).

Dietary fiber alters the morphology of the intestinal mucosa in rats in a manner that could influence lipid digestion and absorption (Cassidy et al., 1986; Tasman-Jones, 1986a,b; Vahouny and Cassidy 1986b). Soluble dietary fiber may also influence serum lipid levels through effects on lipoprotein secretion and metabolism. Mechanisms posited include increased catabolism of LDL cholesterol (Chen and Anderson, 1986) and increased serum acetate, which has been shown to inhibit cholesterol synthesis in hepatocytes (Beynen et al., 1982) and, possibly, to increase peripheral LDL receptors and LDL clearance (LSRO, 1987).

Cancer

Large Intestine

Epidemiologic Studies

The relative lack of cancer of the large intestine in Africa led to the hypothesis that fiber might be protective against a number of chronic diseases common in Western countries (including CHD, diverticulitis, and colorectal cancer) (Burkitt and Trowell, 1975). Most epidemiologic evidence on cancer relates to cancer of the colon, and the correlation between colon cancer rates and fiber consumption has been the subject of several studies. Direct comparisons of fiber intake between two geographic areas with differing colon cancer incidence rates but similar levels of fat intake have been reported for northern and southern India (Malhotra, 1977), for rural Finland and New York (Reddy et al., 1978), and for Denmark and Finland (Jensen et al., 1982). In these studies, the lower risk populations had the higher fiber intake. In contrast, a study in New Zealand showed that Maoris have lower colon cancer rates (and CHD rates) than do whites despite higher fat and lower fiber intakes (Smith et al., 1985).

Early international comparisons did not suggest an inverse association of fiber intake with colon cancer risk. Drasar and Irving (1973) failed to find a correlation between colon cancer incidence in 37 countries and per-capita intake of fiber-containing foods, but they did find a negative association with intake of cereals (Irving and Drasar, 1973). Liu et al. (1979) compared per-capita intake from 1954 to 1965 in 20 industrialized countries with colon cancer mortality from 1967 to 1973. Although fiber intake was inversely correlated with colon cancer mortality, this relationship was no longer significant in a partial correlation analysis controlling for cholesterol intake. This analysis was considered appropriate in light of the low colon cancer rates in Finland where cholesterol intake is high. In a later study of 38 countries, international age-standardized colon cancer rates did not correlate with fiber intake after controlling for intake of fat. However, there was a negative correlation of cereal intake with colon cancer, even after controlling for fat intake (McKeown-Eyssen and Bright-See, 1984). This finding supported three earlier studies showing an inverse association of colon cancer with cereal intake (Armstrong and Doll, 1975; Drasar and Irving, 1973; Knox, 1977).

Intracountry correlation studies in general have produced negative results. For example, Lyon and Sorenson (1978) found little difference in intake of fiber and other dietary constituents between the low-risk population of Utah and the U.S. population as a whole. However, the power of this study was probably low, since no significant differences were found for any of the other dietary items studied. Total fiber intake did not correlate with colon cancer rates among counties in England and Wales, but there was a negative correlation with both vegetable intake (excluding potatoes) and the pentose subfraction of fiber (Bingham et al.,

1979). Subsequently, Bingham and coworkers (1985) reanalyzed the results using data that distinguished more specifically among various fiber fractions and showed that colon cancer mortality in these counties was negatively associated with the uronic acid fraction of fiber (derived largely from fruits and vegetables) rather than with the pentose fraction.

Case-control studies of large bowel cancer have been conducted in a variety of geographic locations and populations using several different techniques for sampling cases and controls. Most did not include indices of fiber intake, and their findings were presented in terms of specific foods or food groups. For these studies, it is difficult to conclude that a particular association with colon cancer indicates an effect of dietary fiber per se rather than an effect of other factors associated with the intake of fiber-rich foods.

Four case-control studies did include indices of total fiber intake, and they provide inconsistent findings. In these studies, total fiber intake was estimated from diet history questionnaires administered to populations consuming diets similar to average diets in the United States. One of these, in Canada, showed no association between colorectal cancer and crude fiber intake or total dietary fiber (Jain et al., 1980; Miller et al., 1983). In a recent reanalysis of those data, which included data on intakes of calories, saturated fat, and dietary fiber, Howe et al. (1986) estimated that the relative risk in the upper two tertiles of fiber consumption was very close to 1.0 with narrow confidence intervals. In a case-control study conducted in South Australia, Potter and McMichael (1986) found *higher* fiber intake by colon cancer cases than by controls, especially among females. In both sexes, a finding of an increased risk associated with high protein and total energy intakes was confined to those consuming a low-fiber diet. In females, adjusting fiber intake for these and other variables attenuated the increase in risk associated with fiber. In Melbourne, Australia, Kune et al. (1987) found high fiber intake to be protective in association with a high vegetable intake. In Utah, Lyon et al. (1987) used an index of crude dietary fiber and found a weak protective effect, especially in females, after adjustment for caloric intake.

The remaing case-control studies did not assess fiber intake per se. In studies conducted in Minnesota (Bjelke, 1978), San Francisco (Dales et al., 1979), and New York State (Graham et al., 1978), the reported frequency of eating foods with a high-fiber content was used rather than a direct index of fiber consumption. All three studies showed that cases consumed less of these foods than did controls. In the New York State study, the protective effect was specifically attributed to vegetables of the *Brassica* genus (e.g., cabbage, cauliflower, Brussels sprouts).

A study in Norway (Bjelke, 1978), conducted in parallel with the Minnesota study, produced similar results. In a case-control study in Puerto Rico, on the other hand, Martinez et al. (1979) found that large bowel cancer cases consumed *greater* amounts of fiber-containing foods (as well as other dietary items) than did controls. They did not study the association of fiber-containing foods and colon cancer risk when other dietary factors were controlled.

Three dietary case-control studies of cancer of the large intestine have been conducted in Mediterranean populations. In Greece (Manousos et al., 1983) and in Marseilles, France (Macquart-Moulin et al., 1986), the consumption of certain vegetables was associated with a protective effect. In the Greek study, the protective effect provided by the consumption of cabbage, lettuce, spinach, and beets persisted in a multivariate analysis that adjusted for age, sex, and meat intake (Manousos et al., 1983). In the French study, vegetables with a *low* fiber content (e.g., cucumbers, zucchini, tomatoes, lettuce, and onion) were protective in a similar multivariate analysis, but, notably, other vegetables with medium or high fiber content were not (Macquart-Moulin et al., 1986). However, the individual contribution of the low-fiber vegetable group and the high-fiber vegetable group to total dietary fiber consumption was not considered in the analysis. In the third study, conducted earlier in Israel, investigators found that a grouping of foods with a crude fiber content of $\geq 0.5\%$ was protective for colon cancer, but not for rectal cancer (Modan et al., 1975). The specific food items found to be protective were primarily vegetables.

Animal Studies

Like epidemiologic studies, laboratory animal studies on dietary fiber and cancer have focused largely on colon cancer. These studies were reviewed by the National Research Council's Committee on Diet, Nutrition, and Cancer (NRC, 1982) and more recently by Jacobs (1986b, 1987), Kritchevsky (1986b), and Reddy (1986). A variety of compounds carcinogenic to the colon, including 1,2-dimethylhydrazine (DMH), azoxymethane

(AOM), 3,2'-dimethyl-4-aminobiphenyl (DMAB), and methylnitrosourea (MNU), have been used in animal models to study the effects of the amount and type of dietary fibers on colon carcinogenesis (Shamsuddin, 1986). The results of these studies are conflicting (Jacobs, 1986b; Kritchevsky, 1986b), possibly reflecting differences in susceptibility across animal species; in the dosages, type, and mode of administration of the carcinogen; in the amount and type of dietary fiber consumed; in the timing of the feeding (i.e., at the stage of initiation or promotion); and in the length of the study.

Several animal studies indicate a protective effect of dietary fiber on colon cancer risk. For example, addition of 15% pectin to a semipurified diet containing 20% fat inhibited AOM-induced, but not MNU-induced, colon carcinogenesis in Fischer 344 rats (Watanabe et al., 1979). The authors hypothesized that pectin interferes with the metabolic activation of AOM in the liver or colon that is necessary for carcinogenesis, but that it has no corresponding effect on the more direct-acting MNU. Addition of 15% wheat bran inhibited both AOM- and MNU-induced colon carcinogenesis. In another study, the same substitution protected against oral and subcutaneous DMH-induced colon cancer (Barbolt and Abraham, 1978). Wheat bran fed with dehydrated citrus fiber at the 15% level with 5% fat also yielded a lower incidence and multiplicity of colon tumors in AOM-challenged Fischer 344 rats (Reddy et al., 1981), whereas wheat bran alone exhibited the same effect in DMAB-challenged animals (Reddy and Mori, 1981). Nigro et al. (1979) reported that diets consisting of 35% beef fat plus 10% wheat bran, alfalfa, or cellulose did not inhibit AOM-induced colon carcinogenesis, whereas diets with 5% fat and 20% or 30% wheat bran or cellulose did. This finding suggests that the promoting effect of fat on colon carcinogenesis can outweigh the protective effect of dietary fiber.

Other animal studies indicate either an enhancing effect or no effect of dietary fiber on colon carcinogenesis (Jacobs, 1987). For example, 20% wheat bran added to the diet of rats did not protect them against DMH-induced colon carcinogenesis in three separate studies (Bauer et al., 1979; Cruse et al., 1978; Jacobs, 1983), nor did the addition of cellulose and guar gum (Bauer et al., 1981; Jacobs and Lupton, 1986).

These findings suggest that type of fiber is important in modulating the effects of a colon carcinogen and that wheat bran has the most consistent inhibiting effect.

Mechanisms of Action

Several plausible biologic mechanisms may explain a protective effect of dietary fiber against colorectal cancer (Jacobs, 1986a,b). Fiber could act as a diluent, increasing fecal bulk and thus reducing exposure to a carcinogen (MacLennan et al., 1978) or may reduce such exposure by decreasing transit time in the gastrointestinal tract (Stephen and Cummings, 1980a). In general, high intakes of insoluble fibers (e.g., cereal fibers) tend to increase fecal bulk (Eastwood and Brydon, 1985) and weight and to decrease transit time (Cummings, 1986), whereas water-soluble fibers such as pectin have variable or little effect (LSRO, 1987). Comparisons between rural Finnish and New York populations suggest that the increased bulk resulting from the intake of certain dietary fibers serves to dilute bile acids, which are believed to promote colon carcinogenesis (Reddy et al., 1978). In addition, certain dietary fibers may decrease the excretion of fecal secondary bile acids, thereby reducing colonic exposure to these substances (Reddy 1986).

As noted earlier in this chapter, dietary fiber can also influence intestinal cell morphology and cell proliferation, which may modify the effects of colon carcinogens. For example, animal studies indicate that diets with 15% fiber produce ultrastructural cell surface changes in the small intestine and colon that may modify risk; the strongest effects are produced by alfalfa, pectin, cellulose, and bran (Cassidy et al., 1981). Paradoxically, diets supplemented with wheat bran or cellulose can increase the growth of epithelial cells in the large bowel of the rat—a phenomenon believed to enhance carcinogenesis (Jacobs, 1984). The process may be mediated by fermentation of fiber in the large bowel, which has been reported to produce short-chain fatty acids capable of stimulating intestinal cell proliferation (Jacobs, 1986b).

Other Cancers

Epidemiologic Studies

The role of dietary fiber in other cancers has not been studied extensively. Two case-control studies suggest that a decreased risk of stomach cancer is associated with high fiber intake. In one of these, conducted in Israel, Modan et al. (1974) did not calculate a specific fiber index but, rather, showed that controls consumed fiber-rich foods more frequently than did the cases. In Canada, Risch et al. (1985) calculated a fiber index that showed a strong protective effect of dietary fiber and "fibrous foods," including vegetables, fruits, soybeans, seeds, and nuts.

Two case-control studies suggest an inverse association between dietary fiber and breast cancer. Adlercreutz et al. (1982) reported that excretion of enterolactone and enterodiol—urinary lignans that correlate with fiber intake and are produced by intestinal microflora acting on precursors in fiber-rich foods—was lower in women with breast cancer than in normal controls. Lubin et al. (1986) found that diets highest in animal fats and protein and low in fiber were associated with increased risk of breast cancer and that the risk was higher in women under the age of 50. Information on intake of specific fiber subfractions was not reported in either study.

Intake of high-fiber foods has also been studied in relation to ovarian cancer (Byers et al., 1983) and endometrial cancer (La Vecchia et al., 1986). Both studies found that consumption of fiber-rich foods provided a protective effect, but that the effect did not persist when other factors were considered.

Animal Studies

The committee found no data on dietary fiber in relation to other cancers.

Diabetes

Epidemiologic Studies

Although the evidence generally suggests that the risk of diabetes mellitus is inversely associated with diets high in fiber-containing foods, the nature of the association has not been established as causal. For example, comparisons of diabetes prevalence in 11 countries and 2 locations in the United States demonstrated an inverse association with total carbohydrate intake (West and Kalbfleisch, 1971). This finding was confirmed in two subsequent studies (West, 1974a,b). A time-trend analysis of diabetes death rates in England and Wales from 1920 to 1970 showed an inverse association with intake of grains and high-fiber flour. Similarly, groups consuming high-fiber diets in Africa were found to have a lower prevalence of diabetes than groups consuming diets with lower levels of fiber (Trowell, 1960; Walker, 1961; Walker et al., 1970). The epidemiologic evidence is not entirely consistent, however. In a comparison of two populations in Micronesia (King et al.,

1984), one at high risk and the other at low risk of noninsulin-dependent diabetes, estimates of dietary fiber intake were of no predictive value in estimating risk of subsequent diabetes. The wide differences in diet, environment, genetic factors, and socioeconomic level among the various groups studied may explain the difference.

Clinical and Metabolic Studies

Although clinical and metabolic studies indicate that some fiber supplements can control glycemic response in diabetics, the relevance of these studies to the prevention of diabetes is unknown. In general, these studies indicate that water-soluble fibers such as guar and pectin are most effective in reducing the postprandial rise in serum glucose after mixed meals or glucose load than are water-insoluble fibers such as wheat, corn bran, soy hulls, and cellulose (Jenkins et al., 1976, 1978b, 1979a; LSRO, 1987; Monnier et al., 1978; Morgan et al., 1979; Poynard et al., 1980). Water-soluble fibers also appear to be more effective in reducing serum insulin response in diabetics (Jenkins et al., 1976, 1978a).

In some studies, diets emphasizing fiber-rich foods (rather than fiber supplements) have also appeared to be effective in reducing fasting serum glucose levels, insulin requirements, and urinary excretion of glucose in insulin-dependent diabetics (Kinmonth et al., 1982; H.C.R. Simpson et al., 1981) and noninsulin-dependent diabetics (Barnard et al., 1983; Karlström et al., 1984; H.C.R. Simpson et al., 1981). Other studies have shown no effect (McCulloch et al., 1985; Pacy et al., 1986). However, the beneficial effect of high-fiber diets noted in most studies cannot be attributed solely to their increased fiber content, since they also differ from average diets in other important respects, such as the content of total calories, fats, and cholesterol, which are usually higher, and in the carbohydrate content, which is usually lower.

Animal Studies

Dietary fiber has been studied in several different animal models of diabetes. Berglund et al. (1982) used two strains of mice with a genetic susceptibility to diabetes to study effects of diets prepared from skim milk and breads made from either whole-rye flour or refined-rye flour. The dietary fiber content of these diets was 13.9 and 4.4 g/100 g, respectively. The non-inbred C57BL/KsJ=ob/ob mice, which develop a moderate hyperglycemia with compensatory β-cell hyperplasia, became more hyperglycemic on the low-fiber diet than on the high-fiber diet, but no effect on serum insulin was observed. C57BL/KsJ=db/db mice, which develop severe diabetes resembling the disease in humans, became obese on the high-fiber diet but began to lose weight at 20 to 25 weeks of age and died at a median age of 28 weeks. The mice on the low-fiber diet had more severe hyperglycemia and less pronounced hyperinsulinemia than did those on the high-fiber diet.

In a study of rats made diabetic by treatment with streptozotocin, Yamashita et al. (1980) found that the addition of 5% fiber reduced fasting blood sugar and triglyceride levels and decreased plasma glucagon levels relative to controls. In another study, Yamashita and Yamashita (1980) found that the addition of 10% dietary fiber lowered fasting blood sugar and increased the level of HDL cholesterol in the same rat model. Madar (1983) also used this rat model to show that dietary soybean fiber was more effective than brown rice in reducing plasma glucose, triglyceride, and glucagon levels. He noted that soybean fiber contains pectins, galactomannans, and arabinogalactans, which are highly viscous, whereas rice fiber consists mainly of cellulose and hemicellulose, which have low viscosity.

These studies provide evidence that dietary fiber can help to delay the development of diabetes in diabetes-prone animals. This finding is consistent with the weaker epidemiologic evidence suggesting a positive association between diabetes prevalence and diets high in fiber-depleted starch.

Diverticulosis

Epidemiologic Studies

Diverticulosis of the colon is an acquired pathological defect characterized by small, saccular herniations of the mucosa through the muscular wall of the colon, most often the sigmoid colon. This defect is common in Western industrialized nations and is estimated to occur in 30 to 40% of people aged 50 and over in the United States (Berkow, 1982). The true prevalence of diverticulosis is unknown, since the great majority of cases are asymptomatic.

Ohi et al. (1983) compared fiber intake in the United States and Japan with subsequent prevalence rates of diverticulosis in the populations of these countries. Although these factors correlate well, many other factors, both dietary and nondietary, changed in these countries during the relevant time periods. Segal and coworkers diagnosed several cases of diverticulosis in black South African residents of Johannesburg, normally a low-risk

population, who had been consuming diets with high levels of refined carbohydrates and low levels of fiber. Dietary fiber intakes were lower in these cases than in matched controls (Segal and Walker, 1982; Segal et al, 1977).

Clinical Studies

As with diabetes, most clinical studies on diet and diverticular disease focus on treatment of existing cases. Several studies demonstrated a beneficial effect of fiber-rich diets in treating uncomplicated diverticular disease (Plumley and Francis, 1973; Tarpila et al., 1978), but others did not (Devroede et al., 1977; Ornstein et al., 1981). Several investigators suggested that the inconsistent study findings may reflect, in part, differences among individuals in response to supplemental fiber (LSRO, 1987; Painter, 1985).

OTHER CHRONIC DISEASES

Hypertension

Epidemiologic studies have demonstrated lower mean blood pressures in vegetarians and other groups consuming diets high in fiber than in nonvegetarians and other groups consuming diets lower in fiber (Armstrong et al., 1977; Rouse et al., 1982; Sacks et al., 1974; Trowell, 1981). Similarly, clinical studies indicate a fairly consistent blood pressure-lowering effect of diets with high levels of fiber from various sources in normal as well as hypertensive subjects (Anderson, 1986; Dodson et al., 1984; Lindahl et al., 1984). However, the diets observed in the majority of studies also differ in other respects that could influence blood pressure (e.g., lower in total calories, fats, and animal protein, and atypical in sodium, potassium, chloride, and calcium content). Thus, no firm conclusions can be drawn about the effect of high levels of dietary fiber on blood pressure. No animal data are available.

Gallstones

Epidemiologic evidence linking dietary fiber to risk of gallstones is indirect. For example, Kameda et al. (1984) contrasted the nearly fivefold increase in gallstone incidence observed in Japan from 1950 to 1975 to the increased intakes of total energy (4%), animal protein (129%), and fats (190%) and decreased intake of carbohydrates (32%) observed during the same period. They suggested that the increase in gallstone incidence was attributable to the increased fat intake and decreased fiber intake. Burkitt (1976) similarly attributed the low rates of gallstones in sub-Saharan Africa to the high-fiber diets prevalent in his study populations. Scragg et al. (1984) in a case-control analysis, noted that fiber was protective against gallstones when they controlled for sugar intake.

Clinical studies in healthy people and in subjects with gallstones indicated that supplemental wheat bran (30 to 50 g/day) can lower both the saturation index (Weschler et al., 1984) and the deoxycholic acid content of bile (McDougall et al., 1978; Watts et al., 1978). Normal subjects fed pectin (12 g/day), cellulose (15 g/day), or lignin (12 g/day) for 4 weeks experienced an 11% drop in their lithogenic index on the pectin diet but not on the other diets. The ratio of primary to secondary bile acids fell on the pectin diet, rose on the cellulose diet, and did not change demonstrably on the lignin diet (Hillman et al., 1986).

The addition of pectin, cellulose, or lignin to semipurified diets known to be lithogenic to hamsters inhibited gallstone formation and reduced the lithogenic index (Rotstein et al., 1981). Pectin, but not cellulose, can also promote regression of gallstones (Kritchevsky et al., 1984).

POTENTIAL UNDESIRABLE EFFECTS OF DIETARY FIBER

Effects on Mineral Bioavailability

Some concern has been expressed that high-fiber diets may lead to decreased absorption of minerals due to binding by fiber. However, vegetarians consuming high-fiber diets have normal levels of hemoglobin and serum transferrin, as well as normal zinc levels in serum, hair, and urine (Anderson et al., 1981; King et al., 1981), copper levels in serum, and copper and selenium levels in urine (Gibson et al., 1983; Shultz and Leklem, 1983). Similarly, levels of iron, calcium, and magnesium in serum and total iron-binding capacity are reported to be no different in diabetics fed a high-fiber diet than in diabetics consuming an average diet (Anderson et al., 1980).

There have been several studies of the effect of supplemental fiber on mineral bioavailability. People who took two tablespoons of bran daily for 6 months had normal total iron-binding capacity and normal serum levels of iron, magnesium, calcium, phosphorus, and zinc (Rattan et al., 1981). Vaaler et al. (1985) placed insulin-dependent diabetics on ordinary diets including low-fiber

bread (15 to 20 g of fiber per day) for 3 months, then gave them supplemental guar gum (29 g/day) for 3 months, and then bran (33 g/day) in the place of guar for another 3 months. These subjects had normal serum concentrations of iron, zinc, selenium, magnesium, calcium, and inorganic phosphate at the end of each 3-month period. Urinary calcium concentrations were somewhat lower after treatment with wheat bran, but urinary concentrations of zinc, magnesium, and inorganic phosphates did not change throughout the study. Addition of whole-wheat bread to meals, however, decreases absorption of nonheme iron in normal subjects (K.M. Simpson et al., 1981). This effect appears to be countered by the addition of protein to the whole-wheat bread (Sandström et al., 1980). When bran, pectin, or cellulose was added to whole-wheat muffins, only bran significantly lowered iron absorption (Cook et al., 1983). Godara et al. (1981) fed female adolescents on low-fiber diets 21 g of cellulose daily for 3 weeks. At the end of this period, fecal excretion of calcium, phosphorus, and iron had increased. Stasse-Wolthuis et al. (1980) compared fecal excretions of calcium and magnesium among four groups fed one of four diets: a low-fiber diet (18 g of fiber per day), a diet containing fruits and vegetables (43 g of fiber per day), a diet containing citrus pectin (28 g of fiber per day), and a diet containing wheat bran (37 g of fiber per day). Subjects fed the wheat bran had an increased fecal excretion of magnesium, but no other differences were noted.

Walker (1985) reviewed mineral deficiencies in populations consuming high-fiber diets in developing countries. He concluded that there is little evidence that high-fiber diets alone induce a mineral deficiency in people who otherwise consume a balanced diet.

OTHER POTENTIAL EFFECTS

Sudden shifts from low-fiber to high-fiber diets, particularly those with increased intakes of wheat bran and guar gum, can produce undesirable gastrointestinal symptoms, including bloating, nausea, increased flatulence, eructation, and vomiting as well as steatorrhea in patients with pancreatic insufficiency (Dutta and Hlasko, 1985; LSRO, 1987); however, these effects seem to be temporary. Studies to investigate the influence of high levels of dietary fiber on the bioavailability of water-soluble and fat-soluble vitamins show no effect, although concern about a possible fiber-associated decrease in the bioavailability of fat-soluble vitamins was originally expressed when dietary fiber was found to affect serum lipid levels (Kasper, 1986; Kelsey, 1982).

Diets containing high levels of unleavened whole-wheat bread have been associated with increased risk of rickets in some populations (Reinhold, 1976), suggesting a deleterious effect on vitamin D metabolism. Infants given wheat bran to treat constipation developed clinical features (e.g., low serum levels of calcium and elevated serum levels of akaline phosphatase) indicative of vitamin D-dependent rickets (Zoppi et al., 1982).

SUMMARY

In general, the evidence for a protective role of dietary fiber per se in CHD, colon and rectal cancers, stomach cancer, female gynecologic cancers, diabetes, diverticulosis, hypertension, and gallstones is inconclusive. Even where the evidence is strongest, it has not been possible to adequately separate the effects of fiber from those of other components of the diet (e.g., total calories, fats, vitamins, minerals, and nonnutritive constituents of fruits and vegetables) and nondietary factors (e.g., socioeconomic status). It is possible that the ranges of fiber intake in most populations studied to date are too small to demonstrate a clear effect. The general lack of data on dietary levels of specific fiber fractions may also have contributed to the inconsistency in study findings.

Total Dietary Fiber

Metabolic and epidemiologic studies indicate that the excretion of fecal mutagens is more prevalent and the concentration of fecal secondary bile acids higher in populations at high risk of colon cancer than in those at low risk. Such studies suggest that dietary fiber, particularly from whole-grain cereals and bread, may be effective in inhibiting production and excretion of fecal mutagens and in decreasing the concentration of fecal secondary bile acids. Clinical studies indicate that dietary fiber can decrease colonic exposure to carcinogens by increasing fecal bulk.

Case-control studies of colon cancer have provided inconsistent findings of a protective effect of dietary fiber per se, but reasonably consistent findings of a protective effect of fiber-rich foods. Such foods may be protective because of factors other than fiber per se—e.g., carotenoids (discussed in Chapter 11) or inducers of microsomal monoxygenase activity, which have been shown to protect against chemical carcinogens. Two studies suggest a protective effect of fiber on gastric cancer. The ability of dietary fiber to reduce risk of other cancers, such as those of the breast, endometrium, and ovaries, has not been adequately documented.

Evidence from epidemiologic and clinical studies suggests that populations consuming high levels of dietary fiber (e.g., vegetarians) have lower blood pressures as well as reduced levels of serum total cholesterol and LDL cholesterol. Clinical studies have shown that high fiber intake decreases insulin requirements and improves glycemic response in diabetics, but the implication of this finding for reduction of diabetes risk is unknown. Descriptive epidemiologic and clinical evidence suggests that high-fiber diets may reduce the risk of diverticulosis. The evidence on dietary fiber and risk of gallstones is inconclusive.

Specific Dietary Fibers

Clinical studies of hyperlipidemics demonstrate that water-soluble fibers, including pectin, guar gum, and oat gum, can markedly reduce serum total cholesterol and LDL cholesterol without affecting serum HDL cholesterol. Water-insoluble fibers have little or no effect in this regard. Animal studies are consistent with these clinical findings. Soluble fiber supplements improve glycemic control and decrease insulin requirements in diabetics, but their potential to prevent diabetes is unknown.

In clinical studies, water-insoluble fibers, including wheat bran and cellulose, have been effective in providing stool bulk and decreasing intestinal transit time. There is no direct evidence from studies in humans to indicate whether or not these fibers affect colon carcinogenesis. However, animal studies suggest that wheat bran in particular is an effective inhibitor of experimentally induced carcinogenesis. Clinical studies show that water-insoluble fibers may relieve symptoms of uncomplicated diverticulosis, but their effect on reducing diverticulosis risk is unknown.

Potential Adverse Effects

There is little evidence that high fiber intake impedes mineral absorption and bioavailability. Although some clinical studies suggest that fiber decreases absorption of iron and zinc, the differences seem too small to pose a major health hazard. The evidence for calcium is further reviewed in Chapter 23.

Therefore, until more detailed information on intake of fiber in general and specific fiber types in particular is available, evidence for a protective role of high fiber intake per se for cancer, CHD, or other diseases must be regarded as inconclusive. However, epidemiologic studies are consistent in showing that a diet with large amounts of fiber-containing foods, including vegetables, and relatively low levels of meat and fat products is beneficial with respect to cancer of the colon and possibly atherogenesis. It is not known whether this is due to the high fiber content of such diets or to the presence or absence of some other dietary factor. Therefore, although it is reasonable to recommend a diet containing high levels of fiber-rich foods, there is little evidence to support direct supplementation of the diet with fiber products.

DIRECTIONS FOR RESEARCH

The committee recommends that the following types of research be undertaken:

• More definitive analytical epidemiologic studies that are designed carefully to include adequate variation of dietary fiber intake in the study population; improved methods for assessing dietary intake in general; improved quality and quantity of data about specific fractions of fiber consumed by the study population; adequate sample size; and collaboration among investigators to adopt a common protocol and method of dietary assessment so that any inconsistencies in results can be related to differences in populations.

• Intervention studies in human populations that could serve to clarify the role of specific fiber components vis-à-vis that of dietary fiber per se.

• Further animal and clinical metabolic studies to define the mechanisms by which dietary fibers protect against chronic diseases. Such definition would serve to identify the appropriate variables on which epidemiologic studies could focus, e.g., the specific fraction of fiber under investigation or the possibility of interaction between fiber subfractions and other food components.

• Studies to examine the long-term effects of increasing the percentage of complex carbohydrates (starches and fibers) in the diet on the risk of and biochemical markers for several diseases, especially stomach and pancreatic cancers, noninsulin-dependent diabetes mellitus, and atherosclerotic cardiovascular diseases. Studies in the elderly should be given a high priority, because the elderly may be prone to more severe adverse effects (e.g., calcium malabsorption).

• Studies to clarify the metabolic role of fiber in colon cancer etiology. As this role becomes known, the new knowledge should be applied in studies of other cancers, CHD, and diabetes.

REFERENCES

Adlercreutz, H., T. Fotsis, R. Heikkinen, J.T. Dwyer, M. Woods, B.R. Goldin, and S.L. Gorbach. 1982. Excretion of the lignans enterolactone and enterodial and of equol in omnivorous and vegetarian postmenopausal women and in women with breast cancer. Lancet 2:1295–1299.

Anderson, B.M., R.S. Gibson, and J.H. Sabry. 1981. The iron and zinc status of long-term vegetarian women. Am. J. Clin. Nutr. 34:1042–1048.

Anderson, J.W. 1986. High-fiber, hypocaloric vs. very-low-calorie diet effects on blood pressure of obese men. Am. J. Clin. Nutr. 43:695.

Anderson, J.W., S.K. Ferguson, D. Karounos, L. O'Malley, B. Sieling, and W.J.L. Chen. 1980. Mineral and vitamin status on high-fiber diets: long-term studies of diabetic patients. Diabetes Care 3:38–40.

Anderson, J.W., L. Story, B. Sieling, W.J.L. Chen, M.S. Petro, and J. Story. 1984. Hypocholesterolemic effects of oat-bran or bean intake for hypercholesterolemic men. Am. J. Clin. Nutr. 40:1146–1155.

Armstrong, B., and R. Doll. 1975. Environmental factors and cancer incidence and mortality in different countries, with special reference to dietary practices. Int. J. Cancer 15:617–631.

Armstrong, B., A.J. Van Merwyk, and H. Coates. 1977. Blood pressure in Seventh-Day Adventist vegetarians. Am. J. Epidemiol. 105:444–449.

Asp, N.G., and C.G. Johansson. 1984. Dietary fibre analysis. Nutr. Abstr. Rev. Clin. Nutr. 54:735–752.

Baird, I.M., R.L. Walters, P.S. Davies, M.J. Hill, B.S. Drasar, and D.A.T. Southgate. 1977. The effects of two dietary fiber supplements on gastrointestinal transit, stool weight and frequency, and bacterial flora, and fecal bile acids in normal subjects. Metab. Clin. Exp. 26:117–128.

Barbolt, T.A., and R. Abraham. 1978. The effect of bran on dimethylhydrazine-induced colon carcinogenesis in the rat. Proc. Soc. Exp. Biol. Med. 157:656–659.

Barnard, R.J., M.R. Massey, S. Cherny, L.T. O'Brien, and N. Pritikin. 1983. Long-term use of a high-complex-carbohydrate, high-fiber, low-fat diet and exercise in the treatment of NIDDM patients. Diabetes Care 6:268–273.

Bauer, H.G., N.G. Asp, R. Öste, A. Dahlqvist, and P.E. Fredlund. 1979. Effect of dietary fiber on the induction of colorectal tumors and fecal β-glucuronidase activity in the rat. Cancer Res. 39:3752–3756.

Bauer, H.G., N.G. Asp, A. Dahlqvist, P.E. Fredlund, M. Nyman, and R. Öste. 1981. Effect of two kinds of pectin and guar gum on 1,2-dimethylhydrazine initiation of colon tumors and on fecal β-glucuronidase activity in the rat. Cancer Res. 41:2518–2523.

Berglund, O., G. Hallmans, C. Nygren, and I.B. Täljedal. 1982. Effects of diets rich and poor in fibres on the development of hereditary diabetes in mice. Acta Endocrinol. 100:556–564.

Berkow, R., ed. 1982. P. 794 in The Merck Manual of Diagnosis and Therapy, 14th ed. Merck, Sharpe & Dohme Research Laboratories, Rahway, N.J.

Beynen, A.C., K.F. Buechler, A.J. Van der Molen, and M.J.H. Geelan. 1982. The effects of lactate and acetate on fatty acid and cholesterol biosynthesis by isolated rat hepatocytes. Int. J. Biochem. 14:165–169.

Bingham S., and J.H. Cummings. 1980. Sources and intakes of dietary fiber in man. Pp. 261–284 in G.A. Spiller and R.M. Kay, eds. Medical Aspects of Dietary Fiber. Plenum Medical Book Co., New York.

Bingham, S., D.R.R. Williams, T.J. Cole, and W.P.T. James. 1979. Dietary fibre and regional large-bowel cancer mortality in Britain. Br. J. Cancer 40:456–463.

Bingham, S.A., D.R.R. Williams, and J.H. Cummings. 1985. Dietary fiber consumption in Britain: new estimates and their relation to large bowel cancer mortality. Br. J. Cancer 52:399–402.

Bjelke, E. 1978. Dietary factors and the epidemiology of cancer of the stomach and large bowel. Aktuel. Ernaehrungsmed. Klin. Prax. Suppl. 2:10–17.

Bolton, R.P., K.W. Heaton, and L.F. Burroughs. 1981. The role of dietary fiber in satiety, glucose, and insulin: studies with fruit and fruit juice. Am. J. Clin. Nutr. 34:211–217.

Burkitt, D.P. 1976. Economic development—not all bonus. Nutr. Today 11:6–13.

Burkitt, D.P., and H.C. Trowell. 1975. Refined Carbohydrate Foods and Disease: Some Implications of Dietary Fibre. Academic Press, London. 356 pp.

Burr, M.L. 1982. Vegetarianism, dietary fiber, and mortality. Am. J. Clin. Nutr. 36:873–877.

Burslem, J., G. Schonfeld, M.A. Howald, S.W. Weidman, and J.P. Miller. 1978. Plasma apoprotein and lipoprotein lipid levels in vegetarians. Metabolism 27:711–719.

Byers, T., J. Marshall, S. Graham, C. Mettlin, and M. Swanson. 1983. A case-control study of dietary and nondietary factors in ovarian cancer. J. Natl. Cancer Inst. 71:681–686.

Cassidy, M.M., F.G. Lightfoot, L.E. Grau, J.A. Story, D. Kritchevsky, and G.V. Vahouny. 1981. Effect of chronic intake of dietary fibers on the ultrastructural topography of rat jejunum and colon: a scanning electron microscopy study. Am. J. Clin. Nutr. 34:218–228.

Cassidy, M.M., L.R. Fitzpatrick, and G.V. Vahouny. 1986. The effect of fiber in the post weaning diet on nutritional and intestinal morphological indices in the rat. Pp. 229–251 in G.V. Vahouny and D. Kritchevsky, eds. Dietary Fiber: Basic and Clinical Aspects. Plenum Press, New York.

Challen, A.D., W.J. Branch, and J.H. Cummings. 1983. The effect of pectin and wheat bran on platelet function and haemostasis in man. Hum. Nutr. Clin. Nutr. 37:209–217.

Chen, W.J.L., and J.W. Anderson. 1986. Hypocholesterolemic effects of soluble fibers. Pp. 275–286 in G.V. Vahouny and D. Kritchevsky, eds. Dietary Fiber: Basic and Clinical Aspects. Plenum Press, New York.

Cook, J.D., N.L. Noble, T.A. Morck, S.R. Lynch, and S.J. Petersburg. 1983. Effect of fiber on nonheme iron absorption. Gastroenterology 85:1354–1358.

Cruse, J.P., M.R. Lewin, and C.G. Clark. 1978. Failure of bran to protect against experimental colon cancer in rats. Lancet 2:1278–1280.

Cummings, J.H. 1986. The effect of dietary fiber on fecal weight and composition. Pp. 211–280 in G.A. Spiller, ed. CRC Handbook of Dietary Fiber in Human Nutrition. CRC Press, Boca Raton, Fla.

Dales, L.G., G.D. Friedman, H.K. Ury, S. Grossman, and S.R. Williams. 1979. A case-control study of relationships of diet and other traits to colorectal cancer in American blacks. Am. J. Epidemiol. 109:132–144.

Devroede, G., J.S. Vobecky, J.M. Vobecky, R. Beaudry, H. Haddad, H. Navert, B. Perey, and J. Poisson. 1977. Medical management of diverticular disease: a random trial. Gastroenterology 72:1157.

Dintzis, F.R. 1982. Dietary fiber analysis—concepts and problems. Pp. 312–332 in D.R. Lineback and G.E. Inglett, eds. Food Carbohydrates: IFT Basic Symposium Series. Avi Publishing Co., Westport, Conn.

Dodson, P.M., P.J. Pacy, P. Bal, A.J. Kubicki, R.F. Fletcher, and K.G. Taylor. 1984. A controlled trial of a high fibre, low fat and low sodium diet for mild hypertension in type 2 (non-insulin-dependent) diabetic patients. Diabetologia 27:522–526.

Drasar, B.S., and D. Irving. 1973. Environmental factors and cancer of the colon and breast. Br. J. Cancer 27:167–172.

Drasar, B.S., D.J.A. Jenkins, and J.H. Cummings. 1976. The influence of a diet rich in wheat fibre on the human faecal flora. J. Med. Microbiol. 9:423–431.

Duncan, K.H., J.A. Bacon, and R.L. Weinsier. 1983. The effects of high and low energy density diets on satiety, energy intake, and eating time of obese and nonobese subjects. Am. J. Clin. Nutr. 37:763–767.

Dutta, S.K., and J. Hlasko. 1985. Dietary fiber in pancreatic disease: effect of high fiber diet on fat malabsorption in pancreatic insufficiency and in vitro study of the interaction of dietary fiber with pancreatic enzymes. Am. J. Clin. Nutr. 41:517–525.

Eastwood, M., and W.G. Brydon. 1985. Physiological effects of dietary fibre on the alimentary tract. Pp. 105–131 in H. Trowell, D. Burkitt, and K. Heaton, eds. Dietary Fibre, Fibre-Depleted Foods and Disease. Academic Press, New York.

Englyst, H., H.S. Wiggins, and J.H. Cummings. 1982. Determination of the non-starch polysaccharides in plant foods by gas-liquid chromatography of constituent sugars as alditol acetates. Analyst 107:307–318.

Finegold, S.M., and V.L. Sutter. 1978. Fecal flora in different populations, with specific reference to diet. Am. J. Clin. Nutr. 31:S116–S122.

Fisher, H., W.G. Siller, and P. Griminger. 1966. The retardation by pectin of cholesterol-induced atherosclerosis in the fowl. J. Atheroscler. Res. 6:292–298.

Gibson, R.S., B.M. Anderson, and J.H. Sabry. 1983. The trace metal status of a group of post-menopausal vegetarians. J. Am. Diet. Assoc. 82:246–250.

Godara, R., A.P. Kaur, and C.M. Bhat. 1981. Effect of cellulose incorporation in a low fiber diet on fecal excretion and serum levels of calcium, phosphorus, and iron in adolescent girls. Am. J. Clin. Nutr. 34:1083–1086.

Graham, S., H. Dayal, M. Swanson, A. Mittelman, and G. Wilkinson. 1978. Diet in the epidemiology of cancer of the colon and rectum. J. Natl. Cancer Inst. 61:709–714.

Grande, F., J.T. Anderson, and A. Keys. 1965. Effect of carbohydrates of leguminous seeds, wheat and potatoes on serum cholesterol concentration in man. J. Nutr. 86:313–317.

Grande, F., J.T. Anderson, and A. Keys. 1974. Sucrose and various carbohydrate-containing foods and serum lipids in man. Am. J. Clin. Nutr. 27:1043–1051.

Hamilton, R.M.G., and K.K. Carroll. 1976. Plasma cholesterol levels in rabbits fed low fat, low cholesterol diets. Effects of dietary proteins, carbohydrates and fibre from different sources. Atherosclerosis 24:47–62.

Hardinge, M.G., and F.J. Stare. 1954. Nutritional studies of vegetarians. 2. Dietary and serum levels of cholesterol. Am. J. Clin. Nutr. 2:83–88.

Hardinge, M.G., A.C. Chambers, H. Crooks, and F.J. Stare. 1958. Nutritional studies in vegetarians. III. Dietary levels of fiber. Am. J. Clin. Nutr. 6:523–525.

Health and Welfare Canada. 1985. Report of the Expert Advisory Committee on Dietary Fibre. Health Protection Branch, Health and Welfare Canada, Ottawa, Canada. 58 pp.

Heaton, K.W. 1980. Food intake regulation and fiber. Pp. 223–238 in G.A. Spiller and R.M. Kay, eds. Medical Aspects of Dietary Fiber. Plenum Medical Book Co., New York.

Hillman, L.C., S.G. Peters, C.A. Fisher, and E.W. Pomare. 1986. Effects of the fibre components pectin, cellulose, and lignin on bile salt metabolism and biliary lipid composition in man. Gut 27:29–36.

Holt, S., R.C. Heading, D.C. Carter, L.F. Prescott, and P. Tothill. 1979. Effect of gel fibre on gastric emptying and absorption of glucose and paracetamol. Lancet 1:636–639.

Howe, G.R., A.B. Miller, and M. Jain. 1986. Re: "Total energy intake: implications for epidemiologic analyses." Am. J. Epidemiol. 124:157–159.

Hudson, G.J., and B.S. Bailey. 1980. Mutual interference effects in the calorimetric methods used to determine the sugar composition of dietary fibre. Food Chem. 5:201–206.

Irving, D., and B.S. Drasar. 1973. Fibre and cancer of the colon. Br. J. Cancer 28:462–463.

Jacobs, L.R. 1983. Enhancement of rat colon carcinogenesis by wheat bran consumption during the stage of 1,2-dimethylhydrazine administration. Cancer Res. 43:4057–4061.

Jacobs, L.R. 1984. Stimulation of rat colonic crypt cell proliferative activity by wheat bran consumption during the stage of 1,2-dimethylhydrazine administration. Cancer Res. 44:2458–2463.

Jacobs, L.R. 1986a. Dietary fiber and gastrointestinal epithelial cell proliferation. Pp. 211–228 in G.V. Vahouny and D. Kritchevsky, eds. Dietary Fiber: Basic and Clinical Aspects. Plenum Press, New York.

Jacobs, L.R. 1986b. Relationship between dietary fiber and cancer: metabolic, physiologic and cellular mechanisms. Proc. Soc. Exp. Biol. Med. 183:290–311.

Jacobs, L.R. 1987. Dietary fiber and cancer. J. Nutr. 117: 1319–1321.

Jacobs, L.R., and J.R. Lupton. 1986. Relationship between colonic luminal pH, cell proliferation, and colon carcinogenesis in 1,2-dimethylhydrazine treated rats fed high fiber diets. Cancer Res. 46:1727–1734.

Jain, M., G.M. Cook, F.G. Davis, M.G. Grace, G.R. Howe, and A.B. Miller. 1980. A case-control study of diet and colo-rectal cancer. Int. J. Cancer 26:757–768.

Jenkins, D.J.A., D.V. Goff, A.R. Leeds, K.G.M.M. Alberti, T.M.S. Wolever, M.A. Gassull, and T.D.R. Hockaday. 1976. Unabsorbable carbohydrates and diabetes: decreased postprandial hyperglycemia. Lancet 2:172–174.

Jenkins, D.J.A., T.M.S. Wolever, A.R. Leeds, M.A. Gassull, P. Haisman, J. Dilawari, D.V. Goff, G.L. Metz, and K.G.M.M. Alberti. 1978a. Dietary fibres, fibre analogues, and glucose tolerance: importance of viscosity. Br. Med. J. 1:1392–1394.

Jenkins, D.J.A., T.M.S. Wolever, R. Nineham, R. Taylor, G.L. Metz, S. Bacon, and T.D.R. Hockaday. 1978b. Guar crispbread in the diabetic diet. Br. Med. J. 2:1744–1746.

Jenkins, D.J.A., R.H. Taylor, R. Nineham, D.V. Goff, S.R. Bloom, D. Sarson, and K.G.M.M. Alberti. 1979a. Combined use of guar and acarbose in reduction of postprandial glycaemia. Lancet 2:924–927.

Jenkins, D.J.A., D. Reynolds, A.R. Leeds, A.L. Waller, and J.H. Cummings. 1979b. Hypocholesterolemic action of dietary fiber unrelated to fecal bulking effect. Am. J. Clin. Nutr. 32:2430–2435.

Jenkins, D.J.A., C.G. Rainey-Macdonald, A.L. Jenkins, and G. Benn. 1986. Fiber in the treatment of hyperlipidemia. Pp. 327–344 in G.A. Spiller, ed. CRC Handbook of Dietary Fiber in Human Nutrition. CRC Press, Boca Raton, Fla.

Jensen, O.M., R. MacLennan, and J. Wahrendorf. 1982. Diet, bowel function, fecal characteristics, and large bowel cancer in Denmark and Finland. Nutr. Cancer 4:5–19.

Judd, P.A., and A.S. Truswell. 1985. Dietary fibre and blood lipids in man. Pp. 23–39 in A.R. Leeds and A. Avenell, eds. Dietary Fibre Perspectives: Reviews and Bibliography. John Libbey and Company Ltd., London.

Kameda, H., F. Ishihara, K. Shibata, and E. Tsukie. 1984. Clinical and nutritional study on gallstone disease in Japan. Jpn. J. Med. 23:109–113.

Karlström, B., B. Vessby, N.G. Asp, M. Boberg, I.B. Gustafsson, H. Lithell, and I. Werner. 1984. Effects of an increased content of cereal fibre in the diet of Type 2 (non-insulin-dependent) diabetic patients. Diabetologia 26: 272–277.

Kasper, H. 1986. Effects of dietary fiber on vitamin metabolism. Pp. 201–208 in G.A. Spiller, ed. CRC Handbook of Dietary Fiber in Human Nutrition. CRC Press, Boca Raton, Fla.

Kay, R.M., and S. Stitt. 1978. Food form, postprandial glycemia, and satiety. Am. J. Clin. Nutr. 31:738–739.

Kay, R.M., and A.S. Truswell. 1980. Dietary fiber: effects on plasma and biliary lipids in man. Pp. 153–173 in G.A. Spiller and R.M. Kay, eds. Medical Aspects of Dietary Fiber. Plenum Medical Book Co., New York.

Kay, R.M., Z.I. Sabry, and A. Csima. 1980. Multivariate analysis of diet and serum lipids in normal men. Am. J. Clin. Nutr. 33:2566–2572.

Kay, R. M., M. Jacobs, M.B. Katan, and B. Lewis. 1985. Relationship between changes in plasma lipoprotein concentrations and fecal steroid excretion in man during consumption of four experimental diets. Atherosclerosis 55:15–23.

Kelsey, J.L. 1982. Effects of fiber on mineral and vitamin bioavailability. Pp. 91–103 in G.V. Vahouny and D. Kritchevsky, eds. Dietary Fiber in Health and Disease. Plenum Press, New York.

Keys, A., J.T. Anderson, and F. Grande. 1960. Diet-type (fats constant) and blood lipids in man. J. Nutr. 70:257–266.

Khaw, K.T., and E. Barrett-Connor. 1987. Dietary fiber and reduced ischemic heart disease mortality rates in men and women: a 12-year prospective study. Am. J. Epidemiol. 126: 1093–1102.

King, H., P. Zimmet, K. Pargeter, L.R. Raper, and V. Collins. 1984. Ethnic differences in susceptibility to non-insulin-dependent diabetes: a comparative study of two urbanized Micronesian populations. Diabetes 33:1002–1007.

King, J.C., T. Stein, and M. Doyle. 1981. Effect of vegetarianism on the zinc status of pregnant women. Am. J. Clin. Nutr. 34:1049–1055.

Kinmonth, A.L., R.M. Angus, P.A. Jenkins, M.A. Smith, and J.D. Baum. 1982. Whole foods and increased dietary fibre improve blood glucose control in diabetic children. Arch. Dis. Child. 57:187–194.

Knox, E.G. 1977. Foods and diseases. Br. J. Prev. Soc. Med. 31:71–80.

Knuiman, J.T., and C.E. West. 1982. The concentration of cholesterol in serum and in various serum lipoproteins in macrobiotic, vegetarian and non-vegetarian men and boys. Atherosclerosis 43:71–82.

Kritchevsky, D. 1964. Experimental atherosclerosis in rabbits fed cholesterol-free diets. J. Atheroscler. Res. 4:103–105.

Kritchevsky, D. 1986a. Dietary fiber and atherosclerosis. Pp. 265–274 in G.V. Vahouny and D. Kritchevsky, eds. Dietary Fiber: Basic and Clinical Aspects. Plenum Press, New York.

Kritchevsky, D. 1986b. Fat, calories and fiber. Pp. 495–515 in C. Ip, D.F. Birt, A.E. Rogers, and C. Mettlin, eds. Dietary Fat and Cancer. Alan R. Liss, New York.

Kritchevsky, D., and J.A. Story. 1986. Influence of dietary fiber on cholesterol metabolism in experimental animals. Pp. 129–142 in G.A. Spiller, ed. Handbook of Dietary Fiber in Human Nutrition. CRC Press, Boca Raton, Fla.

Kritchevsky, D., and S.A. Tepper. 1965. Factors affecting atherosclerosis in rabbits fed cholesterol-free diets. Life Sci. 4:1467–1471.

Kritchevsky, D., S.A. Tepper, D.E. Williams, and J.A. Story. 1977. Experimental atherosclerosis in rabbits fed cholesterol-free diets. Part 7: Interaction of animal or vegetable protein with fiber. Atherosclerosis 26:397–403.

Kritchevsky, D., S.A. Tepper, and D.M. Klurfeld. 1984. Effect of pectin and cellulose on formation and regression of gallstones in hamsters. Experientia 40:350–351.

Kromhout, D., and C. de Lezenne Coulander. 1984. Diet, prevalence and 10-year mortality from coronary heart disease in 871 middle-aged men: the Zutphen Study. Am. J. Epidemiol. 119:733–741.

Kromhout, D., E.B. Bosschieter, and C. de Lezenne Coulander. 1982. Dietary fibre and 10-year mortality from coronary heart disease, cancer, and all causes: the Zutphen Study. Lancet 2:518–522.

Kune, S., G.A. Kune, and L.F. Watson. 1987. Case-control study of dietary etiological factors: the Melbourne Colorectal Cancer Study. Nutr. Cancer 9:21–42.

Kushi, L.H., R.A. Lew, F.J. Stare, C.R. Ellison, M. el Lozy, G. Bourke, L. Daly, I. Graham, N. Hickey, and R. Mulcahy. 1985. Diet and 20-year mortality from coronary heart disease: the Ireland–Boston Diet–Heart Study. N. Engl. J. Med. 312:811–818.

Lanza, E., and R.R. Butrum. 1986. A critical review of food fiber analysis and data. J. Am. Diet. Assoc. 86:732–743.

Lanza, E., D.Y. Jones, G. Block, and L. Kessler. 1987. Dietary fiber intake in the U.S. population. Am. J. Clin. Nutr. 46: 790–797.

La Vecchia, C., A. Decarli, M. Fasoli, and A. Gentile. 1986. Nutrition and diet in the etiology of endometrial cancer. Cancer 57:1248–1253.

Lindahl, O., L. Lindwall, A. Spangberg, A. Stenram, and P.A. Öckerman. 1984. A vegan regimen with reduced medication in the treatment of hypertension. Br. J. Nutr. 52:11–20.

Liu, K., J. Stamler, D. Moss, D. Garside, V. Persky, and I. Soltero. 1979. Dietary cholesterol, fat, and fibre, and colon-cancer mortality. Lancet 2:782–785.

Liu, K., J. Stamler, M. Trevison, and D. Moss. 1982. Dietary lipids, sugar, fiber, and mortality from coronary heart disease: bivariate analysis of international data. Arteriosclerosis 2:221–227.

LSRO (Life Sciences Research Office). 1987. Physiological Effects and Health Consequences of Dietary Fiber. Federation of American Societies for Experimental Biology, Bethesda, Md. 236 pp.

Lubin, F., Y. Wax, and B. Modan. 1986. Role of fat, animal protein, and dietary fiber in breast cancer etiology: a case-control study. J. Natl. Cancer Inst. 77:605–612.

Lyon, J.L., and A.W. Sorenson. 1978. Colon cancer in a low-risk population. Am. J. Clin. Nutr. 31:S227–S230.

Lyon, J.L., A.W. Mahoney, D.W. West, J.W. Gardner, K.R. Smith, A.W. Sorenson, and W. Stanish. 1987. Energy intake: its relationship to colon cancer risk. J. Natl. Cancer Inst. 78:853–861.

MacLennan, R., O.M. Jensen, J. Mosbech, and H. Vuori. 1978. Diet, transit time, stool weight, and colon cancer in two Scandinavian populations. Am. J. Clin. Nutr. 31: S239–S242.

Macquart-Moulin, G., E. Riboli, J. Cornée, B. Charnay, P. Berthezène, and N. Day. 1986. Case-control study on colorectal cancer and diet in Marseilles. Int. J. Cancer 38: 183–191.

Madar, Z. 1983. Effect of brown rice and soybean dietary fiber on the control of glucose and lipid metabolism in diabetic rats. Am. J. Clin. Nutr. 38:388–393.

Malhotra, S.L. 1977. Dietary factors in a study of cancer colon from cancer registry, with special reference to the role of saliva, milk and fermented milk products and vegetable fibre. Med. Hypotheses 3:122–126.

Manousos, O., N.E. Day, D. Trichopoulos, F. Gerovassilis, A. Tzonou, and A. Polychronopoulou. 1983. Diet and colorectal cancer: a case-control study in Greece. Int. J. Cancer 32:1–5.

Martinez, I., R. Torres, Z. Frias, J.R. Colon, and N. Fernandez. 1979. Factors associated with adenocarcinomas of the large bowel in Puerto Rico. Pp. 45–52 in J.M. Birch, ed. Advances in Medical Oncology, Research and Education, Vol. 3: Epidemiology. Pergamon Press, New York.

McCulloch, D.K., R.D. Mitchell, J. Ambler, and R.B. Tattersall. 1985. A prospective comparison of "conventional" and high carbohydrate/high fiber/low fat diets in adults with established type 1 (insulin-dependent) diabetes. Diabetologia 28:208–212.

McDougall, R.M., L. Yakymyshyn, K. Walker, and O.G. Thurston. 1978. Effect of wheat bran on serum lipoproteins and biliary lipids. Can. J. Surg. 21:433–435.

McKeown-Eyssen, G.E., and E. Bright-See. 1984. Dietary factors in colon cancer: international relationships. Nutr. Cancer 6:160–170.

Miller, A.B., G.R. Howe, M. Jain, K.J.P. Craib, and L. Harrison. 1983. Food items and food groups as risk factors in a case-control study of diet and colo-rectal cancer. Int. J. Cancer 32:155–161.

Modan, B., F. Lubin, V. Barell, R.A. Greenberg, M. Modan, and S. Graham. 1974. The role of starches in the etiology of gastric cancer. Cancer 34:2087–2092.

Modan, B., V. Barell, F. Lubin, M. Modan, R.A. Greenberg, and S. Graham. 1975. Low-fiber intake as an etiologic factor in cancer of the colon. J. Natl. Cancer Inst. 55:15–18.

Monnier, L., T.C. Pham, L. Aguirre, A. Orsetti, and J. Mirouze. 1978. Influence of indigestible fibers on glucose tolerance. Diabetes Care 1:83–88.

Morgan, L.M., T.J. Goulder, D. Tsiolakis, V. Marks, and K.G.M.M. Alberti. 1979. The effect of unabsorbable carbohydrate on gut hormones: modification of post-prandial GIP secretion by guar. Diabetologia 17:85–89.

Morris, J.N., J.W. Marr, and D.G. Clayton. 1977. Diet and heart: a postscript. Br. Med. J. 2:1307–1314.

Nigro, N.D., A.W. Bull, B.A. Klopfer, M.S. Pak, and R.L. Campbell. 1979. Effect of dietary fiber on azoxymethane-induced intestinal carcinogenesis in rats. J. Natl. Cancer Inst. 62:1097–1102.

NRC (National Research Council). 1982. Diet, Nutrition, and Cancer. Report of the Committee on Diet, Nutrition, and Cancer, Assembly of Life Sciences. National Academy Press, Washington, D.C. 478 pp.

Ohi, G., K. Minowa, T. Oyama, M. Nagahashi, N. Yamazaki, S.-I. Yamamoto, K. Nagasako, K. Hayakawa, K. Kimura, and B. Mori. 1983. Changes in dietary fiber intake among Japanese in the 20th century: a relationship to the prevalence of diverticular disease. Am. J. Clin. Nutr. 38:115–121.

Ornstein, M.H., E.R. Littlewood, I.M. Baird, J. Fowler, W.R.S. North, and A.G. Cox. 1981. Are fibre supplements really necessary in diverticular disease of the colon: a controlled clinical trial. Br. Med. J. 282:1353–1356.

Pacy, P.J., P.M. Dodson, and R.F. Fletcher. 1986. Effect of a high carbohydrate, low sodium and low fat diet in type 2 diabetics with moderate hypertension. Int. J. Obesity 10:43–52.

Painter, N. 1985. Diverticular disease of the colon. Pp. 145–160 in H. Trowell, D. Burkitt, and K. Heaton, eds. Dietary Fibre, Fibre-Depleted Foods and Disease. Academic Press, New York.

Paul, A.A., and D.A. Southgate. 1978. McCance and Widdowson's The Composition of Foods. Elsevier/North Holland, Amsterdam. 418 pp.

Plumley, P.F., and B. Francis. 1973. Dietary management of diverticular disease. Am. J. Diet. Assoc. 63:527–530.

Pomare, E.W., and K.W. Heaton. 1973. Alteration of bile salt metabolism by dietary fibre (bran). Br. Med. J. 4:262–264.

Pomare, E.W., K.W. Heaton, T.S. Low-Beer, and H.J. Espiner. 1976. The effect of wheat bran upon bile salt metabolism and upon the lipid composition of bile in gallstone patients. Am. J. Dig. Dis. 21:521–536.

Potter, J.C., and A.J. McMichael. 1986. Diet and cancer of the colon and rectum: a case-control study. J. Natl. Cancer Inst. 76:557–569.

Poynard, T., G. Slama, A. Delage, and G. Tchobroutsky. 1980. Pectin efficacy in insulin-treated diabetics assessed by the artificial pancreas. Lancet 1:158.

Prosky, L., N.G. Asp, I. Furda, J.W. DeVries, T.F. Schweizer, and B.F. Harland. 1985. Determination of total dietary fiber in foods and food products: collaborative study. J. Assoc. Off. Anal. Chem. 68:677–679.

Qureshi, A.A., W.C. Burger, D.M. Peterson, and C.E. Elson. 1986. The structure of an inhibitor of cholesterol biosynthesis isolated from barley. J. Biol. Chem. 261:10544–10550.

Rattan, J., N. Levin, E. Graff, N. Weizer, and T. Gilat. 1981. A high-fiber diet does not cause mineral and nutrient deficiencies. J. Clin. Gastroenterol. 3:389–393.

Reddy, B.S. 1986. Diet and colon cancer: evidence from human and animal model studies. Pp. 47–65 in B.S. Reddy and L.A. Cohen, eds. Diet, Nutrition, and Cancer—A Critical Evaluation, Vol. 1: Macronutrients and Cancer. CRC Press, Boca Raton, Fla.

Reddy, B.S., and H. Mori. 1981. Effect of dietary wheat bran and dehydrated citrus fiber on 3,2'-dimethyl-4-aminobiphenyl-induced intestinal carcinogenesis in F344 rats. Carcinogenesis 2:21–25.

Reddy, B.S., A.R. Hedges, K. Laakso, and E.L. Wynder. 1978. Metabolic epidemiology of large bowel cancer: fecal bulk and constituents of high-risk North American and low-risk Finnish population. Cancer 42:2832–2838.

Reddy, B.S., H. Mori, and M. Nichois. 1981. Effect of dietary wheat bran and dehydrated citrus fiber on azoxymethane-induced intestinal carcinogenesis in Fischer 344 rats. J. Natl. Cancer Inst. 66:553–557.

Reinhold, J.G. 1976. Rickets in Asian immigrants. Lancet 2:1132–1133.

Risch, H.A., M. Jain, N.W. Choi, J.G. Fodor, C.J. Pfeiffer, G.R. Howe, L.W. Harrison, K.J.P. Craib, and A.B. Miller. 1985. Dietary factors and the incidence of cancer of the stomach. Am. J. Epidemiol. 122:947–959.

Rotstein, O.D., R.M. Kay, M. Wayman, and S.M. Strasberg. 1981. Prevention of cholesterol gallstones by lignin and lactulose in the hamster. Gastroenterology 81:1098–1103.

Rouse, I.L., B.K. Armstrong, and L.J. Beilin. 1982. Vegetarian diet, lifestyle and blood pressure in two religious populations. Clin. Exp. Pharmacol. Physiol. 9:327–330.

Rydning, A., A. Berstad, T. Berstad, and L. Hertzenberg. 1985. The effect of guar gum and fiber-enriched wheat bran on gastric emptying of a semisolid meal in healthy subjects. Scand. J. Gastroenterol. 20:330–334.

Sacks, F.M., B. Rosner, and E.H. Kass. 1974. Blood pressure in vegetarians. Am. J. Epidemiol. 100:390–398.

Sacks, F.M., W.P. Castelli, A. Donner, and E.H. Kass. 1975. Plasma lipids and lipoproteins in vegetarians and controls. N. Engl. J. Med. 292:1148–1151.

Sandström, B., B. Arvidsson, A. Cederblad, and E. Björn-Rasmussen. 1980. Zinc absorption from composite meals. I. The significance of wheat extraction rate, zinc, calcium, and protein content in meals based on breads. Am. J. Clin. Nutr. 33:739–745.

Schneeman, B.O., and M. Lefevre. 1986. Effects of fiber on plasma lipoprotein composition. Pp. 309–321 in G.V. Vahouny and D. Kritchevsky, eds. Dietary Fiber: Basic and Clinical Aspects. Plenum Press, New York.

Schweizer, T.F., A.R. Bekhechi, B. Koellreutter, S. Reimann, D. Pometta, and B.A. Bron. 1983. Metabolic effects of dietary fiber from dehulled soybeans in humans. Am. J. Clin. Nutr. 38:1–11.

Scragg, R.K.R., A.J. McMichael, and P.A. Baghurst. 1984. Diet, alcohol, and relative weight in gall stone disease: a case-control study. Br. Med. J. 288:1113–1119.

Segal, I., A. Solomon, and J.A. Hunt. 1977. Emergence of diverticular disease in the urban South African black. Gastroenterology 72:215–219.

Segal, I., and A.R.P. Walker. 1982. Diverticular disease in urban Africans in South Africa. Digestion 24:42–46.

Selvendran, R.R. 1984. The plant cell wall as a source of dietary fiber: chemistry and structure. Am. J. Clin. Nutr. 39:320–337.

Selvendran, R.R., and M.S. Du Pont. 1980. Simplified methods for the preparation and analysis of dietary fibre. J. Sci. Food Agric. 31:1173–1182.

Selvendran, R.R., and M.S. Du Pont. 1984. The analysis of dietary fiber. Pp. 1–68 in R.D. King, ed. Food Analysis Techniques, Vol. 3. Applied Science, London.

Shamsuddin, A.K.M. 1986. Carcinoma of the large intestine:

animal models and human disease. Hum. Pathol. 17:451–453.

Shultz, T.D., and J.E. Leklem. 1983. Selenium status of vegetarians, nonvegetarians, and hormone-dependent cancer subjects. Am. J. Clin. Nutr. 37:114–118.

Simpson, H.C.R., R.W. Simpson, S. Lousley, R.D. Carter, M. Geekie, T.D.R. Hockaday, and J.I. Mann. 1981. A high carbohydrate leguminous fibre diet improves all aspects of diabetic control. Lancet 1:1–5.

Simpson, K.M., E.R. Morris, and J.D. Cook. 1981. The inhibitory effect of bran on iron absorption in man. Am. J. Clin. Nutr. 34:1469–1478.

Smith, A.H., N.E. Pearce, and J.G. Joseph. 1985. Major colorectal aetiological hypotheses do not explain mortality trends among Maori and non-Maori New Zealanders. Int. J. Epidemiol. 14:79–85.

Southgate, D.A.T., G.J. Hudson, and H. Englyst. 1978. The analysis of dietary fibre, the choices for the analyst. J. Sci. Food Agric. 29:979–998.

Southgate, D.A.T. 1982. Definitions and terminology of dietary fiber. Pp. 1–7 in G.V. Vahouny and D. Kritchevsky, eds. Dietary Fiber in Health and Disease. Plenum Press, New York.

Stasse-Wolthuis, M., H.F.F. Albers, J.G.C. van Jeveren, J. Wil de Jong, J.G.A.J. Hautvast, R.J.J. Hermus, M.B. Katan, W.G. Brydon, and M.A. Eastwood. 1980. Influence of dietary fiber from vegetables and fruits, bran or citrus pectin on serum lipids, fecal lipids, and colonic function. Am. J. Clin. Nutr. 33:1745–1756.

Stephen, A.M., and J.H. Cummings. 1980a. Mechanism of action of dietary fibre in the human colon. Nature 284:282–284.

Stephen, A.M., and J.H. Cummings. 1980b. The microbial contribution to human faecal mass. J. Med. Microbiol. 13:45–56.

Story, J.A. 1980. Dietary fiber and lipid metabolism: an update. Pp. 137–152 in G.A. Spiller and R.M. Kay, eds. Medical Aspects of Dietary Fiber. Plenum Medical Book Co., New York.

Story, J.A. 1986. Modification of steroid excretion in response to dietary fiber. Pp. 253–264 in G.V. Vahouny and D. Kritchevsky, eds. Dietary Fiber: Basic and Clinical Aspects. Plenum Press, New York.

Tadesse, K. 1982. The effect of dietary fibre on gastric secretion and emptying in man. J. Physiol. 332:102P–103P.

Tarpila, S., T.A. Miettinen, and L. Metsäranta. 1978. Effects of bran on serum cholesterol, faecal mass, fat bile acids and neutral sterols, and biliary lipids in patients with diverticular disease of the colon. Gut 19:137–145.

Tasman-Jones, C. 1986a. Effect of dietary fiber and fiber-rich foods on structure of the upper gastrointestinal tract. Pp. 285–286 in G.A. Spiller, ed. Handbook of Dietary Fiber in Human Nutrition. CRC Press, Boca Raton, Fla.

Tasman-Jones, C. 1986b. Effect of dietary fiber on structure of the colon. Pp. 287–288 in G.A. Spiller, ed. Handbook of Dietary Fiber in Human Nutrition. CRC Press, Boca Raton, Fla.

Theander, O. 1981. Review of the different analytical methods and remaining problems. Pp. 263–276 in W.P.T. James and O. Theander, eds. The Analysis of Dietary Fiber in Food. Marcel Dekker, New York.

Trowell, H. 1972. Crude fibre, dietary fibre and atherosclerosis. Atherosclerosis 16:138–140.

Trowell, H. 1981. Hypertension, obesity, diabetes mellitus and coronary heart disease. Pp. 3–32 in H.C. Trowell and

D.P. Burkitt, eds. Western Diseases: Their Emergence and Prevention. Harvard University Press, Cambridge, Mass.

Trowell, H., D.A.T. Southgate, T.M.S. Wolever, A.R. Leeds, M.A. Gassull, and D.J.A. Jenkins. 1976. Dietary fibre redefined. Lancet 1:967.

Trowell, H., E. Godding, G. Spiller, and G. Briggs. 1978. Fiber bibliographies and terminology. Am. J. Clin. Nutr. 31:1489–1490.

Trowell, H.C. 1960. Non-infective Disease in Africa. Edward Arnold Publishers Ltd., London. 481 pp.

USDA (U.S. Department of Agriculture). 1985. Nationwide Food Consumption Survey. Continuing Survey of Food Intakes of Individuals. Women 19–50 Years and Their Children 1–5 Years, 1 Day, 1985. Report No. 85-1. Nutrition Monitoring Division, Human Nutrition Information Service, Hyattsville, Md. 102 pp.

USDA (U.S. Department of Agriculture). 1986a. Nationwide Food Consumption Survey. Continuing Survey of Food Intakes of Individuals. Low-Income Women 19–50 Years and Their Children 1–5 Years, 1 Day, 1985. Report No. 85-2. Nutrition Monitoring Division, Human Nutrition Information Service, Hyattsville, Md. 186 pp.

USDA (U.S. Department of Agriculture). 1986b. Nationwide Food Consumption Survey. Continuing Survey of Food Intakes of Individuals. Men 19–50 Years, 1 Day, 1985. Report No. 85-3. Nutrition Monitoring Division, Human Nutrition Information Service, Hyattsville, Md. 94 pp.

USDA (U.S. Department of Agriculture). 1987a. Nationwide Food Consumption Survey. Continuing Survey of Food Intakes of Individuals. Women 19–50 Years and Their Children 1–5 Years, 4 Days, 1985. Report No. 85-4. Nutrition Monitoring Division, Human Nutrition Information Service, Hyattsville, Md. 182 pp.

USDA (U.S. Department of Agriculture). 1987b. Nationwide Food Consumption Survey. Continuing Survey of Food Intakes of Individuals. Low-Income Women 19–50 Years and Their Children 1–5 Years, 1 Day, 1986. Report No. 86-2. Nutrition Monitoring Division, Human Nutrition Information Service, Hyattsville, Md. 166 pp.

USDA (U.S. Department of Agriculture). 1988. Nationwide Food Consumption Survey. Continuing Survey of Food Intakes of Individuals. Low-Income Women 19–50 Years and Their Children 1–5 Years, 4 Days, 1985. Report No. 85-5. Nutrition Monitoring Division, Human Nutrition Information Service, Hyattsville, Md. 220 pp.

Vaaler, S., J. Aaseth, K.F. Hanssen, K. Dahl-Jörgensen, W. Frölich, B. Ødegaard, and O. Agenaes. 1985. Trace elements in serum and urine of diabetic patients given bread enriched with wheat bran or guar gum. Pp. 446–449 in International Symposium on Trace Element Metabolism in Man and Animals, TEMA-5. Churchill Livingstone, Edinburgh.

Vahouny, G.V. 1982. Dietary fiber, lipid metabolism, and atherosclerosis. Fed. Proc. 41:2801–2806.

Vahouny, G.V. 1985. Dietary fibers: aspects of nutrition, pharmacology, and pathology. Pp. 207–277 in H. Sidransky, ed. Nutritional Pathology: Pathobiochemistry of Dietary Imbalances. Marcel Dekker, New York.

Vahouny, G.V., and M.M. Cassidy. 1986a. Dietary fiber and intestinal adaptation. Pp. 181–209 in G.V. Vahouny and D. Kritchevsky, eds. Dietary Fiber: Basic and Clinical Aspects. Plenum Press, New York.

Vahouny, G.V., and M.M. Cassidy. 1986b. Effect of dietary fiber on intestinal absorption of lipids. Pp. 121–128 in G.A.

Spiller, ed. Handbook of Dietary Fiber in Human Nutrition. CRC Press, Boca Raton, Fla.

Walker, A. 1985. Mineral metabolism. Pp. 361–375 in H. Trowell, D. Burkitt, and K. Heaton, eds. Dietary Fibre, Fibre-Depleted Foods and Disease. Academic Press, New York.

Walker, A.R.P. 1961. Crude fibre, bowel motility, and pattern of diet. S. Afr. Med. J. 35:114–115.

Walker, A.R.P., B.F. Walker, and B.D. Richardson. 1970. Glucose and fat tolerances in Bantu children. Lancet 2:51–52.

Watanabe, K., B.S. Reddy, C.Q. Wong, and J.H. Weisburger. 1979. Effect of dietary alfalfa, pectin, and wheat bran on azoxymethane- or methylnitrosourea-induced colon carcinogenesis in F344 rats. J. Natl. Cancer Inst. 63:141–145.

Watts, J.M., P. Jablonski, and J. Toouli. 1978. The effect of added bran to the diet in the saturation of bile in people without gallstones. Am. J. Surg. 135:321–324.

Wechsler, J.G., W. Swobodnik, H. Wenzel, T. Heuchemer, W. Nebelung, V. Hutt, and H. Ditschuneit. 1984. Ballaststoffe vom Typ Weizenkleie senken Lithogenität der Galle. Dtsch. Med. Wochenschr. 109:1284–1288.

West, K.M. 1974a. Diabetes in American Indians and other native populations of the New World. Diabetes 23:841–855.

West, K.M. 1974b. Epidemiologic observations on thirteen populations of Asia and the Western Hemisphere. Pp. 34–43 in S.S. Hillebrand, ed. Is the Risk of Becoming Diabetic Affected by Sugar Consumption? Proceedings of the Eighth International Sugar Research Symposium, March 14, Washington, D.C. International Sugar Research Foundation, Bethesda, Md.

West, K.M., and J.M. Kalbfleisch. 1971. Influence of nutritional factors on prevalence of diabetes. Diabetes 20:99–108.

Wilmshurst, P., and J.C.W. Crawley. 1980. The measurement of gastric transit time in obese subjects using ^{24}Na and the effects of energy content and guar gum on gastric emptying and satiety. Br. J. Nutr. 44:1–6.

Yamashita, S., and K. Yamashita. 1980. Effect of high-fiber diet on plasma high density lipoprotein (HDL) cholesterol level in streptozotocin-induced diabetic rats. Endocrinol. Jpn. 27:671–673.

Yamashita, S., K. Yamashita, H. Yasuda, and E. Ogato. 1980. High-fiber diet in the control of diabetes in rats. Endocrinol. Jpn. 27:169–173.

Zoppi, G., L. Gobio-Casali, A. Deganello, R. Astolfi, F. Saccomani, and M. Cecchettin. 1982. Potential complications in the use of wheat bran for constipation in infancy. J. Pediatr. Gastroenterol. Nutr. 1:91–95.

11

Fat-Soluble Vitamins

Small amounts of vitamins are required in the diet to promote growth, reproduction, and health. Vitamins A, D, E, and K are called the fat-soluble vitamins, because they are soluble in organic solvents and are absorbed and transported in a manner similar to that of fats.

DIETARY SOURCES, PATTERNS OF INTAKE, AND LEVELS OF FAT-SOLUBLE VITAMINS

Vitamin A: Carotenoids and Retinoids

Vitamin A is required for the maintenance of normal mucous membranes and for normal vision. It occurs naturally only in foods of animal origin, such as liver, butter, whole milk, and egg yolks, but the body converts certain carotenoids, especially β-carotene, to vitamin A. Only 50 of the more than 500 naturally occurring carotenoids have provitamin A activity (Isler et al., 1971; Olson, 1983, 1984). Carotenoids are present in dark-green, leafy vegetables and in yellow and orange vegetables and fruits. In addition, skim milk, margarines, and certain breakfast cereals are fortified with vitamin A. From food composition tables, one can estimate only the total vitamin activity (vitamin A value) but not the quantity of specific carotenoids or retinoids in

foods (Beecher and Khachik, 1984). However, researchers are now beginning to add carotenoid values to those in the U.S. Department of Agriculture (USDA) data bank.

In 1980 the Recommended Dietary Allowance (RDA) for males 11 years of age and older was 1,000 retinol equivalents (RE), or 5,000 International Units (IU), and for females, 800 RE (4,000 IU) (NRC, 1980). By definition, 1 RE is equal to 1 μg of retinol, 6 μg of β-carotene, or 12 μg of other provitamin A carotenoids. One IU of vitamin A activity is defined as 0.3 μg of retinol and as 0.6 μg of β-carotene. One RE is equal to 3.33 IU of vitamin A activity from retinol and to 10 IU of vitamin A activity from β-carotene. Many food composition tables and most food labels still list vitamin A activity in IU, although the official unit is now RE.

The availability of vitamin A in the food supply rose from 7,300 IU per capita in 1967–1969 to 9,900 IU in 1985, an increase of 37% (see Table 3-3). This increase was due chiefly to new varieties of carrots containing higher amounts of carotenoids.

The 1977–1978 Nationwide Food Consumption Survey, based on 3-day dietary intake reports, indicated that total vitamin A intakes averaged 133% of the RDA. More than two-thirds of the population had intakes of at least 70% of the RDA. Intakes were higher for adults

311

over 64 years of age and for children under 8 than for other age groups. People above poverty levels were more apt to reach the RDA for vitamin A than were those below. Intakes were highest in the western United States and lowest in the South (DHHS–USDA, 1986). According to the 1976–1980 National Health and Nutrition Examination Survey (NHANES II), total mean dietary intake of vitamin A in the U.S. population, excluding infants, was approximately 1,000 RE. Carotenoids and preformed vitamin A contributed 25 and 75%, respectively, of the total intake. Mean serum vitamin A levels measured in NHANES II were within normal ranges for all race, sex, and economic groups.

Vitamin D

The active form of vitamin D promotes intestinal absorption of calcium and phosphorus and influences bone mineralization. Vitamin D occurs in two forms that are equally well utilized in the body. Vitamin D_2 (ergocalciferol) is produced commercially by ultraviolet (UV) irradiation of the plant sterol ergosterol; vitamin D_3 (cholecalciferol) is formed by the action of sunlight on the precursor 7-dehydrocholesterol in the skin. The human body utilizes both forms of vitamin D by hydroxylating first the 25-position in the liver and then the 1α-position in the kidney, producing the biologically active $1\alpha,25$-dihydroxycalciferols.

Vitamin D occurs naturally only in animal foods such as liver, butter, fatty fish (fish containing high levels of cholesterol or fatty acids as glycerides), and egg yolks. Because natural milk is a poor source, it is fortified with vitamin D to provide 10 μg (400 IU) per quart. The amount of vitamin D formed by exposure of skin to sunlight depends upon the length of the UV irradiation, the intensity, which can be diminished by atmospheric pollution, and skin pigmentation. Aging skin may have diminished capacity to synthesize vitamin D (MacLaughlin and Holick, 1985).

The 1980 RDAs for vitamin D are set at 10 μg (400 IU) of cholecalciferol per day during periods of growth (childhood, pregnancy, lactation) and 5 μg (200 IU) per day for nonpregnant, nonlactating adults. National surveys in the United States have never monitored vitamin D intake or nutritional status. Recent studies suggest that some elderly people may exhibit poor vitamin D status (Omdahl et al., 1982; Parfitt et al., 1982).

Vitamin E

Vitamin E is an important antioxidant that is thought to protect polyunsaturated fatty acids from oxidative destruction in cell membranes. Vitamin E activity in foods is due to the presence of tocopherols and tocotrienols—compounds of plant origin. The most important of these is α-tocopherol; less active are β-tocopherol, γ-tocopherol, and α-tocotrienol. Vegetable oils are the richest source of vitamin E. Other good sources include nuts, seeds, whole grains, and wheat germ. The vitamin E content of animal foods is generally low.

The RDA for adults is 8 mg of α-tocopherol equivalents (α-TE) or 12 IU for females age 11 and older and 10 mg of α-TE (15 IU) for males age 15 or older. The need for vitamin E is increased if the polyunsaturated fat intake is high, but in the U.S. food supply, foods with high levels of polyunsaturated fatty acids also have a high vitamin E content.

Vitamin E was not included in national surveys until 1985, when the Continuing Survey of Food Intakes of Individuals was initiated by USDA. In 1985, this survey indicated that on the average, women 19 to 50 years of age consumed 97% of the RDA for vitamin E (USDA, 1987).

Vitamin K

Vitamin K is needed in the liver for formation of several blood clotting factors. Vitamin K_1 (phylloquinone) is synthesized by plants, whereas vitamin K_2 homologs (menoquinones) are synthesized by bacteria. The human body can obtain vitamin K from dietary sources as well as through synthesis by the gut microflora.

Larger amounts of vitamin K are present in dark-green leafy vegetables; lower levels are found in cereals, dairy products, meats, and fruits. A committee of the Food and Nutrition Board estimated the safe and adequate intake range for adults to be 70 to 140 μg per day. The lower end of that range was based on the assumption that half the daily vitamin K intake is supplied by the diet and that half comes from intestinal synthesis. The higher end of the range represents intake derived entirely from diet. The usual diet of the U.S. population contains 300 to 500 μg per day, and there are no reports of vitamin K deficiency or toxicity in the general population; thus, it has been assumed that dietary intake of vitamin K does not need to be monitored (NRC, 1980).

EVIDENCE ASSOCIATING FAT-SOLUBLE VITAMINS WITH CHRONIC DISEASES

Vitamin A: β-Carotene and Other Carotenoids

Cancer

Human Studies of Lung Cancer

Early epidemiologic studies focused generally on foods with vitamin A activity but did not distinguish between β-carotene and retinol (NRC, 1982). A 5-year prospective study of 8,278 Norwegian men indicated that intake of foods with vitamin A activity was inversely associated with incidence of lung cancer independently of cigarette smoking (Bjelke, 1975). This result was extended to women as well as men in the 11-year follow-up of Bjelke's study (Kvåle et al., 1983) and in hospital-based case-comparison studies in the United States (Mettlin et al., 1979) and in the United Kingdom (Gregor et al., 1980). Peto et al. (1981) hypothesized that the relevant dietary exposure was β-carotene rather than retinol. This was subsequently supported by a 19-year prospective study of 1,954 middle-aged men in Chicago (Shekelle et al., 1981) and population-based case-comparison studies in New Jersey (Ziegler et al., 1984), Hawaii (Hinds et al., 1984), and New Mexico (Samet et al., 1985). Two other studies—a 10-year prospective study of 265,118 adults in Japan (Hirayama, 1979) and a hospital-based case-comparison study of Chinese in Singapore (MacLennan et al., 1977)—indicated that lung cancer risk was inversely associated with the frequency of eating green and yellow vegetables.

Retrospective studies of serum β-carotene levels and lung cancer risk are difficult to interpret, because the disease itself may affect the variable under study. In two prospective studies, blood samples were taken from subjects before they developed cancer. One was conducted in men of Japanese ancestry in Hawaii (Nomura et al., 1985) and another in white adults in Washington County, Maryland (Menkes et al., 1986). Blood samples were taken from people apparently free of cancer and stored at −70°C or lower (to prevent oxidative loss of β-carotene). Beta-carotene was subsequently measured by high-performance liquid chromatography (HPLC) in subjects who developed cancer and in controls. In both studies, β-carotene concentrations in serum were associated inversely with lung cancer risk independently of cigarette smoking. Clinical trials to determine the effect of dietary β-carotene supplements on lung cancer are in progress, but results are not yet available.

Human Studies of Cancers Other Than Lung Cancer

As with lung cancer, early studies of other cancers and food intake generally focused on vitamin A activity without making a distinction between β-carotene and retinol. Two case-comparison studies—one in Norway and Minnesota (Bjelke, 1974) and one in Pennsylvania (Stehr et al., 1985)—indicated an inverse association between intake of foods with vitamin A activity and gastric cancer risk. In contrast, a series of case-comparison studies conducted at Roswell Park, reported by Graham and colleagues (1983) (Graham et al., 1960, 1963, 1967, 1978, 1983; Mettlin and Graham, 1979), showed no association between intake of foods with vitamin A activity and gastrointestinal cancer. However, they did find that intake of such foods was inversely associated with cancers of the bladder, mouth, larynx, esophagus, and breast and was positively associated with cancer of the prostate (Graham, 1983; Graham et al., 1983).

In a hospital-based case-comparison study conducted in Italy, dietary intake of β-carotene, but not of retinol, was inversely associated with risk of invasive cervical cancer after adjustment for risk factors such as age at first intercourse, number of sexual partners, and educational status (La Vecchia et al., 1988). This result supports two earlier case-comparison studies in the United States (Marshall et al., 1983; Wylie-Rosett et al., 1984). A 5-year prospective study of 1,271 Massachusetts residents 66 years of age or older demonstrated an inverse association between frequency of eating green and yellow vegetables and risk of death from cancer after adjustment for age, smoking habits, sex, and total food intake (Colditz et al., 1985). A case-comparison study in Israel suggested a strong, graded inverse association between the number of carotene-containing foods eaten daily and risk of gastrointestinal cancer (Modan et al., 1981); however, no association was found with intake of dietary β-carotene itself. The investigators concluded that the association with foods was probably due to factors other than β-carotene.

In three case-comparison studies, intake of foods with vitamin A activity was positively associated with risk of prostate cancer. Two groups of investigators (Graham et al., 1983; Heshmat et al., 1985) did not analyze their data separately for carotenoids and retinoids. A third group (Kolonel et al., 1987) found a positive association with carotenoids and retinoids for men aged 70 or older but not for younger men.

In a prospective study by Nomura et al. (1985), there was no statistically significant association between concentrations of serum β-carotene and 10-year risk of cancers of the colon, stomach, rectum, and urinary bladder, although, as noted above, an inverse association with lung cancer was observed. However, since the statistical test was not particularly powerful and the mean concentrations of serum β-carotene in cases of stomach and colon cancer (22.8 and 23.5 μg/dl, respectively) were lower than those in the comparison group (29.0 μg/dl), these data are consistent with a hypothesis of an inverse association as well as the hypothesis of no association. In another prospective study, Willett et al. (1984) found no association between serum total carotenoid concentration and 5-year risk of cancer. The implications of this evidence for hypotheses specifically about β-carotene are limited, because β-carotene comprises only about 20 to 25% of total carotenoids in serum (Katrangi et al., 1984), and the correlation between concentrations of β-carotene and total carotenoids in serum is only .6 to .7 (Russell-Briefel et al., 1985).

Several clinical trials testing supplemental β-carotene as a chemopreventive agent are currently under way, but no results have yet been published. There has been one study, however, in which dietary supplementation with retinol and β-carotene was found to decrease markedly the proportion of micronucleated buccal mucosal cells in Filipino betel chewers (Stich et al., 1984).

Animal Studies

Only a few studies have explored the potential chemopreventive effects of carotenoids on experimentally induced tumors in animals. The incidence of tumors decreased and the latent period for development of tumors increased in mice fed supplemental β-carotene before inoculation with Moloney's sarcoma virus; the rate of tumor regression markedly increased when β-carotene was fed after tumors were already present (Seifter et al., 1982). Similar results were obtained in mice inoculated with C3HBA adenocarcinoma cells. Injection of β-carotene decreased the incidence of skin cancer in hairless mice exposed to ultraviolet-B (UV-B) radiation (Epstein, 1977a). Both β-carotene and canthaxanthin, a carotenoid without vitamin A activity, decreased the incidence of skin cancer in mice exposed to benzo[a]pyrene and UV

light (Santamaria et al., 1983). β-Carotene, canthaxanthin, and phytoene, another carotenoid without vitamin A activity, decreased the incidence of skin tumors and increased the latent period in mice exposed to UV-B only, but only β-carotene exerted these effects in mice exposed to dimethylbenzanthracene (DMBA) (Mathews-Roth and Krinsky, 1984). In at least one study, growth of tumor cells was not suppressed in mice injected with β-carotene (Tomita, 1983). More information is clearly needed concerning the potential roles of specific carotenoids as chemopreventive agents for specific neoplasms in laboratory animals.

In Vitro Assays: Possible Mechanisms of Action

Peto et al. (1981) suggested several possible mechanisms through which dietary carotenoids might be able to affect cancer risk. These include (1) a direct or indirect retinoid-like effect (as described below) on cellular differentiation in target tissues (including possible conversion to retinoids in the target tissue), (2) their action as antioxidants, thereby protecting against transformation, and (3) protection afforded through some other mechanism (for example, by enhancing some immunologic function). See also Dimitrov (1986) and Willett and MacMahon (1984) for reviews and references. Bendich and Shapiro (1986) reported that T- and B-lymphocyte responses were enhanced in rats fed β-carotene or canthaxanthin. β-Carotene is highly effective in quenching singlet oxygen and in trapping free radicals. These potent antioxidant effects of carotenoids may protect cells against oxidative damage to DNA, thereby exerting a chemopreventive effect against cancer (Dimitrov, 1986).

Hypercarotenemia

The intake of very large quantities of β-carotene can result in elevated plasma carotene levels (hypercarotenemia) and a yellow-orange pigmentation of the skin (carotenodermia). This condition is clinically innocuous and reversible. Furthermore, abnormally elevated plasma levels of vitamin A and clinical evidence of hypervitaminosis A do not result from the consumption of high doses of β-carotene. The medical induction of hypercarotenemia has been used successfully in the treatment of photosensitive conditions in humans (Mathews-Roth, 1982).

Other Diseases

Carotenoids in plants and long-chain retinyl esters in animal tissues are the major natural sources of vitamin A, which is necessary for growth, health, vision, reproduction, and maintenance of differentiated epithelia and mucus secretion. Thus, to the extent that other sources of vitamin A are absent, a decreased intake of carotenoids with vitamin A activity, especially β-carotene, can be a cause of hypovitaminosis A. In her review of carotenoids in medical applications, Mathews-Roth (1982) noted that certain conditions—for example, menstrual disorders and leukopenia—have been observed in persons who habitually consume very large quantities of carotenoid-containing foods. She concluded, however, that these were not effects of β-carotene specifically, because such abnormalities have not been observed in persons taking pure β-carotene.

Vitamin A: Retinol and Other Retinoids

Cancer

Human Studies

Among early studies not distinguishing between retinol and β-carotene, one case-comparison study found that vitamin A supplementation was associated with lower cancer risk (Smith and Jick, 1978), and another found that the inverse association between vitamin A intake and lung cancer risk was due primarily to intake of liver and vitamin A preparations (Gregor et al., 1980). However, the weight of evidence from several studies (e.g., La Vecchia et al., 1988; Samet et al., 1985; Shekelle et al., 1981; Ziegler et al., 1984) indicates that intake of preformed vitamin A, either by diet or by supplementation, is not associated with decreased risk of cancer. In fact, Modan et al. (1981) found that some retinol-containing foods were positively associated with risk of gastrointestinal cancers, but it seems more likely that the association was due to the lipid composition of these foods—eggs, butter, sour cream—than to the vitamin A content. As mentioned earlier, three case-comparison studies (Graham et al., 1983; Heshmat et al., 1985; Kolonel et al., 1987) indicated a positive association between intake of foods with vitamin A activity and risk of prostate cancer. It is not possible, however, to separate clearly the potential effects of dietary carotenoids, retinoids, and other food components in this association.

Prospective studies in London (Wald et al., 1980), Evans County, Georgia (Kark et al., 1981),

and eastern Finland (Salonen et al., 1985) were reported to show that there is an inverse association between serum levels of retinol and subsequent risk of cancer, particularly in the lung. However, a second study of the Evans County population by Peleg et al. (1984) failed to confirm the first study's results. Two large studies, by Friedman et al. (1986) and by Menkes et al. (1986), provide strong evidence that serum retinol concentrations are not associated with risk of lung cancer. Other studies (Nomura et al., 1985; Stähelin et al., 1984; Willet et al., 1984) indicate that serum retinol concentration is not associated with cancer risk generally.

It now seems unlikely that variation in retinol intake or in serum retinol concentrations within the normal range is associated with cancer risk generally or lung cancer risk specifically. Nonetheless, it still is possible that deficiency in vitamin A nutriture may affect the incidence of cancer in populations. Yang et al. (1984) found low average plasma levels of retinol, β-carotene, and α-tocopherol in Linxian, a province in northern China with very high incidence rates of esophageal cancer. Systematic studies of the ecological correlation between vitamin A nutriture and cancer risk have not yet been reported.

Animal Studies

Wolbach and Howe (1925) reported that vitamin A deficiency resulted in a change in cell differentiation and in keratinization of epithelia in the respiratory tract, salivary glands, eyes, and genitourinary tract. Much subsequent work (described below) shows that retinoids profoundly affect the differentiation and proliferation of cells. The activity of retinoids in preventing, suppressing, or retarding experimentally induced cancer in animals has been studied extensively in a variety of animal models; see Moon and Itri (1984) and Sporn and Newton (1981) for reviews and references. Retinoids are highly effective in the prevention of experimental cancer of the skin, breast, and bladder (see, e.g., Bollag, 1975; Davies, 1967; Epstein and Grenkin, 1981; McCormick et al., 1980; Moon et al., 1977; Saffiotti et al., 1967; Schmähl and Habs, 1978; Shklar et al., 1980; Sporn and Newton, 1979). Promising but less definitive results have been obtained in studies of the prevention of carcinogenesis at a number of other sites, including the pancreas, prostate, lung, esophagus, and colon. Not all studies have shown that retinoids decrease susceptibility to experimentally induced cancer, and some studies have reported no effect or even increased susceptibility (Epstein, 1977b; Levij and Polliack, 1968; Nettesheim, 1980; Smith et al., 1975a,b; Ward et al., 1978; Welsch et al., 1981). Wholly satisfactory explanations for these variations are not yet available. Overall, however, the strong preponderance of evidence from experimental animal studies shows that vitamin A deficiency enhances chemically induced carcinogenesis in many animal tissues and that retinoids can exert a protective or preventive effect against many kinds of cancer (NRC, 1982).

In Vitro Assays: Possible Mechanisms of Action

Retinoids have powerful effects on cell differentiation and proliferation (for reviews and references, see Goodman, 1984; Roberts and Sporn, 1984; Sporn and Roberts, 1983, 1984). They have been used extensively in studies in vitro to induce cell differentiation in organ and cell culture systems, especially in the hamster tracheal organ culture system (Sporn and Newton, 1981). Retinoids affect the differentiation of neoplastic and nonneoplastic cells in culture and can act directly on nonneoplastic cells to suppress malignant transformation induced by chemical carcinogens, radiation, or transforming growth factors. Furthermore, they can induce terminal differentiation of neoplastic cells, such as mouse embryonal carcinoma cells (Strickland and Mahdavi, 1978) and human promyelocytic leukemia cells (Breitman et al., 1980). Retinoids also counteract the effects of phorbol esters in a variety of systems. The molecular mechanisms through which retinoids exert these effects are not known. They may relate to signal transduction. It is likely that retinoids affect gene expression in target cells (Roberts and Sporn, 1984).

Other Diseases

Vitamin A deficiency is found frequently among young children in many poor and undernourished populations. Xerophthalmia is the most important clinical effect. Sommer (1982) estimated that approximately 500,000 new cases occur annually in India, Bangladesh, Indonesia, and the Philippines and that half these cases are likely to result in blindness. In the United States, nutrition surveys indicate that frank vitamin A deficiency does not occur frequently; however, borderline serum concentrations of vitamin A and reduced liver stores of vitamin A have been observed at autopsy (Goodman, 1984; Underwood, 1984).

Excess intakes of retinol (hypervitaminosis A) can also have harmful effects on humans and other animals. This topic is discussed in Chapter 18.

Vitamin D

Vitamin D serves to maintain serum calcium concentrations, which in turn influence bone mineralization. Vitamin D as 1,25-dihydroxycholecalciferol [1,25(OH)$_2$D] acts primarily to maintain the cellular calcium transport system in the intestine. Parathyroid hormone (PTH) and vitamin D are interdependent: the renal production of 1,25(OH)$_2$D depends on the prevailing concentration of PTH in the blood, and the ability of PTH to increase plasma calcium depends on a calcium transport system maintained by 1,25(OH)$_2$D.

Vitamin D stimulates an active calcium transport system that increases calcium absorption in the small intestine (DeLuca, 1988; DeLuca et al., 1982; Nicolaysen and Eeg-Larsen, 1953; Wasserman and Feher, 1977). It also acts in bone mineralization primarily by maintaining adequate plasma concentrations of calcium and phosphorus, rather than by having a direct trophic effect on bone (Holtrop et al., 1981; Underwood and DeLuca, 1984; Weinstein et al., 1984). Vitamin D also plays an important role in bone remodeling. The exact mechanism by which vitamin D maintains normal bone development is unknown, but disorders of the vitamin D endocrine system are the leading cause of osteomalacia through decreased bioavailability of vitamin D, abnormal metabolism, and abnormal response of target tissues to the biologically active vitamin D metabolites (Bikle, 1985).

Osteoporosis and Osteomalacia

Human Studies

The term osteoporosis refers to a group of disorders with various etiologies that is characterized by a decrease in bone mass per unit volume. In cases of osteoporosis, bone has a normal ratio of mineral to matrix. Osteomalacia refers to a disorder in which there is abnormal bone mineralization and the ratio of mineral to matrix is diminished due to an excess of unmineralized osteoid.

Two patterns of osteoporosis have been postulated: postmenopausal and senile. Postmenopausal osteoporosis affects predominantly trabecular bone in women and is manifested as vertebral fractures that occur particularly during the 15 to 20 years after menopause. Senile osteoporosis affects cortical and trabecular bone in women and men and results in vertebral and hip fractures after age 75 (Riggs et al., 1982).

In countries with limited sunlight or where the population dresses in a fashion that minimizes sunlight exposure, circulating levels of vitamin D metabolites are often low. This might explain why there is a higher incidence of osteomalacia in Great Britain, Scandinavia, the Middle East, India, and other Muslim countries than in the United States (Bikle, 1985). In the United States, nutritional deficiency of vitamin D is uncommon; however, it may occur in children of vegetarians who avoid milk products (and likely have low stores of vitamin D) and in children who are not weaned to vitamin D-supplemented milk by age 2. The contribution of nutritional vitamin D deficiency to osteomalacia in the elderly is unknown.

One of the many causes of osteoporosis is decreased calcium absorption. There is a dispute whether this decreased absorption can be correlated with decreased circulating levels of 1,25-$(OH)_2D$ (Crilly et al., 1981; Gallagher et al., 1979; Nordin et al., 1979). Nevertheless, calcium absorption markedly improves by administering small doses of 1,25$(OH)_2D$ (Finkelman and Butler, 1985). Riggs et al. (1979) found that treatment of postmenopausal osteoporotic females with as little as 0.5 μg per day greatly improved calcium balance.

Caniggia et al. (1986) noted a dramatic improvement in the intestinal transport of calcium in subjects treated with 1,25$(OH)_2D$, but the increases in bone mineral content were not significant. These results are in agreement with those of Gallagher et al. (1982), who reported that treatment with 1,25$(OH)_2D$ improved net calcium absorption and balance and increased trabecular bone volume in a controlled study in postmenopausal osteoporotic women with one or more traumatic vertebral fractures.

Investigators in Finland reported that serum 25-hydroxycholecalciferol (25-OH-D) concentrations were lower in patients with hip fractures than in age-matched controls (Harju et al., 1985). They attribute this to lack of sunlight exposure and insufficient dietary vitamin D intake. Those authors suggest that elderly disabled persons should be given vitamin D supplements.

Caniggia et al. (1986) reported that serum bone γ-carboxyglutamyl-protein levels increased in postmenopausal osteoporotic women treated with 1,25$(OH)_2D$. They attributed this to osteoblast stimulation, suggesting that the osteoblasts do not

lose their sensitivity to this stimulus during postmenopausal osteoporosis. The implications of this are uncertain.

Animal Studies

Adult rats were fed a calcium-deficient diet for 6 weeks and subsequently fed a combination of 1α-hydroxycholecalciferol (1α-OH-D_3) and optimal levels of calcium (Lindholm et al., 1981) for 6 weeks. Osteoporosis as well as morphological changes of the parathyroids were almost totally reversed. In another study, when calcium-deficient mice were refed calcium alone, reversal of osteoporotic changes was not complete (Sevastikoglou et al., 1977).

In the rat liver, 1α-OH-D_3 is converted to 1,25$(OH)_2D_3$. It is known to promote calcium absorption in the small intestine and to increase resorption of calcium in the kidneys. It may also act through direct or indirect mechanisms on bone tissue to promote new bone formation (Kraft et al., 1979; Kream et al., 1977; Lindholm et al., 1981).

Mechanisms of Action and Interactions

Interaction of vitamin D with other nutrients, particularly calcium, was addressed in the preceding sections; thus, only a brief overview is presented here. The vitamin D endocrine system is an important regulator of calcium homeostasis. The metabolite that plays the most important physiological role in calcium and bone metabolism is 1,25$(OH)_2D$ (both D_2 and D_3 forms), which is also referred to as the hormonal form of vitamin D. This extremely active form does not vary with the amount of vitamin D synthesis or ingestion, and its concentration remains relatively constant over a broad range of 25-OH-D serum concentrations.

1,25$(OH)_2D$ is important in the control of calcium absorption through the small intestine and is involved in both bone calcification and bone resorption. Resorption of bone appears to be tightly coupled to the formation of new bone in vivo and in vitro. A decrease in serum 1,25$(OH)_2D$ has been noted in patients with osteoporosis (Goldsmith, 1984); however, it is unclear if vitamin D deficiency is an important risk factor for bone loss in most aging American women (Tsai et al., 1987). The entire sequence proposed is: estrogen deficiency → increased calcium release from bone → decreased PTH secretion → decreased conversion of 25-OH-D to 1,25$(OH)_2D$ → decreased calcium absorption. Thus, estrogen deficiency may be the primary cause or the trigger of the subsequent events resulting in decreased calcium absorption. Hence, 1,25(OH)$_2$D plays an important role in maintaining normal calcium homeostasis by increasing the intestinal absorption of calcium.

Aging

Low serum calcium levels predispose to osteoporosis. A low calcium intake is a particular hazard in the elderly because they cannot adapt by increasing calcium absorption. This may be due partly to their failure to produce a sufficient amount of 1,25(OH)$_2$D in response to calcium deficiency, perhaps because of an impaired response of renal 1α-hydroxylase to PTH (Raisz and Johannesson, 1984). Increased supplementation with 25-OH-D as a substrate may not result in increased synthesis of 1,25(OH)$_2$D in elderly women. Lukert et al. (1987) observed a negative correlation between serum 25-OH-D and PTH hormone levels in perimenopausal women and elderly men, but not in elderly, postmenopausal women. They also observed a significant negative correlation between bone loss and serum 25-OH-D in elderly postmenopausal women.

Whether or not the serum level of 1,25(OH)$_2$D is decreased in elderly osteoporotic women is uncertain. Gallagher et al. (1982) reported a causal relationship between the osteoporotic state and decreased serum 1,25(OH)$_2$D levels as well as calcium absorption rates. In contrast, Christiansen and Rødbro (1984) reported that serum 1,25(OH)$_2$D concentrations were virtually the same in 44 early postmenopausal women and 28 women 70 years of age with and without osteoporotic fractures. Tsai et al. (1984) suggest that elderly women have abnormal vitamin D metabolism. In their study of pre- and postmenopausal normal and osteoporotic women, they noted that the kidneys of elderly subjects had a decreased ability to synthesize 1,25(OH)$_2$D. They concluded that this may contribute to the pathogenesis of senile osteoporosis. These results were confirmed in another study by Tsai et al. (1987), in which they measured serum levels of 25-OH-D$_2$, 25-OH-D$_3$, and total 25-OH-D and used single and dual photon absorptiometry to measure bone mineral density. They found no association between any of the vitamin D metabolites and any of three skeletal scanning sites; however, they noted that levels of serum total 25-OH-D and serum 25-OH-D$_3$ decrease with age, which may be related to several factors. The elderly are often malnourished and are less likely to be exposed to the sun (Parfitt et al., 1982). In addition, there are decreases in vitamin D absorption (Barragry et al., 1978) and dermal biosynthesis after exposure to sunlight (Holick and MacLaughlin, 1981).

Renal Disease

Metabolic studies indicate that vitamin D acts in the kidney with PTH to stimulate the final resorption of calcium in the distal tubule (DeLuca, 1979; Sutton et al., 1977). This probably leads to the resorption of an additional 1%—7 to 10 g of calcium (DeLuca, 1981). In renal disease, these normal events and the 1α-hydroxylation of 25-OH-D can be impaired.

Vitamin E

Cancer

Human Studies

The prospective epidemiologic studies reviewed below suggest that vitamin E intake is in itself not related to overall risk of cancer, but that low serum levels of vitamin E coupled with low serum levels of selenium may increase the risk of at least some cancers. Additional studies are needed to investigate this hypothesis and to determine whether intake of vitamin E may be related to risk of specific cancers, for example, of the breast and lung.

At entry into the Hypertension Detection and Follow-up Program in 1973–1974, venous blood specimens were collected from 10,940 participants at least 4 hours after their last meal and sera were stored at −70°C (Willett et al., 1984). The investigators subsequently measured retinol, α-tocopherol, and total carotenoids in the serum of 321 participants who were apparently free of cancer at entry. Five years later, 111 of these participants were diagnosed as having cancer [17, lung; 14, breast; 11, prostate; 11, leukemia or lymphoma; 11, gastrointestinal (GI) tract, and 40, other sites excluding nonmelanoma skin cancers]. The other 210 subjects (matched with cases for age, sex, race, smoking history, and other characteristics) did not have a diagnosis of cancer during 5 years of follow-up from the start of the study. The two groups did not differ significantly in mean concentration of serum α-tocopherol; the unadjusted mean values for cases and controls were 1.16 and 1.26 mg/dl [crude difference = −0.10, standard error (SE) = 0.06, p = .23]. After adjustment for total lipids, the difference was −0.05 (SE = 0.06, p = .68). Similar results were obtained when the data were analyzed according to site. These results do not support the hypothesis that low serum vitamin E by itself is associated with overall incidence of cancer. In an earlier paper from this same study, however, Willett et al. (1983) reported that the cancer risk associated with low serum selenium appeared strongest in persons with low serum vitamin E.

Wald et al. (1984) studied 5,004 women aged 28 to 75 in Guernsey, United Kingdom, who gave blood between 1968 and 1975. The plasma was stored at $-20°C$. By the end of 1982, general practitioners reported 39 cases of breast cancer in women whose plasma samples were available for analysis. The stored samples for these women and samples from 78 controls were matched 2-to-1 for menopausal status, parity, family history of breast cancer, and history of benign breast disease. Vitamin E was significantly lower in cases (0.47 mg/dl) than in controls (0.60 mg/dl)—$p < .025$—after adjusting for age of subject and duration of plasma storage. The adjusted relative odds of breast cancer according to plasma levels of vitamin E were only meaningful below 0.5 mg/dl.

In Basel, Switzerland, between 1971 and 1973, Stähelin et al. (1984) measured vitamin E in fresh samples of fasting blood from employed men who volunteered for venipuncture. It is unclear whether or not they excluded subjects with evidence of cancer. They conducted a mortality follow-up of this cohort through 1980. Information regarding cancer in subjects who died during this 7- to 9-year period was obtained from death certificates, autopsies, and a cancer registry. Mean concentrations of plasma vitamin E for men who died with a diagnosis of cancer—notably of lung, stomach, and colon—did not differ significantly from those for age-matched men who were still alive in 1980.

In 1977, Salonen et al. (1985) collected (and stored at $-20°C$) sera from a random 6.7% sample of 30- to 64-year-old people living in two provinces of eastern Finland. Deaths were ascertained through 1980, and diagnoses of cancer on the death certificate were confirmed from hospital records. Serum concentrations of α-tocopherol, selenium, and retinol were measured for 51 persons who died of cancer (18, GI tract; 15, lung; and 18, other sites) and 51 controls matched for sex, age, and number of tobacco products smoked daily. Cases did not differ significantly from controls in either mean concentration of serum α-tocopherol (4.9 and 5.0 mg/dl, respectively) or mean ratio of α-tocopherol to cholesterol (18.9 and 20.8%, respectively). However, multivariate analysis showed a strong interaction between selenium and

α-tocopherol. After adjustment for main effects, the relative risk of fatal cancer for persons in the lower tertile of selenium and of α-tocopherol levels was 11.4.

From 1971 through 1975, as part of the Honolulu Heart Program, nonfasting serum specimens were obtained (and stored at $-75°C$) from 6,860 men of Japanese ancestry who were born between 1900 and 1919 and lived on Oahu (Nomura et al., 1985). Subsequent cancer diagnoses were monitored by continuous surveillance of all general hospitals on Oahu and through the Hawaii Tumor Registry. After 10 years of follow-up, 284 newly diagnosed cases of epithelial cancer, all confirmed histologically, were identified: 81, colon; 74, lung; 70, stomach; 32, rectum; and 27, urinary bladder. Controls (302) were randomly selected from the examined men who did not have any of the cancers that were under study. This sampling was stratified by age group so that the age distribution of all cases combined could be matched. The mean serum concentrations of vitamin E in controls and in men with cancer of the lung, stomach, colon, rectum, and bladder were 12.3, 12.8, 12.2, 12.2, 11.6, and 12.7 mg/dl, respectively; none of the case-control differences was statistically significant.

Menkés and Comstock (1984) noted that serum vitamin E levels were significantly lower ($p = .01$) in 88 persons who subsequently developed lung cancer than in 76 controls matched for age, sex, date of venipuncture, and smoking history.

Animal Studies

Jaffe (1946) reported that wheat germ oil inhibited production of methylcholanthrene-induced tumors in rats. Subsequently, several investigators conducted studies to determine if vitamin E was effective in preventing sarcomas and cancers of the mouth, skin, and breast in animals, but their results have been mixed.

Haber and Wissler (1962) observed some inhibition of sarcoma formation in mice injected with 3-methylcholanthrene, but such inhibition was not found by Epstein et al. (1967), who exposed mice to 3,4,9,10-dibenzpyrene. Constantinides and Harkey (1985) reported that α-tocopherol, administered subcutaneously in a base of soya oil, produced vigorously growing sarcomas at the site of injection in 77% of animals, but they did not determine whether the effect was due to the soya oil, the vitamin E, or the combination.

Shklar (1982) noted that twice-weekly vitamin E supplementation of the diets of hamsters exposed to dimethylbenz[a]anthracene resulted in fewer, smaller, and less invasive oral tumors than in hamsters whose diets were not supplemented with vitamin E. Odukoya et al. (1984) observed fewer and smaller oral tumors in hamsters after topical application of vitamin E than in hamsters to which vitamin E was not topically applied.

Shamberger (1970) found that α-tocopherol reduced the incidence of skin cancer in mice when administered with a promoting agent (croton oil) but not when given simultaneously with 7,12-dimethylbenz[a]anthracene. Slaga and Bracken (1977) noted only minimal effect of vitamin E when measuring epidermal metabolic activity. Pauling et al. (1982) observed no effect of vitamin E supplementation on incidence of squamous cell carcinomas in hairless mice exposed to UV radiation. These results indicate that the role of vitamin E in cancer inhibition is inconclusive at this time.

Mechanisms of Action

Vitamin E is an antioxidant and free-radical scavanger—functions that may be responsible for an antineoplastic effect. Fiddler et al. (1978) and Mergens et al. (1978) reported that vitamin E, by competing for nitrates, blocks formation of nitrosamines and nitrosamides. Vitamin E may also regulate functions of coenzyme Q and of specific enzymes and proteins required for tissue differentiation. The stimulation of immune functions by vitamin E has also been suggested as an anticancer mechanism (Carpenter, 1986; Watson, 1986). Much of this work is speculative, however; anticancer mechanisms for vitamin E have not been definitively demonstrated.

Atherosclerotic Heart Disease

Vogelsang and Shute (1946) reported that large doses of vitamin E had a dramatic effect in the treatment of angina pectoris in an uncontrolled case-series study. That observation was not confirmed, however, in four placebo-controlled clinical trials (Anderson and Reid, 1974; Donegan et al., 1949; Makinson et al., 1948; Rinzler et al., 1950) and two double-blind trials (Anderson and Reid, 1974; Rinzler et al., 1950). Large doses of vitamin E were also tried in the treatment of intermittent claudication with mixed results (Farrell, 1980), but definitive studies of this question have never been done.

Preliminary reports that vitamin E might raise the concentration of high-density lipoprotein cholesterol (Barboriak et al., 1982; Hermann et al., 1979) were not confirmed in a randomized, double-blind, placebo-controlled study by Stampfer et

al. (1983). Others, however, reported that large vitamin E supplements might be associated with modest elevations in plasma triglycerides (Farrell and Bieri, 1975; Tsai et al., 1978). In another study, vitamin E did not appreciably affect the extent or severity of atherosclerosis in cynomolgus and cebus monkeys (Hayes, 1974).

Other Diseases

As an antioxidant, vitamin E may protect against free radicals implicated in cell damage leading to normal aging and to the development of neoplasia, but there are few reports of vitamin E deficiency in humans, except in the premature baby (Hassan et al., 1966; Oski and Barness, 1967). The incidence of retrolental fibroplasia in infants and very young children is decreased by vitamin E supplementation (Johnson et al., 1974). In older children and adults, severe vitamin E deficiency sometimes complicated by deficits of other vitamins—for example folate—have led to muscular function alterations along with creatinuria, encephalomalacia, and hemolytic anemia (Binder et al., 1965). The reduced biliary excretion resulting from chronic intrahepatic obstructive jaundice (primary biliary cirrhosis) leads to steatorrhea and an associated decrease in absorption of fat-soluble vitamins, including vitamin E (Atkinson et al., 1956).

Inadequate vitamin E absorption can be caused not only by intrahepatic cholestasis and extrahepatic biliary atresia but also by extensive therapeutic administration of bile acid-binding agents and the absence of water-soluble vitamin E preparations during therapy. Vitamin E can prevent progressive loss of neurological function in infants and children with prolonged neonatal cholestatic disorders (Guggenheim et al., 1983; Sokol et al., 1985). Morphological and functional alterations in the neuromuscular system result from the loss of antioxidant protection against free-radical-induced peroxidation of unsaturated fatty acyl moieties of membrane phospholipids (Muller et al., 1983; Neville et al., 1983). Slater and Swaiman (1977) suggested that increases in vitamin E intake may also prevent the deposition of ceroid in smooth muscle and pathological changes in the spinal cord unique to patients with cystic fibrosis.

The efficacy of vitamin E in treating certain hematological and malabsorption disorders is no longer in doubt (Bieri et al., 1983). The evidence does not, however, support claims that increased supplements are beneficial for less experimentally documented purposes, for example, the delay of carcinogenesis or cardiovascular diseases and the restoration of male potency (Horwitt, 1986). In premature infants, daily intravenous administration of 50 mg of all-*rac-dl*-tocopheryl acetate with emulsifiers was found to be toxic (Phelps, 1984). Also, megadoses of vitamin E inhibit vitamin K and can create complications in patients being treated with anticoagulants (Farrell and Bieri, 1975).

Vitamin K

Cancer

Human Studies

Chlebowski et al. (1984) conducted extensive research on vitamin K_3 (menadione) and its effect on human and animal cell lines. In their study of a variety of human tumor lines, including explants from breast, colon, kidney, ovary, and lung, the vitamin resulted in decreased tumor colony-forming units. In a comparison of vitamins K_1 and K_3, vitamin K_3 was found to be cytotoxic at much lower doses than the vitamin K_1 preparation.

Animal Studies

Chlebowski et al. (1983) studied the effects of warfarin (a vitamin K antagonist) or vitamin K in conjunction with two standard chemotherapeutic agents, 5-fluorouracil (5-FU) and methotrexate, in L1210 cells. Both the warfarin and the vitamin K inhibited the salvage pathways used by the L1210 cells. These investigators suggest that the cytotoxicity of 5-FU and methotrexate could be enhanced with the addition of either vitamin K or warfarin. Israels et al. (1983) studied the effect of vitamins K_1 and K_3 on ICR/Ha mice. Mice receiving vitamin K_3 developed tumors at a slower rate than did control mice or mice receiving vitamin K_1. Indeed, in some animals, vitamin K_1 was associated with accelerated benzo[a]pyrene tumorigenesis. These researchers indicated that vitamins K_1 and K_3 act at different metabolic sites as evidenced by benzo[a]pyrene activation and detoxification.

Liver Disease

Human Studies

Severe parenchymal liver disease of several different etiologies can produce deficiencies in plasma clotting factors. This may be due to abnormal synthesis, increased utilization, or decreased production of clotting factors. Multiple factors can have a direct effect on hemostasis (Rock, 1984).

For example, the vitamin K-dependent clotting factors II, VII, IX, and X and protein C require vitamin K for the carboxylation of the γ-methylene group of glutamic acid residues. These residues are often located near the amino terminus of the peptide.

In patients with parenchymal liver disease, the vitamin K-dependent carboxylase reaction may be impaired (Atkinson et al., 1979; Blanchard et al., 1981; Malia et al., 1980). Corrigan et al. (1982) reported that since protein synthesis is also altered in liver disease, reduced levels of inactive precursor and functional prothrombin are present, irrespective of activity of the carboxylase system. They also observed reduced levels of prothrombin antigen in patients with substantial liver disease. The more severe the hepatocellular damage, the more severe the reduction in the antigen level. The authors suggest that monitoring the level of factor II antigen seems to offer a more sensitive method than the standard prothrombin time for early detection of recovery from severe hepatic necrosis and dysfunction.

Spontaneous hemorrhage or death has been associated with reduced factor II activity when it is less than 20% of normal (Deutsch, 1965; Tucker et al., 1973). When levels of the antigen are increased out of proportion to the clotting activity (normally coagulant activity closely approximates antigen, so the ratio of coagulant activity to antigen approaches unity), a secondary vitamin K deficiency is likely (Corrigan et al., 1982).

Parenchymal liver disease results in hypoprothrombinemia, because the utilization of vitamin K in the biosynthesis of vitamin K-dependent clotting factors is impaired. This usually results from destruction of the rough endoplasmic reticulum in the hepatocyte (Suttie and Olson, 1984). Diminished synthesis of bile salts by the diseased liver results in steatorrhea and reduced ability to emulsify and absorb fat-soluble vitamins, including vitamin K. The clinical manifestations of the blood clotting disorder associated with vitamin K deficiency include ecchymoses, hematoma, and hemorrhage (Mezey, 1983).

Malabsorption

In addition to malabsorption resulting from liver cirrhosis and biliary diseases, other gastrointestinal disorders (e.g., cystic fibrosis, sprue, celiac disease, ulcerative colitis, regional ileitis, ascaris infection, short-bowel syndrome) can lead to depression of vitamin K-dependent coagulation factors (Suttie and Olson, 1984). Since as much as half the vitamin K found in the adult liver is of the menaquinone (K_2) type (Reitz et al., 1970), which is synthesized by intestinal microflora, a decrease in intestinal production, especially if dietary intake of phylloquinones (K_1) is marginal can lead to problems. In early infancy, when intestinal synthesis is minimal (NRC, 1980), subjects are especially prone to vitamin K deficiency, which is exacerbated by antibiotic therapy for infantile diarrhea. Sulfa drugs, neomycin, and other broad-spectrum antibiotics can markedly decrease gut microflora and induce a hemorrhagic syndrome characteristic of vitamin K deficiency (Suttie and Olson, 1984). For example, apoplectic patients given neomycin and maintained on intravenous fluids deficient in vitamin K had lower than normal levels of clotting factors after 1 month (Frick et al., 1967).

Other drugs that affect vitamin K status include those such as coumarin, which suppresses synthesis of γ-carboxyglutamyl residues in vitamin K-dependent coagulation factors, or those that act indirectly by altering the effectiveness of such anticoagulants. The latter includes oxyphenbutazone, which enhances the effect of warfarin by displacing it from the albumin binding site, and barbiturates, which decrease the effect of warfarin by inducing hepatic inactivation (Young and Solomons, 1983). As pointed out above, high levels of vitamin E can also adversely affect vitamin K functions. This has been documented in laboratory animals—for example, chicks (March et al., 1973)—and in humans (Korsan-Bengsten et al., 1974). Vitamin K deficiency in patients taking megadoses of vitamin E (800 IU/day) has resulted in a hypersensitivity to the coumarin anticoagulants administered to patients (Corrigan and Marcus, 1974).

SUMMARY

The intake of carotenoid-rich foods is inversely associated with risk of lung cancers of the types associated with cigarette smoking. Persons who smoke cigarettes and rarely or never eat carotenoid-rich foods have an appreciably greater risk of lung cancer than do comparable cigarette smokers who usually eat one or more servings of such foods daily. However, the consumption of carotenoid-rich foods does not necessarily serve as a protective factor against lung cancer for persons who smoke. The magnitude of the relative risk of both of these factors has not yet been well characterized. Studies also suggest an inverse association between β-carotene in serum and risk of lung cancer, but the evidence does not yet permit a

conclusion that the association is with β-carotene specifically rather than some other carotenoid. In addition, intake of carotenoid-rich foods may be associated with a decreased risk of carcinomas at other sites—for example, the uterine cervix—but the data are inconclusive.

Neither intake of foods rich in preformed vitamin A nor serum concentrations of retinol appear to be associated with risk of cancer in humans, including cancer of the lung. However, the ability of retinoids to prevent, suppress, or retard some chemically induced cancers at sites such as the pancreas, prostate, lung, esophagus, and colon in animal models is well established.

Evidence regarding anticancer roles for other fat-soluble vitamins is not persuasive. Intake of vitamin E by itself has not been related to overall risk of cancer, but the combination of low serum levels of vitamin E and selenium may be related to increased risk of some cancers, such as breast and lung cancers. Results of animal studies have been inconsistent, and anticancer mechanisms for vitamin E have not been established.

Vitamin D influences bone mineralization by enhancing absorption of calcium from the intestinal tract and maintaining serum calcium concentrations. However, the exact mechanism by which this occurs is unknown. There is a higher incidence of osteomalacia among populations that avoid exposure to sunlight and such people often have low serum levels of vitamin D metabolites. The contribution of vitamin D deficiency to osteomalacia in the elderly is not known.

Vitamin K_2 is synthesized by intestinal microflora. A decrease in this synthesis, especially if dietary intake of vitamin K is low, can lead, for example, to vitamin K deficiency in infants. Vitamins K_1 and K_3 act at different metabolic sites and consequently their roles in the causation or prevention of cancer are not the same. Vitamin K status is affected by certain drugs such as sulfa drugs and other broad spectrum antibiotics. High levels of vitamin E can interfere with the clotting activity of vitamin K.

DIRECTIONS FOR RESEARCH

• More information is needed concerning the potential roles of specific carotenoids as putative chemopreventive agents for specific neoplasms in laboratory animals.

• Further studies, including clinical trials, should be conducted to examine the use of β-carotene in the prevention of cancers of the lung,

GI tract, and cervix. There is also a need for more observational studies on cancers of the GI and genitourinary systems.

- Much of the data on vitamin E are correlational, and anticancer mechanisms for vitamin E have not been definitively demonstrated. Therefore, animal studies are needed to elucidate the association between vitamin E and cancer.

- Research is needed to determine whether vitamin E deficiency in intact animals increases the risk of certain cancers, such as mammary tumors in mice, when combined with a high intake of polyunsaturated fat, and to define the optimal concentration of vitamin E in persons who increase their consumption of polyunsaturated fat.

- The relationship between selenium and α-tocopherol and their possible role in altering cancer risk in humans should be elucidated.

REFERENCES

Anderson, T.W., and D.B. Reid. 1974. A double-blind trial of vitamin E in angina pectoris. Am. J. Clin. Nutr. 27:1174–1178.

Atkinson, M., B.E.C. Nordin, and S. Sherlock. 1956. Malabsorption and bone disease in prolonged obstructive jaundice. Q. J. Med. 25:299–312.

Atkinson, P.M., M.C. Kew, A. Sayed, and B.A. Bradlow. 1979. The use of Dispholidus typus venom in elucidating the cause of a low prothrombin index. Clin. Lab. Haematol. 1:281–290.

Barboriak, J.J., A.Z. Ghatit, K.R. Shetty, and J.H. Kalbfleisch. 1982. Vitamin E supplements and plasma high-density lipoprotein cholesterol. Am. J. Clin. Pathol. 77:371–372.

Barragry, J.M., M.W. France, D. Corless, S.P. Gupta, S. Switala, B.J. Boucher, and R.D. Cohen. 1978. Intestinal cholecalciferol absorption in the elderly and in younger adults. Clin. Sci. Mol. Med. 55:213–220.

Beecher, G.R., and F. Khachik. 1984. Evaluation of vitamin A and carotenoid data in food composition tables. J. Natl. Cancer Inst. 73:1397–1404.

Bendich A., and S.S. Shapiro. 1986. Effect of beta-carotene and canthaxanthin on the immune responses of the rat. J. Nutr. 116:2254–2262.

Bieri, J.G., L. Corash, and V.S. Hubbard. 1983. Medical uses of vitamin E. N. Engl. J. Med. 308:1063–1071.

Bikle, D.D. 1985. Osteomalacia and rickets. Pp. 1425–1431 in J.B. Wyngaarden and L.H. Smith, Jr., eds. Cecil Textbook of Medicine, Vol. 2. Saunders, Philadelphia.

Binder, H.J., D.C. Herting, V. Hurst, S.C. Finch, and H.M. Spiro. 1965. Tocopherol deficiency in man. N. Engl. J. Med. 273:1289–1297.

Bjelke, E. 1974. Epidemiologic studies of cancer of the stomach, colon, and rectum; with special emphasis on the role of diet. Scand. J. Gastroenterol. 9:1–235.

Bjelke, E. 1975. Dietary vitamin A and human lung cancer. Int. J. Cancer 15:561–565.

Blanchard, R.A., B.C. Furie, M. Jorgensen, S.F. Kruger, and B. Furie. 1981. Acquired vitamin K-dependent carboxyla-

tion deficiency in liver disease. N. Engl. J. Med. 305:242–248.

Bollag, W. 1975. Prophylaxis of chemically induced epithelial tumors with an aromatic retinoid acid analog (RO 10-9359). Eur. J. Cancer 11:721–724.

Breitman, T.R., S.E. Selonick, and S.J. Collins. 1980. Induction of differentiation of the human promyelocytic leukemia cell line (HL-60) by retinoic acid. Proc. Natl. Acad. Sci. U.S.A. 77:2936–2940.

Caniggia, A., R. Nuti, M. Galli, F. Loré, V. Turchetti, and G.A. Righi. 1986. Effect of a long-term treatment with 1,25-dihydroxyvitamin D_3 on osteocalcin in postmenopausal osteoporosis. Calcif. Tissue Int. 38:328–332.

Carpenter, M.P. 1986. Effects of vitamin E on the immune system. Pp. 199–211 in F.L. Meyskens, Jr., and K.N. Prasad, eds. Vitamins and Cancer. Humana Press, Clifton, N.J.

Chlebowski, R.T., J.B. Block, M. Dietrich, E. Octay, N. Barth, R. Yanagihara, C. Gota, and I. Ali. 1983. Inhibition of human tumor growth and DNA biosynthetic activity by vitamin K and warfarin: in vitro and clinical results. Proc. Am. Assoc. Cancer Res. 24:165.

Chlebowski, R.T, M. Dietrich, S.A. Akman, and J.B. Block. 1984. Vitamin K_3 (menadione) inhibition of human tumor growth in the soft agar assay system. Proc. Annu. Meet. Am. Soc. Clin. Oncol. 3:93.

Christiansen, C., and P. Rødbro. 1984. Serum vitamin D metabolites in younger and elderly postmenopausal women. Calcif. Tissue Int. 36:19–24.

Colditz, G.A., L.G. Branch, R.J. Lipnick, W.C. Willett, B. Rosner, B.M. Posner, and C.H. Hennekens. 1985. Increased green and yellow vegetable intake and lowered cancer deaths in an elderly population. Am. J. Clin. Nutr. 41:32–36.

Constantinides, P., and M. Harkey. 1985. Initiation of a transplantable fibrosarcoma by the synergism of two non-initiators, alpha-tocopherol and soya oil. Virchows Arch. Pathol. Anat. 405:285–297.

Corrigan, J.J., Jr., and F.I. Marcus. 1974. Coagulopathy associated with vitamin E ingestion. J. Am. Med. Assoc. 230:1300–1301.

Corrigan, J.J., M. Jeter, and D.L. Earnest. 1982. Prothrombin antigen and coagulant activity in patients with liver disease. J. Am. Med. Assoc. 248:1736–1739.

Crilly, R.G., A. Horseman, M. Peacock, and B.E. Nordin. 1981. The vitamin D metabolites in the pathogenesis and management of osteoporosis. Curr. Med. Res. Opin. 7:337–348.

Davies, R.E. 1967. Effect of vitamin A on 7,12-dimethyl-benz(alpha)anthracene-induced papillomas in rhino mouse skin. Cancer Res. 27:237–241.

DeLuca, H.F. 1979. Vitamin D: Metabolism and Function. Monographs on Endocrinology, Vol. 13. Springer-Verlag, Berlin. 80 pp.

DeLuca, H.F. 1981. Recent advances in the metabolism of vitamin D. Annu. Rev. Physiol. 43:199–209.

DeLuca, H.F. 1988. The vitamin D story: a collaborative effort of basic science and clinical medicine. FASEB J. 2:224–236.

DeLuca, H.F., R.T. Franceschi, B.P. Halloran, and E.R. Massaro. 1982. Molecular events involved in 1,25-dihydroxyvitamin D_3 stimulation of intestinal calcium transport. Fed. Proc. 41:66–71.

Deutsch, E. 1965. Blood coagulation changes in liver disease. Prog. Liver Dis. 2:69–83.

DHHS/USDA (Department of Health and Human Services/ U.S. Department of Agriculture). 1986. Nutrition Monitoring in the United States—A Progress Report from the Joint Nutrition Monitoring Evaluation Committee. DHHS Publ. No. (PHS) 86-1255. National Center for Health Statistics, Public Health Service, U.S. Department of Health and Human Services, Hyattsville, Md. 356 pp.

Dimitrov, N.V. 1986. Beta-carotene: biological properties and applications. Pp. 167–202 in J. Bland, ed. 1986: A Year in Nutritional Medicine, 2nd ed. Keats Publishing, New Canaan, Conn.

Donegan, C.K., A.L. Messer, E.S. Orgain, and J.M. Ruffin. 1949. Negative results of tocopherol therapy in cardiovascular disease. Am. J. Med. Sci. 217:294–299.

Epstein, J.H. 1977a. Chemicals and photocarcinogenesis. Australas. J. Dermatol. 18:57–61.

Epstein, J.H. 1977b. Effects of beta-carotene on ultraviolet induced cancer formation in the hairless mouse skin. Photochem. Photobiol. 25:211–213.

Epstein, J.H., and D.A. Grenkin. 1981. Inhibition of ultraviolet-induced carcinogenesis by all-trans retinoic acid. J. Invest. Dermatol. 76:178–180.

Epstein, S.S., S. Joshi, J. Andrea, J. Forsyth, and N. Mantel. 1967. The null effect of antioxidants on the carcinogenicity of 3,4,9,10-dibenzpyrene to mice. Life Sci. 6:225–233.

Farrell, P.M. 1980. Deficiency states, pharmacological effects, and nutrient requirements. Pp. 520–620 in L.J. Machlin, ed. Vitamin E: A Comprehensive Treatise, Basic and Clinical Nutrition, Vol. 1. Marcel Dekker, New York.

Farrell, P.M., and J.G. Bieri. 1975. Megavitamin E supplementation in man. Am. J. Clin. Nutr. 28:1381–1386.

Fiddler, W., J.W. Pensabene, E.G. Piotrowski, J.G. Philips, J. Keating, W.J. Mergens, and H.L. Newmark. 1978. Inhibition of formation of volatile nitrosamines in fried bacon by the use of pure-solubilized alpha-tocopherol. J. Agric. Food Chem. 26:653–656.

Finkelman, R.D., and W.T. Butler. 1985. Vitamin D and skeletal tissues. J. Oral Pathol. 14:191–215.

Frick, P.G., G. Riedler, and H. Brögli. 1967. Dose response and minimal daily requirement for vitamin K in man. J. Appl. Physiol. 23:387–389.

Friedman, G.D., W.S. Blaner, D.S. Goodman, J.H. Vogelman, J.L. Brind, R. Hoover, B.H. Fireman, and N. Orentreich. 1986. Serum retinol and retinol-binding protein levels do not predict subsequent lung cancer. Am. J. Epidemiol. 123:781–789.

Gallagher, J.C., B.L. Riggs, J. Eisman, A. Hamstra, S.B. Arnaud, and H.F. DeLuca. 1979. Intestinal calcium absorption and serum vitamin D metabolites in normal subjects and osteoporotic patients: effect of age and dietary calcium. J. Clin. Invest. 64:729–736.

Gallagher, J.C., C.M. Jerpbak, W.S. Jee, K.A. Johnson, H.F. DeLuca, and B.L. Riggs. 1982. 1,25-Dihydroxy vitamin D_3: short- and long-term effects on bone and calcium metabolism in patients with postmenopausal osteoporosis. Proc. Natl. Acad. Sci. U.S.A. 79:3325–3329.

Goldsmith, R.S. 1984. Vitamin D and osteoporosis. Pp. 49–51 in Osteoporosis, NIH Consensus Development Conference, April 2–4, 1984. National Institute of Arthritis, Diabetes, and Digestive and Kidney Diseases and the Office of Medical Applications of Research, National Institutes of Health, Bethesda, Md.

Goodman, D.S. 1984. Vitamin A and retinoids in health and disease. N. Engl. J. Med. 310:1023–1031.

Graham, S. 1983. Results of case-control studies of diet and cancer in Buffalo, New York. Cancer Res. 43:2409s–2413s.

Graham, S., M. Levin, and A.M. Lilienfeld. 1960. The socioeconomic distribution of cancer of various sites in Buffalo, N.Y., 1948–1952. Cancer 13:180–191.

Graham, S., M.L. Levin, A.M. Lilienfeld, and P. Sheehe. 1963. Ethnic derivation as related to cancer at various sites. Cancer 16:13–27.

Graham, S., A.M. Lilienfeld, and J.E. Tidings. 1967. Dietary and purgation factors in the epidemiology of gastric cancer. Cancer 20:2224–2234.

Graham, S., H. Dayal, M. Swanson, A. Mittelman, and G. Wilkinson. 1978. Diet in the epidemiology of cancer of the colon and rectum. J. Natl. Cancer Inst. 61:709–714.

Graham, S., B. Haughey, J. Marshall, R. Priore, T. Rzepka, C. Mettlin, and J.E. Pontes. 1983. Diet in the epidemiology of carcinoma of the prostate gland. J. Natl. Cancer Inst. 70:687–692.

Gregor, A., P.N. Lee, F.J.C. Roe, M.J Wilson, and A. Melton. 1980. Comparison of dietary histories in lung cancer cases and controls with special reference to vitamin A. Nutr. Cancer 2:93–97.

Guggenheim, M.A., V. Jackson, J. Lilly, and A. Silverman. 1983. Vitamin E deficiency and neurologic disease in children with cholestasis: a prospective study. J. Pediatr. 102:577–579.

Haber, S.L., and R.W. Wissler. 1962. Effect of vitamin E on carcinogenicity of methyl cholanthrene. Proc. Soc. Exp. Biol. Med. 111:774–775.

Harju, E., E. Sotaniemi, J. Puranen, and R. Lahti. 1985. High incidence of low serum vitamin D concentration in patients with hip fracture. Arch. Orthop. Trauma Surg. 103:408–416.

Hassan, H., S.A. Hashim, T.B. VanItallie, and W.W. Sebrell. 1966. Syndrome in premature infants associated with low plasma vitamin E levels and high polyunsaturated fatty acid diet. Am. J. Clin. Nutr. 19:147–157.

Hayes, K.C. 1974. Pathophysiology of vitamin E deficiency in monkeys. Am. J. Clin. Nutr. 27:1130–1140.

Hermann, W.J., Jr., K. Ward, and J. Faucett. 1979. The effect of tocopherol on high-density lipoprotein cholesterol. A clinical observation. Am. J. Clin. Pathol. 72:848–852.

Heshmat, M.Y., L. Kaul, J. Kovi, M.A. Jackson, A.G. Jackson, G.W. Jones, M. Edson, J.P. Enterline, R.G. Worrell, and S.L. Perry. 1985. Nutrition and prostate cancer: a case control study. Prostate 6:7–17.

Hinds, M.W., L.N. Kolonel, J.H. Hankin, and J. Lee. 1984. Dietary vitamin A, carotene, vitamin C and risk of lung cancer in Hawaii. Am. J. Epidemiol. 119:227–237.

Hirayama, T. 1979. Diet and cancer. Nutr. Cancer 1:67–81.

Holick, M.F., and J.A. MacLaughlin. 1981. Aging significantly decreases the capacity of human epidermis to produce vitamin D_3. Clin. Res. 29:408A.

Holtrop, M.E., K.A. Cox, M.B. Clark, M.F. Holick, and C.S. Anast. 1981. 1,25-Dihydroxycholecalciferol stimulates osteoclasts in rat bones in the absence of parathyroid hormone. Endocrinology 108:2293–2301.

Horwitt, M.K. 1986. The promotion of vitamin E. J. Nutr. 116:1371–1377.

Isler, O., H. Gutmann, and U. Solms, eds. 1971. Carotenoids. Birkhäuser-Verlag, Basel. 932 pp.

Israels, L.G., G.A. Walls, D.J. Ollmann, E. Friesen, and E.D. Israels. 1983. Vitamin K as a regulator of benzo(a)pyrene metabolism, mutagenesis and carcinogenesis. J. Clin. Inv. 71:1130–1140.

Jaffe, W. 1946. Influence of wheat germ oil on production of tumors in rats by methylcholanthrene. Exp. Med. Surg. 4:278–282.

Johnson, L., D. Schaffer, and T.R. Boggs, Jr. 1974. The premature infant, vitamin E deficiency and retrolental fibroplasia. Am. J. Clin. Nutr. 27:1158–1173.

Kark, J.D., A.H. Smith, B.R. Switzer, and C.G. Hames. 1981. Serum vitamin A (retinol) and cancer incidence in Evans County, Georgia. J. Natl. Cancer Inst. 66:7–16.

Katrangi, N., L.A. Kaplan, and E.A. Stein. 1984. Separation and quantitation of serum beta-carotene and other carotenoids by high performance liquid chromatography. J. Lipid Res. 25:400–406.

Kolonel, L.N., J.H. Hankin, and C.N. Yoshizawa. 1987. Vitamin A and prostate cancer in elderly men: enhancement of risk. Cancer Res. 47:2982–2985.

Korsan-Bengsten, K., D. Elmfeldt, and T. Holm. 1974. Prolonged plasma clotting time and decreased fibrinolysis after long-term treatment with α-tocopherol. Thromb. Diath. Haemorrh. 31:505–512.

Kraft, D., G. Offermann, and R. Steldinger. 1979. Effect of dihydroxylated vitamin D metabolites on experimental rickets. Pp. 431–434 in A.W. Norman, K. Schaefer, D.V. Herrath, H.G. Grigoleit, J.W. Coburn, H.F. DeLuca, E.B.Mawer, and T. Suda, eds. Vitamin D: Basic Research and Its Clinical Application. Walter de Gruyter, New York.

Kream, B.E., M. Jose, S. Tamada, and H.F. De Luca. 1977. A specific high-affinity binding macromolecule for 1,25-dihydroxyvitamin D_3 in fetal bone. Science 197:1086–1088.

Kvåle, G., E. Bjelke, and J.J. Gart. 1983. Dietary habits and lung cancer risk. Int. J. Cancer 31:397–405.

La Vecchia, C., A. Decarli, M. Fasoli, F. Parazzini, S. Franceschi, A. Gentile, and E. Negri. 1988. Dietary vitamin A and the risk of intraepithelial and invasive cervical neoplasia. Gynecol. Oncol. 30:187–195.

Levij, I.S., and A. Polliack. 1968. Potentiating effect of vitamin A on 9-10 dimethyl 1-2 benzathracene—carcinogenesis in the hamster cheek pouch. Cancer 22:300–306.

Lindholm, T.S., O.S. Nilsson, and S. Eriksson. 1981. Effect of 1α-hydroxycholecalciferol on bone mass and composition of cortical bone in adult male rats. Isr. J. Med. Sci. 17:416–421.

Lukert, B.P., M. Carey, B. McCarty, S. Tiemann, L. Goodnight, M. Helm, R. Hassanein, C. Stevenson, M. Stoskopf, and L. Doolan. 1987. Influence of nutritional factors on calcium-regulating hormones and bone loss. Calcif. Tissue Int. 40:119–125.

MacLaughlin, J., and M.F. Holick. 1985. Aging decreases the capacity of human skin to produce vitamin D_3. J. Clin. Invest. 76:1536–1538.

MacLennan, R., J. Da Costa, N.E. Day, C.H. Law, Y.K. Ng., and K. Shanmugaratnam. 1977. Risk factors for lung cancer in Singapore Chinese, a population with high female incidence rates. Int. J. Cancer 20:854–860.

Makinson, D.H., S. Oleesky, and R.V. Stone. 1948. Vitamin E in angina pectoris. Lancet 1:102.

Malia, R.G., F.E. Preston, and C.D. Holdsworth. 1980. Clinical responses to vitamin K_1. Pp. 342–347 in J.W. Suttie, ed. Vitamin K Metabolism and Vitamin K-Dependent Proteins. University Park Press, Baltimore.

March, B.E., E. Wong, L. Seier, J. Sim, and J. Biely. 1973. Hypervitaminosis E in the chick. J. Nutr. 103:371–377.

Marshall, J.R., S. Graham, T. Byers, M. Swanson, and J. Brasure. 1983. Diet and smoking in the epidemiology of cancer of the cervix. J. Natl. Cancer Inst. 70:847–851.

Mathews-Roth, M.M. 1982. Antitumor activity of beta-carotene, canthaxanthin and phytoene. Oncology 39:33–37.

Mathews-Roth, M.M., and N.I. Krinsky. 1984. Effect of dietary fat level on UV-B induced skin tumors, and anti-tumor action of beta-carotene. Photochem. Photobiol. 40:671–673.

McCormick, D.L., F.J. Burns, and R.E. Albert. 1980. Inhibition of rat mammary carcinogenesis by short dietary exposure to retinyl acetate. Cancer Res. 40:1140–1143.

Menkes, M., and G. Comstock. 1984. Vitamins A and E and lung cancer. Am. J. Epidemiol. 120:491.

Menkes, M.S., G.W. Comstock, J.P. Vuilleumier, K. Helsing, A.A. Rider, and R. Brookmeyer. 1986. Serum beta-carotene, vitamins A and E, selenium, and the risk of lung cancer. N. Engl. J. Med. 315:1250–1254.

Mergens, W.J., J.J. Kamm, H.L. Newmark, W. Fiddler, and J. Pensabene. 1978. Alpha-tocopherol: uses in preventing nitrosamine formation. IARC Sci. Publ. 19:199–212.

Mettlin, C., and S. Graham. 1979. Dietary risk factors in human bladder cancer. Am. J. Epidemiol. 110:255–263.

Mettlin, C., S. Graham, and M. Swanson. 1979. Vitamin A and lung cancer. J. Natl. Cancer Inst. 62:1435–1438.

Mezey, E. 1983. Liver and biliary system. Pp. 13.1–13.18 in D.M. Paige, ed. Manual of Clinical Nutrition. Nutrition Publications, Pleasantville, N.J.

Modan B., H. Cuckle, and F. Lubin. 1981. A note on the role of dietary retinol and carotene in human gastro-intestinal cancer. Int. J. Cancer 28:421–424.

Moon, R.C., and L.M. Itri. 1984. Retinoids and cancer. Pp. 327–371 in M.B. Sporn, A.B. Roberts, and D.S. Goodman, eds. The Retinoids, Vol. 2. Academic Press, New York.

Moon, R.C., C. Grubbs, N. Sporn, and D. Goodman. 1977. Retinyl acetate inhibits mammary carcinogenesis induced by N-methyl-N-nitrosourea. Nature 267:620–621.

Muller, D.P.R., J.K. Lloyd, and O.H. Wolff. 1983. Vitamin E and neurological function. Lancet 1:225–228.

Nettesheim, P. 1980. Inhibition of carcinogenesis by retinoids. Can. Med. Assoc. J. 122:757–765.

Neville, H.E., S.P. Ringel, M.A. Guggenheim, C.A. Wehling, and J.M. Starcevich. 1983. Ultrastructural and histochemical abnormalities of skeletal muscle in patients with chronic vitamin E deficiency. Neurology 33:483–488.

Nicolaysen, R., and N. Eeg-Larsen. 1953. The biochemistry and physiology of vitamin D. Vitam. Horm. 11:29–60.

Nomura, A.M.Y., G.N. Stemmermann, L.K. Heilbrun, R.M. Salkeld, and J.P. Vuilleumier. 1985. Serum vitamin levels and the risk of cancer of specific sites in men of Japanese ancestry in Hawaii. Cancer Res. 45:2369–2372.

Nordin, B.E.C., M. Peacock, R.G. Crilly, G. Taylor, and D.H. Marshall. 1979. Plasma 25-hydroxy and 1,25-dihydroxy vitamin D levels and calcium absorption in postmenopausal women. Pp. 363–373 in I. MacIntyre and M. Szelke, eds. Molecular Endocrinology. Elsevier/North-Holland, Amsterdam.

NRC (National Research Council). 1980. Recommended Dietary Allowances, 9th ed. Report of the Committee on Dietary Allowances, Food and Nutrition Board, Division of Biological Sciences, Assembly of Life Sciences. National Academy Press, Washington, D.C. 185 pp.

NRC (National Research Council). 1982. Diet, Nutrition, and Cancer. Report of the Committee on Diet, Nutrition, and Cancer, Food and Nutrition Board, Commission on Life Sciences. National Academy Press, Washington, D.C. 478 pp.

Odukoya, O., F. Hawach, and G. Shklar. 1984. Retardation

of experimental oral cancer by topical vitamin E. Nutr. Cancer 6:98–104.

Olson, J.A. 1983. Formation and function of vitamin A. Pp. 371–412 in J.W. Porter, ed. Polyisoprenoid Synthesis, Vol. II. Wiley, New York.

Olson, J.A. 1984. Vitamin A. Pp. 1–43 in L.J. Machlin, ed. Handbook of Vitamins: Nutritional, Biochemical, and Clinical Aspects. Marcel Dekker, New York.

Omdahl, J.L., P.J. Garry, L.A. Hunsaker, W.C. Hunt, and J.S. Goodwin. 1982. Nutritional status in a healthy elderly population: vitamin D. Am. J. Clin. Nutr. 36:1225–1233.

Oski, F.A., and L.A. Barness. 1967. Vitamin E deficiency: a previously unrecognized cause of hemolytic anemia in the premature infant. J. Pediatr. 70:211–220.

Parfitt, A.M., J.C. Gallagher, R.P. Heaney, C.C. Johnston, R. Neer, and G.D. Whedon. 1982. Vitamin D and bone health in the elderly. Am. J. Clin. Nutr. 36:1014–1031.

Pauling, L., R. Willoughby, R. Reynolds, B.E. Blaisdell, and S. Lawson. 1982. Incidence of squamous cell carcinoma in hairless mice irradiated with ultraviolet light in relation to intake of ascorbic acid (vitamin C) and of D,L-alpha-tocopheryl acetate (vitamin E). Int. Z. Vitam. Ernährungsforsch. 23:53–82.

Peleg, I., S. Heyden, M. Knowles, and C.G. Hames. 1984. Serum retinol and risk of subsequent cancer: extension of the Evans County, Georgia, study. J. Natl. Cancer Inst. 73:1455–1458.

Peto, R., R. Doll, J.D. Buckley, and M.B. Sporn. 1981. Can dietary beta-carotene materially reduce human cancer rates? Nature 290:201–208.

Phelps, D.L. 1984. E-Ferol: what happened and what now? Pediatrics 74:1114–1116.

Raisz, L.G., and A. Johannesson. 1984. Pathogenesis, prevention and therapy of osteoporosis. J. Med. 15:267–278.

Reitz, P., U. Gloor, and O. Wiss. 1970. Menaquinones from human liver and sludge. Int. Z. Vitaminforsch. 40:351–362.

Riggs, B.L., J.C. Gallagher, and H.F. DeLuca. 1979. Osteoporosis and age-related osteopenia: evaluation of possible role of vitamin D endocrine system in pathogenesis of impaired intestinal calcium absorption. Pp. 107–113 in A.W. Norman, K. Schaefer, D.V. Herrath, H.G. Grigoleit, J.W.Coburn, H.F. DeLuca, E.B. Mawer, and T. Suda, eds. Vitamin D: Basic Research and Its Clinical Application. Walter de Gruyter, New York.

Riggs, B.L., H.W. Wahner, E. Seeman, K.P. Offord, W.L. Dunn, R.B. Mazess, K.A. Johnson, and L.J. Melton III. 1982. Changes in bone mineral density of the proximal femur and spine with aging. J. Clin. Invest. 70:716–723.

Rinzler, S.H., H. Bakst, Z.H. Benjamin, A.L. Bobb, and J. Travell. 1950. Failure of alpha tocopherol to influence chest pain in patients with heart disease. Circulation 1:288–293.

Roberts, A.B., and M.B. Sporn. 1984. Cellular biology and biochemistry of the retinoids. Pp. 209–286 in M.B. Sporn, A.B. Roberts, and D.S. Goodman, eds. The Retinoids, Vol. 2. Academic Press, New York.

Rock, W.A., Jr. 1984. Laboratory assessment of coagulation disorders in liver disease. Clin. Lab. Med. 4:419–442.

Russell-Briefel, R., M.W. Bates, and L.H. Kuller. 1985. The relationship of plasma carotenoids to health and biochemical factors in middle-aged men. Am. J. Epidemiol. 122:741–749.

Saffiotti, U., R. Montesano, A.R. Sellakumar, and S.A. Borg. 1967. Experimental cancer of the lung. Inhibition by vitamin A of the induction of tracheobronchial squamous metaplasia and squamous cell tumors. Cancer 20:857–864.

Salonen, J.T., R. Salonen, R. Lappeteläinen, P.H. Mäenpää, G. Alfthan, and P. Puska. 1985. Risk of cancer in relation to serum concentrations of selenium and vitamins A and E: matched case-control analysis of prospective data. Br. Med. J. 290:417–420.

Samet, J.M., B.J. Skipper, C.G. Humble, and D.P. Pathak. 1985. Lung cancer risk and vitamin A consumption in New Mexico. Am. Rev. Respir. Dis. 131:198–202.

Santamaria L., A. Bianchi, A. Arnaboldi, L. Andreoni, and P. Bermond. 1983. Dietary carotenoids block photocarcinogenic enhancement by benzo(a)pyrene and inhibit its carcinogenesis in the dark. Experientia 39:1043–1045.

Schmähl, D., and M. Habs. 1978. Experiments on the influence of an aromatic retinoid on the chemical carcinogenesis in rats by butyl-butanol-nitrosamine and 1,2-dimethylhydrazine. Arzneim. Forsch. 28:49–51.

Seifter, E., G. Rettura, J. Padawer, and S.M. Levenson. 1982. Moloney murine sarcoma virus tumors in CBA/J mice: chemopreventive and chemotherapeutic actions of supplemental beta-carotene. J. Natl. Cancer Inst. 68:835–840.

Sevastikoglou, J.A., V.T. Thomaidis, and T.S. Lindholm. 1977. Reversibility of osteoporosis induced in adult rats by calcium deficiency. Long- and short-term observations. Calcif. Tissue Res. 22:260–265.

Shamberger, R.J. 1970. Relationship of selenium to cancer. I. Inhibitory effect of selenium on carcinogenesis. J. Natl. Cancer Inst. 44:931–936.

Shekelle, R.B., M. Lepper, S. Liu, C. Maliza, W.J. Raynor, Jr., A.H. Rossof, O. Paul, A.M. Shryock, and J. Stamler. 1981. Dietary vitamin A and risk of cancer in the Western Electric study. Lancet 2:1186–1190.

Shklar, G. 1982. Oral mucosal carcinogenesis in hamsters: inhibition by vitamin E. J. Natl. Cancer Inst. 68:791–797.

Shklar, G., E. Flynn, G. Szabo, and P. Marefat. 1980. Retinoid inhibition of experimental lingual carcinogenesis: ultrastructural observations. J. Natl. Cancer Inst. 65:1307–1316.

Slaga, T.J., and W.M. Bracken. 1977. The effects of antioxidants on skin tumor initiation and aryl hydrocarbon hydroxylase. Cancer Res. 37:1631–1635.

Slater, G.E., and K.F. Swaiman. 1977. Muscular dystrophies of childhood. Pediatr. Ann. 6:170–193.

Smith, D.M., A.E. Rogers, and P.M. Newberne. 1975a. Vitamin A and benzo(a)pyrene carcinogenesis in the respiratory tract of hamsters fed a semisynthetic diet. Cancer Res. 35:1485–1488.

Smith, D.M., A.E. Rogers, B.J. Herndon, and P.M. Newberne. 1975b. Vitamin A (retinyl acetate) and benzo(alpha)pyrene-induced respiratory tract carcinogenesis in hamsters fed a commercial diet. Cancer Res. 35:11–16.

Smith, P.G., and H. Jick. 1978. Cancers among users of preparations containing vitamin A: a case-control investigation. Cancer 808–811.

Sokol, R.J., M.A. Guggenheim, J.E. Heubi, S.T. Iannaccone, N. Butler-Simon, V. Jackson, C. Miller, M. Cheney, W.F. Balistreri, and A. Silverman. 1985. Frequency and clinical progression of the vitamin E deficiency neurologic disorder in children with prolonged neonatal cholestasis. Am. J. Dis. Child. 139:1211–1215.

Sommer, A. 1982. Nutritional blindness: xerophthalmia and keratomalacia. Oxford University Press, New York. 282 pp.

Sporn, M.B., and D.L. Newton. 1979. Chemoprevention of cancer with retinoids. Fed. Proc. 38:2528–2534.

Sporn, M.B., and D.L. Newton. 1981. Retinoids and chemoprevention of cancer. Pp. 71–100 in M.S. Zedeck and M.

Lipkin, eds. Inhibition of Tumor Induction and Development. Plenum Press, New York.

Sporn, M.B., and A.B. Roberts. 1983. Role of retinoids in differentiation and carcinogenesis. Cancer Res. 43:3034–3040.

Sporn, M.B., and A.B. Roberts. 1984. Biological methods for analysis and assay of retinoids—relationships between structure and activity. Pp. 235–279 in M.B. Sporn, A.B. Roberts, and D.S. Goodman, eds. The Retinoids, Vol. 1. Academic Press, New York.

Stähelin, H.B., F. Rösel, E. Buess, and G. Brubacher. 1984. Cancer, vitamins, and plasma lipids: Prospective Basal Study. J. Natl. Cancer. Inst. 73:1463–1468.

Stampfer, M.J., W. Willett, W.P. Castelli, J.O. Taylor, J. Fine, and C.H. Hennekens. 1983. Effect of vitamin E on lipids. Am. J. Clin. Pathol. 79:714–716.

Stehr, P.A., M.F. Gloninger, L.H. Kuller, G.M. Marsh, E.P. Radford, and G.B. Weinberg. 1985. Dietary vitamin A deficiencies and stomach cancer. Am. J. Epidemiol. 121:65–70.

Stich, H.F., M.P. Rosin, and M.O. Vallejera. 1984. Reduction with vitamin A and beta-carotene administration of proportion of micronucleated buccal mucosal cells in Asian betel nut and tobacco chewers. Lancet 1:1204–1206.

Strickland, S., and V. Mahdavi. 1978. The induction of differentiation in teratocarcinoma stem cells by retinoic acid. Cell 15:393–403.

Suttie, J.W., and R.E. Olson. 1984. Vitamin K. Pp. 241–259 in Present Knowledge in Nutrition, 5th ed. The Nutrition Foundation, Washington, D.C.

Sutton, R.A.L., C.A. Harris, N.L.M. Wong, and J.H. Dirks. 1977. Effects of vitamin D on renal tubular calcium transport. Pp. 451–453 in A.W. Norman, K. Schaefer, J.W. Coburn, H.F. DeLuca, D. Fraser, H.G. Grigoleit, and D.V. Herrath, eds. Vitamin D: Biochemical, Chemical and Clinical Aspects Related to Calcium Metabolism. Walter de Gruyter, Berlin.

Tomita, Y. 1983. Immunological role of vitamin A and its related substances in prevention of cancer. Nutr. Cancer 5:187–194.

Tsai, A.C., J.J. Kelly, B. Peng, and N. Cook. 1978. Study on the effect of megavitamin E supplementation in man. Am. J. Clin. Nutr. 31:831–837.

Tsai, K.S., H. Heath III, R. Kumar, and B.L. Riggs. 1984. Impaired vitamin D metabolism with aging in women: possible role in pathogenesis of senile osteoporosis. J. Clin. Invest. 73:1668–1672.

Tsai, K.S., H.W. Wahner, K.P. Offord, L.J. Melton III, R. Kumar, and B.L. Riggs. 1987. Effect of aging on vitamin D stores and bone density in women. Calcif. Tissue Int. 40:241–243.

Tucker, J.S., I.L. Woolf, B.E. Boyes, J.M. Thomson, L. Poller, and I.W. Dymock. 1973. Coagulation studies in acute hepatic failure. Gut 14:418.

Underwood, B.A. 1984. Vitamin A in animal and human nutrition. Pp. 281–392 in M.B. Sporn, A.B. Roberts, and D.S. Goodman, eds. The Retinoids, Vol. 1. Academic Press, New York.

Underwood, J.L., and H. DeLuca. 1984. Vitamin D is not directly necessary for bone growth and mineralization. Am. J. Physiol. 246:E493-E498.

USDA (U.S. Department of Agriculture). 1987. Nationwide Food Consumption Survey. Continuing Survey of Food Intakes by Individuals. Women 19–50 Years and Their Children 1–5 Years, 4 Days, 1985. Report No. 85–4. Nutrition Monitoring Division, Human Nutrition Information Service, U.S. Department of Agriculture, Hyattsville, Md. 182 pp.

Vogelsang A., and E.V. Shute. 1946. Effect of vitamin E in coronary heart disease. Nature (London) 157:772.

Wald, N., M. Idle, J. Boreham, and A. Bailey. 1980. Low serum-vitamin-A and subsequent risk of cancer. Preliminary results of a prospective study. Lancet 2:813–815.

Wald, N.J., J. Boreham, J.L. Hayward, and R.D. Bulbrook. 1984. Plasma retinol, beta-carotene and vitamin E levels in relation to the future risk of breast cancer. Br. J. Cancer 49:321–324.

Ward, J.M., M.B. Sporn, M.L. Wenk, J.M. Smith, D. Feeser, and R.J. Dean. 1978. Dose response to intrarectal administration of N-methyl-N-nitrosourea and histopathologic evaluation of the effect of two retinoids on colon lesions induced in rats. J. Natl. Cancer Inst. 60:1489–1493.

Wasserman, R.H., and J.J. Feher. 1977. Vitamin D-dependent calcium-binding proteins. Pp. 291–302 in R.H. Wasserman, R.A. Corradino, E. Carafoli, R.H. Kretsinger, D.H. MacLennan, and F.L. Siegel, eds. Calcium-Binding Proteins and Calcium Function. Elsevier/North-Holland, Amsterdam.

Watson, R.R. 1986. Retinoids and vitamin E: modulators of immune functions and cancer resistance. Pp. 439–451 in F.L. Meyskens, Jr., and K.N. Prasad, eds. Vitamins and Cancer. Humana Press, Clifton, N.J.

Weinstein, R.S., J.L. Underwood, M.S. Hutson, and H.F. DeLuca. 1984. Bone histomorphometry in vitamin D-deficient rats infused with calcium and phosphorus. Am. J. Physiol. 246:E499-E505.

Welsch, C.W., M. Goodrich-Smith, C.K. Brown, and N. Crowe. 1981. Enhancement by retinyl acetate of hormone-induced mammary tumorigenesis in female GR/A mice. J. Natl. Cancer Inst. 67:935–938.

Willett, W.C., and B. MacMahon. 1984. Diet and cancer—an overview. N. Engl. J. Med. 310:633–638.

Willett, W.C., B.F. Polk, J.S. Morris, M.J. Stampfer, S. Pressel, B. Rosner, J.O. Taylor, K. Schneider, and C.G. Hames. 1983. Prediagnostic serum selenium and risk of cancer. Lancet 2:130–136.

Willett, W.C., B.F. Polk, B.A. Underwood, M.J. Stampfer, S. Pressel, B.Rosner, J.O. Taylor, K. Schneider, and C.G. Hames. 1984. Relation of serum vitamins A and E and carotenoids to the risk of cancer. N. Engl. J. Med. 310:430–434.

Wolbach, S.B., and P.R. Howe. 1925. Tissue changes following deprivation of fat-soluble A vitamin. J. Exp. Med. 42:753–777.

Wylie-Rosett, J.A., S.L. Romney, N.S. Slagle, S. Wassertheil-Smoller, G.L. Miller, P.R. Palan, D.J. Lucido, and C. Duttagupta. 1984. Influence of vitamin A on cervical dysplasia and carcinoma in situ. Nutr. Cancer 6:49–57.

Yang, C.S., Y. Sun, Q. Yang, K.W. Miller, G. Li, S.F. Zheng, A.G. Ershow, W.J. Blot, and J. Li. 1984. Vitamin A and other deficiencies in Linxian, a high esophageal cancer incidence area in northern China. J. Natl. Cancer Inst. 73:1449–1453.

Young, V.R., and N.W. Solomons. 1983. Nonnutrient factors in metabolism. Pp. 3.1–3.13 in D.M. Paige, ed. Manual of Clinical Nutrition. Nutrition Publications, Pleasantville, N.J.

Ziegler, R.G., T.J. Mason, A. Stemhagen, R. Hoover, J.B. Schoenberg, G. Gridley, P.W. Virgo, R. Altman, and J.F. Fraumeni, Jr. 1984. Dietary carotene and vitamin A and risk of lung cancer among white men in New Jersey. J. Natl. Cancer Inst. 73:1429–1435.

12

Water-Soluble Vitamins

The water-soluble vitamins include ascorbic acid (vitamin C), thiamin, riboflavin, niacin, vitamin B_6 (pyridoxine, pyridoxal, and pyridoxamine), folacin, vitamin B_{12}, biotin, and pantothenic acid.

DIETARY SOURCES, PATTERNS OF INTAKE, AND LEVELS OF WATER-SOLUBLE VITAMINS

Vitamin C

Vitamin C is active in the body either as L-ascorbic acid or as dehydroascorbic acid. Its best-known function is as a cofactor for the enzyme required to hydroxylate prolyl and lysyl residues for the synthesis of connective tissue proteins. The 1980 Recommended Dietary Allowance (RDA) for adults—60 mg/day—maintains a body pool of 1.5 g, whereas 10 mg/day is sufficient to prevent or cure scurvy (NRC, 1980).

Since the beginning of the century, the amount of vitamin C in the food supply has increased, partly because of the greater supplies of citrus fruits and dark-green vegetables and partly because of the fortification of some foods. According to the U.S. Department of Agriculture's Continuing Survey of Food Intakes of Individuals (CSFII) in 1985 (USDA, 1987), the mean vitamin C intake for children 1 to 5 years of age was 187% of the RDA, and for women 19 to 50 years of age, it was 125% of the

RDA, based on 4 nonconsecutive days of intake. For men 19 to 50 years of age, the mean intake was 207% of the RDA (USDA, 1986), based on a 1-day intake.

NHANES II—the National Health and Nutrition Examination Survey, conducted from 1976 to 1980—indicated that 3% of the respondents 3 to 74 years of age had low serum vitamin C levels. Therefore, the Joint Nutrition Monitoring Evaluation Committee concluded that this vitamin should be accorded high-priority status for future monitoring (DHHS–USDA, 1986).

The Nationwide Food Consumption Survey (NFCS) of 1977–1978 indicated that 73% of the vitamin C intake came from fruits and vegetables. Mean intakes of vegetables and fruits were decidedly less for women and children under 131% of the poverty level on the basis of 4 nonconsecutive days of intake in 1985 (USDA, 1987).

The highest levels of vitamin C are found in green peppers, broccoli, citrus fruits, strawberries, melons, tomatoes, raw cabbage, and leafy greens such as spinach, turnip, and mustard greens. Losses of vitamin C occur when foods are cooked in large amounts of water, exposed to extensive heating, or exposed to air.

Thiamin

Thiamin functions in the body in the form of thiamin pyrophosphate (TPP), the coenzyme for the transfer of active aldehyde in carbohydrate metabolism and decarboxylation of α-keto acids such as pyruvate. The requirement for thiamin is directly correlated with carbohydrate intake and increases as the metabolic rate increases due to pregnancy, lactation, or increased physical exercise. The 1980 RDA of 0.5 mg/1,000 kcal was set to maintain normal levels of TPP-dependent erythrocyte transketolase activity and urinary excretion. For those whose total caloric intake is less than 2,000 kcal, at least 1.0 mg/day is recommended.

NFCS data for 1977–1978 indicate that 83% of all respondents consumed 70% or more of the thiamin RDA (USDA, 1984). Men and women 19 to 50 years of age in the 1985 survey averaged 0.70 mg/1,000 kcal, whereas children 1 to 5 years old averaged 0.79 mg/1,000 kcal (USDA, 1986, 1987).

Riboflavin

In its coenzyme forms (flavin mononucleotide and flavin adenine dinucleotide), riboflavin functions in oxidation-reduction reactions in energy production, in the respiratory chain, and in many other metabolic pathways. Richest food sources of riboflavin include liver, milk, dark-green leafy vegetables, and enriched breads and cereals.

The 1980 RDA for riboflavin is 0.6 mg/1,000 kcal; a minimum of 1.2 mg/day is recommended for those whose caloric intake is less than 2,000 kcal/day. In 1985 the mean intake for men and women 19 to 50 years of age was 0.82 mg/1,000 kcal and 0.88 mg/1,000 kcal, respectively (USDA, 1986, 1987); for children 1 to 5 years of age, it was 1.12 mg/1,000 kcal (USDA, 1987). Food groups contributing the most riboflavin to diets of women and children in the 1985 and 1986 surveys were enriched grain products, milk and milk products, meat, poultry, and fish.

Niacin

In nutrition literature, the term niacin is used generically to encompass the active forms of this vitamin, nicotinic acid and nicotinamide; however, estimates of niacin requirements take into account preformed niacin as well as that obtained as equivalent (NE) in the body from tryptophan metabolism. For this purpose, it is estimated that when 60 mg of tryptophan are consumed by an adult, enough is oxidized to produce 1 mg of niacin (NRC, 1980).

Hundreds of enzymes in the body require niacin in its coenzyme forms nicotinamide adenine dinucleotide (NAD) and nicotinamide adenine dinucleotide phosphate (NADP). Many reactions utilizing these enzymes are involved in energy metabolism. Hence, the 1980 RDA is set at 6.6 niacin equivalents (NE) per 1,000 kcal, and an intake of not less than 13 NE is recommended when the caloric intake is less than 2,000 kcal. One NE is equal to either 1 mg of niacin or 60 mg of tryptophan.

The 1985 CSFII indicated that the mean intake of preformed niacin for women (USDA, 1987) and men (USDA, 1986) 19 to 50 years was 10.8 NE/1,000 kcal, whereas for children 1 to 5 years it was 9.6 (USDA, 1987). Average diets in the United States have been estimated to furnish 500 to 1,000 mg or more of tryptophan per day, providing 8 to 17 NE (NRC, 1980). Grain products, meat, poultry, and fish were the most important sources of preformed niacin reported in the 1985 and 1986 CSFII; nuts and legumes were identified as good sources.

Vitamin B_6

Vitamin B_6 is the generic term used for pyridoxine, pyridoxal, and pyridoxamine, the coenzyme forms of which are pyridoxal phosphate and pyridoxamine phosphate. Vitamin B_6-dependent enzymes are needed in a wide range of reactions, most of which involve amino acid metabolism. The 1980 RDAs were based on a ratio of 0.02 mg of vitamin B_6 per gram of protein consumed. The allowance for adult females was therefore set at 2.0 mg/day, assuming a protein intake of 100 g/day; for adult males, it was set at 2.2 mg/day, assuming a protein intake of 110 g/day. A lower allowance presumably would be appropriate for those with lower protein intakes.

A major difficulty in assessing vitamin B_6 intake is that values for the B_6 content of food are unreliable. In the 1977–1978 NFCS, on the 3 days studied, 72% of the respondents consumed at least 80% of the desired ratio of vitamin B_6 to protein, whereas only 39% had at least 80% of the vitamin B_6 RDA. The 1985 CSFII indicated that on the 1 day surveyed, men 19 to 50 years of age on average consumed 85% of the B_6 RDA, but that only 27% of women consumed 70% or more of their B_6 RDA (USDA, 1986, 1987). However, the mean ratio of vitamin B_6 to protein was 0.019 for women, despite the fact that 43% of them consumed less than 50% of the RDA (USDA, 1987). Failure to meet the RDA does not denote a deficient diet because actual requirements differ in a population (see Chapter 3). Women in lower income groups had lower intakes of vitamin B_6 than did those of higher income brackets. The major food sources of vitamin B_6 in those surveys were meats, poultry, fish, grain products, fruits, and vegetables. More research is needed on the adequacy of vitamin B_6 intake and the nutritional status of the population for this vitamin (DHHS–USDA, 1986).

Vitamin B_{12}

Vitamin B_{12} substances are physiologically active cobalamins. The coenzyme (5'-deoxyadenosyl) and methyl forms of this vitamin are essential for the recyling of the active folate coenzyme, for the methylation of homocysteine to form methionine, and for metabolism of propionate. Vitamin B_{12} is also essential in the metabolism of fatty acids and aliphatic amino acids through its role in the isomerization of methylmalonyl-CoA to succinyl-CoA.

Vitamin B_{12} is synthesized by bacteria and is found only in animal foods such as meats, milk and milk products, and eggs. The 1980 RDA is 3 μg/day for individuals 7 years of age and older. National surveys indicate that intakes are higher for males than for females and higher for those in higher economic groups. The 1985 CSFII indicated that 60% of women 19 to 50 years of age consumed 100% of the RDA or more (USDA, 1987).

Folacin (Folic Acid or Folate)

Folacin intakes have been studied very little, because values for this vitamin in food composition tables are imputed. In addition, present analytical methods for this vitamin are not very reliable. There is also some concern that the 1980 RDA for folacin is unrealistically high (DHHS–USDA, 1986).

Folacin coenzymes are essential in the body for the transfer of single carbon units. They are needed for the synthesis of purine, methionine, and thymidylate, for the catabolism of histidine, and for the conversion of serine to glycine. The metabolism of folacin and vitamin B_{12} is linked because normal activity of methyl vitamin B_{12} is needed to maintain the metabolically active form of folacin.

The 1980 RDA was set at 400 μg/day for persons 11 years of age and older. The first national survey to report folacin intakes was CSFII in 1985. Women 19 to 50 years of age had average intakes of 189 μg/day (USDA, 1987), whereas intakes for men 19 to 50

years of age averaged 305 μg/day (USDA, 1986). On the basis of limited data, women 20 to 44 years of age were reported in NHANES II to be at greatest risk for folacin deficiency (Senti and Pilch, 1984).

The Joint Nutrition Monitoring Evaluation Committee accorded high priority to monitoring the status of vitamin C, because of some low serum values reported in NHANES II and concluded that thiamin, riboflavin, and niacin warrant continued monitoring. That committee also recommended further investigation of the relationship between dietary intakes and nutritional status for both vitamin B_6 and folacin (DHHS–USDA, 1986).

Following is the evidence relating water-soluble vitamins to chronic diseases.

EVIDENCE ASSOCIATING WATER-SOLUBLE VITAMINS WITH CHRONIC DISEASES

Vitamin C

Cancer

Human Studies

In epidemiologic studies, the association of vitamin C with cancer is mostly indirect, since it is based on the consumption of foods known to contain high or low concentrations of the vitamin rather than on measured ingestion of ascorbic acid.

Meinsma (1964) noted that the consumption of citrus fruits by persons with gastric cancer was lower than that by controls. Similar inverse associations between fresh fruit consumption or vitamin C intake and gastric cancer were reported by Bjelke (1978), Higginson (1966), Haenszel and Correa (1975), and Kolonel et al. (1981). In a case-control study of stomach cancer conducted in Canada, Risch et al. (1985) found that citrus fruit intake was somewhat protective (odds ratio 0.75 per 100 g daily average intake). In a univariate analysis, vitamin C intake was significantly ($p = .0056$) protective against stomach cancer. Risch and colleagues analyzed vitamin C intake from 21 common vegetables along with the intake of nitrate and found that vitamin C consumption had a strong and highly protective effect. In a multiple logistic regression model, however, vitamin C intake did not make a significant contribution to risk reduction beyond a protective effect found for dietary fiber. This could partly be explained by the correlation between the sources of vitamin C and dietary fiber.

Mettlin et al. (1981) found inverse associations of indices of vitamin A and vitamin C consumption with esophageal cancer based on frequency of consumption of selected food items by male cases and controls. The relationship was stronger for vitamin C than for vitamin A, and only the association with vitamin C was statistically significant after controlling for smoking and alcohol use.

In studies of esophageal cancer in the Caspian Littoral of Iran, inverse associations were found between esophageal cancer and consumption of fresh fruits and estimated vitamin C intake based on correlational and case-control data (Cook-Mozaffari, 1979; Cook-Mozaffari et al., 1979; Hormozdiari et al., 1975; Joint Iran–International Agency for Research on Cancer Study Group, 1977). In a study of diet and esophageal cancer conducted in the Calvados region of France, Tuyns et al. (1987b) found further evidence for a protective effect of vitamin C consumption as estimated from food data banks. The estimate of relative risk for moderate consumers of vitamin C was 0.7 and for heavy consumers, 0.4. Similar protective effects were also found for vitamin E, carotene, and some other micronutrients. It is not clear whether the results of this study reflect general nutritional deficiency, particularly in individuals with high alcohol consumption, or a more specific effect of vitamin C.

Jain et al. (1980) found no association between vitamin C consumption, also estimated from food data banks, and colon cancer in a case-control study in Canada. In a case-control study on colorectal cancer in Marseilles, Macquart-Moulin et al. (1986) found a significant protective effect of vitamin C after adjustment for age, caloric intake, and weight. The risk in the highest consumption category relative to the lowest was 0.16. In a multivariate analysis including other macro- and micronutrients, however, vitamin C was no longer significantly protective. The effect of vitamin C was also evaluated in two case-control studies of colorectal cancer in Australia. In one (Potter and McMichael, 1986), vitamin C consumption was associated with a reduced relative risk for rectal cancer in males and females (ages 30–74 years), especially for younger males; the effect disappeared by 70 years of age. No protective effect was found for colon cancer. In another case-control study, conducted in Belgium by Tuyns et al. (1987a), there was no indication of a protective effect of vitamin C.

The effect of vitamin C has also been assessed in several studies of other cancer sites. In a case-control study of laryngeal cancer, Graham et al. (1981) found an inverse relationship between risk and indices of both vitamin C and vitamin A consumption after controlling for cigarette smok-

ing and alcohol consumption. There was a similar relationship for vegetable consumption in general. Wassertheil-Smoller et al. (1981) reported an association between vitamin C consumption and uterine cervical dysplasia in a case-control study in New York. The findings persisted after the investigators controlled for sexual activity. Stähelin et al. (1984) evaluated plasma vitamin C in a cohort of more than 4,000 men primarily studied for the risk of cardiovascular disease. Plasma vitamin C was found to be consistently lower in cancer cases than in controls. The largest differences were for cancers of the lung and stomach. Böing et al. (1985) analyzed regional nutritional data from a national survey on income and food consumption in the Federal Republic of Germany and correlated mortality rates with the food consumption data for 15 nutrients. Significant positive correlations were found between vitamin C and cancers of the breast, prostate, liver, and colon. In a case-control study of lung cancer in Hawaii, however, Hinds et al. (1984) found no association between dietary vitamin C intake and lung cancer risk.

Animal Studies

Ascorbic acid has been reported to prevent the formation of N-nitroso compounds (Mirvish, 1981a; Tannenbaum and Mergens, 1980). Vitamin C is postulated to act by the reduction of nitrite, ultimately preventing formation of nitrosamine or nitrosourea as demonstrated in vitro. (For a review, see Mirvish, 1981b.)

Abdel-Galil (1986) investigated the effect of ascorbic acid given in drinking water on local methylcholanthrene-induced sarcomas in mice and found that test animals had fewer sarcomas compared to the controls. Vitamin C supplementation, however, did not reduce the diameters or weights of the tumors.

Pauling et al. (1985) studied the effect of varying amounts of L-ascorbic acid (between 0.076% and 8.3% of total diet) on the incidence of spontaneous tumors in RIII mice. They reported that as the amount of ascorbic acid in the diet increased, there was a large decrease in the first-order rate constant. Other studies by the same researchers indicated that increased levels of dietary vitamin C delayed the onset of dermal neoplasms induced in hairless mice by ultraviolet (UV) light (Cameron and Pauling, 1979; Pauling et al., 1982). Dunham et al. (1982) also showed that skin carcinogenesis (squamous cell carcinomas and papillomas) in UV light-treated mice was inhibited by vitamin C.

Male Syrian hamsters taking vitamin C supplements were exposed to cigarette smoke and subcutaneous injections of diethylnitrosamine (DEN) (Harada et al., 1985). In comparison with the unsupplemented smoke-exposed hamsters treated with DEN, the vitamin C-supplemented group had a lower incidence of nasal cavity tumors, but tracheal and laryngeal tumors appeared sooner. These results suggest that vitamin C supplementation accelerates the development of certain cancers and inhibits induction at other sites.

The ability of vitamin C (in drinking water) to inhibit induction of renal carcinoma by estrogens was examined in Syrian hamsters (Liehr and Wheeler, 1983). The incidence of renal carcinoma in the vitamin C-supplemented group was considerably lower than in the nonsupplemented group. High doses of vitamin C (525 mg/day) provided in drinking water to Wistar rats largely inhibited benzo[a]pyrene-induced malignant tumors (Kallistratos and Fasske, 1980).

Silverman et al. (1983) explored the possible inhibitory effect of vitamin C (sodium ascorbate) on metastases from two transplantable murine tumors in male Balb/c mice. There was no difference in survival rates or in the number or size of metastases between the treated and control groups. In fact, brain and regional lymph node metastases appeared to be enhanced by ascorbic acid. Divergent effects of vitamin C were also observed in colon carcinogenesis by dimethylhydrazine (DMH) in the rat. Results from Reddy et al. (1982) indicate that 2 to 10 g of vitamin C per kilogram of diet inhibited carcinogenesis, whereas enhancement of carcinogenesis was observed in another study in which vitamin C was administered to Fischer 344 rats at 50 g/kg diet (Shirai et al., 1985). The incidence of DMH-induced large bowel neoplasms was reduced in mice that consumed a diet containing <0.5 g of vitamin C/kg (Jones et al., 1984).

In another study, methylnitrosourea (MNU)-induced colon cancer in rats was not influenced by dietary vitamin C (Reddy et al., 1982). High doses of ascorbic acid administered in the drinking water had no effect on the growth of transplantable mammary tumors induced by dimethylbenzanthracene in rats (Abul-Hajj and Kelliher, 1982). There was either no reduction or enhancement of subcutaneous 3-methylcholanthrene-induced tumors in scorbutic guinea pigs treated with vitamin C (Banic, 1981; Russell et al., 1952).

Vitamin C has also been observed to be a promotor of cancer. Urinary bladder carcinogenesis induced in rats by MNU or n-butyl-n-(4-hydroxybutyl)-nitrosamine (BBN) was promoted when sodium ascorbate was administered at 50 g/kg body weight (Fukushima et al., 1983; Imaida et al., 1984). However, in another study ascorbic acid fed at the same level was observed to have no effect on BBN-induced cancer (Fukushima et al., 1984). The authors speculated that the sodium salts of certain organic acids act as promoters of urinary bladder cancer.

In short-term tests, Krishna et al. (1986) found that ascorbic acid per se did not affect sister chromatid exchanges (SCEs) induced by cyclophosphamide (CPA) and mitomycin E (MME) in bone marrow and spleen cells in mice in vivo. However, increasing concentrations of ascorbic acid caused decreasing levels of CPA- and MME-induced SCEs in both types of cells in vivo.

Atherosclerosis and Coronary Heart Disease

Human Studies

An association between vitamin C and atherosclerosis has been suggested in studies that evaluated the relationship between vitamin C and cholesterol. Dubick et al. (1987) found ascorbic acid levels to be low in tissue samples from 29 patients with abdominal aortic aneurysms and 14 patients with atherosclerotic occlusive disease. Spittle (1972) found that in healthy people under the age of 25, cholesterol levels tended to fall when 1 g of vitamin C per day was added to an otherwise normal diet. In older people, no consistent pattern of serum cholesterol change was seen. Ramirez and Flowers (1980) compared the ascorbic acid level of leukocytes in patients with coronary heart disease (CHD) to that in patients without CHD, as demonstrated by coronary arteriography. Leukocyte ascorbic acid levels were found to be lower in the patients with coronary artery disease. Mayet et al. (1986) studied Indian and black South African patients with diagnoses of cardiac infarction and diabetes mellitus. They found a negative correlation between leukocyte ascorbic acid and serum cholesterol levels in Indians, especially in patients with infarctions.

Animal Studies

Beetens et al. (1984, 1986) reported that a low dose of vitamin C added to a cholesterol-rich diet given to rabbits decreased lipid infiltration and intimal thickening. Altman et al. (1980) found that vitamin C, especially when associated with phospholipids, led to prevention or resolution of atheromatous plaques provoked in rabbits by cholesterol feeding.

The B Vitamins—Thiamin

Cancer

Human Studies

De Reuck et al. (1980) observed severe thiamin deficiency (Wernicke's encephalopathy) in patients with tumors of the lymphoid-hematopoietic system. Since all the patients had gastrointestinal bleeding, hepatic failure, and sepsis, the authors suggested that malabsorption was a probable cause of the thiamin deficiency. Hence, there is probably no direct relationship between thiamin deficiency and tumorigenesis. Rather, thiamin deficiency may be a secondary event related to malnutrition.

Animal Studies

The committee was unable to identify any laboratory studies of thiamin and cancer.

Liver Disease

Human Studies

In the United States, clinical thiamin deficiency is usually the result of alcoholism. The relation between thiamin deprivation and caloric intake appears to determine whether the deficiency is expressed as beriberi, Wernicke's encephalopathy, Korsakoff's syndrome, or alcoholic polyneuritis (Alpers et al., 1983; Schenker et al., 1980). There is no abnormality in the proportion of phosphorylated species of thiamin to total thiamin in well-nourished alcoholics, and the thiamin levels in their organs are maintained (Dancy et al., 1984; Hoyumpa, 1983).

Alcohol has multiple effects on thiamin nurniture. Hepatic storage of thiamin may be reduced due to fatty infiltration of the liver, decreased functional liver mass, or other liver pathology. The mechanism of action is still not clear.

Riboflavin

Cancer

Human Studies

More than 30 years ago, Wynder et al. (1957) observed that Plummer–Vinson disease, often associated with esophageal cancer, was linked with riboflavin deficiency. More recently, diets marginal or deficient in riboflavin, nicotinic acid, magnesium, and zinc have been correlated with esophageal cancer (Thurnham et al., 1982; van Rensburg et al., 1986).

Riboflavin deficiency has also been reported to cause possibly precancerous lesions in the esophageal epithelium of humans (Foy and Mbaya, 1977). However, substances other than riboflavin (e.g., alcoholic beverages or nass—a chewing tobacco product) that contain N-nitroso compounds may contribute independently to the development and progression of esophageal cancer. Low levels of riboflavin, vitamin A, and carotenoids have been found in a population with a high incidence of oral and esophageal cancer (Zaridze et al., 1985). A remarkably high proportion (41%) of the men surveyed were users of nass. The authors suggest that since low levels of riboflavin, vitamin A, and carotenoids were associated with a high incidence of certain cancers, higher levels of these nutrients may have a protective effect against the development of cancer.

Esophageal cancer and riboflavin deficiencies are widespread in Africa, Iran, and China. It has not yet been established, however, that riboflavin deficiency per se plays a role in esophageal cancer, because riboflavin metabolism may be affected by zinc status (Merrill and McCormick, 1980), and zinc deficiency is also associated with esophageal cancer.

In an endoscopic study in Linxian, Hunan Province, China, Thurnham et al. (1982) found that 97% of 527 subjects had ariboflavinosis, based on the erythrocyte glutathione reductase activity coefficients. Blood samples were collected to measure the status of riboflavin and several other nutrients in persons in certain geographic areas of China. In two surveys in China, one in Linxian County (a high-risk area for esophogeal cancer) and the other in Jiaoxian County (a low-risk area), the distribution of erythrocyte glutathione reductase activity coefficient values suggested that riboflavin levels were higher in the low-risk community (Thurnham et al., 1985).

The hypothesis that riboflavin deficiencies are associated with precancerous lesions of the esophagus has been examined by Munoz et al. (1985). A population at high risk for esophageal cancer in China received weekly supplements of retinol, riboflavin, and zinc, or a placebo in a randomized double-blind intervention trial. No differences in the prevalence of esophagitis with or without atrophy or dysplasia were noted in the two groups examined at 13 months. It is not known if different results would have been obtained if the study had been continued.

Animal Studies

Male baboons fed a diet lacking riboflavin developed cutaneous lesions, including hyperkeratosis, gross derangement of keratinization with acanthosis, and impressive pseudocarcinomatous hyperplasia (Foy and Kondi, 1984). The esophageal epithelium was thin and pale in some of the animals, and there was esophagitis and large, chronic, disorganized lesions. The numerous mitotic figures that were commonly encountered were distinguishable from carcinomas only by their disorganized, highly active epithelial growth and by the absence of muscular invasion. Foy and Kondi (1984) noted that this condition may reflect a precursor state that could take years to become invasive.

Rats were fed test diets supplemented with low doses of riboflavin, nicotinic acid, zinc, magnesium, selenium, and molybdenum for 45 days, dosed with N-nitroso-methylbenzylamine (3 mg/kg), and then continued on the test diets for 150 days (van Rensburg et al., 1986). Compared to controls, the supplemented group had fewer tumors (esophageal carcinomas) and tumor-bearing animals. These results indicate that low doses of supplements are helpful in the treatment of premalignant esophageal changes. The effects of high doses of supplements are unknown. The findings of that study, however, are most likely relevant to early prevention of esophageal cancer, since supplementation was started 45 days before dosing with the carcinogen.

Mechanism of Action

Kensler et al. (1941) noted a relationship between the consumption of riboflavin and susceptibility to carcinoma induced by dimethylaminoazobenzene. Numerous studies have confirmed this general phenomenon. (For reviews see Bidlack et al., 1986; Miller and Miller, 1953; Rivlin, 1975). Bidlack et al. (1986), for example, reported that riboflavin deficiency adversely affects liver detoxification mechanisms. In addition, reduced nicotinamide dinucleotide phosphate (NADPH)-cytochrome P-450 reductase activity is decreased, as is the metabolism of aniline, acetaniline, aminopyrine, and ethylmorphine. Riboflavin deficiency appears to increase susceptibility to abnormal processing of potential carcinogens. Lee et al. (1983) found that riboflavin deficiency in rats only modestly decreased cytochrome P-450 but markedly decreased peroxisomal flavoprotein oxidases, which produce hydrogen peroxide; a decrease in liver catalase followed.

Cancer patients frequently metabolize riboflavin in aberrant ways. They excrete lower than normal levels of riboflavin in the urine (Kagan, 1960) and do not excrete larger amounts after oral or intravenous doses (Kagan, 1957, 1960). Riboflavin may be trapped by the tumor or the host. Baker et al. (1981) found that samples of colon adenocarcinoma obtained at autopsy contained nearly twice as much riboflavin and elevated amounts of other water-soluble vitamins as did neighboring tissue. However, liver adenocarcinomas were found to contain about the same levels as liver tissue from controls (and smaller amounts of several other vitamins such as B_{12}). Innis et al. (1985, 1986) reported that immunoglobulins are the major proteins responsible for riboflavin binding in human plasma and that their levels are higher in patients with breast cancer and melanoma. The lower urinary levels and clearance in cancer patients could be due in part to increased plasma binding rather than trapping by tumor tissue.

Liver Disease

Human Studies

Ethanol consumption can reduce intestinal bioavailability of riboflavin, particularly flavin adenine dinucleotide (FAD) (Pinto et al., 1984). The accumulation of fat in the liver in riboflavin-deficient persons resembles changes observed in the liver of chronic alcoholics. In humans with liver cirrhosis, decreased concentrations of riboflavin are found mostly in necrotic regions (Chen and Liao, 1960). Riboflavin deficiency is usually encountered when there is a general lack of B vitamin intake, such as in forms of malnutrition that accompany alcoholism. Changes in the activities of flavoproteins and other hepatic enzymes result from riboflavin deficiency, but it is not known whether all these changes can be fully reversed after supplementation with riboflavin.

Animal Studies

Hepatic concentrations of FAD were reported to be one-third the normal level in rats fed diets deficient in riboflavin (Fass and Rivlin, 1969). Flavokinase activity in rats fed riboflavin-free diets was decreased to about 40% of normal. Riboflavin deficiency has selective effects on the activities of liver enzymes involved in riboflavin metabolism (Lee and McCormick, 1983). It appears to have the greatest effect on flavokinase, which is physiologically rate-limiting in the biosynthesis of flavocoenzymes.

Riboflavin deficiency in mice alters hepatic architecture, including enlargement and distortion of mitochondria, possibly due to defects in oxidative phosphorylation resulting from lack of flavoproteins (Burch et al., 1960; Tandler et al., 1968). Decreased mitotic activity has been observed in fetal liver of the offspring of riboflavin-deficient dams (Miller et al., 1962).

Niacin

Cancer

Human Studies

Warwick and Harington (1973) noted that the incidence of pellagra also often increases in geographic areas where esophageal cancer is becoming more frequent. The authors cautioned, however, that pellagra may reflect an extreme deficiency of niacin complicated by deficiencies of other vitamins and minerals such as riboflavin, magnesium, and zinc. The predisposition to esophageal cancer and cancer of other sites may be due to damaging effects of these deficiencies on the organs (Thurnham et al., 1982; van Rensburg et al., 1986).

Animal Studies

Diets low in protein (5.5%) and high in carbohydrates were used to test the effect of 0, 50, or 500 mg of nicotinamide per kilogram of diet on N-nitrosodimethylamine-induced carcinogenesis in Holtzman albino rats (Miller and Burns, 1984). Both the oxidized and the reduced forms of NAD and NADP were found in lower concentrations in the livers of test animals than in controls. In the kidney, only NADH and NADPH were below normal. After 5 weeks of treatment, all the animals were returned to a standard diet for 85 weeks. The investigators reported that the initial diets had no effect on tumor incidence or tumor type. These results suggest that nicotinamide does not exert a long-term effect on tumorigenesis.

Schoental (1977) reported an increased incidence of kidney neoplasms in rats given nicotinamide (300 to 500 mg/kg of body weight) intraperitoneally before and after each dose of DEN. Rosenberg et al. (1985) reported that nicotinamide (6.7 or 30 mM) in the drinking water of male Fischer 344 rats also receiving DEN (25 mg/kg by intraperitioneal injection) caused a 28 to 59%

increase in the incidence of kidney tumors. There was a 5% incidence of kidney tumors in rats treated with DEN alone, whereas no kidney tumors were found in rats given nicotinamide alone. Grassetti (1986) noted that several analogs of niacin (sulfur-containing, 5- and 6-membered, heterocyclic carboxylic acids) decreased the number of pulmonary metastases in C57B/6 mice implanted with Lewis lung carcinoma. These niacin compounds also inhibited the growth rate of the primary implanted tumor by 50%.

These conflicting results suggest that niacin may be a carcinogen or a cocarcinogen, or it may inhibit carcinogenesis. The precise effect of niacin appears to be influenced by the dose and nature of the niacin compound, time and site of administration, nature of the carcinogen, and type of tumor. For example, in some systems, nicotinamide increased the incidence of tumors of the pancreas but decreased the incidence of kidney tumors (Rakieten et al., 1971). The effects of nicotinamide may be due to increasing the NAD pools, which are depleted by certain carcinogens (Rakieten et al., 1971; Schoental, 1975).

Liver Disease

Human Studies

The human liver contains approximately 60 mg of nicotinic acid (free and covalently bound in coenzymes) per kilogram wet weight—an amount similar to concentrations in other tissues (Wiss and Weber, 1964); it contains no special stores of nicotinic acid or its derivatives. In alcoholics, the degree of liver disease influences the concentrations of nicotinic acid in that organ. For example, the total nicotinic acid content of the cirrhotic liver can fall as low as 80% of normal values (Baker et al., 1964; Jusko and Levy, 1975). The increase in liver lipid content caused by ethanol administration can be reversed by administration of nicotinic acid (Baker et al., 1976), which inhibits the peripheral release of free fatty acid and liver alcohol dehydrogenase. These studies suggest that the condition of the liver influences nicotinic acid concentrations.

Other Diseases

A high nicotinic acid intake has been associated with hepatotoxicity. One-third to one-half of patients taking 3 g of nicotinic acid per day for 5 years had elevated levels of serum glutamic oxaloacetic transaminase (SGOT) and alkaline phosphatase (Coronary Drug Project Research Group,

1975; DiPalma and Ritchie, 1977; Einstein et al., 1975). (The RDA for niacin is 18 mg for males and 13 mg for females.)

Niacin may increase serum uric acid levels (APA, 1973; Coronary Drug Project Research Group, 1975; Ivey, 1979). In the Coronary Drug Project Group (1975), patients on niacin had an increased incidence of acute gouty arthritis and a decrease in nonfatal recurrent myocardial infarction, but there was no decrease in total mortality. It was not known whether this was the result of the cholesterol-lowering effect of nicotinic acid, a direct effect of niacin, or both.

Vitamin B_6

Cancer

Human Studies

Bell (1980) reported that women with breast cancer who excrete less pyridoxic acid than average (one reflection of vitamin B_6 status) have an increased probability of a recurrence of breast cancer. The physiological significance of the relationship between low excretion of pyridoxic acid and risk of recurrence is unknown. Ladner and Salkeld (1988) noted that the 5-year survival rate of patients with stage II endometrial carcinoma was increased by administering pyrodoxine.

Several groups have reported unusual levels of vitamin B_6 metabolites, such as lower plasma pyridoxal 5'-phosphate (PLP), in breast cancer patients despite normal urinary pyridoxic acid (Potera et al., 1977). Chabner et al. (1970) reported low plasma PLP in patients with Hodgkin's disease, as well as abnormalities in tryptophan metabolism in these patients.

Animal Studies

Foy et al. (1974) fed baboons pyridoxine-deprived diets either continually or intermittently for 2 to 6 years. The livers of the intermittently deprived animals developed striking changes suggesting liver neoplasia. The acutely deprived animals died within 6 to 8 months. The surviving animals had lower serum B_6 values and increased tryptophan metabolites in the urine compared to controls. The authors suggest that pyridoxine deficiency may be associated with disturbances in immunologic competence.

In laboratory animals, diets deficient in pyridoxine inhibit the growth of some types of tumors (Kline et al., 1943; Mihich and Nichol, 1959; Tryfiates and Morris, 1974). Ha et al. (1984)

reported that vitamin B_6 deficiency affects host susceptibility to Moloney sarcoma virus-induced tumor growth in mice. However, vitamin B_6 status does not affect the growth of some tumors such as spontaneous mammary tumors in strain C3H mice (Morris, 1947). DiSorbo et al. (1985) observed a 62% reduction in tumor weight, compared with controls, in mice pretreated with PLP for 2 weeks and then injected with B-16 melanoma cells. In mice with established tumors, a 39% reduction in tumor growth was observed when the animals were treated with PLP for 6 days. The exact mechanism by which PLP exerts its inhibitory effect was not determined; however, the authors suggest that vitamin B_6 may act on the plasma membrane to reduce precursor transport into the cell.

Vitamin B_6 is involved in the synthesis of DNA bases; it is a coenzyme in the biosynthesis of thymidine. According to Prior (1985), a dietary B_6 deficiency or an increase in the thymidine requirement at a critical time during cell division could result in initial cell mutations that develop into a tumor. The author suggests that dietary vitamin B_6 supplementation could assist in preventing some cancers.

Liver Disease

Human Studies

Although there is no consensus on the best biochemical marker for the assessment of vitamin B_6 status in humans, plasma PLP is the one most frequently used (Williams et al., 1984). Most dietary vitamin B_6 is rapidly converted by the liver to this active coenzyme form, which has a central role in the metabolism of amino acids.

As measured by PLP levels in plasma, vitamin B_6 deficiency can occur in as many as 30 to 50% of alcoholics without liver disease and in 80 to 100% of those with liver damage (Frank et al., 1971; Spannuth et al., 1978). Inadequate intake may not be the only factor contributing to low plasma levels of PLP. Lumeng and Li (1974) suggest that PLP in erythrocytes is destroyed more rapidly in the presence of acetaldehyde, the first product of ethanol oxidation, perhaps by displacement of PLP from protein and its exposure to phosphatase. Low plasma levels of PLP may also be due to increased breakdown or to poor absorption of dietary vitamin B_6 (Zaman et al., 1986). Thus, abnormal vitamin B_6 metabolism in liver disease may be due to several factors.

Liver and plasma PLP levels are considerably reduced in patients with cirrhosis and other hepatic diseases, even when the patients are given a normal diet (Bonjour, 1980; Henderson et al., 1986; Merrill et al., 1986). In cirrhotics, plasma PLP response to administered pyridoxine is impaired (Henderson et al., 1986; Spannuth et al., 1978). Mitchell et al. (1976) reported that PLP administered intravenously is cleared more rapidly by patients with liver disease than by controls. Cirrhotics are capable of apparently normal PLP synthesis but have increased hepatic dephosphorylation, which may be responsible for low plasma levels of PLP (Merrill and Henderson, 1987; Merrill et al., 1986). This is associated with elevated alkaline phosphatase in the plasma of these patients (Anderson et al., 1980). Attempts to normalize plasma PLP in cirrhotics have had limited success.

Animal Studies

Shane (1982) found that rats receiving approximately 30% of their calories from ethanol metabolized pyridoxine relatively normally and their tissue stores were not decreased. There was, however, an increase in hepatic PLP. In histological examinations, no evidence of liver damage was found. These results differ from most observations reported in human subjects and cannot be fully explained.

Folacin

Cancer

Human Studies

In a randomized trial, Butterworth et al. (1982) administered oral folic acid (10 mg) or ascorbic acid (10 mg) to 87 women with cervical cancer. Their results suggest that oral folate supplements may prevent the progression of cervical dysplasia or promote regression to normalcy.

Animal Studies

An increased incidence of tumors in the liver, colon, and esophagus results from diets deficient in methyl groups (Ghoshal and Farber, 1984; Hoover et al., 1984; Lombardi and Shinozuka, 1979; Mikol et al., 1983; Rogers, 1975). Feeding rats a diet deficient in lipotropes (choline, methionine, folate) and vitamin B_{12} for 15 weeks was found to increase the incidence of hepatic tumors after a single dose of diethylnitrosamine (Hoover et al., 1984).

It has long been recognized that folic acid inhibits tumor growth (Prentice et al., 1985). Early studies in mice by Leuchtenberger et al.

(1945) showed inhibition of spontaneous breast tumors by folate. More recently, Rogers and Newberne (1980) showed that diets deficient in lipotrope and high in fat enhance chemical hepatocarcinogenesis in rats. Severe lipidosis and cell death result from methyl group-deficient diets (Ghoshal et al., 1983; Giambarresi et al., 1982; Shinozuka and Lombardi, 1980).

Liver Disease

Human Studies

Folate deficiency in alcoholics is likely to be caused by impaired intestinal uptake as well as by decreased storage in the damaged liver (Halsted and Tamura, 1979; Hillman, 1980). Leevy et al. (1970) observed a 60% reduction in total liver folate concentration in cirrhotics, while the hepatic intake of ^{3}H-labeled folate in moderate-to-severe cirrhotics was only 10% that of the normal liver. Moreover, administration of nonradioactive folate caused a 10-fold greater displacement of the radioactive form of this vitamin in patients with cirrhosis as compared to subjects with a normal liver. Vitamin therapy also is not successful in raising folacin levels during active necrosis or cirrhosis. Other studies in humans and animals have failed to confirm that alcohol can affect the uptake, storage, reduction, or methylation of labeled folate (Brown et al., 1973; Lane et al., 1976; McGuffin et al., 1975). Lane et al. (1976) suggest that the blocked release of tissue folate stores may result from the rapid depression of serum methyltetrahydropteroylglutamate levels and early induction of megaloblastic erythropoiesis, which has been observed following acute alcohol ingestion. Normal as well as low liver folate levels have been found in patients with chronic hepatitis and nonalcoholic cirrhosis (Kimber et al., 1965; Klipstein and Lindenbaum, 1965; Wu et al., 1975).

Alcoholic cirrhotics can develop megaloblastic anemia due to folate deficiency (Hillman, 1975). Inadequate retention of folate in the liver as well as low dietary intake of folate may contribute to this condition. Healthy subjects receiving a folate-free diet develop megaloblastic anemia after about 22 weeks (Herbert et al., 1963), whereas chronic alcoholics show a similar hematologic picture within 5 to 10 weeks (Eichner and Hillman, 1971; Halstead et al., 1973). Malnourished alcoholics (without liver disease) absorb folic acid less well than their better nourished counterparts (Halsted et al., 1971). Anemia from folic acid deficiency is rare in well-nourished alcoholics (Eichner et al., 1972).

Disordered folate metabolism is also associated with viral hepatitis. An increased excretion of urinary folate due to release of stored folates from the liver has been reported (Retief and Huskisson, 1969; Tamura and Stokstad, 1977). These data suggest that low liver folate levels in alcoholics may be due to some combination of decreased intake, decreased absorption, or increased excretion.

Vitamin B_{12}

Cancer

Human Studies

Kaplan and Rigler (1945) found that patients with pernicious anemia have a higher incidence of gastric carcinoma. This association was confirmed and expanded to other types of cancer, including leukemias, erythremic myelosis, polycythemia vera, and multiple myeloma (Arvanitakis et al., 1979). Ruddell et al. (1978) suggested that the increased gastric cancer risk could be caused by the intragastric formation of carcinogenic N-nitroso compounds. The concentrations of gastric nitrite are increased when the gastric acidity is decreased, as in persons with pernicious anemia. Ahmann and Durie (1984) caution that leukemia can be accelerated by the excessive replacement of vitamin B_{12} in patients with pernicious anemia.

Carmel and Eisenberg (1977) studied 139 patients with several types of malignancies (28 breast, 19 colon, 17 stomach, 12 lung, 8 pancreas, 8 prostate, 8 ovary, and some less prevalent sites) and found that serum levels of vitamin B_{12} and B_{12}-binding proteins were elevated frequently in malignancies other than granulocytic proliferation or hepatic tumors, as had been suggested by other studies (e.g., Carmel, 1975). No correlation between serum vitamin B_{12} and small-cell lung cancer was found by Clamon et al. (1984).

Brain, heart, and lung tumors were found by Sheppard et al. (1984) to have higher cobalamin-binding as well as unsaturated cobalamin-binding capacity, whereas the liver tumors had an increased unsaturated cobalamin-binding capacity and a reduced total binding capacity. The results for liver cancer are consistent with the observation that liver adenocarcinomas had a lower vitamin B_{12} content than did specimens from adjacent, uninvaded liver (Baker et al., 1981). Presently, the relationship between vitamin B_{12} and the etiology of various cancers is not clear.

Areekul et al. (1986) measured serum vitamin B_{12}, red-cell folate, and serum vitamin B_{12}-binding protein in 18 patients with neuroblastoma. The status of vitamin B_{12} in these patients was within normal limits, but low serum and red-cell folate concentrations indicated that these patients were in a state of negative folate balance. Van Tonder et al. (1985) reported that unsaturated vitamin B_{12} binding capacity (UBBC) and vitamin B_{12} activity were slightly elevated in 80% of South African blacks with hepatocellular carcinoma, with and without cirrhosis. Paradinas et al. (1982) reported that only 9% of their patients with hepatocellular carcinomas had increased UBBC but that these patients survived longer than patients without increased UBBC. Serum vitamin B_{12} and UBBC values have been observed to be both elevated (although not dramatically) and normal in cancer patients.

Animal Studies

Chemical carcinogenesis in the liver and sometimes other tissues of rats is enhanced by lipotrope deficiencies (Mikol et al., 1983; Rogers, 1975). Hoover et al. (1984) found that a diet deficient in choline, methionine, folate, and vitamin B_{12} fed to rats for 15 weeks after a single dose of diethylnitrosamine was sufficient to cause a high incidence of hepatic tumors.

Liver Disease

Human Studies

The intake of ethanol affects the storage of vitamin B_{12} in the liver. Vitamin B_{12} deficiency is not common in alcoholics, as indicated by normal serum B_{12} levels in patients with folate deficiency, both with and without cirrhosis (Halsted et al., 1971; Herbert et al., 1963). The degree of liver pathology influences the extent to which liver vitamin B_{12} concentrations are decreased (Baker et al., 1964; Russell, 1979). Acute liver damage causes release of vitamin B_{12} into the plasma, where some of it binds to serum proteins and some remains free. Various liver diseases causing hepatic necrosis, such as viral hepatitis, cirrhosis, malignancy, and obstructive jaundice, result in decreased liver concentrations of vitamin B_{12} and increased plasma concentrations (Jones et al., 1957; Linnell, 1975; Wiss and Weber, 1964). In patients with acute hepatitis and necrosis, free vitamin B_{12} plasma levels are high, whereas the bound form is elevated during chronic liver disease (Jones et al., 1957).

Thus, it appears that liver and plasma levels of vitamin B_{12} can be sharply influenced by ethanol.

It is not clear how vitamin B_{12} supplementation will affect the levels of B_{12} in chronic alcoholics.

Biotin

Cancer

Human Studies

The committee did not identify any studies of humans concerning biotin and cancer.

Animal Studies

Early investigations indicate that when biotin and avidin are given together to rats fed p-dimethyl-aminoazobenzene (DMAB), the possible cocarcinogenic action of biotin is arrested by its binding to avidin to form a complex (Du Vigneaud et al., 1942). Several attempts have been made to retard the growth of various types of neoplasia in human patients and animals by the administration of egg white or avidin (Kaplan, 1944; Kensler et al., 1943; West and Woglom, 1942) but none have been successful. Kline et al. (1945) fed rats DMAB with a highly purified diet containing suboptimal levels of riboflavin. They attempted to alter the effect of egg white by injecting biotin or denaturing the avidin by heat. The results suggest that the beneficial effects of egg white on hepatoma formation are independent of any egg white-biotin relationship but, rather, that they are dependent on optimal levels of riboflavin. These early observations do not appear to have been followed up with additional human or animal studies.

Liver Disease

Animal and Human Studies

Biotin concentrations are higher in the liver than in other organs (Semenza et al., 1959). In the perfused livers of normal and alcohol-fed rats, ethanol did not induce the release of biotin as it did with other vitamins (Sorrell et al., 1974). In cirrhotics, even mild fatty liver infiltration reduced liver biotin levels (Baker et al., 1964). The change in frank cirrhotics was much less.

Pantothenic Acid

Cancer

Human Studies

The committee did not identify any studies concerning pantothenic acid and cancer in humans.

Animal Studies

Sodium ω-methylpantothenate, an antagonist of pantothenic acid, was found by Bulovskaia (1976) to inhibit tumor growth in mice bearing transplanted tumors.

As with many other vitamins, levels of pantothenate in tumors may be higher or lower than in adjacent uninvolved tissues. Primary colon adenocarcinoma in rats was found to contain significantly more of the B vitamins, including pantothenate, than did normal colon tissue (Baker et al., 1981).

Liver Disease

Human Studies

Because pantothenic acid concentrations are several times higher in the liver than in other tissues, the liver is affected by nutritional intake more than other organs. Spontaneous gross pantothenic acid deficiency in humans has seldom been described, although Olson (1984) has suggested that some symptoms, such as malaise and abdominal distress, may be related to deficiency of the vitamin. These symptoms, among others, were observed when volunteers were fed ω-methylpantothenate.

Plasma levels of pantothenic acid vary in patients with diseased as well as nondiseased livers. The reason for this is unclear. Marked elevation of blood pantothenic acid was characteristic of alcoholics hospitalized with acute fatty liver (Cole et al., 1969). Leevy et al. (1960) reported that plasma pantothenic acid levels were normal in 172 alcoholics free of liver disease. Decreased pantothenic acid levels were observed in patients with cirrhotic fatty livers and even in some with normal liver function. In most cases, a nutritious diet and mobilization of liver fat caused levels to return to normal (Leevy et al., 1970).

Hypertension

Human and Animal Studies

Some Japanese populations with endemic pantothenic acid deficiency also have an increased prevalence of hypertension (Koyanagi et al., 1966). Schwabedal et al. (1985) fed a semisynthetic pantothenic acid-deficient diet to rats for 5 weeks. The rats were unilaterally adrenonephrectomized and then given standard rat chow together with 1% sodium chloride in drinking water. The rats developed hypertension; their final blood pressure values were more than 215 mm Hg.

SUMMARY

Epidemiologic studies suggest that vitamin C-containing foods and possibly vitamin C itself either may protect against cancer or have no association with the disease. The strongest evidence for a protective effect seems to be for stomach cancer; the evidence for esophageal cancer is not as strong. Findings are contradictory for cancers of the colon, rectum, and lung. However, frequent consumption of these foods, especially those rich in β-carotene, is strongly associated with a protective effect against lung cancer (see Chapter 11). One problem in drawing conclusions about vitamin C and cancer is that the primary sources of vitamin C—fruits and vegetables—also contain other potentially protective factors, for example, dietary fiber, whose intake is strongly correlated with the intake of vitamin C. Protective effects from other nutrients, such as vitamin A, carotenoids, and vitamin E, cannot be ruled out. In animal models, vitamin C may inhibit the induction of certain cancers, such as dermal neoplasms and renal carcinoma. Possible mechanisms of action for ascorbic acid are the blocking of nitrosamine formation and the reduction of other highly reactive endogenous compounds such as superoxide radicals.

Epidemiologic data derived primarily from China indicate that low riboflavin levels may be associated with a greater risk of esophageal cancer. These data are supported by similar results in animal studies. Moreover, low doses of riboflavin supplements given to animals have been found to be helpful in the treatment of premalignant esophageal changes.

In humans, elevated serum B_{12} and B_{12}-binding protein have been associated with cancer of such sites as the breast, colon, and stomach; however, there is no clearly established relationship between vitamin B_{12} and the etiology of various cancers. Animal studies suggest that vitamin B_{12} is likely to be a cocarcinogen, but the mechanism has not been clarified.

Hepatic disease is often accompanied by hypovitaminosis due to an increased need for vitamins in the face of decreased intake, intestinal malabsorption, and reduced hepatic storage capacity. Liver dysfunction can also prevent conversion of vitamins into their metabolically useful forms. Vitamin B complex depletion is common in hepatocellular disease.

The data on the remaining B vitamins and chronic diseases are too meager to permit any conclusions.

DIRECTIONS FOR RESEARCH

● The role of vitamin C in cancer needs to be defined. In particular, there is a need to identify the mechanisms other than nitrosamine inhibition whereby vitamin C may influence tumorigenesis. It is difficult to identify with certainty the effects due specifically to vitamin C because foods containing that vitamin also contain such potentially protective factors as fiber, carotenoids, and vitamin E.

● The requirements for water-soluble vitamins at all stages of the life cycle need to be determined as they may relate to the prevention of chronic disease, especially cancer and liver disease.

● A better understanding of the interactions among various nutrients (e.g., fiber, vitamin C, lipotropes) in the prevention of cancer and liver disease is needed.

● Greater attention should be directed to epidemiologic studies to gather data on the relationship of the B vitamins to cancer.

REFERENCES

Abdel-Galil, A.M. 1986. Preventive effect of vitamin C (L-ascorbic acid) on methylcholanthrene-induced soft tissue sarcomas in mice. Oncology 43:335–337.

Abul-Hajj, Y.J., and M. Kelliher. 1982. Failure of ascorbic acid to inhibit growth of transplantable and dimethylbenzanthracene induced rat mammary tumors. Cancer Lett. 17:67–73.

Ahmann, F.R., and B.G.M. Durie. 1984. Acute myelogenous leukaemia modulated by B_{12} deficiency: a case with bone marrow blast cell assay corroboration. Br. J. Haematol. 58:91–94.

Alpers, D.H., R.E. Clouse, and W.F. Stenson. 1983. Manual of Nutritional Therapeutics. Little, Brown and Company, Boston. 457 pp.

Altman, R.F., G.M. Schaeffer, C.A. Salles, A.S. Ramos de Souza, and P.M. Cotias. 1980. Phospholipids associated with vitamin C in experimental atherosclerosis. Arzneim. Forsch. 30:627–630.

Anderson, B.B., H. O'Brien, G.E. Griffin, and D.L. Mollin. 1980. Hydrolysis of pyridoxal 5′-phosphate in plasma in conditions with raised alkaline phosphate. Gut 21:192–194.

APA (American Psychiatric Association). 1973. Megavitamin and Orthomolecular Therapy in Psychiatry. A Report of the Task Force on Vitamin Therapy in Psychiatry. American Psychiatric Association, Washington, D.C. 54 pp.

Areekul, S., P. Hathirat, and K. Churdchu. 1986. Folic acid, vitamin B_{12}, and vitamin B_{12} binding proteins in patients with neuroblastoma. Southeast Asian J. Trop. Med. Public Health 17:184–188.

Arvanitakis, C., F.F. Holmes, and E. Hearne III. 1979. A possible association of pernicious anemia with neoplasia. Oncology 36:127–129.

Baker, H., O. Frank, H. Ziffer, S. Goldfarb, C.M. Leevy, and H. Sobotka. 1964. Effect of hepatic disease on liver B-complex vitamin titers. Am. J. Clin. Nutr. 14:1–6.

Baker, H., O. Frank, and M.F. Sorrell. 1976. Nicotinic acid

and alcoholism. Bibl. Nutr. Dieta. 24:32–39.

Baker, H., O. Frank, T. Chen, S. Feingold, B. DeAngelis, and E.R. Baker. 1981. Elevated vitamin levels in colon adenocarcinoma as compared with metastatic liver adenocarcinoma from colon primary and normal adjacent tissue. Cancer 47:2883–2886.

Banic, S. 1981. Vitamin C acts as a cocarcinogen to methylcholanthrene in guinea-pigs. Cancer Lett. 11:239–242.

Beetens, J.R., M.C. Coene, A. Verheyen, L. Zonnekeyn, and A.G. Herman. 1984. Influence of vitamin C on the metabolism of arachidonic acid and the development of aortic lesions during experimental atherosclerosis in rabbits. Biomed. Biochim. Acta 43:S273-S276.

Beetens, J.R., M.C. Coene, A. Verheyen, L. Zonnekeyn, and A.G. Herman. 1986. Vitamin C increases the prostacyclin production and decreases the vascular lesions in experimental atherosclerosis in rabbits. Prostaglandins 32:335–352.

Bell, E. 1980. The excretion of a vitamin B_6 metabolite and the probability of recurrence of early breast cancer. Eur. J. Cancer 16:297–298.

Bidlack, W.R., R.C. Brown, and C. Mohan. 1986. Nutritional parameters that alter hepatic drug metabolism, conjugation, and toxicity. Fed. Proc. 45:142–148.

Bjelke, E. 1978. Dietary factors and the epidemiology of cancer of the stomach and large bowel. Aktuel. Ernaehrungsmed. Klin. Prax. Suppl. 2:10–17.

Böing, H., L. Martinez, R. Frentzel-Beyme, and U. Oltersdorf. 1985. Regional nutritional pattern and cancer mortality in the Federal Republic of Germany. Nutr. Cancer 7:121–130.

Bonjour, J.P. 1980. Vitamins and alcoholism. III. Vitamin B_6. Int. J. Vitam. Nutr. Res. 50:215–230.

Brown, J.P., G.E. Davidson, J.M. Scott, and J. Weir. 1973. Effect of diphenylhydantoin and ethanol feeding on the synthesis of rat liver folates from exogenous pteroylglutamate (3H). Biochem. Pharmacol. 22:3287–3289.

Bulovskaia, L.N. 1976. Acetylation reaction in mice in the normal state and in tumors. Vopr. Onkol. 22:59–63.

Burch, H.B., F.E. Hunter, Jr., A.M. Combs, and B.A. Schutz. 1960. Oxidative enzymes and phosphorylation in hepatic mitochondria from riboflavin-deficient rats. J. Biol. Chem. 235:1540–1544.

Butterworth, C.E., Jr., K.D. Hatch, H. Gore, H. Mueller, and C.L. Krumdieck. 1982. Improvement in cervical dysplasia associated with folic acid therapy in users of oral contraceptives. Am. J. Clin. Nutr. 35:73–82.

Cameron, E., and L. Pauling. 1979. Cancer and Vitamin C. Linus Pauling Institute of Science and Medicine, Menlo Park, Calif. 238 pp.

Carmel, R. 1975. Extreme elevation of serum transcobalamin I in patients with metastatic cancer. N. Engl. J. Med. 292:282–284.

Carmel, R., and L. Eisenberg. 1977. Serum vitamin B_{12} and transcobalamin abnormalities in patients with cancer. Cancer 40:1348–1353.

Chabner, B.A., V.T. DeVita, D.M. Livingston, and V.T. Oliverio. 1970. Abnormalities of tryptophan metabolism and plasma pyridoxal phosphate in Hodgkin's disease. N. Engl. J. Med. 282:838–843.

Chen, C., and T. Liao. 1960. Histochemical study on riboflavin. J. Vitaminol. Osaka 6:171–195.

Clamon, G.H., R. Feld, W.K. Evans, R.S. Weiner, B.S. Kramer, L.L. Lininger, L.B. Gardner, E.C. Wolfe, W.D. DeWys, and F.A. Hoffman. 1984. Serum folate and vitamin B_{12} levels in patients with small cell lung cancer. Cancer 53:306–310.

Cole, M., A. Turner, O. Frank, H. Baker, and C.M. Leevy. 1969. Extraocular palsy and thiamin therapy in Wernicke's encephalopathy. Am. J. Clin. Nutr. 22:44–51.

Cook-Mozaffari, P. 1979. The epidemiology of cancer of the oesophagus. Nutr. Cancer 1:51–60.

Cook-Mozaffari, P.J., F. Azordegan, N.E. Day, A. Ressicaud, C. Sabai, and B. Aramesh. 1979. Oesophageal cancer studies in the Caspian Littoral of Iran: results of a case-control study. Br. J. Cancer 39:293–309.

Coronary Drug Project Research Group. 1975. Clofibrate and niacin in coronary artery disease. J. Am. Med. Assoc. 231:360–381.

Dancy, M., G. Evans, M.K. Gaitonde, and J.D. Maxwell. 1984. Blood thiamine and thiamine phosphate ester concentrations in alcoholic and non-alcoholic liver diseases. Br. Med. J. 289:79–82.

De Reuck, J.L., G.J. Sieben, M.R. Sieben-Praet, P. Ngendahayo, W.J. De Coster, and H.M. Vander Eecken. 1980. Wernicke's encephalopathy in patients with tumors of the lymphoid-hemopoietic systems. Arch. Neurol. 37:338–341.

DHHS–USDA (Department of Health and Human Services and U.S. Department of Agriculture). 1986. Nutrition Monitoring in the United States—A Progress Report from the Joint Nutrition Monitoring Evaluation Committee. DHHS Pub. No. (PHS) 86-1255, Public Health Service, National Center for Health Statistics, Department of Health and Human Services, Hyattsville, Md. 356 pp.

DiPalma, J.R., and D.M. Ritchie. 1977. Vitamin toxicity. Annu. Rev. Pharmacol. Toxicol. 17:133.

DiSorbo, D.M., R. Wagner, Jr., and L. Nathanson. 1985. In vivo and in vitro inhibition of B_{16} melanoma growth by vitamin B_6. Nutr. Cancer 7:43–52.

Dubick, M.A., G.C. Hunter, S.M. Casey, and C.L. Keen. 1987. Aortic ascorbic acid, trace elements, and superoxide dismutase activity in human aneurysmal and occlusive disease. Proc. Soc. Exp. Biol. Med. 184:138–143.

Dunham, W.B., E. Zuckerkandl, R. Reynolds, R. Willoughby, R. Marcuson, R. Barth, and L. Pauling. 1982. Effects of intake of L-ascorbic acid on the incidence of dermal neoplasms induced in mice by ultraviolet light. Proc. Natl. Acad. Sci. U.S.A. 79:7532–7536.

Du Vigneaud, V., J.M. Spangler, D. Burk, C.J. Kensler, K. Sugiura, and C.P. Rhoades. 1942. The procarcinogenic effect of biotin in butter yellow tumor formation. Science 95:174–176.

Eichner, E.R., and R.S. Hillman. 1971. The evolution of anemia in alcoholic patients. Am. J. Med. 50:218–232.

Eichner, E.R., B. Buchanan, J.W. Smith, and R.S. Hillman. 1972. Variations in the hematologic and medical status of alcoholics. Am. J. Med. Sci. 263:35–42.

Einstein, N., A. Baker, J. Galper, and H. Wolfe. 1975. Jaundice due to nicotinic acid therapy. Am. J. Dig. Dis. 20:282–286.

Fass, S., and R.S. Rivlin. 1969. Regulation of riboflavin-metabolizing enzymes in riboflavin deficiency. Am. J. Physiol. 217:988–991.

Foy, H., and A. Kondi. 1984. The vulnerable esophagus: riboflavin deficiency and squamous cell dysplasia of the skin and the esophagus. J. Natl. Cancer Inst. 72:941–948.

Foy, H., and V. Mbaya. 1977. Riboflavin. Prog. Food Nutr. Sci. 2:357–394.

Foy, H., A. Kondi, J.N. Davies, B. Anderson, A. Parker, J. Preston, and F.J. Peers. 1974. Histologic changes in livers of pyridoxine-deprived baboons—relation to alpha l-fetoprotein and liver cancer in Africa. J. Natl. Cancer Inst. 53:1295–1311.

Frank, O., A. Luisada-Opper, M.F. Sorrell, A.D. Thomson, and H. Baker. 1971. Vitamin deficits in severe alcoholic fatty liver of man calculated from multiple reference units. Exp. Mol. Pathol. 15:191–197.

Fukushima, S., K. Imaida, T. Sakata, T. Okamura, M.A. Shibata, and N. Ito. 1983. Promoting effects of sodium L-ascorbate on two-stage urinary bladder carcinogenesis in rats. Cancer Res. 43:4454–4457.

Fukushima, S., Y. Kurata, M.A. Shibata, E. Ikawa, and N. Ito. 1984. Promotion by ascorbic acid, sodium erythorbate and ethoxyquin of neoplastic lesions in rats initiated with N-butyl-N-(4-hydroxybutyl)nitrosamine. Cancer Lett. 23:29–37.

Ghoshal, A.K., and E. Farber. 1984. The induction of liver cancer by dietary deficiency of choline and methionine without added carcinogens. Carcinogenesis 5:1367–1370.

Ghoshal, A.K., M. Ahluwalia, and E. Farber. 1983. The rapid induction of liver cell death in rats fed a choline-deficient methionine-low diet. Am. J. Pathol. 113:309–314.

Giambarresi, L.I., S.L. Katyal, and B. Lombardi. 1982. Promotion of liver carcinogenesis in the rat by a choline-devoid diet: role of liver cell necrosis and regeneration. Br. J. Cancer 46:825–829.

Graham, S., C. Mettlin, J. Marshall, R. Priore, T. Rzepka, and D. Shedd. 1981. Dietary factors in the epidemiology of cancer of the larynx. Am. J. Epidemiol. 113:675–680.

Grassetti, D.R. 1986. The antimetastatic and tumor growth retarding effects of sulfur containing analogs of nicotinamide. Cancer Lett. 31:187–195.

Ha, C., N.I. Kerkvliet, and L.T. Miller. 1984. The effect of vitamin B_6 deficiency on host susceptibility to Moloney sarcoma virus-induced tumor growth in mice. J. Nutr. 114:938–945.

Haenszel, W., and P. Correa. 1975. Developments in the epidemiology of stomach cancer over the past decade. Cancer Res. 35:3452–3459.

Halsted, C.H., and T. Tamura. 1979. Folate deficiency in liver disease. Pp. 91–100 in C.S. Davidson, ed. Problems in Liver Diseases. Stratton, New York.

Halsted, C.H., E.A. Robles, and E. Mezey. 1971. Decreased jejunal uptake of labeled folic acid (3H-PGA) in alcoholic patients: roles of alcohol and nutrition. N. Engl. J. Med. 285:701–706.

Halsted, C.H., E.A. Robles, and E. Mezey. 1973. Intestinal malabsorption in folate-deficient alcoholics. Gastroenterology 64:526–532.

Harada, T., T. Kitazawa, K. Maita, and Y. Shirasu. 1985. Effects of vitamin C on tumor induction by diethylnitrosamine in the respiratory tract of hamsters exposed to cigarette smoke. Cancer Lett. 26:163–169.

Henderson, J.M., M.A. Codner, B. Hollins, M.H. Kutner, and A.H. Merrill. 1986. The fasting B_6 vitamer profile and response to a pyridoxine load in normal and cirrhotic subjects. Hepatology 6:464–471.

Herbert, V., R. Zalusky, and C.S. Davidson. 1963. Correlation of folate deficiency with alcoholism and associated macrocytosis, anemia, and liver disease. Ann. Intern. Med. 58:977–998.

Higginson, J. 1966. Etiological factors in gastrointestinal cancer in man. J. Natl. Cancer Inst. 37:527–545.

Hillman, R.S. 1975. Alcohol and hematopoiesis. Ann. N.Y. Acad. Sci. 252:297–306.

Hillman, R.S. 1980. Vitamin B_{12}, folic acid, and the treatment of megaloblastic anemias. Pp. 1331–1346 in A.G. Gilman, L.S. Goodman, and A. Gilman, eds. The Pharmacological Basis of Therapeutics. Macmillan, New York.

Hinds, M.W., L.N. Kolonel, J.H. Hankin, and J. Lee. 1984. Dietary vitamin A, carotene, vitamin C and risk of lung cancer in Hawaii. Am. J. Epidemiol. 119:227–237.

Hormozdiari, H., N.E. Day, B. Aramesh, and E. Mahboubi. 1975. Dietary factors and esophageal cancer in the Caspian Littoral of Iran. Cancer Res. 35:3493–3498.

Hoover, K.L., P.H. Lynch, and L.A. Poirier. 1984. Profound postinitiation enhancement by short-term severe methionine, choline, vitamin B_{12}, and folate deficiency of hepatocarcinogenesis in F344 rats given a single low-dose diethylnitrosamine injection. J. Natl. Cancer Inst. 73:1327–1336.

Hoyumpa, A.M., Jr. 1983. Alcohol and thiamine metabolism. Alcoholism 7:11–14.

Imaida, K., S. Fukushima, T. Shirai, T. Masui, T. Ogiso, and N. Ito. 1984. Promoting activities of butylated hydroxyanisole, butylated hydroxytoluene and sodium L-ascorbate on forestomach and urinary bladder carcinogenesis initiated with methylnitrosourea in F344 male rats. Gann 75:769–775.

Innis, W.S.A., D.B. McCormick, and A.H. Merrill, Jr. 1985. Variations in riboflavin binding by human plasma: identification of immunoglobulins as the major proteins responsible. Biochem. Med. 34:151–165.

Innis, W.S.A., D.W. Nixon, D.R. Murray, D.B. McCormick, and A.H. Merrill, Jr. 1986. Immunoglobulins associated with elevated riboflavin binding by plasma from cancer patients. Proc. Soc. Exp. Biol. Med. 181:237–241.

Ivey, M. 1979. Nutritional supplement, mineral, and vitamin products. Pp. 141–174 in L.L. Corrigan, J. Welch, M.T. Rasmussen, S.W. Goldstein, and J. Kelly, eds. Handbook of Non-Prescription Drugs, 6th ed. American Pharmaceutical Association, Washington, D.C.

Jain, M., G.M. Cook, F.G. Davis, M.G. Grace, G.R. Howe, and A.B. Miller. 1980. A case-control study of diet and colorectal cancer. Int. J. Cancer 26:757–768.

Joint Iran–International Agency for Research on Cancer Study Group. 1977. Esophageal cancer studies in the Caspian Littoral of Iran: results of population studies—a prodrome. J. Natl. Cancer Inst. 59:1127–1138.

Jones, F.E., R.A. Komorowski, and R.E. Condon. 1984. The effects of ascorbic acid and butylated hydroxyanisole in the chemoprevention of 1,2-dimethylhydrazine-induced large bowel neoplasms. J. Surg. Oncol. 25:54–60.

Jones, P.N., E.H. Mills, and R.B. Capps. 1957. The effect of liver disease on serum vitamin B_{12} concentrations. J. Lab. Clin. Med. 49:910–922.

Jusko, W.J., and G. Levy. 1975. Absorption, protein binding, and elimination of riboflavin. Pp. 99–152 in R.S. Rivlin, ed. Riboflavin. Plenum Press, New York.

Kagan, I.A. 1957. The effect of riboflavin infusion on the vitamin B_2 level in urine in cases of malignant tumors. Patol. Fiziol. Eksp. Ter. 1:44–48.

Kagan, I.A. 1960. Determination of riboflavin in the urine of patients with malignant tumors. Khirurgiya (Moscow) 36:103–108 (Russ.).

Kallistratos, G., and E. Fasske. 1980. Inhibition of benzo(a)pyrene carcinogenesis in rats with vitamin C. J. Cancer Res. Clin. Oncol. 97:91–96.

Kaplan, H.S., and L.G. Rigler. 1945. Pernicious anemia and carcinoma of stomach—autopsy studies concerning their interrelationship. Am. J. Med. Sci. 209:339–348.

Kaplan, I.I. 1944. One-year observations of treatment of cancer with avidin (egg white). Am. J. Med. Sci. 207:733–743.

Kensler, C.J., K. Sugiura, N.F. Young, C.R. Halter, and C.P. Rhoads. 1941. Partial protection of rats by riboflavin with casein against liver cancer caused by dimethylaminazobenzene. Science 93:308–310.

Kensler, C.J., C. Wadsworth, K. Sugiura, C.P. Rhoads, K. Kittmer, and V. Du Vigneaud. 1943. Influence of egg white and avidin feeding on tumor growth. Cancer Res. 3:823–824.

Kimber, C., D.J. Deller, R.N. Ibbotson, and H. Lander. 1965. The mechanism of anaemia in chronic liver disease. Q. J. Med. 34:33–64.

Kline, B.E., H.P. Rusch, C.A. Baumann, and P.S. Lavik. 1943. Effect of pyridoxine on tumor growth. Cancer Res. 3:825–829.

Kline, B.E., J.A. Miller, and H.P. Rusch. 1945. Certain effects of egg white and biotin on carcinogenicity of p-dimethylaminoazobenzene in rats fed sub-protective level of riboflavin. Cancer Res. 5:641–643.

Klipstein, F.A., and J. Lindenbaum. 1965. Folate deficiency in chronic liver disease. Blood 25:443–456.

Kolonel, L.N., J.H. Hankin, J. Lee, S.Y. Chu, A.M.Y. Nomura, and M.W. Hinds. 1981. Nutrient intakes in relation to cancer incidence in Hawaii. Br. J. Cancer 44:332–339.

Koyanagi, T., S. Hareyama, R. Kikuchi, and T. Kimura. 1966. Effect of diet on the pantothenic acid content in serum and on the incidence of hypertension among villagers. Tohoku J. Exp. Med. 88:93–97.

Krishna, G., J. Nath, and T. Ong. 1986. Inhibition of cyclophosphamide and mitomycin C-induced sister chromatid exchanges in mice by vitamin C. Cancer Res. 46:2670–2674.

Ladner, H.A., and R.M. Salkeld. 1988. Vitamin B_6 status in cancer patients: effect of tumor site, irradiation, hormones and chemotherapy. Prog. Clin. Biol. Res. 259:273–281.

Lane, F., P. Goff, R. McGuffin, E.R. Eichner, and R.S. Hillman. 1976. Folic acid metabolism in normal, folate deficient and alcoholic man. Br. J. Haematol. 34:489–500.

Lee, S.S., and D.B. McCormick. 1983. Effect of riboflavin status on hepatic activities of flavin-metabolizing enzymes in rats. J. Nutr. 113:2274–2279.

Lee, S.S., J. Ye, D.P. Jones, and D.B. McCormick. 1983. Correlation of H_2O_2 production and liver catalase during riboflavin deficiency and repletion in mammals. Biochem. Biophys. Res. Commun. 117:788–793.

Leevy, C.M., W.S. George, H. Ziffer, and H. Baker. 1960. Pantothenic acid, fatty liver and alcoholism. J. Clin. Invest. 39:1005.

Leevy, C.M., A. Thompson, and H. Baker. 1970. Vitamins and liver injury. Am. J. Clin. Nutr. 23:493–499.

Leuchtenberger, R., C. Leuchtenberger, D. Laszlo, and R. Lewisohn. 1945. The influence of folic acid on spontaneous breast cancers in mice. Science 101:46.

Liehr, J.G., and W.J. Wheeler. 1983. Inhibition of estrogen-induced renal carcinoma in Syrian hamsters by vitamin C. Cancer Res. 43:4638–4642.

Linnell, J. 1975. The fate of cobalamins in vivo. Pp. 287–333 in B.M. Babior, ed. Cobalamin Biochemistry and Pathophysiology. Wiley, New York.

Lombardi, B., and H. Shinozuka. 1979. Enhancement of 2-acetylaminofluorene liver carcinogenesis in rats fed a choline-devoid diet. Int. J. Cancer 23:565–570.

Lumeng, L., and T.K. Li. 1974. Vitamin B_6 metabolism in chronic alcohol abuse. Pyridoxal phosphate levels in plasma and the effects of acetaldehyde on pyridoxal phosphate synthesis and degradation in human erythrocytes. J. Clin. Invest. 53:693–704.

Macquart-Moulin, G., E. Riboli, J. Cornee, B. Charnay, P. Berthezène, and N. Day. 1986. Case-control study on colorectal cancer and diet in Marseilles. Int. J. Cancer 38:183–191.

Mayet, F.H., M. Sewdarsen, and S.G. Reinach. 1986. Ascorbic acid and cholesterol levels in patients with diabetes mellitus and coronary artery disease. S. Afr. Med. J. 70:661–664.

McGuffin, R., P. Goff, and R.S. Hillman. 1975. The effect of diet and alcohol on the development of folate deficiency in the rat. Br. J. Haematol. 31:185–192.

Meinsma, L. 1964. Nutrition and cancer. Voeding 25:357–365.

Merrill, A.H., Jr., and J.M. Henderson. 1987. Diseases associated with defects in vitamin B_6 metabolism or utilization. Annu. Rev. Nutr. 7:137–156.

Merrill, A.H., Jr., and D.B. McCormick. 1980. Affinity chromatographic purification and properties of flavokinase (ATP:riboflavin 5′-phosphotransferase) from rat liver. J. Biol. Chem. 255:1335–1338.

Merrill, A.H., Jr., J.M. Henderson, E. Wang, M.A. Codner, B. Hollins, and W.J. Millikan. 1986. Activities of the hepatic enzymes of vitamin B_6 metabolism for patients with cirrhosis. Am. J. Clin. Nutr. 44:461–467.

Mettlin, C., S. Graham, R. Priore, J. Marshall, and M. Swanson. 1981. Diet and cancer of the esophagus. Nutr. Cancer 2:143–147.

Mihich, E., and C.A. Nichol. 1959. The effect of pyridoxine deficiency on mouse sarcoma 180. Cancer Res. 19:279–284.

Mikol, Y.B., K.L. Hoover, D. Creasia, and L.A. Poirier. 1983. Hepatocarcinogenesis in rats fed methyl-deficient, amino acid-defined diets. Carcinogenesis 4:1619–1629.

Miller, E.G., and H. Burns, Jr. 1984. N-nitrosodimethylamine carcinogenesis in nicotinamide-deficient rats. Cancer Res. 44:1478–1482.

Miller, J.A., and E.C. Miller. 1953. The carcinogenic aminoazo dyes. Adv. Cancer Res. 1:339–396.

Miller, Z., I. Poncet, and E. Takacs. 1962. Biochemical studies on experimental congenital malformations: flavin nucleotides and folic acid in fetuses and livers from normal and riboflavin-deficient rats. J. Biol. Chem. 237:968–973.

Mirvish, S.S. 1981a. Ascorbic acid inhibition of N-nitroso compound formation in chemical, food and biological systems. Pp. 101–126 in M.S. Zedeck and M. Lipkin, eds. Inhibition of Tumor Induction and Development. Plenum Press, New York.

Mirvish, S.S. 1981b. Inhibition of the formation of carcinogenic N-nitroso compounds by ascorbic acid and other compounds. Pp. 557–587 in J.H. Burchenal and H.P. Oettgen, eds. Cancer 1980: Achievements, Challenges, Projects, Vol. 1. Grune & Stratton, New York.

Mitchell, D., C. Wagner, W.J. Stone, G. Wilkinson, and S. Schenker. 1976. Abnormal regulation of plasma pyridoxal 5′-phosphate in patients with liver disease. Gastroenterology 71:1043–1049.

Morris, H.P. 1947. Effects on genesis and growth of tumors associated with vitamin intake. Ann. N.Y. Acad. Sci. 49:119–140.

Munoz, N., J. Wahrendorf, L.J. Bang, M. Crespi, D.I. Thurnham, N.E. Day, Z.H. Ji, A. Grassi, L.W. Yan, L.G.

Lin, F.Y. Quan, Z. Yun, Z.S. Fang, L.J. Yao, P. Correa, G.T. O'Conor, and X. Bosch. 1985. No effect of riboflavine, retinol, and zinc on prevalance of precancerous lesions of oesophagus. Randomized double-blind intervention study in high-risk population of China. Lancet 2:111–114.

NRC (National Research Council). 1980. Recommended Dietary Allowances, 9th ed. Report of the Committee on Dietary Allowances, Food and Nutrition Board, Division of Biological Sciences, Assembly of Life Sciences. National Academy Press, Washington, D.C. 185 pp.

Olson, R. 1984. Pantothenic acid. Pp. 377–382 in R.E. Olson, H.P. Broquist, C.O. Chichester, W.J. Darby, A.C. Kolbye, Jr., and R.M. Stalvey, eds. Present Knowledge in Nutrition, 5th ed. Nutrition Foundation, Washington, D.C.

Paradinas, F.J., W.M. Melia, M.L. Wilkinson, B. Portmann, P.J. Johnson, I.M. Murray-Lyon, and R. Williams. 1982. High serum vitamin B_{12} binding capacity as a marker of the fibrolamellar variant of hepatocellular carcinoma. Br. Med. J. 285:840–842.

Pauling, L., R. Willoughby, R. Reynolds, B.E. Blaisdell, and S. Lawson. 1982. Int. J. Vitam. Nutr. Res. 23:53–82.

Pauling, L., J.C. Nixon, F. Stitt, R. Marcuson, W.B. Dunham, R. Barth, K. Bensch, Z.S. Herman, B.E. Blaisdell, C. Tsao, M. Prender, V. Andrews, R. Willoughby, and E. Zuckerkandl. 1985. Effect of dietary ascorbic acid on the incidence of spontaneous mammary tumors in RIII mice. Proc. Natl. Acad. Sci. U.S.A. 82:5185–5189.

Pinto, J., Y. Huang, and R. Rivlin. 1984. Selective effects of ethanol and acetaldehyde upon intestinal enzymes metabolizing riboflavin: mechanism of reduced flavin bioavailability due to ethanol. Am. J. Clin. Nutr. 39:685.

Potera, C., D.P. Rose, and R.R. Brown. 1977. Vitamin B_6 deficiency in cancer patients. Am. J. Clin. Nutr. 30:1677–1679.

Potter, J.D., and A.J. McMichael. 1986. Diet and cancer of the colon and rectum: a case-control study. J. Natl. Cancer Inst. 76:557–569.

Prentice, R.L., G.S. Omenn, G.E. Goodman, J. Chu, M.M. Henderson, P. Feigl, G.D. Kleinman, D.B. Thomas, M.L. Hutchinson, B. Lund, and R.W. Day. 1985. Rationale and design of cancer chemoprevention studies in Seattle. Natl. Cancer Inst. Monogr. 69:249–258.

Prior, F.G. 1985. Theoretical involvement of vitamin B_6 in tumour initiation. Med. Hypotheses 16:421–428.

Rakieten, N., B.S. Gordon, A. Beaty, D.A. Cooney, R.D. Davis, and P.S.Schein. 1971. Pancreatic islet cell tumors produced by the combined action of streptozotocin and nicotinamide. Proc. Soc. Exp. Biol. Med. 137:280–283.

Ramirez, J., and N.C. Flowers. 1980. Leukocyte ascorbic acid and its relationship to coronary artery disease in man. Am. J. Clin. Nutr. 33:2079–2087.

Reddy, B.S., N. Hirota, and S. Katayama. 1982. Effect of dietary sodium ascorbate on 1,2-dimethylhydrazine- or methylnitrosourea-induced colon carcinogenesis in rats. Carcinogenesis 3:1097–1099.

Retief, F.P., and Y.J. Huskisson. 1969. Serum and urinary folate in liver disease. Br. Med. J. 1:150–153.

Risch, H.A., M. Jain, N.W. Choi, J.G. Fodor, C.J. Pfeiffer, G.R. Howe, L.W. Harrison, K.J.P. Craib, and A.B. Miller. 1985. Dietary factors and the incidence of cancer of the stomach. Am. J. Epidemiol. 122:947–957.

Rivlin, R.S. 1975. Riboflavin and cancer. Pp. 369–391 in R.S. Rivlin, ed. Riboflavin. Plenum Press, New York.

Rogers, A.E. 1975. Variable effects of a lipotrope-deficient,

high-fat diet on chemical carcinogenesis in rats. Cancer Res. 35:2469–2474.

Rogers, A.E., and P.M. Newberne. 1980. Lipotrope deficiency in experimental carcinogenesis. Nutr. Cancer 2:104–112.

Rosenberg, M.R., D.L. Novicki, R.L. Jirtle, A. Novotny, and G. Michalopoulos. 1985. Promoting effect of nicotinamide on the development of renal tubular cell tumors in rats initiated with diethylnitrosamine. Cancer Res. 45:809–814.

Ruddell, W.S., E.S. Bone, M.J. Hill, and C.L. Waters. 1978. Pathogenesis of gastric cancer in pernicious anemia. Lancet 1:521–523.

Russell, R.M. 1979. Vitamin and mineral supplements in the management of liver disease. Med. Clin. North Am. 63:537–544.

Russell, W.O., L.R. Ortega, and E.S. Wynne. 1952. Studies on methylcholanthrene induction of tumors in scorbutic guinea pigs. Cancer Res. 12:216–218.

Schenker, S., G.I. Henderson, A.M. Hoyumpa, Jr., and D.W. McCandless. 1980. Hepatic and Wernicke's encephalopathies: current concepts of pathogenesis. Am. J. Clin. Nutr. 33:2719–2726.

Schoental, R. 1975. Pancreatic islet-cell and other tumors in rats given heliotrine, a monoester pyrrolizidine alkaloid, and nicotinamide. Cancer Res. 35:2020–2024.

Schoental, R. 1977. The role of nicotinamide and of certain other modifying factors in diethylnitrosamine carcinogenesis: fusaria mycotoxins and "spontaneous" tumors in animals and man. Cancer 40:1833–1840.

Schwabedal, P.E., K. Pietrzik, and W. Wittkowski. 1985. Pantothenic acid deficiency as a factor contributing to the development of hypertension. Cardiology 72:187–189.

Semenza, G., L.S. Prestidge, D. Ménard-Jeker, and M. Bettex-Galland. 1959. Oxalacetat-carboxylase and biotin. Helv. Chim. Acta 42:669–678.

Senti, F.R., and S.M. Pilch, eds. 1984. Assessment of the Folate Nutritional Status of the U.S. Population Based on Data Collected in the Second National Health and Nutrition Examination Survey, 1976–1980. Contract No. FDA 223 83-2384. Life Science Research Office, Federation of American Societies for Experimental Biology, Bethesda, Md. 96 pp.

Shane, B. 1982. Vitamin B-6 metabolism and turnover in the ethanol-fed rat. J. Nutr. 112:610–618.

Sheppard, K., D.A. Bradbury, J.M. Davies, and D.R. Ryrie. 1984. Cobalamin and folate binding proteins in human tumour tissue. J. Clin. Pathol. 37:1336–1338.

Shinozuka, H., and B. Lombardi. 1980. Synergistic effect of a choline-devoid diet and phenobarbital in promoting the emergence of foci of gamma-glutamyltranspeptidase-positive hepatocytes in the liver of carcinogen-treated rats. Cancer Res. 40:3846–3849.

Shirai, T., E. Ikawa, M. Hirose, T. Witaya, and N. Ito. 1985. Modification by five antioxidants of 1,2-dimethylhydrazine-initiated colon carcinogenesis in F344 rats. Carcinogenesis 6:637–639.

Silverman, J., A. Rivenson, and B. Reddy. 1983. Effect of sodium ascorbate on transplantable murine tumors. Nutr. Cancer 4:192–197.

Sorrell, M.F., H. Baker, A.J. Barak, and O. Frank. 1974. Release by ethanol of vitamins into rat liver perfusates. Am. J. Clin. Nutr. 27:743–745.

Spannuth, C.L., D. Mitchell, W.J. Stone, S. Schenker, and C. Wagner. 1978. Vitamin B_6 nutriture in patients with uremia and with liver disease. Pp. 180–192 in Human

Vitamin B₆ Requirements. Proceedings of a Workshop, Committee on Dietary Allowances, Food and Nutrition Board, National Academy Press, Washington, D.C.

Spittle, C.R. 1972. Atherosclerosis and vitamin C. Lancet 1:798.

Stähelin, H.B., F. Rösel, E. Buess, and G. Brubacher. 1984. Cancer, vitamins, and plasma lipids: Prospective Basal Study. J. Natl. Cancer Inst. 73:1463–1468.

Tamura, T., and E.L. Stokstad. 1977. Increased folate excretion in acute hepatitis. Am. J. Clin. Nutr. 30:1378–1379.

Tandler, B., R.A. Erlandson, and E.L. Wynder. 1968. Riboflavin and mouse hepatic cell structure and function, I. Ultrastructural alterations in simple deficiency. Am. J. Pathol. 52:69–96.

Tannenbaum, S.R., and W. Mergens. 1980. Reaction of nitrite with vitamins C and E. Ann. N.Y. Acad. Sci. 355:267–279.

Thurnham, D.I., P. Rathakette, K.M. Hambidge, N. Munoz, and M. Crespi. 1982. Riboflavin, vitamin A and zinc status in Chinese subjects in a high-risk area for oesophageal cancer in China. Hum. Nutr. Clin. Nutr. 36:337–349.

Thurnham, D.I., S.F. Zheng, N. Munoz, M. Crespi, A. Grassi, K.M. Hambidge, and T.F. Chai. 1985. Comparison of riboflavin, vitamin A, and zinc status of Chinese populations at high and low risk for esophageal cancer. Nutr. Cancer 7:131–143.

Tryfiates, G.P., and H.P. Morris. 1974. Effect of pyridoxine deficiency on tyrosine transaminase activity and growth of four Morris hepatomas. J. Natl. Cancer Inst. 52:1259–1262.

Tuyns, A.J., M. Haelterman, and R. Kaaks. 1987a. Colorectal cancer and the intake of nutrients: oligosaccharides are a risk factor, fats are not. A case-control study in Belgium. Nutr. Cancer 10:181–196.

Tuyns, A.J., E. Riboli, G. Doornbos, and G. Péquignot. 1987b. Diet and esophageal cancer in Calvados (France). Nutr. Cancer 9:81–92.

USDA (U.S. Department of Agriculture). 1984. Nationwide Food Consumption Survey. Nutrient Intakes: Individuals in 48 States, Years 1977–1978. Report No. I-2. Consumer Nutrition Division, Human Nutrition Information Service, U.S. Department of Agriculture, Hyattsville, Md. 439 pp.

USDA (U.S. Department of Agriculture). 1986. Nationwide Food Consumption Survey. Continuing Survey of Food Intakes by Individuals. Men 19–50 Years, 1 Day, 1985. Report No. 85-3. Nutrition Monitoring Division, Human Nutrition Information Service, U.S. Department of Agriculture, Hyattsville, Md. 94 pp.

USDA (U.S. Department of Agriculture). 1987. Nationwide Food Consumption Survey. Continuing Survey of Food Intakes by Individuals. Women 19–50 Years and Their Children 1–5 Years, 4 Days, 1985. Report No. 85-4. Nutrition Monitoring Division, Human Nutrition Information Service, U.S. Department of Agriculture, Hyattsville, Md. 182 pp.

van Rensburg, S.J., J.M. Hall, and P.S. Gathercole. 1986. Inhibition of esophageal carcinogenesis in corn-fed rats by riboflavin, nicotinic acid, selenium, molybdenum, zinc, and magnesium. Nutr. Cancer 8:163–170.

van Tonder, S., M.C. Kew, J. Hodkinson, J. Metz, and F. Fernandes-Costa. 1985. Serum vitamin B₁₂ binders in South African blacks with hepatocellular carcinoma. Cancer 56:789–792.

Warwick, G.P., and J.S. Harington. 1973. Some aspects of the epidemiology and etiology of esophageal cancer with particular emphasis on the Transkei South Africa. Pp. 81–229 in G. Klein and S. Weinhouse, eds. Advances in Cancer Research, Vol. 17. Academic Press, New York.

Wassertheil-Smoller, S., S.L. Romney, J. Wylie-Roselt, S. Slagle, G. Miller, D. Lucido, C. Duttagupta, and P.R. Palan. 1981. Dietary vitamin C and uterine cervical dysplasia. Am. J. Epidemiol. 114:714–724.

West, P.M., and W.H. Woglom. 1942. Abnormalities in distribution of biotin in certain tumors and embryo tissues. Cancer Res. 2:324–331.

Williams, R.D., E. Wang, and A.H. Merrill, Jr. 1984. Enzymology of long-chain base synthesis by liver: characterization of serine palmitoyltransferase in rat liver microsomes. Arch. Biochem. Biophys. 228:282–291.

Wiss, O., and F. Weber. 1964. The liver and vitamins. Pp. 145–162 in C.H. Rouiller, ed. The Liver: Morphology, Biochemistry, Physiology, Vol. II. Academic Press, New York.

Wu, A., I. Chanarin, G. Slavin, and A.J. Levi. 1975. Folate deficiency in the alcoholic—its relationship to clinical and haematological abnormalities, liver disease, and folate stores. Br. J. Haematol. 29:469–478.

Wynder, E.L., S. Hultberg, F. Jacobson, and I.J. Bross. 1957. Environmental factors in cancer of the upper alimentary tract; a Swedish study with special reference to Plummer-Vinson (Paterson-Kelly) syndrome. Cancer 10:470–487.

Zaman, S.N., J.M. Tredger, P.J. Johnson, and R. Williams. 1986. Vitamin B₆ concentrations in patients with chronic liver disease and hepatocellular carcinoma. Br. Med. J. 293:175.

Zaridze, D.G., M. Blettner, N.N. Trapeznikov, J.P. Kuvshinov, E.G. Matiakin, B.P. Poljakov, B.K. Poddubni, S.M. Parshikova, V.I. Rottenberg, F.S. Chamrakulov, M.C. Chodjaeva, H.F. Stich, M.P. Rosin, D.I. Thurnham, D. Hoffmann, and K.D. Brunnemann. 1985. Survey of a population with a high incidence of oral and oesophageal cancer. Int. J. Cancer 36:153–158.

13

Minerals

Mineral salts are responsible for structural functions involving the skeleton and soft tissues and for regulatory functions including neuromuscular transmission, blood clotting, oxygen transport, and enzymatic activity. Calcium, phosphorus, and magnesium are required in relatively large amounts and are designated as macrominerals. These are discussed in this chapter. Minerals needed in smaller amounts are called trace elements; these are discussed in Chapter 14.

Calcium is the most abundant mineral in the human body, making up 1.5 to 2% of the total body weight. Approximately 1,200 g of calcium are present in the body of an adult human; more than 99% of that amount is found in bones. All living animals possess powerful mechanisms both to conserve calcium and to maintain constant cellular and extracellular concentrations (Arnaud, 1978, 1988; Exton, 1986). These functions are so vital to survival that during severe dietary deficiency or abnormal losses of calcium from the body, they can demineralize bone to prevent even minor degrees of hypocalcemia (i.e., low plasma calcium). Thus, bone acts as a vital physiological tissue providing a readily available source of calcium for maintenance of normal plasma calcium levels, 50% of which is ionized and physiologically active (Arnaud, 1988).

People need more calcium in their diets when they are forming bone, when intestinal absorption of calcium is impaired, and when there are inordinate losses of calcium to the environment (e.g., through increased renal excretion or lactation). If there is insufficient dietary calcium during bone formation, linear growth will be impeded and peak bone mass may not be achieved. If it is insufficient when intestinal absorption is impaired or when there are inordinate losses, the serum concentration of calcium ion (Ca^{2+}) can be maintained at normal levels only at the expense of bone calcium (Arnaud, 1988).

Phosphorus, along with calcium, is essential for calcification of bones (85% of body phosphorus is located in the skeleton). The remainder of body phosphorus is needed in soft tissues as a cofactor in myriad enzyme systems essential in the metabolism of carbohydrates, lipids, and proteins. In the form of high-energy phosphate compounds, phosphorus contributes to the metabolic potential. The phosphate ion also plays an important role in acid/base balance.

Of total body *magnesium*, 60 to 65% is found in bone and 27% is located in muscles (Shils, 1988). Magnesium is second only to potassium as the most predominant cation within cells and is essential both for the functions of many enzyme systems and for neuromuscular transmission.

Historical trends in the amounts of various minerals present in the food supply have been reported by the U.S. Department of Agriculture

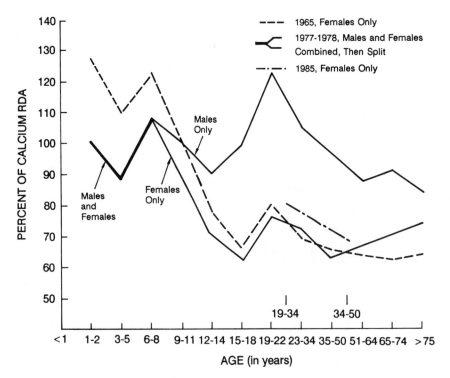

FIGURE 13–1 Mean calcium intakes expressed as percentages of the 1980 RDA (NRC, 1980) for 1965 (females only), 1977–1978 (males and females combined until 8 years of age, then separately for age 9 years and up), and 1985 (females only). Data for 1965 and 1977–1978 are based on one 24-hour recall (USDA, 1984); those for 1985 are based on 4 nonconsecutive days of intake (USDA, 1987).

(USDA) since 1909 (see Table 3–3). These data do not represent actual consumption, however, since they fail to document how much food was wasted. Per-capita calcium availability in the food supply increased 23% from 750 mg/day during 1909–1913 to 920 mg/day in 1985 (see Table 3–3). The change resulted primarily from an increased supply of dairy products during this period. The per-capita availability of phosphorus in the food supply has remained fairly steady at 1,500 mg/day since 1909–1913, and that of magnesium has declined from 380 mg/day during 1909–1913 to 320 mg/day in 1985 (see Table 3–3). The decline resulted primarily from the decreased use of grains and flour and increased practice of low-extraction milling.

Information on current intakes of calcium, phosphorus, and magnesium has been collected in national surveys, including the 1977–1978 Nationwide Food Consumption Survey (USDA, 1984), the second National Health and Nutrition Examination Survey (Carroll et al., 1983), the Continuing Survey of Food Intakes of Individuals (USDA, 1986, 1987), and the Total Diet Study (Pennington et al., 1986) (see Chapter 3). In USDA surveys, calcium intakes have been reported in terms of the 1980 Recommended Dietary Allowance (RDA), which is highest (1,200 mg) at ages 11 to 18 years and is only 800 mg for ages 1 to 10 and 18 and above (NRC, 1980). Mean intakes

below the RDA do not necessarily mean that individuals in the group are malnourished. Nutrient requirements differ from individual to individual, and the RDAs are set at high enough levels to cover the requirements of practically all healthy people in the population. Furthermore, these nationwide surveys do not reflect the usual or habitual intakes of individuals. It is inappropriate, therefore, to conclude that failure to meet the RDA indicates that an individual has an inadequate calcium intake, although the risk that some people will have inadequate intakes increases as the mean intake falls further below the RDA. Percentages of the RDA are reported here only to indicate relative intakes on the days surveyed.

Mean intakes of calcium are lower for females than for males and lower for blacks than for whites. USDA surveys indicate that females ages 9 to 19 had somewhat higher intakes in 1965 than during 1977–1978, but that older women (51 to 75 years of age) had higher intakes during 1977–1978 than in 1965 (Figure 13–1) (USDA, 1984). Mean intakes for women 19 to 50 years old were higher in 1985 than in the previous surveys (USDA, 1987).

The 1985 survey indicated that 22% of women ages 19 to 50 consumed the RDA or more, 24% consumed between 70 and 99%, 26% consumed between 50 and 69%, and 29% consumed less than 50% of the RDA. The mean intake for black women was 55% of the RDA compared with 77% for white women. Calcium intakes were lower among men and women in the older age group (35 to 50 years old) and among those living in poverty. Among children 1 to 5 years of age, 45% consumed 100% or more of the calcium RDA, while 39% consumed 70 to 99%. The 1977–1978 survey based on a 1-day intake indicated that males ages 9 to 18 maintained an average calcium intake at 90% of the RDA or above, whereas females in the same age range had progressively lower calcium intakes. Females ages 9 to 11 years, 12 to 14 years, and 15 to 18 years consumed 89, 72, and 64% of the calcium RDA, respectively. In 1985, men and women ages 19 to 50 reported mean calcium intakes of 360 and 397 mg/1,000 kcal, or 115 and 74% of the RDA, respectively. This reflects the lower caloric intake of women.

Major food sources of calcium include milk and milk products. Although leafy greens such as turnip, collard, and mustard greens are good sources, they are not consumed in large amounts by the U.S. population as a whole. The Joint Nutrition Monitoring Evaluation Committee (JNMEC) concluded that calcium deserves public health monitoring priority because of the low dietary intakes by women and the possible association of low intakes with osteoporosis in elderly women (DHHS/USDA, 1986).

Mean daily intakes of *phosphorus* for men and women 19 to 50 years of age were 1,536 mg and 966 mg, respectively, in 1985, compared with an RDA of 800 mg for this age group. Children ages 1 to 5 years consumed a mean of 992 mg/day (USDA, 1986, 1987). Major food sources of phosphorus in the U.S. diet include milk and milk products, meats, poultry, fish, and grain products. Some forms of dietary phosphorus—such as phytic acid, which is found in cereals and seeds—are not well absorbed. However, dietary deficiency of phosphorus is unlikely because of its wide distribution in foods. JNMEC judged that phosphorus intake by the U.S. population is generally adequate, requiring less monitoring than certain other nutrients (DHHS/USDA, 1986).

Mean intakes of *magnesium* in 1985 were 193 mg/day for children 1 to 5 years of age (115% of 1980 RDA) (USDA, 1987). For adults ages 19 to 50, mean intakes were 207 mg/day for women (67% of the 1980 RDA) (USDA, 1987) and 329 mg/day for men (94% of the 1980 RDA) (USDA, 1986). Major food sources of magnesium include grain products, vegetables, dairy products, meat, poultry, and fish. JNMEC found no association of magnesium intake with any chronic disease (DHHS/USDA, 1986). However, since significant portions of the population have magnesium intakes below recommended levels, they recommend further investigation of the role of magnesium nutritional status in disease and health.

EVIDENCE ASSOCIATING MINERALS WITH CHRONIC DISEASES

Calcium

Osteoporosis

Osteoporosis is a disease characterized by an absolute decrease in bone mass that results in an increased susceptibility to fracture, especially of the wrist, spine, and hip. It is common in postmenopausal women and in the elderly of both sexes and constitutes an important public health problem (Kelsey, 1984, 1987) (see Chapters 5 and 23).

Pathophysiological Relationships Among Dietary Calcium, Intestinal Absorption of Calcium, and Bone Mass

RELATIVE IMPORTANCE OF BONE CELL ACTIVITIES AND MINERAL BALANCE AS DETERMINANTS OF BONE MASS Bone is a metabolically active tissue that is turning over constantly. This process is regulated by cellular activities that resorb (osteoclastic) and form (osteoblastic) bone. In normal adult bone, resorption is precisely balanced by formation. Furthermore, these activities are coupled so that when one increases or decreases, the other shifts in degree and direction so that little or no net change in the amount of bone ensues. The driving forces for changing net bone mass are intrinsic to the cellular processes that govern bone resorption and formation. Thus, functional uncoupling of these cellular processes is required to either increase or decrease bone mass. Calcium balance generally reflects the degree to which coupling of bone formation and resorption is in balance. Negative calcium balances indicate that bone resorption exceeds formation; positive balances indicate the opposite.

In contrast to cellular processes in bone, calcium, phosphorus, and magnesium play a more passive role in any mass changes that occur in bone. They must be present at physiological concentrations in extracellular fluids for bone mineralization (formation) to occur normally. Dietary minerals contribute to this physiological state by helping to replace minerals that have been lost by obligatory processes (in urine, feces, and sweat).

PEAK BONE MASS AS A FACTOR IN MODIFYING OSTEO-
POROSIS RISK The level of bone mass achieved at
skeletal maturity (peak or maximal bone mass) is a
major factor modifying the risk for osteoporosis.
The more bone mass available before age-related
bone loss occurs, the less likely it will decrease to
a level at which fracture will occur (Heaney, 1986;
Marcus, 1982; Parfitt, 1983). Normally, longitudinal bone growth is completed sometime during the
second decade of life. It is axiomatic that positive
calcium balance is needed for this to occur normally, and it is easy to calculate that the required
average daily body retention of calcium during this
20-year period is approximately 110 mg/day for
females and 140 mg/day for males. During the
adolescent growth spurt, the required calcium retention is two to three times higher than these
average values (Garn, 1970; Nordin et al., 1979).
To achieve such retention, the RDA for calcium
has been set at 1,200 mg/day for people 10 to 18
years of age (NRC, 1980). If obligatory calcium
losses in urine, feces, and sweat are not greater
than average, the calcium RDAs are adequate
provided that 50% of the calcium ingested is
absorbed. A lower percentage of absorption or
calcium intakes less than 1,200 mg/day without
compensatory increases in the absorption rate
would not provide adequate quantities of calcium
to achieve peak bone growth. It is not known if
teenagers have such levels of calcium absorption
nor is it known whether absorption rates in teenagers can increase in response to reduced calcium
intakes.

Opinion is mixed as to the age at which peak
bone mass is achieved. The only data concerning
this issue were collected in cross-sectional studies.
These studies suggest that the metacarpal cortical
area (Garn, 1970), phalangeal density (Albanese
et al., 1975), combined cortical thickness (Matkovic et al., 1979), and bone mineral content of
the spine (Krolner and Pors Nielsen, 1982) do not
reach maximum levels until sometime during the
middle of the third or the early part of the fourth
decade of life. Such data suggest that peak bone
mass may not be achieved until 5 to 10 years after
longitudinal bone growth has ceased. During this
period, cortical porosity, which increases during
the adolescent growth spurt, is probably filled in
and bone cortices become thicker. The quantity of
bone mass that can be added is unclear; it has been
variously estimated to range from 5 to 10%
(Parfitt, 1983). The optimum calcium retention
needed to achieve this apparent increment in bone
mass is not yet known but probably ranges from 40

to 60 mg/day (Garn, 1970; Nordin et al., 1979;
Parfitt, 1983). This association of bone mass with
calcium intake is suggested by the results of a
Yugoslavian study in which there was a 5 to 10%
higher metacarpal bone mass in the inhabitants of
a "high-calcium" district starting at age 30 years
and extending at least to age 75 years when the
investigation terminated (Matkovic et al., 1979).

It is a logical extension of the above that the
quantity of dietary calcium required to achieve
peak bone mass would be greater than that required to replace obligatory losses through urine,
feces, and sweat (approximately 200 to 300 mg/
day). Thus, the period during which positive
calcium balance needs to be maintained to achieve
peak bone mass should probably be extended beyond the period of longitudinal bone growth to
perhaps ages 25 to 30 years (Heaney, 1986; Marcus, 1982; Parfitt, 1983).

BONE LOSS AS A FACTOR MODIFYING OSTEOPOROSIS
RISK Another major factor modifying osteoporosis
risk is the rate at which bone is lost as life
progresses. After peak bone mass is achieved, bone
mass appears to be maintained without much
change until 40 to 45 years of age. Subsequently,
bone is lost at a rate of 0.2 to 0.5% per year in men
and women until the eighth or ninth decade of
life. In women, bone loss accelerates to 2 to 5%
per year immediately before and for approximately
10 years after menopause (Heaney, 1986) and then
returns to its former rate—0.2 to 0.5% per year.

DECREASED CALCIUM ABSORPTION AS A FACTOR IN
OSTEOPOROSIS RISK Intestinal calcium absorption
and the ability to adapt to low-calcium diets are
impaired in many postmenopausal women
(Heaney, 1985, 1986; Heaney et al., 1977) and
elderly people of both sexes (Alevizaki et al., 1973;
Avioli et al., 1965; Bullamore et al., 1970; Gallagher et al., 1979; Ireland and Fordtran, 1973;
Nordin et al., 1976). The pathogenesis of these
abnormalities is controversial, but evidence suggests that they may be due either to a functional
decrease in the ability of the kidney to produce the
major biologically active metabolite of vitamin
D—1,25-dihydroxy vitamin D [$1,25(OH)_2D_3$]
(Gallagher et al., 1979; Riggs et al., 1981)—or to
absolute decreases in renal $1,25(OH)_2D_3$ production due to renal diseases such as that occurring in
old age (Tsai et al., 1984) (discussed in Chapter
11). The findings that levels of serum immunoreactive parathyroid hormone (Gallagher et al.,
1980; Insogna et al., 1981; Marcus et al., 1984;

Orwoll and Meier, 1986) and bioactive parathyroid hormone (Forero et al., 1987) increase with age imply that these defects in calcium absorption result in sufficient degrees of hypocalcemia to induce chronic hyperparathyroidism (secondary hyperparathyroidism). It is well established that hyperparathyroidism increases the bone remodeling rate and that a high rate of remodeling leads to accelerated bone loss whenever intrinsic imbalance favors the process of resorption over formation (Parfitt, 1980; Sakhaee et al., 1984).

Thus, it appears that the ability of the intestine to support calcium homeostasis progressively declines with age and that elderly people are increasingly forced to rely on their own bones rather than on the external environment as a source of calcium for maintaining normal extracellular free calcium (Arnaud et al., 1981). The degree to which this occurs depends on the severity of the described defects in calcium absorption, the level and bioavailability of dietary calcium, and whether specific therapeutic means are taken to correct defects in calcium absorption. The quantitative contribution, if any, of this homeostatic mechanism to the decrease in bone mass and the increase in incidence of fractures in the elderly is not known and is the subject of intensive investigation.

Epidemiologic and Clinical Studies

PROBLEMS IN ESTIMATING BONE MASS AND CALCIUM INTAKE   In most epidemiologic studies of the relationship of dietary calcium to bone mass, investigators have used radiograms (measurements of cortical bone width, area, or calculated volume from x-ray images of metacarpal bones). Such measurements are easy to obtain in the field. Moreover, their precision is similar to the more elegant single- or dual-photon absorptiometry and quantitative computed tomography techniques (Cohn, 1981; Mazess, 1983); however, they are less sensitive and specific. In addition, these cortical bone measurements do not accurately reflect bone mass in the trabecular or spongy bone compartment where rapid turnover occurs. Thus, population-based data obtained with cortical width or area measurements may not detect subtle changes that other, more sensitive and specific techniques might easily detect. Such changes that are detected reflect, at best, those that have occurred in cortical bone and not in trabecular bone. Trabecular bone makes up at least 50% of the bone in the spine (Nottestad et al., 1987) and is affected to the greatest extent early in menopause (Riggs and Melton, 1986).

The methods used to assess dietary calcium intake in these studies have varied from "the best available estimates" (Nordin, 1966) to 7-day replicate dietary records and 47-category interviews (Garn, 1970), to chemical analyses of foodstuffs (Matkovic et al., 1979). Most authors have been aware of the inherent inaccuracies of dietary recall data, and because of the even greater inaccuracies of estimates of calcium intake over a lifetime, most have relied on estimates of current calcium intake. Thus, even the most careful approaches to providing accurate calcium intake data can be faulted, and their interpretation must be approached with caution, especially in relation to estimates of bone mass based on a measurement technique with inherent flaws.

CALCIUM INTAKE AND BONE MASS   Published reports have shown either no relationship or only a modestly positive relationship between dietary calcium and cortical bone mass. Garn et al. (1969) found the same rate of loss of metacarpal cortical mass in more than 5,800 subjects from seven countries, despite wide variations in calcium intake between groups. In fact, low calcium intakes by some ethnic groups were associated with bone mass values higher than in groups with high calcium intakes over a lifetime. On the other hand, in a 10-state nutrition survey, Garn et al. (1981) found a statistically significant increase in metacarpal cortical area in people in the highest, as compared to the lowest, percentile of calcium intake. In a similar analysis, using data from the first Health and Nutrition Examination Survey (HANES I), investigators observed a significant positive correlation between calcium intake and metacarpal cortical width for all 2,250 subjects (Carroll et al., 1983; DHEW, 1979). When the 960 white women in the study were excluded, the significance of the correlation disappeared.

Matkovic et al. (1979) investigated metacarpal bone mass and the incidence of hip fracture in two regions of Yugoslavia whose inhabitants ingested greatly different quantities of calcium (500 mg/day compared to 1,100 mg/day largely through dairy products). The inhabitants of the high-calcium district ingested more calories, fats, and protein and less carbohydrates than the low-calcium district. However, the regions were similar in their agrarian economy, and except for a significantly longer lower limb length in the high-calcium district, ages, weights, and other anthropomorphic indices were identical. The inhabitants of the high-calcium district had a 50% lower incidence of hip fractures and a significant increase in metacarpal cortical bone volume as compared with the inhabitants of the low-calcium district. Because the differences in bone mass as a function of age were constant, it is more likely that high lifelong calcium intakes in this population increased peak cortical bone mass than that it prevented bone loss. In contrast to the decreased incidence in hip fractures observed in the high-calcium district, the incidence of fractures of the distal forearm (the distal 3 cm of the radius or ulna) was the same in the two regions. This is of interest because the fracture sites at the hip generally are composed mainly of cortical bone, whereas those at the wrist are mainly of trabecular bone. The results of a correlation study reported by Anderson and Tylavsky (1984) are highly relevant in this regard. Those investigators related current and lifelong calcium intake to bone mineral content (measured by single-photon absorptiometry) at the distal radius (mixture of cortical and trabecular bone) and at the midshaft of the radius (largely cortical bone) in residents of four North Carolina communities. They found a positive correlation of bone mineral content with calcium intake at the midshaft site but no correlation at the distal site.

Several clinical studies have been conducted to examine the relationship between calcium intake and bone mass. Using radiograms, Smith and Frame (1965), Smith and Rizek (1966), and Garn (1970) found no association between current calcium intake and current bone mass. Similarly, Lavel-Jeanet et al. (1984) and Pacifici et al. (1985) observed no correlation of calcium intake with vertebral density as measured by quantitative computed tomography. Most recently, Riggs et al. (1987) found no relationship between the calcium intakes (range, 260 to 2,003 mg/day; mean, 922 mg/day) of 106 normal women ages 23 to 84 years and the rates of change in bone mineral density at the midradius (determined by single-photon absorptiometry) and the lumbar spine (determined by dual-photon absorptiometry) over a mean period of 4.1 years.

In contrast to the negative observations made by Lavel-Jeanet et al. (1984) and by Pacifici et al. (1985) with quantitative computed tomography of the spine, Kanders et al. (1984), using dual-photon absorptiometry, found that the BMC of L2 through L4 vertebrae in young women with a high calcium intake was higher than that in women with a low intake. In a longitudinal study of 76 healthy postmenopausal women, Dawson-Hughes et al. (1987) found, using dual-photon absorptiometry, that women with calcium intakes less than 405 mg/day lost spinal bone density at a significantly greater rate than those with an intake of greater than 777 mg/day ($p < .026$).

CALCIUM INTAKE AND OSTEOPOROSIS Nordin (1966) reported the results of an intercountry comparison of calcium intake and osteoporotic fractures. Despite inconsistency in the methods used to report calcium intakes in the 12 countries surveyed, it was possible to demonstrate an inverse rank-order relationship between frequency of osteoporotic vertebral fracture as determined by spine x-ray and calcium intakes. Japanese women, whose calcium intake averaged 400 mg/day, had the highest frequency of fracture, whereas women in Finland had the highest intake (1,300 mg/day) and the lowest fracture frequency. This relationship did not hold for some countries. For example, in The Gambia and Jamaica, calcium intakes were low but osteoporotic fractures were rare. As reported by Matkovic et al. (1979), the hip fracture incidence in the Yugoslav district with a high calcium intake was 50% lower than in the low calcium district. But no difference was detected in the incidence of fractures around the wrist.

Most clinical studies show lower calcium intakes by osteoporotic patients than by age-matched controls (Hurxthal and Vose, 1969; Lutwak and Whedon, 1963; Nordin, 1961; Riggs et al., 1967; Vinther-Paulsen, 1953). Dietary calcium was lower than 800 mg/day in patients and controls in all these investigations. In another study, intakes were greater than 800 mg/day in patients and controls, and no differences in calcium intake between the two groups were observed (Nordin et al., 1979). The results of that study support the view of Heaney (1986) that low dietary calcium may play a permissive rather than a causative role in the development of osteoporosis and that this role can be demonstrated best when dietary calcium is below a "saturation" level.

Clinical Studies on Calcium Supplementation

EFFECT OF CALCIUM SUPPLEMENTATION ON BONE MASS The long-term effects of calcium supplementation on bone mass are not yet established. The results of short-term investigations (2 years or less) are mixed. In general, they show a slowing of bone loss measured at sites composed mostly of cortical bone but not at sites composed of trabecular bone. All studies in which estrogen treatment was used as a companion protocol have shown that calcium supplementation is inferior to estrogen in slowing cortical bone loss and that estrogen prevents trabecular bone loss completely. Some of these studies were randomized (Lamke et al., 1978; Recker and Heaney, 1985; Recker et al., 1977; Riis et al., 1987; Smith et al., 1981), but only two were blinded (Riis et al., 1987; Smith et al., 1981). In the study by Smith et al. (1981), 40% of the subjects were lost to follow-up.

The results of Recker et al. (1977) reflect those of the others. These investigators showed that after 2 years, a 1.04-g supplement of calcium given as the carbonate salt to 22 women between 55 and 65 years of age resulted in a 0.22% decrease in metacarpal cortical bone area as compared with a 1.18% decrease in 20 placebo-treated age-matched women (p <.05). By contrast, there was no difference in bone mineral content of the distal radius (mixture of trabecular and cortical bone). The reduction of metacarpal cortical bone loss with calcium supplementation was less than the reduction resulting from estrogen treatment of 18 age-matched women, which completely prevented bone loss at the distal radius (Recker et al., 1977).

In a similar but nonrandomized study, Horsman et al. (1977) administered 800 mg of elemental calcium as the gluconate salt to 24 postmenopausal women over a 2-year period and found a significant decrease in bone loss from the ulna (cortical bone) compared to 18 placebo-treated control subjects. However, calcium treatment caused little if any diminution of the bone loss observed at the distal radius or in metacarpal cortices. Similarly, Nilas et al. (1984) found no change in bone mineral content at the distal radius when three groups of women with calcium intakes varying from below 550 mg/day to more than 1,150 mg/day were given a 500-mg elemental calcium supplement daily. In contrast, a randomized and blinded investigation in postmenopausal women by the same group (Riis et al., 1987) showed that daily administration of 2,000 mg of elemental calcium as the carbonate salt for 2 years slowed bone loss at the proximal forearm and slowed calcium loss from the total skeleton, whereas the loss of bone from sites composed predominantly of trabecular bone was no different from that of placebo-treated control subjects. As in previous studies, bone mineral content remained constant at all measurement sites in subjects receiving estrogen.

In a nonrandomized study, Ettinger et al. (1987) observed that calcium supplementation up to 1,500 mg/day as the carbonate salt had no effect on bone mineral content in the spine as assessed by quantitative computed tomography, distal radius, or metacarpal cortical bone mass in 44 postmenopausal women as compared with 25 age-matched women who elected not to receive treatment. By contrast, in 15 women who elected to take low-dose conjugated estrogen (0.3 mg/day) combined with 1,500 mg of calcium per day, there was complete protection against bone loss. This latter observation is of considerable theoretical and practical interest, because this same group of investigators previously demonstrated that conjugated estrogen at the same low dose, given without calcium, failed to prevent vertebral bone loss (Cann et al., 1980). Thus, it is possible that dietary calcium plays a sex hormone-dependent permissive role in the maintenance of bone mass.

Riggs et al. (1976) showed that the increased bone resorption surfaces observed in biopsies of the iliac crest bone from osteoporotic patients are partially restored by combined calcium and vitamin D supplementation. This effect was associated with a decrease in serum immunoreactive parathyroid hormone (iPTH) within the normal range—an event the authors justifiably speculated was responsible for the decrease in resorption surfaces. The results of several other investigations, not involving bone histomorphometry, are consistent with this apparent antiresorption effect of calcium supplementation. Recker et al. (1977) showed that bone resorption, as assessed by kinetic analysis of plasma ^{45}Ca decay curves, was decreased by supplementation of postmenopausal women with calcium carbonate. Horowitz et al. (1984) reported that oral calcium suppresses hydroxyproline excretion, a well-established index of bone resorption, in osteoporotic postmenopausal women.

EFFECT OF CALCIUM SUPPLEMENTATION ON FRACTURE The evidence relating calcium supplementation to fracture prevalence is scanty. The only study of substance comes from the Mayo Clinic, where Riggs et al. (1982) conducted a nonrandomized but prospective assessment of the effect of various treatments of postmenopausal females with generalized osteopenia on the occurrence of future vertebral fractures. In that study, eight subjects received calcium carbonate (1,500 to 2,500 mg/day) and 19 received calcium plus vitamin D (50,000 IU once or twice a week). Both groups had 50% fewer vertebral fractures than did 27 placebo-treated and 18 untreated patients.

SAFETY OF CALCIUM SUPPLEMENTATION Calcium supplementation is safe in the absence of conditions that cause hypercalcemia or nephrolithiasis (Heath and Callaway, 1985). Thus, in normal individuals, calcium intakes ranging from 1,000 to 2,500 mg/day do not result in hypercalcemia (FDA, 1979) and extremely high intakes (>2,500 mg/day) are required to produce hypercalciuria (>300 mg within 24 hours) (Knapp, 1947). Elemental calcium intakes in excess of 3 to 4 g/day should be avoided because they will cause hypercalcemia in most subjects (Ivanovich et al., 1967). Constipation can be a limiting side effect of calcium supplementation in many people and is particularly bothersome in the elderly. Calcium carbonate is currently the favored and cheapest form of supplemental calcium. Other anionic forms (e.g., calcium gluconate, calcium lactate) are equally effective but are generally more expensive.

Animal Studies

There is no completely satisfactory animal model of age-related or postmenopausal osteoporosis. Nevertheless, the animal studies on dietary calcium and bone mass conducted thus far have produced results consistent with those from human studies. However, almost all reports concern young growing or aged animals and thus differ from investigations in humans (Leichsenring et al., 1951; Malm, 1953; Zemel and Linkswiler, 1981), which in general focus on young or middle-aged adults.

Nordin (1960) reviewed the extensive literature describing the many species in which bone mass decreases as a result of calcium deficiency. In all these studies, it is clear that the bone disease produced by calcium deficiency resembles osteoporosis in humans. Low-calcium diets cause a loss of trabecular bone in adult cats (Bauer et al., 1929) and a generalized thinning of bone in dogs (Jaffe et al., 1932). After feeding adult cats a low-calcium diet for 5 months, Jowsey and Gershon-Cohen (1964) found that the animals had decreased skeletal weight, decreased density of bone as determined radiographically, and microradiographic evidence of increased bone resorption. These changes were partially reversed by feeding the animals a diet containing increased calcium. Many investigators have demonstrated that low-calcium diets lead to increased bone resorption typical of hyperparathyroidism and a generalized decrease in bone mass in rats and mice (Bell et al., 1941; de Winter and Steendijk, 1975; Gershon-Cohen et al., 1962; Harrison and Fraser, 1960; Ornoy et al., 1974; Rasmussen, 1977; Salomon, 1972; Salomon and Volpin, 1970; Shah et al., 1967; Sissons et al., 1985).

Of interest in relation to the possible influence of calcium deficiency on fracture is the study by Ferretti et al. (1985), who showed that femora from rats maintained on a low-calcium diet for 5 months had reduced inertial parameters and load resistance in comparison to femora from chronically thyroparathyroidectomized (thyroxine-treated) animals or animals fed a high-calcium diet. Griffiths et al. (1975) showed that rhesus monkeys on a low-calcium diet for several years developed radiological and histological changes in their skeletons that were consistent with hyperparathyroidism and osteoporosis.

Interactions

ESTROGEN   The lack and diminished levels of estrogen are risk factors for osteoporosis. Estrogen replacement therapy reduces the loss of bone mass associated with oophorectomy and markedly reduces risk of hip and vertebral fracture (see Chapter 23). It is not clear whether the addition of calcium supplements to hormone-replacement therapy results in added benefit.

PHOSPHORUS   Although data from animal studies suggest that high levels of dietary phosphorus increase bone loss, detailed studies in humans show little to no effect of high phosphorus intake on calcium balance (see section on Phosphorus, below).

PROTEIN   Studies over the past half century indicate that high intakes of purified isolated protein increase the renal excretion of calcium (see Chapter 8). However, epidemiologic studies have shown no adverse effect of high dietary protein on either rate of hip fracture (Matkovic et al., 1979) or metacarpal cortical bone mass (Garn et al., 1981). As discussed in Chapters 8 and 23, the calciuric effect of protein is considerably reduced when increased protein intake is accompanied by high phosphorus intake—a common occurrence, since most foods in the United States with a high protein content also contain high levels of phosphorus.

FIBER   Dietary fiber has been reported to chelate calcium and other minerals in the gastrointestinal tract (Dobbs and Baird, 1977; Ismail-Beigi et al., 1977; McCance and Widdowson, 1942). This observation led to concern that high-fiber diets may increase risk of bone loss and osteoporotic fracture. However, there is little evidence that high-fiber diets alone induce calcium deficiency in people who otherwise consume a balanced diet (see Chapters 10 and 23).

DRUGS   Although some drugs (e.g., thiazide diuretics) increase renal tubular reabsorption of calcium, they do not appear to influence calcium balance or changes in bone mass (Sakhaee et al., 1985). Phosphate-binding antacids such as the nonprescription aluminum hydroxide gels, if taken chronically even at low doses, can cause phosphate depletion and an accompanying increase in bone resorption and urinary calcium excretion (Maierhofer et al., 1984; Spencer and Lender, 1979; Spencer et al., 1982). It is not clear, however, whether the phosphate-binding type of antacid is related to age-related bone loss, particularly in calcium-deficient people.

Hypertension

Contraction of smooth muscle depends on the interaction among the contractile proteins—actin and myosin—and is the end result of a cascade of reactions initiated by a rise in cytosolic free calcium concentrations (Johansson and Somlyo, 1980). This observation led to the hypothesis that dietary calcium influences blood pressure and possibly risk for hypertension.

Epidemiologic Studies

Within the past decade, considerable new evidence from human studies has suggested a role for dietary calcium in blood pressure regulation. However, views and theories are still in conflict, in part because of the wide range in study findings. For example, in an analysis of data from HANES I, McCarron et al. (1984) concluded that reduced calcium intake was the best predictor of increased blood pressure among all variables analyzed. Similar conclusions were reached in studies conducted in California (Ackley et al., 1983), Puerto Rico (Garcia-Palmieri et al., 1984), and the Netherlands (Kok et al., 1986).

Other investigators have reached different conclusions. For example, Feinleib et al. (1984) reanalyzed the HANES I data studied by McCarron et al. (1984), controlling for age and weight of subjects, and found no significant association between calcium intake and blood pressure. Harlan et al. (1984) found systolic blood pressure and calcium intake to be negatively correlated in women but positively correlated in men. Gruchaw et al. (1985) concluded that dietary calcium was not a significant predictor of blood pressure. In a large prospective study of omnivorous Japanese men in Hawaii, Reed et al. (1985) found inverse associations between intakes of calcium, potassium, protein, and milk (determined from 24-hour dietary recalls) and both systolic and diastolic blood pressure levels, although it was not possible to determine whether any of these dietary components had an independent effect on blood pressure.

The inconsistency among epidemiologic findings may be, in part, a result of the high degree of collinearity among other dietary factors associated with blood pressure (e.g., potassium and protein) and the limitations in the methods of assessing calcium intake in noninstitutionalized populations (Kaplan and Meese, 1986; Lau and Eby, 1985).

Clinical Studies

Acute elevations of serum calcium by intravenous infusions of calcium sharply raises blood pressure (Weidmann et al., 1972). Chronic hypercalcemia due to primary hyperparathyroidism is frequently accompanied by hypertension (Rosenthal and Roy, 1972), which is often reversible after the hyperparathyroidism is cured by removing abnormal parathyroid tissue (Blum et al., 1977). Serum calcium within the normal range has also been shown to correlate with high blood pressure (Bianchetti et al., 1983; Kesteloot, 1984a).

Hypertensive patients have been shown to have mild hypercalciuria (Morris et al., 1983; Strazzullo et al., 1986) and lower levels of serum ionized and ultrafiltrable calcium than normotensive patients, even in the absence of differences in total serum calcium (Folsom et al., 1986). Postnov and Orlov (1985) reported that the cells of hypertensive patients bind calcium less avidly than normotensives, and Erne et al. (1984) found increased calcium levels in platelets from hypertensive patients. Resnick et al. (1986) reported alterations in the serum concentrations of the calcium-regulating hormones (i.e., parathyroid hormone, calcitonin, and calcitriol) in hypertensive patients that are associated with differences in the renin–aldosterone system. Although all these reported changes indicate that calcium metabolism is probably perturbed in primary hypertension, it is not clear whether they are the cause or the result of the hypertension, and taken together, they do not support any single coherent theory of disordered blood pressure regulation.

Most intervention studies of calcium supplementation demonstrate a mild short-term reduction in blood pressure in certain normotensive and hypertensive subjects (Belizan et al., 1983;

Grobbee and Hofman, 1986; McCarron and Morris, 1985; Resnick et al., 1984a; Singer et al., 1985). In some patients with hypertension and high levels of plasma renin, blood pressure may actually rise in response to calcium supplementation (Resnick et al., 1984b). No clinical trial of adequate size and design to test the hypothesis that increasing dietary calcium reduces hypertension risk has yet been reported.

ANIMAL STUDIES   Most animal studies on the relationship of calcium metabolism and hypertension have compared the spontaneously hypertensive rat (SHR) to its normotensive control—the Wistar-Kyoto rat (WKR) (Young et al., 1988). The results are confusing and controversial. Most investigators (Bindels et al., 1987; Lau et al., 1984b; McCarron et al., 1981; Stern et al., 1984; Wright and Rankin, 1982) reported that serum concentrations of ionized calcium [Ca^{2+}] are lower in the SHR than in the WKR. Some (Lau et al., 1984b; McCarron et al., 1981), but not all (Bindels et al., 1987; Hsu et al., 1986), agree that urinary calcium excretion is increased in SHRs. Although difficult to measure, serum iPTH has generally been reported to be slightly increased in the serum of SHRs (Bindels et al., 1987; McCarron et al., 1981; Stern et al., 1984), whereas serum 1,25-dihydroxycholecalciferol has been found to be increased (Bindels et al., 1987; Lau et al., 1986), decreased (Kurtz et al., 1986; Lucas et al., 1986; Merke et al., 1987; Schedl et al., 1986; Young et al., 1986), or unchanged (Kawashima, 1986; Schedl et al., 1984, 1986; Stern et al., 1984), depending to some extent upon the age and sex of the SHRs studied. Measurements of intestinal calcium absorption by a variety of techniques have been inconsistent (Bindels et al., 1987; Gafter et al., 1986; Hsu et al., 1986; Lau et al., 1984b, 1986; Lucas et al., 1986; McCarron et al., 1985, 1986; Roullet et al., 1986; Schedl et al., 1984; Stern et al., 1984; Toraason and Wright, 1981). It is thus difficult to ascribe the hypercalciuria in the SHR to intestinal hyperabsorption of calcium. Interestingly, studies that have measured bone calcium content (Izawa et al., 1985; Lucas et al., 1986) show it to be decreased in older (22 to 52 weeks) SHRs. These data do not help determine if the recorded abnormalities in calcium metabolism observed in the SHR are the cause, the result, or merely associated with its hypertension. However, they do suggest a pathogenic sequence for the changes in mineral and bone metabolism in SHRs. Such a sequence would include hypercalci-

uria due to a renal leak of calcium, leading to a decrease in serum calcium, secondary hyperparathyroidism, and finally, bone demineralization. As discussed above in the section on Clinical Studies, some of these same abnormalities have been observed in hypertensive humans. Thus, whether or not they are ultimately proved to be related etiologically to hypertension, they should be investigated independently in the SHR as a potential animal model of a clinical disorder of mineral and bone metabolism that might coexist with, or be caused by, certain hypertensive states.

Dietary calcium supplementation lowers blood pressure in SHRs (Ayachi, 1979; Kageyama et al., 1986; Lau et al., 1984a; McCarron et al., 1981, 1985). These observations suggest a possible etiologic link between the abnormalities of calcium metabolism and the hypertension found in SHRs; however, they fall well short of the evidence needed to prove a causative relationship.

Cancer

Epidemiologic and Clinical Studies

The relationship of calcium intake to risk of colon cancer has been examined in a number of epidemiologic studies. In one 19-year cohort study of 1,954 people in the United States, the calcium and vitamin D intake of people with colorectal cancer was significantly lower than in those without the disease (Garland et al., 1985). Mean calcium intake was 290 mg/1,000 kcal for colorectal cancer subjects and 328 mg/1,000 kcal for controls.

The results of case-control studies are inconsistent. G.R. Howe (National Cancer Institute of Canada, personal communication, 1989) found no association between dietary calcium and colorectal cancer in a reanalysis of an earlier study by Jain et al. (1980), who examined the role of a number of nutrients in relation to colorectal cancer risk. However, a protective effect of calcium with increasing intake was suggested in a case-control study conducted in Marseilles, France (Macquart-Moulin et al., 1986). The relative risk for the highest quartile of consumption compared to the lowest was 0.7. The association just failed to achieve statistical significance and was not further considered in a multivariate model. In addition, no association between calcium intake and risk of colorectal cancer was found in case-control studies conducted in Belgium (Tuyns et al., 1987a) and in Melbourne, Australia (Kune et al., 1987). In the Melbourne study, however, there was a suggestion of a protective effect in females when calcium intake was considered as a univariate.

Intercountry comparisons of calcium availability and colorectal cancer mortality rates also do not support a protective role for calcium intake. One comparison of 38 countries (G. McKeown-Eyssen, University of Toronto, and E. Bright-See, Ludwig Institute for Cancer Research, personal communication, 1989) gave a correlation of .51 between estimates of per-capita calcium availability and colorectal cancer mortality that was reduced to −.03 when the investigators controlled for fat intake. Studies of colon cancer incidence in rural Finland, other parts of Scandinavia, and New York that show a protective effect of dietary fiber (IARC, 1977; Jensen et al., 1982; Reddy et al., 1978) could also be explained by differences in calcium intake since the main contributor to dietary fat intake in the low-risk areas was milk products. However, there were no direct measurements of calcium intake in those study areas.

In a pilot study of the effect of calcium supplementation on proliferation of colonic cells in patients considered to be at increased risk for colon cancer, Lipkin and Newmark (1985) found that the daily administration of 1.2 g of elemental calcium as calcium carbonate led to a reduction of colonic crypt labeling with tritiated thymidine, in vitro, that approximated the pattern seen in a low-risk control population.

Tuyns et al. (1987b) found a weak protective effect of dietary calcium against risk of esophageal cancer. However, the finding was not statistically significant and was substantially weaker than the protective effect found for vitamin C.

Animal Studies

Dietary calcium has been found to have a significant effect on the colonic epithelium of laboratory animals under several different experimental conditions. Calcium reduces the loss of superficial epithelial cells or the compensatory proliferation of basal crypt cells that occurs in animals exposed to bile and fatty acids or excess dietary fats. This effect has been seen in animals into which bile and fatty acids have been instilled intrarectally (Wargovich et al., 1983), in animals whose colons were perfused with bile acids (Rafrer et al., 1986), in animals whose diets were supplemented with cholic acid (Bird et al., 1986), in animals given oral boluses of fat (Bird, 1986), and in animals fed high-fat diets (Caderni et al., 1988). Two studies that did not show an effect of calcium in reducing the number of colonic tumors

also showed no cancer-promoting effect of high dietary fat (Bull et al., 1987).

Phosphorus

All living organisms require phosphorus to maintain their structure and function. In biologic fluids, it exists as phosphate ion. A major element in hydroxyapatite, phosphorus is a key inorganic constituent of bone. In cells, it is an important part of many life-sustaining compounds, such as phospholipids, phosphoproteins, and nucleic acids; the hormonal second messengers, cyclic adenosine monophosphate, cyclic guanine monophosphate, and inositol polyphosphates; and 2,3-diphosphoglycerate, which is the regulator of oxygen release by hemoglobin. Phosphorus is also the repository of metabolic energy in the form of the high-energy phosphate bond, an allosteric regulator of many enzymes, and an active participant in many physiological buffer systems. Serum concentrations of phosphate serve as one of the regulators of the rate of renal production of $1,25(OH)_2D_3$.

Hypophosphatemia

Hypophosphatemia is a serious complication of many medical disorders (e.g., acute alcoholism, during the withdrawal phase); however, the food supply is so replete with phosphorus that the condition occurs only under the most adverse nutritional conditions. One exception is found in people who chronically ingest phosphate-binding antacids (see the discussion on Interactions in the section on Calcium). The major clinical manifestation of chronic moderate hypophosphatemia is a defective bone mineralization resembling osteomalacia. Severe hypophosphatemia may cause a life-threatening syndrome that includes blood cell, muscular, hepatic, and central and peripheral nervous system dysfunctions.

Excessive Dietary Phosphorus

Spencer et al. (1978) showed that an increase in phosphorus intake from 800 mg/day (the RDA) to 2,000 mg/day in adult males failed to affect calcium balance regardless of the calcium intake, which ranged from 200 to 2,000 mg/day. Similarly, Heaney and Recker (1982) reported that varying phosphorus intake had no effect on overall calcium balance in perimenopausal women. Both groups observed that urinary calcium excretion varied inversely with dietary phosphorus, implying that fecal calcium excretion must have varied directly with dietary phosphorus because there was no change in calcium balance. It thus appears that changes in phosphorus intake by normal adult humans have important effects on calcium metabolism (i.e., decreased intestinal calcium absorption and decreased renal excretion of calcium) but that these effects probably cancel one another so that calcium balance is not affected.

The mechanism by which increased dietary phosphorus might decrease intestinal absorption of calcium has been investigated by Portale et al. (1986). Those investigators showed that increasing dietary phosphorus from a low intake of <500 mg/day to 3,000 mg/day decreased the production rate of $1,25(OH)_2D_3$ so that its serum concentration fell from a level 80% greater than normal to the low-normal range. This observation strongly suggests that the ability to adapt to decreases or increases in dietary phosphorus depends on the ability of the kidney to respond by increasing or decreasing its production of $1,25(OH)_2D_3$, respectively.

There is, therefore, a question whether or not increases in dietary phosphorus might adversely influence calcium economy in people whose kidneys have a limited capacity to produce $1,25(OH)_2D_3$ or in those who need to be in positive calcium balance, such as pregnant and lactating women. Portale et al. (1984) reported that normal dietary phosphorus levels were sufficient to suppress plasma concentrations of $1,25(OH)_2D_3$ in children with moderate renal insufficiency. No studies of the influence of dietary phosphorus on calcium and bone metabolism have been reported in other populations that may be unduly sensitive to increments in dietary phosphorus above the RDA [e.g., the young who are building bone or some elderly people who have a decreased ability to absorb or conserve calcium (Sakhaee et al., 1984)], who have a decreased ability to absorb or conserve calcium (Sakhaee et al., 1984), even though concern has been expressed (Bell et al., 1977; Lutwak, 1975) that high phosphorus intakes may contribute to age-related bone loss in humans.

There is considerable evidence in animals that diets containing phosphorus in relatively larger quantities than calcium cause hyperparathyroidism and bone loss (Draper and Bell, 1979; Draper et al., 1972; Krishnarao and Draper, 1972; Krook, 1968; Miller, 1969; Saville and Krook, 1969). Almost all these reports concern young (growing) or aged animals and differ from other investigations of the influence of high-phosphate diets on calcium metabolism in young or middle-aged adult humans (Bell et al., 1977; Leichsenring et al., 1951; Malm, 1953; Zemel and Linkswiler, 1981).

Magnesium

Magnesium is the fourth most common positively charged ion in the body and is the second most abundant intracellular cation (next to potassium). It plays important roles in osmotic pressure maintenance, enzyme activation, muscular activity, energy metabolism, stabilization of nerve function, and maintenance of bone structure. The average adult body contains about 25 g of magnesium, approximately 50 to 60% of which is found in bone.

Hypomagnesemia

Hypomagnesemia results either from decreased intestinal absorption of magnesium or from increased renal excretion. The disease occurs only rarely as an isolated dietary deficiency. It is more often associated with severe general nutritional deficiency, intestinal malabsorption syndromes, excessive vomiting and diarrhea, genetic defects in the kidney, uncontrolled diabetes, and prolonged diuretic therapy. Severe hypomagnesemia (serum levels <1.0 mg/dl) can produce cardiac arrythmias, coronary spasm, hypocalcemia, low blood potassium, changes in mental status, seizures, anorexia, and weakness (Miller, 1985).

Hypertension

Epidemiologic Studies

Magnesium is a potent inhibitor of vascular smooth-muscle contraction. It decreases peripheral vascular resistance and is a vasodilator that may play a role in the regulation of blood pressure. There are no data linking magnesium intake to the prevalence of hypertension. In case-control studies, serum magnesium levels have variously been reported as both higher and lower in hypertensive, compared to normotensive, people. Sangal and Beevers (1982) found an inverse association between serum magnesium and blood pressure in 73 Danish men and women whose mean age was 60 years. Similar findings have been reported by Albert et al. (1958) and Petersen et al. (1977). Kesteloot et al. (1984b) observed an inverse relationship between urinary magnesium and diastolic blood pressure levels in a subsample of the Belgian population. Resnick et al. (1984a) reported a close inverse correlation between erythrocyte magnesium concentration and both systolic and diastolic blood pressure.

The few intercountry comparisons of magnesium intake and blood pressure show no association. Thulin et al. (1980) reported that magnesium intake was similar in normotensive and hypertensive Scandinavian women. Likewise, no relationship between magnesium excretion and blood pressure was seen in a Korean population (Kesteloot, 1984a) or in the NHANES II population in the United States (Harlan et al., 1984).

Animal Studies

Data from studies in animals show a consistent inverse effect of magnesium intake on blood pressure. An increase in blood pressure and constriction of arteriolar, capillary, and postcapillary blood vessels has been observed in magnesium-deficient rats (Altura et al., 1984). Berthelot and Esposito (1983) noted a more rapid increase in the blood pressure level and heart rate of SHRs fed a magnesium-deficient diet compared with those fed a diet containing a normal amount of magnesium. SHRs fed a magnesium-supplemented diet (1.05%) had a blunted rise in blood pressure and a significantly lower mean blood pressure level as compared with controls after 22 weeks of feeding.

Wallach and Verch (1986) reported that numerous organs from SHRs, including the heart, lungs, kidneys, and bone, had 6 to 10% reductions in their magnesium content as hypertension became manifest. An inverse relationship between arterial blood pressure and tissue magnesium was also noted, but the authors could not determine whether the reduced tissue magnesium was a cause of or a response to the developing hypertension.

Resnick et al. (1986) reported that the higher the intracellular free magnesium in male Wistar rats, the lower the blood pressure. The authors suggest that there is a uniform and tightly coupled relationship between levels of intracellular free magnesium and blood pressure, regardless of pathological subtypes of hypertension or dietary conditions.

Cardiovascular Diseases

Populations in areas with hard water (i.e., water with high levels of minerals, including magnesium) have lower rates of cardiovascular diseases than those in areas with soft water (Neri and Johansen, 1978; Schroeder, 1960). This phenomenon, as well as the relationship between magnesium nutrition and cardiac rhythmicity in ischemic heart disease, has been reviewed extensively by Seelig (1974). She concluded that the role of magnesium in maintaining the normal rhythmicity

of the heart during ischemic insult may explain the decrease in sudden cardiac death rates in areas with hard water as compared with rates in soft-water areas.

SUMMARY

Minerals that are required in relatively large amounts are called macrominerals to distinguish them from trace elements—minerals needed in smaller amounts. Calcium, phosphorus, and magnesium are macrominerals. Low intakes of calcium, which occur commonly, have been associated with age-related osteoporosis. A dietary deficiency of phosphorus is unlikely, due to its wide distribution in foods. The mean population intake of magnesium, although slightly below the RDA, probably does not represent a health hazard.

Maximum bone mass is achieved by approximately 25 to 30 years of age. It is maintained until 35 to 45 years of age and then declines. Decreased skeletal mass is the most important risk factor for fracture of bones and is a significant public health problem in the United States. One of the problems in assessing the relationship of calcium intake to bone mass is the inherent inaccuracy of dietary recall. In addition, metabolic balance studies, although conducted extensively to determine nutritional requirements for calcium, also have important limitations that prevent accurate determination of the amount of dietary calcium needed to achieve balance.

It is important to achieve peak bone mass because the more mass that is available before age-related loss begins, the less likely it will decrease to a level at which fracture will occur. More dietary calcium is required to achieve peak bone mass than to replace obligatory losses of this ion in urine, feces, and sweat. Thus, people under 25 years of age probably need to ingest sufficient calcium to maintain a positive balance. This quantity will vary from person to person, depending on individual efficiencies of intestinal calcium absorption, but 1,200 mg/day probably provides a margin of safety for almost all normal people ages 11 to 25 years.

Once maximum bone mass is achieved, it is maintained without much change for 10 to 20 years. Calcium intake need not be greater than 800 mg/day during this period, because bone building has been completed and intestinal absorption of calcium is normal. However, men and women lose bone at a constant rate of 0.2 to 0.5% per year, starting at ages 40 to 45. For approximately 10 years immediately before, during, and after menopause, women lose bone more rapidly than men (2 to 5% per year). This rapid rate of bone loss in menopausal women returns to the slower rate shared by the sexes after this 10-year period.

Intestinal calcium absorption and the ability to adapt to low-calcium diets are impaired in many postmenopausal women and elderly people of both sexes. The pathogenesis of these abnormalities is controversial, but evidence suggests that they may be due either to a decreased ability of the kidney to produce the major biologically active metabolite of vitamin D, $1,25(OH)_2D_3$, such as after menopause, or to absolute decreases in the production of this metabolite due to renal disease, as in old age. The finding that serum levels of immunoreactive and bioactive parathyroid hormone increase with age implies that defects in calcium absorption are functionally important in that they result in sufficient degrees of hypocalcemia to produce chronic secondary hyperparathyroidism—a condition generally associated with bone demineralization. It appears, therefore, that the ability of the intestine to support calcium homeostasis progressively declines with age and that elderly people are increasingly forced to rely on their own bones rather than on the external environment as a source of calcium for maintaining normal extracellular fluid calcium. The degree to which this homeostatic response is needed depends on the severity of the described defects in calcium absorption, the level and bioavailability of dietary calcium, and whether specific therapeutic means are taken to correct defects in calcium absorption.

There is no direct evidence that the impaired intestinal calcium absorption observed during menopause and aging can be overcome by increased calcium intake. Moreover, the evidence that calcium supplementation prevents the trabecular bone loss associated with the menopause is, at best, weak. Thus, calcium supplementation should not be substituted for sex hormone replacement, which prevents postmenopausal bone loss in most women and appears to restore intestinal calcium absorption toward normal. Women taking estrogen replacement should continue to ingest 800 mg of calcium (the RDA). Those menopausal and postmenopausal women at risk for osteoporosis who are unable or refuse to take estrogen may require at least 1,200 mg of calcium per day. Such intakes could delay cortical bone loss and prevent chronic secondary hyperparathyroidism.

The association between decreased calcium intake and hypertension is suggestive but inconclusive. The epidemiologic and animal evidence relating calcium to colorectal cancer risk is also inconclusive. High-phosphorus diets may decrease calcium bioavailability, but they also reduce urinary calcium excretion and their influence on bone mass and the risk of osteoporosis is unknown. There are no known adverse effects of magnesium in the amounts currently consumed in the United States, although animal studies show a consistent inverse association between magnesium intake and blood pressure.

DIRECTIONS FOR RESEARCH

- The age at which peak bone mass is achieved and the influence of calcium supplementation on peak bone mass need to be determined by longitudinal measurements.

- Additional studies should be conducted to determine the dietary requirement for calcium during and immediately before menopause in different groups of women (e.g., whites, blacks, and Asians). If requirements are known to be increased, investigations can then proceed to determine if therapeutic lowering of the requirement by increasing the fraction of calcium absorbed from the diet will influence the rate at which bone is lost in these patients.

- Long-term studies are needed to determine the effect of calcium supplementation on rate of bone loss in the elderly (65 years and older) in whom intestinal absorption of calcium is decreased.

- Dietary phosphorus, protein, and fiber each have potentially deleterious effects on calcium economy. Their individual and joint effects on calcium balance need to be determined in people such as the elderly who have decreased ability to produce 1,25-dihydroxycholecalciferol and in those such as adolescents who have a need to be in positive calcium balance.

- Continued research is needed to develop noninvasive, quantitative, analytical techniques that can accurately predict individuals at risk for osteoporotic fracture.

- Randomized, prospective, long-term studies in humans should be conducted to determine the influences of calcium supplementation on blood pressure.

- The association between magnesium intake and both blood pressure and cardiovascular diseases in humans needs to be clarified.

REFERENCES

Ackley, S., E. Barrett-Connor, and L. Suarez. 1983. Dairy products, calcium, and blood pressure. Am. J. Clin. Nutr. 38:457–461.

Albanese, A.A., A.H. Edelson, E.J. Lorenze, Jr., M.L. Woodhull, and E.H. Wein. 1975. Problems of bone health in elderly. Ten-year study. N.Y. State J. Med. 75:326–336.

Albert, D.G., Y. Morita, and L.T. Iseri. 1958. Serum magnesium and plasma sodium levels in essential vascular hypertension. Circulation 17:761–764.

Alevizaki, C.C., D.G. Ikkos, and P. Singhelakis. 1973. Progressive decrease of true intestinal calcium absorption with age in normal man. J. Nucl. Med. 14:760–762.

Altura, B.M., B.T. Altura, A. Gebrewold, H. Ising, and T. Gunther. 1984. Magnesium deficiency and hypertension: correlation between magnesium-deficient diets and microcirculatory changes in situ. Science 223:1315–1317.

Anderson, J.J.B., and F.A. Tylavsky. 1984. Diet and osteopenia in elderly caucasian women. Pp. 299–304 in C. Christiansen, C.D. Arnaud, B.E.C. Nordin, A.M. Parfitt, W.A. Peck, and B.L. Riggs, eds. Osteoporosis: Proceedings of the Copenhagen International Symposium on Osteoporosis. Department of Clinical Chemistry, Glostrup Hospital, Copenhagen.

Arnaud, C.D. 1978. Calcium homeostasis: regulatory elements and their integration. Fed. Proc. 37:2557–2560.

Arnaud, C.D. 1988. Mineral and bone homeostasis. Pp. 1469–1479 in J.B. Wyngaarden, L.H. Smith, Jr., and F. Plum, eds. Cecil Textbook of Medicine, 18th ed. W.B. Saunders, Philadelphia.

Arnaud, C.D., J.C. Gallagher, C.M. Jerpbak, and B.L. Riggs. 1981. On the role of parathyroid hormone in the osteoporosis of aging. Pp. 215–225 in H.F. DeLuca, H.M. Frost, W.S.S. Jee, C.C. Johnston, Jr., and A.M. Parfitt, eds. Osteoporosis: Recent Advances in Pathogenesis and Treatment. University Park Press, Baltimore.

Avioli, L.V., J.E. McDonald, and S.W. Lee. 1965. The influence of age on the intestinal absorption of 47-Ca absorption in post-menopausal osteoporosis. J. Clin. Invest. 44:1960–1967.

Ayachi, S. 1979. Increased dietary calcium lowers blood pressure in the spontaneously hypertensive rat. Metabolism 28:1234–1238.

Bauer W., J.C. Aub, and F. Albright. 1929. Studies of calcium and phosphorus metabolism. V. A study of the bone trabeculae as a readily available reserve supply of calcium. J. Exp. Med. 49:145–161.

Belizan, J.M., J. Villar, O. Pineda, A.E. Gonzalez, E. Sainz, G. Garrera, and R. Sibrian. 1983. Reduction of blood pressure with calcium supplementation in young adults. J. Am. Med. Assoc. 249:1161–1165.

Bell, G.H., D.P. Cuthbertson, and J. Orr. 1941. Strength and size of bone in relation to calcium intake. J. Physiol. 100: 299–317.

Bell, R.R., H.H. Draper, D.Y. Tzeng, H.K. Shin, and G.R. Schmidt. 1977. Physiological responses of human adults to foods containing phosphate additives. J. Nutr. 107:42–50.

Berthelot, A., and J. Esposito. 1983. Effects of dietary magnesium on the development of hypertension in the spontaneously hypertensive rat. J. Am. Coll. Nutr. 2:343–353.

Bianchetti, M.G., C. Beretta-Piccoli, P. Weidamn, L. Link, K. Boehringer, C. Ferrier, and J.J. Morton. 1983. Calcium and blood pressure regulation in normal hypertensive subjects. Hypertension 5:II57–II65.

Bindels, R.J., L.A. van den Broek, and M.J. Jougen, W.H. Hackeng, C.W. Lowik, and C.H. van Os. 1987. Increased plasma calcitonin levels in young spontaneously hypertensive rats: role in disturbed phosphate homeostasis. Pflugers Arch. 408:395–400.

Bird, R.P. 1986. Effect of dietary components on the pathobiology of colonic epithelium: possible relationship with colon tumorigenesis. Lipids 21:289–291.

Bird, R.P., R. Schneider, D. Stamp, and W.R. Bruce. 1986. Effect of dietary calcium and cholic acid on the proliferation indices of murine colonic epithelium. Carcinogenesis 7: 1657–1661.

Blum, M., M. Kirsten, and M.H. Worth, Jr. 1977. Reversible hypertension. Caused by the hypercalcemia of hyperparathyroidism, vitamin D toxicity, and calcium infusion. J. Am. Med. Assoc. 237:262–263.

Bull, A., R.P. Bird, W.R. Bruce, N. Nigro, and A. Medline. 1987. Effect of calcium on azoxymethane induced intestinal tumors in rats. Gastroenterology 92:1332.

Bullamore, J.R., R. Wilkinson, J.C. Gallagher, B.E. Nordin, and D.H. Marshall. 1970. Effect of age on calcium absorption. Lancet 2:535–537.

Caderni, G., E.W. Stuart, and W.R. Bruce. 1988. Dietary factors affecting the proliferation of epithelial cells in the mouse colon. Nutr. Cancer 11:147–153.

Cann, C.E., H.K. Genant, B. Ettinger, and G.S. Gordan. 1980. Spinal mineral loss in oophorectomized women. Determined by quantitative computed tomography. J. Am. Med. Assoc. 244:2056–2059.

Carroll, M.D., S. Abraham, and C.M. Dresser. 1983. Dietary Intake Source Data: United States, 1976–1980. Vital and Health Statistics, Series 11, No. 231. DHHS Publ. No. (PHS) 83-1681. National Center for Health Statistics, Public Health Service, U.S. Department of Health and Human Services, Hyattsville, Md. 483 pp.

Cohn, S.H., ed. 1981. Non-Invasive Measurements of Bone Mass and Their Clinical Application. CRC Press, Boca Raton, Fla. 229 pp.

Dawson-Hughes, B., P. Jacques, and C. Shipp. 1987. Dietary calcium intake and bone loss from the spine in healthy postmenopausal women. Am. J. Nutr. 46:685–687.

de Winter, F.R., and R. Steendijk. 1975. The effect of a low-calcium diet in lactating rats; observations on the rapid development and repair of osteoporosis. Calcif. Tissue Res. 17:303–316.

DHEW (U.S. Department of Health, Education, and Welfare). 1979. Dietary Intake Source Data: United States, 1971–74. Vital and Health Statistics, DHEW Publ. No. (PHS) 79-1221. National Center for Health Statistics, Public Health Service, U.S. Department of Health, Education, and Welfare, Hyattsville, Md. 421 pp.

DHHS/USDA (Department of Health and Human Services/ U.S. Department of Agriculture). 1986. Nutrition Monitoring in the United States—A Progress Report from the Joint Nutrition Monitoring Evaluation Committee. DHHS Publ. No. (PHS) 86-1255. National Center for Health Statistics, Public Health Service, U.S. Department of Health and Human Services, Hyattsville, Md. 356 pp.

Dobbs, R.J., and I.M. Baird. 1977. Effect of wholemeal and white bread on iron absorption in normal people. Br. Med. J. 1:1641–1642.

Draper, H.H., and R.R. Bell. 1979. Nutrition and osteoporosis. Pp. 79–106 in H.H. Draper, ed. Advances in Nutritional Research, Vol. 2. Plenum Press, New York.

Draper, H.H., T.L. Sie, and J.G. Bergan. 1972. Osteoporosis in aging rats induced by high phosphorus diets. J. Nutr. 102:1133–1141.

Erne, P., P. Bolli, E. Bürgisser, and F.R. Bühler. 1984. Correlation of platelet calcium with blood pressure. Effect of antihypertensive therapy. N. Engl. J. Med. 310:1084–1088.

Ettinger, B., H.K. Genant, and C.E. Cann. 1987. Postmenopausal bone loss is prevented by treatment with low-dosage estrogen with calcium. Ann. Int. Med. 106:40–45.

Exton, J.H. 1986. Mechanisms involved in calcium-mobilizing agonist responses. Adv. Cyclic Nucleotide Res. 20:211–262.

FDA (Food and Drug Administration). 1979. Vitamin and mineral drug products for over-the-counter human use. Establishment of a monograph; notice of proposed rulemaking–1. Calcium. Fed. Reg. 44:16175–16178.

Feinleib, M., C. Lenfant, and S.A. Miller. 1984. Hypertension and calcium. Science 226:384–389.

Ferretti, J.L., R.D. Tessaro, E.O. Audisio, and C.D. Galassi. 1985. Long-term effects of high or low Ca intakes and lack of parathyroid function on rat femur biomechanics. Calcif. Tissue Int. 37:608–612.

Folsom, A.R., C.L. Smith, R.J. Prineas, and R.H. Grimm, Jr. 1986. Serum calcium fractions in essential hypertensive and matched normotensive subjects. Hypertension 8:11–15.

Forero, M.S., R.F. Klein, R.A. Nissenson, K. Nelson, H. Heath III, C.D. Arnaud, and B.L. Riggs. 1987. Effect of age on circulating immunoreactive and bioactive parathyroid hormone levels in women. J. Bone Min. Res. 2:363–366.

Gafter, U., S. Kathpalia, D. Zikos, and K. Lau. 1986. Ca fluxes across the duodenum and colon of spontaneously hypertensive rats: effect of 1,25(OH)$_2$D$_3$. Am. J. Physiol. 251:F278–F282.

Gallagher, J.C., B.L. Riggs, J. Eisman, A. Hamstra, S.B. Arnaud, and H.F. Deluca. 1979. Intestinal calcium absorption and serum vitamin D metabolites in normal subjects and osteoporotic patients: effect of age and dietary calcium. J. Clin. Invest. 64:729–736.

Gallagher, J.C., B.L. Riggs, C.M. Jerpbak, and C.D. Arnaud. 1980. The effect of age on serum immunoreactive parathyroid hormone in normal and osteoporotic women. J. Lab. Clin. Med. 95:373–385.

Garcia-Palmieri, M.R., R. Costas, Jr., M. Cruz-Vidal, P.D. Sorlie, J. Tillotson, and R.J. Havlik. 1984. Milk consumption, calcium intake, and decreased hypertension in Puerto Rico. Puerto Rico Heart Health Program Study. Hypertension 6:322–328.

Garland, C., R.B. Shekelle, E. Barrett-Connor, M.H. Criqui, A.H. Rossof, and O. Paul. 1985. Dietary vitamin D and calcium and risk of colorectal cancer: a 19-year prospective study in men. Lancet 1:307–309.

Garn, S.M. 1970. The Earlier Gain and Later Loss of Cortical Bone, in Nutritional Perspective. C.C. Thomas, Springfield, Ill. 146 pp.

Garn, S.M., C.G. Rohmann, B. Wagner, G.H. Davila, and W. Ascoli. 1969. Population similarities in the onset and rate of adult endosteal bone loss. Clin. Orthop. 65:51–60.

Garn, S.M., M.A. Solomon, and J. Friedl. 1981. Calcium intake and bone quality in the elderly. Ecol. Food Nutr. 10:131–133.

Gershon-Cohen, J., J.F. McClendon, J. Jowsey, and W.C. Foster. 1962. Osteoporosis produced and cured in rats by low- and high-calcium diets. Radiology 78:251–252.

Griffiths, H.J., R.D. Hunt, R.E. Zimmerman, H. Fineberg, and J. Cuttino. 1975. The role of calcium and fluoride in osteoporosis in rhesus monkeys. Invest. Radiol. 10:263–268.

Grobbee, D.E., and A. Hofman. 1986. Effect of calcium supplementation on diastolic blood pressure in young people with mild hypertension. Lancet 2:703–707.

Gruchaw, H.W., K.A. Sobocinski, and J.J. Barboriak. 1985. Alcohol, nutrient intake, and hypertension in U.S. adults. J. Am. Med. Assoc. 253:1567–1570.

Harlan, W.R., A.L. Hull, R.L. Schmouder, J.R. Landis, F.E. Thompson, and F.A. Larkin. 1984. Blood pressure and nutrition in adults. The National Health and Nutrition Examination Survey. Am. J. Epidemiol. 120:17–28.

Harrison, M., and R. Fraser. 1960. Bone structure and metabolism in calcium-deficient rats. J. Endocrinol. 21:197–205.

Heaney, R.P. 1985. The role of calcium in osteoporosis. J. Nutr. Sci. Vitaminol. 31:S21–S26.

Heaney, R.P. 1986. Calcium, bone health and osteoporosis. Pp. 255–301 in W.A. Peck, ed. Bone and Mineral Research, Annual 4: A Yearly Survey of Developments in the Field of Bone and Mineral Metabolism. Elsevier, New York.

Heaney, R.P., and R.R. Recker. 1982. Effects of nitrogen, phosphorus, and caffeine on calcium balance in women. J. Lab. Clin. Med. 99:46–55.

Heaney, R.P., R.R. Recker, and P.D. Saville. 1977. Calcium balance and calcium requirements in middle-aged women. Am. J. Clin. Nutr. 30:1603–1611.

Heath, H., III. and C.W. Callaway. 1985. Calcium tablets for hypertension? Ann. Intern. Med. 103:946–947.

Horowitz, M., A.C. Need, J.C. Philcox, and B.E. Nordin. 1984. Effect of calcium supplementation on urinary hydroxyproline in osteoporotic postmenopausal women. Am. J. Clin. Nutr. 39:857–859.

Horsman, A., J.C. Gallagher, M. Simpson, and B.E. Nordin. 1977. Prospective trial of oestrogen and calcium in postmenopausal women. Br. Med. J. 2:789–792.

Hsu, C.H., P.S. Chen, D.E. Smith, and C.S. Yang. 1986. Pathogenesis of hypercalciuria in spontaneously hypertensive rats. Miner. Electrolyte Metab. 12:130–141.

Hurxthal, L.M., and G.P. Vose. 1969. The relationship of dietary calcium intake to radiographic bone density in normal and osteoporotic persons. Calcif. Tissue Res. 4:245–256.

IARC (International Agency for Research on Cancer). 1977. Intestinal Microecology Group. Dietary fibre, transit-time, faecal bacteria, steroids and colon cancer in two Scandinavian populations. Lancet 2:207–211.

Insogna, K.L., A.M. Lewis, B.A. Lipinski, C. Bryant, and D.T. Baran. 1981. Effect of age on serum immunoreactive parathyroid hormone and its biological effects. J. Clin. Endocrinol. Metab. 53:1072–1075.

Ireland, P., and J.S. Fordtran. 1973. Effect of dietary calcium and age on jejunal calcium absorption in humans studied by intestinal perfusion. J. Clin. Invest. 52:2672–2681.

Ismail-Beigi, F., J.G. Reinhold, B. Faraji, and P. Abadi. 1977. Effects of cellulose added to diets of low and high fiber content upon the metabolism of calcium, magnesium, zinc and phosphorus by man. J. Nutr. 107:510–518.

Ivanovich, P., H. Fellows, and C. Rich. 1967. The absorption of calcium carbonate. Ann. Intern. Med. 66:917–923.

Izawa, Y., K. Sagara, T. Kadota, and T. Makita. 1985. Bone disorders in spontaneously hypertensive rat. Calcif. Tissue Int. 37:605–607.

Jaffe, H.L., A. Bodansky, and J.P. Chandler. 1932. Ammonium chloride decalcification, as modified by calcium intake: relation between generalized osteoporosis and ostitis fibrosa. J. Exp. Med. 56:823–834.

Jain, M., G.M. Cook, F.G. Davis, M.G. Grace, G.R. Howe, and A.B. Miller. 1980. A case-control study of diet and colo-rectal cancer. Int. J. Cancer 26:757–768.

Jensen, O.M., R. MacLennan, and J. Wahrendorf on behalf of the IARC Large Bowel Cancer Group. 1982. Diet, bowel function, fecal characteristics, and large bowel cancer in Denmark and Finland. Nutr. Cancer 4:5–19.

Johansson, B., and A.P. Somlyo. 1980. Electrophysiology and excitation–contraction coupling. Pp. 301–323 in D.F. Bohr, A.P. Somlyo, and H.V. Sparks, Jr., eds. Handbook of Physiology, Section II: The Cardiovascular System, Vol. II—Vascular Smooth Muscle. American Physiological Society, Bethesda, Md.

Jowsey, J., and J. Gershon-Cohen. 1964. Effect of dietary calcium levels on production and reversal of experimental osteoporosis in cats. Proc. Soc. Exp. Biol. Med. 116:437–441.

Kageyama, Y., H. Suzuki, K. Hayashi, and T. Saruta. 1986. Effects of calcium loading on blood pressure in spontaneously hypertensive rats: attenuation of the vascular reactivity. Clin. Exp. Hypertens. 8:355–370.

Kanders, B., R. Lindsay, D. Dempster, L. Markhard, and G. Valiquette. 1984. Determinants of bone mass in young healthy women. Pp. 337–340 in C. Christiansen, C.D. Arnaud, B.E.C. Nordin, A.M. Parfitt, W.A. Peck, and B.L. Riggs, eds. Osteoporosis: Proceedings of the Copenhagen International Symposium on Osteoporosis. Department of Clinical Chemistry, Glostrup Hospital, Copenhagen.

Kaplan, N.M., and R.B. Meese. 1986. The calcium deficiency hypothesis of hypertension: a critique. Ann. Int. Med. 105:947–955.

Kawashima, H. 1986. Altered vitamin D metabolism in the kidney of the spontaneously hypertensive rat. Biochem. J. 237:893–897.

Kelsey, J.L. 1984. Osteoporosis: Prevalence and Incidence. Pp. 25–28 in Osteoporosis, NIH Consensus Development Conference, April 2–4, 1984. National Institute of Arthritis, Diabetes, and Digestive and Kidney Diseases and the Office of Medical Applications of Research, National Institutes of Health, Bethesda, Md.

Kelsey, J.L. 1987. Epidemiology of osteoporosis and associated fractures. Pp. 409–444 in W.A. Peck, ed. Bone and Mineral Research, Annual 4: A Yearly Survey of Developments in the Field of Bone and Mineral Metabolism. Elsevier, New York.

Kesteloot, H. 1984a. Epidemiological studies on the relationship between sodium, potassium, calcium, and magnesium and arterial blood pressure. J. Clin. Cardiovasc. Pharmacol. 6:S192–S196.

Kesteloot, H. 1984b. Urinary cations and blood pressure—population studies. Ann. Clin. Res. 16 suppl. 43:72–80.

Knapp, E.L. 1947. Factors influencing the urinary excretion of calcium. I. In normal persons. J. Clin. Invest. 26:182–202.

Kok, F.J., J.P. Vandenbroucke, C. Van der Heide-Wessel, and R.M. Van der Heide. 1986. Dietary sodium, calcium, and potassium, and blood pressure. Am. J. Epidemiol. 123:1043–1048.

Krishnarao, G.V., and H.H. Draper. 1972. Influence of dietary phosphate on bone resorption in senescent mice. J. Nutr. 102:1143–1145.

Krolner, B., and S. Pors Nielsen. 1982. Bone mineral content of the lumbar spine in normal and osteoporotic women: cross-sectional and longitudinal studies. Clin. Sci. 62:329–336.

Krook, L. 1968. Dietary calcium-phosphorus and lameness in the horse. Cornell Vet. 58 suppl. 1:59–73.

Kune, S., G.A. Kune, and L.F. Watson. 1987. Case-control study of dietary etiological factors: the Melbourne Colorectal Cancer study. Nutr. Cancer 9:21–42.

Kurtz, T.W., A.A. Portale, and R.C. Morris, Jr. 1986. Evidence for a difference in vitamin D metabolism between spontaneously hypertensive and Wistar-Kyoto rats. Hypertension 8:1015–1020.

Lamke, B., H.E. Sjoberg, and M. Sylven. 1978. Bone mineral content in women with Colles' fracture: effect of calcium supplementation. Acta Orthop. Scand. 49:143–146.

Lau, K., and B. Eby. 1985. The role of calcium in genetic hypertension. Hypertension 7:657–667.

Lau, K., D. Zikos, J. Spirnak, and B. Eby. 1984a. Evidence for an intestinal mechanism in hypercalciuria of spontaneously hypertensive rats. Am. J. Physiol. 247:E625–E633.

Lau, K., S. Chen, and B. Eby. 1984b. Evidence for the role of PO_4 deficiency in antihypertensive action of a high-Ca diet. Am. J. Physiol. 246:H324–H331.

Lau, K., C.B. Langman, U. Gafter, P.K. Dudeja, and T.A. Brasitus. 1986. Increased calcium absorption in prehypertensive spontaneously hypertensive rat. Role of serum 1,25-dihydroxyvitamin D3 levels and intestinal brush border membrane fluidity. J. Clin. Invest. 78:1083–1090.

Lavel-Jeanet, A.M., G. Paul, C. Bergot, J.L. Lamarque, and M.N. Ghiania. 1984. Correlation between vertebral bone density measurement and nutritional status. Pp. 305–309 in C. Christiansen, C.D. Arnaud, B.E.C. Nordin, A.M. Parfitt, W.A. Peck, and B.L. Riggs, eds. Osteoporosis: Proceedings of the Copenhagen International Symposium on Osteoporosis. Department of Clinical Chemistry, Glostrup Hospital, Copenhagen.

Leichsenring, J.M., L.M. Norris, S.A. Lamison, E.D. Wilson, and M.B. Patton. 1951. The effect of level of intake on calcium and phosphorus metabolism in college women. J. Nutr. 45:407–418.

Lipkin, M., and H. Newmark. 1985. Effect of added dietary calcium on colonic epithelial-cell proliferation in subjects at high risk for familial colon cancer. N. Engl. J. Med. 313:1381–1384.

Lucas, P.A., R.C. Brown, T. Drüeke, B. Lacour, J.A. Metz, and D.A. McCarron. 1986. Abnormal vitamin D metabolism, intestinal calcium transport, and bone calcium status in the spontaneously hypertensive rat compared with its genetic control. J. Clin. Invest. 78:221–227.

Lutwak, L. 1975. Metabolic and biochemical considerations of bone. Ann. Clin. Lab. Sci. 5:185–194.

Lutwak, L., and G.D. Whedon. 1963. Disease-a-Month: Osteoporosis. Year Books Medical Publ., Chicago. 39 pp.

Macquart-Moulin, G., E. Riboli, J. Cornee, B. Charnay, P. Berthezene, and N. Day. 1986. Case-control study on colorectal cancer and diet in Marseilles. Int. J. Cancer 38:183–191.

Maierhofer, W.J., R.W. Gray, and J. Lemann, Jr. 1984. Phosphate deprivation increases serum 1,25-$(OH)_2$-vitamin D concentrations in healthy men. Kidney Int. 25:571–575.

Malm, O.J. 1953. On phosphates and phosphoric acid as dietary factors in the calcium balance of man. Scand. Clin. Lab. Invest. 5:75–84.

Marcus, R. 1982. The relationship of dietary calcium to the maintenence of skeletal integrity in man—an interface of endocrinology and nutrition. Metabolism 31:93–102.

Marcus, R., P. Madvig, and G. Young. 1984. Age-related changes in parathyroid hormone and parathyroid hormone action in normal humans. J. Clin. Endocrinol. Metab. 58: 223–230.

Matkovic, V., K. Kostial, I. Simonovic, R. Buzina, A. Brodarec, and B.E. Nordin. 1979. Bone status and fracture rates in two regions of Yugoslavia. Am. J. Clin. Nutr. 32: 540–549.

Mazess, R.B. 1983. The noninvasive measurement of skeletal mass. Pp. 223–279 in W.A. Peck, ed. Bone and Mineral Research, Annual 1: A Yearly Survey of Developments in the Field of Bone and Mineral Metabolism. Excerpta Medica, Amsterdam.

McCance, R.A., and E.M. Widdowson. 1942. Mineral metabolism of healthy adults on white and brown bread dietaries. J. Physiol. 101:44–85.

McCarron, D.A., and C.D. Morris. 1985. Blood pressure response to oral calcium in persons with mild to moderate hypertension. A randomized, double-blind, placebo-controlled, crossover trial. Ann. Int. Med. 103:825–831.

McCarron, D.A., N.N. Yung, B.A. Ugoretz, and S. Krutzik. 1981. Disturbances of calcium metabolism in the spontaneously hypertensive rat. Hypertension 43:I162–I167.

McCarron, D.A., C.D. Morris, H.J. Henry, and J.L. Stanton. 1984. Blood pressure and nutrient intake in the United States. Science 224:1392–1398.

McCarron, D.A., P.A. Lucas, R.S. Schneidman, B. LaCour, and T. Drüeke. 1985. Blood pressure development of the spontaneously hypertensive rat after concurrent manipulations of dietary Ca^{2+} and Na^+: relation to Ca^{2+} intestinal fluxes. J. Clin. Invest. 76:1147–1154.

McCarron, D.A., P. Lucas, B. Lacour, and T. Drueke. 1986. Ca^{2+} efflux rate constant (K°Ca) in isolated SHR enterocytes. Kidney Int. 29:252.

Merke, J., A. Slotkowski, H. Mann, P.H. Lucas, T. Drüeke, and E. Ritz. 1987. Abnormal $1,25(OH)_2D_3$ receptor status in genetically hypertensive rats. Kidney Int. 31:303.

Miller, G. 1985. Magnesium deficiency syndrome. Compr. Ther. 11:58–64.

Miller, R.M. 1969. Nutritional secondary hyperparathyroidism. A review of etiology, symptomatology and treatment in companion animals. Vet. Med. Small Anim. Clin. 64:400–408.

Morris, C.D., H.J. Henry, and D.A. McCarron. 1984. Discordance of hypertensives' dietary Ca^{2+} intake and urinary Ca^{2+} excretion. Clin. Res. 32:57a.

NRC (National Research Council). 1980. Recommended Dietary Allowances, 9th ed. Report of the Committee on Dietary Allowances, Food and Nutrition Board, Division of Biological Sciences, Assembly of Life Sciences. National Academy Press, Washington, D.C. 185 pp.

Neri, L.C., and H.L. Johansen. 1978. Water hardness and cardiovascular mortality. Ann. N.Y. Acad. Sci. 304:203–221.

Nilas, L., C. Christiansen, and P. Rodbro. 1984. Calcium supplementation and postmenopausal bone loss. Br. Med. J. 289:1103–1106.

Nordin, B.E.C. 1960. Osteomalacia, osteoporosis and calcium deficiency. Clin. Orthop. 17:235–258.

Nordin, B.E.C. 1961. The pathogenesis of osteoporosis. Lancet 1:1011–1014.

Nordin, B.E.C. 1966. International patterns of osteoporosis. Clin. Orthop. 45:17–30.

Nordin, B.E.C., R. Wilkinson, D.H. Marshall, J.C. Gallagher, A. Williams, and M. Peacock. 1976. Calcium absorption in the elderly. Calcif. Tissue Res. 21:442–451.

Nordin, B.E.C., A. Horsman, D.H. Marshall, M. Simpson, and G.M. Waterhouse. 1979. Calcium requirement and calcium therapy. Clin. Orthop. 140:216–246.

Nottestad, S.Y., J.J. Baumel, D.B. Kimmel, R.R. Recker, and R.P. Heaney. 1987. The proportion of trabecular bone in human vertebrae. J. Bone Miner. Res. 2:221–229.

Ornoy, A., I. Wolinsky, and K. Guggenheim. 1974. Structure of long bones of rats and mice fed a low calcium diet. Calcif. Tissue Res. 15:71–76.

Orwoll, E.S., and D.E. Meier. 1986. Alterations in calcium, vitamin D, and parathyroid hormone physiology in normal men with aging: relationship to the development of senile osteopenia. J. Clin. Endocrinol. Metab. 63:1262–1269.

Pacifici, R., D. Droke, S. Smith, N. Susman, and L.V. Avioli. 1985. Quantitative computer tomographic (QCT) analysis of vertebral bone mass (VBM) in a female population. Clin. Res. 33:615A.

Parfitt, A.M. 1980. Morphologic basis of bone mineral measurements: transient and steady state effects of treatment in osteoporosis. Miner. Electrolyte Metab. 4:273–287.

Parfitt, A.M. 1983. Dietary risk factors for age-related bone loss and fractures. Lancet 2:1181–1185.

Pennington, J.A., B.E. Young, D.B. Wilson, R.D. Johnson, and J.E. Vanderveen. 1986. Mineral content of foods and total diets: the Selected Minerals in Foods Survey, 1982 to 1984. J. Am. Diet. Assoc. 86:876–891.

Petersen, B., M. Schroll, C. Christiansen, and I. Transbol. 1977. Serum and erythrocyte magnesium in normal elderly Danish people: relationship to blood pressure and serum lipids. Acta Med. Scand. 201:31–34.

Portale, A.A., B.E. Booth, B.P. Halloran, and R.C. Morris, Jr. 1984. Effect of dietary phosphorus on circulation concentrations of 1,25-dihydroxyvitamin D and immunoreactive parathyroid hormone in children with moderated renal insufficiency. J. Clin. Invest. 73:1580–1589.

Portale, A.A., B.P. Halloran, M.M. Murphy, and R.C. Morris, Jr. 1986. Oral intake of phosphorus can determine the serum concentration of 1,25-dihydroxyvitamin D by determining its production rate in humans. J. Clin. Invest. 77:7–12.

Postnov, Y.V., and S.A. Orlov. 1985. Ion transport across plasma membrane in primary hypertension. Physiol. Rev. 65:904–945.

Rafter, J.J., V.W. Eng, R. Furrer, A. Medline, and W.R. Bruce. 1986. Effects of calcium and pH on the mucosal damage produced by deoxycholic acid in the rat colon. Gut 27:1320–1329.

Rasmussen, P. 1977. Calcium deficiency, pregnancy, and lactation in rats. Microscopic and microradiographic observations on bones. Calcif. Tissue Res. 23:95–102.

Recker, R.R., and R.P. Heaney. 1985. The effect of milk supplements on calcium metabolism, bone metabolism and calcium balance. Am. J. Clin. Nutr. 41:254–263.

Recker, R.R., P.D. Saville, and R.P. Heaney. 1977. Effect of estrogens and calcium carbonate on bone loss in postmenopausal women. Ann. Intern. Med. 87:649–655.

Reddy, B.S., A.R. Hedges, K. Laakso, and E.L. Wynder. 1978. Metabolic epidemiology of large bowel cancer: fecal bulk and constituents of high-risk North American and low-risk Finnish populations. Cancer 42:2832–2838.

Reed, D., D. McGee, K. Yano, and J. Hankin. 1985. Diet, blood pressure, and multicollinearity. Hypertension 7:405–410.

Resnick, L.M., R.K. Gupta, and J.H. Laragh. 1984a. Intracellular free magnesium in erythrocytes of essential hypertension: relation to blood pressure and serum divalent cations. Proc. Natl. Acad. Sci. U.S.A. 81:6511–6515.

Resnick, L.M., J.P. Nicholson, and J.H. Laragh. 1984b. Outpatient therapy of essential hypertension with dietary calcium supplementation. J. Am. Coll. Cardiol. 3:616.

Resnick, L.M., F.B. Muller, and J.H. Laragh. 1986. Calcium-regulating hormones in essential hypertension. Relation to plasma renin activity and sodium metabolism. Ann. Intern. Med. 105:649–654.

Riggs, B.L., and L.J. Melton III. 1986. Involutional osteoporosis. N. Engl. J. Med. 314:1676–1686.

Riggs, B.L., P.J. Kelley, W.R. Kinney, D.A. Scholz, and A.J. Bianco, Jr. 1967. Calcium deficiency and osteoporosis. Observations in one hundred and sixty-six patients and critical review of the literature. J. Bone Jt. Surg., Am. Vol. 49:915–924.

Riggs, B.L., J. Jowsey, P.J. Kelly, D.L. Hoffman, and C.D. Arnaud. 1976. Effects of oral therapy with calcium and vitamin D in primary osteoporosis. J. Clin. Endocrinol. Metab. 42:1139–1144.

Riggs, B.L., A. Hamstra, and H.F. DeLuca. 1981. Assessment of 25-hydroxyvitamin D 1 alpha-hydroxylase reserve in postmenopausal osteoporosis by administration of parathyroid extract. J. Clin. Endocrinol. Metab. 53:833–835.

Riggs, B.L., E. Seeman, S.F. Hodgson, D.R. Taves, and W.M. O'Fallon. 1982. Effect of the fluoride/calcium regimen on vertebral fracture occurrence in postmenopausal osteoporosis: comparison with conventional therapy. N. Engl. J. Med. 306:446–450.

Riggs, B.L., H.W. Wahner, L.J. Melton III, L.S. Richelson, H.L. Judd, and W.M. O'Fallon. 1987. Dietary calcium intake and rates of bone loss in women. J. Clin. Invest. 80:979–982.

Riis, B., K. Thomsen, and C. Christiansen. 1987. Does calcium supplementation prevent postmenopausal bone loss? A double-blind, controlled clinical study. N. Engl. J. Med. 316:173–177.

Rosenthal, F.D., and S. Roy. 1972. Hypertension and hyperparathyroidism. Br. Med. J. 4:396–397.

Roullet, C., T. Drüeke, B. Lacour, and D. McCarron. 1986. Ca^{2+} influx of isolated enterocytes in adult SHRs and WKYs. Circulation 74:II-331.

Sakhaee, K., M.J. Nicar, K. Glass, J.E. Zerwekh, and C.Y. Pak. 1984. Reduction in intestinal calcium absorption by hydrochlorothiazide in postmenopausal osteoporosis. J. Clin. Endocrinol. Metab. 59:1037–1043.

Sakhaee, K., M.J. Nicar, K. Glass, J.E. Zerwekh, and C.Y. Pak. 1985. Postmenopausal osteoporosis as a manifestation of renal hypercalciuria with secondary hyperparathyroidism. J. Clin. Endocrinol. Metab. 61:368–373.

Salomon, C.D. 1972. Osteoporosis following calcium deficiency in rats. Calcif. Tissue Res. 8:320–333.

Salomon, C.D., and G. Volpin. 1970. Fine structure of bone resorption in experimental osteoporosis caused by calcium deficient diet in rats. An electron microscopic study of compact bone. Calcif. Tissue Res. 4:80–82.

Sangal, A.K., and D.G. Beevers. 1982. Serum calcium and blood pressure. Lancet 2:493.

Saville, P.D., and L. Krook. 1969. Gravimetric and isotopic studies in nutritional hyperparathyroidism in beagles. Clin. Orthop. 62:15–24.

Schedl, H.P., D.L. Miller, J.M. Pape, R.L. Horst, and H.D. Wilson. 1984. Calcium and sodium transport and vitamin D metabolism in the spontaneously hypertensive rat. J. Clin. Invest. 73:980–986.

Schedl, H.P., D.L. Miller, R.L. Horst, H.D. Wilson, K. Natarajan, and T. Conway. 1986. Intestinal calcium transport in the spontaneously hypertensive rat: response to calcium depletion. Am. J. Physiol. 250:G412–G419.

Schroeder, H.A. 1960. Relation between mortality from cardiovascular disease and treated water supplies: variations in states and 163 largest municipalities of the United States. J. Am. Med. Assoc. 172:1902–1908.

Seelig, M.S. 1974. Magnesium interrelationships in ischemic heart disease: a review. Am. J. Clin. Nutr. 27:59–79.

Shah, B.G., G.V. Krishnarao, and H.H. Draper. 1967. The relationship of Ca and P nutrition during adult life and osteoporosis in aged mice. J. Nutr. 92:30–42.

Shils, M.E. 1988. Magnesium. Pp. 159–192 in M.E. Shils and V.R. Young, eds. Modern Nutrition in Health and Disease, 7th ed. Lea & Febiger, Philadelphia.

Singer, D.R.J., N.D. Markandu, F.P. Cappuccio, G.W. Beynon, A.C. Shore, S.J. Smith, and G.A. MacGregor. 1985. Does oral calcium lower blood pressure: a double-blind study. J. Hypertension 3:661.

Sissons, H.A., G.J. Kelman, and G. Marotti. 1985. Bone resorption in calcium-deficient rats. Bone 6:345–347.

Smith, E.L., Jr., W. Reddan, and P.E. Smith. 1981. Physical activity and calcium modalities for bone mineral increase in aged women. Med. Sci. Sports Exerc. 13:60–64.

Smith, R.W., Jr., and B. Frame. 1965. Concurrent axial and appendicular osteoporosis: its relation to calcium consumption. N. Engl. J. Med. 273:73–78.

Smith, R.W., Jr., and J. Rizek. 1966. Epidemiologic studies of osteoporosis in women of Puerto Rico and Southeastern Michigan with special reference to age, race, national origin and to other related or associated findings. Clin. Orthop. 45:31–48.

Spencer, H., and M. Lender. 1979. Adverse effects of aluminum-containing antacids on mineral metabolism. Gastroenterology 76:603–606.

Spencer, H., L. Kramer, D. Osis, and C. Norris. 1978. Effect of phosphorus on the absorption of calcium and on the balance in man. J. Nutr. 108:447–457.

Spencer, H., L. Kramer, C. Norris, and D. Osis. 1982. Effect of small doses of aluminum-containing antacids on calcium and phosphorus metabolism. Am. J. Clin. Nutr. 36:32–40.

Stern, N., D.B. Lee, V. Silis, F.W. Beck, L. Deftos, S.C. Manolagas, and J.R. Sowers. 1984. Effects of high calcium intake on blood pressure and calcium metabolism in young SHR. Hypertension 6:639–646.

Strazzullo, P., A. Siani, S. Guglielmi, A. Di Carlo, F. Galletti, M. Cirillo, and M. Mancini. 1986. Controlled trial of long-term oral calcium supplementation in essential hypertension. Hypertension 8:1084–1088.

Thulin, T., M. Abdulla, I. Dencker, M. Jagerstad, A. Melander, N. Schersten, and B. Akesson. 1980. Comparison of energy and nutrient intakes in women with high and low blood pressure levels. Acta Med. Scand. 208:367–373.

Toraason, M.A., and G.L. Wright. 1981. Transport of calcium by duodenum of spontaneously hypertensive rats. Am. J. Physiol. 241:G344–G347.

Tsai, K.S., H. Heath III, R. Kumar, and B.L. Riggs. 1984. Impaired vitamin D metabolism with aging in women. Possible role in pathogenesis of senile osteoporosis. J. Clin. Invest. 73:1668–1672.

Tuyns, A.J., M. Haelterman, and R. Kaaks. 1987a. Colorectal cancer and the intake of nutrients: oligosaccharides are a risk factor, fats are not. A case-control study in Belgium. Nutr. Cancer 10:181–196.

Tuyns, A.J., E. Riboli, G. Doornbos, and G. Pequignot. 1987b. Diet and esophageal cancer in Calvados (France). Nutr. Cancer 10:81–92.

USDA (U.S. Department of Agriculture). 1984. Nationwide Food Consumption Survey. Nutrient Intakes: Individuals in 48 States, Year 1977–78. Report No. I-2. Consumer Nutrition Division, Human Nutrition Information Service, Hyattsville, Md. 439 pp.

USDA (U.S. Department of Agriculture). 1986. Nationwide Food Consumption Survey. Continuing Survey of Food Intakes of Individuals. Men 19–50 Years, 1 Day, 1985. Report No. 85-3. Nutrition Monitoring Division, Human Nutrition Information Service, Hyattsville, Md. 94 pp.

USDA (U.S. Department of Agriculture). 1987. Nationwide Food Consumption Survey. Continuing Survey of Food Intakes of Individuals. Women 19–50 Years and Their Children 1–5 Years, 4 Days, 1985. Report No. 85-4. Nutrition Monitoring Division, Human Nutrition Information Service, Hyattsville, Md. 182 pp.

Vinther-Paulsen, N. 1953. Calcium and phosphorus intake in senile osteoporosis. Geriatrics 8:76–79.

Wallach, S., and R.L. Verch. 1986. Tissue magnesium in spontaneously hypertensive rats. Magnesium 5:33–38.

Wargovich, M.J., V.W. Eng, H.L. Newmark, and W.R. Bruce. 1983. Calcium ameliorates the toxic effect of deoxycholic acid on colonic epithelium. Carcinogenesis 4:1205–1207.

Weidmann, P., S.G. Massry, J.W. Coburn, M.H. Maxwell, J. Atleson, and C.R. Kleeman. 1972. Blood pressure effects of acute hypercalcemia. Studies in patients with chronic renal failure. Ann. Intern. Med. 76:741–745.

Wright, G.L., and G.O. Rankin. 1982. Concentrations of ionic and total calcium in plasma of four models of hypertension. Am. J. Physiol. 243:H365–H370.

Young, E.W., S.R. Patel, and C.H. Hsu. 1986. Plasma $1,25(OH)_2D_3$ response to parathyroid hormone, cyclic adenosine monophosphate, and phosphorus depletion in the spontaneously hypertensive rat. J. Lab. Clin. Med. 6:562–566.

Young, E.W., R.D. Bukoski, and D.A. McCarron. 1988. Calcium metabolism in experimental hypertension. Proc. Soc. Exp. Biol. Med. 187:123–124.

Zemel, M.B., and H.M. Linkswiler. 1981. Calcium metabolism in the young adult male as affected by levels and form of phosphorus intake and level of calcium intake. J. Nutr. 111:315–324.

14

Trace Elements

Trace elements (or trace metals) are minerals present in living tissues in small amounts. Some of them are known to be nutritionally essential, others may be essential (although the evidence is only suggestive or incomplete), and the remainder are considered to be nonessential. Trace elements function primarily as catalysts in enzyme systems; some metallic ions, such as iron and copper, participate in oxidation–reduction reactions in energy metabolism. Iron, as a constituent of hemoglobin and myoglobin, also plays a vital role in the transport of oxygen.

All trace elements are toxic if consumed at sufficiently high levels for long enough periods. The difference between toxic intakes and optimal intakes to meet physiological needs for essential trace elements is great for some elements but is much smaller for others.

This chapter is a summary of the role of the following essential trace elements in the etiology and prevention of chronic diseases: iron, zinc, fluoride, selenium, copper, chromium, iodine, manganese, and molybdenum. Also discussed are aluminum, cadmium, mercury, arsenic, and lead; these elements have not been demonstrated to be essential for humans but were reviewed by the committee because they are frequently ingested as contaminants in food or water. Interactions between the various trace elements are also briefly considered.

Epidemiologic data on the relationship between many of the trace elements and the incidence of diseases such as cancer, cardiovascular disease, and hypertension are incomplete. Most such studies have focused on cadmium, chromium, and selenium. Furthermore, most of the evidence is not related to dietary exposure but focuses, for example, on inhalation exposure in the workplace. Data from animal feeding experiments are also incomplete. The committee identifies such gaps in knowledge and suggests directions for research.

EVIDENCE ASSOCIATING TRACE ELEMENTS WITH CHRONIC DISEASES

Iron

Iron is present in all body cells. As a component of hemoglobin and myoglobin, it functions as a carrier of oxygen in the blood and muscles. Because of iron losses during menstruation, women in their reproductive years require higher iron intakes than men. Therefore, the Recommended Dietary Allowance (RDA) for women 11 to 50 years of age is 18 mg/day, but for men 19 years and older is only 10 mg/day. Women have difficulty achieving this high intake, because they generally have a relatively low caloric intake, and the usual U.S. diet provides only 6 to 7 mg of iron per 1,000 kcal. Since the need for iron is greater during periods of rapid growth, children from infancy through adolescence, as well as pregnant women, may fail to consume sufficient iron to meet their needs.

Iron absorption is affected by many factors. Heme iron is present in meats, poultry, and fish and is more efficiently absorbed than inorganic (nonheme) iron, which is found in plant as well as animal foods. Ascorbic acid facilitates the absorption of nonheme iron, but dietary fiber, phytates, and certain trace elements may diminish it. Food composition data provide no indicators concerning the efficiency with which the body absorbs iron from a given food. The publication *Recommended Dietary Allowances* (NRC, 1980) provides directions on how to calculate available iron.

The availability of iron in the food supply has increased since 1909, chiefly because of the enrichment of flour and cereal products. The 1977–1978 Nationwide Food Consumption Survey (NFCS) indicates that on the average respondents of both sexes from 1 to 18 years old and females from 19 to 64 years old failed to meet their RDA for iron (USDA, 1984). The Continuing Survey of Food Intakes of Individuals (CSFII) conducted in 1985 and 1986 (USDA, 1987a,b) supports these findings. By itself, however, failure to meet the RDA is not an indicator of poor iron status.

Using data from the National Health and Nutrition Examination Survey (NHANES II), conducted from 1976 to 1980, an expert scientific group of the Federation of American Societies for Experimental Biology (FASEB) assessed iron status (LSRO, 1984a). Five indicators in three different models were used in the assessment. A relatively high prevalence of impaired iron status was found in children 1 to 2 years old, males 11 to 14 years old, and females 25 to 44 years old. Among those whose incomes were below poverty level, impaired iron status was highest in children 1 to 5 years old and females 25 to 54 years old (LSRO, 1984a).

Cancer

Epidemiologic and Clinical Studies

Iron deficiency is a risk factor for the Plummer–Vinson (Paterson–Kelly) syndrome, which was once common in parts of Sweden but has been almost eliminated through improved nutritional status, especially with regard to dietary iron and vitamins (Larsson et al., 1975; Wynder et al., 1957). This condition is associated with an increased risk for cancers of the upper alimentary tract, especially the esophagus and stomach, suggesting that the underlying iron deficiency might

be one of the factors that contribute to the occurrence of these cancers. However, epidemiologic studies have not implicated low dietary iron intake per se as a risk factor for cancers at these sites (Schottenfeld and Fraumeni, 1982).

In a correlation analysis of nutrition survey data and cancer mortality rates for 11 regions of the Federal Republic of Germany, Böing et al. (1985) found a positive association between estimated iron intake and mortality from colorectal and pancreatic cancer in men and from gallbladder cancer in women. In a prospective cohort of 21,513 Chinese men in Taiwan, ferritin levels were considerably higher in men over age 50 who developed cancer, especially primary hepatocellular carcinoma (PHC), than in controls without cancer, whereas serum transferrin levels were lower in the men who developed cancer (excluding PHC) (Stevens et al., 1986). These findings probably reflect an association of cancer risk with increased body iron stores, although iron stores were not directly assessed.

Occupational inhalation exposure to iron oxides has been associated with an increased risk for lung cancer in hematite miners and foundry workers (Kazantzis, 1981). In these occupational settings, however, there were other exposures to carcinogens, including ionizing radiation, polycyclic aromatic hydrocarbons (PAHs), and cigarette smoke. Thus, the increased cancer risk cannot be attributed specifically to iron (Doll, 1981; Kazantzis, 1981).

Clinical studies of patients with idiopathic hemochromatosis, a condition that includes abnormal deposition of iron in the liver and frequently cirrhosis, show a highly increased risk for hepatocellular carcinoma (Ammann et al., 1980; Bomford and Williams, 1976; Strohmeyer et al., 1988).

Overall, these studies in humans do not provide strong evidence for a role of iron exposure, whether by diet or by other routes, in the etiology of human cancer.

Animal Studies

Iron-deficient rats given 1,2-dimethylhydrazine (DMH) developed neoplastic liver lesions within 4 months, compared to 6 months in an iron-sufficient group (Vitale et al., 1978). The authors noted that severe lack of iron appeared to promote carcinogenesis.

The effect of iron deficiency on tumor growth and host survival was studied in BALB/c mice with transplanted Merwin Plasma Cell-II tumors (Benbassat et al., 1981). Iron deficiency resulted in retardation of body growth and tumor growth in weanling mice, but not in adults. The reason for this difference in response was not determined. Mammary tumors induced by the intragastric administration of dimethylbenz[a]anthracene (DMBA) and fibrosarcomas induced by subcutaneous injections of methylcholanthrene (MCA) were studied in iron-deficient female Wistar rats (Webster, 1981). There was no difference in induction time, tumor site, total number of tumors, or incidence of metastases in the iron-deficient rats compared with controls. In this study, a lack of iron did not appear to inhibit carcinogenesis, as it did in the study by Benbassat et al. (1981). In a later study, albino iron-deficient rats were painted with 4NQO oral carcinogen and left untreated (Prime et al., 1986). These investigators also saw no difference in tumor development or epithelial dysplasia between the iron-deficient and iron-sufficient animals.

Isolated perfused rabbit lung was used to investigate the effects of a cocarcinogen, ferric oxide, on the metabolism of benzo[a]pyrene (BaP) (Warshawsky et al., 1984). The data suggest that ferric oxide increased the production of dihydrodiols from BaP, which may be further metabolized to the ultimate carcinogenic forms. DBA-2 mice fed supplemental doses of iron (24 mg/kg body weight) and inoculated with L1210 cells eventually developed more tumor cells than did the controls. Animals treated at still higher levels of supplemental iron (250 mg/kg body weight) and inoculated with L1210 cells died sooner than untreated but inoculated controls (Bergeron et al., 1985). The authors concluded that high doses of supplemental iron may increase neoplastic proliferation or metastasis in vivo. Iron overload has frequently been associated with an enhanced incidence of malignancy in animals (Weinberg, 1983).

In contrast to epidemiologic studies, animal studies suggest that depending on the conditions, iron can either enhance or inhibit tumor development. Reports disagree as to the effects of iron deficiency on tumor growth, and certain iron compounds may act as cocarcinogens. The route of administration, dose, and specific iron compound all seem to affect the outcome.

Short-Term Tests

Brusick et al. (1976) found that Fe[II] as iron sulfate induced reverse mutations in *Salmonella typhimurium* strains TA1537 and TA1538, with and without metabolic activation by the S9 fraction. In another study, 45 metal salts were evalu-

ated for their capacity to induce morphological tranformation of Syrian hamster fetal cells in vivo. Iron was among the trace elements for which positive transformation assays were obtained (DiPaolo and Casto, 1979).

Coronary Heart Disease

Epidemiologic Studies

The greater prevalence of iron deficiency among women, compared to men, has been proposed as an explanation for the lower coronary heart disease (CHD) rate among premenopausal women (Sullivan, 1986); however, no epidemiologic evidence supports this hypothesis.

Iron-Deficiency Anemia

Epidemiologic Studies

Iron-deficiency anemia is the state in which the amount of iron in the body is less than that required for normal formation of hemoglobin, iron enzymes, and other functioning iron compounds. It is the most widespread nutritional deficiency in the world (Dallman et al., 1979) and is the major cause of anemia in Western countries. In the United States, however, the overall prevalence is low. NHANES II showed that the highest prevalence (9.3%) occurred among children 1 to 2 years old; next came women age 15 to 19 (7.2%) and 20 to 44 (6.3%). Men between the ages of 15 and 64 had a prevalence of less than 1% (LSRO, 1984a).

Iron-deficiency anemia is usually due to inadequate iron nutriture in infants and small children and to blood loss or pregnancy in adults. The most frequent causes of anemia among older people are infections and chronic diseases—not iron deficiency. The prevalence of iron-deficiency anemia varies widely, depending on criteria for diagnosis (Charlton and Bothwell, 1982; Reeves et al., 1983); it can be affected by physiological, pathological, and nutritional factors.

In some segments of the population, the amount of dietary iron has decreased with increases in caloric intake from fats and refined sugar. Where caloric intake has declined, iron intake has also declined. For example, iron-deficiency anemia occurs more commonly among women than among men, even in the absence of pathological blood loss. Women eat less food and are therefore able to absorb less iron, but their requirements for iron are greater because they lose iron through menstruation. Preventive approaches include iron supplementation, fortification, and alteration of eating habits, for example, increasing intake of nutrients and foods stimulating iron absorption (e.g., vitamin C, meat, and fish) or reducing intake of foods inhibiting iron absorption (e.g., phytates).

Older, but still useful, methods for evaluating body iron stores include determination of the plasma iron level and iron-binding capacity. Measurement of serum ferritin and free erythrocyte protoporphyrin concentration provide a more accurate assessment of iron stores.

Animal Studies

Experimentally induced iron-deficiency anemia produced striking morphological changes in the hearts of rats. These changes were characterized by marked cellular hypertrophy together with distinct cellular degeneration and interstitial fibrosis (Rossi and Carillo, 1983). In other studies, Rossi and colleagues treated iron-deficient anemic rats with reserpine (Rossi and Carillo, 1982; Rossi et al., 1981). The hearts of anemic rats not given reserpine were marked by cardiac hypertrophy, as indicated by increases in both heart weight and size of muscle cells. The hearts of reserpine-treated animals were not enlarged. The researchers speculated that noradrenaline may play a key role in the cardiac hypertrophy of iron-deficiency anemia.

Zinc

Zinc, a constituent of more than 200 enzymes, plays an important role in nucleic acid metabolism, cell replication, tissue repair, and growth through its function in nucleic acid polymerases. These zinc-dependent enzymes include the potentially rate-limiting enzymes involved in DNA synthesis. Zinc also has many recognized and biologically important interactions with hormones and plays a role in production, storage, and secretion of individual hormones. Severe, moderate, and marginal zinc deficiencies have been reported in the United States (Hambidge et al., 1986).

The richest sources of zinc are shellfish (especially oysters), beef, and other red meats. Poultry, eggs, hard cheeses, milk, yogurt, legumes, nuts, and whole-grain cereals are also good sources. Many dietary factors, including other minerals, phytates, and dietary fiber, may adversely affect zinc absorption (Hambidge et al., 1986). Food sources of zinc have changed since the turn of the century. Until the middle 1930s, people obtained about equal amounts of zinc from foods of animal and plant origin, but since 1960, people have obtained approximately 70% of food-supply zinc from animal foods. Zinc from animal sources appears to be better absorbed than that from plant sources.

The 1980 RDA for zinc is 15 mg/day for people 11 years of age and older (NRC, 1980), but zinc available in the food supply amounts to only 12.3 mg per capita (see Table 3–5). Zinc intakes have been estimated in national surveys only since 1984. According to the 1985 NFCS, men and women 19 to 50 years of age consumed an average of 94 and 56% of their RDA, respectively, and children 1 to 5 years of age consumed 73% of their RDA of 10 mg/day (USDA 1986, 1987b).

Data from NHANES II were evaluated by a FASEB group (LSRO, 1984b), which concluded that serum zinc levels are inadequate for assessing the nutritional status of zinc in individuals, but that low values may aid in identifying groups whose zinc status should be further investigated.

Atherosclerotic Cardiovascular Diseases

Epidemiologic and Clinical Studies

On the basis of knowledge concerning the relationships of zinc and copper to several risk factors for CHD, including elevated serum cholesterol and hypertension, Klevay (1975) hypothesized that an excess of zinc relative to copper may underlie this disease. For example, supplementation of the diet of 12 adult men with more than 10 times the RDA of zinc for 5 weeks while they took in normal levels of copper led to a significant decrease in high-density-lipoprotein (HDL) cholesterol but no change in total cholesterol (Hooper et al., 1980). This hypothesis and the controversial evidence pertaining to it are discussed in the section on copper.

Animal Studies

The committee found no animal studies on the relationship between zinc and cardiovascular diseases.

Cancer

Epidemiologic and Clinical Studies

Few epidemiologic studies have been conducted to examine the relationship between exposure to zinc, especially dietary zinc, and cancer risk. In correlation analyses, zinc levels in soil, food, or blood have been positively associated with several different cancers (Schrauzer et al., 1977a,b; Stocks and Davies, 1964).

In an effort to identify etiologic factors for esophageal cancer in the very-high-risk area of Linxian in Hunan Province, China, blood and hair samples from a random sample of 58 men and 53 women who had undergone esophagoscopy with biopsy were analyzed for zinc, riboflavin, and vitamin A components (Thurnham et al., 1982). Zinc levels in plasma and hair were not significantly different between subjects with normal histology and those with lesions presumed to be precursors of cancer (e.g., esophagitis, dysplasia, acanthosis). No differences in zinc levels in blood and hair were found in another study of a similar random sample from a low-risk area in Shandong Province (Thurnham et al., 1985).

Dietary zinc was assessed in only one case-control study of cancer. Kolonel et al. (1988) found that patients with prostate cancer who were 70 years old and older ingested more zinc (from supplements but not from food) prior to the onset of cancer than did matched population controls. Occupational studies of workers exposed to zinc by inhalation (usually in the presence of other trace elements such as copper, lead, arsenic, and chromium) have not implicated zinc as a risk factor for cancer (Gerhardsson et al., 1986).

In many clinical studies, serum or tissue levels of zinc in cancer patients have been compared with those in controls. In most of these studies, sample sizes were small; controls were not well matched to the cases, even on age; and potential confounding factors were not considered in the analyses. The results have been mixed. In studies of patients with cancers at several different sites, investigators have found both decreased serum zinc levels in patients (Atukorala et al., 1979; Davies et al., 1968; Lin et al., 1977; Mellow et al., 1983; Sharma et al., 1984; Whelan et al., 1983) and higher zinc levels in the patients (Adler et al., 1981) compared to controls. In other studies, no differences were found between patients and controls (Feustel and Wennrich, 1986; Manousos et al., 1981; Smith et al., 1971; Strain et al., 1972; Thurnham et al., 1982). In many of these studies, serum copper levels were also measured; they were generally and consistently higher in the patients than in the controls, leading to lowered zinc-to-copper ratios. The possibility that the zinc findings in these studies were a consequence rather than a cause of the cancers is suggested by the observation of Sharma

et al. (1984), who reported that the depressed serum zinc levels in lymphoma patients returned to normal following chemotherapy.

The prostate normally contains the highest concentrations of zinc in the body and is therefore of great interest in studies of zinc and cancer (Hambidge et al., 1986). In several studies, investigators have compared zinc levels in prostate tissue from healthy subjects and from patients with benign prostatic hypertrophy (BPH) and cancer. Zinc concentrations were lowest in carcinomatous tissue, highest in BPH tissue, and intermediate in normal tissue (Feustel and Wennrich, 1984; Feustel et al., 1982; Györkey et al., 1967).

Zinc interacts with other trace elements and is an antagonist to copper (Mertz, 1982) (see discussion below under Zinc–Copper Interactions). Zinc also interacts with vitamin A (Solomons and Russell, 1980). Thus, the findings on zinc in human studies could reflect fundamental relationships between other nutrients and the diseases of interest. In general, however, human studies provide no evidence that zinc intake plays an important role in the etiology of cancer.

Animal Studies

Investigators have reported both enhancing and retarding effects of zinc on tumor growth in animals. Several have suggested that a zinc-deficient diet strongly inhibits the growth of transplanted tumors and prolongs survival (Barr and Harris, 1973; Beach et al., 1981; DeWys and Pories, 1972; DeWys et al., 1970; Fenton et al., 1980; Mills et al., 1984; Minkel et al., 1979). These findings suggest that rapidly growing tumor cells require zinc for growth. Zinc deficiency is not recommended as a therapeutic modality, however, because serious zinc deficiency, with or without concomitant malignancies, is itself lethal.

In contrast to transplanted tumors, chemically induced carcinogenesis appears to be enhanced by zinc deficiency. For example, Gabrial et al. (1982) observed that the incidence of esophageal tumors induced by nitrosomethylbenzylamine was much higher in zinc-deficient rats than in control rats. Still other studies indicate that a zinc intake well above nutritional requirements suppresses the carcinogenesis of dimethylbenzylamine in Syrian hamsters (Poswillo and Cohen, 1971) and of azo dyes in rats (Duncan and Dreosti, 1975). On the other hand, Schrauzer (1979) demonstrated that high concentrations of zinc (200 mg/liter) in the drinking water of C3H mice countered the protective effect of selenium against spontaneous mammary carcinoma and resulted in a great increase in tumor growth.

The two different effects of zinc deficiency on carcinogenesis were elucidated in a study by Beach et al. (1981) in which BALB/c mice were fed diets containing four levels of zinc beginning at 6, 3, 1, and 0 weeks before injection of Moloney sarcoma virus (MSV). Mice fed marginal and moderately zinc-deficient diets had greater sarcoma growth than did control mice, whereas those fed a diet severely deficient in zinc had a lower incidence of and smaller sarcomas. Feeding low-zinc diets for 6 weeks before MSV injection caused fewer sarcomas to be initiated and slower progression of the tumors. After sufficient severity and duration of zinc deprivation, mice also had a longer tumor latency and shorter tumor regression time.

These apparently contradictory effects of zinc deficiency—the enhancement of tumor growth at some levels and the inhibition of growth at others—may indicate that there are two different mechanisms of action (Beach et al., 1981). Zinc deprivation has been shown to alter many facets of immunocompetence in experimental animals (Beach et al., 1979; Fernandes et al., 1979) as well as in humans (Golden et al., 1978). Thus, alterations in host immunologic function through zinc deprivation may contribute to changes in host-tumor interactions. However, zinc is also known to influence many aspects of host and tumor metabolism, including nucleic acid and protein synthesis, and tissues in the phase of rapid growth are most severely affected by zinc deprivation (Hurley, 1981). Thus, zinc is also necessary for tumor growth. Altered DNA synthesis by neoplastic tissue contributes to the inhibition of tumor growth in zinc-deficient animals. Zinc deficiency also causes chromosome aberrations in pregnant and fetal rats (Bell et al., 1975).

It is difficult to assess the relative roles of host immune responsiveness and the interaction of host and tumor metabolism. Nevertheless, it appears that the influence of zinc nutrition on carcinogenesis reflects, at least in part, the interaction of the host and tumor. In contrast to human studies, studies in animals show that zinc can either enhance or inhibit tumor growth, perhaps by its effects on host immunocompetence, as stated above, or on nucleic acid synthesis.

Short-Term Tests

Zinc can affect both the tumor cell and the host, interfering with mechanisms that may be important for metastasis. It also promotes the adhesion of leukocytes to the endothelium (Hoover et al., 1980) and inhibits the procoagulant activity of polymorphonuclear leukocytes (Gazdy et al., 1981). Erkell et al. (1986) observed that preincubating B16 tumor cells in 0.1 M zinc caused a dramatic decrease in their intravenous transplantability. They postulated that this may be due to an impairment of cell adhesion.

Other Diseases

Epidemiologic and Clinical Studies

The relationship between diabetes and zinc metabolism has been the subject of recent research. In humans, hyperzincuria is frequently found in diabetics. This condition is not entirely reversed following insulin treatment and does not seem to be compensated for by increased intestinal absorption (Kinlaw et al., 1983; Hallmans and Lithner, 1980; Levine et al., 1983). The increased loss of urinary zinc in diabetics is positively related to glycosuria (McNair et al., 1981; Pidduck et al., 1970).

Stunted growth observed in many diabetic children suggests that the diabetes-induced change in zinc metabolism could be functionally important (Canfield et al., 1984). It is possible that the teratogenicity of diabetes may be due in part to the induction of zinc deficiency in the embryo or fetus. The observation that the offspring of diabetic rats have low zinc concentrations in their livers, compared to controls, supports this suggestion (Uriu-Hare et al., 1985).

Although there is considerable evidence that abnormal zinc metabolism occurs in diabetics, the role of zinc, if any, in the etiology of diabetes is unknown. In a study of children with diabetes mellitus (Hägglöf et al., 1983), hair zinc levels were found to be normal, whereas serum levels were lower and urinary levels were higher than in controls. The serum levels, but not the urinary levels, returned to normal after the diabetes was treated with insulin, suggesting that these two parameters reflect different metabolic processes or defects.

Since zinc is part of the mineral content of bone, it might play a role in osteoporosis; however, there was no difference in the zinc content of bone samples taken from the iliac crest of 88 subjects with normal mineral status and 50 subjects with osteoporosis. Variations in zinc concentrations were best predicted by the copper and fluoride content of the bone (Lappalainen et al., 1982). An opposite finding was reported in a small study of 10 male patients with senile osteoporosis and 12 male controls with degenerative osteoarthritis of the hip joint; the zinc concentrations in serum and bone tissue from the head of the femur were much lower in the patients with osteoporosis (Atik, 1983).

Zinc–Copper Interactions

Excessive intakes of zinc interfere with the absorption and utilization of iron and copper in animals. Campbell and Mills (1974) fed diets with a low or marginal copper content to weanling rats and found that 300 μg of additional zinc per gram of diet reduced plasma ceruloplasmin activity; more zinc, up to 1,000 μg, caused growth depression, hair depigmentation, and depressed copper levels in the liver. In sows, the addition of 5,000 μg of zinc per gram of diet increased zinc and depressed copper concentrations in plasma and liver (Hill et al., 1983). In sheep, increases in dietary zinc also result in copper deficiency, which is manifested by reduced plasma levels of copper, ceruloplasmin, and amine oxidase (Campbell and Mills, 1979).

An antagonistic effect of dietary zinc on copper concentrations in maternal and fetal tissues was observed in pregnant rats fed diets with various levels of copper and zinc (Reinstein et al., 1984). The authors concluded that in zinc-deficient diets, the high copper-to-zinc ratio potentiates the teratogenic effects of zinc deficiency.

In humans, prolonged use of oral zinc supplements, even at relatively modest levels, may have adverse clinical consequences. For example, copper deficiency, evidenced by microcytic anemia, neutropenia, and decreased levels of plasma copper and ceruloplasmin, was found in a man who had been taking 150 mg of zinc daily for 2 years (Prasad et al., 1978).

Fluoride

Fluoride is an integral part of the food chain. Kumpulainen and Koivistoinen (1977) reported that the measured fluoride content of the diet is three times higher in communities with fluoridated water than in those where the water is not fluoridated. Singer and Ophaug (1979) found that the fluoride content of dry cereals is strongly influenced by the fluoride content of the water in which they were processed. They also reported that baby foods contain high levels of fluoride (Singer and Ophaug, 1979). Fluoride is also consumed unintentionally from two major sources: products con-

taining mechanically boned meat and fluoridated dentifrices. The highest daily average consumption (equivalent to 0.3 mg of fluoride) is reported for children under the age of 5 (Barnhart et al., 1974).

The interaction of fluoride with other dietary ions could influence its bioavailability. Aluminum-containing antacids cause a negative fluoride balance by markedly increasing fluoride excretion (Spencer and Kramer, 1985; Spencer et al., 1981). For infants not drinking fluoridated water, and for those receiving human or cow milk (both low in fluoride) rather than infant formula, fluoride supplements of 0.25 mg/day are advised (Forbes and Woodruff, 1985).

Fluoride could be involved in the growth and maintenance of a normal skeleton (see below and Chapter 23, Osteoporosis). Modest accumulations of fluoride in the bone mineral complex result in increased bone crystallinity and decreased solubility. The net result is the formation of a more stable mineral system that is less susceptible to bone resorption (Spencer and Kramer, 1985).

Dental Caries

Epidemiologic Studies

Fluoride therapy has been used since 1949 to prevent dental caries (Dunning, 1979). In the late 1930s, large-scale epidemiologic studies first elucidated the relationship between fluoride in water supplies and reduced prevalance of dental caries (Brown and König, 1977; Dean, 1936; Dean and Elvove, 1935; Levine, 1976). More recently, Burt et al. (1986) determined that children who have lived for a few years in a community with optimal water fluoride have a 30 to 40% lower caries incidence than children who have lived continuously in low-fluoride communities. Similar reductions in dental caries incidence were observed by Driscoll et al. (1981).

For fluoride, there is a narrow range of safe and adequate intake and therefore much concern among health activists about its potential toxicity. The level of fluoride commonly maintained in municipal water supplies is 1 part per million (ppm). At 2 ppm, such undesirable effects as dental fluorosis (i.e., mottling of teeth) have been observed (Pollack and Kravitz, 1985). A fluoride concentration of 4 ppm has been associated with an increased incidence of caries (Ericsson, 1977; Jenkins, 1978).

Although the increased consumption of dietary sugars has led to increases in dental caries prevalence internationally (Taylor, 1980; Yassin and

Low, 1975), World Health Organization data indicate that caries is decreasing in Western countries and increasing in developing countries (WHO, 1988). Reports from the National Institute of Dental Research (NIDR) substantiate this observation (NIDR, 1981). The decline in caries incidence in the United States has been attributed primarily to the widespread use of fluoride in many forms (Dunning, 1979; Newbrun, 1975; Shaw, 1954), to improved oral hygiene, and to the increased use of antibiotics. The role of fluoride in dental caries is discussed more fully in Chapter 26.

Animal Studies

Developing teeth are extremely sensitive to fluoride. Abnormalities in permanent dentition are the most obvious signs of excessive fluoride ingestion. The tooth becomes mottled, perhaps with hypoplasia (thin enamel), and is subject to more rapid wear and possible erosion of the enamel (NRC, 1971). Brown et al. (1960) established that developing incisors in cattle are vulnerable up to 30 months of age. Shupe et al. (1962) fed young dairy heifers various levels of fluoride for 7.5 years. They reported that dental and bone lesions were correlated with the amount of fluoride ingested, the amount of fluoride in the bone, the age of the cow, and the duration of exposure. Milk production in cows given a higher level of fluoride was reduced.

Fluoride concentrations appear to be higher during the matrix-forming secretory stage of enamel formation than in the rapidly mineralizing maturation stage. An in vitro study by Crenshaw et al. (1978) suggests that selective binding of fluoride by newly synthesized matrix proteins may in large measure account for the enhanced uptake. Drinkard et al. (1982) found that fluoride also delays deposition of the matrix proteins in rat molars during the secretory stage of enamel development. It has not been established, however, whether these fluoride–protein interactions contribute to the fluoride-induced changes in enamel crystallinity.

Cancer

Epidemiologic Studies

Epidemiologic studies have focused on the health effects of fluoride in public water supplies—the major source of fluoride for most people. Early reports found no association between fluoride and mortality in communities with and without naturally high fluoride levels in their water supplies

(Hagan et al., 1954; Nixon and Carpenter, 1974), which led the way to the introduction of water fluoridation in many communities.

In the 1970s, attention was abruptly redirected to the possibility of an increased risk for cancer by a well-publicized analysis of cancer mortality rates in 10 fluoridated and 10 nonfluoridated cities in the United States (Yiamouyiannis and Burk, 1977). Although these investigators claimed that cancer mortality was higher in the fluoridated cities, their analysis failed to include necessary and routine adjustments for such demographic differences among populations as age, sex, and racial composition. Subsequently, different investigators reanalyzed in a more appropriate fashion the same data, as well as more comprehensive data sets in the United States, and all concluded that there was no evidence of an increased risk for mortality from cancer overall or at any specific site (Chilvers, 1983; Doll and Kinlen, 1977; Erickson, 1978; Hoover et al., 1976; Kinlen and Doll, 1981; Oldham and Newell, 1977; Rogot et al., 1978; Taves, 1979). Similar ecological studies have been conducted in Great Britain, Canada, Australia, New Zealand, Austria, and Norway, and all have yielded negative results. These studies have been exhaustively reviewed in several recent reports (Clemmesen, 1983; IARC, 1982a,b; Knox, 1985; NRC, 1977b).

Short-Term Tests

Fluoride-induced chromosome changes have been repeatedly demonstrated in mammalian cells. For example, Mukherjee and Sobels (1968) showed that both irradiated and fluoride-treated sperm cells had more chromosome aberrations than did controls.

Jagiello and Lin (1974) found that in vitro exposure to sodium fluoride sharply reduced the percentage of cow and ewe oocytes undergoing meiotic division. In cells of bone and testes of mice, the number of chromosome breaks and abnormalities increased with increasing fluoride levels in drinking water (Mohamed and Weitzenkamp-Chandler, 1976). Similar mutagenic effects and dose responses were observed when bone cells of white rats were exposed to inorganic fluoride (Gileva et al., 1972; Voroshilin et al., 1975). In general, fluoride interacts with DNA and RNA and alters biologic activity in mammalian cells (Clark and Taylor, 1981; Emsley et al., 1981, 1982; Greenberg, 1982).

Tsutsui et al. (1984) produced anaplastic fibrosarcomas by treating hamster embryo cells with fluoride concentrations ranging from 75 to 125 ppm and later injecting the cells into newborn Syrian hamsters. The dose levels used in these experiments were much higher than those to which humans are normally exposed; it is not known what results would be observed at lower doses.

Hypertension and Cardiac Effects

Epidemiologic Studies

The committee found no studies in humans that examine possible effects of fluoride on hypertension or cardiac function.

Animal Studies

Fluoride has caused a decrease in blood pressure and induced cardiac changes in several studies in animals. For example, Leone et al. (1956) subjected dogs to intravenous infusion of fluoride at doses of 20 and 30.6 mg/kg body weight. There was a dose-related depression of the respiratory rate and a conversion to atrioventricular nodal or ventricular rhythm with terminal ventricular fibrillation. Lu et al. (1965) observed the same response in monkeys.

Osteoporosis

Epidemiologic and Clinical Studies

The use of fluoride to reverse or delay the progression of osteoporosis and hence to reduce the risk of fractures has been reviewed by Kanis and Meunier (1984). Methodological limitations and inconsistencies in results of the various studies prevented firm conclusions from being drawn (Kanis and Meunier, 1984). Fluoride may actually increase the risk of femoral fractures at the same time that it decreases the risk of vertebral fractures in some patients (Power and Gay, 1986). Riggs et al. (1982) reported a decrease in the rate of spinal fracture associated with the use of fluoride. However, it is unclear as to whether vertebral fractures are reduced among lifelong residents of areas with highly fluoridated drinking water (Alffram et al., 1969; Bernstein et al., 1966).

Reports of effects of fluoride therapy on bone mass are reasonably consistent. Trabecular bone volume is increased in patients given fluoride (Hanson and Roos, 1978; Ivey and Baylink, 1981; Jowsey, 1979). Other studies show that trabecular bone mass increases in only 60% of patients receiving fluoride therapy (Riggs et al., 1980, 1982). It is not possible to predict which patients

will respond favorably to fluoride, because the factors influencing the response have not been identified. Many questions regarding the use of fluoride to reduce osteoporosis and fractures remain unanswered.

Animal Studies

Miller et al. (1977) reported that the bones of cows with osteoporosis resulting from environmental exposure to fluoride had higher calcium levels and a somewhat lower phosphorus content than the bones of cows not exposed to fluoride. Henrikson et al. (1970) studied the ash of osteoporotic bones from dogs and found that fluoride caused a slight decrease in the calcium content and an increase in phosphorus. The mineral mass also increased with increasing dietary fluoride, but there was no improvement in the degree of osteoporosis. These studies suggest that fluoride may indirectly affect osteoporosis by increasing bone mineral mass; however, the data on calcium are inconsistent, and it is not certain if dogs are an appropriate model for osteoporosis.

Selenium

In the 1950s, recognition of the economic importance of selenium deficiency in food animals led to the mapping of selenium distributions in the soils, forages, and blood of humans in several continents. Extreme differences in exposure were found, even within countries. This knowledge enabled investigators to make epidemiologic correlations of diseases in humans and animals and to conduct laboratory experiments to test hypotheses. In 1980, a committee of the National Research Council set the estimated safe and adequate daily intake of selenium at 10 to 40 µg/day for infants, 20 to 200 µg/day for children, and 50 to 200 µg/day for those over 11 years of age (NRC, 1980). Studies based on saturation of plasma glutathione peroxidase activity suggest that the selenium requirement of Chinese men is about 40 µg/day (G. Q. Yang et al., 1987). After adjusting for differences in body weight and incorporating a safety factor, a dietary recommendation of 70 and 55 µg/day can be calculated for North American men and women, respectively (Levander, 1987). The average dietary selenium intake for U.S. men was 108 µg/day between 1974 and mid-1982 (Pennington et al., 1984).

At present, the only well-characterized biochemical function for selenium in mammals is its role in the peroxide-destroying enzyme glutathione peroxidase (Hoekstra, 1975). However, other selenium-containing proteins in mammals have been described (J. G. Yang et al., 1987). Selenium is also known to participate in several important metabolic interactions with a variety of hazardous elements such as mercury, cadmium, and arsenic, which may be important to public health (Levander and Cheng, 1980).

Atherosclerotic Cardiovascular Diseases

Epidemiologic and Clinical Studies

Several reports on the relationship of serum selenium to the risk of cardiovascular diseases have been published by investigators in Finland—a country with reportedly low selenium intakes. In two prospective cohorts, Salonen et al. (1982, 1985b) found that selenium levels were lower in the serum of subjects who died from cardiovascular diseases, including CHD specifically, than in control subjects matched on daily tobacco consumption and other risk factors for CHD. In two other Finish cohort studies (Miettinen et al., 1983; Virtamo et al., 1985), investigators found no association of serum selenium with CHD, although Virtamo et al. (1985) did find an inverse association with cardiovascular diseases generally and possibly with stroke. In a similar analysis of a large cohort in the Netherlands, where selenium intake is higher than in Finland, Kok et al. (1987b) found no significant association between serum selenium level and mortality from CHD or stroke, although the findings for stroke suggested an inverse association.

Thus, the results of these cohort studies are equivocal. The inconsistencies in findings could reflect, in part, such methodological concerns as reliance on single serum measurements or the possibility of a threshold in serum selenium level above which there is no associated risk of cardiovascular diseases. The observation that regional variations in mean serum levels of selenium within Finland do not correlate inversely with CHD mortality suggests that selenium is unlikely to be a major determinant of risk for this disease (Virtamo et al., 1985).

Ellis et al. (1984) studied the relationship of blood selenium levels to smoking and alcohol consumption in healthy male volunteers. They found much lower selenium levels in the whole blood and serum of cigarette smokers than of nonsmokers, independent of alcohol use. In addition, selenium was not associated with other risk factors for CHD (including blood pressure, serum total and HDL cholesterol, and obesity). Whether the lower selenium concentration in smokers was a metabolic consequence of smoking or was secondary to differences in the dietary patterns of smokers could not be determined from this study.

Clinical studies based on tissue and serum concentrations of selenium generally show no association between coronary artery disease or hypertension and selenium levels (Aro et al., 1986; Masironi and Parr, 1976; Shamberger et al., 1978; Westermarck, 1977), although a few investigators reported inverse associations (Moore et al., 1984; Oster et al., 1986).

A cardiomyopathy (degeneration of the heart muscle), known as Keshan disease, primarily affects young children and women during reproductive years in certain regions of China where the soil levels of selenium are low. The poor soil content is reflected in the very low selenium levels in locally grown cereals, which can explain why mean selenium levels in blood, urine, and hair are substantially lower in the affected areas than in other parts of China.

Trials in children given diets supplemented with sodium selenite provided convincing evidence that selenium deficiency is a major etiologic factor in this disease. These findings are reviewed and discussed by Yang et al. (1984). Since most cardiovascular mortality in Western countries occurs in adults and results from disease of the coronary arteries, not the myocardium, the observations on Keshan disease do not implicate selenium deficiency as a likely risk factor for cardiovascular diseases in the United States, and its role in the etiology of atherosclerotic cardiovascular diseases remains uncertain.

Animal Studies

Cardiomyopathy has been observed in several species of animals fed diets deficient in both vitamin E and selenium (NRC, 1983). Although selenium deficiency clearly is involved in impaired heart function under these conditions, this disease should not be confused with the diseases of coronary arteries prevalent in the West.

No animal model suggestive of a role for selenium in human cardiovascular diseases has been developed; however, biochemical studies show that the production of thromboxane by platelets is increased and biosynthesis of prostacyclin by aortic tissue is decreased in selenium-deficient rats (Schoene et al., 1986). Alterations in the thromboxane-to-prostacyclin ratio in vivo might influence the course of human cardiovascular diseases

(Patrono et al., 1984), but the significance of these animal experiments to human health has not yet been established.

Cancer

Epidemiologic Studies

Many correlation studies suggest that a deficiency of dietary selenium might increase the risk of cancer in humans (Clark, 1985; Cowgill, 1983; Shamberger and Frost, 1969; Shamberger and Willis, 1971; Shamberger et al., 1976). These studies correlated selenium levels in forage crops with corresponding cancer mortality rates by geographic area (states, counties, or cities in the United States) and found an inverse relationship with cancers of several different sites (including the lung, colon, rectum, bladder, esophagus, pancreas, female breast, ovary, and cervix). In the report by Clark (1985), liver and stomach cancers, Hodgkin's disease, and leukemia were positively associated. Schrauzer and colleagues (1977a) estimated per-capita selenium intakes for more than 20 countries on the basis of food disappearance data and found an inverse association between consumption levels and mortality from leukemia and certain other cancers. In other geographic correlation studies, investigators have found inverse associations between pooled blood selenium levels and total cancer mortality as well as mortality from cancer at various sites (Schrauzer et al., 1977a,b; Yu et al., 1985).

Many investigators have compared blood selenium levels in cancer patients with corresponding levels in controls (Broghamer et al., 1976, 1978; Calautti et al., 1980; Clark et al., 1984; Goodwin et al., 1983; McConnell et al., 1975, 1980; Robinson et al., 1979; Schrauzer et al., 1985; Shamberger et al., 1973; Sundström et al., 1984; Thimaya and Ganapathy, 1982). In general, these investigators found lower selenium levels in patients than in controls for all cancers combined, and for cancers of selected sites, but the findings are not entirely consistent among the different reports. These studies are limited by the generally small sample sizes, the failure to adjust for other risk factors, and the possibility that the selenium levels were a consequence, not an antecedent, of the cancers.

The issue of cause and effect is best addressed in prospective studies that determine selenium exposure before clinical manifestations of the cancer are observed. In five cohort studies conducted in Finland, the Netherlands, and the United States,

investigators analyzed stored prediagnostic serum from cancer cases and a group of matched controls (Kok et al., 1987b; Menkes et al., 1986; Salonen et al., 1984, 1985a; Willett et al., 1983). In the two investigations conducted in Finland, significantly lower selenium levels were found in patients than in controls for all cancers combined (Salonen et al., 1984, 1985a). In the more recent study, Salonen et al. (1985a) reported that the risk was restricted to men, particularly smokers. In the Netherlands, Kok et al. (1987a) also found lower selenium intake to be significantly associated with increased mortality from cancer among men only. In the United States, Willett et al. (1983) reported the same inverse association to be limited to smokers, males, and blacks (whose levels were lower than those of the whites in the study). Analyses by specific site in these studies were based on very few cases, but did suggest that cancers of the respiratory and gastrointestinal tracts are influenced most strongly by selenium.

The report of Menkes et al. (1986) contrasts with the others. In their analysis of prediagnostic serum from lung cancer cases and matched controls, these investigators found a *positive* association between selenium level and cancer risk, especially for squamous cell carcinomas. This finding is consistent with the results of a case-control study by Goodwin et al. (1983), who found higher selenium concentrations in the plasma of patients with cancers of the oral cavity and oropharynx than in controls.

Although the analysis of selenium in the prediagnostic serum of subjects in prospective cohorts has the advantage of precise measurement and the proper temporal relationship to the disease, the results could still be misleading for several reasons: Single serum measurements may not accurately represent long-term mean levels; serum selenium levels may only be markers of the intake of other more directly related components of the food sources of selenium; and the relevant determination may actually be tissue rather than blood concentrations of selenium. An additional complexity in these studies is the interaction of selenium with other micronutrients, including certain antioxidant vitamins and possibly other trace metals. Willett et al. (1983) found that selenium-associated risk was enhanced by low serum retinol and low vitamin E levels, whereas Salonen et al. (1985a) also found enhancement by low levels of vitamin E but not of retinol.

It is particularly difficult to assess selenium intake from dietary histories, because plants are highly sensitive to soil concentrations of selenium, leading to great variation in the selenium content of foods. Thus, estimates of consumption may not reliably reflect actual intake. This may account for the low correlations reported between individual estimates of dietary selenium and serum or hair levels (Goodwin et al., 1983; Thimaya and Ganapathy, 1982).

In summary, low selenium intakes or decreased selenium concentrations in blood or tissues are associated with increased risk of cancer in humans. It is not yet clear which cancers may be most affected by selenium, although respiratory and gastrointestinal tumors have been implicated most often. Nevertheless, because of inconsistencies in the findings regarding certain sites, such as the respiratory system (Menkes et al., 1986; Salonen et al., 1985a) and the skin (Clark et al., 1984; Salonen et al., 1984), and the lack of studies based on direct dietary assessment, a firm conclusion on the role of selenium in human cancer risk is not justified at present.

Animal Studies

Several feeding or drinking water studies conducted from the 1940s to the 1970s showed that high levels of selenium induced or enhanced tumor formation (Nelson et al., 1943; Schroeder and Mitchener, 1971; Volgarev and Tscherkes, 1967). Critical review, however, reveals serious drawbacks in the experimental designs, including such conditions as near toxic levels of selenium (5 μg/g and higher), low protein levels in the diet (12%), and a pneumonia epidemic in one of the rat colonies.

More recent animal studies demonstrate that under some conditions, elevated selenium intake protects against numerous types of chemically induced, spontaneous (presumably virally induced), and transplantable tumors in rats and mice (extensively reviewed by Ip, 1985, and Milner, 1985). The incidence of skin cancer induced in hairless mice by ultraviolet light could also be decreased by giving them drinking water containing high selenium concentrations (Overvad et al., 1985). In all these experiments, the amount of selenium given to the animals exceeded 0.25 mg/kg body weight—the level of dietary selenium considered by most investigators to be the upper limit for animal nutrition studies (Clark and Combs, 1986; Clark et al., 1984).

Relatively few experiments have been performed to investigate the effect of selenium deficiency on cancer in animals. Selenium deficiency increased the yield of mammary tumors induced by DMBA in rats fed diets with a high polyunsaturated fat content but not in rats fed diets with low levels of fat or high levels of saturated fat (Ip and Sinha, 1981). Pence and Buddingh (1985) observed that selenium deficiency had no influence on colon tumors induced in rats by DMH.

Some reports indicate that cancer incidence is reduced in animals deficient in dietary selenium. For example, Shamberger (1970) painted three groups of selenium-deficient mice with BaP. In the unsupplemented group, only 40% (14 of 35) developed papillomas. In another group, whose deficient diet was supplemented with selenium at 0.1 mg/kg diet as sodium selenite, 61% (22 of 36) developed papillomas. A higher level of selenium supplementation in a third group (1.0 mg/kg) resulted in a 24% (8 of 33) incidence of papillomas. In another study, Reddy and Tanaka (1986) showed that the incidence of colon tumors induced in male rats by azoxymethane was inhibited by selenium deficiency.

Under some conditions, high dietary selenium levels have little or no protective effect against tumors in animals (reviewed by Levander, 1987). Included in this category are certain chemically induced tumors of the trachea, forestomach, liver, small bowel, and pancreas. The reason for these negative results is unknown, but the data suggest that selenium may not protect against all forms of cancer.

Short-Term Tests

Selenium blocked the mutagenicity of malonaldehyde—a chemical shown to be mutagenic in the Ames *Salmonella* assay—in seven mutant strains used to detect various types of frameshift mutagens (Jacobs et al., 1977; Shamberger et al., 1978), but selenium itself was also shown to be a mutagen. For example, five selenium compounds noted for their ability to induce chromosome aberrations in cultured human leukocytes and for their reactivity with DNA by a *rec*-assay system yielded positive results. Damage to DNA was produced by selenites, but not by selenates (Lo et al., 1978; Nakamura et al., 1976). Nakamura also showed that selenates had the capacity to induce a small but significant DNA-repair synthesis.

Mechanisms of Action

A combination of different biochemical mechanisms may be involved in the expression of the various effects of selenium observed in different animal model tumor systems. These include protection against carcinogen-induced oxidative damage, changes in carcinogen metabolism, and cytotoxicity toward rapidly dividing cells (Combs and Clark, 1985).

The increased tumorigenicity of DMBA in selenium-deficient rats was seen only in animals subjected to the prooxidant stress of a diet with high levels of polyunsaturated fat (Ip and Sinha, 1981). The antitumorigenic effect of selenium in this system may involve its antioxidant function at nutritional levels (dietary selenium equal to or less than 0.1 mg/kg). The biochemical mechanism by which selenium deficiency protects against experimental cancer under some conditions may be related to the increase in non-selenium-dependent glutathione peroxidase activity that occurs in selenium-deficient animals. This enzymatic activity is now known to be due to the xenobiotic conjugating glutathione-S-transferases, certain subunits of which increase in rats made deficient in selenium (Mehlert and Diplock, 1985).

Ip and colleagues conducted a series of experiments to investigate the interaction of selenium with vitamin E in rats given DMBA and fed diets with high levels of polyunsaturated fat to provoke an oxidant stress (Ip, 1986). Vitamin E supplementation alone had no prophylactic effect, but high dietary levels potentiated the protective effect of selenium when fed during the postinitiation or the promotion phase. Moreover, vitamin E deficiency attenuated the anticarcinogenic efficacy of selenium. Although vitamin E was a much more effective antioxidant than selenium, as indicated by its suppression of systemic lipid peroxidation, it was inferior to selenium in terms of anticarcinogenic potency. These studies raise doubts about the hypothesis that high dietary levels of vitamin E and selenium protect against cancer by counteracting oxidant stress.

Thus, the anticarcinogenic effect of high dietary levels of selenium appears unrelated to its antioxidant role in glutathione peroxidase activity (Ip, 1986; Medina, 1986). Selenium is an effective chemopreventive agent when given during either the initiation or the promotion phase of chemical carcinogenesis, but effects of selenium on carcinogen metabolism or DNA-adduct formation do not seem to account for its inhibition of tumorigenesis (Ip, 1986). Elevations in the intracellular ratio of oxidized to reduced glutathione (GSSG/GSH) may account for the antiproliferative effect of selenium by retarding all synthetic stages of the cell cycle (LeBoeuf et al., 1985). Selenodiglutathione (GSSeSG)—a reaction product of selenite and GSH—has been found to inhibit tumor growth (Vernie, 1984). This compound may interfere with certain aspects of protein biosynthesis. It has, however, been questioned whether the intracellular concentration of this metabolite could ever increase to levels high enough to inhibit protein synthesis (Combs and Clark, 1985).

In general, animal studies are contradictory concerning the effect of high levels of selenium on cancer and are confusing with regard to the relationship of selenium deficiency to cancer. Although some studies indicate that selenium deficiency enhances susceptibility to cancer, others suggest that deficiency inhibits it.

Copper

Copper is an essential nutrient that is widely distributed in food and water. In 1980, the National Research Council set the estimated safe and adequate daily dietary intake at 0.5 to 1.0 mg/day for infants, 1.0 to 2.5 mg/day for children, and 2.0 to 3.0 mg/day for those over 11 years of age (NRC, 1980). Pennington et al. (1984) estimated that men consumed a mean of 1.60 mg/day, based on data collected in 1981 and 1982. From data gathered from 1982 to 1984, Pennington et al. (1986) estimated that the mean intakes of 25- to 30-year-old women and men were 0.93 mg/day and 1.24 mg/day, respectively. Intakes of older women and men were lower (0.86 mg/day and 1.17 mg/day, respectively). In 1985, the CSFII indicated that copper intakes averaged 0.8 mg/day for children 1 to 5 years old and 1.0 mg/day for women 19 to 50 years old, based on 4 nonconsecutive days of intake (USDA, 1987a). The mean intake for men 19 to 50 years old, based on 1 day's intake, was 1.6 mg/day. Schrauzer et al. (1977b) reported copper intakes in 28 countries varying from 1.6 to 3.3 mg/day.

Cartwright and Wintrobe (1964) estimate that the healthy adult body contains 80 mg of copper. Individual tissues differ greatly in their susceptibility to variations in dietary copper intakes. Subnormal levels of dietary copper are reflected in subnormal blood copper concentrations. Elements such as zinc, cadmium, and iron depress copper absorption and can reduce plasma copper concentrations when ingested at high dietary levels. Copper also plays a key role in iron absorption and mobilization. Elevated plasma copper levels are characteristic of most acute and chronic infections.

Atherosclerotic Cardiovascular Diseases

Epidemiologic and Clinical Studies

The metabolism of copper is negatively influenced by zinc, and many researchers have used zinc-to-copper ratios to interpret their results. Klevay (1975, 1984) hypothesized that the major risk factor for CHD is a low ratio of copper to zinc. Although some data on the relationship of copper and zinc to established risk factors for CHD support the hypothesis, other data do not (Fischer and Collins, 1981; Klevay, 1975; Mertz, 1982).

Insufficient dietary copper leads to elevated blood lipid levels (hypercholesterolemia) and impaired heart function, including electrocardiographic anomalies, myocardial cellular atrophy, and fibrosis (Allen and Klevay, 1978; Klevay, 1980; Klevay and Viestenz, 1981). Electrocardiogram irregularities disappeared following copper supplementation in human subjects consuming a diet low in copper (Klevay, 1984). In a study by Reiser et al. (1985), subjects fed a diet low in copper (1.03 mg/day per 2,850 kcal) containing 20% fructose or starch exhibited heart-related abnormalities, including arrhythmias, and had to be removed from the study. These results confirm that copper is an essential trace element.

Animal Studies

Studies of low dietary copper levels in animals show degradation of heart muscle, including hypertrophy, degeneration of the muscle fibers, and chronic inflammation. The ventricular apex is the most severely affected. The hypertrophy and myopathy observed in animals consuming a low-copper diet are aggravated by sucrose or fructose ingestion (Fields, 1985).

Kopp et al. (1983) fed male weanling rats a copper-deficient diet for 49 days. In vivo cardiological assessment revealed irregularities, including electrocardiographic anomalies and gross pathology, reconfirming earlier studies (Klevay and Viestenz, 1981). Hypercholesterolemia was also observed. Microscopic examination of heart tissue revealed extensive disruption of mitochondrial fine structure and other changes. The authors concluded that these changes represent the appearance of a copper-dependent cardiomyopathy. Furthermore, they suggest that mitochondrial electron transport activity was inadequately sustained. Indeed, dietary copper deficiency has been shown to decrease cytochrome oxidase activity in cardiac and hepatic tissue (Kitano, 1980; O'Dell, 1976).

Cancer

Epidemiologic and Clinical Studies

Both the absorption and the metabolism of copper are negatively influenced by zinc, and observed associations between copper and cancer or other chronic diseases may reflect the opposite effects of zinc. In many studies, therefore, investigators have reported zinc-to-copper ratios.

Epidemiologic evidence that dietary exposure to copper is etiologically related to cancer is not compelling. Blood levels of copper in pooled samples from healthy donors in 19 U.S. states were weakly but positively correlated with corresponding mortality rates from cancers of the breast, lung, thyroid, and intestine (Schrauzer et al., 1977b). Per-capita estimates of dietary copper in 27 countries were positively correlated with leukemia and cancers of the intestine, breast, and skin (Schrauzer et al., 1977b). In 12 districts of England and Wales, copper levels in the soil of vegetable gardens near houses in which people died from cancer differed little from the levels near houses in which people died from noncancer causes. However, higher zinc levels were associated with deaths from gastric cancer (but not other cancers). Thus, a lower copper-to-zinc ratio was associated with risk for this cancer (Stocks and Davies, 1964).

In many clinical reports, investigators have compared copper levels in tumor tissue or serum of cancer patients with levels in normal tissues from the same subjects or unmatched controls. These studies have generally associated higher copper levels with solid tumors at many sites, including the colorectum, pancreas, stomach, cervix, endometrium, ovary, prostate, and lung (Feustel et al., 1986; Gregoriadis et al., 1983; Jendryczko et al., 1986; Manousos et al., 1981; Margalioth et al., 1983; Schwartz, 1975; Sharma et al., 1984). The associations were sometimes shown to be specific for copper rather than for the other trace elements analyzed, such as magnesium, manganese, and zinc. In cancer patients, however, the abnormal copper levels may have been a consequence of the disease. This speculation is supported by the findings in some studies that copper levels increase with advancing stage or grade of the tumor, that the disease increases copper absorption, and that chemotherapy in lymphoma patients returns low serum copper levels to normal (Braganza et al., 1981; Fabris et al., 1985; Sharma et al., 1984).

Occupational studies of inhalation exposure to copper compounds offer little further evidence that copper may be carcinogenic in humans. Some investigators have reported increased mortality from cancers of the lung and gastrointestinal tract among workers in vineyards where Bordeaux mixture (a fungicide containing copper sulfate and lime) was sprayed and in copper mines or refineries (Logue et al., 1982; Newman et al., 1976; Pimentel and Menezes, 1977); however, the evidence is sparse, and other risk factors such as cigarette smoking have not been ruled out as being responsible for the associations.

Animal Studies

Several independent studies demonstrate that high levels of copper salts added to the diets of animals provide various degrees of protection against liver tumors induced by a variety of different carcinogens (Brada and Altman, 1977). Since these effects were obtained with extremely high concentrations of copper (from 0.3 to 0.6% copper acetate) in the diet and since similar effects were produced when manganese or nickel was substituted for copper (Yamane and Sakai, 1973), copper may have been acting as a nonspecific toxicant.

Carlton and Price (1973) studied the influence of a copper-deficient diet on carcinogenesis. Rats fed the deficient diets and given dimethylnitrosamine in drinking water or acetylaminofluorene in chow had a higher incidence of lung tumors than did copper-sufficient controls. However, copper deficiency had no effect on the initiation and progression of hepatomas.

Other Diseases

Epidemiologic Studies

Copper deficiency secondary to chronic diarrhea or inadequate diet has been associated with anemia, particularly in young children (Danks, 1980). This form of anemia is corrected by the addition of copper to the diet.

Excess exposure to copper, based on hepatic copper levels, has been implicated in a unique childhood cirrhosis of very young children in India (Pandit and Bhave, 1983). Epidemiologic observations in this population are consistent with the hypothesis that the children are exposed to copper in milk stored in brass vessels. However, it has not yet been demonstrated that the risk for this disease is lowered when alternative milk storage methods are adopted.

Copper-containing intrauterine devices have been used by women as contraceptives for several years in the United States. Copper may be lost from these devices and may be absorbed parenterally. No adverse long-term effects from this additional copper exposure have been reported (NRC, 1977c).

Chromium

Chromium is an essential trace element needed for normal carbohydrate metabolism. The biologic function of chromium is closely associated with that of insulin. Most chromium-stimulated reactions are also insulin dependent. For example, chromium functions in carbohydrate and lipid metabolism as a potentiator of insulin action.

It has been difficult to determine the extent and importance of chromium deficiency in humans, partly because analytical techniques are not sufficiently sensitive. Glucose intolerance is usually one of the first signs of chromium deficiency. Among the heavy metals, chromium is the only one whose tissue levels continually decrease throughout life (Schroeder et al., 1962, 1970a). The chromium content of diets ranges from 5 to 150 µg/day in the United States to more than 200 µg/day in Japan (Pi-Sunyer and Offenbacher, 1984). The National Research Council (1980) has set 50 to 200 µg/day as a safe and adequate level for adolescents and adults and 10 to 120 µg for infants and children.

The richest sources of chromium include liver and other organ meats, brewer's yeast, whole grains, and nuts. Acidic foods promote chromium leaching from stainless steel cookware, but it has not been determined whether this is a nutritionally useful chromium source (Offenbacher and Pi-Sunyer, 1983). The amount of chromium in foods tends to decrease with processing (Schroeder, 1968). In general, chromium intake is about 50% of the suggested level (Anderson and Kozlovsky, 1985). This is exacerbated by increased chromium losses due to stress (Anderson, 1986). For example, urinary losses of chromium are usually elevated following physical injury and strenuous exercise (Anderson et al., 1982; Borel et al., 1984). Various forms of stress that affect glucose metabolism often also influence chromium metabolism. At present, it is unclear whether the estimated safe and adequate levels for chromium are unrealistically high.

Atherosclerotic Cardiovascular Diseases

Epidemiologic and Clinical Studies

An inverse association between chromium levels in drinking water and cardiovascular disease rates has been found in some populations (Punsar and Karvonen, 1979; Punsar et al., 1975; Voors, 1971) but not in others (Crawford et al., 1968; Sauer et al., 1971; Schroeder, 1966). In addition, inverse associations between chromium levels in serum or aortic tissue and atherosclerotic cardiovascular diseases have been reported (Mertz, 1982; Schroeder et al., 1970a; Simonoff et al., 1984a, 1984b), and chromium levels in hair samples from men with atherosclerotic cardiovascular diseases were lower than levels in normal controls (Cote et al., 1979).

Most other evidence regarding chromium and cardiovascular diseases pertains to its effects on established cardiovascular disease risk factors, particularly elevated serum cholesterol. As the trivalent ion in chromium chloride or glucose tolerance factor (GTF), chromium lowered serum total cholesterol and raised the HDL fraction in healthy participants in supplementation trials (Anderson, 1986; Riales and Albrink, 1981; Simonoff, 1984). Since elevated serum cholesterol and decreased HDL cholesterol are established risk factors for CHD, these findings offer indirect evidence for a beneficial effect of chromium. However, other trials show no effects of chromium supplementation on lipids or lipoproteins (Anderson et al., 1983; Rabinowitz et al., 1983; Uusitupa et al., 1984). These differences may be explained by the dose or the form (inorganic or organic) of chromium and perhaps by differing chromium status among subjects.

There is little evidence that chromium influences high blood pressure—another risk factor for CHD. Preliminary data from an international correlation study by the World Health Organization suggest that serum chromium levels are lower in hypertensive than in normal subjects (Masironi, 1974). A study of normotensive young adults yielded no correlation between hair chromium concentration and blood pressure (Medeiros et al., 1983), but this outcome cannot rule out an effect at elevated blood pressure levels.

In patients sustained on total parenteral nutrition without added chromium, symptoms such as impaired glucose tolerance, hyperglycemia, and relative insulin resistance were observed (Freund et al., 1979; Jeejeebhoy et al., 1977). These symptoms were reversed upon chromium repletion.

Animal Studies

Mertz and Schwarz (1955) reported that rats fed a low-chromium diet consisting of torula yeast had impaired glucose tolerance. Rats fed a chromium-poor diet had severely impaired glucide metabolism and a diabetes-like syndrome with elevated cholesterol levels (Schroeder, 1968). In another study, Schroeder et al. (1970a) noted increased serum cholesterol levels and the deposition of aortic plaques in rats fed a chromium-poor diet. They also observed that the feeding of chromium at normal levels prevented both the formation of plaques and the increase in serum cholesterol with age. Rats and monkeys fed a low-chromium diet develop glucose intolerance that can be reversed by administering inorganic chromium salts (Davidson and Blackwell, 1968; Mertz, 1979). In rabbits fed a high-cholesterol diet, subsequent intraperitoneal administration of 20 μg of potassium chromate per day led to a reduction in the size of aortic plaques and a decrease in aortic cholesterol concentrations (Abraham et al., 1980).

Several biochemical mechanisms might explain the postulated association between marginal chromium deficiency and cardiovascular diseases. As noted above, marginal chromium deficiency may lead to impaired glucose tolerance, high circulating insulin levels, and impaired lipid metabolism. Chromium supplementation may also lower plasma insulin levels or the response of plasma insulin to glucose (Offenbacher and Pi-Sunyer, 1980; Riales and Albrink, 1981; Uusitupa et al., 1984). These factors have been linked to the development of atherosclerotic cardiovascular diseases. Chromium may also play a role in the maintenance of normal serum lipids, either independently or through changes in glucose and insulin metabolism (Mertz, 1979).

Cancer

Epidemiologic Studies

No epidemiologic studies have shown any increased cancer risk associated with dietary exposure to inorganic or organic chromium. However, occupational exposure by inhalation of hexavalent chromium has been causally related to lung cancer risk (Doll et al., 1981), but its possible association with gastrointestinal cancers has not been established (Doll et al., 1981; Sheffet et al., 1982). Occupational exposure to trivalent chromium, one of the biologically active forms, has not been associated with an increase in cancer risk (Axelsson et al., 1980).

Animal Studies

In a long-term study of rats exposed to a range of chromium-containing materials by the intrabronchial implantation technique, Levy and Venitt (1986) found that the incidence of squamous cell metaplasia increased in all rats exposed to chromium[VI] materials or to the reference carcinogen 20-methylcholanthrene, but not in those exposed to chromium[III] material.

In a study by Maruyama (1983), chromium chloride was more effective than dipotassium chromate in decreasing the hemoglobin level and red blood cell count of rats when administered to them in drinking water. Although other evidence suggests that chromium[VI] compounds are carcinogenic, no tumors were noted in this study.

Short-Term Tests

Potassium chromate induced in-vivo cross-linking of proteins to DNA in intact Novikoff ascite hepatoma cells (Wedrychowski et al., 1985) and induced lambda prophage in *Escherichia coli* WP2S (lambda) (Rossman et al., 1984); sodium chromate induced DNA lesions and breaks in the rat organ nuclei (Tsapakos et al., 1983); and chromate[VI] ions were found to be mutagenic in platelet incorporation and fluctuation assays (Arlauskas et al., 1985). Chromium[VI] compounds were mutagenic in *Salmonella typhimurium* strains, whereas chromium[III] compounds were inactive in all strains (Bennicelli et al., 1983). In other experiments, Warren et al. (1981) showed that chromium[III] can be genetically toxic.

Some salts of chromium[VI] promote the morphological transformation of hamster embryo cells exposed to organic carcinogens (Rivedal and Sanner, 1981) and induce forward mutations in the thymidine locus in L51784 mouse lymphoma cells (Oberly et al., 1982). Levis, Majone, and colleagues (Levis and Majone, 1979, 1981; Majone and Levis, 1979; Majone et al., 1983) studied the clastogenic effects of numerous chromium[II], [III], [IV], and [VI] compounds on cell cultures derived from several cell types and lymphocytes. They concluded that the state of oxidation is the most important parameter affecting the mutagenic activity of chromium compounds.

Diabetes

Clinical Studies

In several studies, chromium supplementation has been found to improve glucose tolerance (in hypo- as well as hyperglycemic subjects) and to lower blood insulin levels (Anderson, 1986; Riales and Albrink, 1981; Simonoff, 1984). However, other reports on chromium supplementation in diabetic subjects do not clearly show a beneficial effect on blood glucose or insulin levels (Anderson, 1986; Rabinowitz et al., 1983). Chromium supplementation of patients being treated for diabetes led to a great increase in HDL cholesterol (Mossop, 1983)—an effect also observed in nondiabetic subjects. It is not known whether the apparent chromium deficiency in some diabetic subjects is a consequence or an antecedent of the disease (Simonoff, 1984).

Animal Studies

The relationship between chromium and glucose/insulin response in animal studies is discussed above under Atherosclerotic Cardiovascular Diseases.

Iodine

Iodine is an essential micronutrient and an integral component of thyroid hormones. In food and water, iodine occurs largely as inorganic iodide and is absorbed from all levels of the gastrointestinal tract.

Dietary deficiency of iodine is associated with enlargement of the thyroid gland and endemic goiter. This is rare in the United States at present, since the mean daily intake is estimated to be much higher than the RDA for all sex and age groups (Fisher and Carr, 1974; Pennington et al., 1986). High intakes are due to the use of iodine in disinfectants, the addition of iodate to dough conditioners, the use of iodophors in the dairy industry, the presence of iodine in alginates, and the use of iodized table salts. No adverse effects are known to result from the present level of iodine in the U.S. diet, but the National Research Council recommends that additional increased intakes should be of concern (NRC, 1980).

Cancer

Epidemiologic Studies

Cancers of two sites, thyroid and breast, have been associated with dietary iodine. In neither instance, however, is the evidence compelling. Although rates of thyroid cancer in some areas with endemic goiter (i.e., with low iodine intake) have been observed to be higher than in nongoiter areas (Wahner et al., 1966), most investigators have found no correlation of regional thyroid cancer mortality rates with corresponding endemic goiter rates or with levels of dietary iodine (Clements, 1954; Pendergrast et al., 1961; Sambade et al., 1983). Furthermore, secular trend analyses in the United States (Pendergrast et al., 1961) and Switzerland (Hedinger, 1981) show no apparent decline in thyroid cancer following the introduction of iodized salt, despite dramatic reductions in endemic goiter rates.

There is evidence that exposure to iodine may have different effects on the main histological types of thyroid cancer. Williams et al. (1977) found higher rates of papillary carcinoma and a higher ratio of papillary-to-follicular carcinoma in the population of Iceland (high iodine intake) than in northeast Scotland (average iodine intake). Wahner et al. (1966) reported a lower ratio of papillary-to-follicular carcinoma in Cali, Colombia (a low-iodine area), compared with other areas of the world. In Switzerland, despite little evidence of a change in overall thyroid cancer incidence following the introduction of iodized table salt (as noted above), the relative frequency of papillary carcinoma increased and that of follicular carcinoma decreased substantially (Hedinger, 1981).

Thus, a high intake of dietary iodine may increase the risk for papillary carcinoma and decrease the risk for follicular carcinoma, whereas low iodine intake may have the opposite effects. Not all data support this hypothesis, however. For example, Sambade et al. (1983) found no significant difference in the ratio of papillary-to-follicular carcinoma between an area of high iodine intake and an area of endemic goiter in Portugal.

Breast cancer incidence in females may be influenced by abnormalities of thyroid function (Ito and Maruchi, 1975; Mittra et al., 1974). However, the role of dietary iodine in determining the risk for breast cancer is unclear. Bogardus and Finley (1961) found a direct correlation between mortality from breast cancer by state in the United States and corresponding prevalence rates of endemic goiter. Stadel (1976) suggested that a low iodine intake might be causally related not only to breast cancer but also to endometrial and ovarian cancers with which breast cancer is highly correlated. However, support for this hypothesis is lacking. For example, all three cancers are rare in sub-Saharan Africa, where iodine intake is low (Edington, 1976), and breast cancer incidence is high in Hawaii and Iceland, where iodine intake is high (Waterhouse et al., 1976).

Animal Studies

Aquino and Eskin (1972), Eskin et al. (1967), and Eskin (1977) reported that iodine deficiency produces hyperplastic changes in the breast tissue of female rats during puberty. The changes, aggravated by estrogen treatment, advanced to preneoplastic and neoplastic conditions and were reversible by supplementation with inorganic iodine. They were not reversed by thyroxine, which in higher doses increased the dysplastic changes. Eskin (1977) proposed that iodine deficiency itself rather than hypothyroidism was responsible for these effects. He demonstrated similar changes by blocking iodine uptake with perchlorate. Upon termination of the blockade or dietary iodine supplementation, most but not all the hyperplastic tissue changes returned to normal. Iodine-deficient prepubescent rats were also susceptible to early appearance of DMBA-induced mammary tumors, suggesting a carcinogenic effect of iodine deficiency (Eskin, 1977). Exposure of iodine-deficient animals to a carcinogen such as 2-acetylaminofluorene or to thyroid irradiation has been reported to increase yields of malignant thyroid tumors (Bieschowsky, 1944; Doniach, 1958).

Ohshima and Ward (1984) reported that rats injected intravenously with the carcinogen N-methyl-N-nitrosourea (MNU) and fed an iodine-deficient diet for 33 weeks had a significant increase in incidence of thyroid carcinoma of the follicular or papillary type, as well as diffuse pituitary thyrotropic hyperplasia, hypertrophy, and vacuolar degeneration. Thus, iodine-deficient diets seem to act as tumor promoters in this system.

Longer-term experiments have confirmed this observation. Ohshima and Ward (1986) reported that MNU-treated rats fed iodine-deficient diets for 52 weeks had increased thyroid gland weight and an increased incidence of both thyroid follicular cell carcinoma and diffuse pituitary thyrotropic hyperplasia, whereas rats fed an iodine-deficient diet alone (without MNU injection) had a lower incidence of thyroid follicular adenomas and a 10% increase of follicular carcinoma. This experiment shows that an iodine-deficient diet, in addition to being a potent promoter of thyroid tumors, can also be carcinogenic.

Endemic Goiter

Epidemiologic Studies

Dietary iodine deficiency is an established, but not exclusive, cause of endemic goiter in human populations (Stanbury and Hetzel, 1980). Endemic goiter is no longer a major public health problem in the United States and will not be considered further in this report; however, the disease still occurs throughout the world in developed as well as developing countries (European Thyroid Association, 1985; Stanbury and Hetzel, 1980).

Manganese

Manganese functions both as a cofactor activating a large number of enzymes that form metal–enzyme complexes and as an integral part of certain metalloenzymes. It is also involved in the metabolism of biogenic amines and participates in the regulation of carbohydrate metabolism (Hurley and Keen, 1987).

Estimates of the human requirement for manganese are based on balance studies. Approximately 0.035 to 0.070 mg/kg body weight per day results in positive balance (McLeod and Robinson, 1972; Schlage and Wortberg, 1972). The daily dietary intake in the United States has been estimated to be between 2 and 4 mg (Kazantzis, 1981). The current safe and adequate intake is 0.5 to 1.0 mg/day for infants, 1.0 to 3.0 mg/day for children up to 10 years of age, and 2.5 to 5.0 mg/day for adolescents and adults (NRC, 1980). The best sources of manganese are plant foods, especially cereals, which contain between 10 and 100 mg/kg (Kazantzis, 1981). Manganese toxicity has been observed in humans, but the route of exposure was inhalation in an occupational setting (Ulrich et al., 1979); dietary manganese appears to be nontoxic.

Cancer

Epidemiologic and Clinical Studies

No studies have specifically addressed dietary exposure to manganese and cancer risk. In a clinical study, Gregoriadis et al. (1983) found no differences in the manganese content of cancerous tissue and adjacent normal tissue at various locations in the large bowel in patients with colorectal cancer.

Animal Studies

No toxic effects were observed in rhesus monkeys that had inhaled the combustion products of methylcyclopentadienyl manganese tricarbonyl, a product found in gasoline, in concentrations of 100 μg of manganese per cubic meter of air for up to 66 weeks (Cooper, 1984). Manganese chloride, given in a single injection to mice, enhanced cell-mediated cytotoxicity (Smialowicz et al., 1984), an effect apparently mediated by interferon.

In some instances, an anticarcinogenic role has been ascribed to manganese. In a study of an experimental tumor system, increased concentrations of manganese were found in malignant tissues, especially in the nuclear fraction of the cancerous cells (Ranade et al., 1979). The investigators suggest the use of transition metals (manganese, copper, and zinc) as markers of malignancy.

Short-Term Tests

Miyaki et al. (1979) reported that manganese was mutagenic in cultured V79 Chinese hamster cells. Hsi et al. (1979) found manganese to be mutagenic in the Chinese hamster ovary cell. Other researchers observed that manganese caused chromosome aberrations or possible transformations in several in vitro systems (DiPaolo and Casto, 1979; Umeda and Nishimura, 1979). The addition of soluble manganese salts altered the fidelity of DNA synthesis in vitro (Dube and Loeb, 1975; Sirover and Loeb, 1976, 1977; Van de Sande et al., 1982). Enhanced viral transformation of hamster embryo cells was demonstrated with manganese chloride (Casto et al., 1979). Manganese salts were comutagenic with ultraviolet exposure in Escherichia coli WP2 (Rossman and Molina, 1986). Mutagenesis was detected in the lacI gene of E. coli in cells grown in the presence of manganese (Zakour and Glickman, 1984). Manganese chloride induced lambda prophage in E. coli WP2S (lambda) (Rossman et al., 1984). Thus, various compounds of manganese have been found to be genotoxic and mutagenic in short-term tests.

Diabetes

Clinical Studies

A relationship between dietary manganese and carbohydrate metabolism in humans was suggested by Rubenstein et al. (1962). They described the case of a diabetic patient resistant to insulin therapy who responded to oral doses of manganese chloride (but not other trace elements) with a consistent drop in blood glucose levels.

Animal Studies

In laboratory animals, an essential role of manganese in carbohydrate metabolism was demonstrated by Everson and Shrader (1968), who found that guinea pigs born to manganese-deficient dams and fed manganese-deficient diets from birth to 60 days of age had abnormal glucose tolerance curves and decreased utilization of glucose. Histological examination showed that the deficient animals had hypertrophied pancreatic islet tissue with degranulated β-cells and an increased number of α-cells. All these signs of manganese deficiency were reversed following dietary manganese supplementation for 2 months. A similar observation was reported by Shani et al. (1972), who found that the sand rat, whose natural diet is high in manganese, developed an insulin-resistant diabetes when fed a commercial rat feed containing relatively low levels of manganese. The diabetic condition cleared up after the manganese-rich natural diet was reintroduced.

Baly et al. (1984) observed that the adult manganese-deficient offspring of manganese-deficient rats also had diabetic-like glucose tolerance curves, but that their plasma insulin levels were not commensurate with their high plasma glucose levels. Pancreatic manganese, insulin concentration, and insulin output from the perfused pancreas of these deficient rats were lower than in controls. Insulin synthesis as well as release was impaired by manganese deficiency, indicating a role for manganese in insulin biosynthesis, whereas pancreatic glucagon release was not affected by manganese deficiency (Baly et al., 1984).

Manganese deficiency may also help influence carbohydrate metabolism through effects on phosphoenolpyruvate carboxykinase, for which manganese is a cofactor, or pyruvate carboxylase, a manganese metalloenzyme. Baly et al. (1985) found that pyruvate carboxylase activity in the liver of adult manganese-deficient rats was normal in the fed state but lower than that of controls after they fasted for 48 hours.

Alzheimer's Disease

Markesbery et al. (1984) sampled the manganese content of tissue samples from various regions of the brain and found no differences between patients with Alzheimer's disease and a control group of nondemented adults. (This contrasts with the findings regarding another trace element, aluminum, described below.) The manganese content of the control samples also showed no relationship to age.

Coronary Heart Disease

In male patients with and without CHD, as demonstrated by angiography, Manthey et al. (1981) found a progressive increase in serum manganese levels corresponding to the severity of the disease. The investigators reported a similar relationship for copper and an opposite relationship for magnesium. Serum manganese was also positively correlated with blood pressure. On the other hand, a comparison of drinking water sources in two regions of Finland with different rates of mortality from coronary heart disease in men showed no significant difference in the mean concentration of manganese, whereas differences were found for certain other trace elements, including copper and chromium (Punsar et al., 1975).

Molybdenum

The requirement for molybdenum can only be estimated from balance studies (Golden et al., 1985). The estimated safe and adequate intake set by a committee of the National Research Council's Food and Nutrition Board is 0.15 to 0.5 mg for adults (NRC, 1980). High intakes of molybdenum (above 0.5 mg) can compromise copper balance (Nielsen and Mertz, 1984). Intakes of 10 to 15 mg/day have been associated with gout in the Soviet Union (Koval'skii et al., 1961). Diet-induced molybdenum deficiency has been found in one patient on total parenteral nutrition (Abumrad et al., 1981). The role of molybdenum in animal and human nutrition has been reviewed by Hainline and Rajagopalan (1983).

Cancer

Epidemiologic Studies

No epidemiologic reports have clearly associated molybdenum with cancer risk. However, the soil content of molybdenum (and other trace elements) has been inversely correlated with esophageal cancer mortality rates in high-risk areas for this cancer in China and Africa, and low molybdenum levels in water supplies have been correlated with excess esophageal cancer mortality in the United States (Lu and Lin, 1982; NRC, 1982). Supplementation of soil in the high-risk region of China has altered the chemical composition of locally produced grains and vegetables, but as yet there have been no reports of an associated reduction in esophageal cancer incidence or mortality.

Animal Studies

Luo et al. (1981, 1983) found that molybdenum supplementation tended to reduce the induction of tumors by gastric intubation of N-nitrososarcosine ethyl ester in the esophagus and forestomach of Sprague-Dawley rats. They also observed that 200 ppm concentrations of dietary tungsten countered the inhibitory effect of molybdenum at natural dietary levels (Luo et al., 1983). Later, Wei et al. (1985) observed that molybdenum added to the drinking water inhibited mammary carcinoma induced in female rats by intravenous injection of N-methyl-N-nitrosourea (MNU) and that the effect was countered by tungsten.

Sprague-Dawley rats received either selenium as sodium selenite in drinking water, low or high doses of molybdenum as sodium molybdate in drinking water, or distilled, deionized water before being given methylbenzylnitrosamine intragastrically. Most rats on each regimen had precancerous lesions, and all had papillomas. Molybdenum was not observed to be a cocarcinogen (Bogden et al., 1986).

Molybdenum given intraperitoneally as molybdenum oxide was shown to induce a large increase in the number of lung adenomas in strain A mice (Stoner et al., 1976). These differing results cannot be reconciled at this time.

Other Diseases

Adding molybdenum to a diet containing sodium fluoride reduced dental caries in rats (Büttner, 1963).

Aluminum

Aluminum is the second most plentiful element in the earth's crust. Its concentrations in seawater and freshwater are usually quite low but are increasing in some surface waters because of acid rain.

Ingestion of aluminum in foods ranges from 3 to 5 mg/day (Gorsky et al., 1979; Greger and Baier, 1983). Dietary sources include aluminum used as a filler in pickles and cheese or as a major component of some types of baking powder. Aluminum is also leached from cooking utensils during preparation of acid foods. Drinking water is another source; the U.S. Environmental Protection Agency reported that some municipal waters contain as much as 2 to 4 mg/liter (Miller et al., 1984). Little of the ingested aluminum is actually absorbed, however, so that the total body content is extremely low and does not increase with age (Alfrey, 1986).

Cancer

Epidemiologic Studies

Exposure to aluminum from food or water has not been associated with an increase in cancer risk for humans in any reports. In a few epidemiologic studies, workers in aluminum smelters were found to have an increased risk for cancer, particularly of the lung and bladder (Gibbs, 1985; Rockette and Arena, 1983; Simonato, 1981). In a case-control study of bladder cancer among aluminum smelter workers, the authors concluded that exposure to polycyclic aromatic hydrocarbons (PAHs), not aluminum, was probably the source of the increased risk (Thériault et al., 1984). At present, there is no reliable evidence that aluminum is carcinogenic in humans.

Animal Studies

Aluminum nitrilotriacetate was tested in male Wistar rats for nephrotoxicity and carcinogenicity (Ebina et al., 1986). No tumors developed. Thus, the authors suggest that aluminum is not related to renal carcinogenicity. In mice pretreated with aluminum, administration of dimethylnitrosamine by intraperitoneal injection once a week for 3 weeks resulted in a lower incidence of lung tumors than in untreated mice (Yamane et al., 1981). The incidence of lung tumors was also lower in groups pretreated with aluminum and then subjected to nitroquinoline oxide (Kobayashi et al., 1970).

Pigott et al. (1981) exposed rats to two types of alumina fibers by inhalation. They recorded minimal pulmonary reaction, supporting the contention that the alumina fibers were inert.

Short-Term Tests

Rat alveolar macrophages containing ingested aluminum oxide were incubated for 24 hours with dimethylbenzanthracene (DMBA) (Palmer and Creasia, 1984). The aluminum oxide did not act as a cocarcinogen with the DMBA.

Alzheimer's Disease

Epidemiologic and Clinical Studies

Incidence rates of Alzheimer's disease were positively correlated with the concentration of aluminum in county district water supplies in England and Wales (Martyn et al., 1989). In patients with Alzheimer's disease, higher levels of intracellular aluminum have been found in the neurofibrillary tangles of the hippocampal region than in other areas of the brain or in nonaffected control patients (Perl and Brody, 1980). Similar increases in neuronal aluminum have been found in members of the Chamorro population on Guam afflicted with amyotrophic lateral sclerosis or parkinsonian dementia (Garruto et al., 1984; Perl, 1985). In two other areas of the Pacific with similar neurological disorders (parts of southern Japan and New

Guinea), the soil and water are rich in aluminum and poor in calcium and magnesium (Perl, 1985). This suggests that aluminum could be a common etiologic factor in several related neurological conditions.

However, present evidence does not exclude the possibility that the accumulation of aluminum in brain tissue is secondary to the degeneration in the affected neurons (Shore and Wyatt, 1983). Supporting this view is the finding that the use of aluminum-containing antacids by patients with Alzheimer's disease was not higher than in matched controls (Heyman et al., 1984), nor were there differences between patients and controls in serum, cerebrospinal fluid, or hair levels of aluminum (Shore and Wyatt, 1983). Furthermore, there are no reports of increased risks for Alzheimer's disease among workers in aluminum smelters (Perl, 1985).

Animal Studies

Troncoso et al. (1986) postulated that aluminum may produce damage by altering patterns of neurofilament phosphorylation, as has been recently observed in Alzheimer's disease. Antibodies against phosphorylated and nonphosphorylated neurofilament epitopes were used for immunocytochemical analysis of spinal cord sections from aluminum-treated rabbits. Proximal axons of affected motor neurons showed striking accumulations of immunoactivity of one phosphorylated epitope. This pathological finding was similar, but not identical, to the patterns observed in the neurofibrillary tangles in Alzheimer's disease. Benuck et al. (1985) have reported similar findings. De Boni (1985) reported that in cultured human cells, aluminum interacts with acidic nuclear proteins, decreases steroid binding, and produces a form of neurofibrillary degeneration.

The primary lesion in Alzheimer's disease is postulated to be an impaired permeability of the blood–brain barrier that allows neurotoxins such as aluminum to reach the central nervous system (Banks and Kastin, 1983; Crapper et al., 1980). Intraperitoneal injection of aluminum chloride into rats increased the permeability of the blood–brain barrier to certain peptides by 60 to 70% (Banks and Kastin, 1983). Direct injection of aluminum into the cerebrospinal fluid of cats resulted in a progressive encephalopathy with neurofibrillary degeneration and increased intranuclear aluminum content (Crapper et al., 1980).

Cadmium

Cadmium is known to be toxic at certain levels but may also have a physiological function (Schwarz, 1977). It is absent from the human body at birth and accumulates over the years to approximately 50 years of age (Underwood, 1977). The most recent data from a large-scale survey on the mean cadmium intake from food and water in the United States comes from the Food and Drug Administration's marketbasket survey conducted during 1968–1974. These data indicate that the mean cadmium intake from birth to 50 years of age ranges from 26 to 38 μg/day, adjusted for calories and age (Mahaffey et al., 1975; Ryan et al., 1982). Most foodstuffs contain less than 0.05 mg of cadmium per kilogram, but considerably higher amounts may be found in certain types of seafood and in beef liver and kidney (Elinder, 1985).

Cadmium accumulates in the fiber-rich parts of plants and the cotyledon (Moldrup, 1984). The cadmium content of plants varies with the type of plant and soil characteristics, particularly pH. An extensive report on cadmium uptake by plants has been published (CAST, 1980), and the potential hazard of increasing cadmium levels in plants through crop fertilization is being comprehensively evaluated (Bingham, 1979; Ryan et al., 1982; Yost, 1979). In addition to diet, people may be exposed to cadmium through their occupation, household dust, or smoking (Elinder, 1985; Nordberg et al., 1985).

Cancer

Epidemiologic Studies

The human health effects of exposure to cadmium have been extensively reviewed (Friberg et al., 1985b); however, few investigators have focused on exposure to cadmium in food and drinking water. Most of these studies have been based on ecologic correlations. Cadmium levels in drinking water supplies in the United States and Canada have been positively correlated with incidence or mortality rates of prostate and other cancers (Bako et al., 1982; Berg and Burbank, 1972). Similarly, per-capita cadmium intakes (based on food disappearance data) in more than 20 countries and cadmium levels in pooled blood samples in the United States have been positively correlated with cancers at several different sites (Schrauzer et al., 1977a,b). In a case-control study, Kolonel (1976) found a positive association between renal cancer and combined exposure to cadmium from diet, cigarette smoking, and occupation.

In contrast to these positive associations between cadmium intake and cancer risk, Inskip et al. (1982) found no evidence that mortality from cancer at any site was increased in a village with a high soil cadmium content in Britain, and Shigematsu (1984) found no difference in prostate cancer mortality between cadmium-polluted and control areas in Japan.

Prostate tissue levels of cadmium were higher in men with prostatic cancer than in men with benign prostatic hypertrophy (BPH) or normal prostates (Feustel et al., 1982), but such tissue differences may reflect a secondary accumulation of cadmium in malignant tissue. The increased cadmium levels found in lung tissue from patients with bronchogenic carcinoma (Gerhardsson et al., 1986) are undoubtedly a reflection of the association of this cancer with tobacco use, since cigarette smoke contains cadmium (IARC, 1976).

Although several studies of workers occupationally exposed to cadmium indicate increased risks for prostate cancer (Adams et al., 1969; Kipling and Waterhouse, 1967; Kjellström et al., 1979; Lemen et al., 1976; Potts, 1965), other reports, including updated analyses of some of the earlier studies, have not supported this association (Armstrong and Kazantzis, 1983; Kolonel and Winkelstein, 1977; Sorahan and Waterhouse, 1983; Thun et al., 1985).

Animal Studies

Subcutaneous injections of cadmium as sulfide, oxide, sulfate, or chloride induced sarcomas and Leydig cell tumors of (WI/Cbi) Wistar rats (Haddow et al., 1964; Kazantzis and Hanbury, 1966; Roe et al., 1964). Intratesticularly administered cadmium chloride also induced teratomas in white leghorn cockerels (Guthrie, 1964) and sarcomas in Wistar rats and albino mice (Gunn et al., 1963, 1964, 1967). Lung carcinomas were found in rats exposed to cadmium chloride aerosols (Takenaka et al., 1983). Exposure of experimental animals to soluble forms of cadmium causes renal, hepatic, pulmonary, hematopoietic, and testicular damage as well as chromosome aberrations and immunotoxicity (Friberg et al., 1979).

Intratracheal instillation of cadmium oxide at 75% of the LD$_{50}$ caused mammary tumors in rats (Sanders and Mahaffey, 1984), whereas injection of cadmium chloride into the prostate induced tumors of the prostate (Scott and Aughey, 1978) or the pancreatic islet cells (Poirier et al., 1983).

No carcinogenic response has been observed in mice given cadmium at 5 mg/liter drinking water (Schroeder et al., 1964, 1965) or in rats fed cadmium chloride at concentrations up to 50 mg/g diet for 2 years (Löser, 1980).

Short-Term Tests

Various salts of cadmium decreased the fidelity of avian myeloblastosis virus AMV/DNA polymerase for replication of synthetic polynucleotide templates (Sirover and Loeb, 1976). Cadmium salts were mutagenic to *Escherichia coli* (Yagi and Nishioka, 1977) and *Salmonella typhimurium* and were positive in the *Bacillus subtilis* rec-assay (Nishioka, 1975). In vitro treatment of human lymphocytes with cadmium sulfide and cadmium[II] induced chromosome aberrations (Andersen, 1983; Shiraishi et al., 1972). Cadmium[II] induced the formation of morphologically altered colonies in Syrian hamster fetal cells (Casto et al., 1976; Rivedal and Sanner, 1981). Cadmium[II] also induced forward mutations in the thymidine kinase locus in certain strains of mouse lymphoma cells (Oberly et al., 1982). Other researchers found that cadmium[II] is not clastogenic (Ohno et al., 1982; Umeda and Nishimura, 1979). Short-term tests thus indicated that cadmium can be mutagenic and possibly clastogenic. The relationship of these data to human risk remains to be determined.

Hypertension

Epidemiologic Studies

There is little evidence on the relationship of dietary cadmium intake to hypertension in humans. Two studies based on samples of residents of two different communities in the United States indicated a positive correlation between cadmium in drinking water and blood pressure levels (Folsom and Prineas, 1982). In another study, conducted in the United Kingdom, mortality from hypertension was moderately increased among males but not among females in a village with high levels of cadmium in the soil (Inskip et al., 1982). In another, the prevalence of hypertension in areas of Japan where drinking water and rice are heavily contaminated with cadmium was not greater than in control areas (Shigematsu et al., 1979).

In several studies, the levels of cadmium in blood, hair, and renal tissue in normotensive and hypertensive subjects have been compared, but the findings have not been consistent (Adamska-Dyniewska et al., 1982; Beevers et al., 1980; Cummins et al., 1980; Ewers et al., 1985; Lener and Bibr, 1971; Medeiros and Pellum,.1984; Ostergaard, 1978). The results of these studies are difficult to interpret, however, because most investigators did not adequately address such concerns as the accumulation of cadmium in tissues with age, exposure to cadmium through smoking, the poor correlation of blood levels of cadmium with long-term exposure, and the possibility of artificially low cadmium levels in the tissues of hypertensive subjects secondary to renal damage and urinary loss of stores.

Most studies of occupational groups exposed to cadmium have shown no increase in mortality from hypertension (Armstrong and Kazantzis, 1983; Sorahan and Waterhouse, 1983; Thun et al., 1985). Cigarette smoking, an important source of exposure to cadmium (IARC, 1976), also was not associated with hypertension (Friedman et al., 1982).

Animal Studies

Despite some evidence linking cadmium exposure to hypertension in animals, the mechanism of action is poorly understood. Doses insufficient to produce other signs of cadmium toxicity induced hypertension in animal models, whereas high doses chronically administered produced toxicity but no hypertension (Kopp et al., 1980, 1983; Perry et al., 1980; Schroeder et al., 1962). However, not all investigators were able to demonstrate cadmium-induced hypertension in feeding studies in rats and dogs (Eakin et al., 1980; Fingerle et al., 1982; Perry et al., 1980; Whanger, 1979). According to Perry and Kopp (1983), the presence of other elements such as selenium, copper, and zinc may have counteracted the hypertension-inducing action of cadmium. Talwar et al. (1985) demonstrated that cadmium produced a biphasic response in rats over time, i.e., an initial fall followed by a sustained increase in blood pressure. Cadmium-induced hypertension has also been associated with an increase in plasma noradrenalin (Revis et al., 1983).

Carmignani and Boscolo (1984) studied hemodynamics and cardiovascular reactivity to various physiological agonists in rats given cadmium. Cadmium exposure from the environment reduced the pressor effects of intravenous norepinephrine, angiotensin, and elevated doses of epinephrine, and also reduced the depressor effects of bradykinin. The exposed rats also had an increased vascular responsiveness to the β-adrenoceptor-stimulating effects of lower doses of epinephrine. That study suggests that cadmium affects several neuro-humoral mechanisms that regulate cardiovascular function.

Renal Diseases

The kidney is the first organ affected by long-term exposure to cadmium. Severe renal cadmium poisoning may affect the glomerular filtration rate and cause tubular damage (Adams et al., 1969; Friberg et al., 1985a). It is unlikely that humans would ever encounter dietary exposures sufficiently high to produce these effects, except for an unusual contamination of foods.

Bone Diseases

Renal dysfunction secondary to long-term human exposure to high concentrations of cadmium in food or air may eventually lead to osteomalacia (Friberg et al. 1985b). Studies in rats show that under certain experimental conditions, cadmium can induce osteomalacia or osteoporosis (Kawamura et al., 1978; Nogawa et al., 1981; Takashima et al., 1980). A contributing factor may be the suppression of 1,25-dihydroxycholecalciferol by exposures to high levels of dietary cadmium (Lorentzon and Larsson, 1977). Chronic cadmium toxicosis was also reported to result in osteoporosis and nephrocalcinosis in horses (Gunson et al., 1982).

Mercury

In nature, mercury is found mainly in low concentrations as sulfides in the earth's crust, except for rich focal deposits where it may also be present in metallic form. Soil levels of metallic mercury are low (Kazantzis, 1981). Methyl mercury, completely absorbed from the gastrointestinal tract as a lipid-soluble compound, readily accumulates in the brain. Its half-life in the body is estimated to be approximately 70 days (Chisolm, 1985).

Occupational exposure occurs most commonly through inhalation of metallic mercury vapor or of a variety of inorganic mercury compounds such as aerosols and alkyl mercurials. The provisional tolerable weekly intake established by the World Health Organization (WHO, 1972) is 0.3 mg of total mercury, of which not more than 0.2 mg should be present as methyl mercury.

Cancer

Epidemiologic Studies

The major form of mercury in food is methyl mercury, which is ingested primarily through marine products. There is no epidemiologic evidence that such exposure is associated with cancer in humans. In a retrospective cohort analysis, occupational exposure to elemental mercury was not clearly associated with increased mortality from cancer at any site, although there was a small increase in deaths from renal cancer (Cragle et al., 1984).

Animal Studies

Mercuric chloride was reported to induce murine renal cell carcinoma in mice (Herr et al., 1981). Female Swiss mice were exposed to mercury concentrations of 1.0 to 2.0 µg/ml as methyl mercury in the drinking water. After 3 weeks all mice were given 1.5 mg/g of methyl mercury intraperitoneally per gram of body weight. Twelve weeks later, the incidence of pulmonary adenomas was significantly higher in the mice initially given the higher doses. Mercury at the levels given in the drinking water did not cause any clinical manifestations (Blakley, 1984).

Short-Term Tests

Mercuric chloride at acutely cytotoxic doses caused a rapid induction of DNA single-strand breaks in cultured Chinese hamster ovary cells (Cantoni and Costa, 1983) and inhibited the repair of these breaks, but the authors suggest that the compound was not severely mutagenic or carcinogenic.

Skerving et al. (1970) observed dose-related chromosome aberrations in the lymphocytes of people who consumed methyl mercury-contaminated fish. At blood methyl mercury levels of 100 µg/liter, they found an increase of aneuploidy, unstable chromosome-type aberrations, and cells with chromatid-type aberrations.

Other Diseases

Epidemiologic Studies

The primary organ affected by chronic exposure to inorganic or organic mercury is the brain, although renal damage may also occur (Berlin, 1979). In 1953 and 1965, in the Kumamoto and Niigata prefectures of Japan, respectively, severe poisoning occurred from the ingestion of fish heavily contaminated with methyl mercury. This disease, known as Minamata disease, is characterized by a spectrum of neurological symptoms and signs (Tsubaki and Irukayama, 1977). In a comparison of Minamata disease patients and residents of an unaffected area in Japan, a higher prevalence of hypertension was found in the patients, perhaps secondary to renal damage (Tsubaki and Irukayama, 1977). An occupational group exposed to elemental mercury had no evidence of increased mortality from nonmalignant diseases of the brain, kidney, liver, or lung (Cragle et al., 1984).

Arsenic

Schwarz (1977) postulated that arsenic is essential for growth in animals, and the evidence for essentiality of very low levels has grown considerably (Anke, 1986; Nielsen, 1982). Small amounts of this element are widely distributed throughout the soils and waters of the world, and trace amounts occur in foods (especially seafood) and in some meats and vegetables. Arsenic may be present in food as a contaminant (e.g., the unintentional residue of the insecticides calcium arsenate or lead arsenate). Daily intakes of arsenic in the United States are estimated to range from 10 to 130 µg (Buchet et al., 1983).

Absorption, retention, and excretion of arsenic are influenced by the chemical form and the amount in which it is ingested. Rats, unlike other mammals, concentrate arsenic in their blood and appear unique in their metabolic management of arsenic (Dutkiewiez, 1977). Thus, experimental findings from rats may not be applicable to other species.

Atherosclerotic Cardiovascular Diseases

Epidemiologic Studies

Chronic exposure to arsenic through drinking water has been associated with peripheral vascular disease in Taiwan, Mexico, and Chile (NRC, 1977a; Tseng, 1977; Zaldivar and Ghai, 1980). Exposure of vintners, probably through consumption of contaminated wine as well as inhalation of dusts contaminated with arsenical insecticides, has also been associated with peripheral vascular disease (NRC, 1977a). However, exposure of U.S. populations in Alaska and Oregon to contaminated well water (at levels much lower than those found in Taiwan and Chile) was not associated with signs or symptoms of peripheral vascular disease (Harrington et al., 1978; Morton et al., 1976). Although excess mortality from cardiovascular, mainly cerebrovascular, diseases was found in a cohort of Swedish copper smelter workers exposed to arsenic, it was not possible to attribute the risk to arsenic exposure in particular (Wall, 1980).

Animal Studies

The committee did not find information regarding arsenic and cardiovascular diseases in animal models.

Cancer

Epidemiologic Studies

Inorganic arsenic has been identified as a human carcinogen, associated with malignancies of the lung, skin, and possibly liver (Landrigan, 1981; NRC, 1977a; Pershagen, 1981). Because most epidemiologic studies of arsenic have been carried out in occupational settings, the potential carcinogenic effects of human exposure through food sources—particularly seafoods, which contain primarily organic arsenic (Pershagen, 1981)—have not been well studied. In Japan, population exposures to arsenic through food (powdered milk, soy sauce) and well-water contamination were not associated with the occurrence of cancers of the skin, lung, or other sites (Tsuchiya, 1977).

The primary source of ingested inorganic arsenic is drinking water. In areas where populations have high exposures through water sources, such as artesian wells in the southwest region of Taiwan, arsenic has been associated with nonmelanotic skin cancers and possibly with cancers of the lung, bladder, and liver (Chen et al., 1985, 1986; NRC, 1977a,b). Studies of exposed populations in the western United States were negative, possibly because the levels of exposure were much lower than in Taiwan (Calabrese, 1983; Harrington et al., 1978; Morton et al., 1976). Reports of increased risks for cancer of the skin, lung, and liver among vineyard workers in the Federal Republic of Germany and in France, who were exposed to arsenic through pesticide use, suggest that contaminated grapes or wine may be another potable source of exposure (NRC, 1982). However, these workers were exposed by inhalation as well as by ingestion. Thus, more research is necessary to establish the association as causal.

Smelter workers exposed to airborne inorganic arsenic are at increased risk for lung cancer (Lee-Feldstein, 1986; Pershagen et al., 1981; Wall, 1980). Medicinal use of arsenic, particularly as Fowler's solution (potassium arsenite), has been associated with nonmelanotic skin cancer and angiosarcomas of the liver in several case reports, but not in a follow-up study on 478 subjects treated with arsenic (Cuzick et al., 1982; Roat et al., 1982).

Animal Studies

Epidemiologic evidence of the carcinogenicity of arsenic in humans has not been confirmed in most animal studies (Furst, 1983; Leonard and Lauwerys, 1980; Pershagen, 1981). Several earlier long-term studies in rats and mice given arsenic or its salts in food or drinking water failed to show that it is either a carcinogen or a cocarcinogen (Baroni et al., 1963; Boutwell, 1963; Furst, 1977; Hueper and Payne, 1962).

Arsenic administered as arsenite at a level of 100 μg/liter drinking water for 15 months reduced mammary tumor incidence in female mice; however, once the tumors were established, arsenite enhanced their growth rate (Schrauzer and Ishmael, 1974). Shirachi et al. (1983) suggested that sodium arsenite increases the incidence of diethylnitrosamine-initiated renal tumors in rats by acting as a promoter.

Arsenic compounds were weakly carcinogenic in hamsters (Ishinihsi and Yamamoto, 1983). In dogs, a 2-year feeding study failed to show that sodium arsenite or arsenate was carcinogenic (Byron et al., 1967).

Short-Term Tests

Arsenic[III] yielded positive results in a *Bacillus subtilis rec*-assay (Nishioka, 1975). Later reports by Rossman and colleagues (Rossman, 1981a,b; Rossman et al. 1980) and Simonato (1981) indicate that arsenic[III] does not induce mutations in tryptophan auxotrophic strains of *Escherichia coli*. Tiedemann and Einbrodt (1982) reported negative results for arsenic[III] and [V] in the Ames *Salmonella* microsome assay. Arsenic[III] transformed Syrian hamster cells in vitro and enhanced the susceptibility of these cells to transformation by simian adenovirus (Casto et al., 1976). Larramendy et al. (1981) found that sodium arsenite elevates the sister chromatid exchange frequency from 11 to 19 in Syrian hamster cells.

Chromosome aberrations were found in leukocytes and fibroblasts in humans after exposure to arsenic compounds (Paton and Allison, 1972; Petres and Berger, 1972). Arsenic also appeared to enhance the clastogenic effect of cigarette smoking in lymphocytes of smelter workers (Nordenson et al., 1978).

Lead

Lead is not known to be essential to human nutrition. However, trace amounts of lead (29 ng/

g diet) have been reported to be essential in rats to maintain growth, reproduction, and hematopoiesis (Reichlmayr-Lais and Kirchgessner, 1981). Humans are exposed to oxides and salts of lead through various environmental sources, such as automobile exhausts, atmospheric dust, paint, or contaminated drinking water, food, and whiskey. Formerly, the main contributor was the lead that leached into canned foods (Chisolm, 1985), but the food canning industry has since converted from lead-soldered to lead-free cans. At present, the major source of lead exposure is likely to be dust particles from paint or the soil carried into homes.

The World Health Organization/Food and Agriculture Organization (WHO, 1978) recommended a permissible level of lead intake for adults up to 490 μg of lead per day or 7 μg/kg body weight per day. There is no comparable standard for infants and children. In metabolic balance studies, however, Ziegler et al. (1978) found that a daily lead intake exceeding 5 μg/kg per day is associated with positive lead balance in infants up to 24 months of age. Excess lead intakes by children (blood lead levels >20 μg/dl) have been associated with impairment of a variety of enzymatic and neurophysiological processes (Mahaffey et al., 1982; Otto et al., 1985; Piomelli et al., 1982).

Atherosclerotic Cardiovascular Diseases

Epidemiologic Studies

(See section on Hypertension, below.)

Animal Studies

Signs of cardiac disease are frequently observed as part of the syndrome of lead intoxication in animals. Neonatal animals are particularly susceptible to small doses of lead (Williams et al., 1983); rats given ≤1 μg of lead per milliliter of drinking water for 25 weeks developed ultrastructural changes in the cardiac mitochondria, including the loss of regular spacing and orientation of the cristae (Moore et al., 1975).

Cancer

Epidemiologic Studies

There is little information on cancer risks associated with dietary exposure to lead, and the data are not specific. Berg and Burbank (1972) correlated the levels of lead and seven other trace elements in the water supplies of 10 regions of the United States with corresponding cancer mortality rates in the population. The levels of lead and several other elements were positively correlated with several malignancies, including gastrointestinal and hematopoietic cancers.

In an analysis of cancerous and surrounding noncancerous tissues taken from several locations in the large bowel of patients with colorectal cancer who had no special occupational exposures, Gregoriadis et al. (1983) found increased concentrations of lead (as well as nickel and copper, but not zinc or manganese) in the cancerous tissue; however, this trace metal accumulation could have been a consequence rather than a precursor of the cancers.

Most epidemiologic evidence pertaining to the possible carcinogenic effects of lead is based on occupational exposures. Studies of workers in smelters and plants producing or utilizing lead have generally shown no increase in mortality from cancer (Davies, 1984; Dingwall-Fordyce and Lane, 1963; Robinson, 1976; Selevan et al., 1985). However, in a follow-up study on two cohorts of workers exposed to lead (smelter and battery plant workers), the investigators observed increased mortality from cancers of the lung and stomach, but they did not control for cigarette smoking and other exposures that are potentially carcinogenic for these sites (Cooper et al., 1985). Evidence for an association between Wilms's tumor in children and possible occupational exposure to lead by the fathers has not been consistent (Kantor et al., 1979; Wilkins and Sinks, 1984a,b).

Animal Studies

Swiss mice fed 0.1% lead subacetate had a much higher frequency of renal tumors than did untreated controls (Van Esch and Kroes, 1969). In long-term feeding studies, the number of renal tumors in Wistar rats increased after treatment with lead acetate (Hass et al., 1967; Hiasa et al., 1983; Ito, 1973; Ito et al., 1971; Mao and Molnar, 1967; Van Esch and Kroes, 1969). Lead nitrate and lead powder were not carcinogenic when fed to Long Evans or Fischer rats (Furst et al., 1976; Schroeder et al., 1970b).

Rats fed lead at 2,600 ppm in their diet for 76 weeks had an 81% incidence of renal tumors, whereas those fed 2,600 ppm in combination with ethylurea and sodium nitrite had a 50% incidence of tumors (Koller et al., 1985). Lead did not appear to be syncarcinogenic to the activity of ethylnitrosourea—the carcinogen formed by oral exposure to ethylurea and sodium nitrite. The lead-induced renal neoplasms were histologically similar to those that occur spontaneously in humans and therefore may serve as an animal model to study human disease. Lead in the form of lead acetate was found to accelerate the onset and development of all renal lesions in rats exposed to N-(4'-fluoro-4-biphenyl)acetamide (Tanner and Lipsky, 1984). Lead acetate was also a promoter of 2-(ethylnitrosamino)ethanol-induced renal carcinomas in Fischer 344 rats (Shirai et al., 1984). Male rats were injected close to the prostate with either 50 μg of lead acetate, 50 μg of cadmium chloride, or 25 μg of both. After daily injections for 1 month, lead and cadmium exerted a synergistic effect on testicular damage and prostatic cytology. Although no tumor formation was observed in the prostate, tissue changes were suggestive of progressive precancerous changes (Fahim and Khare, 1980).

Short-Term Tests

Lead[II] reacted with phosphate groups of DNA bases to yield stable complexes (Sissoëff et al., 1976; Venugopal and Luckey, 1978). Lead chloride diminished the fidelity of DNA polymerase (Sirover and Loeb, 1976).

Lead acetate was negative in the Ames *Salmonella* assay test and in the *Escherichia coli* pol A assay for DNA-modifying effects (Rosenkranz and Poirier, 1979); in the host-mediated assay in Swiss Webster mice with Ames *Salmonella* strains and *Saccharomyces cerevisiae* D3 (Simmon, 1979); and in the *Bacillus subtilis rec* assay (Kada et al., 1980; Kanematsu et al., 1980; Nishioka, 1975). Long-term exposure to subtoxic doses of lead nitrate facilitated the induction of lambda prophage in *E. coli* WP2S (lambda) (Rossman et al., 1984).

There were more achromatic lesions in Chinese hamster ovary cells treated with lead acetate than in untreated controls (Bauchinger and Schmid, 1972). Morphological transformations of Syrian hamster embryo cells were observed after exposure to lead acetate (1 to 2.5 g/liter of medium), which produced fibrosarcomas (DiPaolo et al., 1978). Increased rates of sister chromatid exchanges were observed in human lymphocytes and macrophages exposed to lead[II] (Andersen, 1983). Lead increases misincorporation of nucleotide bases in the daughter strand of DNA that is synthesized in vitro from polynucleotide templates by microbial DNA polymerases (Zakour et al., 1981a,b).

Hypertension

Epidemiologic and Clinical Studies

Several studies of patients with hypertension have suggested a possible association with lead. In an area of Scotland with relatively high levels of lead in water supplies, blood lead levels of hypertensive patients were higher than those of normotensive controls (Beevers et al., 1980). Levels of lead (and of cadmium and zinc) in the hair of hypertensive black women in the United States were higher than corresponding levels in normotensive controls (Medeiros and Pellum, 1984). Batuman et al. (1983) studied patients with essential hypertension (some of whom had evidence of renal impairment) and controls and found higher lead levels in the patients, independent of renal impairment.

Data on the relationship of lead to blood pressure levels in primarily normotensive populations are conflicting. Weiss et al. (1986) and Pirkle et al. (1985) found positive correlations between blood lead levels and blood pressure among U.S. white males. Pirkle's study was based on NHANES II. In contrast, Pocock et al. (1984) found no correlation in a representative group of British men similar to the NHANES II sample. Similarly, there was no correlation between the lead content of drinking water and blood pressure levels in two areas of the United States and one area of Finland, but there was a modest correlation in another area of Finland (Calabrese and Tuthill, 1978; Punsar et al., 1975). Some of these conflicting results may be attributed to the exposure measures used, since blood levels of lead do not reflect the body burden (Batuman et al., 1983) and therefore may not be meaningful indicators of chronic exposure. Most occupational studies have shown no association between lead exposure and hypertension (Beevers et al., 1980; Lilis et al., 1984; Robinson, 1976; Selevan et al., 1985), but two of them suggest an increased risk (Cooper et al., 1985; Lilis et al., 1982).

Animal Studies

Hypertension was found in rat pups whose mothers were fed lead during gestation and lactation and was associated with defects in the renin-angiotensin system (Victery et al., 1982). Tarugi et al. (1982) reported lead-induced elevation of plasma lipoproteins and cholesterol esters in rats.

Renal Diseases

Epidemiologic and Clinical Studies

One plausible mechanism for the effect of lead on hypertension is through kidney damage and consequent impaired renal control of blood pressure. Although evidence of renal damage was not found in many of the reports cited (see section on Hypertension, above), slight degrees of impairment are likely to have been missed in most such studies (Meyer et al., 1984).

Animal Studies

Chronic exposures of rats to lead at 0.5 to 250 mg/g body weight per day for as long as 9 months resulted in pathological changes in the kidney, principally in the epithelium of the proximal convoluted tubules. These changes included intranuclear inclusion bodies, mitochondrial damage, tubular swelling, atrophy, fibrosis, and hyperuricemia. Renal lead levels of 5 mg/g were associated with a blood lead concentration of 11 µg/dl and with cytomegaly and karyomegaly in renal proximal tubule cells (Fowler et al., 1980).

Chronic Effects of Lead Exposure on Children

Debate persists regarding the blood lead level at which deficits in children's learning and behavior become apparent (Smith, 1985; Yule and Rutter, 1985). Several investigators concluded that blood lead levels persistently elevated above 60 µg/dl in preschool children carry a substantial risk of permanent central nervous system injury (DHSS, 1980; Rutter, 1980). However, a review of other studies by the U.S. Environmental Protection Agency (EPA) (Ernhart et al., 1981; Needleman et al., 1979) neither confirms nor refutes the hypothesis that low-level lead exposure causes permanent neuropsychological deficits in children (Marshall, 1983). The EPA in its proposed drinking water regulations has stated that fetal exposure at blood levels around 10 to 15 µl/dl appears to be associated with delays in early mental and physical development (EPA, 1988). The Centers for Disease Control established 25 µg/dl as the blood lead level above which medical intervention is necessary for children (CDC, 1985).

In a prospective cohort study assessing the relationship between prenatal and postnatal lead exposure and early cognitive development, Bellinger et al. (1987) found that the fetus may be adversely affected at maternal blood lead concentrations well below the CDC guideline of 25 µg/dl. They did not find that cognitive test scores were related to the postnatal blood lead levels of the infants.

SUMMARY

Essential as well as nonessential trace elements have been implicated in the risk of certain chronic diseases in humans, but the evidence is weak in most instances. Some trace elements have been associated with an increased risk of cancer at certain sites, most notably chromium with lung cancer and arsenic with cancers of the lung and skin, but the evidence is based primarily on respiratory rather than dietary exposure. Animal data provide little support for these associations, and no conclusions regarding dietary intake of these elements and cancer risk are warranted at present. In several epidemiologic studies, selenium has been inversely associated with risk of cancer at several different sites, but the data are not entirely consistent and some animal studies do not show this inverse finding. The role of selenium in cancer etiology is unclear. The effects of zinc deficiency on tumor growth are also equivocal; however, zinc deprivation has been shown to alter immunocompetence in experimental animals as well as in humans.

The effects of dietary trace elements on cardiovascular disease risk are not well established. Some epidemiologic studies suggest that copper and chromium may be inversely associated and arsenic directly associated with these diseases or certain of their known risk factors, and some animal evidence supports the findings; however, the data are inconclusive.

Certain other associations of trace elements with chronic diseases have been established with certainty. The ingestion of fluoride in water is clearly associated with a reduction in dental caries. Dietary iodine deficiency is a cause of endemic goiter. Iron deficiency leads to the commonest form of anemia in the United States.

Most other reported relationships between trace elements and chronic diseases are much more weakly supported. Examples include positive associations of aluminum with Alzheimer's disease and of lead with hypertension.

DIRECTIONS FOR RESEARCH

• *Interactions with Other Dietary Components* Literature on the chronic effects resulting from the dietary exposure of humans to most trace elements is limited. Further research in this area could yield potentially important information, particularly on the interaction of these elements with other dietary and nondietary risk factors for conditions such as cancer, atherosclerotic cardiovascular diseases, and diabetes mellitus. Such research would be greatly facilitated by the identification of optimal markers of long-term dietary exposure to these elements.

• *Selenium and Cancer*   Selenium is being promoted to the public as a protective factor against cancer, despite inconclusive scientific evidence. Because there are some reports that selenium may enhance cancer risk at certain sites, it is important that the role of this trace element in human cancer be clarified through further epidemiologic and experimental study.

• *Nutritional Requirements*   There are still fundamental gaps in knowledge about nutritional requirements for trace elements, partly because assessment methods are poor. In particular, the development of better methods for determining zinc nutriture in individuals would permit a more adequate study of the relationship of this nutrient to health and disease.

• *Immune System*   The effects of certain trace elements, such as zinc and copper, on the immune system should be studied in order to offer plausible mechanisms for their associations with chronic diseases in humans.

REFERENCES

Abraham, A.S., M. Sonnenblick, M. Eini, O. Shemesh, and A.P. Batt. 1980. The effect of chromium on established atherosclerotic plaques in rabbits. Am. J. Clin. Nutr. 33:2294–2298.

Abumrad, N.N., A.J. Schneider, D. Steel, and L.S. Rogers. 1981. Amino acid intolerance during prolonged total parenteral nutrition reversed by molybdate therapy. Am. J. Clin. Nutr. 34:2551–2559.

Adams, R.G., J.F. Harrison, and P. Scott. 1969. The development of cadmium-induced proteinuria, impaired renal function and osteomalacia in alkaline battery workers. Q. J. Med. 38:425–443.

Adamska-Dyniewska, H., T. Bala, H. Florczak, and B. Trojanowska. 1982. Blood cadmium in healthy subjects and in patients with cardiovascular diseases. Cor Vasa 24:441–447.

Adler, A.L., B. Safai, Y.B. Wang, C. Menendez-Botet, and R.A. Good. 1981. Serum zinc levels in patients with basal-cell carcinoma. J. Dermatol. Surg. Oncol. 7:911–914.

Alffram, P.A., J. Hernborg, and B.E.R. Nilsson. 1969. The influence of a high fluoride content in the drinking water on the bone mineral mass in man. Acta Orthop. Scand. 40:137–142.

Alfrey, A.C. 1986. Aluminum. Pp. 399–413 in W. Mertz, ed. Trace Elements in Human and Animal Nutrition, Vol. 2, 5th ed. Academic Press, Orlando, Fla.

Allen, K.G.D., and L.M. Klevay. 1978. Cholesterolemia and cardiovascular abnormalities in rats caused by copper deficiency. Atherosclerosis 29:81–93.

Ammann, R.W., E. Müller, J. Bansky, G. Schüler, and W.H. Häcki. 1980. High incidence of extrahepatic carcinomas in idiopathic hemochromatosis. Scand. J. Gastroenterol. 15:733–736.

Andersen, O. 1983. Effects of coal combustion products and metal compounds on sister chromatid exchange in a macrophage cell line. Environ. Health Perspect. 47:239–253.

Anderson, R.A. 1986. Chromium metabolism and its role in disease processes in man. Clin. Physiol. Biochem. 4:31–41.

Anderson, R.A., and A.S. Kozlovsky. 1985. Chromium intake, absorption and excretion of subjects consuming self-selected diets. Am. J. Clin. Nutr. 41:1177–1183.

Anderson, R.A., M.M. Polansky, N.A. Bryden, E.E. Raginski, K.Y. Patterson, and D.C. Reamer. 1982. Effect of exercise (running) on serum glucose, insulin, glucagon, and chromium excretion. Diabetes 31:212–216.

Anderson, R.A., M.M. Polansky, N.A. Bryden, E.E. Roginski, W. Mertz, and W. Glinsmann. 1983. Chromium supplementation of human subjects: effects on glucose, insulin, and lipid variables. Metabolism 32:894–899.

Anke, M. 1986. Arsenic. Pp. 347–372 in W. Mertz, ed. Trace Elements in Human and Animal Nutrition, Vol. 2, 5th ed. Academic Press, Orlando, Fla.

Aquino, T.I., and B.A. Eskin. 1972. Rat breast structure in altered iodine metabolism. Arch. Pathol. 94:280–285.

Arlauskas, A., R.S. Baker, A.M. Bonin, R.K. Tandon, P.T. Crisp, and J. Ellis. 1985. Mutagenicity of metal ions in bacteria. Environ. Res. 36:379–388.

Armstrong, B.G., and G. Kazantzis. 1983. The mortality of cadmium workers. Lancet 1:1425–1427.

Aro, A., G. Alfthan, S. Soimakallio, and E. Voutilainen. 1986. Se concentrations in serum and angiographically defined coronary artery disease are uncorrelated. Clin. Chem. 32:911–912.

Atik, O.S. 1983. Zinc and senile osteoporosis. J. Am. Geriatr. Soc. 31:790–791.

Atukorala, S., T.K. Basu, J.W. Dickerson, D. Donaldson, and A. Sakula. 1979. Vitamin A, zinc and lung cancer. Br. J. Cancer 40:927–931.

Axelsson, G., R. Rylander, and A. Schmidt. 1980. Mortality and incidence of tumours among ferrochromium workers. Br. J. Ind. Med. 37:121–127.

Bako, G., E.S. Smith, J. Hanson, and R. Dewar. 1982. The geographical distribution of high cadmium concentrations in the environment and prostate cancer in Alberta. Can. J. Public Health 73:92–94.

Baly, D.L., D.L. Curry, C.L. Keen, and L.S. Hurley. 1984. Effect of manganese deficiency on insulin secretion and carbohydrate homeostasis in rats. J. Nutr. 114:1438–1446.

Baly, D.L., C.L. Keen, and L.S. Hurley. 1985. Pyruvate carboxylase and phosphoenolpyruvate carboxykinase activity in developing rats: effect of manganese deficiency. J. Nutr. 115:872–879.

Banks, W.A., and A.J. Kastin. 1983. Aluminium increases permeability of the blood-brain barrier to labelled DSIP and beta-endorphin: possible implications for senile and dialysis dementia. Lancet 2:1227–1229.

Barnhart, W.E., L.K. Hiller, G.J. Leonard, and S.E. Michaels. 1974. Dentifrice usage and ingestion among four age groups. J. Dent. Res. 53:1317–1322.

Baroni, C., G.J. van Esch, and U. Saffiotti. 1963. Carcinogenesis tests of two inorganic arsenicals. Arch. Environ. Health 7:668–674.

Barr, D.H., and J.W. Harris. 1973. Growth of the P388 leukemia as an ascites tumor in zinc-deficient mice. Proc. Soc. Exp. Biol. Med. 144:284–287.

Batuman, V., E. Landy, J.K. Maesaka, and R.P. Wedeen. 1983. Contribution of lead to hypertension with renal impairment. N. Engl. J. Med. 309:17–21.

Bauchinger, M., and E. Schmid. 1972. Chromosomenanalysen in Zellkulturen des chinesischen Hamsters nach Applikation von Bleiacetat. Mutat. Res. 14:95–100.

Beach, R.S., M.E. Gershwin, and L.S. Hurley. 1979. Altered thymic structure and mitogen responsiveness in postnatally zinc-deprived mice. Dev. Comparat. Immunol. 3:725–738.

Beach, R.S., M.E. Gershwin, and L.S. Hurley. 1981. Dietary zinc modulation of Moloney sarcoma virus oncogenesis. Cancer Res. 41:552–559.

Beevers, D.G., J.K. Cruickshank, W.B. Yeoman, G.F. Carter, A. Goldberg, and M.R. Moore. 1980. Blood–lead and cadmium in human hypertension. J. Environ. Pathol. Toxicol. 4:251–260.

Bell, L.T., M. Branstrator, C. Roux, and L.S. Hurley. 1975. Chromosomal abnormalities in maternal and fetal tissues of magnesium- or zinc-deficient rats. Teratology 12:221–226.

Bellinger, D., A. Leviton, C. Waternaux, H. Needleman, and M. Rabinowitz. 1987. Longitudinal analyses of prenatal and postnatal lead exposure and early cognitive development. N. Engl. J. Med. 316:1037–1043.

Benbassat, J., C. Hershko, R. Laskov, and M. Eliakim. 1981. Effect of iron deficiency on transplantable murine plasmacytoma. Nutr. Cancer 3:20–26.

Bennicelli, C., A. Camoirano, S. Petruzzelli, P. Zanacchi, and S. De Flora. 1983. High sensitivity of salmonella TA102 in detecting hexavalent chromium mutagenicity and its reversal by liver and lung preparations. Mutat. Res. 122:1–5.

Benuck, M., K. Iqbal, H.M. Wisniewski, and A. Lajtha. 1985. Proteolytic activity in brains of rabbits treated with aluminum. Neurochem. Res. 10:729–736.

Berg, J.W., and F. Burbank. 1972. Correlations between carcinogenic trace metals in water supplies and cancer mortality. Ann. N.Y. Acad. Sci. 199:249–264.

Bergeron, R.J., R.R. Streiff, and G.T. Elliott. 1985. Influence of iron on in vivo proliferation and lethality of L1210 cells. J. Nutr. 115:369–374.

Berlin, M. 1979. Mercury. Pp. 503–530 in L. Friberg, G.F. Nordberg, and V.B. Vouk, eds. Handbook on the Toxicology of Metals. Elsevier/North Holland Biomedical Press, Amsterdam.

Bernstein, D.S., N. Sadowsky, D.M. Hegsted, C.D. Guri, and F.J. Stare. 1966. Prevalence of osteoporosis in high- and low-fluoride areas in North Dakota. J. Am. Med. Assoc. 198:499–504.

Bielschowsky, F. 1944. Tumors of the thyroid produced by 2-acetylaminofluorene and allylthiourea. Br. J. Exp. Pathol. 25:90–95.

Bingham, F.T. 1979. Bioavailability of CD to food crops in relation to heavy metal content to sludge-amended soil. Environ. Health Perspect. 28:39–43.

Blakley, B.R. 1984. Enhancement of urethan-induced adenoma formation in Swiss mice exposed to methylmercury. Can. J. Comp. Med. 48:299–302.

Bogardus, G.M., and J.W. Finley. 1961. Breast cancer and thyroid disease. Surgery 49:461–468.

Bogden, J.D., H.R. Chung, F.W. Kemp, K. Holding, K.S. Bruening, and Y. Naveh. 1986. Effect of selenium and molybdenum on methylbenzylnitrosamine-induced esophageal lesions and tissue trace metals in the rat. J. Nutr. 116: 2432–2442.

Böing, H., L. Martinez, R. Frentzel-Beyme, and U. Oltersdorf. 1985. Regional nutritional pattern and cancer mortality in the Federal Republic of Germany. Nutr. Cancer 7: 121–130.

Bomford, A., and R. Williams. 1976. Long term results of venesection therapy in idiopathic haemochromatosis. Q. J. Med. 45:611–623.

Borel, J.S., T.C. Majerus, M.M. Polansky, P.B. Moser, and R.A. Anderson. 1984. Chromium intake and urinary chromium excretion of trauma patients. Biol. Trace Element Res. 6:317–326.

Boutwell, R.K. 1963. A carcinogenicity evaluation of potassium arsenite and arsanilic acid. J. Agric. Food Chem. 11: 381–385.

Brada, Z., and N.H. Altman. 1977. The inhibitory effect of copper on ethionine carcinogenesis. Adv. Exp. Med. Biol. 91:193–206.

Braganza, J.M., H.J. Klass, M. Bell, and G. Sturniolo. 1981. Evidence of altered copper metabolism in patients with chronic pancreatitis. Clin. Sci. 60:303–310.

Broghamer, W.L., K.P. McConnell, and A.J. Blotcky. 1976. Relationship between serum selenium levels and patients with carcinoma. Cancer 37:1384–1388.

Broghamer, W.L., Jr., K.P. McConnell, M. Grimaldi, and A.J. Blotcky. 1978. Serum selenium and reticuloendothelial tumors. Cancer 41:1462–1466.

Brown, W.A.B., P.V. Christofferson, M. Massler, and M.B. Weiss. 1960. Postnatal tooth development in cattle. Am. J. Vet. Res. 21:7–34.

Brown, W.E., and K.G. König, eds. 1977. Cariostatic mechanisms of fluorides. Caries Res. 11 Suppl. 1:1–327.

Brusick, D., F. Gletten, D.R. Jagannath, and U. Weeks. 1976. The mutagenic activity of ferrous sulfate for *Salmonella typhimurium*. Mutat. Res. 38:386–387.

Buchet, J.P., R. Lauwerys, A. Vandevoorde, and J.M. Pycke. 1983. Oral daily intake of cadmium, lead, manganese, copper, chromium, mercury, calcium, zinc and arsenic in Belgium: a duplicate meal study. Food Chem. Toxicol. 21: 19–24.

Burt, B.A., S.A. Eklund, and W.J. Loesche. 1986. Dental benefits of limited exposure to fluoridated water in childhood. J. Dent. Res. 65:1322–1325.

Büttner, W. 1963. Action of trace elements on the metabolism of fluoride. J. Dent. Res. 42:453–460.

Byron, W.R., G.W. Bierbower, J.B. Brouwer, and W.H. Hansen. 1967. Pathologic changes in rats and dogs from two-year feeding of sodium arsenite or sodium arsenate. Toxicol. Appl. Pharmacol. 10:132–147.

Calabrese, E.J. 1983. Role of epidemiologic studies in deriving drinking water standards for metals. Environ. Health Perspect. 52:99–106.

Calabrese, E., and R.W. Tuthill. 1978. Elevated blood pressure levels and community drinking water characteristics. J. Environ. Sci. Health, Part A A13:781–802.

Calautti, P., G. Moschini, B.M. Stievano, L. Tomio, F. Calzavara, and G. Perona. 1980. Serum selenium levels in malignant lymphoproliferative diseases. Scand. J. Haematol. 24:63–66.

Campbell, J.K., and C.F. Mills. 1974. Effects of dietary cadmium and zinc on rats maintained on diets low in copper. Proc. Nutr. Soc. 33:15A–16A.

Campbell, J.K., and C.F. Mills. 1979. The toxicity of zinc to pregnant sheep. Environ. Res. 20:1–13.

Canfield, W.K., K.M. Hambidge, and L.K. Johnson. 1984. Zinc nutriture in type I diabetes mellitus: relationship to growth measures and metabolic control. J. Pediatr. Gastroenterol. Nutr. 3:577–584.

Cantoni, O., and M. Costa. 1983. Correlations of DNA strand breaks and their repair with cell survival following acute exposure to mercury (II) and x-rays. Mol. Pharmacol. 24:84–89.

Carlton, W.W., and P.S. Price. 1973. Dietary copper and the induction of neoplasms in the rat by acetylaminofluorene and dimethylnitrosamine. Food Cosmet. Toxicol. 11:827–840.

Carmignani, M., and P. Boscolo. 1984. Cardiovascular responsiveness to physiological agonists of male rats made hypertensive by long-term exposure to cadmium. Sci. Total Environ. 34:19–33.

Cartwright, G.E., and M.M. Wintrobe. 1964. Copper metabolism in normal subjects. Am. J. Clin. Nutr. 14:224–232.

CAST (Council for Agricultural Science and Technology). 1980. Effects of Sewage Sludge on the Cadmium and Zinc Content of Crops. Report No. 83. CAST, Ames, Iowa. 77 pp.

Casto, B.C., W.J. Pieczynski, R.L. Nelson, and J.A. DiPaolo. 1976. *In vitro* transformation and enhancement of viral transformation with metals. Proc. Am. Assoc. Cancer Res. 17:12.

Casto, B.C., J.D. Meyers, J.A. DiPaolo. 1979. Enhancement of viral transformation for evaluation of the carcinogenic or mutagenic potential of inorganic metal salts. Cancer Res. 39:193–198.

CDC (Centers for Disease Control). 1985. Preventing Lead Poisoning in Young Children. A Statement by the Centers for Disease Control, January 1985. Publ. No. 99-2230. Environmental Health Service Division, Bureau of State Services, Public Health Service, U.S. Department of Health and Human Services, Atlanta. 35 pp.

Charlton, R.W., and T.H. Bothwell. 1982. Definition, prevalence and prevention of iron deficiency. Clin. Haematol. 11:309–325.

Chen, C.J., Y.C. Chuang, T.M. Lin, and H.Y. Wu. 1985. Malignant neoplasms among residents of a blackfoot disease-endemic area in Taiwan: high-arsenic artesian well water and cancers. Cancer Res. 45:5895–5899.

Chen, C.J., Y.C. Chuang, S.L. You, T.M. Lin, and H.Y. Wu. 1986. A retrospective study on malignant neoplasms of bladder, lung and liver in blackfoot disease endemic area in Taiwan. Br. J. Cancer 53:399–405.

Chilvers, C. 1983. Cancer mortality and fluoridation of water supplies in 35 U.S. cities. Int. J. Epidemiol. 12:397–404.

Chisolm, J.J., Jr. 1985. Pediatric exposures to lead, arsenic, cadmium, and methyl mercury. Pp. 229–262 in R.K. Chandra, ed. Trace Elements in Nutrition of Children. Raven Press, New York.

Clark, J.H., and J.S. Taylor. 1981. I.R. evidence for a strong hydrogen bond in the fluoride-uracil system. J. Chem. Soc. Commun. 41:466–468.

Clark, L.C. 1985. The epidemiology of selenium and cancer. Fed. Proc. 44:2584–2589.

Clark, L.C., and G.F. Combs, Jr. 1986. Selenium compounds and the prevention of cancer: research needs and public health implications. J. Nutr. 116:170–173.

Clark, L.C., G.F. Graham, R.G. Crounse, R. Grimson, B. Hulka, and C.M. Shy. 1984. Plasma selenium and skin neoplasms: a case-control study. Nutr. Cancer 6:3–21.

Clements, F.W. 1954. The relationship of thyrotoxicosis and carcinoma of the thyroid to endemic goitre. Med. J. Aust. 2:894–897.

Clemmesen, J. 1983. The alleged association between artificial fluoridation of water supplies and cancer: a review. Bull. W.H.O. 61:871–883.

Combs, G.F., Jr., and L.C. Clark. 1985. Can dietary selenium modify cancer risk? Nutr. Rev. 43:325–331.

Cooper, W.C. 1984. The health implications of increased manganese in the environment resulting from the combustion of fuel additives: a review of the literature. J. Toxicol. Environ. Health 14:23–46.

Cooper, W.C., O. Wong, and L. Kheifets. 1985. Mortality among employees of lead battery plants and lead-producing plants, 1947–1980. Scand. J. Work Environ. Health 11:331–345.

Cote, M., L. Munan, M. Gagne-Billon, A. Kelly, O. di Pietro, and D. Shapcott. 1979. Hair chromium concentration and arteriosclerotic heart disease. Pp. 223–228 in D. Shapcott and J. Hubert eds. Chromium in Nutrition and Metabolism: Developments in Nutrition and Metabolism, Vol. 2. Elsevier/North-Holland Biomedical Press, Amsterdam.

Cowgill, U.M. 1983. The distribution of selenium and cancer mortality in the continental United States. Biol. Trace Element Res. 5:345–361.

Cragle, D.L., D.R. Hollis, J.R. Qualters, W.G. Tankersley, and S.A. Fry. 1984. A mortality study of men exposed to elemental mercury. J. Occup. Med. 26:817–821.

Crapper, D.R., S. Quittkat, S.S. Krishnan, A.J. Dalton, and U. De Boni. 1980. Intranuclear aluminum content in Alzheimer's disease, dialysis encephalopathy, and experimental aluminum encephalopathy. Acta Neuropathol. 50:19–24.

Crawford, M.D., M.J. Gardner, and J.N. Morris. 1968. Mortality and hardness of local water supplies. Lancet 1:827–831.

Crenshaw, M.A., A. Wennberg, and J.W. Bawden. 1978. Flouride-binding by the organic matrix of developing bovine enamel. Arch. Oral Biol. 23:285–287.

Cummins, P.E., J. Dutton, C.J. Evans, W.D. Morgan, A. Sivyer, and P.C. Elwood. 1980. An in-vivo study of renal cadmium and hypertension. Eur. J. Clin. Invest. 10:459–461.

Cuzick, J., S. Evans, M. Gillman, and D.A. Price Evans. 1982. Medicinal arsenic and internal malignancies. Br. J. Cancer 45:904–911.

Dallman, P.R., M.A. Siimes, and A. Stekel. 1979. Iron Deficiency in Infancy and Childhood. A Report for the International Nutritional Anemia Consultive Group. The Nutrition Foundation, Washington, D.C. 49 pp.

Danks, D.M. 1980. Copper deficiency in humans. Ciba Found. Symp. 79:209–225.

Davidson, I., and W. Blackwell. 1968. Changes in carbohydrate metabolism of squirrel monkeys with chromium dietary supplementation. Proc. Soc. Exp. Biol. Med. 127:66–70.

Davies, I.J., M. Musa, and T.L. Dormandy. 1968. Measurements of plasma zinc. II. In malignant disease. J. Clin. Pathol. 21:363–365.

Davies, J.M. 1984. Lung cancer mortality among workers making lead chromate and zinc chromate pigments at three English factories. Br. J. Ind. Med. 41:158–169.

Dean, H.T. 1936. Chronic endemic dental fluorosis (mottled enamel). J. Am. Med. Assoc. 107:1269–1273.

Dean, H.T., and E. Elvove. 1935. Studies on the minimal threshold of the dental sign of chronic endemic fluorosis (mottled enamel). Public Health Rep. 50:1719–1729.

De Boni, U. 1985. Cultured cells of the nervous system, including human neurones, in the study of the neurodegenerative disorder, Alzheimer's disease: an overview. Xenobiotica 15:643–647.

DeWys, W., and W. Pories. 1972. Inhibition of a spectrum of

animal tumors by dietary zinc deficiency. J. Natl. Cancer Inst. 48:375–381.

DeWys, W., W.J. Pories, M.C. Richter, and W.H. Strain. 1970. Inhibition of Walker 256 carcinosarcoma growth by dietary zinc deficiency. Proc. Soc. Exp. Biol. Med. 135:17–22.

DHSS (Department of Health and Social Security). 1980. Lead and Health: the Report of a DHSS Working Party on Lead in the Environment. Her Majesty's Stationary Office, London. 128 pp.

Dingwall-Fordyce, I., and R.E. Lane. 1963. A follow-up study of lead workers. Br. J. Ind. Med. 20:313–315.

DiPaolo, J.A., and B.C. Casto. 1979. Quantitative studies on in vitro morphological transformation of Syrian hamster cells by inorganic metal salts. Cancer Res. 39:1008–1013.

DiPaolo, J.A., R.L. Nelson, and B.C. Casto. 1978. In vitro neoplastic transformation of Syrian hamster cells by lead acetate and its relevance to environmental carcinogenesis. Br. J. Cancer 38:452–455.

Doll, R., and L. Kinlen. 1977. Fluoridation of water and cancer mortality in the U.S.A. Lancet 1:1300–1302.

Doll, R., L. Fishbein, P. Infante, P. Landrigan, J.W. Lloyd, T.J. Mason, E. Mastromatteo, T. Norseth, G. Pershagen, U. Saffiotti, and R. Saracci. 1981. Problems of epidemiological evidence. Environ. Health Perspect. 40:11–20.

Doniach, I. 1958. Experimental induction of tumours of the thyroid by radiation. Br. Med. Bull. 14:181–183.

Drinkard, C.R., M.A. Crenshaw, and J.W. Bawden. 1982. F Effect on protein/phosphorus in developing rat molar enamel. J. Dent. Res. (sp. iss.) 61:216.

Driscoll, W.S., S.B. Heifetz, and J.A. Brunelle. 1981. Caries-preventive effects of fluoride tablets in schoolchildren four years after discontinuation of treatments. J. Am. Dent. Assoc. 103:878–881.

Dube, D.K., and L.A. Loeb. 1975. Manganese as a mutagenic agent during in vitro DNA synthesis. Biochem. Biophys. Res. Commun. 67:1041–1046.

Duncan, J.R., and I.E. Dreosti. 1975. Zinc intake, neoplastic DNA synthesis, and chemical carcinogenesis in rats and mice. J. Natl. Cancer Inst. 55:195–196.

Dunning, J.M. 1979. Water fluoridation. Pp. 377–414 in Principles of Dental Public Health, 3rd ed. Harvard University Press, Cambridge, Mass.

Dutkiewiez, T. 1977. Experimental studies on arsenic absorption routes in rats. Environ. Health Perspect. 19:173–176.

Eakin, D.J., L.A. Schroeder, P.D. Whanger, and P.H. Weswig. 1980. Cadmium and nickel influence on blood pressure, plasma renin, and tissue mineral concentrations. Am. J. Physiol. 238:E53–E61.

Ebina, Y., S. Okada, S. Hamazaki, F. Ogino, J.L. Li, and O. Midorikawa. 1986. Nephrotoxicity and renal cell carcinoma after use of iron- and aluminum-nitrilotriacetate complexes in rats. J. Natl. Cancer Inst. 76:107–113.

Edington, G.M. 1976. Dietary iodine and risk of breast, endometrial, and ovarian cancer. Lancet 1:1413–1414.

Elinder, C.G. 1985. Cadmium: uses, occurrence and intake. Pp. 23–64 in L. Friberg, C.G. Elinder, T. Kjellström, and G.F. Nordberg, eds. Cadmium and Health: A Toxicological and Epidemiological Appraisal, Vol. I. Exposure, Dose, and Metabolism. CRC Press, Boca Raton, Fla.

Ellis, N.I., B. Lloyd, R.S. Lloyd, and B.E. Clayton. 1984. Selenium and vitamin E in relation to risk factors for coronary heart disease. J. Clin. Pathol. 37:200–206.

Emsley, J., D.J. Jones, J.M. Miller, R.E. Overill, and R.A. Waddilove. 1981. An unexpectedly strong hydrogen bond: ab initio calculations and spectroscopic studies of amide-fluoride systems. J. Am. Chem. Soc. 103:24–28.

Emsley, J., D.J. Jones, and R.E. Overill. 1982. The uracil fluoride interaction Ab-initio calculations including solvation. J. Chem. Soc. Chem. Commun. (9):476–478.

EPA (Environmental Protection Agency). 1988. Proposed drinking water regulations. Fed. Reg. 53:31523.

Erickson, J.D. 1978. Mortality in selected cities with fluoridated and non-fluoridated water supplies. N. Engl. J. Med. 298:1112–1116.

Ericsson, S.Y. 1977. Cariostatic mechanisms of fluorides: clinical observations. Caries Res. 11 Suppl. 1:2–41.

Erkell, L.J., W. Ryd, and B. Hagmar. 1986. Effects of zinc on tumor transplantability. Invasion Metastasis 6:112–122.

Ernhart, C.B., B. Landa, and N.B. Schell. 1981. Subclinical levels of lead and developmental deficit—a multivariate follow-up reassessment. Pediatrics 67:911–919.

Eskin, B.A. 1977. Iodine and mammary cancer. Adv. Exp. Med. Biol. 91:293–304.

Eskin, B.A., D.G. Bartuska, M.R. Dunn, G. Jacob, and M.B. Dratman. 1967. Mammary gland dysplasia in iodine deficiency. J. Am. Med. Assoc. 200:691–695.

European Thyroid Association. 1985. Report of the Subcommittee for the Study of Endemic Goitre and Iodine Deficiency. Goitre and iodine deficiency in Europe. Lancet 1: 1289–1293.

Everson, G.J., and R.E. Shrader. 1968. Abnormal glucose tolerance in manganese-deficient guinea pigs. J. Nutr. 94: 89–94.

Ewers, U., A. Brockhaus, R. Dolgner, I. Freier, E. Jermann, A. Bernard, R. Stiller-Winkler, R. Hahn, and N. Manojlovic. 1985. Environmental exposure to cadmium and renal function of elderly women living in cadmium-polluted areas of the Federal Republic of Germany. Int. Arch. Occup. Environ. Health 55:217–239.

Fabris, C., R. Farini, G. Del Favero, G. Gurrieri, A. Piccoli, G.C. Sturniolo, A. Panucci, and R. Naccarato. 1985. Copper, zinc and copper/zinc ratio in chronic pancreatitis and pancreatic cancer. Clin. Biochem. 18:373–375.

Fahim, M.S., and N.K. Khare. 1980. Effects of subtoxic levels of lead and cadmium on urogenital organs of male rats. Arch. Androl. 4:357–362.

Fenton, M.R., J.P. Burke, F.D. Tursi, and F.P. Arena. 1980. Effect of a zinc-deficient diet on the growth of an IgM-secreting plasmacytoma (TEPC-183). J. Natl. Cancer Inst. 65:1271–1272.

Fernandes, G., M. Nair, K. Onoe, T. Tanaka, R. Floyd, and R.A. Good. 1979. Impairment of cell-mediated immunity functions by dietary zinc deficiency in mice. Proc. Natl. Acad. Sci. U.S.A. 76:457–461.

Feustel, A., and R. Wennrich. 1984. Determination of the distribution of zinc and cadmium in cellular fractions of BPH, normal prostate and prostatic cancers of different histologies by atomic and laser absorption spectrometry in tissue slices. Urol. Res. 12:253–256.

Feustel, A., and R. Wennrich. 1986. Zinc and cadmium plasma and erythrocyte levels in prostatic carcinoma, BPH, urological malignancies, and inflammations. Prostate 8:75–79.

Feustel, A., R. Wennrich, D. Steiniger, and P. Klauss. 1982. Zinc and cadmium concentration in prostatic carcinoma of different histological grading in comparison to normal prostate tissue and adenofibromyomatosis (BPH). Urol. Res. 10: 301–303.

Fields, M. 1985. Newer understanding of copper metabolism. Arch. Intern. Med. 6:91–98.

Fingerle, H., G. Fischer, and H.G. Classen. 1982. Failure to produce hypertension in rats by chronic exposure to cadmium. Food Chem. Toxicol. 20:301–306.

Fischer, P.W., and M.W. Collins. 1981. Relationship between serum zinc and copper and risk factors associated with cardiovascular disease. Am. J. Clin. Nutr. 34:595–597.

Fisher, K.D., and C.J. Carr. 1974. Iodine in Foods: Chemical Methodology and Sources of Iodine in the Human Diet. Life Sciences Research Office, Federation of American Societies for Experimental Biology, Bethesda, Md. 105 pp.

Folsom, A.R., and R.J. Prineas. 1982. Drinking water composition and blood pressure: a review of the epidemiology. Am. J. Epidemiol. 115:818–832.

Forbes, G.B., and C.W. Woodruff. 1985. Pediatric Nutrition Handbook, 2nd ed. Committee on Nutrition, American Academy of Pediatrics, Elk Grove Village, Ill. 421 pp.

Fowler, B.A., C.A. Kimmel, J.S. Woods, E.E. McConnell, and L.D. Grant. 1980. Chronic low-level lead toxicity in the rat. III. An integrated assessment of long-term toxicity with special reference to the kidney. Toxicol. Appl. Pharmacol. 56:59–77.

Freund, H., S. Atamian, and J. Fisher. 1979. Chromium deficiency during total parenteral nutrition. J. Am. Med. Assoc. 241:496–498.

Friberg, L., T. Kjellström, G. Nordberg, and G.M. Piscator. 1979. Cadmium. Pp. 355–381 in L. Friberg, G.F. Nordberg, and V.B. Vouk, eds. Handbook on the Toxicology of Metals. Elsevier/North-Holland Biomedical Press, Amsterdam.

Friberg, L., C.G. Elinder, T. Kjellström, and G.F. Nordberg, eds. 1985a. Cadmium and Health: A Toxicological and Epidemiological Appraisal, Vol. I. Exposure, Dose, and Metabolism. CRC Press, Boca Raton, Fla. 209 pp.

Friberg, L., C.G. Elinder, T. Kjellström, and G.F. Nordberg, eds. 1985b. Cadmium and Health: A Toxicological and Epidemiological Appraisal, Vol. II. Effects and Response. CRC Press, Boca Raton, Fla. 307 pp.

Friedman, G.D., A.L. Klatsky, and A.B. Siegelaub. 1982. Alcohol, tobacco, and hypertension. Hypertension 4: III143–III150.

Furst, A. 1977. Inorganic agents as carcinogens. Pp. 209–229 in H.F. Kraybill and M.A. Mehlman, eds. Environmental Cancer: Advances in Modern Toxicology, Vol. 3. Wiley, New York.

Furst, A. 1983. A new look at arsenic carcinogenesis. Pp. 151–165 in W.H. Lederer and R.J. Fensterheim, eds. Arsenic: Industrial Biomedical Environmental Perspectives. Van Nostrand Reinhold Co., New York.

Furst, A., M. Schlauder, and D.P. Sasmore. 1976. Tumorigenic activity of lead chromate. Cancer Res. 36:1779–1783.

Gabrial, G.N., T.F. Schrager, and P.M. Newberne. 1982. Zinc deficiency, alcohol, and retinoid: association with esophageal cancer in rats. J. Natl. Cancer Inst. 68:785–789.

Garruto, R.M., R. Fukatsu, R. Yanagihara, D.C. Gajdusek, G. Hook, and C.E. Fiori. 1984. Imaging of calcium and aluminum in neurofibrillary tangle-bearing neurons in Parkinsonism-dementia of Guam. Proc. Natl. Acad. Sci. U.S.A. 81:1875–1879.

Gazdy, E., H. Csernyanszky, and T. Szilagyi. 1981. The effect of zinc ions (Zn^+) on the procoagulent activity of PMN leukocytes. Acta Physiol. Acad. Sci. Hung. 57:29–35.

Gerhardsson, L., D. Brune, G.F. Nordberg, and P.O. Wester. 1986. Distribution of cadmium, lead and zinc in lung, liver and kidney in long-term exposed smelter workers. Sci. Total Environ. 50:65–85.

Gibbs, G.W. 1985. Mortality of aluminum reduction plant workers, 1950 through 1977. J. Occup. Med. 27:761–770.

Gileva, E.A., E.G. Plotko, and E.Z. Gatiiatullina. 1972. Mutagenic activity of inorganic flourine compounds. Gig. Sanit. 37:9–12.

Golden, M.H.N., B.E. Golden, P.S.E.G. Harland, and A.A. Jackson. 1978. Zinc and immunocompetence in protein-energy malnutrition. Lancet 1:1226–1228.

Golden, M.H.N., B.E. Golden, and F.I. Bennett. 1985. Relationship of trace element deficiencies to malnutrition. Pp. 185–207 in R.K. Chandra, ed. Trace Elements in Nutrition of Children. Raven Press, New York.

Goodwin, W.J., Jr., H.W. Lane, K. Bradford, M.V. Marshall, A.C. Griffin, H. Geopfert, and R.H. Jesse. 1983. Selenium and glutathione peroxidase levels in patients with epidermoid carcinoma of the oral cavity and oropharynx. Cancer 51:110–115.

Gorsky, J.E., A.A. Dietz, H. Spencer, and D. Osis. 1979. Metabolic balance of aluminum studied in six men. Clin. Chem. 25:1739–1743.

Greenberg, S.R. 1982. Leucocyte response in young mice chronically exposed to fluorides. Fluoride 15:119–133.

Greger, J.L., and M.J. Baier. 1983. Excretion and retention of low or moderate levels of aluminum by human subjects. Food Chem. Toxicol. 21:473–476.

Gregoriadis, G.C., N.S. Apostolidis, A.N. Romanos, and T.P. Paradellis. 1983. A comparative study of trace elements in normal and cancerous colorectal tissues. Cancer 52:508–519.

Gunn, S.A., T.C. Gould, and W.A.D. Anderson. 1963. Cadmium-induced interstitial cell tumors in rats and mice and their prevention by zinc. J. Natl. Cancer Inst. 31:745–759.

Gunn, S.A., T.C. Gould, and W.A.D. Anderson. 1964. Effect of zinc on cancerogenesis by cadmium. Proc. Soc. Exp. Biol. Med. 115:653–657.

Gunn, S.A., T.C. Gould, and W.A.D. Anderson. 1967. Specific response of mesenchymal tissue to cancerigenesis by cadmium. Arch. Pathol. 83:493–499.

Gunson, D.E., D.F. Kowalczyk, C.R. Shoop, and C.F. Ramberg, Jr. 1982. Environmental zinc and cadmium pollution associated with generalized osteochondrosis, osteoporosis, and nephrocalcinosis in horses. J. Am. Vet. Med. Assoc. 180:295–299.

Guthrie, J. 1964. Histological effects of intra-testicular injections of cadmium chloride in domestic fowl. Br. J. Cancer 18:255–260.

Györkey, F., K.W. Min, J.A. Huff, and P. Györkey. 1967. Zinc and magnesium in human prostate gland: normal, hyperplastic and neoplastic. Cancer Res. 27:1348–1353.

Haddow, A., F.J.C. Roe, C.E. Dukes, and B.C.V. Mitchley. 1964. Cadmium neoplasia: sarcomata at the site of injection of cadmium sulphate in rats and mice. Br. J. Cancer 18:667–673.

Hagan, T.L., M. Pasternack, and G.C. Scholz. 1954. Waterborne fluorides and mortality. Public Health Rep. 69:450–454.

Hägglöf, B., G. Hallmans, G. Holmgren, J. Ludvigsson, and S. Falkmer. 1983. Prospective and retrospective studies of zinc concentrations in serum, blood clots, hair and urine in young patients with insulin-dependent diabetes mellitus. Acta Endocrinol. 102:88–95.

Hainline, B.E., and K.V. Rajagopalan. 1983. Molybdenum in animal and human health. Pp 150–166 in J. Rose, ed. Trace Elements in Health: A Review of Current Issues. Butterworths, London.

Hallmans, G., and F. Lithner. 1980. Early changes in zinc and copper metabolism in rats with alloxan diabetes of short duration after local traumatization with heat. Upsala J. Med. Sci. 85:59–66.

Hambidge, K.M., C.E. Casey, and N.F. Krebs. 1986. Zinc. Pp. 1–137 in W. Mertz, ed. Trace Elements in Human and Animal Nutrition, Vol. 2, 5th ed. Academic Press, Orlando, Fla.

Hanson, T., and B. Roos. 1978. Effect of combined therapy with sodium fluoride, calcium, and vitamin D on the lumbar spine in osteoporosis. Am. J. Roentgenol., Radium Ther. Nucl. Med. 126:1294–1297.

Harrington, J.M., J.P. Middaugh, D.L. Morse, and J. Housworth. 1978. A survey of a population exposed to high concentrations of arsenic in well water in Fairbanks, Alaska. Am. J. Epidemiol. 108:377–385.

Hass, G.M., J.H. McDonald, R. Oyasu, H.A. Battifora, and J.T. Paloucek. 1967. Renal neoplasia induced by combinations of dietary lead subacetate and N-2-fluorenylacetamide. Pp. 377–412 in J.S. King, Jr., ed. Renal Neoplasia. J. & A. Churchill Ltd., London.

Hedinger, C. 1981. Geographic pathology of thyroid diseases. Pathol. Res. Pract. 171:285–292.

Henrikson, P.A., L. Lutwak, L. Krook, R. Skogerboe, F. Kallfelz, L.F. Bélanger, J.R. Marier, B.E. Sheffy, B. Romanus, and C. Hirsch. 1970. Fluoride and nutritional osteoporosis: physicochemical data on bones from an experimental study in dogs. J. Nutr. 100:631–642.

Herr, H.W., E.L. Kleinert, and W.F. Whitmore, Jr. 1981. Mercury-induced necrosis of murine renal cell carcinoma. J. Surg. Oncol. 18:95–99.

Heyman, A., W.E. Wilkinson, J.A. Stafford, M.J. Helms, A.H. Sigmon, and T. Weinberg. 1984. Alzheimer's disease: a study of epidemiological aspects. Ann. Neurol. 15:335–341.

Hiasa, Y., M. Ohshima, Y. Kitahori, T. Fujita, T. Yuasa, and A. Miyashiro. 1983. Basic lead acetate: promoting effect on the development of renal tubular cell tumors in rats treated with N-ethyl-N-hydroxyethylnitrosamine. J. Natl. Cancer Inst. 70:761–765.

Hill, G.M., E.R. Miller, P.A. Whetter, and D.E. Ullney. 1983. Concentration of minerals in tissues of pigs from dams fed different levels of dietary zinc. J. Anim. Sci. 57:130–138.

Hoekstra, W.G. 1975. Biochemical function of selenium and its relation to vitamin E. Fed. Proc. 34:2083–2089.

Hooper, P.L., L. Visconti, P.J. Garry, and G.E. Johnson. 1980. Zinc lowers high-density lipoprotein-cholesterol levels. J. Am. Med. Assoc. 244:1960–1961.

Hoover, R.N., F.W. McKay, and J.F. Fraumeni, Jr. 1976. Fluoridated drinking water and the occurrence of cancer. J. Natl. Cancer Inst. 57:757–768.

Hoover, R.L., R. Folger, W.A. Haering, B.R. Ware, and M.J. Karnovsky. 1980. Adhesion of leukocytes to endothelium: roles of divalent cations, surface charge, chemotactic agents and substrate. J. Cell Sci. 45:73–86.

Hsi, A., N.P. Johnson, J. San Sebastian, J.P. O'Neill, R.O. Rahn, and N.L. Forbes. 1979. Quantitative mammalian cell mutagenesis and a study of mutagenic potential of metallic compounds. Pp. 55–69 in Kharasch, ed. Trace Metals in Health and Disease. Raven Press, New York.

Hueper, W.C., and W.W. Payne. 1962. Experimental studies in metal carcinogenesis: chromium, nickel, iron, arsenic. Arch. Environ. Health 5:445–462.

Hurley, L.S. 1981. Teratogenic aspects of manganese, zinc, and copper nutrition. Physiol. Rev. 61:249–295.

Hurley, L.S., and C.L. Keen. 1987. Manganese. Pp. 185–223 in W. Mertz, ed. Trace Elements in Human and Animal Nutrition, Vol. I. Academic Press, New York.

IARC (International Agency for Research on Cancer). 1976. Cadmium and cadmium compounds. Pp. 39–74 in IARC Monographs on the Evaluation of Carcinogenic Risk of Chemicals to Man, Vol. 11. Cadmium, Nickel, Some Epoxides, Miscellaneous Industrial Chemicals and General Considerations on Volatile Anaesthetics. IARC, Lyon, France.

IARC (International Agency for Research on Cancer). 1982a. Inorganic fluorides used in drinking-water and dental preparations. Pp. 237–303 in IARC Monographs on the Evaluation of the Carcinogenic Risk of Chemicals to Humans, Vol. 27. Some Aromatic Amines, Anthraquinones and Nitroso Compounds, and Inorganic Fluorides Used in Drinking-Water and Dental Preparations. IARC, Lyon, France.

IARC (International Agency for Research on Cancer). 1982b. Iron dextran complex (group 3). Pp. 145–146 in IARC Monographs on the Evaluation of the Carcinogenic Risk of Chemicals to Human, Suppl. 4. Chemical, Industrial Processes and Industries Associated with Cancer in Humans. IARC, Lyon, France.

Inskip, H., V. Beral, and M. McDowall. 1982. Mortality of Shipham residents: 40-year follow-up. Lancet 1:896–899.

Ip, C. 1985. Selenium inhibition of chemical carcinogenesis. Fed. Proc. 44:2573–2578.

Ip, C. 1986. The chemopreventive role of selenium in carcinogenesis. Adv. Exp. Med. Biol. 206:431–447.

Ip, C., and D.K. Sinha. 1981. Enhancement of mammary tumorigenesis by dietary selenium deficiency in rats with high polyunsaturated fat intake. Cancer Res. 41:31–34.

Ishinihsi, N., and A. Yamamoto. 1983. Discrepancy between epidemiological evidence and animal experimental result. Sangyo Ika Daigaku Zasshi J. UOEH, Suppl. 5:109–116.

Ito, K., and N. Maruchi. 1975. Breast cancer in patients with Hashimoto's thyroiditis. Lancet 2:1119–1121.

Ito, N. 1973. Experimental studies on tumors of the urinary system of rats induced by chemical carcinogens. Acta Pathol. Jpn. 23:87–109.

Ito, N., Y. Hiasa, Y. Kamakoto, S. Makiura, and S. Sugihara. 1971. Histopathological analysis of kidney tumors in rats induced by chemical carcinogens. Gann 62:435–444.

Ivey, J.L., and D.J. Baylink. 1981. Postmenopausal osteoporosis: proposed roles of defective coupling and estrogen deficiency. Metab. Bone Dis. Relat. Res. 3:3–7.

Jacobs, M.M., T.S. Matney, and A.C. Griffin. 1977. Inhibitory effects of selenium on the mutagenicity of 2-acetylaminofluorene (AAF) and AAF derivatives. Cancer Lett. 2:319–322.

Jagiello, G., and J.S. Lin. 1974. Sodium fluoride as potential mutagen in mammalian eggs. Arch. Environ. Health 29:230–235.

Jeejeebhoy, K.N., R.C. Chu, E.B. Marliss, G.R. Greenberg, and A. Bruce-Robertson. 1977. Chromium deficiency, glucose intolerance, and neuropathy reversed by chromium supplementation, in a patient receiving long-term total parenteral nutrition. Am. J. Clin. Nutr. 30:531–538.

Jendryczko, A., M. Crozdz, J. Tomala, and K. Magner. 1986. Copper and zinc concentrations, and superoxide dismutase activities in malignant and nonmalignant tissues of female reproductive organs. Neoplasma 33:239–244.

Jenkins, G.N. 1978. Fluoride. Pp. 466–500 in The Physiology and Biochemistry of the Mouth, 4th ed. Blackwell Scientific Publications, Oxford.

Jowsey, J. 1979. The long-term treatment of osteoporosis with fluoride, calcium, and vitamin D. Pp. 123–134 in U.S. Barzel, ed. Osteoporosis II. Grune & Stratton, New York.

Kada, T., K. Hirano, and Y. Shirasu. 1980. Screening of environmental chemical mutagens by the rec-assay system with Bacillus subtilis. Pp. 149–173 in F.J. de Serres and A. Hollaender, eds. Chemical Mutagens: Principles and Methods for Their Detection, Vol. 6. Plenum Press, New York.

Kanematsu, N., M. Hara, and T. Kada. 1980. Rec assay and mutagenicity studies on metal compounds. Mutat. Res. 77: 109–116.

Kanis, J.A., and P.J. Meunier. 1984. Should we use fluoride to treat osteoporosis? A review. Q. J. Med. 53:145–164.

Kantor, A.F., M.G. Curnen, J.W. Meigs, and J.T. Flannery. 1979. Occupations of fathers of patients with Wilms's tumour. J. Epidemiol. Community Health 33:253–256.

Kawamura, J., O. Yoshida, K. Nishino, and Y. Itokawa. 1978. Disturbances in kidney functions and calcium and phosphate metabolism in cadmium poisoned rats. Nephron 20: 101–110.

Kazantzis, G. 1981. Role of cobalt, iron, lead, manganese, mercury, platinum, selenium, and titanium in carcinogenesis. Environ. Health Perspect. 40:143–161.

Kazantzis, G., and W.J. Hanbury. 1966. The induction of sarcoma in the rat by cadmium sulphide and by cadmium oxide. Br. J. Cancer 20:190–199.

Kinlaw, W.B., A.S. Levine, J.E. Morley, S.E. Silvis, and C.J. McClain. 1983. Abnormal zinc metabolism in type II diabetes mellitus. Am. J. Med. 75:273–277.

Kinlen, L., and R. Doll. 1981. Fluoridation of water supplies and cancer mortality. III. A re-examination of mortality in cities in the USA. J. Epidemiol. Community Health 35: 239–244.

Kipling, M.D., and J.A.H. Waterhouse. 1967. Cadmium and prostatic carcinoma. Lancet 1:730–731.

Kitano, S. 1980. Membrane and contractile properties of rat vascular tissue in copper-deficient conditions. Circ. Res. 46: 681–689.

Kjellström, T., L. Friberg, and B. Rahnster. 1979. Mortality and cancer morbidity among cadmium-exposed workers. Environ. Health Perspect. 29:199–204.

Klevay, L.M. 1975. Coronary heart disease: the zinc/copper hypothesis. Am. J. Clin. Nutr. 28:764–774.

Klevay, L.M. 1980. Interactions of copper and zinc in cardiovascular disease. Ann. N.Y. Acad. Sci. 355:140–151.

Klevay, L.M. 1984. The role of copper, zinc, and other chemical elements in ischemic heart disease. Pp. 129–157 in O.M. Rennert and W.Y. Chan, eds. Metabolism of Trace Metals in Man, Vol I. Developmental Aspects. CRC Press, Boca Raton, Fla.

Klevay, L.M., and K.E. Viestenz. 1981. Abnormal electrocardiograms in rats deficient in copper. Am. J. Physiol. 240: H185–H189.

Knox, E.G., ed. 1985. Fluoridation of Water and Cancer: A Review of the Epidemiological Evidence. Report of the Working Party on the Fluoridation of Water and Cancer. Her Majesty's Stationary Office, London. 115 pp.

Kobayashi, N., H. Katsuki, and Y. Yamane. 1970. Inhibitory effect of aluminum on the development of experimental lung tumor in mice induced by 4-nitroquinone 1-oxide. Gann 61: 239–244.

Kok, F.J., A.M. de Bruijn, A. Hofman, R. Vermeeren, and H.A. Valkenburg. 1987a. Is serum selenium a risk factor for cancer in men only? Am. J. Epidemiol. 125:12–16.

Kok, F., A.M. de Bruijn, R. Vermeeren, A. Hofman, A. van Laar, M. de Bruin, R.J. Hermus, and H.A. Valkenburg. 1987b. Serum selenium, vitamin antioxidants, and cardiovascular mortality: a 9-year follow-up study in the Netherlands. Am. J. Clin. Nutr. 45:462–468.

Koller, L.D., N.I. Kerkvliet, and J.H. Exon. 1985. Neoplasia induced in male rats fed lead acetate, ethyl urea, and sodium nitrite. Toxicol. Pathol. 13:50–57.

Kolonel, L.N. 1976. Association of cadmium with renal cancer. Cancer 37:1782–1787.

Kolonel, L.N., and W. Winkelstein, Jr. 1977. Cadmium and prostatic carcinoma. Lancet 2:566–567.

Kolonel, L.N., C.N. Yoshigama, and J.H. Hankin. 1988. Diet and prostatic cancer: a case-control study in Hawaii. Am. J. Epidemiol. 127:999-1012.

Kopp, S.J., T. Glonek, M. Erlanger, E.F. Perry, M. Barany, and H.M. Perry, Jr. 1980. Altered metabolism and function of rat heart following chronic low level cadmium/lead feeding. J. Mol. Cell Cardiol. 12:1407–1425.

Kopp, S.J., L.M. Klevay, and J.M. Feliksik. 1983. Physiological and metabolic characterization of a cardiomyopathy induced by chronic copper deficiency. Am. J. Physiol. 245: H855–H866.

Koval'skii, V.V., G.A. Iarovaia, and D.M. Shmavonian. 1961. Modification of human and animal purine metabolism in conditions of various molybdenum bio-geochemical areas. Zh. Obshch. Biol. 22:179–191.

Kumpulainen, J., and P. Koivistoinen. 1977. Fluorine in foods. Residue Rev. 68:37–57.

Landrigan, P.J. 1981. Arsenic—state of the art. Am. J. Ind. Med. 2:5–14.

Lappalainen, R., M. Knuuttila, S. Lammi, E.M. Alhava, and H. Olkkonen. 1982. Zn and Cu content in human cancellous bone. Acta Orthop. Scand. 53:51–55.

Larramendy, M.L., N.C. Popescu, and J.A. DiPaolo. 1981. Induction by inorganic metal salts of sister chromatid exchanges and chromosome aberrations in human and Syrian hamster cell strains. Environ. Mutagen 3:597–606.

Larsson, L.G., A. Sandström, and P. Westling. 1975. Relationship of Plummer–Vinson disease to cancer of the upper alimentary tract in Sweden. Cancer Res. 35:3308–3316.

LeBoeuf, R.A., B.A. Laishes, and W.G. Hoekstra. 1985. Effects of selenium on cell proliferation in rat liver and mammalian cells as indicated by cytokinetic and biochemical analysis. Cancer Res. 45:5496–5504.

Lee-Feldstein, A. 1986. Cumulative exposure to arsenic and its relationship to respiratory cancer among copper smelter employees. J. Occup. Med. 28:296–302.

Lemen, R.A., J.S. Lee, J.K. Wagoner, and H.P. Blejer. 1976. Cancer mortality among cadmium production workers. Ann. N.Y. Acad. Sci. 271:273–279.

Lener, J., and B. Bibr. 1971. Cadmium and hypertension. Lancet 1:970.

Leonard, A., and R.R. Lauwerys. 1980. Carcinogenicity,

mutagenicity, and teratogenicity of arsenic. Mutat. Res. 75: 49–62.

Leone, N.C., E.F. Geever, and N.C. Moran. 1956. Acute and subacute toxicity studies of sodium fluoride in animals. Public Health Rep. 71:459–467.

Levander, O.A. 1987. A global view of selenium nutrition. Annu. Rev. Nutr. 7:227–250.

Levander, O.A., and L. Cheng, eds. 1980. Micronutrient interactions: vitamins, minerals, and hazardous elements. Ann. of N.Y. Acad. Sci. 355:1–372.

Levine, R.S. 1976. The action of fluoride in caries prevention. A review of current concepts. Br. Dent. J. 140:9–14.

Levine, A.S., C.J. McClain, B.S. Handwerger, D.M. Brown, and J.E. Morley. 1983. Tissue zinc status of genetically diabetic and streptozotocin-induced diabetic mice. Am. J. Clin. Nutr. 37:382–386.

Levis, A.G., and F. Majone. 1979. Cytotoxic and clastogenic effects of soluble chromium compounds on mammalian cell cultures. Br. J. Cancer 40:523–533.

Levis, A.G., and F. Majone. 1981. Cytotoxic and clastogenic effects of soluble and insoluble compounds containing hexavalent and trivalent chromium. Br. J. Cancer. 44:219–235.

Levy, L.S., and S. Venitt. 1986. Carcinogenicity and mutagenicity of chromium compounds: the association between bronchial metaplasia and neoplasia. Carcinogenesis 7:831–835.

Lilis, R., J.A. Valciukas, S. Kon, L. Sarkosi, C. Campbell, and I.J. Selikoff. 1982. Assessment of lead health hazards in a body shop of an automobile assembly plant. Am. J. Ind. Med. 3:33–51.

Lilis, R., J.A. Valciukas, J.P. Weber, J. Malkin, and I.J. Selikoff. 1984. Epidemiologic study of renal function in copper smelter workers. Environ. Health Perspect. 54:181–192.

Lin, H.J., W.C. Chan, Y.Y. Fong, and P.M. Newberne. 1977. Zinc levels in serum, hair and tumors from patients with esophageal cancer. Nutr. Rep. Int. 15:634–643.

Lo, L.W., J. Koropatnick, and H.F. Stich. 1978. The mutagenicity and cytotoxicity of selenite, "activated" selenite and selenate for normal and DNA repair-deficient human fibroblasts. Mutat. Res. 49:305–312.

Logue, J.N., M.D. Koontz, and M.A. Hattwick. 1982. A historical prospective mortality study of workers in copper and zinc refineries. J. Occup. Med. 24:398–408.

Lorentzon, R., and S.E. Larsson. 1977. Vitamin D metabolism in adult rats at low and normal calcium intake and the effect of cadmium exposure. Clin. Sci. Mol. Med. 53:439–446.

Löser, E. 1980. A 2 year oral carcinogenicity study with cadmium on rats. Cancer Lett. 9:191–198.

LSRO (Life Sciences Research Office). 1984a. Assessment of the Iron Nutritional Status of the U.S. Population Based on Data Collected in the Second National Health and Nutrition Examination Survey, 1976–1980. Federation of American Societies for Experimental Biology, Bethesda, Md. 120 pp.

LSRO (Life Sciences Research Office). 1984b. Assessment of the Zinc Nutritional Status of the U.S. Population Based on Data Collected in the Second National Health and Nutrition Examination Survey, 1976–1980. Federation of American Societies for Experimental Biology, Bethesda, Md. 82 pp.

Lu, F.C., R.S. Grewal, W.B. Rice, R.C.B. Graham, and M.G. Allmark. 1965. Acute toxicity of sodium fluoride for rhesus monkeys and other laboratory animals. Acta Pharmacol. Toxicol. 22:99–106.

Lu, S.H., and P. Lin. 1982. Recent research on the etiology of esophageal cancer in China. Z. Gastroenterol. 20:361–367.

Luo, X.M., H.J. Wei, G.G. Hu, A.L. Shang, Y.Y. Liu, S.M. Lu, and S.P. Yang. 1981. Molybdenum and esophageal cancer in China. Fed. Proc. 40:928.

Luo, X.M., H.J. Wei, and S.P. Yang. 1983. Inhibitory effects of molybdenum on esophageal and forestomach carcinogenesis in rats. J. Natl. Cancer Inst. 71:75–80.

Mahaffey, K.R., P.E. Corneliussen, C.F. Jelinek, and J.A. Fiorino. 1975. Heavy metal exposure from foods. Environ. Health Perspect. 12:63–69.

Mahaffey, K.R., J.F. Rosen, R.W. Chesney, J.T. Peeler, C.M. Smith, and H.F. DeLuca. 1982. Association between age, blood lead concentration, and serum 1,25-dihydroxycholecalciferol levels in children. Am. J. Clin. Nutr. 35: 1327–1331.

Majone, F., and A.G. Levis. 1979. Chromosome aberrations and sister-chromatid exchanges in Chinese hamster cells treated in vivo with hexavalent chromium compounds. Mutat. Res. 67:231–238.

Majone, F., A. Montaldi, F. Ronchese, A. DeRossi, L. Chieco-Bianchi, and A.G. Levis. 1983. Sister-chromatid exchanges induced in vivo and in vitro by chemical carcinogens in mouse lymphocytes carrying endogenous Maloney leukemia virus. Carcinogenesis 4:33–37.

Manousos, O., D. Trichopoulos, A. Koutselinis, C. Papadimitriou, and X. Zavitsanos. 1981. Epidemiologic characteristics and trace elements in pancreatic cancer in Greece. Cancer Detect. Prev. 4:439–442.

Manthey, J., M. Stoeppler, W. Morgenstern, E. Nüssel, D. Opherk, A. Weintraut, H. Wesch, and W. Kübler. 1981. Magnesium and trace metals: risk factors for coronary heart disease? Association between blood levels and angiographic findings. Circulation 64:722–729.

Mao, P., and J.J. Molnar. 1967. The fine structure and histochemistry of lead-induced renal tumors in rats. Am. J. Pathol. 50:571–603.

Margalioth, E.J., J.G. Schenker, and M. Chevion. 1983. Copper and zinc levels in normal and malignant tissues. Cancer 52:868–872.

Markesbery, W.R., W.D. Ehmann, T.I. Hossain, and M. Alauddin. 1984. Brain manganese concentrations in human aging and Alzheimer's disease. Neurotoxicology 5:49–57.

Marshall, E. 1983. EPA faults classic lead poisoning study. A review questions a study linking lead in teeth with low IQ scores: EPA finds other grounds for regulation. Science 222: 906–907.

Martyn, C.N., D.J.P. Barker, C. Osmond, E.C. Harris, J.A. Edwardson, and R.F. Lacey. 1989. Geographical relation between Alzheimer's disease and aluminium in drinking water. Lancet 1:59–62.

Maruyama, Y. 1983. The health effect of mice given oral administration of trivalent and hexavalent chromium over a long-term. Gifu Daigaku Igakubu Kiyo 31:25–46.

Masironi, R., ed. 1974. Trace Elements in Relation to Cardiovascular Diseases; Status of the Joint WHO/IAEA Research Programme. WHO Offset Publ. No. 5. World Health Organization, Geneva. 45 pp.

Masironi, R., and R. Parr. 1976. Selenium and cardiovascular diseases: preliminary results of the WHO/IAEA joint research programme. Pp. 316–325 in Proceedings of the Symposium on Selenium–Tellurium in the Environment. Industrial Health Foundation, Pittsburgh.

McConnell, K.P., W.L. Broghamer, Jr., A.J. Blotcky, and

O.J. Hurt. 1975. Selenium levels in human blood and tissues in health and disease. J. Nutr. 105:1026–1031.

McConnell, K.P., R.M. Jager, K.I. Bland, and A.J. Blotcky. 1980. The relationship of dietary selenium and breast cancer. J. Surg. Oncol. 15:67–70.

McLeod, B.E., and M.F. Robinson. 1972. Dietary intake of manganese by New Zealand infants during the first six months of life. Br. J. Nutr. 229–232.

McNair, P., S. Kiilerich, C. Christiansen, M.S. Christensen, S. Madsbad, and I. Transbol. 1981. Hyperzincuria in insulin treated diabetes mellitus—its relation to glucose homeostasis and insulin administration. Clin. Chem. Acta 112: 343–348.

Medeiros, D.M., and L.K. Pellum. 1984. Elevation of cadmium, lead, and zinc in the hair of adult black female hypertensives. Bull. Environ. Contam. Toxicol. 32:525–532.

Medeiros, D.M., L.K. Pellum, and B.J. Brown. 1983. The association of selected hair minerals and anthropometric factors with blood pressure in a normotensive adult population. Nutr. Res. 3:51–60.

Medina, D. 1986. Mechanisms of selenium inhibition of tumorigenesis. Adv. Exp. Med. Biol. 206:465–472.

Mehlert, A., and A.T. Diplock. 1985. The glutathione S-transferases in selenium and vitamin E deficiency. Biochem. J. 227:823–831.

Mellow, M.H., E.A. Layne, T.O. Lipman, M. Kaushik, C. Hostetler, and J.C. Smith, Jr. 1983. Plasma zinc and vitamin A in human squamous carcinoma of the esophagus. Cancer 51:1615–1620.

Menkes, M.S., G.W. Comstock, J.P. Vuilleumier, K.J. Helsing, A.A. Rider, and R. Brookmeyer. 1986. Serum beta-carotene, vitamins A and E, selenium, and the risk of lung cancer. N. Engl. J. Med. 315:1250–1254.

Mertz, W. 1979. Chromium—an overview. Pp. 1–14 in D. Shapcott and J. Hubert, eds. Chromium and Metabolism. Elsevier/North-Holland, Amsterdam.

Mertz, W. 1982. Trace minerals and atherosclerosis. Fed. Proc. 41:2807–2812.

Mertz, W., and K. Schwarz. 1955. Impaired intravenous glucose tolerance as an early sign of dietary necrotic liver degeneration. Arch. Biochem. Biophys. 58:504–506.

Meyer, B.R., A. Fischbein, K. Rosenman, Y. Lerman, D.E. Drayer, and M.M. Reidenberg. 1984. Increased urinary enzyme excretion in workers exposed to nephrotoxic chemicals. Am. J. Med. 76:989–998.

Miettinen, T.A., G. Alfthan, J.K. Huttunen, J. Pikkarainen, V. Naukkarinen, S. Mattila, and T. Kumlin. 1983. Serum selenium concentration related to myocardial infarction and fatty acid content of serum lipids. Br. Med. J. 287:517–519.

Miller, G.W., M.N. Egyed, and J.L. Shupe. 1977. Alkaline phosphatase activity, fluoride citric acid, calcium, and phosphorus content in bones of cows with osteoporosis. Fluoride 10:76–82.

Miller, R.G., F.C. Kopfler, K.C. Kelty, J.A. Stober, and N.S. Ulmer. 1984. The occurrence of aluminum in drinking water. J. Am. Water Works Assoc. 77:84–91.

Mills, B.J., W.L. Broghamer, P.J. Higgins, and R.D. Lindeman. 1984. Inhibition of tumor growth by zinc depletion in rats. J. Nutr. 114:746–752.

Minkel, D.T., P.J. Dolhun, B.L. Calhoun, L.A. Saryan, and D.H. Petering. 1979. Zinc deficiency and growth of Ehrlich ascites tumor. Cancer Res. 39:2451–2456.

Mittra, I., J.L. Hayward, and A.S. McNeilly. 1974. Hypothalamic–pituitary–prolactin axis in breast cancer. Lancet 1: 885–889.

Miyake, M., N. Akamatsu, T. Ono, and H. Koyama. 1979. Mutagenicity of metal cations in cultured cells from Chinese hamster. Mutat. Res. 68:259–263.

Mohamed, A.H., and M.E.W. Chandler. 1976. Cytological effects of sodium fluoride on mitotic and meiotic chromosomes of mice. Presented at American Chemical Society, 172nd National Meeting, San Francisco, August 29–September. 3 pp.

Moldrup, A.M. 1984. Cadmium in Foods With a Special Emphasis on Cadmium in Grain Products. Ph.D. thesis, University of Copenhagen.

Moore, J.A., R. Noiva, and I.C. Wells. 1984. Selenium concentrations in plasma of patients with arteriographically defined coronary atherosclerosis. Clin. Chem. 30:1171–1173.

Moore, M.R., P.A. Meredith, A. Goldberg, K.E. Carr, P.G. Toner, and T.D.V. Lawrie. 1975. Cardiac effects of lead in drinking water of rats. Clin. Sci. Mol. Med. 49:337–341.

Morton, W., G. Starr, D. Pohl, J. Stoner, S. Wagner, and D. Weswig. 1976. Skin cancer and water arsenic in Lane County, Oregon. Cancer 37:2523–2532.

Mossop, R.T. 1983. Effects of chromium III on fasting blood glucose, cholesterol and cholesterol HDL levels in diabetics. Cent. Afr. J. Med. 29:80–82.

Mukherjee, R.W., and F.H. Sobels. 1968. The effects of sodium fluoride and iodoacetamide on mutation induction by x-irradiation in mature spermatozoa of Drosophila. Mutat. Res. 6:217–225.

Nakamuro, K., K. Yoshikawa, Y. Sayato, H. Kurata, M. Tonomura, and A. Tonomura. 1976. Studies on selenium-related compounds. V. Cytogenetic effect and reactivity with DNA. Mutat. Res. 40:177–183.

Needleman, H.L., C. Gunnoe, A. Leviton, R. Reed, H. Peresie, C. Maher, and P. Barrett. 1979. Deficits in psychological and classroom performance of children with elevated dentine lead levels. N. Engl. J. Med. 300:689–695.

Nelson, A.A., O.G. Fitzhugh, and H.O. Calvery. 1943. Liver tumors following cirrhosis caused by selenium in rats. Cancer Res. 3:230–236.

Newbrun, E., ed. 1975. Fluorides and Dental Caries, 2nd ed: Contemporary Concepts for Practitioners and Students. C.C. Thomas, Springfield, Ill. 181 pp.

Newman, J.A., V.E. Archer, G. Saccomanno, M. Kuschner, O. Auerbach, R.D. Grondahl, and J.C. Wilson. 1976. Histologic types of bronchogenic carcinoma among members of copper-mining and smelting communities. Ann. N.Y. Acad. Sci. 271:260–268.

NIDR (National Institute of Dental Research). 1981. The Prevalence of Dental Caries in United States Children: 1979–1980. NIH Publ. No. 82-2245. National Caries Program, National Institutes of Health, Public Health Service, U.S. Department of Health and Human Services, Bethesda, Md. 159 pp.

Nielsen, F.H. 1982. Possible future implications of nickel, arsenic, silicon, vanadium, and other ultratrace elements in human nutrition. Pp. 379–404 in A.S. Prasad, ed. Clinical, Biochemical, and Nutritional Aspects of Trace Elements: Current Topics in Nutrition and Disease, Vol. 6. Alan R. Liss, New York.

Nielsen, F.H., and W. Mertz. 1984. Other trace elements. Pp. 607–618 in R.E. Olson, H.P. Broquist, C.O. Chichester, W.J. Darby, A.C. Kolbye, Jr., and R.M. Stalvey, eds.

Nutrition Reviews' Present Knowledge in Nutrition. The Nutrition Foundation, Washington, D.C.

Nishioka, H. 1975. Mutagenic activities of metal compounds in bacteria. Mutat. Res. 31:185–189.

Nixon, J.M., and R.G. Carpenter. 1974. Mortality in areas containing natural fluoride in their water supplies, taking account of socioenvironmental factors and water hardness. Lancet 2:1068–1071.

Nogawa, K., E. Kobayashi, and F. Konishi. 1981. Comparison of bone lesions in chronic cadmium intoxication and vitamin D deficiency. Environ. Res. 24:233–249.

Nordberg, G.F., T. Kjellström, and M. Nordberg. 1985. Kinetics and metabolism. Pp. 103–178 in L. Friberg, C.G. Elinder, T. Kjellström, and G.F. Nordberg, eds. Cadmium and Health: A Toxicological and Epidemiological Appraisal, Vol. I. Exposure, Dose, and Metabolism. CRC Press, Boca Raton, Fla.

Nordenson, I., G. Beckman, L. Beckman, and S. Nordström. 1978. Occupational and environmental risks in and around a smelter in northern Sweden. II. Chromosomal aberrations in workers exposed to arsenic. Hereditas 88:47–50.

NRC (National Research Council). 1971. Fluorides. Report of the Committee on Biologic Effects of Atmospheric Pollutants. National Academy of Sciences, Washington, D.C. 295 pp.

NRC (National Research Council). 1977a. Arsenic. Report of the Committee on Medical and Biologic Effects of Environmental Pollutants, Division of Medical Sciences, Assembly of Life Sciences. National Academy of Sciences, Washington, D.C. 332 pp.

NRC (National Research Council). 1977b. Drinking Water and Health, Vol. 1. Report of the Safe Drinking Water Committee, Advisory Center on Toxicology, Assembly of Life Sciences, National Academy of Sciences, Washington, D.C. 939 pp.

NRC (National Research Council). 1977c. Medical and Biological Effects of Environmental Pollutants: Copper. Report of the Committee on Medical and Biologic Effects of Environmental Pollutants, Division of Medical Sciences, Assembly of Life Sciences, National Academy of Sciences, Washington, D.C. 115 pp.

NRC (National Research Council). 1980. Magnesium. Pp. 134–136 in Recommended Dietary Allowances, 9th ed. Report of the Committee on Dietary Allowances, Food and Nutrition Board, Division of Biological Sciences, Assembly of Life Sciences. National Academy Press, Washington, D.C.

NRC (National Research Council). 1982. Diet, Nutrition, and Cancer. Report of the Committee on Diet, Nutrition, and Cancer, Assembly of Life Sciences. National Academy Press, Washington, D.C. 478 pp.

NRC (National Research Council). 1983. Selenium in Nutrition, rev. ed. Report of the Subcommittee on Selenium, Committee on Animal Nutrition, Board on Agriculture. National Academy Press, Washington, D.C. 174 pp.

Oberly, T.J., C.E. Piper, and D.S. McDonald. 1982. Mutagenicity of metal salts in the C51784 mouse lymphoma assay. J. Toxicol. Environ. Health 9:367–376.

O'Dell, B.L. 1976. Biochemistry of copper. Med. Clin. North Am. 60:687–703.

Offenbacher, E.G., and F.X. Pi-Sunyer. 1980. Beneficial effect of chromium-rich yeast on glucose tolerance and blood lipids. Diabetes 29:919–925.

Offenbacher, E.G., and F.X. Pi-Sunyer. 1983. Temperature and pH effects on the release of chromium from stainless steel into water and fruit juices. J. Agric. Food Chem. 31:89–92.

Ohno, H., F. Hanaoka, and M.A. Yamada. 1982. Inducibility of sister chromatid exchanges by heavy metal ions. Mutat. Res. 104:141–145.

Ohshima, M., and J.M. Ward. 1984. Promotion of N-methyl-N-nitrosourea-induced thyroid tumors by iodine deficiency in F344/NCr rats. J. Natl. Cancer Inst. 73:289–296.

Ohshima, M., and J.M. Ward. 1986. Dietary iodine deficiency as a tumor promoter and carcinogen in male F344/NCr rats. Cancer Res. 46:877–883.

Oldham, P.D., and D.J. Newell. 1977. Fluoridation of water supplies and cancer—a possible association? Appl. Statist. 26:125–135.

Oster, O., M. Drexler, J. Schenk, T. Meinertz, W. Kasper, C.J. Schuster, and W. Prellwitz. 1986. The serum selenium concentration of patients with acute myocardial infarction. Ann. Clin. Res. 18:36–42.

Ostergaard, K. 1978. Renal cadmium concentration in relation to smoking habits and blood pressure. Acta Med. Scand. 203:379–383.

Otto, D., G. Robinson, S. Baumann, S. Schoeder, P. Mushak, D. Kleinbaum, and L. Boone. 1985. 5-year follow-up study of children with low-to-moderate lead absorption: electrophysiological evaluation. Environ. Res. 38:168–186.

Overvad, K., E.B. Thorling, P. Bjerring, and P. Ebbesen. 1985. Selenium inhibits UV-light-induced skin carcinogenesis in hairless mice. Cancer Lett. 27:163–170.

Palmer, W.G., and D.A. Creasia. 1984. Metabolism of 7,12-dimethylbenz(a)anthracene by alveolar macrophages containing ingested ferric oxide, aluminum oxide or carbon particles. J. Environ. Pathol. Toxicol. Oncol. 5:261–270.

Pandit, A.N., and S.A. Bhave. 1983. Cooper and Indian childhood cirrhosis. Indian Pediatr. 20:893–899.

Paton, G.R., and A.C. Allison. 1972. Chromosome damage in human cell cultures induced by metal salts. Mutat. Res. 16:332–336.

Patrono, C., F.E. Preston, and J. Vermylen. 1984. Platelet and vascular arachidonic acid metabolites: can they help detect a tendency towards thrombosis? Br. J. Haematol. 57:209–212.

Pence, B.C., and F. Buddingh. 1985. Effect of dietary selenium deficiency on incidence and size of 1,2-dimethylhydrazine-induced colon tumors in rats. J. Nutr. 115:1196–1202.

Pendergrast, W.J., B.K. Milmore, and S.C. Marcus. 1961. Thyroid cancer and thyrotoxicosis in the United States: their relation to endemic goiter. J. Chronic Dis. 13:22–38.

Pennington, J.A., D.B. Wilson, R.F. Newell, B.F. Harland, R.D. Johnson, and J.E. Vanderveen. 1984. Selected minerals in foods surveys, 1974 to 1981/82. J. Am. Diet. Assoc. 84:771–780.

Pennington, J.A., D.E. Young, D.B. Wilson, R.D. Johnson, and J.E. Vanderveen. 1986. Mineral content of foods and total diets: the Selected Minerals in Foods Survey, 1982 to 1984. J. Am. Diet. Assoc. 86:876–891.

Perl, D.P. 1985. Relationship of aluminum to Alzheimer's disease. Environ. Health Perspect. 63:149–153.

Perl, D.P., and A.R. Brody. 1980. Alzheimer's disease: x-ray spectrometric evidence of aluminum accumulation in neurofibrillary tangle-bearing neurons. Science 208:297–299.

Perry, H.M., Jr., and S.J. Kopp. 1983. Does cadmium contribute to human hypertension. Sci. Total Environ. 26:223–232.

Perry, H.M., Jr., E.F. Perry, and M.W. Erlanger. 1980. Possible influence of heavy metals in cardiovascular disease: introduction and overview. J. Environ. Pathol. Toxicol. 4:195–203.

Pershagen, G. 1981. The carcinogenicity of arsenic. Environ. Health Perspect. 40:93–100.

Pershagen, G., S. Wall, A. Taube, and L. Linnman. 1981. On the interaction between occupational arsenic exposure and smoking and its relationship to lung cancer. Scand. J. Work Environ. Health 7:302–309.

Petres, J., and A. Berger. 1972. The effect of inorganic arsenic on DNA-synthesis of human lymphocytes in vitro. Arch. Dermatol. Forsch. 242:343–352.

Pidduck, H.G., P.J. Wren, and D.A. Evans. 1970. Hyperzincuria of diabetes mellitus and possible genetical implications of this observation. Diabetes 19:240–247.

Pigott, G.H., B.A. Gaskell, and J. Ishmael. 1981. Effects of long term inhalation of alumina fibres in rats. Br. J. Exp. Pathol. 62:323–331.

Pimentel, J.C., and A.P. Menezes. 1977. Liver disease in vineyard sprayers. Gastroenterology 72:275–283.

Piomelli, S., C. Seaman, D. Zullow, A. Curran, and B. Davidow. 1982. Threshold for lead damage to heme synthesis in urban children. Proc. Natl. Acad. Sci. U.S.A. 79: 3335–3339.

Pirkle, J.L., J. Schwartz, J.R. Landis, and W.R. Harlan. 1985. The relationship between blood lead levels and blood pressure and its cardiovascular risk implications. Am. J. Epidemiol. 121:246–258.

Pi-Sunyer, F.X., and E.G. Offenbacher. 1984. Chromium. Pp. 571–586 in R.E. Olson, H.P. Broquist, C.O. Chichester, W.J. Darby, A.C. Kolbye, Jr., and R.M. Stalvey, eds. Nutrition Reviews' Present Knowledge in Nutrition. Nutrition Foundation, Washington, D.C.

Pocock, S.J., A.G. Shaper, D. Ashby, T. Delves, and T.P. Whitehead. 1984. Blood lead concentration, blood pressure, and renal function. Br. Med. J. 289:872–874.

Poirier, L.A., K.S. Kasprzak, K.L. Hoover, and M.L. Wenk. 1983. Effects of calcium and magnesium acetates on the carcinogenicity of cadmium chloride in Wistar rats. Cancer Res. 43:4575–4581.

Pollack, R.L., and E. Kravitz, eds. 1985. Nutrition in Oral Health and Disease. Lea & Febiger, Philadelphia. 483 pp.

Poswillo, D.E., and B.Cohen. 1971. Inhibition of carcinogenesis by dietary zinc. Nature 231:447–448.

Potts, C.L. 1965. Cadmium proteinuria—the health of battery workers exposed to cadmium oxide dust. Ann. Occup. Hyg. 8:55–61.

Power, G.R., and J.D. Gay. 1986. Sodium fluoride in the treatment of osteoporosis. Clin. Invest. Med. 9:41–43.

Prasad, A.S., G.J. Brewer, E.B. Schoomaker, and P. Rabbani. 1978. Hypocupremia induced by zinc therapy in adults. J. Am. Med. Assoc. 240:2166–2168.

Prime, S.S., D.G. MacDonald, D.R. Sawyer, and J. Rennie. 1986. The effect of iron deficiency on early oral carcinogenesis in the rat. J. Oral Pathol. 15:265–267.

Punsar, S., and M.J. Karvonen. 1979. Drinking water quality and sudden death: observations from west and east Finland. Cardiology 64:24–34.

Punsar, S., O. Erametsa, M.J. Karvonen, A. Ryhanen, P. Hilska, and H. Vornamo. 1975. Coronary heart disease and drinking water. A search in two Finnish male cohorts for epidemiologic evidence of a water factor. J. Chronic Dis. 28: 259–287.

Rabinowitz, M.B., H.C. Gonick, S.R. Levin, and M.B. Davidson. 1983. Effects of chromium and yeast supplements on carbohydrate and lipid metabolism in diabetic men. Diabetes Care 6:319–327.

Ranade, S.S., S. Shah, and P. Haria. 1979. Transition metals in an experimental tumor system. Experientia 35:460–461.

Reddy, B.S., and T. Tanaka. 1986. Interactions of selenium deficiency, vitamin E, polyunsaturated fat, and saturated fat on azoxymethane-induced colon carcinogenesis in small F344 rats. J. Natl. Cancer Inst. 76:1157–1162.

Reeves, J.D., E. Vichinsky, J. Addiego, Jr., and B.H. Lubin. 1983. Iron deficiency in health and disease. Adv. Pediatr. 30:281–320.

Reichlmayr-Lais, A.M., and M. Kirchgessner. 1981. Essentiality of lead for growth and metabolism. Z. Tierphysiol. Tierernahr. Futtermittelkd. 46:1–8.

Reinstein, N.H., B. Lönnerdal, C.L. Keen, and L.S. Hurley. 1984. Zinc–copper interactions in the pregnant rat: fetal outcome and maternal and fetal zinc, copper and iron. J. Nutr. 114:1266–1279.

Reiser, S., J.C. Smith, W. Mertz, J.T. Holbrook, D.J. Scholfield, A.S. Powell, W.K. Canfield, and J.J. Canary. 1985. Indices of copper status in humans consuming a typical American diet containing either fructose or starch. Am. J. Clin. Nutr. 42:242–253.

Revis, N.W., T.C. Major, and C.Y. Horton. 1983. The response of the adrenergic system in the cadmium induced hypertension. J. Am. Coll. Toxicol. 2:165.

Riales, R., and M.J. Albrink. 1981. Effect of chromium chloride supplementation on glucose tolerance and serum lipids including high-density lipoprotein of adult men. Am. J. Clin. Nutr. 34:2670–2678.

Riggs, B.L., S.F. Hodgson, D.L. Hoffman, P.J. Kelly, K.A. Johnson, and D. Taves. 1980. Treatment of primary osteoporosis with fluoride and calcium. Clinical tolerance and fracture occurrence. J. Am. Med. Assoc. 243:446–449.

Riggs, B.L., E. Seeman, S.F. Hodgson, D.R. Taves, and W.M. O'Fallon. 1982. Effect of the fluoride/calcium regimen on vertebral fracture occurrence in postmenopausal osteoporosis. Comparison with conventional therapy. N. Engl. J. Med. 306:446–450.

Rivedal, E., and T. Sanner. 1981. Metal salts as promoters of in vitro morphological transformation of hamster embryo initiated by benzoapyrene. Cancer Res. 41:2950–2958.

Roat, J.W., A. Wald, H. Mendelow, and K.I. Pataki. 1982. Hepatic angiosarcoma associated with short-term arsenic ingestion. Am. J. Med. 73:933–936.

Robinson, M.F., P.J. Godfrey, C.D. Thomson, H.M. Rea, and A.M. van Rij. 1979. Blood selenium and glutathione peroxidase activity in normal subjects and in surgical patients with and without cancer in New Zealand. Am. J. Clin. Nutr. 32:1477–1485.

Robinson, T.R. 1976. The health of long service tetraethyl lead workers. J. Occup. Med. 18:31–40.

Rockette, H.E., and V.C. Arena. 1983. Mortality studies of aluminum reduction plant workers: potroom and carbon department. J. Occup. Med. 25:549–557.

Roe, F.J.C., C.E. Dukes, K. M. Cameron, R.C.B. Pugh, and B.C.V. Mitchley. 1964. Cadmium neoplasia: testicular atrophy and Leydig cell hyperplasia and neoplasia in rats and mice following the subcutaneous injection of cadmium salts. Br. J. Cancer 18:674–681.

Rogot, E., A.R. Sharrett, M. Feinleib, and R.R. Fabsitz. 1978. Trends in urban mortality in relation to fluoridation status. Am. J. Epidemiol. 107:104–112.

Rosenkranz, H.S., and L.A. Poirier. 1979. Evaluation of the mutagenicity and DNA-modifying activity of carcinogens and noncarcinogens in microbial systems. J. Natl. Cancer Inst. 62:873–892.

Rossi, M.A., and S.V. Carillo. 1983. Electron microscopic study on the cardiac hypertrophy induced by iron deficiency anaemia in the rat. Br. J. Exp. Pathol. 64:373–387.

Rossi, M.A., S.V. Carillo, and J.S. Oliveira. 1981. The effect of iron deficiency anemia in the rat on catecholamine levels and heart morphology. Cardiovasc. Res. 15:313–319.

Rossman, T.G. 1981a. Effect of metals on mutagenesis and DNA repair. Environ. Health Perspect. 40:187–195.

Rossman, T.G. 1981b. Enhancement of UV-mutagenesis by low concentrations of arsenite in E. coli. Mutat. Res. 91: 207–211.

Rossman, T.G., and M. Molina. 1986. The genetic toxicology of metal compounds. II. Enhancement of ultraviolet light-induced mutagenesis in Escherichia coli WP2. Environ. Mutagen 8:263–271.

Rossman, T.G., D. Stone, M. Molina, and W. Troll. 1980. Absence of arsenite mutagenicity in E. coli and Chinese hamster cells. Environ. Mutagen 2:371–379.

Rossman, T.G., M. Molina, and L.W. Meyer. 1984. The genetic toxicology of metal compounds. I. Induction of lambda prophage in E. coli WP2s (lambda). Environ. Mutagen 6:59–69.

Rubenstein, A.H., N.W. Levin, and G.A. Elliott. 1962. Manganese-induced hypoglycemia. Lancet 2:1348–1351.

Rutter, M. 1980. Raised lead levels and impaired cognitive/behavioral functioning: a review of the evidence. Dev. Med. Child. Neurol. Suppl. 42:1–36.

Ryan, J.A., H.R. Pahren, and J.B. Lucas. 1982. Controlling cadmium in the human food chain: a review and rationale based on health effects. Environ. Res. 28:251–302.

Salonen, J.T., G. Alfthan, J.K. Huttunen, J. Pikkarainen, and P. Puska. 1982. Association between cardiovascular death and myocardial infarction and serum selenium in a matched-pair longitudinal study. Lancet 2:175–179.

Salonen, J.T., G. Alfthan, J.K. Huttunen, and P. Puska. 1984. Association between serum selenium and the risk of cancer. Am. J. Epidemiol. 120:342–349.

Salonen, J.T., R. Salonen, R. Lappeteläinen, P.H. Mäenpää, G. Alfthan, and P. Puska. 1985a. Risk of cancer in relation to serum concentrations of selenium and vitamins A and E: matched case-control analysis of prospective data. Br. Med. J. 290:417–420.

Salonen, J.T., R. Salonen, I. Penttilä, J. Herranen, M. Jauhiainen, M. Kantola, R. Lappeteläinen, P.H. Mäenpää, G. Alfthan, and P. Puska. 1985b. Serum fatty acids, apolipoproteins, selenium and vitamin antioxidants and the risk of death from coronary artery disease. Am. J. Cardiol. 56:226–231.

Sambade, M.C., V.S. Gonçalves, M. Dias, and M.A. Sobrinho-Simoes. 1983. High relative frequency of thyroid papillary carcinoma in Northern Portugal. Cancer 51:1754–1759.

Sanders, C.L., and J.A. Mahaffey. 1984. Carcinogenicity of single and multiple intratracheal instillations of cadmium oxide in the rat. Environ. Res. 33:227–233.

Sauer, H.I., D.W. Parke, and M. Neill. 1971. Associations between drinking water and death rates. Pp. 318–325 in D.D. Hemphill, ed. Trace Substances in Environmental Health. University of Missouri Press, Columbia, Mo.

Schlage, C., and B. Wortberg. 1972. Manganese in the diet of healthy preschool and school children. Acta Paediatr. Scand. 61:648–652.

Schoene, N.W., V.C. Morris, and O.A. Levander. 1986. Altered arachidonic acid metabolism in platelets and aortas from selenium-deficient rats. Nutr. Res. 6:75–83.

Schottenfeld, D., and J.F. Fraumeni, Jr., eds. 1982. Cancer Epidemiology and Prevention. W.B. Saunders, Philadelphia. 1173 pp.

Schrauzer, G.N. 1979. Trace elements in carcinogenesis. Pp. 219–244 in H.H. Draper, ed. Advances in Nutritional Research, Vol. 2. Plenum Press, New York.

Schrauzer, G.N., and D. Ishmael. 1974. Effects of selenium and of arsenic on the genesis of spontaneous mammary tumors in inbred C3H mice. Ann. Clin. Lab. Sci. 4:441–447.

Schrauzer, G.N., D.A. White, and C.J. Schneider. 1977a. Cancer mortality correlation studies. III. Statistical associations with dietary selenium intakes. Bioinorg. Chem. 7:23–34.

Schrauzer, G.N., D.A. White, and C.J. Schneider. 1977b. Cancer mortality correlation studies. IV. Associations with dietary intakes and blood levels of certain trace elements, notably Se-antagonists. Bioinorg. Chem. 7:35–56.

Schrauzer, G.N., T. Molenaar, S. Mead, K. Kuehn, H. Yamamoto, and E. Araki. 1985. Selenium in the blood of Japanese and American women with and without breast cancer and fibrocystic disease. Jpn. J. Cancer Res. 76:374–377.

Schroeder, H.A. 1966. Municipal drinking water and cardiovascular death rates. J. Am. Med. Assoc. 195:125–129.

Schroeder, H.A. 1968. The role of chromium in mammalian nutrition. Am. J. Clin. Nutr. 21:230–244.

Schroeder, H.A., and M. Mitchener. 1971. Selenium and tellurium in rats: effect on growth, survival and tumors. J. Nutr. 101:1531–1540.

Schroeder, H.A., J.J. Balassa, and I.H. Tipton. 1962. Abnormal trace metals in man. J. Chronic Dis. 15:941–964.

Schroeder, H.A., J.J. Balassa, and W.H. Vinton, Jr. 1964. Chromium, lead, cadmium, nickel and titanium in mice: effect on mortality, tumors and tissue levels. J. Nutr. 83: 239–250.

Schroeder, H.A., J.J. Balassa, and W.H. Vinton, Jr. 1965. Chromium, cadmium and lead in rats: effects on life span, tumors and tissue levels. J. Nutr. 86:51–66.

Schroeder, H.A., A.P. Nason, and I.H. Tipton. 1970a. Chromium deficiency as a factor in artherosclerosis. J. Chronic Dis. 23:123–142.

Schroeder, H.A., M. Mitchener, and A.P. Nason. 1970b. Zirconium, niobium, antimony, vanadium and lead in rats: life term studies. J. Nutr. 100:59–68.

Schwartz, M.K. 1975. Role of trace elements in cancer. Cancer Res. 35:3481–3487.

Schwarz, K. 1977. Essentiality versus toxicity of metals. Pp. 3–22 in S.S. Brown, ed. Clinical Chemistry and Chemical Toxicology of Metals. Elsevier/North-Holland Biomedical Press, Amsterdam.

Scott, R., and E. Aughey. 1978. Methyl cholanthrene and cadmium induced changes in rat prostate. Br. J. Urol. 50: 25–28.

Selevan, S.G., P.J. Landrigan, F.B. Stern, and J.H. Jones. 1985. Mortality of lead smelter workers. Am. J. Epidemiol. 122:673–683.

Shamberger, R.J. 1970. Relationship of selenium to cancer. I. Inhibitory effect of selenium on carcinogenesis. J. Natl. Cancer Inst. 44:931–936.

Shamberger, R.J., and D.V. Frost. 1969. Possible protective effect of selenium against human cancer. Can. Med. Assoc. J. 100:682.

Shamberger, R.J., and C.E. Willis. 1971. Selenium distribution and human cancer mortality. Crit. Rev. Clin. Lab. Sci. 2:211–221.

Shamberger, R.J., E. Rukovena, A.K. Longfield, S.A. Tytko, S. Deodhar, and C.E. Willis. 1973. Antioxidants and cancer. I. Selenium in the blood of normals and cancer patients. J. Natl. Cancer Inst. 50:863–870.

Shamberger, R.J., S.A. Tytko, and C.E. Willis. 1976. Antioxidants and cancer. Part VI. Selenium and age-adjusted human cancer mortality. Arch. Environ. Health 31:231–235.

Shamberger, R.J., K.D. Beaman, C.L. Corlett, and B.L. Kasten. 1978. Effect of selenium and other antioxidants on the mutagenicity of malonaldehye. Fed. Proc. 37:261.

Shani, J., Z. Ahronson, F.G. Sulman, W. Mertz, G. Frenkel, and P.F. Kraicer. 1972. Insulin-potentiating effect of salt bush (*Atriplex halimus*) ashes. Isr. J. Med. Sci. 8:757–758.

Sharma, V.P., V. Parikh, and L.M. Bhandari. 1984. Serum copper and zinc levels in patients with solid tumours. Indian J. Cancer 21:1–6.

Shaw, J.H., ed. 1954. Fluoridation as a Public Health Measure. American Association for the Advancement of Science, Washington, D.C. 240 pp.

Sheffet, A., I. Thind, A.M. Miller, and D.B. Louria. 1982. Cancer mortality in a pigment plant utilizing lead and zinc chromates. Arch. Environ. Health 37:44–52.

Shigematsu, I. 1984. The epidemiological approach to cadmium pollution in Japan. Ann. Acad. Med. Singapore 13:231–236.

Shigematsu, I., M. Minowa, T. Yoshida, and K. Miyamoto. 1979. Recent results of health examinations on the general population in cadmium-polluted and control areas in Japan. Environ. Health Perspect. 28:205–210.

Shirachi, D.Y., M.G. Johansen, J.P. McGowan, and S.H. Tu. 1983. Tumorigenic effect of sodium arsenite in rat kidney. Proc. West. Pharmacol. Soc. 26:413–415.

Shirai, T., M. Ohshima, A. Masuda, S. Tamano, and N. Ito. 1984. Promotion of 2-(ethylnitrosamino)ethanol-induced renal carcinogenesis in rats by nephrotoxic compounds: positive responses with folic acid, basic lead acetate, and N-(3,5-dichlorophenyl)succinimide but not with 2,3-dibromo-1-propanol phosphate. J. Natl. Cancer Inst. 72:477–482.

Shiraishi, Y., H. Kurahashi, and T.H. Yosida. 1972. Chromosomal aberrations in cultured human leukocytes induced by cadmium sulfide. Proc. Jpn. Acad. 48:133–137.

Shore, D., and R.J. Wyatt. 1983. Aluminum and Alzheimer's disease. J. Nerv. Ment. Dis. 171:553–558.

Shupe, J.L., M.L. Miner, D.A. Greenwood, L.E. Harris, and G.E. Stoddard. 1962. The effect of fluorine on dairy cattle. II. Clinical and pathologic effects. Am. J. Vet. Res. 24:964–979.

Simmon, V.F. 1979. In vitro assays for recombinogenic activity of chemical carcinogens and related compounds with Saccharomyces cerevisiae D₃. J. Natl. Cancer Inst. 62:901–909.

Simonato, L. 1981. Carcinogenic risk in the aluminum production industry: an epidemiological overview. Med. Lav. 72:266–276.

Simonoff, M. 1984. Chromium deficiency and cardiovascular risk. Cardiovasc. Res. 18:591–596.

Simonoff, M., Y. Llabador, G.N. Simonoff, P. Besse, and C. Conri. 1984a. Cineangiographically determined coronary artery disease and plasma chromium level for 150 subjects. Nucl. Instrum. Methods 231:368–372.

Simonoff, M., Y. Llabador, C. Hamon, P.A. MacKenzie, and G.N. Simonoff. 1984b. Low plasma chromium in patients with coronary artery and heart diseases. Biol. Trace Element Res. 26:431–439.

Singer, L., and R. Ophaug. 1979. Total fluoride intake of infants. Pediatrics 63:460–466.

Sirover, M.A., and L.A. Loeb. 1976. Infidelity of DNA synthesis in vitro: screening for potential metal mutagens or carcinogens. Science 194:1434–1436.

Sirover, M.A., and L.A. Loeb. 1977. On the fidelity of DNA replication: effect of metal activators during synthesis with avian myeloblastosis virus DNA polymerase. J. Biol. Chem. 252:3606–3610.

Sissoëff, I., J. Grisvard, and E. Guillé. 1976. Studies on metal ions–DNA interactions: specific behaviour of reiterative DNA sequences. Prog. Biophys. Mol. Biol. 31:165–199.

Skerving, S., K. Hansson, and J. Lindsten. 1970. Chromosome breakerage in humans exposed to methyl mercury through fish consumption. Arch. Environ. Health 21:133–139.

Smialowicz, R.J., R.R. Rogers, M.M. Riddle, R.W. Luebke, D.G. Rowe, and R.J. Garner. 1984. Manganese chloride enhances murine cell-mediated cytotoxicity: effects on natural killer cells. J. Immunopharmacol. 6:1–23.

Smith, J.C., Jr., H.H. Hansen, M.P. Howard, L.D. McBean, and J.A. Halsted. 1971. Plasma-zinc concentration in patients with bronchogenic cancer. Lancet 2:1323.

Smith, M. 1985. Recent work on low level exposure and its impact on behavior, intelligence, and learning: a review. J. Am. Acad. Child. Psychiatry 24:24–32.

Solomons, N.W., and R.M. Russell. 1980. The interaction of vitamin A and zinc: implications for human nutrition. Am. J. Clin. Nutr. 33:2031–2040.

Sorahan, T., and J.A. Waterhouse. 1983. Mortality study of nickel-cadmium battery workers by the method of regression models in life tables. Br. J. Ind. Med. 40:293–300.

Spencer, H., and L. Kramer. 1985. Osteoporosis: calcium, fluoride, and aluminum interactions. J. Am. Coll. Nutr. 4:121–128.

Spencer, H., L. Kramer, C. Norris, and E. Wiatrowski. 1981. Effect of aluminum hydroxide on plasma fluoride and fluoride excretion during a high fluoride intake in man. Toxicol. Appl. Pharmacol. 58:140–144.

Stadel, B.V. 1976. Dietary iodine and risk of breast, endometrial, and ovarian cancer. Lancet 1:890–891.

Stanbury, J.B., and B.S. Hetzel, eds. 1980. Endemic Goiter and Endemic Cretinism: Iodine Nutrition in Health and Disease. Wiley, New York. 606 pp.

Stevens, R.G., R.P. Beasley, and B.S. Blumberg. 1986. Iron-binding proteins and risk of cancer in Taiwan. J. Natl. Cancer Inst. 76:605–610.

Stocks, P., and R.I. Davies. 1964. Zinc and copper content of soils associated with the incidence of cancer of the stomach and other organs. Br. J. Cancer 18:14–24.

Stoner, G.D., M.B. Shimkin, M.C. Troxell, T.L. Thompson, and L.S. Terry. 1976. Test for carcinogenicity of metallic compounds by the pulmonary tumor response in strain A mice. Cancer Res. 36:1744–1747.

Strain, W.H., E.G. Mansour, A. Flynn, W.J. Pories, A.J. Tomaro, and O.A. Hill, Jr. 1972. Plasma-zinc concentration in patients with bronchogenic cancer. Lancet 1:1021–1022.

Strohmeyer, G., C. Niederau, and W. Stremmel. 1988. Survival and causes of death in hemochromatosis: observations in 163 patients. Ann. N.Y. Acad. Sci. 526:245–257.

Sullivan, J.L. 1986. Sex, iron, and heart disease. Lancet 2: 1162.

Sundström, H., E. Yrjänheikki, and A. Kauppila. 1984. Low serum selenium concentration in patients with cervical or endometrial cancer. Int. J. Gynaecol. Obstet. 22:35–40.

Takashima, M., S. Moriwaki, and Y. Itokawa. 1980. Osteomalacic change induced by long-term administration of cadmium to rats. Toxicol. Appl. Pharmacol. 54:223–228.

Takenaka, S., H. Oldiges, H. Koenig, D. Hochrainer, and G. Oberdoerster. 1983. Carcinogenicity of cadmium chloride aerosols in W-rats. J. Natl. Cancer Inst. 70:367–371.

Talwar, S.J., S. Qadry, K.K. Pillai, and R.G. Arora. 1985. Cadmium zinc antagonism in the hypertensive rat (abstract 004). Indian J. Pharm. 17 suppl. 1.

Tanner, D.C., and M.M. Lipsky. 1984. Effect of lead acetate on N-(4'-fluoro-4-biphenyl)acetamide-induced renal carcinogenesis in the rat. Carcinogenesis 5:1109–1113.

Tarugi, P., S. Calandra, P. Borella, and G.F. Vivoli. 1982. Heavy metals and experimental atherosclerosis. Effect of lead intoxication on rabbit plasma lipoproteins. Atherosclerosis 45:221–234.

Taves, D.R. 1979. Claims of harm from fluoridation. Pp. 295–321 in E. Johansen, D.R. Taves, and T.O. Olsen, eds. Continuing Evaluation of the Use of Fluorides. Westview Press, Boulder, Colo.

Taylor, C. 1980. Oral health status in primary school children in two areas of Papua New Guinea 1979: primary results. J. Dent. Res. 59:1773.

Thériault, G., C. Tremblay, S. Cordier, and S. Gingras. 1984. Bladder cancer in the aluminum industry. Lancet 1: 947–950.

Thimaya, S., and S.N. Ganapathy. 1982. Selenium in human hair in relation to age, diet, pathological condition and serum levels. Sci. Total Environ. 24:41–49.

Thun, M.J., T.M. Schnorr, A.B. Smith, W.E. Halperin, and R.A. Lemen. 1985. Mortality among a cohort of U.S. cadmium production workers—an update. J. Natl. Cancer Inst. 74:325–333.

Thurnham, D.I., P. Rathakette, K.M. Hambidge, N. Munoz, and M. Crespi. 1982. Riboflavin, vitamin A and zinc status in Chinese subjects in a high-risk area for oesophageal cancer in China. Hum. Nutr. Clin. Nutr. 36:337–349.

Thurnham, D.I., S.F. Zheng, N. Munoz, M. Crespi, A. Grassi, K.M. Hambidge, and T.F Chai. 1985. Comparison of riboflavin, vitamin A, and zinc status of Chinese populations at high and low risk for esophageal cancer. Nutr. Cancer 7:131–143.

Tiedemann, G., and H.J. Einbrodt. 1982. Mutagen reaction of inorganic arsenic compounds. Wiss. Umwelt. 3:170–173.

Troncoso, J.C., N.H. Sternberger, L.A. Sternberger, P.N. Hoffman, and D.L. Price. 1986. Immunocytochemical studies of neurofilament antigens in the neurofibrillary pathology induced by aluminum. Brain Res. 364:295–300.

Tsapakos, M.J., T.H. Hampton, and K.E. Wetterhahn. 1983. Chromium(VI)-induced DNA lesions and chromium distribution in rat kidney, liver, and lung. Cancer Res. 43:5662–5667.

Tseng, W.P. 1977. Effects and dose-response relationships of skin cancer and blackfoot disease with arsenic. Environ. Health Perspect. 19:109–119.

Tsubaki, T., and K. Irukayama, eds. 1977. Minamata Disease: Methylmercury Poisoning in Minamata and Niigata, Japan. Elsevier Scientific Publishing Co., New York. 317 pp.

Tsuchiya, K. 1977. Various effects of arsenic in Japan depending on type of exposure. Environ. Health Perspect. 19:35–42.

Tsutsui, T., N. Suzuki, and M. Ohmori. 1984. Sodium fluoride induced morphological and neoplastic transformation, chromosome aberrations, sister chromatid exchanges and unscheduled DNA synthesis in cultured Syrian hamster embryo cells. Cancer Res. 44:938–941.

Ulrich, C.E., W. Rinehart, and W. Busey. 1979. Evaluation of the chronic inhalation toxicity of a manganese oxide aerosol. 1. Introduction, experimental design and aerosol generation methods. Am. Ind. Hyg. Assoc. J. 40:238–244.

Umeda, M., and M. Nishimura. 1979. Inducibility of chromosomal aberrations by metal compounds in cultured mammalian cells. Mutat. Res. 67:221–229.

Underwood, E.J. 1977. Trace Elements in Human and Animal Nutrition, 4th ed. Academic Press, New York. 545 pp.

Uriu-Hare, J.Y., J.S. Stern, G.M. Reaven, and C.L Keen. 1985. The effect of maternal diabetes on trace element status and fetal development in the rat. Diabetes 34:1031–1040.

USDA (U.S. Department of Agriculture). 1984. Nationwide Food Consumption Survey. Nutrient Intakes: Individuals in 48 States, Year 1977–78. Report No. I-2. Consumer Nutrition Division, Human Nutrition Information Service, Hyattsville, Md. 439 pp.

USDA (U.S. Department of Agriculture). 1986. Nationwide Food Consumption Survey. Continuing Survey of Food Intakes of Individuals. Men 19–50 Years, 1 Day, 1985. Report No. 85-3. Nutrition Monitoring Division, Human Nutrition Information Service, Hyattsville, Md. 94 pp.

USDA (U.S. Department of Agriculture). 1987a. Nationwide Food Consumption Survey. Continuing Survey of Food Intakes of Individuals. Women 19–50 Years and Their Children 1–5 Years, 1 Day, 1986. Report No. 86-1. Nutrition Monitoring Division, Human Nutrition Information Service, Hyattsville, Md. 98 pp.

USDA (U.S. Department of Agriculture). 1987b. Nationwide Food Consumption Survey. Continuing Survey of Food Intakes of Individuals. Women 19–50 Years and Their Children 1–5 Years, 4 Days, 1985. Report No. 85-4. Nutrition Monitoring Division, Human Nutrition Information Service, Hyattsville, Md. 182 pp.

Uusitupa, M.I.J., J.T. Kumpulainen, E. Voutilainen, K. Hersio, H. Sarlund, P.K. Pyorala, P.E. Kovistoinen, and J.T. Lehto. 1984. Effect of inorganic chromium supplementation on glucose tolerance, insulin response, and serum lipids in noninsulin-dependent diabetics. Am. J. Clin. Nutr. 38:404–410.

Van de Sande, J., L.P. McIntosh, and T.M. Jovin. 1982. Mn and other transition metals at low concentration induce the right-to-left helical transformation poly(dG–dC). Eur. Mol. Biol. Org. J. 1:777–782.

Van Esch, G.J., and R. Kroes. 1969. The induction of renal tumours by feeding basic lead acetate to mice and hamsters. Br. J. Cancer 23:765–771.

Venugopal, B., and T.D. Luckey. 1978. Lead. Pp. 185–195 in Metal Toxicity in Mammals, 2. Chemical Toxicity of Metals and Metalloids. Plenum Press, New York.

Vernie, L.N. 1984. Selenium in carcinogenesis. Biochim. Biophys. Acta 738:203–217.

Victery, W., A.J. Vander, J.M. Shulak, P. Schoeps, and S. Julius. 1982. Lead, hypertension, and the renin-angiotensin system in rats. J. Lab. Clin. Med. 99:354–362.

Virtamo, J., E. Valkeila, G. Alfthan, S. Punsar, J.K. Huttunen, and M.J. Karvonen. 1985. Serum selenium and the risk of coronary heart disease and stroke. Am. J. Epidemiol. 122:276–282.

Vitale, J.J., S.A. Broitman, E. Vavrousek-Jakuba, P.W. Rodday, and L.S. Gottlieb. 1978. The effects of iron deficiency and the quality and quantity of fat on chemically induced cancer. Adv. Exp. Med. Biol. 91:229–242.

Volgarev, M.N., and L.A. Tscherkes. 1967. Further studies in tissue changes associated with sodium selenate. Pp. 179–184 in O.H. Muth, J.E. Oldfield, and P.H. Weswig, eds. Symposium: Selenium in Biomedicine. First International Symposium, Oregon State University, 1966. AVI Publishing Co., Westport, Conn.

Voors, A.W. 1971. Minerals in the municipal water and atherosclerotic heart death. Am. J. Epidemiol. 93:259–266.

Voroshilin, S.I., E.G. Plotko, and V.I. Nikiforova. 1975. Mutagennoe deistvie ftoristogo vodoroda na zhivotnykh. Tsitol. Genet. 9:42–44.

Wahner, H.W., C. Cuello, P. Correa, L.F. Uribe, and E. Gaitan. 1966. Thyroid carcinoma in an endemic goiter area, Cali, Colombia. Am. J. Med. 40:58–66.

Wall, S. 1980. Survival and mortality pattern among Swedish smelter workers. Int. J. Epidemiol. 9:73–87.

Warren, G., P. Schultz, D. Bancroft, K. Bennett, E.H. Abbott, and S. Rogers. 1981. Mutagenicity of a series of hexacoordinate chromium (III) compounds. Mutat. Res. 90: 111–118.

Warshawsky, D., E. Bingham, and R.W. Niemeier. 1984. The effects of a cocarcinogen, ferric oxide, on the metabolism of benzo[a]pyrene in the isolated perfused lung. J. Toxicol. Environ. Health 14:191–209.

Waterhouse, J., C. Muir, P. Correa, and J. Powell, eds. 1976. Cancer Incidence in Five Continents, Vol. 3. IARC Scientific Publ. No. 15. International Agency for Research on Cancer, Lyon, France.

Webster, D.J. 1981. Tumour induction by carcinogens in iron deficient rats. Anticancer Res. 1:293–294.

Wedrychowski, A., W.S. Ward, W.N. Schmidt, and L.S. Hnilica. 1985. Chromium-induced cross-linking of nuclear proteins and DNA. J. Biol. Chem. 260:7150–7155.

Wei, H.J., X.M. Luo, and S.P. Yang. 1985. Effects of molybdenum and tungsten on mammary carcinogenesis in SD rats. J. Natl. Cancer Inst. 74:469–473.

Weinberg, E.D. 1983. Iron in neoplastic disease. Nutr. Cancer 4:223–233.

Weiss, S.T., A. Muñoz, A. Stein, D. Sparrow, and F.E. Speizer. 1986. The relationship of blood lead to blood pressure in a longitudinal study of working men. Am. J. Epidemiol. 123:800–808.

Westermarck, T. 1977. Selenium content of tissues in Finnish infants and adults with various diseases, and studies on the effects of selenium supplementation in neuronal ceroid lipofuscinosis patients. Acta Pharmacol. Toxicol. 41:121–128.

Whanger, P.D. 1979. Cadmium effects in rats on tissue iron, selenium, and blood pressure: blood and hair cadmium in some Oregon residents. Environ. Health Perspect. 28:115–121.

Whelan, P., B.E. Walker, and J. Kelleher. 1983. Zinc, vitamin A and prostatic cancer. Br. J. Urol. 55:525–528.

WHO (World Health Organization). 1972. Evaluation of Certain Food Additives and the Contaminants Mercury,

Lead, and Cadmium. Sixteenth Report of the Joint FAO/WHO Expert Committee on Food Additives. Technical Report Series No. 505. World Health Organization, Geneva. 32 pp.

WHO (World Health Organization). 1978. Evaluation of Certain Food Additives and Contaminants. Twenty-Second Report of the Joint FAO/WHO Expert Committee on Food Additives. Technical Reports Series No. 631. World Health Organization, Geneva. 39 pp.

WHO (World Health Organization). 1988. The Work of WHO 1986–1987. Biennial Report of the Director General to the World Health Assembly and to the United Nations. World Health Organization, Geneva. 250 pp.

Wilkins, J.R., III, and T.H. Sinks, Jr. 1984a. Occupational exposures among fathers of children with Wilms' tumor. J. Occup. Med. 26:427–435.

Wilkins, J.R., III, and T.H. Sinks, Jr. 1984b. Paternal occupation and Wilms' tumour in offspring. J. Epidemiol. Community Health 38:7–11.

Willett, W.C., B.F. Polk, J.S. Morris, M.J. Stampfer, S. Pressel, B. Rosner, J.O. Taylor, K. Schneider, and C.G. Hames. 1983. Prediagnostic serum selenium and the risk of cancer. Lancet 2:130–134.

Williams, B.J., M.R. Hejtmancik, and M. Abreu. 1983. Cardiac effects of lead. Fed. Proc. 42:2989–2993.

Williams, E.D., I. Doniach, O. Bjarnason, and W. Michie. 1977. Thyroid cancer in an iodide rich area: a histopathological study. Cancer 39:215–222.

Wynder, E.L., S. Hultberg, F. Jacobsson, and I.J. Bross. 1957. Environmental factors in cancer of the upper alimentary tract: a Swedish study with special reference to Plummer-Vinson (Paterson-Kelly) syndrome. Cancer 10:470–487.

Yagi, T., and H. Nishioka. 1977. DNA damage and its degradation by metal compounds. Sci. Eng. Rev. Doshisha Univ. 18:63–70.

Yamane, Y., and K. Sakai. 1973. Suppressive effect of concurrent administration of metal salts on carcinogenesis by 3'-methyl-4-(dimethylamino)azobenzene, and the effect of these metals on aminoazo dye metabolism during carcinogenesis. Gann 64:563–573.

Yamane, Y., K. Sakai, M. Ohtawa, N. Murata, T. Yarita, and G. Ide. 1981. Suppressive effect of aluminum chloride administration on mouse lung carcinogenesis by dimethylnitrosamine. Gann 72:992–996.

Yang, G.Q., J.S. Chen, Z.M. Wen, K.Y. Ge, L.Z. Zhu, X.C. Chen, and X.S. Chen. 1984. The role of selenium in Keshan disease. Adv. Nutr. Res. 6:203–231.

Yang, G.Q., P.C. Qian, L.Z. Zhu, J.H. Huang, S.J. Liu, M.D. Lu, and L.Z. Gu. 1987. Human selenium requirement in China. Pp. 589–607 in G.F. Combs, Jr., O.A. Levander, J.E. Spallholz, and J.E. Oldfield, eds. Selenium in Biology and Medicine. Van Nostrand Reinhold Co., New York.

Yang, J.G., J. Morrison-Plummer, and R.F. Burk. 1987. Purification and quantitation of a rat plasma selenoprotein distinct from glutathione perioxidase using monoclonal antibodies. J. Biol. Chem. 262:13372–13375.

Yassin, I., and T. Low. 1975. Caries prevalence in different racial groups of schoolchildren in West Malaysia. Community Dent. Oral Epidemiol. 3:179–183.

Yiamouyiannis, J., and D. Burk. 1977. Fluoridation and cancer: age-dependence of cancer mortality related to artificial fluoridation. Fluoride 10:102–125.

Yost, K.J. 1979. Some aspects of cadmium flow in the U.S. Environ. Health Perspect. 28:5–16.

Yu, S.Y., Y.J. Chu, X.L. Gong, and C. Hou. 1985. Regional variation of cancer mortality incidence and its relation to selenium levels in China. Biol. Trace Element Res. 7:21–29.

Yule, W., and M. Rutter. 1985. Effect of lead on children's behavior and cognitive performance: a critical review. Pp. 211–259 in K.R. Mahaffey, ed. Dietary and Environmental Lead: Human Health Effects. Topics in Environmental Health, Vol. 7. Elsevier Press, Amsterdam.

Zakour, R.A., and B.W. Glickman. 1984. Metal-induced mutagenesis in the lacI gene of Escherichia coli. Mutat. Res. 126:9–18.

Zakour, R.A., T.A. Kunkel, and L.A. Loeb. 1981a. Metal-induced infidelity of DNA synthesis. Environ. Health Perspect. 40:197–205.

Zakour, R.A., L.K. Tkeshelashvili, C.W. Shearman, R.M. Koplitz, and L.A. Loeb. 1981b. Metal-induced infidelity of DNA synthesis. J. Cancer Res. Clin. Oncol. 99:187–196.

Zaldivar, R., and G.L. Ghai. 1980. Clinical epidemiological studies on endemic chronic arsenic poisoning in children and adults, including observations on children with high- and low-intake of dietary arsenic. Zentralbl. Bakteriol. B 170:409–421.

Ziegler, E.E., B.B. Edwards, R.L. Jensen, K.R. Mahaffey, and S.J. Fomon. 1978. Absorption and retention of lead by infants. Pediatr. Res. 12:29–34.

15

Electrolytes

Sodium, potassium, and their attendant anions are important components of all body fluids. Sodium is the major cation of extracellular fluid, and potassium, of intracellular fluid. Complex mechanisms regulate electrolyte concentrations in the body fluids and the volume of both the extracellular and the intracellular fluid compartments. The processes that maintain gradient concentrations of these cations across cell membranes require energy; at least three transport systems seem to be involved. Regulation of fluid volumes and concentrations involves the cardiovascular and endocrine systems, the central nervous system, and the autonomic nervous system; all act chiefly by regulating the rate at which water and electrolytes are excreted by the kidneys.

Archaeological and anthropological studies show that the diets of hunter–gatherers during the Paleolithic period and the diets of present-day traditional societies outside the dominant culture have, with few exceptions, had high levels of potassium and very low levels of sodium (Denton, 1982). Salt has historically been scarce in most regions, and it was highly prized by early humans and by many ancient cultures in Asia, Africa, and Europe. It was used in rituals and for the preservation of food in many primitive cultures. In areas with a scarcity of salt, a mechanism to preserve extracellular fluid volume in the face of dehydration, trauma, hemorrhage, pregnancy, and lacta-

tion would be biologically useful. Thus, the physiology of mammals evolved to foster the conservation of salt by the kidneys, gastrointestinal tract, and sweat glands and to develop a taste for sodium chloride in the tongue and the salt appetite centers in the brain (Denton, 1982).

There is evidence for the existence of salt appetite centers in the central nervous system of some mammals, and a mechanism to taste salt is found in humans and many mammals. Craving for salt develops during acute salt depletion and hypovolemia. Some recent evidence suggests that two ranges of salt appetite exist: the physiological range of salt intake necessary to preserve body fluid volume and maintain sufficient arterial pressure to perfuse tissues adequately; and the higher range of salt appetite, which is determined by a learned desire to ingest salt in excess of physiological need (Beauchamp et al., 1985). Deprivation of these higher levels of salt for several months results in a preference for less salt.

Neolithic agricultural societies developed various methods for preserving and storing foods. For meat and dairy products, they usually used salt. Most modern processing methods, including the processing of grains and refined flours, increase sodium content and reduce potassium, whether needed for preservation or not. More sodium is added during the preparation of foods for the table and at the table itself.

413

EVIDENCE ASSOCIATING ELECTROLYTES WITH CHRONIC DISEASES

Physiological regulating mechanisms normally maintain close control over the concentrations of sodium, potassium, and chloride as well as the total body content of several electrolytes. Failure of regulation profoundly affects body fluid volumes, blood pressure, cardiovascular function, and acid-base balance. Most perturbations in regulation and balance result from disease processes rather than from variations in dietary intake.

Sodium

Physiologic Requirements

In foods, sodium is present mainly in salt (sodium chloride). Sodium bicarbonate, sodium citrate, sodium glutamate, and other sodium salts are also consumed in small amounts. The quantity of dietary sodium is often expressed as milligrams of sodium or sodium chloride. In chemical terms, it may be expressed as mEq of ionized sodium or as mmol of sodium chloride. In this chapter, it is also expressed as milligrams of salt. Since potassium exists in the body in association with various chemicals and the chloride salt of potassium is not predominant, potassium is expressed in grams of elemental potassium and in chemical terms, as mEq.

The basal sodium requirement for growing and adult humans is no greater than 8 to 10 mmol/day (500 mg of sodium chloride) (AAP, 1974; Dahl, 1958) and may be lower. Dahl (1958) reported a mean sodium chloride intake of 10,340 mg (range, 4,000 to 24,200 mg) for 71 working men in New York based on a single 24-hour measurement of urinary excretion. Sanchez-Castillo et al. (1987a,b) performed metabolic balance studies using a lithium chloride marker to trace use of salt in cooking and at the table. Daily sodium chloride excretion over a 12-day period by men was 10,600 ± 0.550 mg and by women was 7,400 ± 2,900 mg. Ten percent of the salt came from the natural salt content of foods, 75% from processing and manufacturing, and 15% from discretionary addition of salt (both in cooking and at the table). Sweat and fecal excretion of sodium in these studies were found to contribute only 2 to 5% of total excretion; the remainder was excreted in the urine (Sanchez-Castillo et al., 1987a). Salt excretion was higher by men than by women and was directly proportional to body weight.

James et al. (1987) reported that the total salt excretion is similar in northern Europe and the United States; the lowest known intake is that of the Yanomami Indians of Brazil, who excrete an average of 1.5 mEq/day (87 mg of sodium chloride) in their urine (Oliver et al., 1975) and presumably lose some additional salt through sweating and lactation. Because the physiologic mechanisms for conserving salt are very efficient, chronic deficiencies do not ordinarily occur, even in populations such as the Yanomami and others on very-low-sodium diets (Page, 1976, 1979). Nevertheless, it is likely that people subsisting on very-low-salt diets are slightly more vulnerable to acute losses resulting from diarrhea, trauma, or blood loss (Gothberg et al., 1983).

Acute depletion of salt resulting in heat exhaustion and cardiovascular collapse may follow heavy sweating in people who have a high-salt intake and in whom adrenal mechanisms for conserving sodium have not been sufficiently activated (Conn, 1949). Healthy Caucasian men, after adaptation to heat and a moderately low-salt intake for 1 week, maintain sodium balance on an intake of 90 mEq/day (5,200 mg of sodium chloride), even while sweating 9 liters/day (Conn, 1949). Lower salt intakes have not been tested under similar laboratory conditions. Normal men with salt intakes varying from 10 to 1,500 mEq/day (580 to 87,000 mg of sodium chloride) maintained sodium balance without acute ill effects for 3 days (Luft et al., 1979, 1982). Despite these apparently wide tolerances, variations in salt intake among populations are associated with substantial variations in blood pressure and, therefore, occurrence of hypertension.

Hypertension

Primary hypertension, or high blood pressure, is a major risk factor for cardiovascular disease and death in the United States (Pooling Project Research Group, 1978). Definitions of high blood pressure are arbitrary and vary substantially. Average levels of both systolic and diastolic blood pressure in populations vary with age and sex (see Chapter 20). The prevalence of hypertension increases with age and is present in approximately 15% of the U.S. population age 30 and over (WHO, 1978). Criteria for adults, recommended by an expert committee of the World Health Organization (WHO, 1978), are as follows:

- Normotensives: systolic ≤ 140 mm Hg
  diastolic ≤ 90 mm Hg

- Borderline: systolic 141–159 mm Hg
    diastolic 91–94 mm Hg
- Hypertensives: systolic ≥ 160 mm Hg
    diastolic ≥ 95 mm Hg

Additional definitions of hypertension are discussed in Chapter 5.

No single factor causes hypertension, which involves the renal, cardiovascular, endocrine, and central and autonomic nervous systems. It is generally agreed that different factors play greater or lesser roles in different people and that there are variations in the rapidity of onset and degree of severity. Hypertension is usually asymptomatic but increases the risk for stroke, heart attack, and other cardiovascular events.

There is a genetic predisposition to hypertension, but there are no known reliable specific genetic markers. The inherited susceptibility appears to be expressed as a result of interaction with other factors: obesity, alcohol, and a variety of nutrients, including sodium and potassium (Denton, 1982; Folkow, 1982). Intake of polyunsaturated and saturated fats and calcium and exposure to psychological stress may also have roles in the expression of hypertension (Kaplan et al., 1985; see also Chapter 13).

Although studies of the relationship of sodium to hypertension have been conducted since the beginning of the twentieth century (Folkow, 1982; Porter, 1983), there is still some controversy about the importance of salt in regulation of blood pressure and about the mechanisms by which salt influences blood pressure. By far the greatest difference of opinion, and the most strongly held opinions, relate to the desirability of recommending to the general public that dietary sodium intake should be restricted. Numerous research studies, reviews, symposia, and books on these topics provide an abundance of data and a wide range of interpretations. There is little likelihood that these controversies will be entirely resolved in the foreseeable future.

Epidemiologic Evidence

Methods for estimating salt intake have varied, and timed urine collections and dietary intake recalls frequently do not match. Liu et al. (1979) found wide day-to-day variations in repeated measurements of sodium excretion by urban workers. Such intraindividual variability will tend to obscure real associations. Multiple urine collections are necessary to obtain consistent results, but even these collections and meticulous attention to

methods may fail to give reproducible results (Cooper et al., 1982). In addition, other variables known to affect blood pressure, such as genetically determined salt sensitivity, obesity, alcohol intake, and emotional stress, can obscure the relationship of salt to blood pressure (Jacobs et al., 1979; Liu et al., 1979).

Studies of blood pressure and sodium intake or excretion in individuals within populations have often failed to show a statistically significant relationship (Dawber et al., 1967; Holden et al., 1983; Karvonen and Punsar, 1977; Ljungman et al., 1981; Schlierf et al., 1980), but most studies based on a single 24-hour urine collection have not had sufficient statistical power to detect a slope of 0.1 mm Hg/mmol sodium (Watt et al., 1983). Significant intrapopulation correlations have been observed by some investigators (Cooper et al., 1980; Kesteloot et al., 1980; Khaw and Barrett-Connor, 1987, 1988; Page et al., 1981; Tao et al., 1984; Voors et al., 1983).

Secondary analyses of results from cross-sectional surveys of various populations have generally shown a positive correlation between intake of sodium and level of systolic and diastolic blood pressures (Froment et al., 1979; Gleibermann, 1973; Simpson, 1985). However, interpretation of these results has been complicated because the data came from separate, individual studies with unstandardized measurements of sodium and blood pressure and because results were usually not adjusted for confounding factors other than age and sex.

The Intersalt Cooperative Research Group (1988) studied both intra- and interpopulation associations between 24-hour urinary excretion of electrolytes and blood pressure in 10,079 men and women, 20 to 59 years of age, who were sampled in groups of about 200 at each of 52 centers in 32 countries around the world. The investigators used a highly standardized protocol with central training of observers, a central laboratory, and extensive quality control procedures. Median systolic blood pressure varied from 95 to 132 mm Hg, median diastolic blood pressure from 61 to 82 mm Hg, and prevalence of hypertension (defined as systolic blood pressure ≥ 140 mm Hg, or diastolic blood pressure ≥ 90 mm Hg, or use of antihypertensive agents) from 0 to 33%. Median daily excretion of sodium chloride varied from 0.2 mmol (11.6 mg) in the Yanomami Indians of Brazil to 242.1 mmol (14,043 mg) in Tianjin, northern China, but the distribution within this range was not even. Four geographically isolated centers had mean values below 57 mmol/day, no center was between 57 and 103, 4 were between 104 and 138, and 44 were higher. Thus, data are limited on the association between sodium excretion and blood pressure for populations with mean sodium excretion less than 138 mmol/day (8 g/day).

Among individuals within centers, 24-hour sodium excretion was positively and significantly associated with level of systolic blood pressure, and this association persisted after adjustment for age, sex, body mass index, alcohol consumption, and urinary excretion of potassium. A similar association was observed for diastolic blood pressure after adjustment for age and sex, but the regression coefficient was nearly zero and not statistically significant after adjustment also for body mass index, alcohol consumption, and urinary potassium. Sodium to potassium ratio was positively and significantly associated with both systolic and diastolic blood pressure after adjustment for age, sex, body mass index, and alcohol consumption.

In cross-center analyses involving all 52 centers, median sodium excretion was positively and significantly associated with median systolic blood pressure after adjustment for age, sex, body mass index, and alcohol consumption. As customarily happens when the range of a regressor is truncated, the regression coefficient was reduced in magnitude (and was no longer statistically significant) when the four centers with lowest median values for sodium excretion were excluded from the analysis. Associations with diastolic blood pressure were smaller and not statistically significant.

Median sodium excretion was positively and significantly associated with the age-related rise in systolic and diastolic blood pressure in all 52 centers and also in the 48 centers with the highest median values for sodium excretion. These associations persisted after adjustment for sex, body mass index, and alcohol consumption. The adjusted results for all 52 centers indicated that an increment of 100 mmol/day of sodium was associated with an increment of 10 mm Hg in mean systolic blood pressure and 6 mm Hg in mean diastolic blood pressure between the ages of 25 and 55.

Median sodium excretion was positively and significantly associated with prevalence of hypertension in cross-center analyses involving all 52 centers, but the association was not significant when the four centers with lowest median values for sodium excretion were excluded. Similarly, the ratio of sodium to potassium was positively associated with the slope of blood pressure with age and with the prevalence of hypertension, but these associations were statistically significant only in the analyses including all 52 centers.

These results indicate that in unacculturated populations where habitual salt intake is less than 4,500 mg/day, blood pressure does not rise with age, average adult blood pressure is low, and hypertension is rare or absent (Page, 1979). In the four Intersalt populations with median sodium excretion under 60 mmol/day (3,480 mg/day), age had little or no association with blood pressure, while in the populations with median sodium excretion of 100 mmol/day (5,800 mg/day) or higher, age was positively associated with blood pressure, and the rate of rise with age was proportional to the median sodium excretion. An absence of hypertension despite high intake of sodium has been reported in India (Malhotra, 1970) and among Buddhist farmers in Thailand (Henry and Cassel, 1969), but further examination of both cases indicated that the data were inadequate to support any conclusions about sodium intake and hypertension (Denton, 1982; Prineas and Blackburn, 1985).

Since blood pressure must rise with age for hypertension to become prevalent in a population, these results indicate that the average consumption of sodium is an important factor in determining the prevalence of hypertension in populations. The relatively weaker associations observed in the Intersalt populations between median sodium excretion and median levels of blood pressure may have been due to factors such as climate, physical activity, or other dietary components, which, while varying among centers, were similar within centers and could have biased comparisons of medians across centers without biasing the slope of blood pressure with age or other within-center associations. The committee recognizes that the results of Intersalt and other epidemiologic investigations of this topic are subject to various interpretations, but concludes that the weight of evidence supports the contention that intake of sodium is an important factor in the occurrence of hypertension.

A significant intrapopulation correlation has been found within other populations, at least for systolic blood pressures in Iran (Page et al., 1981), China (Tao et al., 1984), and Korea (Intersalt Cooperative Research Group, 1988; Kesteloot et al., 1980; Khaw and Barrett-Connor, 1987, 1988). Cooper et al. (1980) reported a slope of 0.06 mm Hg/mmol sodium in children, using seven consecutive 24-hour urine collections.

A positive correlation between blood pressure and salt intake among individuals might occur only in people with a genetic susceptibility to hypertension. American blacks account for an unusually high proportion of those genetically susceptible, and Voors et al. (1983) found a positive correlation between salt intake and blood pressure in black teenagers.

Clinical Studies

Several investigators have studied responses to changes in sodium intake and sodium depletion in an attempt to identify people who are sensitive or resistant to the effects of salt on blood pressure. Salt loading acutely lowers forearm vascular resistance in healthy, normal people, but it increases resistance in those with borderline hypertension (Mark et al., 1975). Luft et al. (1982) fed normotensive men six successively higher levels of salt, ranging from 10 to 1,500 mEq (580 to 87,000 mg of sodium chloride per day), each for a period of 3 days. The subjects maintained sodium balance, but nearly all subjects developed some increase in blood pressure as levels of salt increased. Hofman et al. (1983) compared two groups of newborn infants fed formulas with two different salt levels. One formula contained 6.3 mEq (370 mg) of sodium chloride per liter, approximately equal to that in human milk. The other contained 19.2 mEq (1,100 mg) of sodium chloride per liter, approximately equal to the level in cow's milk. At the end of the study, systolic pressure was 2.1 mmHg higher in those on the higher sodium formula, but no residual difference in blood pressure was found after 1 year. Weight and growth rate were the same in the two groups. Studies such as these indicate that short-term changes in sodium intake influence blood pressure. Long-term prospective controlled trials of variations in sodium intake have not been conducted.

Arterial blood pressure at any time is the result of a complex interplay of dynamic variables. Any satisfactory theory must consider short-term and long-term effects as well as the influence of heredity, body fluid volumes, cardiac and vascular factors, regulatory mechanisms mediated through the central and autonomic nervous systems, the endocrine system, and the kidneys. It must also take into account the other factors known to influence blood pressure, including race, body mass, psychosocial stresses, and nutrients other than sodium. Only selected facets of this large subject are presented herein, specifically those that seem most relevant to the long-term effects of habitual sodium intake on blood pressure in human populations.

Tobian and Binion (1952, 1954) reported increased intracellular sodium in the arteries of hypertensive patients. Recently, increased permeability of cell membranes to sodium has been found in several animal models of hypertension (Tobian et al., 1986) and in many patients with primary hypertension (Page, 1976). Abnormalities in membrane lipids and in calcium binding have also been found both in hypertensive humans and in animals (Tobian et al., 1985a). The possible role of calcium in hypertension is discussed in Chapter 13.

Animal Studies

For 50 million years, almost all mammals have lived in a world where foodstuffs tend to have quite a low sodium content. The saltiest foods available to most mammals are other animal tissues; however, even completely carnivorous animals still have a salt intake substantially lower than that of most modern humans.

Studies suggest that a high-salt diet increases blood pressure in some animals, but not in others. When a high-salt diet raises blood pressure in animals, there is usually some defect in the ability of the kidneys to excrete salt rapidly. The combination of a high-salt intake and defective salt excretion tends to increase the salt content of the body, which appears to trigger a rise in blood pressure (Tobian, 1983; Tobian et al., 1977). In turn, the increased pressure entering the renal artery encourages a more rapid natriuresis, which tends to normalize the defect in salt excretion. Evidence suggests that two processes are involved. One process appears to be the interaction of a high-salt intake with a diminished renal capacity to excrete salt rapidly, which tends to cause sodium retention. The other process triggers a rise in blood pressure in response to increased body sodium, but the mechanism for this is not entirely clear. However, there is recent evidence that this sodium chloride signal is perceived in brain tissue around the third brain ventricle (Tobian, 1988).

Salt-induced high blood pressure can be observed in studies comparing Dahl S and Dahl R rats—now designated DS and DR (Dahl et al., 1962). When these two strains consume a low-salt diet, both have blood pressure well within the normal range, although the DS rat has a slightly higher blood pressure and some evidence of defective renal salt excretion. When dietary salt was increased, the blood pressure of the DR rat did not rise, whereas the blood pressure of the DS rat rose markedly over a 2-month period (Dahl et al., 1962). When salt excretion was facilitated by a thiazide diuretic, DS rats had little rise in blood pressure (Tobian et al., 1979).

Kyoto spontaneously hypertensive rats (SHRs) are hypertensive on a fairly low salt diet. SHRs fed very low amounts of salt in the diet do not develop high blood pressure unless salt intake is too low to allow normal growth of the animal (Toal and Leenen, 1983; Wilczynski and Leenen, 1987).

A continuous excess of aldosterone or deoxycorticosterone intake causes rats and pigs to retain sodium and develop hypertension (Kaplan and Lieberman, 1986; Tobian, 1986), but hypertension does not occur when the same amount of deoxycorticosterone or aldosterone is combined with a very low salt diet. Continued high blood pressure tends to cause kidney damage, which further reduces sodium excretion by the kidney. Hypertension is aggravated in the rat by removal of one kidney.

A sodium-dependent type of hypertension can also be induced in rats by subtotal nephrectomy (Chanutin and Ferris, 1932). Hypertension supervenes when reduction in renal mass is accompanied by a high salt intake, but a low salt intake induces little or no hypertension. A similar type of hypertension was induced in dogs by Coleman and Guyton (1969). If the high-salt diet is discontinued, blood pressure returns to normal levels in the dog. A high-salt diet also increases blood pressure in some strains of monkeys (Srinivasan et al., 1984) and chickens (Sapirstein et al., 1950).

Muirhead et al. (1975) fed rats a high-salt diet and injected them with angiotensin, which stimulates the adrenal gland to secrete aldosterone and also stimulates renal proximal tubule sodium reabsorption. When angiotensin is combined with a high-salt diet, these rats develop "angiotensin-salt" hypertension. Hypertension does not occur if the angiotensin injections are combined with a low-salt diet.

In DS rats made hypertensive by high salt intake, postsalt hypertension occurs after resumption of normal salt intake (Tobian et al., 1975). This is related to changes in the kidney, including destruction of nephrons and damage to glomeruli and tubules in the surviving nephrons. Tobian et al. (1986) reported that high-salt diets consumed for 20 days caused little rise of blood pressure but reduced intrinsic filtration capacity of the kidney to 50% below normal.

Destruction of certain parts of the central nervous system (CNS) can prevent salt-induced hypertension, suggesting that the CNS is involved in salt-induced hypertension (Tobian et al., 1982).

In summary, the combination of a high-salt diet and a diminished capacity for sodium excretion increases blood pressure in many animals. Studies suggest that this combination may also lead to hypertension in humans (Grim et al., 1979).

Hereditary Factors Interacting with Sodium

Familial aggregation of blood pressure has been demonstrated repeatedly (Feinleib et al., 1975; Hamilton et al., 1954; Zinner et al., 1976), but the mode of inheritance has not been determined. A bimodal blood pressure distribution, originally proposed by Platt (1947), has received some recent support in an analysis by McManus (1983). Most studies support a polygenic mode of inheritance (Hamilton et al., 1954; Miller and Grim, 1983). The term *hypertension* is used in these studies to designate the upper end of the biologic distribution curve for blood pressure in a normal population.

Many kinds of evidence support a hereditary, polygenic predisposition to hypertension (Folkow, 1982; Miall and Oldham, 1963; Pickering, 1968), although the prediction of hypertension based on the blood pressure of first-degree relatives is imperfect and qualitative. For example, Feinleib et al. (1975) showed closer correlations in blood pressure in monozygotic than in dizygotic twins. Consequently, many efforts have been made to identify genetic markers in individuals likely to develop hypertension in response to excess sodium intake or other environmental variables, but these efforts have not been successful. In recent years, several ion transport systems have been described, and there have been attempts to identify abnormalities in such systems that might represent markers for genetic susceptibility to hypertension (Weissberg et al., 1983).

A polygenic predisposition to primary hypertension would have important implications. For example, it would indicate that several or many components of the cardiovascular control mechanisms are involved and that a variety of constellations in genetically controlled responses to environmental influences are likely to be present in human populations. It would also help to explain the apparent heterogeneity of mechanisms in the genesis of hypertension and make it unlikely that one hypothesis will apply to all cases. Furthermore, it complicates efforts to identify genetic markers that could reliably predict who is or is not at risk for development of hypertension.

Mechanisms for Development of Hypertension

The maintenance of high-concentration gradients for sodium and potassium across cell mem-

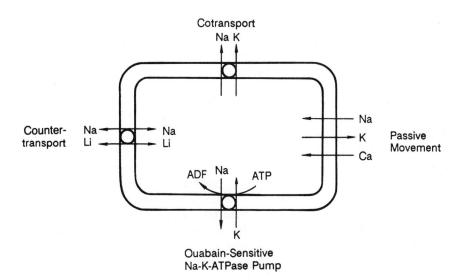

Cotransport
Na K

Counter-
transport

Na → Na
Li → Li

Na
K
Ca

Passive
Movement

ADF Na ATP

K

Ouabain-Sensitive
Na-K-ATPase Pump

FIGURE 15–1 Four sodium transport mechanisms that have been demonstrated in red blood cells. From Kaplan and Lieberman (1986).

branes requires expenditure of energy. Several separate systems for maintaining high concentrations of sodium outside cells and high concentrations of potassium inside cells have been described (Hilton, 1986). Many studies of ion transport systems have tested the hypothesis that they reflect the action of one or more genes that determine hereditary susceptibility to hypertension and, thus, may be used to identify people at risk prior to onset of the disease. Figure 15–1 is a schematic diagram of the most important ion transport systems.

In the sodium–potassium adenosine triphosphatase (ATP-ase) pump, a membrane-bound enzyme (ATP-ase) releases energy from ATP to transport sodium and potassium in opposite directions across the cell membrane. The system is inhibited by ouabain and other digitalis glycosides. The activity of this sodium pump is decreased in hypertensives and some of their relatives (Swales et al., 1982). Plasma from hypertensives inhibits this mechanism in the white cells of normotensives (Poston et al., 1981). Abnormalities in this system have been observed in spontaneous and induced hypertension in animals (Overbeck et al., 1981). Variations in activity of this system occur in different racial groups (Beutler et al., 1983) and can be induced by changes in weight and diet (Bradlaugh et al., 1984; De Luise et al., 1980). Thus, the sodium–potassium ATP-ase pump does not appear to be a reliable specific genetic marker for hypertension.

The sodium–potassium cotransport system brings about simultaneous inward or outward coupled transport of sodium and potassium. This system is inhibited by furosemide and was reported to be decreased in patients with hypertension and in their first-degree relatives (Garay and Meyer,

1979). Subsequent results have been inconsistent (Weissberg et al., 1983). Thus, this system has proved to be a disappointing candidate as a genetic marker.

An increased rate of sodium–lithium countertransport has been observed in hypertensives (Canessa et al., 1980) and in many normotensive relatives of white hypertensives, but no relationship to blood pressure has been found in black hypertensives (Weissberg et al., 1983). Countertransport cannot alter the net concentration of sodium within cells. Nevertheless, numerous studies of the sodium–lithium countertransport system have shown consistently increased activity in variable proportions of Caucasian hypertensives studied in different laboratories (Motulsky et al., 1987). Familial aggregation and higher concordance of sodium–lithium countertransport in monozygotic, but not in dizygotic, twins has been demonstrated in several studies (Dadone et al., 1984; Woods et al., 1982). The system is unaffected by sodium restriction and antihypertensive medications (Burke et al., 1984; Cooper et al., 1984). Motulsky et al. (1987) tested several different genetic models for their control of increased countertransport and found that results were most consistent with a major gene determining increased sodium–lithium countertransport activity superimposed on a background of polygenic control of blood pressure. The findings thus support the thesis that hypertension has a heterogeneous genetic basis. Further investigation on genetic linkage relationships for this putative gene may clarify the role of at least one possible genetic marker for hypertension.

Studies of Sodium Sensitivity in Humans

In several studies, acute or short-term sodium loading and sodium depletion have been used to classify types of genetic susceptibility to salt-induced hypertension. Their duration has ranged from hours to days, or at most, to a few weeks. Most of the studies have shown considerable variation in responsiveness of hypertensive patients to salt, without a clear separation between salt-sensitive and salt-resistant subjects (Bittle et al., 1985; Fujita et al., 1980; Kawasaki et al., 1978). A variety of procedures and protocols have been used by different investigators to identify sodium sensitivity in hypertensives (Logan, 1986). The proportion of hypertensives identified by these investigators as sodium sensitive has varied from 35 to 73%.

Weinberger et al. (1986) showed that acute responses to variations in sodium intake occurred in both hypertensive and normotensive subjects. Responses were somewhat greater in the hypertensives, but there was considerable overlap. Greater increases in blood pressure and lesser natriuretic responses after sodium loading have been reported in blacks under 40 years of age and in blacks and whites older than 40 years (Luft et al., 1979).

The studies cited above fail to show clear-cut differences in sodium sensitivity between hypertensive and normotensive subjects, although quantitative differences were noted in response to the procedures used. All studies were designed to show responses to acute changes in sodium; none were analogous to the changes observed during primary hypertension, where blood pressure rises slowly over many years. These studies do not convincingly demonstrate the presence of sharply defined hereditary sodium sensitivity in the genesis of chronic hypertension.

At present, knowledge of blood pressure in first-degree relatives is the most superior method for predicting the development of hypertension. Although epidemiologic studies provide strong evidence that sensitivity to excess sodium chloride is an important factor in initiating hypertension, there is no certain method to predict individual responses or even for estimating the percentage of a susceptible group of individuals that become hypertensive as a result of excess sodium intake. Other environmental influences, such as psychosocial stresses, obesity, and habitual alcohol intake, may elevate blood pressure singly or in combination with sodium intake, depending on the genetic profile of the individual. Body mass and obesity, and heavy use of ethanol, are powerful determinants of blood pressure in population studies (see Chapter 20). Nevertheless, among the nutrients, indirect evidence is strongest and most extensive for the role of sodium chloride.

Reduced Sodium Intake in the Treatment of Hypertension

Although treatment of established hypertension by sodium chloride restriction is relevant to dietary recommendations, neither a response to such treatment nor the absence of response is adequate to prove or disprove the role of sodium in the etiology of hypertension. Diets with very low levels of sodium chloride, such as a rice diet, were shown to be effective in treating moderate and severe hypertension before modern drug treatment was available (Kempner, 1948). Most studies of moderate sodium restrictions in the treatment of mild to moderate hypertension have been small, brief, and flawed by lack of blinding or absence of appropriate controls. Larger trials over a longer period are needed to clarify the importance of salt restriction in the treatment of hypertension.

Patients whose hypertension had been maintained in the normotensive range by medication over a 5-year period in a large intervention trial (HDFP, 1979a,b) subsequently participated in a second trial (Langford et al., 1985). Eligible subjects were randomized into control and discontinued-medication groups, with and without dietary intervention. Interventions were weight loss or sodium reduction to 40 mEq/day. Both dietary interventions, continued for 56 weeks, increased the likelihood of remaining normotensive without medication. The highest success rate was obtained in nonoverweight, mild hypertensives on sodium restriction. That study demonstrates the value of salt restriction in preventing recurrence of hypertension in previously hypertensive patients. Studies such as that by Langford et al. (1985) also demonstrate the feasibility and safety of prolonged moderate sodium restriction. Clinical trials of hypertension prevention using different levels of dietary salt in normotensive subjects over an extended period would provide additional evidence on the etiologic role of sodium chloride in hypertension.

Gastric Cancer

Studies in Humans

Correa et al. (1985) reported a high urinary excretion of sodium in Colombian populations with elevated gastric cancer mortality rates and with documented high prevalence of atrophic gastritis. Correa (1982) postulated that salt is important in the development of precursors of stomach cancer, particularly atrophic gastritis. Nevertheless, cross-sectional and time-trend correlation analyses do not show consistent associations between per-capita salt consumption and gastric cancer mortality rates in Japan (Howson et al., 1986; Kono et al., 1983). Difficulties in obtaining valid estimates of salt intake have limited similar analyses in other countries. Some investigators have reported a positive correlation between gastric cancer mortality and stroke incidence and mortality, which they took as a surrogate measure of salt intake (Joossens, 1980; Joossens and Geboers, 1981; Tuomilehto et al., 1984), but others have reported no association (Harrington, 1981; Walker, 1982; Whelton and Goldblatt, 1982).

The association of salt with gastric cancer becomes stronger and more uniform when salt intake from salted, smoked, and pickled foods is considered (Joossens and Geboers, 1984; NRC, 1982; West, 1984). Consumption of salted, smoked, and pickled fish products and other salted products, such as salt-cured ham, sausage, and salami, has been associated with increased gastric cancer risk (Bjelke, 1974; Correa et al., 1983, 1985; Haenszel et al., 1972; Hara et al., 1985; Hirayama, 1979; Ishiwata et al., 1975; Kolonel et al., 1980; Sato et al., 1959, 1961). Similar foods may account for the elevated gastric cancer rates observed in Iceland, Chile, Portugal, and the Adriatic coast of Yugoslavia (Alderson, 1981; Howson et al., 1986).

A concurrence of declining gastric cancer mortality and decreasing consumption of salted, dried fish and salted vegetables in Japan has been noted in time-trend analyses (Japan Ministry of Health and Welfare, 1980). One clinical study indicated that consumption of gherkins pickled in high-salt soy sauce led to abnormal changes in gastric mucosa (MacDonald et al., 1967).

Animal Studies

Salt alone has not been carcinogenic in the gastrointestinal tract in a variety of animal bioassays or in short-term studies in rodents (Ohgaki et al., 1984; Takahashi et al., 1983; Tatematsu et al., 1975). In rodents, however, a high salt intake increased absorption of polycyclic aromatic hydrocarbons (PAHs), which are known to be gastric carcinogens (Capoferro and Torgersen, 1974). High-salt diets in the presence of other gastric carcinogens have also been reported to facilitate both gastric cancer initiation (Kodama et al.,

1984; Takahashi et al., 1983) and promotion (Hanawa et al., 1980; Ohgaki et al., 1984; Takahashi, 1986), although the evidence for the latter is not consistent (Takahashi et al., 1983).

In addition to salt, salted, smoked, and dried fish contain PAHs (Stewart, 1967) as well as nitrosated products (Kodama et al., 1982; Yano, 1981), which include at least one as yet unidentified substance that can induce glandular stomach tumors in rats (Weisburger, 1981; Weisburger et al., 1980). In one study, mice fed a diet of dried cod containing 7% sodium chloride developed lesions characteristic of acute and chronic gastritis (Sato et al., 1959). In humans, chronic gastritis is suspected of being a precursor to gastric cancer (Correa, 1982).

Mechanism of Action

Despite the lack of direct evidence that dietary salt is a gastric carcinogen per se, experimental evidence suggests that a high salt intake may enhance tumor initiation by irritating and damaging the gastric mucosal barrier, thereby facilitating mutation of the target cell by a suitable carcinogen (Howson et al., 1986). If such enhancement occurs, it may be related in part to a salt-induced reduction in the viscosity of hyaluronic acid, one of the mucopolysaccharides that protect the gastric mucosa (Takahashi et al., 1983).

In summary, stomach cancer is associated with diets containing large amounts of foods preserved with salt and possibly also containing precursors of nitrosamines.

Potassium

Evidence that potassium is important in human nutrition has grown steadily in the past four decades. Prehistoric humans and hominids ate only the food that they could obtain by hunting or collecting vegetation such as roots, fruits, tubers, nuts, grains, and seeds. Such foods contain small amounts of sodium and large amounts of potassium (Denton, 1982; Eaton and Konner, 1985). Studies indicate that present-day hunter–gatherers consume between 200 and 285 mEq (7.8 and 11.0 g of elemental potassium per day) (Denton, 1982; Eaton and Konner, 1985). Today, most people consume less than one-quarter of the potassium eaten by prehistoric hunter–gatherers. Urban whites in the United States eat about 2.5 g of elemental potassium per day (Khaw and Barrett-Connor, 1987). Lower intakes have been observed in blacks, whose average excretion rate has been reported to be 25 to 30 mEq/day (0.98 to 1.17 g/day) (Grim et al., 1980; Langford, 1985). There is a wide diversity in habitual daily potassium intake among various populations of the world.

Hypertension, Cardiovascular Diseases, and Stroke

Epidemiologic Studies

A substantial body of evidence in humans and animals indicates that dietary potassium exerts a beneficial effect on hypertension. This is partly because of its effect on lowering blood pressure and partly because of its separate, protective effect against vascular damage and stroke. Several studies have shown that supplemental potassium decreases the blood pressure of hypertensive patients (Addison, 1928; Iimura et al., 1981; Kaplan et al., 1985; MacGregor et al., 1982; Morino et al., 1978; Priddle, 1931; Svetkey et al., 1986).

Populations with habitually low-potassium diets appear to have an increased incidence of various cardiovascular morbid events. In the United States, for example, blacks consume less potassium than do whites (Cushman and Langford, 1983; Dai et al., 1984; Frate and Langford, 1985; Grim et al., 1980; Voors et al., 1983; Walker et al., 1979; Watson et al., 1980; Zinner et al., 1976). These differences in potassium intake may be related to the higher frequency of hypertension and related complications in blacks. Blacks in the southeastern part of the United States who eat a very low-potassium diet appear to have a higher stroke rate than any other geographic or ethnic group in the United States (Langford, 1985). Blacks also have a very high incidence of end-stage renal disease caused by hypertension. The incidence of hypertensive renal damage is 18 times higher in blacks than in whites (Rostand et al., 1982) and is correlated with differences in potassium intake.

Diets in Scotland are relatively low in potassium, averaging about 46 mEq of elemental potassium per day (1.80 g). There is a considerably greater incidence of cardiovascular diseases in Scotland than in France, Italy, or southern England, where higher levels of potassium are consumed (Tobian, 1986). Sasaki et al. (1959) described two adjoining prefectures in northern Japan with contrasting diets. The Aamori diet provides a greater potassium and a lower sodium intake, and the Aamori population has a much lower stroke rate than do people in Akita.

Langford (1985) studied 101 black women about 20 years of age and found no significant correlation between blood pressure and sodium excretion. However, he found a modest positive correlation between the urinary sodium–potassium ratio and diastolic blood pressure. In a study by the Intersalt Cooperative Research Group (1988), potassium excretion was negatively correlated with blood pressure after adjustment for confounding variables.

Walker et al. (1979) found no meaningful correlation between blood pressure and sodium intake in a large cohort in Baltimore, Maryland. However, a negative correlation was found between potassium excretion and recumbent diastolic blood pressure.

Page et al. (1981) found a correlation between blood pressure and sodium intake in men among pastoral nomads in Iran. Women of the same tribe did not show a correlation between blood pressure and sodium excretion, but their blood pressure was positively correlated with the urinary sodium–potassium ratio. Langford (1985) observed a very high correlation between mean urinary sodium–potassium ratio and mean diastolic blood pressure in Norwegian populations from three different areas (Langford, 1985).

In several recent studies (Khaw and Barrett-Connor, 1984; Khaw and Rose, 1982; Reed et al., 1985), investigators found a positive correlation of blood pressure with the dietary sodium–potassium ratio and a negative correlation with the urinary potassium–creatinine ratio and with potassium in the diet. Similarly, potassium intake was inversely correlated with blood pressure (Kromhout et al., 1985). In the Intersalt study, the sodium–potassium ratio followed a pattern similar to that of sodium (Intersalt Cooperative Research Group, 1988).

Khaw and Barrett-Connor (1987) showed that over a period of 12 years the incidence of stroke-related deaths in people over 50 years of age in a retirement community was negatively correlated with the daily intake of potassium. Results were unchanged when the correlation of potassium with death from stroke was adjusted for age, caloric intake, systolic or diastolic blood pressure, and fiber, magnesium, and calcium in the diet. No similar relationship of potassium to coronary artery events was found in this study. The corrected data suggest that an increase of 10 mEq (400 mg) of elemental potassium per day would lead to an approximately 40% decrease in the incidence of stroke-related deaths over the 12 years of the study; this amounts to only one or two extra servings of fruits, fruit juices, vegetables, or potatoes per day.

In this study, the protective effect of added potassium in the diet appeared to be independent of any change in blood pressure.

In summary, evidence from epidemiologic studies suggests that a diet with high levels of potassium and low levels of sodium may be beneficial in lowering blood pressure and that a high potassium intake may be independently protective against death from stroke. An intake of ≥3.5 g/day of elemental potassium is associated with a beneficial effect, and no threshold for this effect is known.

Animal Studies

DS rats fed a diet with 4% sodium chloride and 0.75% potassium developed hypertension, a gradual, progressive destruction of the kidney tubules, and an increase in the wall thickness of the renal arterioles. With supplemental potassium (2.11%), control DS rats had fewer lesions in the renal cortex, outer medulla, and papillae, and the average thickness of their renal arterioles was not greater than that of normotensive DR rats, although there was no lowering of blood pressure in the salt-fed rats (Tobian et al., 1984). Added potassium salts attenuated the expected thickening of the arteriolar walls and resulted in a lowering of renal lesions (Tobian et al., 1984).

In SHRSP rats (a stroke-prone substrain of spontaneously hypertensive rats), a Japanese rat chow diet markedly increased the incidence of stroke compared to that of a U.S. rat chow diet, mainly because the Japanese diet had a 40% lower potassium content than the U.S. diet and a lower concentration of glycine and sulfur-containing amino acids (Tobian et al., 1985a,b). SHRSP rats surviving on 0.75% potassium intake (normal level) had much more histopathological evidence of brain infarcts than did SHRSP animals given a 2.11% high-potassium diet.

Moderately severe hypertension can cause rents, irregularities, and severe stretching in a tense arterial endothelial layer, which could increase the permeability of the endothelial lining (Goldby and Beilin, 1972). If potassium reduces such endothelial irregularities in cerebral arteries, it could also reduce the incidence of strokes.

A protective effect of high-potassium diets against endothelial cell damage could explain both intimal and medial protection, since it is associated with diminished release of endothelial, macrophage, and platelet-derived growth factors. This in turn may result in reduced medial hypertrophy and intimal hypercellularity. Ratios of heart weight to body weight were reduced in hypertensive rats on high-potassium diets, even though blood pressures were the same in animals without potassium supplements.

Potassium added to the diet of the SHRSP preserves normal function in the arterial endothelial cells, including those with chronically high intraarterial pressure. It also prevents thickening of the intimal layer (Tobian, 1986). Moreover, high-potassium diets preserve the full degree of endothelium-dependent relaxation of the arterial wall, whereas the normal potassium diet allows two-thirds of this relaxation to disappear in the SHRSP rats. Those studies suggest that a high-potassium diet protects the arterial endothelial cells against hypertensive damage.

Meneely and Ball (1958) reported that the addition of potassium substantially prolonged the survival rate in Sprague-Dawley rats on high-salt diets, although blood pressure was not reduced below control levels. Gordon and Drury (1956) produced renal hypertension in rabbits by narrowing a renal artery. Supplements of potassium did not reduce blood pressure in these rabbits, but greatly reduced the frequency of mesenteric hemorrhages.

Although the mechanism by which additional dietary potassium reduces deaths is not known, the evidence suggests that it exerts a protective effect partly through reducing blood pressure and partly through an effect on the vascular system independent of blood pressure (Khaw and Barrett-Conner, 1987; Tobian et al., 1985a).

Chloride

Hypertension

It appears from several studies that both sodium and chloride are necessary to produce hypertension, but the matter remains unresolved. In DS rats, nonchloride-containing sodium salt did not raise blood pressure as much as equimolar amounts of sodium chloride (Whitescarver et al., 1984). Similar observations have been made in studies of other animal models with deoxycorticosterone hypertension (Kurtz and Morris, 1985). Conversely, severe hypertension has been reported in Dahl S rats given supplements of sodium citrate (Tobian et al., 1984). Kurtz et al. (1987) studied five hypertensive men who were selected because their blood pressure was normalized after 7 days of sodium chloride restriction to 10 mmol/day (600 mg). Dietary supplements of sodium chloride at 240 mmol/day (14,000 mg), given in capsules, increased blood pressure by 16/8 mm Hg; equimolar sodium citrate induced no rise in blood pressure. More studies on the effects of different sodium salts are needed.

Salt Substitutes

Many salt substitutes are now commercially available. They include mixtures of sodium chloride and potassium chloride and mixtures of nonsodium salts, 5'-nucleotides, and herbs. The moderate use of these substances for flavoring food does not harm healthy people. Because of the rapid absorption of the potassium, they may be dangerous if used in large amounts by people with renal insufficiency or certain diseases of the endocrine system. The regular use of these condiments warrants medical supervision.

SUMMARY

Epidemiologic data strongly indicate that habitual sodium intake is an important determinant of blood pressure in humans, but that there is wide variation in genetic susceptibility to salt-induced hypertension. Reliable genetic markers for susceptibility to the effect of sodium have not been identified. Blood pressure rises slowly with age in susceptible people. Once induced by a high sodium intake, blood pressure is not necessarily corrected by resumption of a moderately low intake. Evidence points to the kidney as responsible for this elevation of blood pressure.

Studies of hypertension in a variety of animal species and under various experimental conditions confirm the importance of both sodium and potassium intake as determinants of both normal blood pressure and hypertension. Animal models have contributed in several important ways to present understanding of hypertension. Hereditary susceptibility to the effects of sodium has been demonstrated in rodents, pigs, and primates. In the salt-sensitive DS rats, heredity alone does not produce hypertension, but blood pressure increases progressively during and following sodium loading. In SHRs, hypertension occurs as a result of genetic susceptibility alone and without sodium loading, but the hypertension is greatly aggravated by increased sodium intakes.

Hypertension develops to a greater extent in rats or pigs given deoxycorticosterone or aldosterone than in those given high-salt diets. The mechanisms by which salt causes hypertension in animals have not been fully elucidated and appear to vary somewhat from one animal model to another. A common feature is a reduced ability to excrete sodium, which may result from alterations in regulatory mechanisms or from damage to the kidneys. An important role for the central and autonomic nervous systems in modifying the response to salt loading has been demonstrated in some animal models.

Experimental data indicate that a high salt intake can damage stomach mucosa and induce severe gastritis. These data combined with the consistent epidemiologic findings linking salted, dried, and pickled foods to increased gastric cancer risk suggest that salt can act as a cocarcinogen, perhaps by compromising the gastric mucosal barrier and facilitating initiation by a gastric carcinogen.

Diets with a high sodium content tend to be low in potassium, whereas those with high potassium levels have a low sodium content. An important role for potassium in regulation of blood pressure and in modification of the sequelae of hypertension has been documented in humans and animals. Data strongly indicate that a high potassium intake is protective against fatal stroke in humans and in SHRSP and DS rats. It also protects against arterial hypertrophy and injury in animals. This effect is exerted partly through modulation or reduction of blood pressure, but high potassium intake reduces cardiovascular mortality and morbidity due to hypertension, even apart from its effects on blood pressure. In animal models, potassium also prevents strokes as well as hypertrophy and intimal damage of blood vessels without reducing blood pressure.

Epidemiologic studies suggest that dietary potassium protects against death from strokes in humans. Some studies have shown that potassium supplements lower blood pressure, but others—in human populations and in animal models—suggest that potassium exerts a protective effect against stroke that is unrelated to blood pressure.

Anions appear to modify the effects of cations on blood pressure in some studies, but no recommendation concerning anion nutrient content of the diet is warranted at present.

DIRECTIONS FOR RESEARCH

Recommendations for research and the rationale for them are presented below.

• Epidemiologic, clinical, and animal studies indicate a wide genetic variability in blood pressure and in the susceptibility of individuals to the effects of electrolyte intake and other environmental variables. Except for such crude indices as race and family history, however, there are no reliable genetic markers for susceptibility to hypertension. More specific markers are needed for genetic susceptibility to sodium chloride and the modifying effect of potassium. The availability of such markers may make possible the targeting of specific dietary recommendations to susceptible people rather than only to the general public.

• Long-term prospective studies of dietary intervention to prevent hypertension in normotensives would be of great value. Such studies should include variables such as sodium restriction, potassium supplementation, weight control, and possibly other variables such as calcium supplementation or variation in protein and polyunsaturated fat. These studies should be conducted in children as well as in adults.

• Research on the fundamental cellular and physiological mechanisms leading to hypertension and vascular injury from hypertension is currently widely pursued and should be encouraged. Such research should include studies of the interactions of sodium, potassium, and their attendant anions and of the relationships between these dietary electrolytes and minerals such as calcium.

• Further research is needed on the interrelationships between electrolytes, other nutrients, and obesity in the fundamental pathogenesis of hypertension. Special attention should be given to the interactions of nutrients and other environmental factors in different age, sex, and racial groups.

• Anionic composition of sodium salts in human hypertension deserves further study. Sodium and chloride are highly correlated in the urine of humans, and it would be difficult to devise a diet for humans in which the major sodium salt would not be sodium chloride. The principal relevance of studies on anions at present is the possibility that the results could be used as a probe for mechanisms of blood pressure regulation.

REFERENCES

AAP (American Academy of Pediatrics). 1974. Salt intake and eating patterns of infants and children. Pediatrics 53: 115–121.

Addison, W.L.T. 1928. Use of sodium chloride, potassium chloride, sodium bromide, and potassium bromide in cases of arterial hypertension which are amenable to potassium chloride. Can. Med. Assoc. J. 18:281–285.

Alderson, M.R. 1981. International Mortality Statistics. Facts on File, New York. 524 pp.

Beauchamp, G.K., M. Bertino, and K. Engelman. 1985.

Sensory basis for human salt consumption. Pp. 113–124 in M.J. Horan, M. Blaustein, J.B. Dunbar, W. Kachadorian, N.M. Kaplan, and A.P. Simopoulos, eds. NIH Workshop on Nutrition and Hypertension: Proceedings from a Symposium. Biomedical Information Corp., New York.

Beutler, E., W. Kuhl, and P. Sacks. 1983. Sodium–potassium–ATPase activity is influenced by ethnic origin and not by obesity. N. Engl. J. Med. 309:756–760.

Bittle, C.C., Jr., D.J. Molina, and F.C. Bartter. 1985. Salt sensitivity in essential hypertension as determined by the Cosinor Method. Hypertension 7:989–994.

Bjelke, E. 1974. Epidemiologic studies of cancer of the stomach, colon, and rectum; with special emphasis on the role of diet. Scand. J. Gastroenterol. 31:1–235.

Bradlaugh, R., A.M. Heagerty, R.F. Bing, J.D. Swales, and H. Thurston. 1984. Rat thymocyte sodium transport. Effects of changes in sodium balance and experimental hypertension. Hypertension 6:454–459.

Burke, W., S. Hornung, B.R. Copeland, C.E. Furlong, and A.G. Motulsky. 1984. Red cell sodium–lithium countertransport in hypertensives. Pp. 88–99 in H. Villarreal and M.P. Sambhi, eds. Topics in Pathophysiology of Hypertension. Martinus Nijhoff, Boston.

Canessa, M., N. Adragna, H.S. Solomon, T.M. Connolly, and D.C. Tosteson. 1980. Increased sodium–lithium countertransport in red cells of patients with essential hypertension. N. Engl. J. Med. 302:772–776.

Capoferro, R., and O. Torgersen. 1974. The effect of hypertonic saline on the uptake of tritiated 7,12-dimethylbenz[a]-anthracene by the gastric mucosa. Scand. J. Gastroenterol. 9:343–349.

Chanutin, A., and E.B. Ferris, Jr. 1932. Experimental renal insufficiency produced by partial nephrectomy; control diet. Arch. Intern. Med. 49:767–787.

Coleman, T.G., and A.C. Guyton. 1969. Hypertension caused by salt loading in the dog. III. Onset transients of cardiac output and other circulatory variables. Circ. Res. 25: 153–160.

Conn, J.W. 1949. The mechanisms of acclimatization to heat. Adv. Intern. Med. 3:373–393.

Cooper, R., I. Soltero, K. Liu, D. Berkson, S. Levinson, and J. Stamler. 1980. The association between urinary sodium excretion and blood pressure in children. Circulation 62:97–104.

Cooper, R., K. Liu, M. Trevisan, W. Miller, and J. Stamler. 1982. Urinary sodium excretion and blood pressure in children: absence of a reproducible association. Hypertension 5:135–139.

Cooper, R., M. Trevisan, L. Van Horn, E. Larbi, K. Liu, S. Nanas, H. Ueshima, C. Sempos, D. Ostrow, and J. Stamler. 1984. Effect of dietary sodium reduction on red blood cell sodium concentration and sodium–lithium countertransport. Hypertension 6:731–735.

Correa, P. 1982. Precursors of gastric and esophageal cancer. Cancer 50 Suppl. 11:2554–2565.

Correa, P., C. Cuello, L.F. Fajardo, W. Haenszel, O Bolaños, and B. de Ramirez. 1983. Diet and gastric cancer: nutrition survey in a high-risk area. J. Natl. Cancer Inst. 70:673–678.

Correa, P., G. Montes, C. Cuello, W. Haenszel, G. Liuzza, G. Zarama, E. de Marin, and D. Zavala. 1985. Urinary sodium-to-creatinine ratio as an indicator of gastric cancer risk. Natl. Cancer Inst. Monogr. 69:121–123.

Cushman, W.C., and H.G. Langford. 1983. Urinary electrolyte differences in black and white hypertensives: for Veterans Administration Cooperative Study Group on Antihypertensive Agents. Clin. Res. 31:843A.

Dadone, M.M., S.J. Hasstedt, S.C. Hunt, J.B. Smith, O.K. Ash, and R.R. Williams. 1984. Genetic analysis of sodium–lithium countertransport in 10 hypertension-prone kindreds. Am. J. Med. Genet. 17:565–577.

Dahl, L.K. 1958. Salt intake and salt need. N. Engl. J. Med. 258:1152–1157.

Dahl, L.K., M. Heine, and L. Tassinari. 1962. Effects of chronic excess salt ingestion: evidence that genetic factors play an important role in susceptibility to experimental hypertension. J. Exp. Med. 115:1173–1190.

Dai, W.S., L.H. Kuller, and G. Miller. 1984. Arterial blood pressure and urinary electrolytes. J. Chronic Dis. 37:75–84.

Dawber, T.R., W.B. Kannel, A. Kagan, R.K. Donabedian, P.M. McNamara, and G. Pearson. 1967. Environmental factors in hypertension. Pp. 255–288 in J. Stamler, R. Stamler, and T.N. Pullman, eds. The Epidemiology of Hypertension: Proceedings of an International Symposium Sponsored by the Chicago Heart Association and the American Heart Association, Chicago, Illinois, February 3–7, 1964. Grune and Stratton, New York.

De Luise, M., G.L. Blackburn, and J.S. Flier. 1980. Reduced activity of red-cell sodium–potassium pump in human obesity. N. Engl. J. Med. 303:1017–1022.

Denton, D. 1982. The Hunger for Salt: An Anthropological, Physiological and Medical Analysis. Springer-Verlag, Berlin. 650 pp.

Eaton, S.B., and M. Konner. 1985. Paleolithic nutrition: a consideration of its nature and current implications. N. Engl. J. Med. 312:283–289.

Feinleib, M., R. Garrison, N. Borhani, R. Rosenman, and J. Christian. 1975. Studies of hypertension in twins. Pp. 3–20 in O. Paul, ed. Epidemiology and Control of Hypertension. Stratton Intercontinental Medical Book Co., New York.

Folkow, B. 1982. Physiological aspects of primary hypertension. Physiol. Rev. 62:347–504.

Frate, D.A., and H.G. Langford. 1985. Potassium and Hypertension. Pp. 147–153 in M.J. Horan, M. Blaustein, J.B. Dunbar, W. Kachadorian, N.M. Kaplan, and A.P. Simopoulos, eds. NIH Workshop on Nutrition and Hypertension: Proceedings from a Symposium. Biomedical Information Corp., New York.

Froment, A., H. Milon, and C. Gravier. 1979. Relation entre consommation sodée et hypertension artérielle. Contribution de l'épidémiologie géographique. Rev. Epidemiol. Sante Publique 27:437–454.

Fujita, T., W.L. Henry, F.C. Bartter, C.R. Lake, and C.S. Delea. 1980. Factors influencing blood pressure in salt-sensitive patients with hypertension. Am. J. Med. 69:334–344.

Garay, R.P., and P. Meyer. 1979. A new test showing abnormal net Na^+ and K^+ fluxes in erythrocytes of essential hypertensive patients. Lancet 1:349–353.

Gleibermann, L. 1973. Blood pressure and dietary salt in human populations. Ecol. Food Nutr. 2:143–156.

Goldby, F.S., and L.J. Beilin. 1972. Relationship between arterial pressure and the permeability of arterioles to carbon particles in acute hypertension in the rat. Cardiovasc. Res. 6:384–390.

Gordon, D.B., and D.R. Drury. 1956. The effect of potassium on the occurrence of petechial hemorrhages in renal hypertensive rabbits. Circ. Res. 4:167–172.

Gothberg, G., S. Lundin, M. Aurell, and B. Folkow. 1983.

Responses to slow, graded bleeding in salt-depleted rats. J. Hypertension Suppl. 2:24–26.

Grim, C.E., F.C. Luft, J.Z. Miller, P.L. Brown, M.A. Gannon, and M.H. Weinberger. 1979. Effects of sodium loading and depletion in normotensive first-degree relatives of essential hypertensives. J. Lab. Clin. Med. 94:764–771.

Grim, C.E., F.C. Luft, J.Z. Miller, G.R. Meneely, H.D. Battarbee, C.G. Hames, and L.K. Dahl. 1980. Racial differences in blood pressure in Evans County, Georgia: relationship to sodium and potassium intake and plasma renin activity. J. Chronic Dis. 33:87–94.

Haenszel, W., M. Kurihara, M. Segi, and R.K.C. Lee. 1972. Stomach cancer among Japanese in Hawaii. J. Natl. Cancer Inst. 49:969–988.

Hamilton, M., G.W. Pickering, J.A.F. Roberts, and G.S.C. Sowry. 1954. Aetiology of essential hypertension: role of inheritance. Clin. Sci. 13:273–304.

Hanawa, K., S. Yamada, H. Suzuki, et al. 1980. Effects of sodium chloride on gastric cancer induction by N-methyl-N'-nitro-N-nitrosoguanidine (MNNG) in rats. P. 49 in Proceedings of the Thirty-ninth Annual Meeting of the Japanese Cancer Association. Japanese Cancer Association, Tokyo.

Hara, N., K. Sakata, M. Nagai, Y. Fujita, T. Hashimoto, and H. Yanagawa. 1985. Geographical difference of mortality of digestive cancers and food consumption. Gan No Rinsho 30:1665–1674.

Harrington, J.S. 1981. Advances in cancer epidemiology in South Africa. S. Afr. Cancer Bull. 25:9–18.

HDFP (Hypertension Detection and Follow-up Program Cooperative Group). 1979a. Five-year findings of the hypertension detection and follow-up program. I. Reduction in mortality of persons with high blood pressure, including mild hypertension. J. Am. Med. Assoc. 242:2562–2571.

HDFP (Hypertension Detection and Follow-up Program Cooperative Group). 1979b. Five-year findings of the hypertension detection and follow-up program. II. Mortality by race-sex and age. J. Am. Med. Assoc. 242:2572–2577.

Henry, J.P., and J.C. Cassel. 1969. Psychosocial factors in essential hypertension. Recent epidemiologic and animal experimental evidence. Am. J. Epidemiol. 90:171–200.

Hilton, P.J. 1986. Cellular sodium transport in essential hypertension. N. Engl. J. Med. 314:222–229.

Hirayama, T. 1979. Diet and cancer. Nutr. Cancer 1:67–81.

Hofman, A., A. Hazebroek, and H.A. Valkenburg. 1983. A randomized trial of sodium intake and blood pressure in newborn infants. J. Am. Med. Assoc. 250:370–373.

Holden, R.A., A.M. Ostfeld, D.H. Freeman, Jr., K.G. Hellenbrand, and D.A. D'Atri. 1983. Dietary salt intake and blood pressure. J. Am. Med. Assoc. 250:365–369.

Howson, C.P., T. Hiyama, and E.L. Wynder. 1986. The decline in gastric cancer: epidemiology of an unplanned triumph. Epidemiol. Rev. 8:1–27.

Iimura, O., T. Kijima, K. Kikuchi, A. Miyama, T. Ando, T. Nakao, and Y. Takigami. 1981. Studies on the hypotensive effect of high potassium intake in patients with essential hypertension. Clin. Sci. 61:77s–80s.

Intersalt Cooperative Research Group. 1988. Intersalt: an international study of electrolyte excretion and blood pressure. Results for a 24 hour urinary sodium and potassium excretion. Br. Med. J. 297:319–328.

Ishiwata, H., P. Boriboon, Y. Nakamura, M. Harada, A. Tanimura, and M. Ishidate. 1975. Studies on in vivo formation of nitroso compounds. II. Changes of nitrite and nitrate concentrations in human saliva after ingestion of vegetables or sodium nitrate. J. Food Hyg. Soc. 16:19–24.

Jacobs, D.R., Jr., J.T. Anderson, and H. Blackburn. 1979. Diet and serum cholesterol: do zero correlations negate the relationship? Am. J. Epidemiol. 110:77–87.

James, W.P., A. Ralph, and C.P. Sanchez-Castillo. 1987. The dominance of salt in manufactured food in the sodium intake of affluent societies. Lancet 1:426–429.

Japan Ministry of Health and Welfare. 1980. Kosei-no-shihyo "Cancer." Health and Welfare Statistics Association, Japan Ministry of Health and Welfare, Tokyo.

Joossens, J.V. 1980. Stroke, stomach cancer and salt: a possible clue to the prevention of hypertension. Pp. 489–508 in H. Kesteloot and J.V. Joossens, eds. Epidemiology of Arterial Blood Pressure. Martinus Nijhoff, The Hague.

Joossens, J.V., and J. Geboers. 1981. Nutrition and gastric cancer. Proc. Nutr. Soc. 40:37–46.

Joossens, J.V., and J. Geboers. 1984. Diet and environment in the etiology of gastric cancer. Pp. 167–183 in B. Levin and R.H. Riddell, eds. Frontiers in Gastrointestinal Cancer. Elsevier, New York.

Kaplan, N.M., and E. Lieberman. 1986. Clinical Hypertension, 4th ed. Williams & Wilkins, Baltimore. 492 pp.

Kaplan, N.M., A. Carnegie, P. Raskin, J.A. Heller, and M. Simmons. 1985. Potassium supplementation in hypertensive patients with diuretic-induced hypokalemia. N. Engl. J. Med. 312:746–749.

Karvonen, M.J., and S. Punsar. 1977. Sodium excretion and blood pressure of West and East Finns. Acta Med. Scand. 202:501–507.

Kawasaki, T., C.S. Delea, F.C. Bartter, and H. Smith. 1978. The effect of high-sodium and low-sodium intakes on blood pressure and other related variables in human subjects with idiopathic hypertension. Am. J. Med. 64:193–198.

Kempner, W. 1948. Treatment of hypertensive vascular disease with rice diet. Am. J. Med. 4:545–577.

Kesteloot, H., B.C. Park, C.S. Lee, E. Brems-Heyns, J. Claessens, and J.V. Joossens. 1980. A comparative study of blood pressure and sodium intake in Belgium and in Korea. Eur. J. Cardiol. 11:169–182.

Khaw, K.T., and E. Barrett-Connor. 1984. Dietary potassium and blood pressure in a population. Am. J. Clin. Nutr. 39:963–968.

Khaw, K.T., and E. Barrett-Connor. 1987. Dietary potassium and stroke-associated mortality. A 12-year prospective population study. N. Engl. J. Med. 316:235–240.

Khaw, K.T., and E. Barrett-Connor. 1988. The association between blood pressure, age, and dietary sodium and potassium: a population study. Circulation 77:53–61.

Khaw, K.T., and G. Rose. 1982. Population study of blood pressure and associated factors in St. Lucia, West Indies. Int. J. Epidemiol. 11:372–377.

Kodama, M., H. Saito, and Z. Yamaizumi. 1982. Formation of alkylureas in the environment. Pp. 131–136 in H. Bartsch, I.K. O'Neill, M. Castegnaro, M. Okada, and W. Davis, eds. *N*-Nitroso Compounds: Occurrence and Biological Effects—Proceedings of the VIIth International Symposium on *N*-Nitroso Compounds Held in Tokyo, 28 September–1 October 1981. IARC Scientific Publ. No. 41. International Agency for Research on Cancer, Lyon, France.

Kodama, M., T. Kodama, H. Suzuki, and K. Kondo. 1984. Effect of rice and salty rice diets on the structure of mouse stomach. Nutr. Cancer 6:135–147.

Kolonel, L.N., M.W. Hinds, and J.H. Hankin. 1980. Cancer patterns among migrant and native-born Japanese in Hawaii in relation to smoking, drinking, and dietary habits. Pp. 327–340 in H.B. Gelboin, B. MacMahon, T. Matsushima, T. Sugimura, S. Takayama, and H. Takebe, eds. Genetic and Environmental Factors in Experimental and Human Cancer: Proceedings of the 10th International Symposium of the Princess Takamatsu Cancer Research Fund, Tokyo, 1979. Japan Scientific Societies Press, Tokyo.

Kono, S., M. Ikeda, and M. Ogata. 1983. Salt and geographical mortality of gastric cancer and stroke in Japan. J. Epidemiol. Community Health 37:43–46.

Kromhout, D., E.B. Bosschieter, and C.D. Coulander. 1985. Potassium, calcium, alcohol intake and blood pressure: the Zutphen Study. Am. J. Clin. Nutr. 41:1299–1304.

Kurtz, T.W., and P.C. Morris. 1985. Dietary chloride as a determinant of "sodium dependent" hypertension and hypercalemia. Pp. 137–146 in M.J. Horan, M. Blaustein, J.B. Dunbar, W. Kachadorian, N.M. Kaplan, and A.P. Simopoulos, eds. NIH Workshop on Nutrition and Hypertension: Proceedings from a Symposium. Biomedical Information Corp., New York.

Kurtz, T.W., H.H. Al-Bander, and R.C. Morris, Jr. 1987. "Salt-sensitive" essential hypertension in men. Is the sodium ion alone important? N. Engl. J. Med. 317:1043–1048.

Langford, H.G. 1985. Dietary potassium and hypertension. Pp. 147–153 in M.J. Horan, M. Blaustein, J.B. Dunbar, W. Kachadorian, N.M. Kaplan, and A.P. Simopoulos, eds. NIH Workshop on Nutrition and Hypertension: Proceedings from a Symposium. Biomedical Information Corp., New York.

Langford, H.G., M.D. Blaufox, A. Oberman, C.M. Hawkins, J.D. Curb, G.R. Cutter, S. Wassertheil-Smoller, S. Pressel, C. Babcock, J.D. Abernethy, J. Hotchkiss, and M. Tyler. 1985. Dietary therapy slows the return of hypertension after stopping prolonged medication. J. Am. Med. Assoc. 253:657–664.

Liu, K., R. Cooper, J. McKeever, P. McKeever, R. Byington, I. Soltero, R. Stamler, F. Gosch, E. Stevens, and J. Stamler. 1979. Assessment of the association between habitual salt intake and high blood pressure: methodological problems. Am. J. Epidemiol. 110:219–226.

Ljungman, S., M. Aurell, M. Hartford, J. Wikstrand, L. Wilhelmsen, and G. Berglund. 1981. Sodium excretion and blood pressure. Hypertension 3:318–326.

Logan, A.G. 1986. Sodium manipulation in the management of hypertension. The view against its general use. Can. J. Physiol. Pharmacol. 64:793–802.

Luft, F.C., C.E. Grim, N. Fineberg, and M.C. Weinberger. 1979. Effects of volume expansion and contraction in normotensive whites, blacks, and subjects of different ages. Circulation 59:643–650.

Luft, F.C., M.C. Weinberger, and C.E. Grimm. 1982. Sodium sensitivity and resistance in normotensive humans. Am. J. Med. 72:726–736.

MacDonald, W.C., F.H. Anderson, and S. Hashimoto. 1967. Histological effect of certain pickles on the human gastric mucosa: a preliminary report. Can. Med. Assoc. J. 96:1521–1525.

MacGregor, G.A., S.J. Smith, N.D. Markandu, R.A. Banks, and G.A. Sagnella. 1982. Moderate potassium supplementation in essential hypertension. Lancet 2:567–570.

Malhotra, S.L. 1970. Dietary factors causing hypertension in India. Am. J. Clin. Nutr. 23:1353–1363.

Mark, A.L., W.J. Lawton, F.M. Abboud, A.E. Fitz, W.E.

Connor, and D.D. Heistad. 1975. Effects of high and low sodium intake on arterial pressure and forearm vascular resistance in borderline hypertension. A preliminary report. Circ. Res. 36 Suppl. 1:1–194 to 1–198.

McManus, I.C. 1983. Bimodality of blood pressure levels. Stat. Med. 2:253–258.

Meneely, G.R., and C.O.T. Ball. 1958. Experimental epidemiology of chronic sodium chloride toxicity and the protective effect of potassium chloride. Am. J. Med. 25:713–725.

Miall, W.E., and P.D. Oldham. 1963. The heredity factor in arterial blood pressure. Br. Med. J. 1:75–80.

Miller, J.Z., and C.E. Grim. 1983. Heritability of blood pressure. Pp. 79–90 in T.A. Kotchen and J.M. Kotchen, eds. Clinical Approaches to High Blood Pressure in the Young. John Wright, PSG Inc., Boston.

Morino, T., R. McCaa, and H.G. Langford. 1978. Effect of potassium loading on blood pressure, sodium excretion and plasma renin activity in hypertensive patients. Clin. Res. 26:805A.

Motulsky, A.G., W. Burke, P.R. Billings, and R.H. Ward. 1987. Hypertension and the genetics of red cell membrane abnormalities. Pp. 150–166 in G. Bock and G.M. Collins, eds. Molecular Approaches to Human Polygenic Disease: Ciba Foundation Symposium 130. Wiley, Chicester, United Kingdom.

Muirhead, E.E., B.E. Leach, J.O. Davis, F.B. Armstrong, Jr., J.A. Pitcock, and W.L. Brosius. 1975. Pathophysiology of angiotensin-salt hypertension. J. Lab. Clin. Med. 85:734–745.

NRC (National Research Council). 1982. Diet, Nutrition, and Cancer. Report of the Committee on Diet, Nutrition, and Cancer, Assembly of Life Sciences. National Academy Press, Washington, D.C. 478 pp.

Ohgaki, H., T. Kato, K. Morino, N. Matsukura, S. Sato, S. Takayama, and T. Sugimura. 1984. Study of the promoting effect of sodium chloride on gastric carcinogenesis by *N*-methyl-*N'*-nitro-*N*-nitrosoguanidine in inbred Wistar rats. Gann 75:1053–1057.

Oliver, W.J., E.L. Cohen, and J.V. Neel. 1975. Blood pressure, sodium intake and sodium related hormones in the Yanomamo Indians, a "no-salt" culture. Circulation 52:146–151.

Overbeck, H.W., D.D. Ku, and J.P. Rapp. 1981. Sodium pump activity in arteries of Dahl salt-sensitive rats. Hypertension 3:306–312.

Page, L.B. 1976. Epidemiologic evidence on the etiology of human hypertension and its possible prevention. Am. Heart J. 91:527–534.

Page, L.B. 1979. Hypertension and atherosclerosis in primitive and acculturating societies. Pp. 1–12 in J.C. Hunt, ed. Hypertension Update, Vol. 1. Health Learning Systems, Lyndhurst, N.J.

Page, L.B., D.E. Vandevert, K. Nader, N.K. Lubin, and J.R. Page. 1981. Blood pressure of Qash'qai pastoral nomads in Iran in relation to culture, diet, and body form. Am. J. Clin. Nutr. 34:527–538.

Pickering, G. 1968. High Blood Pressure, 2nd ed. Grune & Stratton, New York. 717 pp.

Platt, R. 1947. Heredity in hypertension. Q. J. Med. 16:111–133.

Pooling Project Research Group. 1978. Relationship of blood pressure, serum cholesterol, smoking habit, relative weight and ECG abnormalities to incidence of major coronary events: final report of the Pooling Project. J. Chronic Dis. 31:201–306.

Porter, G.A. 1983. Chronology of the sodium hypothesis and hypertension. Ann. Intern. Med. 98:720–723.

Poston, L., R.B. Sewell, S.P. Wilkinson, P.J. Richardson, R. Williams, E.M. Clarkson, G.A. MacGregor, and H.E. De Wardener. 1981. Evidence for a circulating sodium transport inhibitor in essential hypertension. Br. Med. J. 282:847–849.

Priddle, W.W. 1931. Observations on the management of hypertension. Can. Med. Assoc. J. 25:5–8.

Prineas, R.J., and H. Blackburn. 1985. Clinical and epidemiologic relationships between electrolytes and hypertension. Pp. 63–85 in M.J. Horan, M. Blaustein, J.B. Dunbar, W. Kachadorian, N.M. Kaplan, and A.P. Simopoulos, eds. NIH Workshop on Nutrition and Hypertension: Proceedings from a Symposium. Biomedical Information Corp., New York.

Reed, D., D. McGee, K. Yano, and J. Hankin. 1985. Diet, blood pressure, and multicollinearity. Hypertension 7:405–410.

Rostand, S.G., K.A. Kirk, E.A. Rutsky, and B.A. Pate. 1982. Racial differences in the incidence of treatment for end-stage renal disease. N. Engl. J. Med. 306:1276–1279.

Sanchez-Castillo, C.P., S. Warrender, T.P. Whitehead, and W.P. James. 1987a. An assessment of the sources of dietary salt in a British population. Clin. Sci. 72:95–102.

Sanchez-Castillo, C.P., W.J. Branch, and W.P. James. 1987b. A test of the validity of the lithium-marker technique for monitoring dietary sources of salt in men. Clin. Sci. 72:87–94.

Sapirstein, L.A., W.L. Brandt, and D.R. Drury. 1950. Production of hypertension in the rat by substituting hypertonic sodium chloride solutions for drinking water. Proc. Soc. Exp. Biol. Med. 73:82–85.

Sasaki, N., T. Mitsuhashi, and S. Fukushi. 1959. Effects of the ingestion of large amounts of apples on blood pressure of farmers in Akita prefecture. Igaku To Seibutsugaku 51:103–105.

Sato, T., T. Fukuyama, T. Suzuki, J. Takayanagri, T. Murakami, N. Shiotsuki, R. Tanaka, and R. Tsuji. 1959. Studies of the causation of gastric cancer. 2. The relation between gastric cancer mortality rate and salted food intake in several places in Japan. Koshu Eisei In Kenkyu Hokoku 8:187–198.

Sato, T., T. Fukuyama, T. Suzuki, J. Takayangai, and Y. Sakai. 1961. Studies of the causation of gastric cancer: intake of highly brined foods in several places with high mortality rate in Europe. Koshu Eisei In Kenkyu Hokoku 10:9–17.

Schlierf, G., L. Arab, B. Schellenberg, P. Oster, R. Mordasini, H. Schmidt-Gayk, and G. Vogel. 1980. Salt and hypertension: data from the "Heidelberg Study." Am. J. Clin. Nutr. 33:872–875.

Simpson, F.O. 1985. Blood pressure and sodium intake. Pp. 175–190 in C.J Bulpitt, ed. Handbook of Hypertension, Vol. 6. The Epidemiology of Hypertension. Elsevier Science Publ., New York.

Srinivasan, S.R., E.R. Dalferes, Jr., R.H. Wolf, B. Radhakrishnamurthy, T.A. Foster, and G.S. Berenson. 1984. Variability in blood pressure response to dietary sodium intake among African green monkeys (*Cercopithecus aethiops*). Am. J. Clin. Nutr. 39:792–796.

Stewart, H.L. 1967. Experimental alimentary tract cancer. Natl. Cancer Inst. Monogr. 25:199–217.

Svetkey, L.P., W.E. Yarger, J.R. Feussner, E. DeLong, and P.E. Klotman. 1986. Placebo-controlled trial of oral potassium in the treatment of mild hypertension. Clin. Res. 34:487A.

Swales, J.D., R.F. Bing, A. Heagerty, J.E. Pohl, G.I. Russell, and H. Thurston. 1982. Treatment of refractory hypertension. Lancet 1:894–896.

Takahashi, M. 1986. Enhancing effect of a high salt diet on gastrointestinal carcinogenesis. Gan No Rinsho 32:667–673.

Takahashi, M., T. Kokubo, F. Furukawa, Y. Kurokawa, M. Tatematsu, and Y. Hayashi. 1983. Effect of high salt diet on rat gastric carcinogenesis induced by N-methyl-N'-nitro-N-nitrosoguanidine. Gann 74:28–34.

Tatematsu, M., M. Takahashi, S. Fukushima, M. Hananouchi, and T. Shirai. 1975. Effects in rats of sodium chloride on experimental gastric cancers induced by N-methyl-N'-nitro-N-nitrosoguanidine or 4-nitroquinoline-1-oxide. J. Natl. Cancer Inst. 55:101–106.

Tao, S.C., R.S. Tsai, Z.G. Hong, and J. Stamler. 1984. Timed overnight sodium and potassium excretion and blood pressure in steel workers in Peoples' Republic of China, (PRC)-North. CVD Epidemiol. Newsletter (AHA) 35:64.

Toal, C.B., and F.H. Leenen. 1983. Dietary sodium restriction and development of hypertension in spontaneously hypertensive rats. Am. J. Physiol. 245:H1081–H1084.

Tobian, L. 1983. Human essential hypertension: implications of animal studies. Ann. Intern. Med. 98:729–734.

Tobian, L. 1986. High potassium diets markedly protect against stroke deaths and kidney disease in hypertensive rats, a possible legacy from prehistoric times. Can. J. Physiol. Pharmacol. 64:840–848.

Tobian, L. 1988. The Volhard lecture: potassium and sodium in hypertension. J. Hypertens. Suppl. 4:S12–S24.

Tobian, L., Jr., and J.T. Binion. 1952. Tissue cations and water in arterial hypertension. Circulation 5:754–758.

Tobian, L., Jr., and J. Binion. 1954. Artery wall electrolytes in renal and DCA hypertension. J. Clin. Invest. 33:1407–1414.

Tobian, L., M.A. Johnson, J. Lange, and S. Magraw. 1975. Effect of varying perfusion pressures on the output of sodium and renin and the vascular resistance in kidneys of rats with "post-salt" hypertension and Kyoto spontaneous hypertension. Circ. Res. 36 Suppl. 1:1–162 to 1–170.

Tobian, L., J. Lange, S. Azar, J. Iwai, D. Koop, and K. Coffee. 1977. Reduction of intrinsic natriuretic capacity in kidneys of Dahl hypertension-prone rats. Trans. Assoc. Am. Physicians 90:401–406.

Tobian, L., J. Lange, J. Iwai, K. Hiller, M.A. Johnson, and P. Goossens. 1979. Prevention with thiazide of NaCl-induced hypertension in Dahl "S" rats: evidence for a Na-retaining humoral agent in "S" rats. Hypertension 1:316–323.

Tobian, L., M. Ganguli, A. Goto, T. Ikeda, M.A. Johnson, and J. Iwai. 1982. The influence of renal prostaglandins, central nervous system and NaCl on hypertension in Dahl S rats. Clin. Exp. Pharmacol. Physiol. 9:341–353.

Tobian, L., D. MacNeill, M.A. Johnson, M.C Ganguli, and J. Iwai. 1984. Potassium protection against lesions of the renal tubules, arteries, and glomeruli and nephron loss in salt-loaded hypertensive Dahl S rats. Hypertension 6:I–170 to I–176.

Tobian, L., J. Lange, K. Ulm, L. Wold, and J. Iwai. 1985a. Potassium reduces cerebral hemorrhage and death rate in hypertensive rats, even when blood pressure is not lowered. Hypertension 7 Suppl I:I–110 to I–114.

Tobian, L., Y. Uehara, and J. Iwai. 1985b. Prostaglandin alterations in barely hypertensive Dahl S rats. Trans. Assoc. Am. Physicians XCVIII:378–383.

Tobian, L., J. Lange, K. Ulm, L. Wold, and J. Iwai. 1986. NaCl feeding in Dahl S rats markedly reduces GFR and RBF in isolated kidneys perfused at normotensive inflow pressures. J. Hypertension 4 Suppl. 6:S370–S372.

Tuomilehto, J., J. Geboers, J.V. Joossens, J.T. Salonen, and A. Tanskanen. 1984. Trends in stomach cancer and stroke in Finland. Comparison to Northwest Europe and USA. Stroke 15:823–828.

Voors, A.W., E.R. Dalferes, Jr., G.C. Frank, G.G. Aristimuno, and G.S. Berenson. 1983. Relation between ingested potassium and sodium balance in young blacks and whites. Am. J. Clin. Nutr. 37:583–594.

Walker, A.R. 1982. Changing disease patterns in South Africa. S. Afr. Med. J. 61:126–129.

Walker, W.G., P.K. Whelton, H. Saito, R.P. Russell, and J. Hermann. 1979. Relation between blood pressure and renin, renin substrate, angiotensin II, aldosterone and urinary sodium and potassium in 574 ambulatory subjects. Hypertension 1:287–301.

Watson, R.L., H.G. Langford, J. Abernethy, T.Y. Barnes, and M.J. Watson. 1980. Urinary electrolytes, body weight, and blood pressure: pooled cross-sectional results among four groups of adolescent females. Hypertension 2:93–98.

Watt, G.C., C.J. Foy, and J.T. Hart. 1983. Comparison of blood pressure, sodium intake, and other variables in offspring with and without a family history of high blood pressure. Lancet 1:1245–1248.

Weinberger, M.H., J.Z. Miller, F.C. Luft, C.E. Grimm, and N.S. Fineberg. 1986. Definitions and characteristics of sodium sensitivity and blood pressure resistance. Hypertension 8 Suppl. II:II–127 to II–134.

Weisburger, J.H. 1981. N-Nitroso compounds: diet and cancer trends. An approach to the prevention of gastric cancer. Pp. 305–317 in R.A. Scanlan and S.R. Tannenbaum, eds. N-Nitroso Compounds. Based on a Symposium Cosponsored by the Divisions of Agricultural and Food Chemistry and Pesticide Chemistry of the 181st Meeting of the American Chemical Society, Atlanta, Georgia, March 31–April 1, 1981. ACS Symposium Series 174. American Chemical Society, Washington, D.C.

Weisburger, J.H., H. Marquardt, N. Hirota, H. Mori, and G.M. Williams. 1980. Induction of cancer of the glandular stomach in rats by an extract of nitrite-treated fish. J. Natl. Cancer Inst. 64:163–167.

Weissberg, P.L., M.R. Wilkins, and L.J. Kricka. 1983. Test for circulating Na$^+$-K$^+$ ATPase inhibitors. Lancet 1:1219.

West, R.C., ed. 1984. European Collaborative Study on the Role of Diet and Other Factors in the Aetiology of Atrophic Gastritis: A Precancerous Lesion of Gastric Cancer. Euro-Nut, The Netherlands.

Whelton, P.K., and P. Goldblatt. 1982. An investigation of the relationship between stomach cancer and cerebrovascular disease: evidence for and against the salt hypothesis. Am. J. Epidemiol. 115:418–427.

Whitescarver, S.A., C.E. Ott, B.A. Jackson, G.P. Guthrie, Jr., and T.A. Kotchen. 1984. Salt-sensitive hypertension:

contribution of chloride. Science 223:1430–1432.

WHO (World Health Organization). 1978. Arterial Hypertension. Report of a WHO Expert Committee. Technical Report Series 628. World Health Organization, Geneva. 58 pp.

Wilczynski, E.A., and F.H. Leenen. 1987. Dietary sodium intake and age in spontaneously hypertensive rats: effects on blood pressure and sympathetic activity. Life Sci. 41:707–715.

Woods, J.W., R.J. Falk, A.W. Pittman, P.J. Klemmer, B.S. Watson, and K. Namboodiri. 1982. Increased red-cell sodium–lithium countertransport in normotensive sons of hypertensive parents. N. Engl. J. Med. 306:593–595.

Yano, K. 1981. Alkylating activity of processed fish products treated with sodium nitrite in simulated gastric juice. Gann 72:451–454.

Zinner, S.H., H.S. Margolius, B. Rosner, H.R. Keiser, and E.H. Kass. 1976. Familial aggregation of urinary kallikrein concentration in childhood: relation to blood pressure, race and urinary electrolytes. Am. J. Epidemiol. 104:124–132.

16

Alcohol

Alcohol consumption is difficult to quantify accurately, and there is no universally acceptable classification system or standard for the safe level of drinking. In 1862, the British established a daily upper limit of 1.5 oz as the safe level of alcohol consumption (O'Brien and Chafetz, 1982). The equivalence in drinks can be calculated from Table 16–1 (Baum-Baicker, 1985a). The Fourth Special Report of the U.S. Congress on Alcohol and Health considered the moderate drinker as one who consumed 0.22 to 0.99 oz of ethanol per day and the light drinker as one who consumed 0.01 to 0.21 oz/day (NIAAA, 1981). Accordingly, Turner et al. (1981) proposed that to qualify as moderate, one's alcohol consumption should not exceed 0.8 g/kg of body weight (bw) per day (an absolute limit of 80 g of alcohol) or an average of 0.7 g/kg bw in a 3-day period, as shown in Table 16–2 (Baum-Baicker, 1985a). People exceeding these limits are considered heavy drinkers (Klatsky et al., 1979). By this standard, 24% of all adults in the United States can be considered moderate drinkers, one-third as light drinkers, 9% as heavy drinkers, and about one-third as abstainers (NIAAA, 1987).

The best indicator of drinking is the blood alcohol level (BAL) at any time. At a BAL of 0.05 (5 parts of alcohol to 10,000 parts of blood), generally reached after one or two drinks, many people experience positive sensations such as re-laxation, euphoria, and well-being (Hales and Hales, 1986). Above this mark, a person starts feeling worse and gradually loses control of speech, balance, and emotions. When BAL reaches 0.1, a person is considered to be drunk (i.e., experiences symptoms of frequent headaches, nausea, stomach pain, heartburn, gas, fatigue, weakness, muscle cramps, irregular or rapid heartbeats, dramatic mood swings, and depression and paranoia); at 0.2, some people pass out; at 0.3, some collapse into a coma; and at 0.4, a person can die (Hales and Hales, 1986).

PATTERNS OF ALCOHOL CONSUMPTION IN THE UNITED STATES

In 1985, 18 million adults 18 years of age and over had problems with alcohol use (NIAAA, 1986). Forty-one percent of these (7.3 million) were alcohol abusers, defined by the National Institute on Alcohol Abuse and Alcoholism (NIAAA) as drinkers who experienced at least one severe or moderately severe consequence of alcohol abuse, such as job loss, arrest, or illness, during the previous year. The remaining 59% (10.6 million) were alcoholics, defined as drinkers who, during the past year, experienced at least one symptom of alcohol withdrawal or one loss-of-control symptom plus one other symptom of de-

TABLE 16-1   Amount of Ethanol in a Drink[a]

Beverage Type	Ethanol Content (%)	Unit of Measure	Ethanol in a Drink [oz and (ml)]
Whiskey (80 proof)	40	1-oz shot (30 ml)	0.40 (11.83)
Table wine	12.1[b]	3.5-oz glass (104 ml)	0.42 (12.42)
U.S. beer	3.5[c]	12-oz bottle (355 ml)	0.42 (12.42)

[a]From Baum-Baicker (1985a).
[b]Most table wines contain 11 to 13% ethanol. Fortified wines, such as sherry and port, contain approximately 20% ethanol.
[c]Most U.S. brands contain 3.2 to 4.0% ethanol.

pendence. Although alcohol abusers and alcoholics were defined as separate groups, they were not considered to be mutually exclusive. Many alcoholics also reported consequences of alcohol abuse, and some counted as alcohol abusers may have had alcohol dependence.

Alcohol consumption peaks in the 20- to 40-year age group; alcohol abuse is most frequent in youth and middle age. A national study by Schoenborn and Cohen (1986) showed that 70% of people between the ages of 20 and 34 consumed alcohol.

In a 1985 survey, 66% of the high school seniors interviewed reported that they had consumed alcohol in the past month and 5% described themselves as daily drinkers. Thirty-seven percent of them had had five or more drinks on at least one occasion during the 2 weeks before the survey (NIAAA, 1987).

Alcohol use decreases in the elderly. Among those 65 to 74 years of age, 43% consumed alcohol. The percentage fell to 30% after age 75. The national survey of Cahalan et al. (1967) showed that 15% of those under 40 years and 5% of the elderly were heavy drinkers.

The lower percentage of alcoholics among the elderly is believed to be the consequence of attri-

tion, as younger alcoholics die from accidents, cirrhosis, or other medical complications. It is also more difficult to define alcohol abuse among the elderly, because many of the criteria for such a classification (e.g., inability to hold a job, drunken driving, or other consequences of drinking) are less likely to apply to the elderly. Furthermore, family members may underreport excess alcohol use to protect the dignity of their elderly relatives.

Alcoholism affects nearly 18% of the institutionalized elderly (Schuckit and Miller, 1976), who are more likely to have medical problems. As many as 28% of the elderly residents of psychiatric institutions have had problems with alcohol use. Blose (1978) also found that 40 to 60% of nursing home patients had a history of alcohol-related problems. These figures are especially important in light of the increasingly high percentage of older people in the U.S. population.

Males are more likely to drink alcohol (Table 16-3) and to drink more heavily than females. Nevertheless, the proportion of women who drink has increased in the past 25 years. Through the 1970s, more women than men were abstainers and light drinkers, and fewer women were heavy drinkers. By 1981, the percentage of women who were

TABLE 16-2   Upper Limits of Allowable Daily Alcohol Consumption[a]

Weight of Individual		0.8 g/kg bw per day[b]				0.7 g/kg bw[b]			
(kg)	(lb)	Ethanol (g)	80-Proof Spirits (oz)	12% Table Wine (oz)	3.6%[c] Beer (oz)	Ethanol (g)	80-Proof Spirits (oz)	12% Table Wine (oz)	3.6%[c] Beer (oz)
50	110	40	4.3	14	38	35	3.7	13	33
60	132	48	5.1	17	46	42	4.5	15	40
70	154	56	6.0	20	53	49	5.2	18	47
80	176	64	6.9	23	61	56	6.0	20	53
90	198	72	7.7	26	69	63	6.7	23	60
100	220	80	8.6	29	76	70	7.5	25	67

[a]From Baum-Baicker (1985a). Conversions: 1 oz = 23.34 g or 29.574 ml.
[b]Turner et al. (1981) defined moderate intake as no more than 0.8 g/kg bw per day or an average of 0.7 g/kg bw over a 3-day period. See text.
[c]By weight, or 4.5% by volume.

TABLE 16–3 Estimated Numbers of Adult Alcohol Abusers and Alcoholics, 1985[a]

Sex	Alcohol Abusers[b]		Alcoholics[b]		Total	
	Percent of Groups	Number	Percent of Population	Number	Percent of Total	Number
Male	5.61	4,849,810	8.40	7,296,979	14.01	12,146,789
Female	2.53	2,446,354	3.50	3,327,213	6.03	5,773,567
Both	3.97	7,296,164	5.79	10,624,192	9.76	17,920,356

[a]From NIAAA (1986).
[b]See definitions in text.

heavy drinkers and the percentage of women ages 35 to 44 who were drinkers had increased (Wilsnack et al., 1984).

Rates of excessive drinking and self-reported drinking problems for the adult black population are similar to rates in the general U.S. population (NIAAA, 1987). Black youths have higher abstention rates and lower rates of heavy drinking than white youths. Native Americans, on the average, are more likely to be heavy drinkers than the general population. Some tribes have lower percentages of drinking adults than the U.S. population (30% versus 67%), whereas the percentage of drinkers in other tribes reaches 80% (NIAAA, 1987). Little is known about drinking practices or alcohol-related problems among Asian Americans, although they are generally believed to have a lower prevalence than found in other groups (see Chapter 4 of this report).

GENETICS AND ALCOHOLISM

Studies of families, twins, adoptees, and animals suggest that alcoholism results from an interaction between heredity and environment (NIAAA, 1987). Research is now focused on identifying physiological, psychological, and biochemical markers for susceptibility to alcohol (see Chapter 4).

CULTURAL ASPECTS OF ALCOHOL USE

Historical Perspective

Ethnographic Review

Ancient Egyptians believed that beer (or *bouza*) was invented by the goddess Osiris (Ghalioungui, 1979). Beer, produced by malting, was considered food and drink and was the beverage of common people at festivals. Wine was also produced in ancient Egypt and used in religious celebrations and as a medicine. In contrast with beer, wine was considered an aristocrat's drink (Ghalioungui, 1979). In Mesopotamia 3000 years B.C., beer was the drink of the cereal-growing south, whereas wine was the choice of the vine-growing north (Ghalioungui, 1979). Accounts of drunkenness in ancient Greece and Rome are well documented (Roe, 1979). Greeks ate cabbage to avoid inebriety—a custom later adopted by the Arabs (Ghalioungui, 1979). In the Bible, however, the beneficial references to drinking appear to be related to unfermented grape juice (Wilkerson, 1978).

In pre-Islamic Arabia, beer, fermented dates, milk, and wine were commonly consumed (Gawad, 1968). Drinking took place in houses, taverns, and dancing places and along caravan routes. With the advent of Islam, abstinence became the rule in Arabia. In other Middle Eastern cities, such as Baghdad, Cairo, Damascus, and Tehran, drinking was not banned but was unpopular, and today it is barely tolerated (Ghalioungui, 1979). *Chicha* (beer made from maize) played important religious, economic, and political roles in the Andean South American society during the Incan empire (Morris, 1979). Alcohol had a similar place among the Aztecs of Mexico (Paredes, 1975) and the Mayans of Central America (Gonçalves de Lima et al., 1977).

In medieval Europe, drunkenness was prevalent among the lower orders of clergy (Roe, 1979). In medieval England, wine became plentiful after grapes were imported from France at the end of the fourteenth century. Throughout the Middle Ages, drunkenness was largely associated with revelry, feasting, and religious celebrations. Alcoholism did not become a social problem until distilled beverages became available around 1100 A.D. (Singer et al., 1956). Until the sixteenth century, fortified wine was produced only on a small scale in monasteries. Franciscus Sylvius, a seventeenth-century professor of medicine at the University of Leiden, may be the first to have distilled alcohol from grain and to have named the result *aqua vitae* (Lucia, 1963). The English, who called it gin, imported it during the reign of William III. By 1700, gin was produced from excess corn (Dorothy George, 1931) to compete with French liquors (Hirsch, 1949). In the first half of the eighteenth century in England, especially 1720 to 1750, lower-income people drank large quantities of alcohol, and the adverse nutritional consequences of alcoholism were first recognized at that time (Roe, 1979). The Gin Act of 1751 imposed a duty on spirits and stopped distillers, chandlers, and grocers from retailing liquor. This legislation brought excessive alcohol consumption under control several years later (Webb and Webb, 1903).

Rum was developed in the Caribbean in 1650 as a by-product of the sugarcane industry and was distributed to the British Royal Navy in 1892. It was believed to confer strength and offer protection against scurvy (Chalke, 1976).

Puritans in the American colonies believed that alcoholic drinks were wholesome and strengthening. In the eighteenth century, when rum and whiskey became available, alcohol abuse became evident. Black slaves and American Indians were considered too irresponsible to be trusted with the alcohol (Roe, 1979), but the colonists nevertheless used alcoholic beverages to appease the Indians and to motivate the slaves to perform unpleasant tasks.

Alcohol and Nutritional Disorders

The relationship between alcohol abuse and nutritional disorders was reported as early as the eighteenth century (Sedgewick, 1725). In the United States, Benjamin Rush observed in 1809 that approximately 4,000 people died annually from the use of rum (Rush, 1818). He described such effects of hard drinking as loss of appetite, jaundice, dropsy, diabetes, redness of face, fetid breath, epilepsy, gout, and madness. Bynuum (1968) observed that the concept of chronic alcoholism as a disease, instead of as a vice or a cause of other diseases, began about the turn of the eighteenth century, when the phrase *habitual drunkenness*, the equivalent of today's chronic alcoholism, was coined. Fuchs (1848) described alcohol as a poison. Huss (1852) attributed the effects of chronic alcohol abuse to tissue damage and believed that alcohol's toxic effects were similar to those caused by intoxicating foods. Jolliffe (1940) described the role of alcohol in the development of nutritional deficiencies.

Alcohol in Medicine

In the middle of the nineteenth century, alcohol was commonly used to treat certain diseases and to alleviate symptoms (Roe, 1979). In 1864, a committee of the National Academy of Sciences, in response to a request from the Surgeon General of the U.S. Army, recommended that in military hospitals whiskey be replaced with alcohol, medicated with additives appropriate for the intended objective (Parker, 1978). A strong reaction to its use as a drug occurred early in the nineteenth century and paralleled the growth of the temperance movement (Horsley and Sturge, 1915).

From antiquity, wine, beer, and, later, spirits were considered to be food for the sick when solid foods could not be tolerated (Roe, 1979) and, in many societies, to have nutritional value (Steinkraus, 1979). Although alcohol has been used clinically as an appetite stimulant, as a sedative–hypnotic drug, and as a calorie source for intravenous administration, these uses have not been subjected to controlled medical evaluation (Becker et al., 1974). Ethanol is unusual among drugs in that it has a biphasic impact on the nervous system. In small amounts, it stimulates; but as it accumulates in the body it depresses, and the amount that makes the difference is minute for most people. Many effects of drinking are determined less by the quantity consumed than by one's expectations (Heath, in press).

Transcultural Anthropological Perspective

Alcohol and drinking are perceived differently among Western and non-Western cultures. Some insights into the cultural role of alcohol can be discerned by comparing these cultures.

Western Societies

In Western societies, the frequency of alcoholism is not uniform among various ethnic groups. For example, most Jews drink, but few become alcoholics; ascetic Protestants rarely drink, but those who do so generally drink heavily (Heath, 1975). Bales (1946) explained that Jews regard drinking as a family sacrament, since wine is introduced to children in a sacred ritual context. In contrast, the Irish perceive drinking in a convivial secular context whereby adult men prove their manhood. Since the 1970s, however, Jews have been showing patterns of alcohol abuse (Heath, 1987), presumably because of growing distance from traditional orthodoxy and from the moral authority of their faith (Douglas, 1987). Comparative ethnic studies also show changes in drinking patterns among Italians, Poles, and Portuguese after they migrated to America (Heath, 1987).

Non-Western Literate Societies

Among non-Western literate societies, there are wide differences in consumption of alcoholic beverages. For example, although prohibition of alcoholic beverages is supposed to characterize the Islamic world, alcohol-related problems are now recognized in Saudi Arabia (Al-Qthami, 1978) and in Bahrein (Alsafar, 1974). In India, some groups of Hindus espouse drunkenness as religious duty, whereas others practice complete abstinence (Heath, 1975).

Nonliterate Societies

Among nonliterate societies, the Camba of eastern Bolivia esteem drunkenness and actively pursue it, but there is no alcoholism in the sense that they do not suffer any alcohol-related economic, social, or psychological problems nor do they engage in aggressive behavior (Heath, 1975). Among African tribal societies, beer drinking is an integral part of most social activities among men. Beer is used as an offering to appease the gods, as a pledge of agreement between parties following adjudication, as a reward for help in working one's land in a system of reciprocal labor exchange, and as a medicine. Pathological addiction or aggressive behavior does not occur in these groups (Heath, 1975).

North American Indians also vary widely in their reactions to alcoholic beverages and have changed their attitudes over time. In the first decades of contact with whites, the Iroquois of upstate New York and southeastern Canada consumed distilled liquors in moderation and drinking became an integral part of their religion. In the early eighteenth century, however, aggression became part of their drunken behavior, following the example of white trappers and traders. By 1800, drunkenness had become a serious problem and eventually led to abstinence (Dailey, 1968). Kunitz et al. (1971) suggest that cirrhosis mortality rates are much higher among the Navaho than among the Hopi because the Hopi condemn drinking and reject the drunk, whereas the Navaho expect young men to be heavy drinkers and never force them into isolation or fail to welcome them back into the community.

Some populations show no reactions to alcohol such as hangovers, blackouts, and addiction, even when drunkenness is commonplace, e.g., among the Peruvian Quechua, Bolivian Camba, Salish, Polynesians, and Tarahumara (Heath, 1975). It is not known whether this lack of reaction is due to differences in thresholds to pain, physiological reactions to alcohol, attitudes toward or expected effects of alcohol, or other biologic or cultural factors.

Cross-Cultural Studies

Alcoholic beverages have been used to foster social integration in many societies, such as Finnish Lapps, Bolivian Camba, and many American Indian and South African tribes (Heath, 1975). In other societies, they have been used to appease gods, to pay fines or taxes, to mobilize agricultural labor, to overcome shyness and gain courage, to symbolize social unity, to promote social cohesion or conviviality, to relieve anxieties and pressures due to conflict with a dominant culture, to enhance social status and prestige, to mark personal identity and boundaries between ethnic groups, and to serve as a mode of recreation (Douglas, 1987; Heath, 1975, in press).

Social problems are related more frequently to consumption of alcohol in Western societies than non-Western societies. Alcoholism is rare in non-Western societies, even where most adults of at least one sex drink regularly and where drunkenness is valued (Heath, 1975).

Several generalizations can be derived from cross-cultural studies:

- In most societies, drinking is a social act embedded in a context of values, attitudes, and other norms, all of which influence the expression of effects, regardless of biochemical, physiological, or pharmacokinetic factors.
- Drinking is governed by rules tied to strong emotions and sanctions, determining such things as who may or may not drink, how much of what they may drink, in what context, and with whom.
- Alcohol promotes relaxation and sociability in various populations.
- Physical, economic, psychological, social, or other problems associated with drinking are rare in many cultures.
- When alcohol-related problems occur, they are linked with modalities, attitudes, and norms regarding drinking.
- Attempts at prohibition are not successful unless embedded in sacred or religious values (Heath, 1987).

EVIDENCE ASSOCIATING ALCOHOL CONSUMPTION WITH CHRONIC DISEASES

Assessment of Alcohol Consumption

The accurate assessment of alcohol consumption is difficult in population-based studies, and evidence regarding validity and reliability of the estimates has rarely been obtained. Some people are likely to underreport actual consumption, and the frequency of such underreporting varies with the social undesirability of consuming alcohol. In many epidemiologic studies, particularly the earlier ones, participants were simply asked to report an average number of drinks of beer, wine, and liquor or cocktails per day without regard for the complexities of drinking behavior or for the interview techniques needed to obtain information. Investigators have reported alcohol consumption in different units (e.g., number of drinks per day or volume of alcohol per month) and have used different formulas for converting the reported drinking behavior into these units. As a result, it is often difficult to summarize the results of such studies. Some writers have tried to circumvent this problem by using such terms as *light*, *moderate*, and *heavy* drinking, but such descriptive words are not satisfactory for scientific purposes. Where possible, alcohol consumption is reported herein as grams of ethanol per week, but these figures should be considered approximations and interpreted cautiously. Difficulties in assessing published statistics related to alcohol and drug abuse have been highlighted in a recent editorial (Barnes, 1988).

Obesity

Ethanol may contribute to obesity because, depending on the level of intake, it can serve as an important energy source. The carbohydrate content is negligible for whiskey, cognac, and vodka; however, it is 2 to 10 g of carbohydrate/liter for red or dry white wine, 30 g/liter for beer or dry sherry, and as much as 120 g/liter for sweetened white or port wines (Pekkanen and Forsander, 1977).

National consumption data show that, on the average, alcohol contributes 4.5% of total calories to the energy intake of Americans (Scheig, 1970). The heavy drinker may derive as much as half, or more, of the daily calories from ethanol. Although the combustion of ethanol in a bomb calorimeter yields a value of 7.1 kcal/g, its biologic value may be less when compared in vivo to an equivalent carbohydrate intake. Metabolic ward subjects given additional calories as alcohol failed to gain weight (Lieber et al., 1965). No additional weight was gained by 17 hospitalized alcoholics who were given 1,800 alcohol-derived calories in addition to their 2,600-calorie diet (Mezey and Faillace, 1971). In metabolic ward studies, isocaloric substitution of ethanol for carbohydrates as 50% of total calories in a balanced diet resulted in a decline in body weight, and when given as additional calories, ethanol caused less weight gain than did calorically equivalent carbohydrates or fats (Pirola and Lieber, 1972). Crouse and Grundy (1984) reported variable responses to additional calories given as ethanol: no weight gain in lean individuals and some weight gain in half the obese individuals.

The view that ethanol increases metabolic rate is supported by the observation that ethanol ingestion increases oxygen consumption in normal subjects and that this effect is much greater in alcoholics (Tremolieres and Carre, 1961). Substitution of ethanol for carbohydrates increases the metabolic rate of humans and rodents (Stock and Stuart, 1974; Stock et al., 1973). A 15% increase in thermogenesis was seen in rats fed ethanol for 10 days (Stock and Stuart, 1974). In humans, diet-induced thermogenesis was also increased (Stock and Stuart, 1974). In rats, some, but not most, of the energy wastage was attributable to brown-fat thermogenesis (Rothwell and Stock, 1984). One postulated mechanism of energy wastage is oxidation without phosphorylation by the microsomal ethanol-oxidizing system (Pirola and Lieber, 1972). This pathway was induced by chronic ethanol consumption (Pirola and Lieber, 1975, 1976). Israel et al. (1975) explained energy wastage as the uncoupling of mitochondrial nicotinamide adenine dinucleotide (NADH) reoxidation, perhaps abetted by catecholamine release or a hyperthyroid state. However, the implication of the hyperthyroid state is unresolved (Teschke et al., 1983).

As a calorie source, alcohol is not as efficient as carbohydrates, especially when consumed chronically in large amounts. Thus, ethanol may contribute to excess energy intake, but is not a common primary cause of obesity. Moderate alcohol intake (i.e., 16% of total calories) was associated with a slightly elevated energy intake (Gruchow et al., 1985a). Despite comparable levels of physical activity there was no weight gain, perhaps because of the metabolic considerations discussed above. This and a slightly higher level (23%) of alcohol intake

(Hillers and Massey, 1985) were associated with a substitution of alcohol for carbohydrates as a source of calories. When the percentage of calories from alcohol exceeds 30%, large decreases in protein and fat intake occur.

Cancer

Epidemiologic Studies

Because the associations between alcohol consumption and cancer vary by site, the committee considered the evidence separately for each site.

Oral Cavity and Pharynx

Mortality from oropharyngeal cancer is higher among people in occupations providing ready access to alcohol and among alcoholics, whereas risks are lower among alcohol abstainers such as Seventh-Day Adventists and Mormons in the United States (de Lint and Levinson, 1975; Lyon et al., 1976). In 14,000 Danish brewery workers who were not alcoholics, but who did have an above-average consumption of beer, the incidence of pharyngeal cancer was twice as high as that in the general population (Jensen, 1979).

In a study of 543 men with cancer of the lip, oral cavity, and pharynx and 207 controls, Wynder et al. (1957a,b) found an association of these cancers with alcohol drinking. Rothman and Keller (1972) reanalyzed information on consumption of alcohol and use of tobacco obtained by Keller and Terris (1965). The risk for oropharyngeal cancer increased with increasing alcohol consumption at every level of smoking. In agreement with the findings of Wynder et al. (1957b), the analysis showed multiplicative interactions between alcohol and tobacco in their effects on oral-cavity cancer.

Evidence for the role of alcohol and tobacco in cancer of the oral cavity also comes from a study in France (Schwartz et al., 1962). The average daily consumption of alcohol was significantly increased in patients with cancers of the tongue, buccal cavity, oral pharynx, and hypopharynx. Case-control studies in Puerto Rico (Martinez, 1969) and in the United States (Graham et al., 1977) have confirmed the role of alcohol in cancer of the oral cavity.

Larynx

Early clinical and occupational studies showed an association between access to alcoholic beverages or heavy alcohol drinking and laryngeal cancer (Kennaway and Kennaway, 1947; Kirchner

and Malkin, 1953). Most studies of alcoholics indicate an excess of laryngeal cancer (Monson and Lyon, 1975; Schmidt and de Lint, 1972). The risk of laryngeal cancer among male Danish brewery workers was twice as high as expected (Jensen, 1979).

Several case-control studies have examined the interaction of alcohol and tobacco. Wynder et al. (1957a) reported that the risk of laryngeal cancer increased with the amount of whiskey consumed, even after adjusting for tobacco. Later, Wynder et al. (1976) confirmed the dose–response relationship, although the increase in risk was less than in the earlier studies. Other studies in the United States (Graham et al., 1981), Denmark (Olsen et al., 1985), and Canada (Burch et al., 1981) confirmed the dual role of alcohol and tobacco in increasing the risk of laryngeal cancer. In most of these analyses, the two factors were found to have a synergistic effect.

Esophagus

A high prevalence of alcoholism has been found among patients with esophageal cancer (Piquet and Tison, 1937). Furthermore, the incidence of esophageal cancer was greater among people employed in the production or distribution of alcoholic beverages than in the general population (Jensen, 1979).

Wynder and Bross (1961) reported a dose–response relationship between esophageal cancer and consumption of whiskey and beer by smokers of 16 to 34 cigarettes per day. The risk was approximately 25 times higher among drinkers of seven or more units of whiskey per day than among light whiskey consumers. A dose–response relationship was also found among beer consumers.

In Paris, Schwartz et al. (1962) found that average alcohol consumption was much higher among patients with esophageal cancer than among traffic accident victims. Martinez (1969) reported a clear dose–response relationship between esophageal cancer and daily consumption of alcohol in Puerto Rico. In France, Tuyns et al. (1977, 1979, 1982) found dose–response associations between the consumption of alcohol, after adjusting for tobacco, and the risk of esophageal cancer. Alcohol and tobacco combined had a synergistic effect: There was a very high risk among people who both drank and smoked heavily. Those studies also indicated that the risk of esophageal cancer was pronounced for consumers of apple cider distillates. In a later study, Tuyns (1983) examined the risk associated with alcohol consumption among 74 men and women with esophageal cancer who never smoked. In both sexes, the risk increased with increased daily alcohol consumption. Similar associations were also found in Singapore (De Jong et al., 1974). A case-control study of black men in Washington, D.C., by Pottern et al. (1981) indicated that risk was higher among consumers of hard liquor than among beer drinkers (relative risks of 7.3 and 2.7, respectively).

Stomach

Although no increased stomach cancer risk was found among Finnish alcoholics or Danish brewery workers (Hakulinen et al., 1974; Jensen, 1979), Sundby (1967) reported a mortality ratio of 1.6 for stomach cancer among alcoholics in Norway. Studies in France (Audigier and Lambert, 1974) and in Japan (Hirayama, 1972) also suggested that alcohol may be associated with cancer at this site. One case-control study showed an association between stomach cancer and wine drinking (Hoey et al., 1981), but other case-control studies have not supported such an association (Acheson and Doll, 1964; Graham et al., 1972; Haenszel et al., 1972; Schwartz et al., 1962; Tuyns et al., 1982).

Colon and Rectum

Breslow and Enstrom (1974) reported an association between beer sales and rectal cancer in 41 states in the United States and in 24 countries. However, when consumption data for fats were taken into account, the correlation with colon cancer disappeared, whereas the positive correlation between beer consumption and rectal cancer remained (Schrauzer, 1976). In Denmark, no increased risk of either colon or rectal cancer was found among brewery workers (Jensen, 1979), but a similar study among brewery workers in Ireland showed a doubling of the risk of rectal cancer (Dean et al., 1979). There was a moderately nonsignificant increased risk of rectal cancer in one case-control study by Tuyns et al. (1982).

In a case-control study conducted in Australia, Kune et al. (1987) found little evidence of an association of any alcoholic beverages with colon cancer, but beer was a risk factor for rectal cancer. The effect was more marked in males than in females. The relative risk for the highest consumption levels in quartiles compared to the lowest was approximately 2. The risk of rectal cancer varied with beer-drinking patterns in the previous 15 to 20 years. Nevertheless, in other case-control studies, either no association or only a weak associa-

tion was found between the risk of colorectal cancer, colon cancer, or rectal cancer and the consumption of alcohol or beer (Dales et al., 1979; Graham et al., 1978; Miller et al., 1983). By contrast, in cohort studies conducted in Norway (Bjelke, 1978) and in Hawaii (Pollack et al., 1984), there was a dose–response relationship between risk of rectal cancer and consumption of alcohol, especially with regard to frequency of beer consumption.

Pancreas

Some studies suggest an association between pancreatic cancer and alcohol consumption (Burch and Ansari, 1968; Cubilla and Fitzgerald, 1978); however, most studies of alcoholics have not shown an increased risk for cancer at this site (Hakulinen et al., 1974; Monson and Lyon, 1975). Similarly, no cohort or case-control studies have confirmed an increased risk (Jensen, 1979; MacMahon et al., 1981; Tuyns et al., 1982).

Liver

In North America and western Europe, cirrhosis of the liver is related mainly to alcohol consumption, and there is a firm association between cirrhosis of the liver and primary liver cancer (Tuyns, 1982). However, not all studies of alcoholics suggest an increased risk of primary liver cancer (Nicholls et al., 1974; Schmidt and de Lint, 1972). Studies of male Danish brewery workers, however, provide a clear association between primary liver cancer and cirrhosis of the liver (Jensen, 1979). In Finland, a significant excess ($p < .05$) of primary liver cancer was found among alcohol abusers (Hakulinen et al., 1974). Some studies suggest that primary liver cancer may be increased in alcoholics, even in the absence of cirrhosis (Lieber et al., 1979).

Accumulating evidence links viral hepatitis and hepatocellular carcinoma in alcoholics. Serologic markers of viral hepatitis are more frequent in alcoholics (Chevilotte et al., 1983; Gluud et al., 1982; Hislop et al., 1981; Mills et al., 1979; Orholm et al., 1981). Prevalence of anti-HBV (hepatitis virus B) antibodies was also found to be higher in an unselected outpatient alcoholic population (Gluud et al., 1984). Bréchot et al. (1982) reported that 19 of 51 subjects with various stages of alcoholic liver disease had one or more serologic markers of HBV in their serum. Eight of the 51 subjects had HBV–DNA in their livers. In five of these subjects, the DNA was integrated into the genome. Whether this increased incidence of positive cases is due to the socioeconomic status of the alcoholic, increased exposure to hepatitis infection from blood transfusions, or enhanced susceptibility to infection remains to be determined.

Bréchot et al. (1982) evaluated 20 subjects with alcoholic cirrhosis and hepatocellular carcinoma for evidence of HBV infection. Only 9 of 16 tested serologically had markers of HBV infection, but in all 20 subjects, HBV–DNA was integrated into the genome of the neoplastic liver cells. However, among alcoholic cirrhotics, Omata et al. (1979) found no difference in the frequency of hepatitis infection between those with and those without hepatocellular carcinoma. Goudeau et al. (1981) reported HBV markers in 31% of 125 asymptomatic alcoholics, 55% of 163 alcoholics with cirrhosis, and 22% of 46 with hepatocellular carcinoma. Yarrish et al. (1980) noted similar rates of HBV infection in both alcoholic and nonalcoholic subjects with hepatocellular carcinoma. Of their alcoholic subjects with hepatocellular carcinoma, 88% were seropositive for HBV markers, compared to 69% of nonalcoholic subjects with hepatocellular carcinoma.

In summary, most studies indicate an increased prevalence of HBV infection among alcoholics with cirrhosis and an association between the infection and a high frequency of liver cell cancer.

Breast

Most of the studies conducted on this subject suggest that breast cancer risk is related to alcohol consumption (Graham, 1987; Schatzkin et al., 1987). There was a positive correlation between alcohol consumption and breast cancer in 41 states in the United States, but not in 24 other countries (Breslow and Enstrom, 1974). Breast cancer mortality was twofold higher among 2,070 people admitted to mental hospitals in the United Kingdom with a diagnosis of alcoholism (Adelstein and White, 1976). The Third National Cancer Survey in the United States indicated a relative risk of 1.5 for breast cancer from consumption of hard liquor and wine. There was also a dose–response relationship with total alcohol consumption (Williams and Horm, 1977). In one case-control study, Rosenberg et al. (1982) found increased risk of breast cancer for drinkers compared with nondrinkers; the association was evident for beer, wine, and spirits. In another, conducted in France by Lê et al. (1984), there was an increased risk of breast cancer in subjects who consumed alcoholic beverages with meals. The association was significant for beer (relative risk, 2.2) and for wine (relative risk,

1.5). In a cohort study of more than 96,000 women in a multiphasic health examination program in the United States, breast cancer incidence was increased in those who had reported consuming more than three drinks a day (Hiatt and Bawol, 1984). In a 4-year follow-up study of nearly 90,000 U.S. nurses ages 34 to 59, a significant dose–response relationship was found between alcohol consumption and breast cancer risk (Willett et al., 1987). Among women consuming 5 to 14 g of alcohol daily (about 3 to 9 drinks/week), the age-adjusted relative risk of breast cancer was 1.3 (95% confidence interval, 1.1–1.7). Among those consuming 15 g of alcohol or more per day, the relative risk was 1.6 (range, 1.3–2.0). Adjustment for known breast cancer risk factors (e.g., parity, age at first birth, history of maternal breast cancer, prior breast disease, and relative weight) and a variety of nutritional variables (including estimated consumption of total calories, total fat, saturated fat, polyunsaturated fat, cholesterol, carotene, preformed vitamin A, and vitamin E) did not alter this association.

Several other studies, however, have provided no evidence of an association between alcohol and breast cancer (Byers and Funch, 1982; Webster et al., 1983) or only limited evidence (Begg et al., 1983). These conflicting findings are not easy to reconcile, but could be partly explained by methodological differences. For example, although nutritional variables were evaluated in the study by Willett et al. (1987), the data were obtained from a self-administered questionnaire, and it was not possible to evaluate confounding by variables, which may have masked an association. In that study, therefore, increased alcohol consumption could have been a marker for other factors that increase the risk of breast cancer.

In a detailed review of the epidemiologic findings concerning alcohol consumption and breast cancer, Longnecker et al. (1988) concluded that there was sufficient evidence to support an association.

Animal Studies

Over the past 20 years, animal studies have shown that ethanol, either applied topically or administered as part of the diet, has cocarcinogenic effects. Examples of these experiments include the enhanced carcinogenesis of 7,12-dimethylbenzanthracene applied either to the cheek epithelium of young hamsters (Elzay, 1966, 1969) or to the skin of mice (Stenbäck, 1969), esophageal tumors induced in rats by diethylnitrosamine

(DEN) (Gibel, 1967), liver tumors induced by vinyl chloride (Radike et al., 1981), nasopharyngeal cancers initiated in pair-fed hamsters by nitrosopyrrolidine (McCoy et al., 1981), and rectal cancers initiated by dimethylhydrazine in rats (Seitz et al., 1984). However, the simultaneous addition of DEN and ethanol in drinking water (25%) did not modify DEN induction of hepatocarcinogenesis (Habs and Schmähl, 1981), nor did consumption of diets containing ethanol (35% total calories) affect the number of liver tumors induced by dimethylnitrosamine (DMN) (Teschke et al., 1983) or modify the development of preneoplastic hepatic foci by aflatoxin B_1 in rats (Misslbeck et al., 1984). Similar results were obtained by Schwarz et al. (1983) using DEN or N-nitrosomorpholin as carcinogens and 10% ethanol in drinking water.

The association of alcohol consumption with cancers at sites that do not come into contact with high ethanol concentrations suggests that mechanisms other than, or in addition to, the direct cytotoxic effects of ethanol play a role in carcinogenesis. These are discussed in the following sections.

Activation of Chemical Carcinogens

Ethanol may act as a cocarcinogen at remote sites through its capacity to induce the microsomal cytochrome P450-dependent biotransformation system. Ethanol administration to rats increases hepatic benzpyrene hydroxylase (Rubin et al., 1970). Likewise, activation of nitrosopyrrolidine was substantially increased (Farinati et al., 1985a). Ethanol induces microsomal DMN N-demethylase activity, which functions at low DMN concentrations (Garro et al., 1981). This effect contrasts with those of other microsomal enzyme inducers and may be due to the induction by ethanol of a specific form of cytochrome P450 (Koop et al., 1982; Ohnishi and Lieber, 1977), which differentially affects the activation of various carcinogens. Indeed, a selective affinity for DMN has been demonstrated with the ethanol-induced form of cytochrome P450 (Yang et al., 1985), and an active form of this isozyme (now called P450 IIE1) has been purified from human liver (Lasker et al., 1987). Furthermore, in studies using microsomes of ethanol-fed animals, enhanced mutagenicity was demonstrated at low DMN concentrations (Garro et al., 1981).

A growing body of evidence indicates that ethanol acts as a cocarcinogen. For example, the combined action of DMN and alcohol increased the incidence of olfactory neuroepitheliomas in mice (Griciute et al., 1981). Takada et al. (1986) noted neoplastic changes in the liver of rats treated with alcohol and DEN or with phenobarbital and DEN, suggesting that ethanol, as well as phenobarbitol, is a promoter of hepatocarcinogenesis.

The intestinal metabolism of xenobiotic substances may also be altered by ethanol consumption. Elevated cytochrome P450 levels and microsomal enzyme activities have been observed in the esophagus (Farinati et al., 1985a) and in the upper small intestine of rats after chronic ethanol ingestion (Seitz et al., 1979). In the Salmonella typhimurium test system, chronic ingestion of ethanol enhanced the capacity of intestinal microsomes to activate benzo[a]pyrene to a mutagen (Seitz et al., 1978) and the capacity of intestinal microsomes to activate 2-aminofluorene and tryptophan pyrolysate (Seitz et al., 1981).

Enhanced activation of benzo[a]pyrene to mutagenic derivatives has been mediated by lung microsomes in ethanol-fed rats (Seitz et al., 1981). Ethanol also enhanced the induction of nasopharyngeal tumors in hamsters treated with nitrosopyrrolidine (McCoy et al., 1981) and increased the activation of nitrosopyrrolidine to a mutagen by microsomes isolated from hepatic, pulmonary, and esophageal tissues (Farinati et al., 1985a; McCoy and Wynder, 1979).

In the rats treated with 1,2-dimethylhydrazine (DMH), chronic ethanol consumption enhanced the appearance of rectal tumors but not tumors in the distal or proximal colon (Seitz et al., 1984). This effect did not relate to the cytochrome P450-dependent oxidizing system in the liver or in the colonic mucosa or to changes in the fecal bile acids. However, colonic mucosal alcohol dehydrogenase (ADH) was increased by 47% in rats fed ethanol, but it is not clear whether this local increase is associated with the observed enhancement of carcinogenesis.

Effects of Ethanol on DNA Metabolism

Obe and colleagues reported that acetaldehyde, the first metabolite of ethanol, induces sister chromatid exchanges (SCEs) in cells grown in tissue culture (Obe and Beck, 1979; Obe and Ristow, 1977) and concluded that there is an elevation of chromosome aberrations in alcoholics (Obe and Ristow, 1979). Alcohol may also inhibit the capacity of cells to repair carcinogen-induced DNA damage. O^6-methylguanine transferase (O^6-MeGT) is the enzyme responsible for repairing O^6-methylguanine (O^6-MeG) and O^6-ethylguanine adducts. After 4 weeks on a diet containing ethanol as 36% of total calories, O^6-MeGT activity was reduced by approximately 40% relative to controls. In other experiments in rats, 50 mM of ethanol, a concentration corresponding to blood levels in alcohol abusers, directly inhibited O^6-MeGT activity (Farinati et al., 1985b). Even minute amounts of acetaldehyde noticeably inactivate the enzyme (Espina et al., 1988). Since alkylation at the O^6 position of guanine is associated with both mutagenesis and carcinogenesis (Kleihues et al., 1979; Lewis and Swenberg, 1980; Newbold et al., 1980), the apparent decrease in O^6-MeGT activity in alcohol-fed rats could be a mechanism of cancer induction.

Some studies failed to detect an effect of dietary ethanol in the repair of DMN-induced O^6-MeG adducts (Belinsky et al., 1982; Schwarz et al., 1982). In one of these, however, O^6-MeG levels were examined only until 4 hours after DMN administration (Schwarz et al., 1982). The differences in experimental results may be due to differences in feeding protocols.

Local Effects of Ethanol on Cancer Induction

Ethanol ingestion produced overt tissue damage in the mucosa of the stomach (Dinoso et al., 1976; Eastwood and Kirchner, 1974; Gottfried et al., 1978) and the small intestine (Baraona et al., 1974; Perlow et al., 1977). The damage was followed by cell proliferation when the administration of alcohol was stopped (Baraona et al., 1974; Willems et al., 1971). Ethanol also stimulated cell proliferation in the germinative epithelium of the rat esophagus in the absence of overt mucosal damage (Mak et al., 1987). Stimulation of cell replication would sensitize the esophagus to chemical carcinogens.

Congeners

In addition to the local effects of ethanol, some congeners (nonalcoholic components) in alcoholic beverages may play an etiologic role in the development of cancer. Esophageal cancer has been produced in animals by administering relatively large amounts of nitrosamines, which may occur as congeners in some alcoholic beverages (Lijinsky and Epstein, 1970; Lowenfels, 1974). Ethanol catalyzes the production of nitrosamines from nitrites and secondary amines under conditions present in the upper gastrointestinal tract (Pignatelli et al., 1976).

Alcoholic beverages contain a variety of carcinogens such as polycyclic aromatic hydrocarbons (e.g., phenanthrene, fluoranthrene, benzanthracene, benzopyrene, chrysene) (Masuda et al., 1966). Asbestos fibers derived from filters have been detected in beer, wine, sherry, and vermouth (Bignon et al., 1977; Biles and Emerson, 1968; Cunningham and Pontefract, 1971).

Carcinogenic Effects of Dietary Deficiencies Combined with Alcohol Abuse

Ethanol consumption combined with vitamin A deficiency increases the incidence of squamous metaplasia of the trachea (Mak et al., 1984). Drugs that induce liver microsomes decrease hepatic vitamin A (Leo et al., 1984). A similar effect was also observed in baboons and rats given ethanol (Sato and Lieber, 1981) and other xenobiotic substances, including carcinogens, that interact with liver microsomes (Innami et al., 1976; Kato et al., 1978; Reddy and Weisburger, 1980). Similar observations have been made in humans. For example, patients with alcoholic liver disease had very low hepatic vitamin A levels at all stages of their disease (Leo and Lieber, 1982).

Retinol can compete with DMN for its activation (presumably to carcinogens) in liver microsomes (Leo et al., 1986b). Lowering hepatic vitamin A by diminishing this inhibition may indirectly favor chemical carcinogenesis. Ethanol also may exert a direct stimulatory effect on cell proliferation independent of vitamin A status (Mak et al., 1987).

A Plummer-Vinson-like syndrome was observed among female patients with oral cancer (Wynder et al., 1957a). Hyperplasia was observed on the skin of riboflavin-deficient mice (Wynder and Chan, 1970).

Vitamin B_6 plays an important role in the production of antibody response to various antigens (Axelrod and Trakatellis, 1964). This effect may influence tumor development indirectly by affecting the consequences of exposure to HBV. Wynder (1976) reported that pyridoxine deficiency is associated with enhanced liver tumor formation.

Vitamin E and other antioxidants, such as butylated hydroxytoluene (BHT), propylgallate, and ethoxyquin, have reduced the induction of tumors by certain carcinogens in several target organs (Ulland et al., 1973; Wattenberg, 1972a,b). The protective effect of BHT against chemically induced carcinogenesis may be offset, at least in part, by its potentiation of ethanol-induced vitamin A depletion (Leo et al., 1987b).

Gabrial et al. (1982) reported that zinc deficiency enhanced esophageal tumor induction by methylbenzyl nitrosamine in rats.

Atherosclerotic Cardiovascular Diseases

Hypertension and Stroke

Epidemiologic studies have usually indicated that people who regularly consume on average two drinks or more of alcohol per day (>30 ml of ethanol) have higher mean blood pressure levels and a higher prevalence of hypertension than do people who drink smaller quantities (Criqui, 1987). This association was observed in a representative sample of the U.S. adult population (Gruchow et al., 1985b; Harlan et al., 1984) and in subgroups of the U.S. adult population (Clark et al., 1967; Criqui et al., 1982; D'Alonzo and Pell, 1968; Dyer et al. 1977; Fortmann et al., 1983; Kagan et al., 1981; Kannel and Sorlie, 1974; Klatsky et al., 1977, 1981a,b, 1986; Wallace et al., 1981). It has also been observed in Australia (MacMahon et al., 1984), Finland (Tuomilehto et al., 1984), South Africa (Steyn et al., 1986), France (Cambien et al., 1985), New Zealand (Jackson et al., 1985), Great Britain (Cruickshank et al., 1985; Shaper et al., 1987), Japan (Ueshima et al., 1984a,b), and the Federal Republic of Germany (Cairns et al., 1984).

In a cross-sectional study in Canada, no association was observed between self-reported consumption of alcohol and blood pressure (Coates et al., 1985), but the sample was small and the highest level of consumption was four or more drinks per day. In London, Bulpitt et al. (1987) found no increase in mean blood pressure in subjects consuming less than seven drinks per day. In Italy, Trevisan et al. (1987) found no significant association (i.e., $p > .05$) between alcohol consumption and blood pressure among 203 schoolchildren—a sample in which 50% of the boys and 39% of the girls reported a mean regular alcohol consumption of 57 g/week and 42 g/week, respectively, i.e., less than one 4-oz drink of table wine per day.

The incidence of hypertension has rarely been studied in prospective epidemiologic studies. Determining when persistent elevation of blood pressure occurs usually cannot be done well in such studies, and the definitions of hypertension are substantially different from those customarily used in treatment programs. After 8 years of follow-up in the Framingham Offspring Study (Garrison et al., 1987), alcohol consumption was associated with risk of hypertension in women but not in men after adjustment for adiposity and other variables. The reason for the difference between men and women is not clear.

In cross-sectional studies, the association between alcohol consumption and blood pressure is weaker in women than in men (e.g., Fortmann et al., 1983; Jackson et al., 1985; MacMahon et al., 1984), perhaps because women consume less alcohol than men or underreport consumption more frequently or because female sex hormones modify the effect. The association apparently is not due to confounding by age, race, or ratio of body weight to height. The shape of the association between abstainers and people who consume 200 to 300 g of alcohol per week is uncertain. Mean blood pressures for light drinkers may be higher, lower, or the same as those in abstainers. See, for instance, the different results obtained for men and women by age in the Lipid Research Clinics (LRC) Prevalence Study (Wallace et al., 1982).

In cross-sectional studies, regular daily consumption of 200 to 300 g of alcohol or more is generally associated with increases in blood pressure and elevated blood pressure is the major risk factor for hemorrhagic stroke and cerebral infarction. Thus, it is reasonable to expect that habitual alcohol consumption is associated with increased risk of stroke.

In the Honolulu Heart Program—a prospective study of 8,000 middle-aged men of Japanese ancestry—alcohol consumption was positively associated with risk of hemorrhagic stroke but not of thromboembolic stroke (Donahue et al., 1986; Kagan et al., 1980, 1981). Age-adjusted relative risks of hemorrhagic stroke were determined during 12 years of follow-up for men who at entry reportedly consumed 1 to 14, 15 to 39, and 40 or more ounces of alcohol per month (1 to 79, 80 to 214, and 215 or more g of alcohol/week). In comparison to 2,916 abstainers, their risks were 2.2, 2.9, and 4.7, with 95% confidence intervals of 1.1 to 4.2, 1.4 to 5.9, and 2.4 to 9.5, respectively. After adjustment for hypertension status, cigarette smoking, and other variables in addition to age, the relative risks were 2.3, 2.5, and 2.9—all significantly greater than unity. The association appeared stronger for subarachnoid than intracerebral hemorrhage. Corresponding age-adjusted relative risks for thromboembolic stroke were 1.0, 1.3, and 1.3, with 95% confidence intervals of 0.9 to 1.5, 0.9 to 1.4, and 0.9 to 1.7, respectively.

Gordon and Kannel (1983) reported a similar finding for women in the Framingham Study—i.e., alcohol consumption was positively associated with risk of hemorrhagic stroke but not with thromboembolic stroke, at least in univariate analyses—but they found no association with either category of stroke for men. In a later paper, however, Friedman and Kimball (1986) reported that the data on alcohol consumption used in those earlier studies were seriously faulty, so it is unclear what weight should be given to the reported findings.

Case-comparison studies indicate that recent drinking, particularly heavy drinking (e.g., more than 300 g/week), is associated with increased risk of stroke (Gill et al., 1986; Gorelick et al., 1987; Taylor et al., 1984; von Arbin et al., 1985). Gorelick et al. (1987) concluded that the association is probably due to confounding effects of cigarette smoking, but this has not been established.

In summary, the epidemiologic evidence is generally consistent with the hypothesis that chronic alcohol consumption is associated with increased blood pressure and with increased risk of hemorrhagic stroke but not of cerebral infarction. The latter association appears to be independent of blood pressure. These associations are clearly present at levels of 200 to 300 g of alcohol per week. The shape of the dose–response curves is uncertain, but results from the Honolulu Heart Program indicate an increased risk of stroke even at lower levels of consumption. The evidence also supports the hypothesis that recent heavy alcohol consumption is associated with increased risk of stroke due to cerebral infarction as well as hemorrhage.

Hyperlipidemia

In humans, ethanol consumption consistently results in hyperlipidemia. Serum triglyceride concentrations increase the most due to elevation of very low-density lipoproteins (VLDLs) and chylomicrons, but there is also some elevation of serum cholesterol levels. Upon alcohol withdrawal, triglycerides decrease more rapidly than cholesterol and phospholipids. Postprandial hyperlipidemia was greatly exaggerated by fat-containing meals (Wilson et al., 1970). When 300 g of alcohol were administered daily to humans for several weeks, the initial severalfold increase in triglycerides gradually returned to normal (Lieber et al., 1963). Hyperlipidemia is usually absent with severe liver injury (e.g., cirrhosis), whereas hypolipidemia may result (Borowsky et al., 1980; Guisard et al., 1971; Marzo et al., 1970). In hospitalized alcoholics, serum total cholesterol was not significantly increased (Böttiger et al., 1976). However, in approximately 30% of alcoholics seeking medical attention (Johansson and Laurell, 1969), and in 86% of patients after a recent drinking bout (Johansson and Medhus, 1974), plasma high-density lipoproteins (HDL) were increased but returned to normal after about 2 weeks of abstinence (Devenyi et al., 1980; Johansson and Medhus, 1974). The rise in HDL associated with alcohol has been demonstrated experimentally in rats (Baraona and Lieber, 1970; Baraona et al., 1983). It also has been observed in teenagers (Glueck et al., 1981) and in both older and younger men (Barrett-Connor and Suarez, 1982), but only in inactive men—not in runners whose HDL levels were already increased (Hartung et al., 1983).

Alcohol intake was positively associated in cross-sectional epidemiologic studies with blood levels of HDL cholesterol in the United States (Barrett-Connor and Suarez, 1982; Castelli et al., 1977; Donahue et al., 1986; Gordon et al., 1981), France (Jacqueson et al., 1983), Japan (Chiba et al., 1983), and Norway (Brenn, 1986). In samples of Chinese men in Shanghai matched for age, occupation, and body weight, mean HDL cholesterol was slightly higher (60.2 mg/dl) for those who consumed 6 to 30 g of alcohol per day than in those who abstained (58.5 mg/dl), but the difference was not statistically significant (Chen et al., 1983). Alcohol intake was also positively associated with serum levels of apolipoprotein AI (Phillips et al., 1982) and of both Apo AI and AII (Camargo et al., 1985; Donahue et al., 1986; Fraser et al., 1983; Poynard et al., 1986). The increase in HDL after alcohol consumption involved HDL_2 (Ekman et al., 1981; Taskinen et al., 1982, 1985). These observations were made in people whose alcohol intake was relatively high. After one 40-g dose of ethanol (equivalent to 4 oz of 86-proof beverage), there was a transient increase in both HDL_2 and HDL_3 (Goldberg et al., 1984). Haskell et al. (1984) reported that a moderate dose—12 to 51 g (0.5 to 2.2 oz) of ethanol per day—raised levels of HDL_3 but not HDL_2, and that upon abstention, levels of HLD_3, but not HDL_2, decreased (Haskell et al., 1984). The relationship between alcohol and HDL_3 levels at these alcohol intakes was confirmed by two more recent studies (Haffner et al., 1985; Williams et al., 1985). Williams et al. (1985) reported a correlation between dietary components, such as alcohol and starch, and HDL_3 (but not HDL_2). With progression of alcoholic liver injury, the HDL fractions decreased and abnormal lipoproteins appeared in the blood (Borowsky et al., 1980; Denvenyi et al., 1980; Poynard et al., 1986; Sabesin et al., 1977).

There is some evidence for an inverse association of alcohol intake with the level of low-density lipoproteins (LDL) (Castelli et al., 1977; Hulley and Gordon, 1981). In the LRC Coronary Primary Prevention Trial, change in alcohol intake was associated inversely with change in LDL cholesterol levels among men in the placebo group after adjustment for change in body mass index and dietary lipids (Glueck et al., 1986).

Coronary Heart Disease

Since LDL levels are positively associated with risk of coronary heart disease (CHD) and HDL levels are inversely associated with risk of CHD, the results described above imply that alcohol consumption should be inversely associated with risk of CHD. Investigation of this hypothesis is complicated, however, by the substantial difficulties involved in assessing alcohol intake in population-based studies. Studies based solely on 24-hour recalls, e.g., the Puerto Rico Heart Program (Kittner et al., 1983), have not been included here because a large proportion of drinkers was misclassified as nondrinkers. Studies that did not describe results in sufficient detail, e.g., the London Busmen Study (Morris et al., 1966), were also excluded.

Investigation of this hypothesis has been complicated further by the positive correlations of alcohol with the number of cigarettes smoked (e.g., Friedman and Kimball, 1986), by the level of blood pressure (discussed above), by the many other effects of alcohol on the cardiovascular system, and by the associations of alcohol with risk of death from some cancers, trauma, cirrhosis, and other causes.

Current interest in alcohol and CHD risk began with the observation of Klatsky et al. (1974) that the percentage of teetotalers was larger (32.4%) in a group of 405 patients with first myocardial infarction than in a comparison group (24.7%) matched for 10 coronary risk factors. Since then, the association has been investigated in a number of cohort studies, most of which indicate that middle-aged men who report that they abstain from alcohol have a somewhat higher risk of CHD than those who regularly consume less than 100 g of alcohol per week. These studies include the Honolulu Heart Program (Blackwelder et al., 1980; Kagan et al., 1981; Yano et al., 1977, 1984), the Whitehall Study of British civil ser-

vants (Marmot et al., 1981), the Western Electric Study (Dyer et al., 1977), the urban sample from the Yugoslavia Cardiovascular Disease Study (Kozarevic et al., 1982), the Busselton Study (Cullen et al., 1982), the Albany Study of New York civil servants (Gordon and Doyle, 1985), and the British Regional Heart Study (Shaper et al., 1987). In some studies, such as the Western Electric Study and the British Regional Heart Study, the difference was small and not statistically significant, but in several others (e.g., Friedman and Kimball, 1986; Kozarevic et al., 1982; Yano et al., 1984), the association was highly significant and showed a dose response after adjustment for coronary risk factors such as cigarette smoking, serum cholesterol, and blood pressure.

An especially important aspect of the Honolulu Heart Program is its large number of lifetime abstainers (2,744), which provides a stable base against which to compare the effects in 4,026 current drinkers, who were categorized into four groups of about 1,000 men according to usual amount consumed: 1 to 6, 7 to 15, 16 to 39, and 40 or more ounces of alcohol per month (i.e., 1 to 36, 37 to 83, 84 to 209, and 210 or more g/week) (Yano et al., 1977). The 6-year age-adjusted incidence rates of CHD (coronary death, myocardial infarction, coronary insufficiency, and angina pectoris) were 46 per 1,000 for abstainers and 41, 31, 27, and 21 per 1,000 for the four drinking groups in order of increased consumption. The rate for 821 former drinkers was 56 per 1,000. The association was not specific to any particular type of alcoholic beverage, but was noted for wine, beer, and spirits separately. Similar results were obtained in population-based case-comparison studies (Hennekens et al., 1978, 1979; Klatsky et al., 1986; Scragg et al., 1987; Siscovick et al., 1986).

A subsequent report from the Honolulu Heart Program (Kagan et al., 1981) indicated that risk of CHD death was higher in men consuming 60 oz of alcohol or more per month (315 g/week) than in men consuming 40 to 59 oz/month. An increased risk of CHD among heavy drinkers was also observed in the Albany Study (Gordon and Doyle, 1985), in the Western Electric Study (Dyer et al., 1977), and among nonsmokers in the Framingham Study (Friedman and Kimball, 1986). These groups were usually small and the differences not statistically significant. "Problem" drinking, history of inebriation, and registration with temperance boards have also been associated with increased risk of CHD, coronary death, or sudden coronary death (Dyer et al., 1977; Kozarevic et al.,

1983; Pell and D'Alonzo, 1973; Poikolainen, 1983; Wilhelmsen et al., 1973).

There are few data on the elderly. In a population-based sample of people age 66 years or older (62% females) in Massachusetts, Colditz et al. (1985) observed that the age-adjusted relative risks of CHD death during 5 years of follow-up associated with consuming 0.1 to 8.9, 9 to 34, and >34 g of alcohol per day were 0.3, 0.6, and 1.3, respectively, in comparison to abstainers. The corresponding 95% confidence intervals for the relative risks were 0.2 to 0.8, 0.3 to 1.7, and 0.3 to 4.8.

There are also some data on women. In the Framingham Study (Friedman and Kimball, 1986), a U-shaped association was observed for women smokers, but the trend was not statistically significant. No association was apparent for nonsmoking women. However, statistically significant inverse associations between alcohol consumption and CHD risk were observed among women in at least three case-comparison studies (La Vecchia et al., 1987; Ross et al., 1981; Scragg et al., 1987).

Some inconsistencies have also been observed. The Yugoslavia Cardiovascular Disease Study selected samples of men from two rural areas and two urban areas. The association between alcohol consumption and CHD risk differed greatly among the areas. A strong statistically significant inverse association was observed in the urban areas; a slight negative association was observed in one rural area and a slight positive association in the other, but neither was statistically significant. The rural samples were characterized by low levels of serum cholesterol (186 mg/dl) as compared to 214 mg/dl for the two urban samples. This circumstance might modify an association between alcohol consumption and CHD risk, especially if that association resulted from effects of alcohol on concentrations of blood lipids.

In the Framingham Study (Friedman and Kimball, 1986), the association of alcohol with 24-year risk of coronary death may have been modified by cigarette smoking; no association was apparent for men who smoked less than one pack of cigarettes per day, although an inverse association was observed both for nonsmokers and for heavier smokers. However, it is not clear whether this variation was inconsistent with random sampling error.

In patients undergoing coronary angiography, mean coronary occlusion score was inversely associated with consumption of alcohol (<1, 1 to 6, 6 to 12, 12 to 24, and >24 oz/week) for men as well as women (Anderson et al., 1978; Barboriak et al., 1979a,b). An inverse association between con-

sumption of alcohol and severity of coronary atherosclerosis was observed in one population-based autopsy study (Okumiya et al., 1985), but not in later ones (Reed et al., 1987; Rhoads et al., 1978). In the Rhoads study, however, consumption of alcohol was inversely associated with presence of myocardial scarring (Rhoads et al., 1978).

Some studies indicate that per-capita alcohol consumption is negatively correlated with national CHD death rates (Popham et al., 1983). The contrast between a negative correlation for wine (La Porte et al., 1981; Nanji and French, 1985; St. Leger et al., 1979) and a positive correlation for beer (Nanji and French, 1985), however, suggests that the correlations do not directly reflect causal associations with alcohol per se. In addition, consumption of alcohol among cohorts in the Seven Countries Study was not associated in 15 years of follow up with rates for total mortality (Keys et al., 1986). Cohorts with the highest rates of CHD—in Finland, the United States, and the Netherlands—obtained 3 to 5% of calories from alcohol, whereas cohorts with the lowest risks—in Japan and Greece—obtained 4 to 8% of their calories from alcohol. In California, CHD death rates among Seventh-Day Adventists, who abstain from both tobacco and alcohol, were 20 to 50% lower than for age-matched groups in the total population of California (Phillips et al., 1978). In the British Regional Heart Study, the proportion of heavy drinkers among 22 communities was positively correlated with CHD mortality (Shaper et al., 1987).

The many biologic, psychological, and social effects of alcohol indicate that no account of the association between alcohol and health would be complete without considering total mortality. A U-shaped association has been observed in many cohorts, e.g., the Honolulu Heart Program (Blackwelder et al., 1980), the Whitehall Study of British civil servants (Marmot et al., 1981), the Western Electric Study (Dyer et al., 1977), the Yugoslavia Cardiovascular Disease Study (Kozarevic et al., 1983), the Framingham Study (Friedman and Kimball, 1986), and the Nutrition Canada Survey (Johansen et al., 1987).

In summary, epidemiologic evidence indicates that people who abstain from alcohol—lifetime abstainers as well as former drinkers—have a somewhat higher risk of CHD than persons who consume 1 to 99 g of alcohol per week, at least in populations with mean serum cholesterol levels over 200 mg/dl. The graded nature of this association, its consistency in many different populations, and its continued strength after adjustment for potentially confounding factors support the inference that consumption of small amounts of alcohol—that is, 1 to 99 g distributed throughout a week—may reduce susceptibility to CHD. The mechanism for this has not been determined. Postmortem studies suggest that the effect is not due to an association with severity of coronary atherosclerosis. The evidence also indicates that heavy or so-called problem drinking, e.g., more than 500 g/week, is associated with increased risk of CHD. Moreover, heavy drinking is associated with increased risk of total mortality in many populations. However, the findings in certain religious groups, e.g., Seventh-Day Adventists, indicate that abstaining from alcohol is compatible with low overall risk of CHD. Results from the Seven Countries Study show that populations with moderate per-capita intake, i.e., 3 to 5% of calories from alcohol, may have very low or very high rates of CHD.

Other Cardiovascular Diseases

Alcohol intake was inversely associated with incidence of intermittent claudication in the Framingham Study, but was not associated with risk of congestive heart failure (Gordon and Kannel, 1983). Segel et al. (1984) described alcoholic cardiomyopathy in people with alcoholism and heart disease. This syndrome is typically found in men ages 30 to 44 years who have been ingesting 30 to 40% of their calories as alcohol for 10 to 15 years and is frequently accompanied by arrhythmias. Coronary artery disease, hypertension, valvular abnormalities, and congenital heart disease must be excluded before this disorder is diagnosed. A recent case-comparison study indicated that consumption of more than 85 g of alcohol per day, regardless of type of beverage, was a strong risk factor for dilated cardiomyopathy (Komajda et al., 1986).

Metabolic Disorders

Hyperglycemia and Diabetes

In large population studies, alcohol intake has been correlated with hyperglycemia (Gerard et al. 1977). Aside from patients with chronic pancreatitis and endocrine (insulin) insufficiency, there is no ready explanation for this association. Impairment of glucose tolerance has been suspected (Phillips and Safrit, 1971; Rehfield et al., 1973), but is difficult to prove, because the elevated insulin levels that accompany alcohol intake could

reflect insulin resistance due to alcohol or the augmentation of insulin release, which alcohol itself causes (Dornhorst and Ouyang, 1971; Metz et al. 1969; Nikkilä and Taskinen, 1975). Insulin resistance caused by alcohol has recently been demonstrated in healthy subjects by measuring glucose utilization with the insulin clamp technique during glucose infusions at steady blood glucose and insulin levels (Yki-Järvinen and Nikkilä, 1985).

In animals and humans, administration of large doses of alcohol after meals results in hyperglycemia (Forsander et al., 1958; Krusius et al., 1958; Matunaga, 1942), which is caused by the release of glucose from the glycogen reserves of the liver into the blood and is mediated mostly by the adrenal medulla and the sympathetic nervous system (Ammon and Estler, 1968; Matunaga, 1942). Decreased peripheral utilization of glucose may also contribute to the hyperglycemia (Lochner et al., 1967).

Hypoglycemia

After eating, when liver glycogen is abundant, glycogenolysis maintains blood glucose levels. In the fasting state, hypoglycemia following alcohol administration is a normal reaction in humans and in laboratory animals (Field et al., 1963; Freinkel et al., 1965). Hypoglycemia results from decreased reserves of hepatic glycogen and inhibition of hepatic gluconeogenesis from various precursors as a consequence of the increased ratio of NADH to NAD (Krebs et al., 1969). Glucogenesis from amino acids and the formation of glucose from glycerol, lactate, and galactose are slowed down by concomitant metabolism of alcohol (Krebs et al., 1969; Madison et al., 1967). The increase in the ratio of NADH to NAD due to hepatic metabolism of alcohol is partly responsible for these metabolic changes. Changes in the activity of enzymes involved in gluconeogenesis have also been described (Duruibe and Tejwani, 1981; Stifel et al., 1976). Hypoglycemia is an important complication of acute alcohol abuse and may be responsible for some of the unexplained sudden deaths resulting from acute alcoholic intoxication. A prompt diagnosis and initiation of therapy is mandatory in view of the reported mortality rate of 11% in adults and 25% in children (Madison et al., 1967). Hypoglycemia may be present when an alcohol drinker exhibits altered mental state even when fed, especially in children. In clinical practice, however, severe alcoholic hypoglycemia is uncommon.

In several conditions, refractiveness to alcohol-induced hypoglycemia can be demonstrated: in nondiabetic obese subjects (Arky et al., 1968), in some alcoholics with a diabetic serum glucose pattern (Hed and Nygren, 1968), and in subjects undergoing steroid therapy (Arky and Freinkel, 1966). Refractiveness has also been demonstrated in chronic malnourished alcoholics (Salaspuro, 1971a,b). This refractiveness may be due to the attenuation of alcohol-induced hepatic redox changes after chronic alcohol consumption (Salaspuro et al., 1981). Alcohol-induced hypoglycemia can also be suppressed by 4-methylpyrazole (an alcohol dehydrogenase inhibitor) (Salaspuro et al., 1977).

Hyperuricemia

Excessive drinking of alcoholic beverages is associated with acute gouty arthritis (Newcombe, 1972). The hyperuricemia that accompanies bouts of intense alcohol intake occurs in patients without known disorders of uric acid metabolism or renal function (Lieber et al., 1962). An important mechanism leading to hyperuricemia is decreased urinary excretion of uric acid secondary to elevated serum lactate. Alcoholic hyperuricemia can be readily differentiated from the primary variety because of its reversibility upon discontinuation of alcohol use. Alcohol-associated ketosis or starvation may also further promote hyperuricemia (MacLachlan and Rodan, 1967).

An increase in urate production, partly explained by an increase in adenosine nucleotide turnover, caused hyperuricemia in volunteers with gout (Faller and Fox, 1982). Urinary urate clearance was increased, and levels of urinary urate and oxypurines were higher. This effect was observed at serum alcohol levels lower than those in lactate-related renal hyperuricemia and those usually seen in patients with alcohol-related hyperuricemia. The purine content (guanosine) of some beers may also contribute to hyperuricemia and gout in alcoholic subjects (Gibson et al., 1984).

Chronic Renal Disease

Altered renal function in alcoholics with liver disease is attributable primarily to impaired hepatic function (hepatorenal syndrome). Since the majority of patients with liver disease and associated renal dysfunction in the United States are alcoholics (Epstein, 1985a,b, 1986, 1987a,b), the alterations in renal function may be the effects of alcohol.

Most alcoholics with mild liver disease have enlarged kidneys at autopsy, and rats given ethanol develop morphological changes and increased lipid accumulation in the kidneys. Alcohol has been proposed both to induce renal sodium retention and to provoke natriuresis (Kalbfleisch et al., 1963; Nicholson and Taylor, 1938; Ogata et al., 1968). Certain conditions (such as degree of hydration or volume status) determine the response. This area requires additional study.

Ethanol also modulates renin–angiotensin responsiveness in humans. These effects vary with the amount of ethanol administered (Linkola et al., 1979). Alcohol can also render the patients susceptible to acute renal failure through several mechanisms, including rhabdomyolysis and volume contraction (Epstein, in press).

Chronic Liver Disease

Epidemiology of Alcoholic Liver Disease

MORTALITY AND PREVALENCE Most cases of cirrhosis are due to alcohol consumption (Lelbach, 1975; Martini and Bode, 1970). The role of alcohol in liver cirrhosis is more important in North and South America than in Europe (66 and 42%, respectively). In Asia its contribution is only 11% (Lelbach, 1975), although this appears to be rising. Cirrhosis is the third leading cause of death for those 25 to 64 years of age in New York City (Department of Health, City of New York, 1984).

The progression to more severe liver injury is accelerated in women (Rankin, 1977). Wilkinson et al. (1969) found that women were more susceptible than men to alcoholic cirrhosis. In more recent studies, the prevalence of chronic advanced liver disease was higher among women than men with a similar history of alcohol abuse (Maier et al., 1979; Morgan and Sherlock, 1977; Nakamura et al., 1979). Studies by Pequignot et al. (1974, 1978) show that daily intake of alcohol as low as 40 g by men and 20 g by women resulted in an increased incidence of cirrhosis in a well-nourished population.

RELATION OF LIVER DISEASE TO ALCOHOL CONSUMPTION Despite the high prevalence of alcoholism and cirrhosis throughout the world, the incidence of cirrhosis among alcoholics is low. Autopsies of alcoholics show that the prevalence of cirrhosis is approximately 18%. In liver biopsies of alcoholics, the range was found to be 17 to 31% (Leevy, 1968; Lelbach, 1966, 1967). Alcoholic cirrhosis is correlated both with the magnitude and the duration of alcohol consumption. Pequignot (1958) and Pequignot et al. (1974) estimated that the average cirrhogenic alcohol consumption is 180 g of ethanol per day consumed regularly for approximately 25 years; the risk is increased five times at a level of consumption between 80 and 160 g/day and 25 times if daily ethanol consumption exceeds 160 g. A close correlation exists between per-capita alcohol consumption and cirrhosis mortality (Jolliffe and Jellinek, 1941; Lelbach, 1976; Schmidt, 1975, 1977).

Role of Nutritional Factors in Alcoholic Liver Injury

On the basis of some animal experiments, it was believed until 20 years ago that liver disease among alcoholics was due exclusively to malnutrition and not to direct toxic effects of alcohol itself. Alcoholics undoubtedly suffer from malnutrition for a variety of reasons (Lieber, 1988). Alcohol has a high caloric value, but alcoholic beverages are usually devoid of minerals, vitamins, and proteins. Because alcohol may provide a large portion of the daily caloric intake, high alcohol intake may result in a decreased intake of other nutrients, and maldigestion and malabsorption may contribute to malnutrition. During the past 20 years, however, experiments in animals have shown that ethanol can also affect the liver independently of malnutrition.

The culmination of these studies was the reproduction of the spectrum of alcoholic liver disease, including cirrhosis, in baboons chronically fed a liquid diet containing alcohol and a sufficient amount of protein and other nutrients (Lieber and DeCarli, 1974; Lieber et al., 1975; Popper and Lieber, 1980). In order to quench their thirst or satisfy their hunger, the animals had to ingest the alcohol. The amount of ethanol consumed by baboons was increased to 50% of total energy, and by rats to 36%—proportions comparable to heavy alcohol intake by humans. Isocaloric replacement of sucrose or other carbohydrates by ethanol produced a progressive increase in hepatic lipid content during the first month of an experiment in rats (Lieber et al., 1963, 1965). Fatty liver, however, did not develop when ethanol intake was decreased from 36 to 20% of the total dietary energy. It has not been possible to produce more advanced alcohol-induced liver injury in rats because of the short life and lower alcohol intake of the rat compared to the baboon.

Animal experiments and epidemiologic studies demonstrate that ethanol plays a major role in the pathogenesis of alcoholic liver disease. Multiple and often complex nutrient abnormalities in human alcoholics, however, may contribute to such liver disease and many of its complications.

The deleterious effect of alcohol on the liver has also been confirmed in controlled studies with volunteers in metabolic ward studies. Morphologically and biochemically, an increase in hepatic lipid was demonstrated when ethanol was given either as a supplement or as an isocaloric substitute for carbohydrates together with an otherwise nutritionally adequate diet. Hepatic steatosis was produced, even with a high-protein, vitamin-supplemented diet and was accompanied by major ultrastructural liver changes and by elevations of hepatic transaminases in blood (Lane and Lieber, 1966; Lieber et al., 1963, 1965).

If dietary fat was decreased from 35 to 25% of total calories, hepatic triglyceride accumulation greatly decreased (Lieber and DeCarli, 1970). Replacement of dietary triglycerides containing long-chain fatty acids by fat containing medium-chain fatty acids markedly reduced the capacity of alcohol to produce fatty liver in rats (Lieber et al., 1967).

In rats and in humans, protein deficiency may result in decreased hepatic alcohol dehydrogenase activity (Bode et al., 1971), which in turn prevents some acute metabolic effects of alcohol such as the inhibition of the citric acid cycle, the increase in the ratio of lactate to pyruvate (Salaspuro and Mäenpää, 1966), fasting hypoglycemia (Salaspuro, 1971a,b), and the inhibition of galactose elimination (Salaspuro and Kesäniemi, 1973). However, chronic alcohol consumption combined with a protein- and lipotropic-deficient diet led to more pronounced hepatic steatosis than either deficiency alone (Klatskin et al., 1954; Lieber et al., 1969). In other studies, alcohol consumption along with protein deficiency greatly increased the mortality of laboratory animals without demonstrable differences in hepatic fat accumulation (Best et al., 1949; Koch et al., 1968; Porta and Gomez-Dumm, 1968).

Deficiencies in the lipotropic factors (choline and methionine) produced fatty liver and cirrhosis in growing rats (Best et al., 1949), but primates were less susceptible to protein and lipotrope deficiency than were rodents (Hoffbauer and Zaki, 1965). Moreover, fatty liver, as well as fibrosis (including cirrhosis) with major ultrastructural changes (Arai et al., 1984), developed in baboons (*Papio papio* or *Papio hamadryas*) despite liberal supplementation with methionine (Lieber and De-Carli, 1974). The capacity of ethanol to produce fatty liver, despite choline and methionine supplementation, was also confirmed in four well-fed macaques (*Macaca radiata*) by Mezey et al. (1983); but they failed to produce fibrosis. They postulated that ethanol-produced fibrosis in the baboon might be at least partly due to the lower choline content of the baboon diet. However, Rogers et al. (1981), who fed these animals the exact diet given to the baboon, failed to produce cirrhosis or fibrosis in alcohol-fed rhesus monkeys (*Macaca mulatta*). The amount of lipotrope fed to the baboons was not low enough to account for the absence of cirrhosis. Additional choline failed to prevent the development of fibrosis but caused some liver toxicity (Lieber et al., 1985). Thus, the failure of Mezey et al. (1983) to produce fibrosis in the macaques was probably not due to the higher choline content of the diet, but may have been due to a lower alcohol intake. Because macaques are smaller than baboons and have a higher metabolic rate, the same amount of alcohol does not produce comparable effects in the two species. Furthermore, clinical data from patients with alcoholic liver disease as well as experiments in volunteers have shown the ineffectiveness of lipotropic factors in the prevention of alcohol-associated liver injury (Olson, 1964; Rubin and Lieber, 1968).

Diseases of the Nervous System

Wernicke–Korsakoff Syndrome

The Wernicke–Korsakoff syndrome includes two diseases: Wernicke's encephalopathy, characterized by weakness of eye movements, gait disturbance, and confusion, and Korsakoff's psychosis, a permanent brain disorder characterized by marked abnormalities in cognitive function, particularly the inability to learn new information or to remember recent events. Although severe alcoholics may have both diseases, it is not certain if all Korsakoff patients go through a Wernicke phase (NIAAA, 1987). Avitaminosis, especially of thiamin, is widely regarded as the primary cause of this syndrome, but a direct toxic effect of alcohol has also been implicated in its etiology (NIAAA, 1987). Variations in clinical manifestation, and the finding that most patients with thiamin deficiency do not have the syndrome, suggest that genetic variations may be involved in the etiology of this syndrome (Blass and Gibson, 1977). Since alcohol inhibits the active transfer and not the passive transport of thiamin, it has been postulated that thiamin supplementation in amounts larger than the Recommended Dietary Allowance

(RDA) may overcome the thiamin malabsorption caused by alcohol (Lieber, 1983, 1988).

Alcoholic Peripheral Neuropathy

Alcoholic peripheral neuropathy is a mixed motor sensory neuropathy affecting the distal regions, primarily the lower extremities. It occurs in more than 80% of patients with severe neurological disorders, such as Wernicke's encephalopathy (Victor et al., 1971). Recovery from alcoholic peripheral neuropathy is slow and often incomplete. As in the Wernicke–Korsakoff syndrome, thiamin deficiency is regarded as the primary cause of this neuropathy, although the direct toxic effect of alcohol may also play a role (Behse and Buchthal, 1977).

Alcoholic Dementia

Alcoholic dementia is a cognitive dysfunction associated with alcoholism. It is attributed to a combination of thiamin deficiency and a direct toxic effect of alcohol on the brain (Nakada and Knight, 1984).

Fetal Alcohol Syndrome (FAS)

The deleterious effects of maternal alcoholism on the fetus have been known for centuries. Only since the late 1960s and early 1970s, however, following reports from France (Lemoine et al., 1968) and the United States (Jones and Smith, 1973), has there been wide recognition of the fetal alcohol syndrome (FAS)—a distinct pattern of physical and behavioral anomalies characterized by craniofacial, limb, and cardiovascular defects, as well as persistent growth deficiency and developmental delay. The prevalence of FAS varies with the geographic location and the population under study, but a commonly accepted general estimate is 1 to 3 cases per 1,000 live births (NIAAA, 1987).

Epidemiologic surveys show a high prevalence of FAS in some American Indian populations (May et al., 1983), in people from lower socioeconomic backgrounds, and in children born to alcoholic mothers. These results suggest that alcohol abuse may be higher among these subgroups (Streissguth, 1978). Only a small percentage of women who drink abusively during pregnancy deliver babies with FAS-related birth defects, indicating that other factors modify the impact of alcohol on prenatal development. The most relevant factors are persistent drinking during pregnancy, history of excessive alcohol consumption, number of previous deliveries, and race (Sokol et al., 1986). Such factors can increase the probability of FAS by

50%. Alcohol-related neurological and biologic effects have been observed less frequently in subjects with moderate levels of alcohol consumption (NIAAA, 1987). Mills et al. (1984) reported lower than average birth weights for infants whose mothers consumed just one drink a day during pregnancy.

FAS is presently attributed to the toxic effect of alcohol or its metabolites. In one study of pregnant women, it was observed that alcoholics had lower levels of zinc in their serum and fetal cord blood than did nonalcoholic controls (Flynn et al., 1981). This observation suggests that nutritional factors may play a role in the development of FAS.

Contribution to Nutrient Deficiencies

The potential for alcoholism to undermine nutritional status is generally accepted. Iber (1971) estimated that 20,000 alcoholics were suffering major illnesses due to malnutrition in the United States each year, accounting for 7.5 million days of hospitalization. Patients admitted to hospitals for medical complications of alcoholism had inadequate dietary protein (Patek et al., 1975) as well as signs of protein malnutrition (Iber, 1971; Mendenhall et al., 1985). In hospitalized patients, anthropometric measurements indicated impaired nutrition; for example, height-to-weight ratio was lower (Morgan, 1981), muscle mass estimated by creatinine/height index was reduced (Mendenhall et al., 1984; Morgan, 1981), and triceps skinfolds were thinner (Mendenhall et al., 1984; Morgan, 1981; Simko et al., 1982). Continued drinking was associated with weight loss, whereas abstinence was associated with weight gain (World et al., 1984a,b), in patients with and without liver disease (Simko et al., 1982).

Many patients who drink to excess are clearly not malnourished or are malnourished to a lesser extent than those hospitalized for medical problems. Patients with moderate alcohol intake (Bebb et al., 1971), and even those admitted for alcohol rehabilitation (Neville et al., 1968) rather than for medical problems, did not differ nutritionally from controls (matched for socioeconomic and health history), except that alcoholic women had a lower level of thiamin saturation (Neville et al., 1968). When calories from alcohol exceeded 30%, there were large decreases in intakes of protein and vitamins A and C; an intake of thiamin below the RDA (Gruchow et al., 1985a,b); and appreciably lower intakes of calcium, iron, and fiber (Hillers and Massey, 1985). Thiamin levels in the organs are maintained in laboratory animals (Shaw et al.,

1981) and in well-nourished alcoholics who take in average or greater-than-average amounts of thiamin (Hoyumpa, 1983). Nevertheless, in the United States, profound effects of thiamin deficiency are very often present in alcoholics and are responsible for the Wernicke–Korsakoff syndrome, beriberi, heart disease, and possibly polyneuropathy.

The folic acid status of alcoholics is compromised when the intensity of drinking increases. Among alcoholics, 38% had low serum folate levels and 18% had low red blood cell folate levels (World et al., 1984b). Malnourished alcoholics without liver disease absorbed folic acid less efficiently than did their better-nourished counterparts (Halsted et al., 1971). In well-nourished alcoholics, folic acid deficiency was only a rare cause of anemia (Eichner et al., 1972).

Normal serum B_{12} levels were common in alcoholic patients with folate deficiency, either with cirrhosis (Herbert et al., 1963; Klipstein and Lindenbaum, 1965) or without cirrhosis (Halsted et al., 1971; Racusen and Krawitt, 1977). The low incidence of clinically significant B_{12} deficiency is probably due to the large vitamin stores in the body and the reserve capacity for absorption. Alcohol ingestion caused reduced absorption in volunteers after several weeks (as measured by the Schilling test) (Lindenbaum and Lieber, 1975).

The incidence of pyridoxine deficiency, as measured by low plasma pyridoxal-5'-phosphate (PLP), was more than 50% in alcoholics without abnormal hematologic indices of abnormal liver function (Lumeng and Li, 1974). Inadequate intake may not be the only factor contributing to low plasma levels of PLP. PLP is more rapidly destroyed in erythrocytes in the presence of acetaldehyde, the first product of ethanol oxidation, perhaps by displacement of PLP from protein and its exposure to phosphatase (Lumeng, 1978; Lumeng and Li, 1974). Riboflavin deficiency is usually encountered when there is a general lack of vitamin B intake. Its exact incidence in the alcoholic patient is not known, but evidence of deficiency was found in 50% of a small group of alcoholics with medical complications severe enough to warrant hospitalization (Rosenthal et al., 1973).

Vitamin A ingestion was not considerably below normal in Americans who consumed up to a mean of 400 kcal of alcohol per day (or less than 20% of total calories) (Gruchow et al., 1985a), since the vitamin A density of the nonalcoholic portion of the diet approximated that eaten by control populations. Americans consuming 24 to 28% of their energy as alcohol ingest 75% of the RDA for vitamin A (Hillers and Massey, 1985). Severe alcoholism, in which 50% or more of energy intake is derived from alcohol, is probably associated with even less vitamin A intake in the United States, as shown for wine drinkers in Chile, where consumption of 150 g of alcohol daily was associated with an intake of only 25% of the RDA for vitamin A (Bunout et al., 1983). Elderly American men who consume alcohol regularly had lower vitamin A intakes compared to their abstinent counterparts (Barboriak et al., 1978).

Althausen et al. (1960) reported that alcohol inhibited vitamin A absorption in humans. Vitamin A absorption is reduced even further in the presence of fat malabsorption due to chronic alcoholic pancreatis. In humans with alcoholic liver disease, hepatic vitamin A levels progressively decreased with increasing severity of liver injury (Leo and Lieber, 1982). Enhancement of hepatic vitamin A degradation due to alcohol consumption is a likely explanation for vitamin A depletion. The metabolism of retinoic acid to 4-hydroxy and 4-oxoretinoic acid and other polar metabolites occurs through the action of microsomal enzymes, which are inducible by ethanol consumption (Sato and Lieber, 1982), but they probably do not have sufficient activity to be largely responsible for depleting vitamin A stores.

Newly discovered microsomal pathways for oxidation of retinol to polar metabolites (Leo and Lieber, 1985) and to retinol (Leo et al., 1987a) are also inducible by alcohol (Leo et al., 1986a) and are more likely mechanisms for hepatic vitamin A depletion. In addition, alcohol promotes vitamin A mobilization from the liver (Leo et al., 1986a, 1988). The clinical consequences of altered vitamin A status include the increased incidence of night blindness (xerophthalmia) due to lowered tissue vitamin A levels. Abnormal dark adaptation occurred in 15% of alcoholics without cirrhosis and in 50% of alcoholics with cirrhosis (Bonjour, 1981).

Alcoholics also have illnesses related to abnormalities of calcium, phosphorus, and vitamin D homeostasis as well as decreased bone density (Saville, 1965), decreased bone mass (Gascon-Barré, 1985), increased susceptibility to fractures (Nilsson, 1970), and increased osteonecrosis (Solomon, 1973). Low blood levels of calcium, phosphorus, magnesium, and 25-hydroxy vitamin D have also been reported in alcoholics (Gascon-Barré, 1985). Vitamin D deficiency in alcoholic liver disease probably is due to decreased vitamin D

substrate as a result of poor dietary intake, malabsorption due to cholestasis, pancreatic insufficiency, diminished sunlight, or all these conditions.

Vitamin E deficiency is not a recognized complication of alcoholism. In some studies, however, abnormally low blood levels of vitamin E have been reported in alcoholics (Losowsky and Leonard, 1967; Myerson, 1968).

The diet of many Americans is marginal in zinc (Sandstead, 1973), and alcoholics probably are among those with marginal intake. For example, zinc absorption was low in alcoholic cirrhotics, but not in patients with cirrhosis from other causes (Valberg et al., 1985), and alcoholics with (Vallee et al., 1956) and without (Sullivan and Lankford, 1962) cirrhosis had hyperzincuria and reduced zinc levels. Some instances of night blindness not fully responsive to vitamin A replacement responded to zinc replacement (Leo et al., 1988).

POLICY IMPLICATIONS

The evidence suggests that moderate alcohol consumption reduces stress; increases feelings of happiness, euphoria, and conviviality; decreases tension, depression, and self-consciousness; improves certain types of cognitive performance, such as problem solving and short-term memory; improves psychological well-being; and produces other positive effects, such as increases in HDL levels (Baum-Baicker, 1985a,b). On the other hand, alcohol consumption may lead to addiction (Roe, 1979), and it influences the likelihood of virtually all types of injury: almost half of fatally injured drivers, people killed by falls, drowning, assault, and suicides, and a large percentage of adult passengers and pedestrians killed in motor vehicle crashes have blood alcohol levels of 0.1% or higher (NRC, 1985). Moreover, alcohol can have deleterious effects on the fetus. Attempts to prohibit alcohol consumption through taxation and prohibition have always failed, except when they have been based on religious grounds (Heath, 1975). Thus, prudence suggests a lowering of or abstention from alcohol consumption.

SUMMARY

Of the estimated 18 million alcoholics in the United States, 7.3 million (or 41%) are considered abusers and 10.6 million (59%) are considered alcohol dependent. Alcohol consumption peaks in the 20- to 40-year age group and decreases with advancing age. Although more males than females consume alcohol, the percentage of female drinkers is on the rise. The rate of excessive alcohol consumption among blacks and whites in the general U.S. population is similar. American Indians are three times more likely to be heavier drinkers than the general population, but there is wide variation from tribe to tribe.

Hospitalized alcoholics show signs of protein malnutrition. Those who derive more than 30% of their calories from alcohol have decreases in protein intake; lower calcium and iron intakes; intakes less than the RDAs for vitamins A, C, and thiamin; and deficiencies of pyridoxine and riboflavin. Alcoholics also exhibit abnormalities of calcium, phosphorus, and vitamin D homeostasis as well as reduced zinc absorption. Alcohol consumption, however, is not a primary cause of obesity.

There is consistent evidence that alcohol intake increases the risk of cancer of the oral cavity, pharynx, esophagus, and larynx, where alcohol interacts synergistically with tobacco. There is also a consistent association between alcohol intake and primary liver cancer, although it is unclear whether alcohol increases the risk of primary liver cancer in the absence of liver cirrhosis. Associations have also been found between increasing alcohol consumption and cancers of the pancreas, rectum, and breast. At present, however, there is little or no evidence of a causal relationship. Furthermore, alcoholism is associated with (and perhaps promotes) HBV infection, another factor that independently favors the development of hepatocellular carcinoma. The etiologic role of viruses in the pathogenesis of some tumors has been established. It is conceivable that suppression of immune responsiveness may be important in virus-induced tumors such as hepatocellular carcinoma, which has been associated with HVB infections.

Chronic alcohol abuse may contribute to carcinogenesis through a variety of mechanisms, including the induction of microsomal enzymes that activate procarcinogens, effects on DNA metabolism and DNA repair resulting from alkylation, association with virus hepatitis B, general mechanisms of tissue injury and regeneration, alterations of immune responsiveness, contact-related local effects, the effects of congeners, and the impact of nutritional deficiencies.

Among the dietary deficiencies associated with chronic ethanol abuse, lack of retinoids probably plays a prominent role, because vitamin A depletion favors carcinogenesis in a variety of tissues.

This effect is magnified in the liver, where ethanol promotes vitamin A depletion even in the presence of vitamin A-rich diets. Hepatic depletion is due to enhanced catabolism and to mobilization of vitamin A from the liver to peripheral tissues where vitamin A content then increases; these effects are exacerbated when severe vitamin A depletion is superimposed on chronic alcohol consumption. Hepatic vitamin A stores are then depleted to a level precluding extensive mobilization; as a result, there is a general lack of vitamin A in hepatic and nonhepatic tissues.

Epidemiologic studies associate chronic alcohol consumption with high blood pressure and increased risk of hemorrhagic stroke; acute consumption is linked with increased risk of stroke due to cerebral infarction and hemorrhage. Heavy drinking is associated with increased risk of CHD, but light and moderate drinking are generally associated with a CHD risk that is lower than that for abstainers.

Alcohol consumption is associated with hyperglycemia in humans and animals. Alcohol-induced hypoglycemia, although rare, has also been reported, as has refractiveness to this state. Excessive alcohol consumption has also been associated with gouty arthritis and with ketosis, with minimal or no acidosis. Alcohol also affects renal function, as shown by enlarged kidneys in autopsied alcoholic patients with mild liver disease, by modulating renin–angiotensin responsiveness and by rendering patients susceptible to renal failure.

Alcohol is a causative factor in fatty liver, alcoholic hepatitis, and cirrhosis. Most cases of liver cirrhosis are caused by alcohol consumption: 66% of the cases in North America, 42% in Europe, and 11% in Asia. Women are more susceptible than men. Liver diseases can be due either to alcohol-induced malnutrition or to the toxic effects of alcohol on the metabolic processes of the liver leading to disorders such as decreased fatty acid oxidation, hyper- or hypoglycemia, alteration of the cytochrome P450-dependent oxidizing system, increased production of acetaldehyde, and possibly a direct effect on the metabolism of collagen leading to cirrhosis.

Alcohol has also been implicated as an etiologic agent in nervous system diseases such as Wernicke–Korsakoff syndrome, alcoholic peripheral neuropathy, and alcoholic dementia. Thiamin deficiency is, however, suspected to be the primary cause of those syndromes. Pregnant women who consume high levels of alcohol develop fetuses with a distinct pattern of physical and behavioral abnormalities referred to as fetal alcohol syndrome, characterized by a higher incidence of birth defects.

Moderate alcohol consumption is associated with some beneficial effects. It, however, carries the risk of addictiveness and increases the likelihood of virtually all types of injury, suggesting prudence in alcohol consumption and even abstention.

DIRECTIONS FOR RESEARCH

● *Genetic Determinants of Susceptibility to Alcoholism* Certain genetic variations in enzymes involved in alcohol metabolism influence susceptibility to alcohol addiction. Other genetic variations determine the susceptibility of target organs, such as the liver, to the deleterious effects of alcohol. Therefore, further research in the following topics is warranted:

—Identification of genes or of markers for genes involved in alcohol metabolism to enable the identification of high-risk individuals for intensive preventive efforts.

—Elucidation of the structure and function of these genes and their products to permit more rational and effective means of treating alcoholism and its sequelae. This research is now feasible and is likely to be highly productive.

● *Effects of Alcohol on Chronic Diseases* There is strong evidence that alcohol influences the risk of CHD, hypertension, stroke, osteoporosis, and some types of cancer.

—Investigation of the metabolic mechanisms by which alcohol influences the above diseases would be helpful in planning prevention and treatment strategies. There is sufficient knowledge of the physiological and biochemical processes involved in alcohol metabolism and in the pathogenesis of those diseases to make such research feasible and productive.

REFERENCES

Acheson, E.D., and R. Doll. 1964. Dietary factors in carcinoma of the stomach: a study of 100 cases and 200 controls. Gut 5:126–131.

Adelstein, A., and G. White. 1976. Alcoholism and mortality. Popul. Trends 6:7–13.

Al-Qthami, H. 1978. Pp. 10–12 in Alcohol and Drugs in Saudi Arabia. Proceedings of the Alcohol and Drug Problems Association of North America, Washington, D.C.

Alsafar, J.A. 1974. Alcoholism in Bahrain. Drink. Drugs Pract. Surv. 9:8 et. seq.

Althausen, T.L., K. Uyeyama, and M.R. Loran. 1960. Effects of alcohol on absorption of vitamin A in normal and in gastrectomized subjects. Gastroenterology 38:942–945.

Ammon, H.P., and C.J. Estler. 1968. Inhibition of ethanol-induced glycogenolysis in brain and liver by adrenergic beta-blockade. J. Pharm. Pharmacol. 20:164–165.

Anderson, A.J., J.J. Barboriak, and A.A. Rimm. 1978. Risk factors and angiographically determined coronary occlusion. Am. J. Epidemiol. 107:8–14.

Arai, M., M.A. Leo, M. Nakano, E.R. Gordon, and C.S. Lieber. 1984. Biochemical and morphological alterations of baboon hepatic mitochondria after chronic ethanol consumption. Hepatology 4:165–174.

Arky, R.A., and N. Freinkel. 1966. Alcohol hypoglycemia. V. Alcohol infusion to test gluconeogenesis in starvation, with special reference to obesity. N. Engl. J. Med. 274:426–433.

Arky, R.A., E.A. Abramson, and N. Freinkel. 1968. Alcohol hypoglycemia. VII. Further studies on the refractoriness of obese subjects. Metabolism 17:977–987.

Audigier, J.C., and R. Lambert. 1974. Epidémiologie des cancers du tube digestif. Arch. Fr. Mal. Appar. Dig. 63:413–432.

Axelrod, A.E., and A.C. Trakatellis. 1964. Relationship of pyridoxine to immunological phenomena. Vitamin. Horm. (N.Y.) 22:591–607.

Bales, R.F. 1946. Cultural differences in rates of alcoholism. Q. J. Stud. Alcohol 6:480–499.

Baraona, E., and C.S. Lieber. 1970. Effects of chronic ethanol feeding on serum lipoprotein metabolism in the rat. J. Clin. Invest. 49:769–778.

Baraona, E., R.C. Pirola, and C.S. Lieber. 1974. Small intestinal damage and changes in cell population produced by ethanol ingestion in the rat. Gastroenterology 66:226–234.

Baraona, E., M. Savolainen, C. Karsenty, M.A. Leo, and C.S. Lieber. 1983. Pathogenesis of alcoholic hypertriglyceridemia and hypercholesterolemia. Trans. Assoc. Am. Physicians 96:306–315.

Barboriak, J.J., C.B. Rooney, T.H. Leitschus, and A.J. Anderson. 1978. Alcohol and nutrient intake of elderly men. J. Am. Diet. Assoc. 72:493–495.

Barboriak, J.J., A.J. Anderson, A.A. Rimm, and F.E. Tristani. 1979a. Alcohol and coronary arteries. Alcoholism 3:29–32.

Barboriak, J.J., A.J. Anderson, and R.G. Hoffmann. 1979b. Interrelationship between coronary artery occlusion, high-density lipoprotein cholesterol, and alcohol intake. J. Lab. Clin. Med. 94:348–353.

Barnes, D.M. 1988. Drugs: running the numbers [news]. Science 240:1729–1731.

Barrett-Connor, E., and L. Suarez. 1982. A community study of alcohol and other factors associated with the distribution of high density lipoprotein cholesterol in older vs. younger men. Am. J. Epidemiol. 115:888–893.

Baum-Baicker, C. 1985a. The health benefits of moderate alcohol consumption: a review of the literature. Drug Alcohol Depend. 15:207–227.

Baum-Baicker, C. 1985b. The psychological benefits of moderate alcohol consumption: a review of the literature. Drug Alcohol Depend. 15:305–322.

Bebb, H.T., H.B. Houser, J.C. Witschi, A.S. Littell, and R.K. Fuller. 1971. Calorie and nutrient contribution of alcoholic beverages to the usual diets of 155 adults. Am. J. Clin. Nutr. 24:1042–1052.

Becker, C.E., R.L. Roe, and R.A. Scott. 1974. Alcohol as a Drug: A Curriculum on Pharmacology, Neurology and Toxicology. Medcom Press, New York. 99 pp.

Begg, C.B., A.M. Walker, B. Wessen, and M. Zelen. 1983. Alcohol consumption and breast cancer. Lancet 1:293–294.

Behse, F., and F. Buchthal. 1977. Alcoholic neuropathy: clinical, electrophysiological, and biopsy findings. Ann. Neurol. 2:95–110.

Belinsky, S.A., M.A. Bedell, and J.A. Swenberg. 1982. Effect of chronic ethanol diet on the replication, alkylation, and repair of DNA from hepatocytes and nonparenchymal cells following dimethylnitrosamine administration. Carcinogenesis 3:1293–1297.

Best, C.H., W.S. Hartroft, C.C. Lucas, and J.H. Ridout. 1949. Liver damage produced by feeding alcohol or sugar and its prevention by choline. Br. Med. J. 2:1001–1006.

Bignon, J., M. Bientz, G. Bonnaud, and P. Sebastien. 1977. Evaluation numérique des fibres d'amiante dans des échantillons de vins. Nouv. Presse Med. 6:1148–1149.

Biles, B., and T.R. Emerson. 1968. Examination of fibres in beer. Nature (London) 219:93–94.

Bjelke, E. 1978. Dietary factors and the epidemiology of cancer of the stomach and large bowel. Aktuel. Ernaehrungsmed. Klin. Prax. Suppl. 2:10–17.

Blackwelder, W.C., K. Yano, G.G. Rhoads, A. Kagan, T. Gordon, and Y. Palesch. 1980. Alcohol and mortality: the Honolulu Heart Study. Am. J. Med. 68:164–169.

Blass, J.P., and G.E. Gibson. 1977. Abnormality of a thiamine-requiring enzyme in patients with Wernicke-Korsakoff syndrome. N. Engl. J. Med. 297:1367–1370.

Blose, I.L. 1978. The relationship of alcohol to aging and the elderly. Alcoholism 2:17–21.

Bode, C., B. Buchwald, and H. Goebell. 1971. Hemmung des Athanolabbaues durch Proteinmangel beim Menschen. Dtsch. Med. Wochenschr. 96:1576–1577.

Bonjour, J.P. 1981. Vitamin and alcoholism. IX. Vitamin A. Int. J. Vitam. Nutr. Res. 51:166–177.

Borowsky, S.A., W. Perlow, E. Baraona, and C.S. Lieber. 1980. Relationship of alcoholic hypertriglyceridemia to stage of liver disease and dietary lipid. Dig. Dis. Sci. 25:22–27.

Böttiger, L.E., L.A. Carlson, E. Hultman, and V. Romanus. 1976. Serum lipids in alcoholics. Acta Med. Scand. 199:357–361.

Bréchot, C., B. Nalpas, A. Couroucé, G. Duhamel, P. Callard, F. Carnot, P. Tiollais, and P. Berthelot. 1982. Evidence that hepatitis B virus has a role in liver-cell carcinoma in alcoholic liver disease. N. Engl. J. Med. 306:1384–1387.

Brenn, T. 1986. The Tromsø heart study: alcoholic beverages and coronary risk factors. J. Epidemiol. Community Health 40:249–256.

Breslow, N.E., and J.E. Enstrom. 1974. Geographic correlations between cancer mortality rates and alcohol–tobacco consumption in the United States. J. Natl. Cancer Inst. 53:631–639.

Bulpitt, C.J., M.J. Shipley, and A. Semmence. 1987. The contribution of a moderate intake of alcohol to the presence of hypertension. J. Hypertens. 5:85–91.

Bunout, D., V. Gattás, H. Iturriaga, C. Pérez, T. Pereda, and G. Ugarte. 1983. Nutritional status of alcoholic patients: its possible relationship to alcoholic liver damage. Am. J. Clin.

Nutr. 38:469–473.

Burch, G.E., and A. Ansari. 1968. Chronic alcoholism and carcinoma of the pancreas: a correlative hypothesis. Arch. Intern. Med. 122:273–275.

Burch, J.D., G.R. Howe, A.B. Miller, and R. Semenciw. 1981. Tobacco, alcohol, asbestos, and nickel in the etiology of cancer of the larynx: a case-control study. J. Natl. Cancer Inst. 67:1219–1224.

Byers, T., and D.P. Funch. 1982. Alcohol and breast cancer. Lancet 1:799–800.

Bynum, W.F. 1968. Chronic alcoholism in the first half of the 19th century. Bull. Hist. Med. 42:160–185.

Cahalan, D., I.H. Cisin, and H.M. Crossley. 1967. American Drinking Practices; A National Survey of Drinking Behavior and Attitudes Related to Alcoholic Beverages. Report No. 3. Social Research Group, George Washington University. College and University Press, New Haven, Conn. 355 pp.

Cairns, V., U. Keil, D. Kleinbaum, A. Doering, and J. Stieber. 1984. Alcohol consumption as a risk factor for high blood pressure. Munich Blood Pressure Study. Hypertension 6:124–131.

Camargo, C.A., Jr., P.T. Williams, K.M. Vranizan, J.J. Albers, and P.D. Wood. 1985. The effect of moderate alcohol intake on serum apolipoproteins A-I and A-II. J. Am. Med. Assoc. 253:2854–2857.

Cambien, F., A. Jacqueson, J.L. Richard, J.M. Warnet, and P. Ducimetière. 1985. Pression artérielle, corpulence et consommation de graisse et d'alcool. Arch. Mal. Coeur 78:1607–1610.

Castelli, W.P., J.T. Doyle, T. Gordon, M.G. Hjortland, A. Kagan, C.G. Hames, S.B. Hulley, and W.J. Zukel. 1977. Alcohol and blood lipids. The cooperative lipoprotein phenotyping study. Lancet 2:153–155.

Chalke, H.D. 1976. Alcohol and history. J. Alcohol. 11:128–149.

Chen, H., H. Zhuang, and Q. Han. 1983. Serum high density lipoprotein cholesterol and factors influencing its level in healthy Chinese. Atherosclerosis 48:71–79.

Chevilotte, G., J.P. Durbec, A. Gerolami, P. Berthezene, J.M. Bidart, and R. Camatte. 1983. Interaction between hepatitis B virus and alcohol consumption in liver cirrhosis. An epidemiologic study. Gastroenterology 85:141–145.

Chiba, K., A. Koizumi, M. Kumai, T. Watanabe, and M. Ikeda. 1983. Nationwide survey of high-density lipoprotein cholesterol among farmers in Japan. Prev. Med. 12:508–522.

Clark, V.A., J.M. Chapman, and A.H. Coulson. 1967. Effects of various factors on systolic and diastolic blood pressure in the Los Angeles heart study. J. Chronic Dis. 20:571–581.

Coates, R.A., P.N. Corey, M.J. Ashley, and C.A. Steele. 1985. Alcohol consumption and blood pressure: analysis of data from the Canada Health Survey. Prev. Med. 14:1–4.

Colditz, G.A., L.G. Branch, R.J. Lipnick, W.C. Willett, B. Rosner, B. Posner, and C.H. Hennekens. 1985. Moderate alcohol and decreased cardiovascular mortality in an elderly cohort. Am. Heart J. 109:886–889.

Criqui, M.H. 1987. Alcohol and hypertension: new insights from population studies. Eur. Health J. 8 Suppl. B:19–26.

Criqui, M.H., L.D. Cowan, H.A. Tyroler, S. Bangdiwala, G. Heiss, R.B. Wallace, and C.E. Davis. 1982. Cigarette smoking, alcohol consumption and cardiovascular mortality. The Lipid Research Clinics Follow-Up Study. Circulation 66:II235.

Crouse, J.R., and S.M. Grundy. 1984. Effects of alcohol on

plasma lipoproteins and cholesterol and triglyceride metabolism in man. J. Lipid Res. 25:486–496.

Cruickshank, J.K., S.H. Jackson, D.G. Beevers, L.T. Bannan, M. Beevers, and V.L. Stewart. 1985. Similarity of blood pressure in blacks, whites, and Asians in England: the Birmingham Factory Study. J. Hypertens. 3:365–371.

Cubilla, A.L., and P.J. Fitzgerald. 1978. Pancreas cancer (non-endocrine): a review—Part II. Clin. Bull. 8:143–155.

Cullen, K., N.S. Stenhouse, and K.L. Wearne. 1982. Alcohol and mortality in the Busselton Study. Int. J. Epidemiol. 11:67–70.

Cunningham, H.M., and R. Pontefract. 1971. Asbestos fibres in beverages and drinking water. Nature (London) 232:332–333.

Dailey, R.C. 1968. The role of alcohol among North American Indian tribes as reported in the Jesuit relations. Anthropologica 10:45–57.

Dales, L.G., G.D. Friedman, H.K. Ury, S. Grossman, and S.R. Williams. 1979. A case-control study of relationships of diet and other traits to colorectal cancer in American blacks. Am. J. Epidemiol. 109:132–144.

D'Alonzo, C.A., and S. Pell. 1968. Cardiovascular disease among problem drinkers. J. Occup. Med. 10:344–350.

Dean, G., R. MacLennan, H. McLoughlin, and E. Shelley. 1979. Causes of death of blue-collar workers at a Dublin brewery, 1954–1973. Br. J. Cancer 40:581–589.

De Jong, U.W., N. Breslow, J.G. Goh, M. Sridharan, and K. Shanmugaratnam. 1974. Aetiological factors in oesophageal cancer in Singapore Chinese. Int. J. Cancer 13:291–303.

de Lint, J., and T. Levinson. 1975. Mortality among patients treated for alcoholism: a 5-year follow-up. Can. Med. Assoc. J. 113:385–387.

Department of Health, City of New York. 1984. Summary of Vital Statistics 1983. Bureau of Health Statistics and Analysis, Department of Health, City of New York. 16 pp.

Devenyi, P., G.M. Robinson, and D.A. Roncari. 1980. Alcohol and high-density lipoproteins. Can. Med. Assoc. J. 123:981–984.

Dinoso, V.P., Jr., S. Ming, and J. McNiff. 1976. Ultrastructural changes of the canine gastric mucosa after topical application of graded concentrations of ethanol. Am. J. Dig. Dis. 21:626–632.

Donahue, R.P., R.D. Abbott, D.M. Reed, and K. Yano. 1986. Alcohol and hemorrhagic stroke. The Honolulu Heart Program. J. Am. Med. Assoc. 255:2311–2314.

Dornhorst, A., and A. Ouyang. 1971. Effect of alcohol on glucose tolerance. Lancet 2:957–959.

Dorothy George, M. 1931. England in Transition. Life and Work in the 18th Century. G. Rutledge and Sons, Ltd., London. 93 pp.

Douglas, M. 1987. A distinctive anthropological perspective. Pp. 3–15 in M. Douglas, ed. Constructive Drinking: Perspectives on Drink from Anthropology. Cambridge University Press, Cambridge, Mass.

Duruibe, V., and G.A. Tejwani. 1981. The effect of ethanol on the activities of the key gluconeogenic and glycolytic enzymes of rat liver. Mol. Pharmacol. 20:621–630.

Dyer, A.R., J. Stamler, O. Paul, D.M. Berkson, M.H. Lepper, H. McKean, R.B. Shekelle, H.A. Lindberg, and D. Garside. 1977. Alcohol consumption, cardiovascular risk factors, and mortality in two Chicago epidemiologic studies. Circulation 56:1067–1074.

Eastwood, G.L., and J.P. Kirchner. 1974. Changes in the fine structure of mouse gastric epithelium produced by ethanol and urea. Gastroenterology 67:71–84.

Eichner, E.R., B. Buchanan, J.W. Smith, and R.S. Hillman. 1972. Variations in the hematologic and medical status of alcoholics. Am. J. Med. Sci. 263:35–42.

Ekman, R., G. Fex, B.G. Johansson, P. Nilsson-Ehle, and J. Wadstein. 1981. Changes in plasma high density lipoproteins and lipolytic enzymes after long-term, heavy ethanol consumption. Scand. J. Clin. Lab. Invest. 41:709–715.

Elzay, R.P. 1966. Local effect of alcohol in combination with DMBA on hamster cheek pouch. J. Dent. Res. 45:1788–1795.

Elzay, R.P. 1969. Effect of alcohol and cigarette smoke as promoting agents in hamster pouch carcinogenesis. J. Dent. Res. 48:1200–1205.

Epstein, M. 1985a. Derangements of renal water handling in liver disease. Gastroenterology 89:1415–1425.

Epstein, M. 1985b. Hepatorenal syndrome. Pp. 3138–3149 in J.E. Berk, ed. Bockus Gastroenterology, 4th ed., Vol. 5. W.B. Saunders, Philadelphia.

Epstein, M. 1986. The sodium retention of cirrhosis: a reappraisal. Hepatology 6:312–315.

Epstein, M. 1987a. Pathogenesis of sodium retention in liver disease. Pp. 299–333 in B.M. Brenner and J.H. Stein, eds. Body Fluid Homeostasis. Contemporary Issues in Nephrology, Vol. 16. Churchill Livingstone, New York.

Epstein, M. 1987b. Renal complications in liver disease. Pp. 903–923 in L. Schiff and E.R. Schiff, eds. Diseases of the Liver, 6th ed. J.B. Lippincott Co., Philadelphia.

Epstein, M. In press. In Medical and Nutritional Disorders of Alcoholism. Plenum Press, New York.

Espina, N., V. Lima, C.S. Lieber, and A.J. Garro. 1988. In vitro and in vivo inhibitory effect of ethanol and acetaldehyde on O^6-methylguanine transferase. Carcinogenesis 9:761–766.

Faller, J., and I.H. Fox. 1982. Ethanol-induced hyperuricemia: evidence for increased urate production by activation of adenine nucleotide turnover. N. Engl. J. Med. 307:1598–1602.

Farinati, F., C.S. Lieber, and A.J. Garro. 1985a. The effects of chronic ethanol consumption on carcinogen metabolizing systems in rat upper alimentary tract. Gastroenterology 88:1378.

Farinati, F., N. Espina, C.S. Lieber, and A.J. Garro. 1985b. In vivo inhibition by chronic ethanol exposure of methylguanine transferase activity and DNA repair. Ital. J. Gastroenterol. 17:48–49.

Field, J.B., H.E. Williams, and G.E. Mortimore. 1963. Studies on the mechanism of ethanol-induced hypoglycemia. J. Clin. Invest. 42:497–506.

Flynn, A., S.I. Miller, S.S. Martier, N.L. Golden, R.J. Sokol, and B.C. Del Villano. 1981. Zinc status of pregnant alcoholic women: a determinant of fetal outcome. Lancet 1:572–574.

Forsander, O., K.O. Vartia, and F.E. Krusius. 1958. Experimentelle Studien über die biologische Wirkung von Alkohol. 1. Alkohol und Blutzucker. Ann. Med. Exp. Biol. Fenn. 36:416–423.

Fortmann, S.P., W.L. Haskell, K. Vranizan, B.W. Brown, and J.W. Farquhar. 1983. The association of blood pressure and dietary alcohol: differences by age, sex, and estrogen use. Am. J. Epidemiol. 118:497–507.

Fraser, G.E., J.T. Anderson, N. Foster, R. Goldberg, D. Jacobs, and H. Blackburn. 1983. The effect of alcohol on serum high density lipoprotein (HDL). A controlled experiment. Atherosclerosis 46:275–286.

Freinkel, N., R.A. Arky, D.L. Singer, A.K. Cohen, S.J. Bleicher, and J.B. Anderson. 1965. Alcohol hypoglycemia. IV. Current concepts of its pathogenesis. Diabetes 14:350–361.

Friedman, L.A., and A.W. Kimball. 1986. Coronary heart disease mortality and alcohol consumption in Framingham. Am. J. Epidemiol. 124:481–489.

Fuchs, C.H. 1848. Lehrbuch der Speziellen Nosologie und Therapie, Vol. 2. Göttingen, Germany. (various pagings)

Gabrial, G.N., T.F. Schrager, and P.M. Newberne. 1982. Zinc deficiency, alcohol, and a retinoid: association with esophageal cancer in rats. J. Natl. Cancer Inst. 68:785–789.

Garrison, R.J., W.B. Kannel, J. Stokes III, and W.P. Castelli. 1987. Incidence and precursors of hypertension in young adults: the Framingham Offspring Study. Prev. Med. 16:235–251.

Garro, A.J., H.K. Seitz, and C.S. Lieber. 1981. Enhancement of dimethylnitrosamine metabolism and activation to a mutagen following chronic ethanol consumption. Cancer Res. 41:120–124.

Gascon-Barré, M. 1985. Influence of chronic ethanol consumption on the metabolism and action of vitamin D. J. Am. Coll. Nutr. 4:565–574.

Gawad, A. 1968. Pp. 666–669 in Al-Mufassal fi tarikh el-Arab Kabl al Islam, Vol. 4. Al-Nahda, Baghdad, Iraq.

Gerard, M.J., A.L. Klatsky, A.B. Siegelaub, G.D. Friedman, and R. Feldman. 1977. Serum glucose levels and alcohol-consumption habits in a large population. Diabetes 26:780–785.

Ghalioungui, P. 1979. Fermented beverages in antiquity. Pp. 3–19 in C.F. Gastineau, W.J. Darby, and T.B. Turner, eds. Fermented Food Beverages in Nutrition. Academic Press, New York.

Gibel, W. 1967. Experimentelle Untersuchungen zur Synkarzinogenese beim Eosophaguskarzinom. Arch. Geschwulstforsch. 30:181–189.

Gibson, T., A.V. Rodgers, H.A. Simmonds, and P. Toseland. 1984. Beer drinking and its effect on uric acid. Br. J. Rheumatol. 23:203–209.

Gill, J.S., A.V. Zezulka, M.J. Shipley, S.K. Gill, and D.G. Beevers. 1986. Stroke and alcohol consumption. N. Engl. J. Med. 315:1041–1046.

Glueck, C.J., G. Heiss, J.A. Morrison, P. Khoury, and M. Moore. 1981. Alcohol intake, cigarette smoking and plasma lipids and lipoproteins in 12–19-year-old children. The Collaborative Lipid Research Clinics Prevalence Study. Circulation 64:48–56.

Glueck, C.J., D.J. Gordon, J.J. Nelson, C.E. Davis, and H.A. Tyroler. 1986. Dietary and other correlates of changes in total and low density lipoprotein cholesterol in hypercholesterolemic men: the Lipid Research Clinics Coronary Primary Prevention Trial. Am. J. Clin. Nutr. 44:489–500.

Gluud, C., J. Aldershvile, J. Henriksen, P. Kryger, and L. Mathiesen. 1982. Hepatitis B and A virus antibodies in alcoholic steatosis and cirrhosis. J. Clin. Pathol. 35:693–697.

Gluud, C., B. Gluud, J. Aldershvile, A. Jacobsen, and O. Dietrichson. 1984. Prevalence of hepatitis B virus infection in out-patient alcoholics. Infection 12:72–74.

Goldberg, C.S., A.R. Tall, and S. Krumholz. 1984. Acute inhibition of hepatic lipase and increase in plasma lipoproteins after alcohol intake. J. Lipid Res. 25:714–720.

Gonçalves de Lima, O., J. Francisco de Mello, I.L. D'Albu-

querque, F.D. Monache, G.B. Marini-Bettolo, and M. Sousa. 1977. Contribution to the knowledge of the Maya ritual wine: Balché. Lloydia 40:195–200.

Gordon, T., and J.T. Doyle. 1985. Drinking and coronary heart disease: the Albany Study. Am. Heart J. 110:331–334.

Gordon, T., and W.B. Kannel. 1983. Drinking habits and cardiovascular disease: the Framingham Study. Am. Heart J. 105:667–673.

Gordon, T., N. Ernst, M. Fisher, and B.M. Rifkind. 1981. Alcohol and high-density lipoprotein cholesterol. Circulation 64:63–67.

Gorelick, P.B., M.B. Rodin, P. Langenberg, D.B. Hier, J. Costigan, I. Gomez, and S. Spontak. 1987. Is acute alcohol ingestion a risk factor for ischemic stroke? Results of a controlled study in middle-aged and elderly stroke patients at three urban medical centers. Stroke 18:359–364.

Gottfried, E.B., M.A. Korsten, and C.S. Lieber. 1978. Alcohol-induced gastric and duodenal lesions in man. Am. J. Gastroenterol. 70:587–592.

Goudeau, A., P. Maupas, F. Dubois, P. Coursaget, and P. Bougnoux. 1981. Hepatitis B infection in alcoholic liver disease and primary hepatocellular carcinoma in France. Prog. Med. Virol. 27:26–34.

Graham, S. 1987. Alcohol and breast cancer. N. Engl. J. Med. 316:1211–1213.

Graham, S., W. Scholtz, and P. Martino. 1972. Alimentary factors in the epidemiology of gastric cancer. Cancer 30:927–928.

Graham, S., H. Dayal, T. Rohrer, M. Swanson, H. Sultz, D. Shedd, and S. Fischman. 1977. Dentition, diet, tobacco, and alcohol in the epidemiology of oral cancer. J. Natl. Cancer Inst. 59:1611–1618.

Graham, S., H. Dayal, M. Swanson, A. Mittelman, and G. Wilkinson. 1978. Diet in the epidemiology of cancer of the colon and rectum. J. Natl. Cancer Inst. 61:709–714.

Graham, S., C. Mettlin, J. Marshall, R. Priore, T. Rzepka, and D. Shedd. 1981. Dietary factors in the epidemiology of cancer of the larynx. Am. J. Epidemiol. 113:675–680.

Griciute, L., M. Castegnaro, and J.C. Bereziat. 1981. Influence of ethyl alcohol on carcinogenesis with N-nitrosodimethylamine. Cancer Lett. 13:345–352.

Gruchow, H.W., K.A. Sobocinski, J.J. Barboriak, and J.G. Scheller. 1985a. Alcohol consumption, nutrient intake and relative body weight among U.S. adults. Am. J. Clin. Nutr. 42:289–295.

Gruchow, H.W., K.A. Sobocinski, and J.J. Barboriak. 1985b. Alcohol, nutrient intake, and hypertension in U.S. adults. J. Am. Med. Assoc. 253:1567–1570.

Guisard, D., J.P. Gonand, J. Laurent, and G. Debry. 1971. Etude de l'épuration plasmatique des lipides chez les cirrhotiques. Nutr. Metab. 13:222–229.

Habs, M., and D. Schmähl. 1981. Inhibition of the hepatocarcinogenic activity of diethylnitrosamine (DENA) by ethanol in rats. Hepatogastroenterology 28:242–244.

Haenszel, W., M. Kurihara, M. Segi, and R.K.C. Lee. 1972. Stomach cancer among Japanese in Hawaii. J. Natl. Cancer Inst. 49:969–988.

Haffner, S.M., D. Applebaum-Bowden, P.W. Wahl, J.J. Hoover, G.R. Warnick, J.J. Albers, and W.R. Hazzard. 1985. Epidemiological correlates of high density lipoprotein subfractions, apolipoproteins A-I, A-II, and D, and lecithin cholesterol acyltransferase. Arteriosclerosis 5:169–177.

Hakulinen, T., L. Lehtimäki, M. Lehtonen, and L. Teppo.

1974. Cancer morbidity among two male cohorts with increased alcohol consumption in Finland. J. Natl. Cancer Inst. 52:1711–1714.

Hales, D., and R.E. Hales. 1986. Alcohol: better than what we thought? Am. Health 5:38–43.

Halsted, C.H., E.A. Robles, and E. Mezey. 1971. Decreased jejunal uptake of labeled folic acid (₃H-PGA) in alcoholic patients: roles of alcohol and nutrition. N. Engl. J. Med. 285:701–706.

Harlan, W.R., A.L. Hull, R.L. Schmouder, J.R. Landis, F.A. Larkin, and F.E. Thompson. 1984. High blood pressure in older Americans. The First National Health and Nutrition Examination Survey. Hypertension 6:802–809.

Hartung, G.H., J.P. Foreyt, R.E. Mitchell, J.G. Mitchell, R.S. Reeves, and A.M. Gotto, Jr. 1983. Effect of alcohol intake on high-density lipoprotein cholesterol levels in runners and inactive men. J. Am. Med. Assoc. 249:747–750.

Haskell, W.L., C. Camargo, Jr., P.T. Williams, K.M. Vranizan, R.M. Krauss, F.T. Lindgren, and P.D. Wood. 1984. The effect of cessation and resumption of moderate alcohol intake on serum high-density-lipoprotein subfractions. A controlled study. N. Engl. J. Med. 310:805–810.

Heath, D.B. 1975. A critical review of ethnographic studies of alcohol use. Pp. 1–93 in R.J. Gibbins, Y. Israel, H. Kalant, R.E. Popham, W. Schmidt, and R.G. Smart, eds. Research Advances in Alcohol and Drug Problems, Vol. 2. Wiley, New York.

Heath, D.B. 1987. A decade of development in anthopological study of alcohol use: 1970–1980. Pp. 16–69 in M. Douglas, ed. Constructive Drinking: Perspectives on Drink from Anthropology. Cambridge University Press, Cambridge.

Heath, D.B. In press. Anthropological and sociocultural perspectives on alcohol as a reinforcer. In W. Miles Cox, ed. Why People Drink: Parameters of Alcohol as a Reinforcer. Gardner Press, New York.

Hed, R., and A. Nygren. 1968. Alcohol-induced hypoglycaemia in chronic alcoholics with liver disease. Acta Med. Scand. 183:507–510.

Hennekens, C.H., B. Rosner, and D.S. Cole. 1978. Daily alcohol consumption and fatal coronary heart disease. Am. J. Epidemiol. 107:196–200.

Hennekens, C.H., W. Willett, B. Rosner, D.S. Cole, and S.L. Mayrent. 1979. Effects of beer, wine, and liquor in coronary deaths. J. Am. Med. Assoc. 242:1973–1974.

Herbert, V., R. Zalusky, and C.S. Davidson. 1963. Correlation of folate deficiency with alcoholism and associated macrocytosis, anemia, and liver disease. Ann. Intern. Med. 58:977–988.

Hiatt, R.A., and R.D. Bawol. 1984. Alcoholic beverage consumption and breast cancer incidence. Am. J. Epidemiol. 120:676–683.

Hillers, V.N., and L.K. Massey. 1985. Interrelationships of moderate and high alcohol consumption with diet and health status. Am. J. Clin. Nutr. 41:356–362.

Hirayama, T. 1972. Epidemiology of stomach cancer. Pp. 3–19 in T. Murakami, ed. Early Gastric Cancer. Gann Monograph on Cancer Research, No. 11. University Park Press, Baltimore.

Hirsch, J. 1949. Enlightened eighteenth century views of the alcohol problem. J. Hist. Med. 4:230–236.

Hislop, W.S., E.A. Follet, I.A. Bouchier, and R.N. MacSween. 1981. Serological markers of hepatitis B in patients with alcoholic liver disease: a multi-centre survey. J. Clin. Pathol. 34:1017–1019.

Hoey, J., C. Montvernay, and R. Lambert. 1981. Wine and tobacco: risk factors for gastric cancer in France. Am. J. Epidemiol. 113:668–674.

Hoffbauer, F.W., and F.G. Zaki. 1965. Choline deficiency in baboon and rat compared. Arch. Pathol. 79:364–369.

Horsley, V., and M.D. Sturge. 1915. Alcohol and the Human Body; an Introduction to the Study of the Subject, and a Contribution to National Health, 5th ed. MacMillan and Co., Ltd., London. 339 pp.

Hoyumpa, A.M., Jr. 1983. Alcohol and thiamine metabolism. Alcoholism 7:11–14.

Hulley, S.B., and S. Gordon. 1981. Alcohol and high-density lipoprotein cholesterol: causal inference from diverse study designs. Circulation 64:57–63.

Huss, M. 1852. Chronische Alkoholskrankheit; Oder, Alcoholismus Chronicus. C.E. Fritze, Stockholm. 574 pp.

Iber, F.L. 1971. In alcoholism, the liver sets the pace. Nutr. Today 6:2–9.

Innami, S., A. Nakamura, M. Miyazaki, S. Nagayama, and E. Nishide. 1976. Further studies on the reduction of vitamin A content in the livers of rats given polychlorinated biphenyls. J. Nutr. Sci. Vitaminol. 22:409–418.

Israel, Y., L. Videla, and J. Bernstein. 1975. Liver hypermetabolic state after chronic ethanol consumption: hormonal interrelations and pathogenic implications. Fed. Proc. 34:2052–2059.

Jackson, R., A. Stewart, R. Beaglehole, and R. Scragg. 1985. Alcohol consumption and blood pressure. Am. J. Epidemiol. 122:1037–1044.

Jacqueson, A., J.L. Richard, P. Ducimetière, J.M. Warnet, and J.R. Claude. 1983. High density lipoprotein cholesterol and alcohol consumption in a French male population. Atherosclerosis 48:131–138.

Jensen, O.M. 1979. Cancer morbidity and causes of death among Danish brewery workers. Int. J. Cancer 23:454–463.

Johansen, H., R. Semenciw, H. Morrison, Y. Mao, P. Verdier, M.E. Smith, and D.T. Wigle. 1987. Important risk factors for death in adults: a 10-year follow-up of the Nutrition Canada survey cohort. Can. Med. Assoc. J. 136:823–828.

Johansson, B.G., and C.B. Laurell. 1969. Disorders of serum alpha-lipoproteins after alcoholic intoxication. Scand. J. Clin. Lab. Invest. 23:231–233.

Johansson, B.G., and A. Medhus. 1974. Increase in plasma alpha-lipoproteins in chronic alcoholics after acute abuse. Acta Med. Scand. 195:273–277.

Jolliffe, N. 1940. Influence of alcohol on adequacy of B vitamins in American diet. Q. J. Stud. Alcohol 1:74–84.

Jolliffe, N., and E.M. Jellinek. 1941. Vitamin deficiencies and liver cirrhosis in alcoholism; cirrhosis of liver. Q. J. Stud. Alcohol 2:544–583.

Jones, K.L., and D.W. Smith. 1973. Recognition of the fetal alcohol syndrome in early infancy. Lancet 2:999-1001.

Kagan, A., J.S. Popper, and G.G. Rhoads. 1980. Factors related to stroke incidence in Hawaii Japanese men. The Honolulu Heart Study. Stroke 11:14–21.

Kagan, A., K. Yano, G.G. Rhoads, and D.L. McGee. 1981. Alcohol and cardiovascular disease: the Hawaiian experience. Circulation 64:27–31.

Kalbfleisch, J.M., R.D. Lindemann, H.E. Ginn, and W.O. Smith. 1963. Effects of ethanol administration on urinary excretion of magnesium and other electrolytes in alcoholic and normal subjects. J. Clin. Invest. 42:1471–1475.

Kannel, W.B., and P. Sorlie. 1974. Hypertension in Framingham. Pp. 553–592 in O. Paul, ed. Epidemiology and Control of Hypertension. Stratton Intercontinental Medical Book Co., New York.

Kato, N., M. Kato, T. Kimura, and A. Yoshida. 1978. Effect of dietary addition of PCB, DDT or BHT and dietary protein on vitamin A and cholesterol metabolism. Nutr. Rep. Int. 18:437–445.

Keller, A.Z., and M. Terris. 1965. The association of alcohol and tobacco with cancer of the mouth and pharynx. Am. J. Public Health 55:1578–1585.

Kennaway, E.L., and N.M. Kennaway. 1947. Further study of incidence of cancer of lung and larynx. Br. J. Cancer 1:260–298.

Keys, A., A. Menotti, M.J. Karvonen, C. Aravanis, H. Blackburn, R. Buzina, B.S. Djordjevic, A.S. Dontas, F. Fidanza, M.H. Keys, D. Kromhout, S. Nedeljkovic, S. Punsar, F. Seccareccia, and H. Toshima. 1986. The diet and 15-year death rate in the seven countries study. Am. J. Epidemiol. 124:903–915.

Kirchner, J.A., and J.S. Malkin. 1953. Cancer of larynx; 30-year survey at New Haven Hospital. Arch. Otolaryngol. 58:19–30.

Kittner, S.J., M.R. Garcia-Palmieri, R. Costas, Jr., M. Cruz-Vidal, R.D. Abbott, and R.J. Havlik. 1983. Alcohol and coronary heart disease in Puerto Rico. Am. J. Epidemiol. 117:538–550.

Klatskin, G., W.A. Krehl, and H.O. Conn. 1954. Effect of alcohol on choline requirement; changes in rat's liver following prolonged ingestion of alcohol. J. Exp. Med. 100:605–614.

Klatsky, A.L., G.D. Friedman, and A.B. Siegelaub. 1974. Alcohol consumption before myocardial infarction. Results from the Kaiser-Permanente epidemiologic study of myocardial infarction. Ann. Intern. Med. 81:294–301.

Klatsky, A.L., G.D. Friedman, A.B. Siegelaub, and M.J. Gerard. 1977. Alcohol consumption and blood pressure. Kaiser-Permanente Multiphasic Health Examination data. N. Engl. J. Med. 296:1194–1200.

Klatsky, A.L., G.D. Friedman, and A.B. Siegelaub. 1979. Alcohol use, myocardial infarction, sudden cardiac death, and hypertension. Alcoholism 3:33–39.

Klatsky, A.L., G.D. Friedman, and A.B. Siegelaub. 1981a. Alcohol and mortality. A ten-year Kaiser-Permanente experience. Ann. Intern. Med. 95:139–145.

Klatsky, A.L., G.D. Friedman, and A.B. Siegelaub. 1981b. Alcohol use and cardiovascular disease: the Kaiser-Permanente experience. Circulation 64:32–41.

Klatsky, A.L., G.D. Friedman, and M.A. Armstrong. 1986. The relationships between alcoholic beverage use and other traits to blood pressure: a new Kaiser-Permanente study. Circulation 73:628–636.

Kleihues, P., G. Doerjer, L.K. Keefer, J.M. Rice, P.P. Roller, and R.M. Hodgson. 1979. Correlation of DNA methylation by methyl(acetoxymethyl)nitrosamine with organ-specific carcinogenicity in rats. Cancer Res. 39:5136–5140.

Klipstein, F.A., and J. Lindenbaum. 1965. Folate deficiency in chronic liver disease. Blood 25:443–456.

Koch, O.R., E.A. Porta, and W.S. Hartroft. 1968. A new experimental approach in the study of chronic alcoholism. 3. Role of alcohol versus sucrose or fat-derived calories in hepatic damage. Lab. Invest. 18:379–386.

Komajda, M., J.L. Richard, J.B. Bouhour, A. Sacrez, C. Bour-

donnec, A. Gerbaux, L. Rozensztajn, J.M. Lablanche, D. Matinat, P. Morand, and Y. Grosoogeat. 1986. Dilated cardiomyopathy and the level of alcohol consumption: a planned multicentre case-control study. Eur. Heart J. 7:512–519.

Koop, D.R., E.T. Morgan, G.E. Tarr, and M.J. Coon. 1982. Purification and characterization of a unique isozyme of cytochrome P-450 from liver microsomes of ethanol-treated rabbits. J. Biol. Chem. 257:8472–8480.

Kozarevic, D., J. Demirovic, T. Gordon, C.T. Kaelber, D. McGee, and W.J. Zukel. 1982. Drinking habits and coronary heart disease: the Yugoslavia cardiovascular disease study. Am. J. Epidemiol. 116:748–758.

Kozarevic, D., N. Vojvodic, T. Gordon, C.T. Kaelber, D. McGee, and W.J. Zukel. 1983. Drinking habits and death. The Yugoslavia cardiovascular disease study. Int. J. Epidemiol. 12:145–150.

Krebs, H.A., R.A. Freedland, R. Hems, and M. Stibbs. 1969. Inhibition of hepatic gluconeogenesis by ethanol. Biochem. J. 112:117–124.

Krusius, F.E., K.O. Vartia, and O. Forsander. 1958. Experimentelle Studien über die biologische Wirkung von Alkohol. 2. Alkohol und Nebennierenrinden-Funktion. Ann. Med. Exp. Biol. Fenn. 36:424–434.

Kune, S., G.A. Kune, and L.F. Watson. 1987. Case-control study of alcoholic beverages as etiological factors: the Melbourne Colorectal Cancer Study. Nutr. Cancer 9:43–56.

Kunitz, S.J., J.E. Levy, C.L. Odoroff, and J. Bollinger. 1971. The epidemiology of alcoholic cirrhosis in two southwestern Indian tribes. Q. J. Stud. Alcohol 32:706–720.

Lane, B.P., and C.S Lieber. 1966. Ultrastructural alterations in human hepatocytes following ingestion of ethanol with adequate diets. Am. J. Pathol. 49:593–603.

Lasker, J.M., J. Raucy, S. Kubota, B.P. Bloswick, M. Black, and C.S. Lieber. 1987. Purification and characterization of human liver cytochrome P-450-ALC. Biochem. Biophys. Res. Commun. 148:232–238.

La Porte, R., L. Valvo-Gerard, L. Kuller, W. Dai, M. Bates, J. Cresanta, K. Williams, and D. Palkin. 1981. The relationship between alcohol consumption, liver enzymes and high-density lipoprotein cholesterol. Circulation 64:67–72.

La Vecchia, C., S. Franceschi, A. Decarli, S. Pampallona, and G. Tognoni. 1987. Risk factors for myocardial infarction in young women. Am. J. Epidemiol. 125:832–843.

Lê, M.G., C. Hill, A. Kramar, and R. Flamanti. 1984. Alcoholic beverage consumption and breast cancer in a French case-control study. Am. J. Epidemiol. 120:350–357.

Leevy, C.M. 1968. Cirrhosis in alcoholics. Med. Clin. North Am. 52:1445–1455.

Lelbach, W.K. 1966. Leberschäden bei chronischem Alkoholismus. Ergebnisse einer klinischen, klinisch-chemischen und bioptisch-histologischen Untersuchung an 526 Alkoholkranken während der Entziehungskur in einer offenen Trinkerheilstätte. Teil I: Klinische Ergebnisse. Acta Hepatosplen. 13:321–349.

Lelbach, W.K. 1967. Leberschäden bei chronischem Alkoholismus. Ergebnisse einer klinischen, klinisch-chemischen und bioptisch-histologischen Untersuchung an 526 Alkoholkranken während der Entziehungskur in einer offenen Trinkerheilstätte. Teil III: Bioptisch-Histologische Ergebnisse. Acta Hepatosplen. 14:9–39.

Lelbach, W.K. 1975. Cirrhosis in the alcoholic and its relation to the volume of alcohol abuse. Ann. N.Y. Acad. Sci. 252:85–105.

Lelbach, W.K. 1976. Epidemiology of alcoholic liver disease.

Pp. 494–515 in H. Popper and F. Schaffner, eds. Progress in Liver Diseases, Vol. 5. Grune & Stratton, New York.

Lemoine, P., H. Harrousseau, J.P. Borteyru, and J.C. Menuet. 1968. Les enfants de parents alcooliques: anomalies observées, apropos de 127 cas. Quest Med. 21:476–482.

Leo, M.A., and C.S. Lieber. 1982. Hepatic vitamin A depletion in alcoholic liver injury. N. Engl. J. Med. 307:597–601.

Leo, M.A., and C.S. Lieber. 1985. New pathway for retinol metabolism in liver microsomes. J. Biol. Chem. 260:5228–5231.

Leo, M.A., N. Lowe, and C.S. Lieber. 1984. Decreased hepatic vitamin A after drug administration in men and in rats. Am. J. Clin. Nutr. 40:1131–1136.

Leo, M.A., C. Kim, and C.S. Lieber. 1986a. Increased vitamin A in esophagus and other extrahepatic tissues after chronic ethanol consumption in the rat. Alcohol. Clin. Exp. Res. 10:487–492.

Leo, M.A., N. Lowe, and C.S. Lieber. 1986b. Interaction of drugs and retinol. Biochem. Pharmacol. 35:3949–3953.

Leo, M.A., C. Kim, and C.S. Lieber. 1987a. NAS$^+$-dependent retinol dehydrogenase in liver microsomes. Arch. Biochem. Biophys. 259:241–249.

Leo, M.A., N. Lowe, and C.S. Lieber. 1987b. Potentiation of ethanol-induced hepatic vitamin A depletion by phenobarbital and butylated hydroxytoluene. J. Nutr. 117:70–76.

Leo, M.A., C. Kim, and C.S. Lieber. 1988. Alcohol, vitamin A, and zinc. Nutr. Rev. 46:32.

Lewis, J.G., and J.A. Swenberg. 1980. Differential repair of O(6)-methylguanine in DNA of rat hepatocytes and non-parenchymal cells. Nature (London) 288:185–241.

Lieber, C.S. 1983. Interactions of alcohol and nutrition. Alcohol. Clin. Exp. Res. 7:2–4.

Lieber, C.S. 1988. The influence of alcohol on nutritional status. Nutr. Rev. 46:241–254.

Lieber, C.S., and L.M. DeCarli. 1970. Quantitative relationship between amount of dietary fat and severity of alcoholic fatty liver. Am. J. Clin. Nutr. 23:474–478.

Lieber, C.S., and L.M. DeCarli. 1974. An experimental model of alcohol feeding and liver injury in the baboon. J. Med. Primatol. 3:153–163.

Lieber, C.S., D.P. Jones, M.S. Losowsky, and C.S. Davidson. 1962. Interrelation of uric acid and ethanol metabolism in man. J. Clin. Invest. 41:1863–1870.

Lieber, C.S., D.P. Jones, J. Mendelson, and L.M. DeCarli. 1963. Fatty liver, hyperlipemia, and hyperuricemia produced by prolonged alcohol consumption, despite adequate dietary intake. Trans. Assoc. Am. Physicians 76:289–300.

Lieber, C.S., D.P. Jones, and L.M. DeCarli. 1965. Effects of prolonged ethanol intake: production of fatty liver despite adequate diets. J. Clin. Invest. 44:1009–1021.

Lieber, C.S., A. Lefèvre, N. Spritz, L. Feinman, and L.M. DeCarli. 1967. Difference in hepatic metabolism of long- and medium-chain fatty acids: the role of fatty acid chain length in the production of the alcoholic fatty liver. J. Clin. Invest. 46:1451–1460.

Lieber, C.S., N. Spritz, and L.M. DeCarli. 1969. Fatty liver produced by dietary deficiencies: its pathogenesis and potentiation by ethanol. J. Lipid Res. 10:283–287.

Lieber, C.S., L.M. DeCarli, and E. Rubin. 1975. Sequential production of fatty liver, hepatitis, and cirrhosis in subhuman primates fed ethanol with adequate diets. Proc. Natl. Acad. Sci. U.S.A. 72:437–441.

Lieber, C.S., H.K. Seitz, A.J. Garro, and T.M. Worner.

1979. Alcohol-related diseases and carcinogenesis. Cancer Res. 39:2863–2886.

Lieber, C.S., M.A. Leo, K.M. Mak, L.M. DeCarli, and S. Sato. 1985. Choline fails to prevent liver fibrosis in ethanol-fed baboons but causes toxicity. Hepatology 5:561–572.

Lijinsky, W., and S.S. Epstein. 1970. Nitrosamines as environmental carcinogens. Nature (London) 225:21–23.

Lindenbaum, J., and C.S. Lieber. 1975. Effects of chronic ethanol administration on intestinal absorption in man in the absence of nutritional deficiency. Ann. N.Y. Acad. Sci. 252:228–334.

Linkola, J., F. Fyhrquist, and R. Ylikahri. 1979. Renin, aldosterone and cortisol during ethanol intoxication and hangover. Acta Physiol. Scand. 106:75–82.

Lochner, A., J. Wulff, and L.L. Madison. 1967. Ethanol-induced hypoglycemia. I. The acute effects of glucose output and peripheral glucose utilization in fasted dogs. Metabolism 16:1–18.

Longnecker, M.P., J.A. Berlin, M.J. Orza, and T.C. Chalmers. 1988. A meta-analysis of alcohol consumption in relation to risk of breast cancer. J. Am. Med. Assoc. 260:652–656.

Losowsky, M.S., and P.J. Leonard. 1967. Evidence of vitamin E deficiency in patients with malabsorption or alcoholism and the effects of therapy. Gut 8:539–543.

Lowenfels, A.B. 1974. Alcohol and cancer. N.Y. State J. Med. 74:56–59.

Lucia, S.P. 1963. The antiquity of alcohol in diet and medicine. Pp. 171–172 in S.P. Lucia, ed. Alcohol and Civilization. McGraw-Hill, New York.

Lumeng, L. 1978. The role of acetaldehyde in mediating the deleterious effect of ethanol on pyridoxal 5'-phosphate metabolism. J. Clin. Invest. 62:286–293.

Lumeng, L., and T.K. Li. 1974. Vitamin B metabolism in chronic alcohol abuse. Pyridoxal phosphate levels in plasma and the effects of acetaldehyde on pyridoxal phosphate synthesis and degradation in human erythrocytes. J. Clin. Invest. 53:693–704.

Lyon, J.L., M.R. Klauber, J.W. Gardner, and C.R. Smart. 1976. Cancer incidence in Mormons and non-Mormons in Utah, 1966–1970. N. Engl. J. Med. 294:129–133.

MacLachlan, M.J., and G.P. Rodan. 1967. Effect of food, fast and alcohol on serum uric acid and acute attacks of gout. Am. J. Med. 42:38–57.

MacMahon, B., S. Yen, D. Trichopoulos, K. Warren, and G. Nardi. 1981. Coffee and cancer of the pancreas. N. Engl. J. Med. 304:630–633.

MacMahon, S.W., R.B. Blacket, G.J. Macdonald, and W. Hall. 1984. Obesity, alcohol consumption and blood pressure in Australian men and women. The National Heart Foundation of Australia Risk Factor Prevalence Study. J. Hypertens. 2:85–91.

Madison, L.L., A. Lochner, and J. Wulff. 1967. Ethanol-induced hypoglycemia. II. Mechanism of suppression of hepatic gluconeogenesis. Diabetes 16:252–258.

Maier, K.P., D. Seitzer, G. Haag, B.M. Peskar, and W. Gerok. 1979. Verlaufsformen alkoholischer Lebererkrankungen. Klin. Wochenschr. 57:311–317.

Mak, K.M., M.A. Leo, and C.S. Lieber. 1984. Ethanol potentiates squamous metaplasia of the rat trachea caused by vitamin A deficiency. Trans. Assoc. Am. Physicians 97:210–221.

Mak, K.M., M.A. Leo, and C.S. Lieber. 1987. Effect of ethanol and vitamin A deficiency on epithelial cell proliferation and structure in the rat esophagus. Gastroenterology 93:362–370.

Marmot, M.G., G. Rose, M.J. Shipley, and B.J. Thomas. 1981. Alcohol and mortality: a U-shaped curve. Lancet 1:580–583.

Martinez, I. 1969. Factors associated with cancer of the esophagus, mouth and pharynx in Puerto Rico. J. Natl. Cancer Inst. 42:1069–1094.

Martini, G.A., and C. Bode. 1970. The epidemiology of cirrhosis of the liver. Pp. 315–335 in A. Engel and T. Larsson, eds. Alcoholic Cirrhosis and Other Toxic Hepatopathias: Skandia International Symposia. Nordiska Bokhandelns Förlag, Stockholm.

Marzo, A., P. Ghirardi, D. Sardini, D. Pradini, and A. Albertini. 1970. Serum lipids and total fatty acids in chronic alcoholic liver disease at different stages of cell damage. Klin. Wochenschr. 48:949–950.

Masuda, Y., K. Mori, T. Hirohata, and M. Kuratsune. 1966. Carcinogenesis in the esophagus. 3. Polycyclic aromatic hydrocarbons and phenols in whiskey. Gann 57:549–557.

Matunaga, H. 1942. Experimentelle Untersuchungen über den Einfluss des Alkohols auf den Kohlehydratstoffwechsel. I. Mitteilung. Über die Wirkung des Alkohols auf den Blutzuckerspiegel und den Glykogengehalt der Leber, mit besonderer Berücksichtigung seines Wirkungsmechanismus. Tohoku J. Exp. Med. 44:130–157.

May, P.A., K.J. Hymbaugh, J.M. Aase, and J.M. Samet. 1983. Epidemiology of fetal alcohol syndrome among American Indians of the Southwest. Soc. Biol. 30:374–387.

McCoy, G.D., and E.L. Wynder. 1979. Etiological and preventive implications in alcohol carcinogenesis. Cancer Res. 39:2844–2850.

McCoy, G.D., S.S. Hecht, S. Katayama, and E.L. Wynder. 1981. Differential effect of chronic ethanol consumption on the carcinogenicity of N-nitrosopyrrolidine and N'-nitrosonornicotine in male Syrian golden hamsters. Cancer Res. 41:2849–2854.

Mendenhall, C.L., S. Anderson, R.E. Weesner, S.J. Goldberg, and K.A. Crolic. 1984. Protein–calorie malnutrition associated with alcohol hepatitis. Veterans Administration Cooperative Study Group on Alcoholic Hepatitis. Am. J. Med. 76:211–222.

Mendenhall, C., G. Bongiovanni, S. Goldberg, B. Miller, J. Moore, S. Rouster, D. Schneider, C. Tamburro, T. Tosch, and R. Weesner. 1985. VA cooperative study on alcoholic hepatitis. III: Changes in protein–calorie malnutrition associated with 30 days of hospitalization with and without enteral nutritional therapy. J. Parenter. Enteral Nutr. 9:590–596.

Metz, R., S. Berger, and M. Mako. 1969. Potentiation of the plasma insulin response to glucose by prior administration of alcohol. An apparent islet-priming effect. Diabetes 18:517–522.

Mezey, E., and L.A. Faillace. 1971. Metabolic impairment and recovery time in acute ethanol intoxication. J. Nerv. Ment. Dis. 153:445–452.

Mezey, E., J.J. Potter, S.W. French, T. Tamura, and C.H. Halsted. 1983. Effect of chronic ethanol feeding on hepatic collagen in the monkey. Hepatology 3:41–44.

Miller, A.B., G.R. Howe, M. Jain, K.J. Craib, and L. Harrison. 1983. Food items and food groups as risk factors in a case-control study of diet and colo-rectal cancer. Int. J. Cancer 32:155–161.

Mills, J.L., B.I. Graubard, E.E. Harley, G.G. Rhoads, and H.W. Berendes. 1984. Maternal alcohol consumption and birth weight. How much drinking during pregnancy is safe? J. Am. Med. Assoc. 252:1875–1879.

Mills, P.R., T.H. Pennington, P. Kay, R.N. MacSween, and G. Watkinson. 1979. Hepatitis Bs antibody in alcoholic cirrhosis. J. Clin. Pathol. 32:778–782.

Misslbeck, N.G., T.C. Campbell, and D.A. Roe. 1984. Effect of ethanol consumed in combination with high or low fat diets on the postinitiation phase of hepatocarcinogenesis in the rat. J. Nutr. 114:2311–2323.

Monson, R.R., and J.L. Lyon. 1975. Proportional mortality among alcoholics. Cancer 36:1077–1079.

Morgan, M.Y. 1981. Enteral nutrition in chronic liver disease. Acta Chir. Scand., Suppl. 507:81–90.

Morgan, M.Y., and S. Sherlock. 1977. Sex-related differences among 100 patients with alcoholic liver disease. Br. Med. J. 1:939–941.

Morris, C. 1979. Maize beer in the economics, politics, and religion of the Inca empire. Pp. 21–34 in C.F. Gastineau, W.J. Darby, and T.B. Turner, eds. Fermented Food Beverages in Nutrition. Academic Press, New York.

Morris, J.N., A. Kagan, D.C. Pattison, and M.J. Gardner. 1966. Incidence and prediction of ischaemic heart-disease in London busmen. Lancet 2:553–559.

Myerson, R.M. 1968. Acute effects of alcohol on the liver with special reference to the Zieve syndrome. Am. J. Gastroenterol. 49:304–311.

Nakada, T., and R.T. Knight. 1984. Alcohol and the central nervous system. Med. Clin. North Am. 68:121–131.

Nakamura, S., Y. Takezawa, T. Sato, K. Kera, and T. Maeda. 1979. Alcoholic liver disease in women. Tohoku J. Exp. Med. 129:351–355.

Nanji, A.A., and S.W. French. 1985. Hepatocellular carcinoma. Relationship to wine and pork consumption. Cancer 56:2711–2712.

Neville, J.N., J.A. Eagles, G. Samson, and R.E. Olson. 1968. Nutritional status of alcoholics. Am. J. Clin. Nutr. 21:1329–1340.

Newbold, R.F., W. Warren, A.S. Medcalf, and J. Amos. 1980. Mutagenicity of carcinogenic methylating agents is associated with a specific DNA modification. Nature (London) 283:596–599.

Newcombe, D.S. 1972. Ethanol metabolism and uric acid. Metab. Clin. Exp. 21:1193–1203.

NIAAA (National Institute on Alcohol Abuse and Alcoholism). 1981. The Fourth Special Report to the U.S. Congress on Alcohol and Health from the Secretary of Health and Human Services. DHHS Publ. No. (ADM) 81-1080. National Institutes of Health, Public Health Service, U.S. Department of Health and Human Services, Rockville, Md. 206 pp.

NIAAA (National Institute on Alcohol Abuse and Alcoholism). 1986. Toward a National Plan to Combat Alcohol Abuse and Alcoholism: A report to the United States Congress. National Institutes of Health, Public Health Service, U.S. Department of Health and Human Services, Rockville, Md. 81 pp.

NIAAA (National Institute on Alcohol Abuse and Alcoholism). 1987. The Sixth Special Report to the U.S. Congress on Alcohol and Health from the Secretary of Health and Human Services. DHHS Publ. No. (ADM) 87-1519. National Institutes of Health, Public Health Service, U.S. Department of Health and Human Services. U.S. Government Printing Office, Washington, D.C. 147 pp.

Nicholls, P., G. Edwards, and E. Kyle. 1974. Alcoholics

admitted to four hospitals in England. II. General and cause-specific mortality. Q. J. Stud. Alcohol 35:841–855.

Nicholson, W.M., and H.M. Taylor. 1938. Effect of alcohol on water and electrolyte balance in man. J. Clin. Invest. 17:279–285.

Nikkilä, E.A., and M.R. Taskinen. 1975. Ethanol-induced alterations of glucose tolerance, postglucose hypoglycemia, and insulin secretion in normal, obese, and diabetic subjects. Diabetes 24:933–943.

Nilsson, B.E. 1970. Conditions contributing to fracture of the femoral neck. Acta Chir. Scand. 136:383–384.

NRC (National Research Council). 1985. Injury in America: A Continuing Public Health Problem. Report of the Committee on Trauma Research, Commission on Life Sciences. National Academy Press, Washington, D.C. 164 pp.

Obe, G., and B. Beck. 1979. Mutagenic activity of aldehydes. Drug Alcohol Depend. 4:91–94.

Obe, G., and H. Ristow. 1977. Acetaldehyde, but not ethanol, induces sister chromatid exchanges in Chinese hamster cells in vitro. Mutat. Res. 56:211–213.

Obe, G., and H. Ristow. 1979. Mutagenic, cancerogenic and teratogenic effects of alcohol. Mutat. Res. 65:229–259.

O'Brien, R., and M. Chafetz. 1982. The Encyclopedia of Alcoholism. Facts on File, Inc., New York. 378 pp.

Ogata, M., J.H. Mendelson, and N.K. Mellow. 1968. Electrolyte and osmolality in alcoholics during experimentally induced intoxication. Psychosom. Med. 30:463–488.

Ohnishi, K., and C.S. Lieber. 1977. Reconstitution of the microsomal ethanol-oxidizing system. Qualitative and quantitative changes of cytochrome P-450 after chronic ethanol consumption. J. Biol. Chem. 252:7124–7131.

Okumiya, N., K. Tanaka, K. Ueda, and T. Omae. 1985. Coronary atherosclerosis and antecedent risk factors: pathologic and epidemiologic study in Hisayama, Japan. Am. J. Cardiol. 56:62–66.

Olsen, J., S. Sabreo, and U. Fasting. 1985. Interaction of alcohol and tobacco as risk factors in cancer of the laryngeal region. J. Epidemiol. Community Health 39:165–168.

Olson, R.E. 1964. Nutrition in alcoholism. Pp. 779–795 in M.G. Wohl and R.S. Goodhart, eds. Modern Nutrition in Health and Disease, 3rd ed. Lea & Febiger, Philadelphia.

Omata, M., M. Ashcavai, C.T. Liew, and R.L. Peters. 1979. Hepatocellular carcinoma in the U.S.A, etiologic considerations. Localization of hepatitis B antigens. Gastroenterology 76:279–287.

Orholm, M., J. Aldershvile, U. Tage-Jensen, P. Schlichting, J.O. Nielsen, F. Hardt, and P. Christoffersen. 1981. Prevalence of hepatitis B virus infection among alcoholic patients with liver disease. J. Clin. Pathol. 34:1378–1380.

Paredes, A. 1975. Social control of drinking among the Aztec Indians of Mesoamerica. Q. J. Stud. Alcohol 36:1139–1153.

Parker, H.S. 1978. Committee rejects whiskey—recommends straight alcohol. P. 3 in ALS Lifelines, Vol. 4, No. 2. Newsletter of the Assembly of Life Sciences, National Research Council. National Academy of Sciences, Washington, D.C.

Patek, A.J., Jr., I.G. Toth, M.G. Saunders, G.A.M. Castro, and J.J. Engel. 1975. Alcohol and dietary factors in cirrhosis. An epidemiological study of 304 alcoholic patients. Arch. Intern. Med. 135:1053–1057.

Pekkanen, L., and O. Forsander. 1977. Nutritional implications of alcoholism. Nutr. Bull. 4:91–102.

Pell, S., and C.A. D'Alonzo. 1973. A five-year mortality study

of alcoholics. J. Occup. Med. 15:120–125.

Pequignot, G. 1958. Enquête par interrogatoire sur les circonstances diététiques de la cirrhose alcoolique en France. Bull. Inst. Natl. Hyg. 3:719–739.

Pequignot, G., C. Chabert, H. Eydoux, and M.A. Courcoul. 1974. Augmentation de risque de cirrhose en fonction de la ration d'alcool. Rev. Alcool. 20:191–202.

Pequignot, G., A.J. Tuyns, and J.L. Berta. 1978. Ascitic cirrhosis in relation to alcohol consumption. Int. J. Epidemiol. 7:113–120.

Perlow, W., E. Baraona, and C.S. Lieber. 1977. Symptomatic intestinal disaccharidase deficiency in alcoholics. Gastroenterology 72:680–684.

Phillips, G.B., and H.F. Safrit. 1971. Alcoholic diabetes. Induction of glucose intolerance with alcohol. J. Am. Med. Assoc. 217:1513–1519.

Phillips, N.R., R.J. Havel, and J.P. Kane. 1982. Serum apolipoprotein A-I levels: relationship to lipoprotein lipid levels and selected demographic variables. Am. J. Epidemiol. 116:302–313.

Phillips, R.L., F.R. Lemon, W.L. Beeson, and J.W. Kuzma. 1978. Coronary heart disease mortality among Seventh-Day Adventists with differing dietary habits: a preliminary report. Am. J. Clin. Nutr. 31 Suppl. 10:S191–S198.

Pignatelli, B., M. Castegnaro, and E.A. Walker. 1976. Effects of gallic acid and of ethanol on formation of nitrosodiethylamine. IARC Sci. Publ. 14:173–178.

Piquet, J., and Tison. 1937. Alcool et cancer de l'oesophage. Bull. Acad. Natl. Med., Paris 117:236–239.

Pirola, R.C., and C.S. Lieber. 1972. The energy cost of the metabolism of drugs, including ethanol. Pharmacology 7:185–196.

Pirola, R.C., and C.S. Lieber. 1975. Energy wastage in rats given drugs that induce microsomal enzymes. J. Nutr. 105:1544–1548.

Pirola, R.C., and C.S. Lieber. 1976. Hypothesis. Energy wastage in alcoholism and drug abuse: possible role of hepatic microsomal enzymes. Am. J. Clin. Nutr. 29:90–93.

Poikolainen, K. 1983. Inebriation and mortality. Int. J. Epidemiol. 12:151–155.

Pollack, E.S., A.M. Nomura, L.K. Heilbrun, G.N. Stemmermann, and S.B. Green. 1984. Prospective study of alcohol consumption and cancer. N. Engl. J. Med. 310:617–621.

Popham, R.E., W. Schmidt, and Y. Israel. 1983. Variation in mortality from ischemic heart disease in relation to alcohol and milk consumption. Med. Hypotheses 12:321–329.

Popper, H., and C.S. Lieber. 1980. Histogenesis of alcoholic fibrosis and cirrhosis in the baboon. Am. J. Pathol. 98:695–716.

Porta, E.A., and C.L. Gomez-Dumm. 1968. A new experimental approach in the study of chronic alcoholism. I. Effects of high alcohol intake in rats fed a commercial laboratory diet. Lab. Invest. 18:352–364.

Pottern, L.M., L.E. Morris, W.J. Blot, R.G. Ziegler, and J.F. Fraumeni, Jr. 1981. Esophageal cancer among black men in Washington, D.C. I. Alcohol, tobacco, and other risk factors. J. Natl. Cancer Inst. 67:777–783.

Poynard, T., A. Abella, J.P. Pignon, S. Naveau, R. Leluc, and J.C. Chaput. 1986. Apolipoprotein A-I (APO-A-I) and alcoholic liver disease. Hepatology 6:1391–1395.

Racusen, L.C., and E.L. Krawitt. 1977. Effect of folate deficiency and ethanol ingestion on intestinal folate absorption. Am. J. Dig. Dis. 22:915–920.

Radike, M.J., K.L. Stemmer, and E. Bingham. 1981. Effect of

ethanol on vinyl chloride carcinogenesis. Environ. Health Perspect. 41:59–62.

Rankin, J.G. 1977. The natural history and management of the patient with alcoholic liver disease. Pp. 365–381 in M.M. Fisher and J.G. Rankin, eds. Alcohol and the Liver. Plenum Press, New York.

Reddy, T.V., and E.K. Weisburger. 1980. Hepatic vitamin A status of rats during feeding of hepatocarcinogen 2-aminoanthraquinone. Cancer Lett. 10:39–44.

Reed, D.M., C.J. MacLean, and T. Hayashi. 1987. Predictors of atherosclerosis in the Honolulu Heart Program. I. Biologic, dietary, and lifestyle characteristics. Am. J. Epidemiol. 126:214–225.

Rehfield, J.F., E. Juhl, and M. Hilden. 1973. Carbohydrate metabolism in alcohol-induced fatty liver. Evidence for an abnormal insulin response to glucagon in alcoholic liver disease. Gastroenterology 64:445–451.

Rhoads, G.G., W.C. Blackwelder, G.N. Stemmermann, T. Hayashi, and A. Kagan. 1978. Coronary risk factors and autopsy findings in Japanese-American men. Lab. Invest. 38:304–311.

Roe, D.A. 1979. Alcohol and the Diet. AVI Publishing Co., Westport, Conn. 229 pp.

Rogers, A.E., J.G. Fox, and L.S. Gottlieb. 1981. Effects of ethanol and malnutrition on nonhuman primate liver. Pp. 167–175 in P.D. Berk and T.C. Chalmers, eds. Frontiers in Liver Disease. Thieme-Stratton, Inc., New York.

Rosenberg, L., D. Slone, S. Shapiro, D.W. Kaufman, S.P. Helmrich, O.S. Miettinen, P.D. Stolley, M. Levy, N.B. Rosenshein, D. Schottenfeld, and R.L. Engle, Jr. 1982. Breast cancer and alcoholic-beverage consumption. Lancet 1:267–270.

Rosenthal, W.S., N.F. Adham, R. Lopez, and J.M. Cooperman. 1973. Riboflavin deficiency in complicated chronic alcoholism. Am. J. Clin. Nutr. 26:858–860.

Ross, R.K., A. Paganini-Hill, T.M. Mack, M. Arthur, and B.E. Henderson. 1981. Menopausal oestrogen therapy and protection from death from ischaemic heart disease. Lancet 1:858–860.

Rothman, K., and A. Keller. 1972. The effect of joint exposure to alcohol and tobacco on risk of cancer of the mouth and pharynx. J. Chronic Dis. 25:711–716.

Rothwell, N.J., and M.J. Stock. 1984. Influence of alcohol and sucrose consumption on energy balance and brown fat activity in the rat. Metabolism 33:768–771.

Rubin, E., and C.S. Lieber. 1968. Alcohol-induced hepatic injury in nonalcoholic volunteers. N. Engl. J. Med. 278:869–876.

Rubin, E., P. Bacchin, H. Gang, and C.S. Lieber. 1970. Induction and inhibition of hepatic microsomal and mitochondrial enzymes by ethanol. Lab. Invest. 22:569–580.

Rush, B. 1818. Medical Inquiries and Observations, 5th ed. M. Carey & Son, Philadelphia. (various pagings)

Sabesin, S.M., H.L. Hawkins, L. Kuiken, and J.B. Ragland. 1977. Abnormal plasma lipoproteins and lecithin-cholesterol acyltransferase deficiency in alcoholic liver disease. Gastroenterology 72:510–518.

Salaspuro, M.P. 1971a. Influence of ethanol on the metabolism of the pathological liver. Pp. 163–182 in Y. Israel and J. Mardones, eds. Biological Basis of Alcoholism. Wiley-Interscience, New York.

Salaspuro, M. 1971b. Influence of the unchanged redox state of the liver during ethanol oxidation, on galactose and glucose metabolism in protein deficiency. Pp. 58–67 in W.

Gerok, K. Sickinger, and H.H. Hennekeuser, eds. Alcohol and the Liver. F.K. Schattauer Verlag, Stuttgart, Federal Republic of Germany.

Salaspuro, M.P., and Y.A. Kesäniemi. 1973. Intravenous galactose elimination tests with and without ethanol loading in various clinical conditions. Scand. J. Gastroenterol. 8:681–686.

Salaspuro, M.P., and P.H. Mäenpää. 1966. Influence of ethanol on the metabolism of perfused normal, fatty and cirrhotic rat livers. Biochem. J. 100:768–778.

Salaspuro, M.P., P. Pikkarainen, and K. Lindros. 1977. Ethanol-induced hypoglycemia in man: its suppression by the alcohol dehydrogenase inhibitor 4-methylpyrazole. Eur. J. Clin. Invest. 7:487–490.

Salaspuro, M.P., S. Shaw, E. Jayatilleke, W.A. Ross, and C.S. Lieber. 1981. Attenuation of the ethanol-induced hepatic redox change after chronic alcohol consumption in baboons: metabolic consequences in vivo and in vitro. Hepatology 1:33–38.

Sandstead, H.H. 1973. Zinc as an unrecognized limiting nutrient. Am. J. Clin. Nutr. 26:790–791.

Sato, M., and C.S. Lieber. 1981. Hepatic vitamin A depletion after chronic ethanol consumption in baboons and rats. J. Nutr. 111:2015–2025.

Sato, M., and C.S. Lieber. 1982. Increased metabolism of retinoic acid after chronic ethanol consumption in rat liver microsomes. Arch. Biochem. Biophys. 213:557–564.

Saville, P.D. 1965. Changes in bone mass with age and alcoholism. J. Bone Jt. Surg., Am. Vol. 47:492–499.

Schatzkin, A., D. Y. Jones, R.N. Hoover, P.R. Taylor, L.A. Brinton, R.G. Ziegler, E.B. Harvey, C.L. Carter, L.M. Licitra, M.C. Dufour, and D.B. Larson. 1987. Alcohol consumption and breast cancer in the Epidemiologic Follow-Up Study of the first National Health and Nutrition Examination Survey. N. Engl. J. Med. 316:1169–1173.

Scheig, R. 1970. Effects of ethanol on the liver. Am. J. Clin. Nutr. 23:467–473.

Schmidt, W. 1975. Agreement, disagreement in experimental, clinical and epidemiological evidence on the etiology of alcoholic liver cirrhosis: a comment. Pp. 19–30 in J.M. Khanna, Y. Israel, and H. Kalant, eds. Alcoholic Liver Pathology. Addition Research Foundation of Ontario, Toronto.

Schmidt, W. 1977. The epidemiology of cirrhosis of the liver: a statistical analysis of mortality data with special reference to Canada. Pp. 1–26 in M.M. Fisher and J.G. Rankin, eds. Alcohol and the Liver. Plenum Press, New York.

Schmidt, W., and J. de Lint. 1972. Causes of death of alcoholics. Q. J. Stud. Alcohol 33:171–185.

Schoenborn, C.A., and B.H. Cohen. 1986. Trends in Smoking, Alcohol Consumption, and Other Health Practices Among U.S. Adults, 1977 and 1983. DHHS Publ. No. (PHS) 86-1250. Division of Health Interview Statistics, National Center for Health Statistics, Public Health Service, U.S. Department of Health and Human Services, Hyattsville, Md. 16 pp.

Schrauzer, G.N. 1976. Cancer mortality correlation studies. II. Regional associations of mortalities with the consumptions of foods and other commodities. Med. Hypotheses 2:39–49.

Schuckit, M.A., and P.L. Miller. 1976. Alcoholism in elderly men: a survey of a general medical ward. Ann. N.Y. Acad. Sci. 273:558–571.

Schwartz, D., J. Lellouch, R. Flamant, and P.F. Denoix.

1962. Alcohol and cancer. Results of a retrospective investigation. Rev. Fr. Etud. Clin. Biol. 7:590–604.

Schwarz, M., G. Weisback, J. Hummel, and W. Kunz. 1982. Effect of ethanol on dimethylnitrosamine activation and DNA synthesis in rat liver. Carcinogenesis 3:1071–1075.

Schwarz, M., A. Buchmann, G. Wiesbeck, and W. Kunz. 1983. Effect of ethanol on early stages in nitrosamine carcinogenesis in the rat liver. Cancer Lett. 20:305–312.

Scragg, R., A. Stewart, R. Jackson, and R. Beaglehole. 1987. Alcohol and exercise in myocardial infarction and sudden coronary death in men and women. Am. J. Epidemiol. 126:77–85.

Sedgewick, J. 1725. A New Treatise on Liquors wherein the Use and Abuse of Wine, Malt Drinks, Water, etc. Are Particularly Considered in Many Diseases, Constitutions and Ages with the Proper Manner of Using Them Hot or Cold Either as Physick, Diet or Both. Rivington, London. (various pagings)

Segel, L.D., S.C. Klausner, J.T. Gnadt, and E.A. Amsterdam. 1984. Alcohol and the heart. Med. Clin. North Am. 68:147–161.

Seitz, H.K., A.J. Garro, and C.S. Lieber. 1978. Effect of chronic ethanol ingestion on intestinal metabolism of and mutagenicity of benzo(alpha)pyrene. Biochem. Biophys. Res. Commun. 85:1061–1066.

Seitz, H.K., M.A. Korsten, and C.S. Lieber. 1979. Ethanol oxidation by intestinal microsomes: increased activity after chronic ethanol administration. Life Sci. 25:1443–1448.

Seitz, H.K., A.J. Garro, and C.S. Lieber. 1981. Sex dependent effect of chronic ethanol consumption in rats on hepatic microsome mediated mutagenicity of benzo(alpha)pyrene. Cancer Lett. 13:97–102.

Seitz, H.K., P. Czygan, R. Waldherr, S. Veith, R. Raedsch, H. Kässmodel, and B. Kommerell. 1984. Enhancement of 1,2-dimethylhydrazine-induced rectal carcinogenesis following chronic ethanol consumption in the rat. Gastroenterology 86:886–891.

Shaper, A.G., A.N. Phillips, S.J. Pocock, and M. Walker. 1987. Alcohol and ischaemic heart disease in middle aged British men. Br. Med. J. 294:733–737.

Shaw, S., B.D. Gorkin, and C.S. Lieber. 1981. Effects of chronic alcohol feeding on thiamin status: biochemical and neurological correlates. Am. J. Clin. Nutr. 34:856–860.

Simko, V., A.M. Connell, and B. Banks. 1982. Nutritional status in alcoholics with and without liver disease. Am. J. Clin. Nutr. 35:197–203.

Singer, C., E.J. Holmyard, A.R. Hall, and T.I. Williams, eds. 1956. A History of Technology, Vol. 2. The Mediterranean Civilizations and the Middle Ages c. 700 B.C. + c. A.D. 1500. Claredon Press, Oxford.

Siscovick, D.S., N.S. Weiss, and N. Fox. 1986. Moderate alcohol consumption and primary cardiac arrest. Am. J. Epidemiol. 123:499–503.

Sokol, R.J., J. Ager, S. Martier, S. Debanne, C. Ernhart, J. Kuzma, and S.I. Miller. 1986. Significant determinants of susceptibility to alcohol teratogenicity. Ann. N.Y. Acad. Sci. 477:87–102.

Solomon, L. 1973. Drug-induced arthropathy and necrosis of the femoral head. J. Bone Jt. Surg., Br. Vol. 55:246–261.

Steinkraus, K.H. 1979. Nutritionally Significant Indigenous Foods Involving an Alcoholic Fermentation. Pp. 35–59 in C.F. Gastineau, W.J. Darby, and T.B. Turner, eds. Fermented Food Beverages in Nutrition. Academic Press, New York.

Stenbäck, F. 1969. The tumorigenic effect of ethanol. Acta Pathol. Microbiol. Scand. 77:325–326.

Steyn, K., P.L. Jooste, J.M. Fourie, C.D. Parry, and J.E. Rossouw. 1986. Hypertension in the coloured population of the Cape Peninsula. S. Afr. Med. J. 69:165–169.

Stifel, F.B., H.L. Greene, E.G. Lufkin, M.R. Wrensch, L. Hagler, and R.H. Herman. 1976. Acute effects of oral and intravenous ethanol on rat hepatic enzyme activities. Biochim. Biophys. Acta 428:633–638.

St. Leger, A.S., A.L. Cochrane, and F. Moore. 1979. Factors associated with cardiac mortality in developed countries with particular reference to the consumption of wine. Lancet 1:1017–1020.

Stock, A.L., M.J. Stock, and J.A. Stuart. 1973. The effect of alcohol (ethanol) on the oxygen consumption of fed and fasting subjects. Proc. Nutr. Soc. 32:40A–41A.

Stock, M.J., and J.A. Stuart. 1974. Thermic effects of ethanol in the rat and man. Nutr. Metabol. 17:297–305.

Streissguth, A.P. 1978. Fetal alcohol syndrome: an epidemiologic perspective. Am. J. Epidemiol. 107:467–478.

Sullivan, J.F., and H.G. Lankford. 1962. Urinary excretion of zinc in alcoholism and postalcoholic cirrhosis. Am. J. Clin. Nutr. 10:153–157.

Sundby, P. 1967. Alcoholism and Mortality. Universitetsforlaget, Oslo. 207 pp.

Takada, A., J. Nei, S. Takase, and Y. Matsuda. 1986. Effects of ethanol on experimental hepatocarcinogenesis. Hepatology 6:65–72.

Taskinen, M.R., M. Välimäki, E.A. Nikkilä, T. Kuusi, C. Ehnholm, and R. Ylikahri. 1982. High density lipoprotein subfractions and postheparin plasma lipases in alcoholic men before and after ethanol withdrawal. Metabolism 31:1168–1174.

Taskinen, M.R., M. Välimäki, E.A. Nikkilä, T. Kuusi, and R. Ylikahri. 1985. Sequence of alcohol-induced initial changes in plasma lipoproteins (VLDL and HDL) and lipolytic enzymes in humans. Metabolism 34:112–119.

Taylor, J.R., T. Combs-Orme, D. Anderson, D.A. Taylor, and C. Koppenol. 1984. Alcohol, hypertension, and stroke. Alcoholism 8:283–286.

Teschke, R., M. Minzlaff, H. Oldiges, and H. Frenzel. 1983. Effect of chronic alcohol consumption on tumor incidence due to dimethylnitrosamine administration. J. Cancer Res. Clin. Oncol. 106:58–64.

Tremolières, J., and L. Carré. 1961. Etudes sur les modalités d'oxydation de l'alcool chez l'homme normal et alcoolique. Rev. Alcool. 7:202–227.

Trevisan, M., P. Strazzulo, F. Cappuccio, V. Krogh, A. Siani, S. De Colle, M.R. Di Muro, A. Albolino, and M. Mancini. 1987. Alcohol consumption and blood pressure in school children. Int. J. Pediatr. Nephrol. 8:25–28.

Tuomilehto, J., P. Puska, A. Nissinen, J. Salonen, A. Tanskanen, P. Pietinen, and E. Wolf. 1984. Community-based prevention of hypertension in North Karelia, Finland. Ann. Clin. Res. 16 Suppl. 43:18–27.

Turner, T.B., V.L. Bennett, and H. Hernandez. 1981. The beneficial side of moderate alcohol use. Johns Hopkins Med. J. 148:53–63.

Tuyns, A.J. 1982. Alcohol. Pp. 293–303 in D. Schottenfeld and J.F. Fraumeni, Jr., eds. Cancer Epidemiology and Prevention. W.B. Saunders, Philadelphia.

Tuyns, A.J. 1983. Oesophageal cancer in non-smoking drinkers and in non-drinking smokers. Int. J. Cancer 32:443–444.

Tuyns, A.J., G. Péquignot, and O.M. Jensen. 1977. Le cancer de l'oesophage en Ille-et-Vilaine en fonction des niveaux de consommation d'alcool et de tabac. Des risques qui se multiplient. Bull. Cancer 64:45–60.

Tuyns, A.J., G. Péquignot, and J.S. Abbatucci. 1979. Oesophageal cancer and alcohol consumption; importance of type of beverage. Int. J. Cancer 23:443–447.

Tuyns, A.J., G. Péquignot, M. Gignoux, and A. Valla. 1982. Cancers of the digestive tract, alcohol and tobacco. Int. J. Cancer 30:9–11.

Ueshima, H., T. Ohsaka, K. Tatara, and S. Asakura. 1984a. Alcohol consumption, blood pressure and stroke mortality in Japan. J. Hypertens., Suppl. 2:S191–S195.

Ueshima, H., T. Shimamoto, M. Iida, M. Konishi, M. Tanigaki, M. Doi, K. Tsujioka, E. Nagano, C. Tsuda, H. Ozawa, S. Kojima, and Y. Komachi. 1984b. Alcohol intake and hypertension among urban and rural Japanese populations. J. Chronic Dis. 37:585–592.

Ulland, B.M., J.H. Weisburger, R.S. Yamamoto, and E.K. Weisburger. 1973. Antioxidants and carcinogenesis: butylated hydroxytoluene, but not diphenyl-*p*-phenylenediamine, inhibits cancer induction by *N*-2-fluorenylacetamide and by *N*-hydroxy-*N*-2-fluorenylacetamide in rats. Food Cosmet. Toxicol. 11:199–207.

Valberg, L.S., P.R. Flanagan, C.N. Ghent, and M.J. Chamberlain. 1985. Zinc absorption and leukocyte zinc in alcoholic and nonalcoholic cirrhosis. Dig. Dis. Sci. 30:329–333.

Vallee, B.C., W.E.C. Wacker, A.F. Bartholomay, and E.D. Robin. 1956. Zinc metabolism in hepatic dysfunction. I. Serum zinc concentration in Laënnec's cirrhosis and their validation by sequential analysis. N. Engl. J. Med. 255:403–408.

Victor, M., R.D. Adams, and G.H. Collins. 1971. The Wernicke-Korsakoff Syndrome: A Clinical and Pathological Study of 245 Patients, 82 with Post-Mortem Examinations. F.A. Davis, Philadelphia. 206 pp.

von Arbin, M., M. Britton, V. de Faire, and A. Tisell. 1985. Circulatory manifestations and risk factors in patients with acute cerebrovascular disease and in matched controls. Acta Med. Scand. 218:373–380.

Wallace, R.B., C.F. Lynch, P.R. Pomrehn, M.H. Criqui, and G. Heiss. 1981. Alcohol and hypertension: epidemiologic and experimental considerations. The Lipid Research Clinics Program. Circulation 64:41–47.

Wallace, R.B., E. Barrett-Connor, M. Criqui, P. Wahl, J. Hoover, D. Hunninghake, and G. Heiss. 1982. Alteration in blood pressures associated with combined alcohol and oral contraceptive use—the lipid research clinics prevalence study. J. Chronic Dis. 35:251–257.

Wattenberg, L.W. 1972a. Dietary modification of intestinal and pulmonary aryl hydrocarbon hydroxylase activity. Toxicol. Appl. Pharmacol. 23:741–748.

Wattenberg, L.W. 1972b. Inhibition of carcinogenic and toxic effects of polycyclic hydrocarbons by phenolic antioxidants and ethoxyquin. J. Natl. Cancer Inst. 48:1425–1430.

Webb, S., and B. Webb. 1903. The History of Liquor Licensing in England, Principally from 1700 to 1830. Longmans, Green & Co., London. (various pagings)

Webster, L.A., P. Layde, P.A. Wingo, and H.W. Ory. 1983. Alcohol consumption and risk of breast cancer. Lancet 2: 724–726.

Wilhelmsen, L., H. Wedel, and G. Tibblin. 1973. Multivariate analysis of risk factors for coronary heart disease. Circulation 48:950–958.

Wilkerson, D. 1978. Sipping Saints. Fleming H. Revell, Old Tappan, N.J. 128 pp.

Wilkinson, P., J.N. Santamaria, and J.G. Rankin. 1969. Epidemiology of alcoholic cirrhosis. Aust. Ann. Med. 18: 222–226.

Willems, G., Y. Vansteenkiste, and P.H. Smets. 1971. Effects of ethanol on the cell proliferation kinetics in the fundic mucosa of dogs. Am. J. Dig. Dis. 16:1057–1063.

Willett, W.C., M.J. Stampfer, G.A. Colditz, B.A. Rosner, C.H. Hennekens, and F.E. Speizer. 1987. Moderate alcohol consumption and the risk of breast cancer. N. Engl. J. Med. 316:1174–1180.

Williams, P.T., R.M. Kraus, P.D. Wood, J.J. Albers, D. Dreon, and N. Ellsworth. 1985. Associations of diet and alcohol intake with high-density lipoprotein subclasses. Metabolism 34:524–530.

Williams, R.R., and J.W. Horm. 1977. Association of cancer sites with tobacco and alcohol consumption and socioeconomic status of patients: interview study from the Third National Cancer Survey. J. Natl. Cancer Inst. 58:525–547.

Wilsnack, S.C., A.D. Klassen, and R.W. Wilsnack. 1984. Drinking and reproductive dysfunction among women in a 1981 national survey. Alcoholism 8:451–458.

Wilson, D.E., P.H. Schreibman, A.C. Brewster, and R.A. Arky. 1970. The enhancement of alimentary lipemia by ethanol in man. J. Lab. Clin. Med. 75:264–274.

World, M.J., P.R. Ryle, O.E. Pratt, and A.D. Thomson. 1984a. Alcohol and body weight. Alcohol Alcohol. 19:1–6.

World, M.J., P.R. Ryle, D. Jones, G.K. Shaw, and A.D. Thomson. 1984b. Differential effect of chronic alcohol intake and poor nutrition on body weight and fat stores. Alcohol Alcohol. 19:281–290.

Wynder, E.L. 1976. Nutrition and cancer. Fed. Proc. 35: 1309–1315.

Wynder, E.L., and I.J. Bross. 1961. A study of etiological factors in cancer of the esophagus. Cancer 14:389–413.

Wynder, E.L., and P.C. Chan. 1970. The possible role of riboflavin deficiency in epithelial neoplasia. II. Effect on skin tumor development. Cancer 26:1221–1224.

Wynder, E.L., S. Hultberg, F. Jacobson, and I.J. Bross. 1957a. Environmental factors in cancer of the upper alimentary tract: a Swedish study with special reference to Plummer-Vinson (Paterson–Kelly) syndrome. Cancer 10:470–487.

Wynder, E.L., I.J. Bross, and R.M. Feldmann. 1957b. A study of the etiological factors in cancer of the mouth. Cancer 10: 1300–1323.

Wynder, E.L., L.S. Covey, K. Mabuchi, and M. Mushinski. 1976. Environmental factors in cancer of the larynx: a second look. Cancer 38:1591–1601.

Yang, C.S., Y.Y. Tu, D.R. Koop, and M.J. Coon. 1985. Metabolism of nitrosamines by purified rabbit liver cytochrome P-450 isozymes. Cancer Res. 45:1140–1145.

Yano, K., G.G. Rhoads, and A. Kagan. 1977. Coffee, alcohol and risk of coronary heart disease among Japanese men living in Hawaii. N. Engl. J. Med. 297:405–409.

Yano, K., D.M. Reed, and D.L. McGee. 1984. Ten-year incidence of coronary heart disease in the Honolulu Heart Program. Relationship to biologic and lifestyle characteristics. Am. J. Epidemiol. 119:653–666.

Yarrish, R.L., B.G. Werner, and B.S. Blumberg. 1980. Association of hepatitis B virus infection with hepatocellular carcinoma in American patients. Int. J. Cancer 26:711–715.

Yki-Järvinen, H., and E.A. Nikkilä. 1985. Ethanol decreases glucose utilization in healthy man. J. Clin. Endocrinol. Metab. 61:941–945.

17

Coffee, Tea, and Other Nonnutritive Dietary Components

Many different nonnutritive substances are commonly consumed in the daily diet. These include the beverages coffee and tea, direct and indirect food additives such as noncaloric sweeteners and food packaging materials, environmental contaminants such as polycyclic aromatic hydrocarbons (PAHs) and pesticides, and naturally occurring toxicants such as aflatoxins and hydrazines. The complete range of nonnutritive dietary constituents of possible significance to human health is not known.

Evaluation of the health effects of nonnutritive dietary substances is complicated for many reasons. It is necessary to consider both average and peak exposures, the potency or level of activity of the substances, and the quality of the experimental and epidemiologic data. Most additives and known contaminants are present in minute quantities in the average diet; however, many of them have not been studied for their long-term effects on health. This is partly because of the large number of such substances and partly because some food constituents are complex, poorly defined mixtures of natural origin. Furthermore, very little is known about the chronic effects of low levels of chemicals on human health and even less is known about their potential synergistic and antagonistic interactions in the diet and in the body. In the following sections, examples of substances in each class of nonnutritive components are used in an attempt to

provide an overall perspective on their significance to human health. Unlike the preceding chapters, data on occurrence and exposure are presented separately for each category of substances before discussions of health effects because of the large number and diversity of these compounds. These discussions are prefaced by a summary of food safety regulations pertinent to the use of these substances in the United States.

FOOD SAFETY LAWS

In 1938, the U.S. Congress passed the Food, Drug, and Cosmetic Act, which contained food-related provisions such as tolerances for unavoidable toxic substances and prohibited the marketing of any food containing such substances (U.S. Congress, 1938). In 1948, the Miller Pesticide Amendment was passed by Congress to streamline procedures for setting safety limits for pesticide residues in raw agricultural commodities (U.S. Congress, 1948). The Food Additive Amendment, known as the Delaney Clause, was passed on September 6, 1958 (U.S. Congress, 1958). That amendment specifically states that no additive is to be permitted in any amount if it has been shown to produce cancer in animal studies or in other appropriate tests, and that—even if not shown to be carcinogenic—it may be permitted only in the smallest amount necessary to produce the intended effect. The amendment does not apply to all food ingredients, since it excludes substances classified as Generally Recognized as Safe (NRC, 1984). The Color Additive Amendment, enacted in 1960, allowed the Food and Drug Administration (FDA) to regulate the conditions of safe use for color additives in foods, drugs, and cosmetics, and to require manufacturers to perform tests to establish safety (U.S. Congress, 1960).

The Food, Drug, and Cosmetic Act and its various amendments are administered by the FDA. These regulations affect approximately 60% of the food produced in the United States. The remaining 40% is under state regulations, which in many cases are tailored after federal legislation (McCutcheon, 1975).

COFFEE AND TEA

Patterns of Intake

Coffee and tea are among the most commonly consumed beverages in the world. Tea came into use in approximately 350 A.D. in China, whereas the consumption of coffee as a hot beverage is more recent—approximately 1000 A.D. In the United States, coffee and tea consumption is monitored in several different surveys, including the Nationwide Food Consumption Survey (NFCS) and the Continuing Survey of Food Intakes of Individuals (CSFII) of the U.S. Department of Agriculture (USDA) (Pao et al., 1982; USDA, 1986, 1987a) and surveys conducted by the Market Research Corporation of America (Abrams, 1977), the International Coffee Organization (ICO, 1986), and the FDA (Gilbert, 1981). The ICO surveys indicate that in the United States on average, 1.74 cups of coffee were consumed per person per day in 1986. This is a 5% decrease from 1.83 cups/day in 1985 and a 44% decrease from 3.12 cups/day in 1962. Males consumed a slightly higher amount than females (1.8 compared to 1.68 cups/person per day). The percentage of the population drinking coffee decreased from 74.7% in 1962 to 52.4% in 1986. Consumption was highest (77.8%) among those over 60 years old, 67% among those between 30 and 59 years old, 38.4% among 20- to 29-year-olds, and 40.1% among 10- to 19-year-olds. Regular coffee continued to be most frequently selected by coffee drinkers, accounting for nearly 8 out of 10 cups consumed. Consumption of decaffeinated coffee increased from 0.10 cups/day per person in 1962 to 0.41 cups/day per person in 1986. In 1986, approximately 48% of all coffee was consumed at breakfast, slightly more than one-third between meals (0.6 cups/person per day), and the remainder ($\approx$17%) at other meals. The home continued to be the location where most coffee was consumed (accounting for 71% of total consumption), consumption at work accounted for 18%, and eating places accounted for 8%. That year, coffee was the second most popular beverage in the United States (52% of the population drank it), outranked only by soft drinks (consumed by 58.4% of the population). Coffee was followed by milk (consumed by 48.3% of the population), juices (consumed by 45.3% of the population), and tea (consumed by 31% of the population). Overall U.S. coffee consumption was highest in the North Central and the Northeast regions (56.3%), followed by the West (51.9%) and the South (50.3%) (ICO, 1986). In the 1985 NFCS (USDA, 1986, 1987a), mean daily coffee intake was estimated to be 1 g for 1- to 5-year-old children born to low-income women, 300 g for low-income women 19 to 50 years old, and 327 g for men 19 to 50 years old. The mean daily intake of tea was 29 g for children, 144 g for women, and 194 g for men (USDA, 1986, 1987a).

Coffee and tea are the greatest contributors to daily intake of caffeine, the alkaloid 1,3,7-trimethylxanthine, accounting for approximately 20% of the intake by adults. Other less important sources of caffeine in the U.S. diet are soft drinks, which contribute approximately 5% of total caffeine intake, and chocolate, which provides approximately 1.5%. Among teenagers, younger children, and infants, however, tea and soft drinks provide a substantially larger percentage of total caffeine intake. Among the heaviest consumers (90th–100th percentile), caffeine intake has been estimated to be approximately 7 mg/kg body weight, or nearly 500 mg/person per day from all sources (Abrams, 1977).

Caffeine intake has also been estimated in several surveys. The ICO estimated that caffeine intake by coffee drinkers averaged 217 mg/day. By comparison, the NFCS estimated that average daily caffeine intake by coffee drinkers ranged from 212 to 283 mg in the over-19 age group and that daily caffeine intake from tea ranged from 69 to 87 mg among tea drinkers over age 19 (Pao et al., 1982). The results of other surveys (Gilbert, 1981; Graham, 1978) support these general estimates of caffeine consumption for the average drinker.

Coffee contains a considerable amount of burned material, including the mutagen (Kasai et al., 1982) and carcinogen (Nagao et al., 1986a) methylglyoxal at approximately 500 to 1,000-µg/cup. It also contains the natural mutagen chlorogenic acid (Stich et al., 1981c), the highly toxic atractylosides (Nagao et al., 1986b), the glutathione transferase inducers kahweal palmitate and cafestol palmitate (Lam et al., 1982), and about 100 mg of caffeine (Ames, 1983).

Evidence Associating Coffee and Tea with Chronic Diseases

Cancer

Epidemiologic Studies

BLADDER CANCER Several cohort studies have been conducted to assess the risk of bladder cancer from coffee consumption. Because of the relative rarity of this disease, results are generally based on small numbers of observed cases. In a cohort study of nearly 24,000 Seventh-Day Adventists, Snowdon and Phillips (1984) found a positive association between deaths from bladder cancer and coffee consumption by people who never smoked. In two other large cohort studies, one in Norway (Jacobsen et al., 1986) and one in Hawaii (Nomura et al., 1986), investigators failed to find an association.

Case-control studies provide more meaningful data. In two early studies in the United States (Cole, 1971; Fraumeni et al., 1971), elevated risks for bladder cancer were found among coffee drinkers. In the study by Cole, these risks were restricted to females; in the study by Fraumeni and colleagues, the risks applied to black females; in neither study was there evidence of a dose–response relationship. A finding similar to that of Cole (1971) was reported by Simon et al. (1975), who conducted a case-control study among women in Boston. In two other case-control studies, one in Canada (Howe et al., 1980) and one in the United States (Mettlin and Graham, 1979), elevated risks from coffee were found among males; there was less evidence for an effect among females, but in neither study was a dose–response relationship observed. In contrast, no overall effects of coffee drinking were found in case-control studies conducted in the United States, Great Britain, and Japan (Morrison et al., 1982b; Ohno et al., 1985); in Copenhagen (Jensen et al., 1986); and in Canada (Risch et al., 1988). In three case-control studies, associations were found between coffee consumption and risk of bladder

cancer: in Greece (Rebelakos et al., 1985), in Connecticut (Marrett et al., 1983), and in a 10-center study in the United States (Hartge et al., 1983). In Connecticut, there was a statistically significant association in males and some evidence of a dose–response relationship. In the 10-center study, based on nearly 3,000 cases and 6,000 controls, there was a statistically significant overall relative risk of 1.4, but there was no evidence of a dose–response relationship.

Thus, the epidemiologic studies relating coffee drinking to risk of bladder cancer are inconsistent. In the positive studies, the observed relative risk is small and there is an absence of a dose–response relationship, leading to the conclusion that this association is unlikely to be causal. Residual confounding by cigarette smoking is the most likely explanation for the findings (Morrison et al., 1982b). In this context, a case-control study among nonsmokers that failed to find an association between coffee drinking and bladder cancer (Kabat et al., 1986) is particularly relevant.

Lack of an association between tea consumption and bladder cancer risk has been reported consistently in cohort and case-control studies (Hartge et al., 1983; Heilbrun et al., 1986; Howe et al., 1980; Miller et al., 1983; Morgan and Jain, 1974; Sullivan, 1982).

COLON CANCER In the cohort study of nearly 24,000 Seventh-Day Adventists by Snowdon and Phillips (1984), no association was observed during the first 10 years, but a positive association was found between coffee consumption and fatal colon cancer during the last 11 years of follow-up. People consuming two or more cups of coffee a day had a relative risk of 1.7 (95% confidence interval, range 1.1 to 2.5) compared to those consuming less than one cup a day. There was a dose–response relationship in the last 11 years, which persisted when meat consumption was included in a multivariate analysis. A statistically significant but small excess risk was found for colon cancer but not for rectal cancer in the case-control study by Graham et al. (1978). In neither of these studies were detailed dietary data collected. It is therefore possible that the association with coffee reflects confounding with another factor, such as dietary fats, that could not be evaluated.

Two case-control studies showed no statistically significant association between tea consumption and colorectal cancer (Phillips and Snowdon, 1985; Tajima and Tominaga, 1985) as did a Canadian case-control study for consumption of combined beverages (tea, coffee, or colas) (Miller et al., 1983). Results of an international geographical correlation study showed a very slight negative association with rectal cancer but a strong positive association with colon cancer (Stocks, 1970). Heilbrun et al. (1986), however, showed a strong dose–response relationship and a positive association of tea consumption with rectal cancer risk over a 16- to 19-year follow-up period, but the mechanism was not apparent and no higher risks were reported at any other sites.

PANCREATIC CANCER Although a correlation between coffee drinking and rates of death from pancreatic cancer has been found in various countries (Binstock et al., 1983), two large cohort studies—one in the United States (Whittemore et al., 1983) and one in Norway (Heuch et al., 1983)—have failed to find evidence for an association.

In contrast, MacMahon et al. (1981) in a case-control study of pancreatic cancer in Boston found a highly significant dose–response relationship between coffee consumption and increased risk of pancreatic cancer. In a second study conducted by some of the same authors (Hsieh et al., 1986), however, the evidence for this association was substantially weaker; in particular, a dose-response relationship was no longer apparent. In other case-control studies (Gold et al., 1985; Mack et al., 1986; Norell et al., 1986; Wynder et al., 1983), investigators also failed to find any consistent evidence of an association between coffee drinking and risk of pancreatic cancer.

Tea consumption has been negatively associated with pancreatic cancer (Heilbrun et al., 1986; Mack et al., 1986; MacMahon et al., 1981). One case-control study using data collected in England and Wales during the 1950s showed a positive association between tea intake and risk of pancreatic cancer in men (Kinlen and McPherson, 1984). In the studies of MacMahon et al. (1981) and Kinlen and McPherson (1984), hospital controls were used. Some or all of these controls had cancers of sites other than the pancreas. Potential selection factors among these controls may account for the differences in the results.

BREAST CANCER In three case-control studies—in Israel (Lubin et al., 1985), the United States (Rosenberg et al., 1985), and France (Lê, 1985)—investigators examined evidence for a possible relationship between coffee drinking and risk of breast cancer. No evidence of such an association was found in any of those studies.

OVARIAN CANCER In two case-control studies—one in Italy (La Vecchia et al., 1984) and one in Greece (Trichopoulos et al., 1981)—evidence was found for an association between coffee drinking and increased risk of ovarian cancer. In contrast, in North America, Byers et al. (1983) and Miller et al. (1987) failed to find any association. Thus, the evidence is inconsistent for coffee.

For tea, however, Miller et al. (1987) found that its consumption did not influence the risk of ovarian cancer in a case-control study in the United States and Canada.

OTHER SITES A weak negative association between tea intake and prostate cancer was reported in a geographical correlation study by Stocks (1970). Another weak negative association between tea consumption and liver cancer risk in men was reported in a prospective study by Heilbrun et al. (1986). Thus, there is no convincing evidence relating tea consumption to any type of cancer.

Animal Studies

Several studies in rats showed no correlation between coffee consumption and tumor induction (Bauer et al., 1977; Dews et al., 1984; NCI, 1978a; Palm et al., 1984; Würzner et al., 1977; Zeitlin, 1972). Caffeine is found in coffee, tea, cola and other carbonated soft drinks, and several over-the-counter drugs. A positive correlation between caffeine intake and cancer in Wistar rats was demonstrated by Takayama (1981). Because of confounding by the presence of other diseases in the test animals, the results were deemed to be inconclusive. In a later study by Takayama in the same rat strain, no statistically significant differences in the rate, type, or number of tumors were observed in the caffeine-treated rats as compared to the controls (Oser and Ford, 1981).

Challis and Bartlett (1975) reported that readily oxidized phenolic compounds that are constituents of coffee catalyze nitrosamine formation from nitrite and secondary amines at gastric pH. On the other hand, caffeic acid (3,4-dihydroxycinnamic acid) was reported to inhibit formation of N-nitroso compounds in vivo (Kuenzig et al., 1984).

Small amounts of tannins are present naturally in coffee and tea. When administered subcutaneously, tannic acid produced liver and bile duct tumors in rats (Korpássy and Mosonyi, 1950). Condensed tannins produced sarcomas at the injection site and liver tumors in rats and mice; extracts of hydrolyzable tannins caused liver tumors in mice (Kirby, 1960). Brewed tea caused skin cancers in mice when applied to the neck (Kaiser, 1967), and the tannin-containing fraction of tea produced histiocytomas at the injection site in mice (Kapadia et al., 1976). In general, high doses were used in these animal studies. Lower doses of tannic acid produced no liver damage or liver cancer in mice and only a slight excess of other cancers in experimental animals as compared to control animals (Bichel and Bach, 1968). The lack of adequate oral feeding studies, the inconsistencies in the studies, and the short duration (each study typically spanned 3 to 10 months) cast doubt on the relationship between tea intake and cancer risk.

Short-Term Tests

Brewed, instant, and decaffeinated coffees were found to be mutagenic to *Salmonella typhimurium* strain TA100 (Aeschbacher and Würzner, 1980; Aeschbacher et al., 1980a; Nagao et al., 1979) and to *Escherichia coli* (Kosugi et al., 1983). Roasted coffee was highly mutagenic in the L-arabinose resistance test in *S. typhimurium* (Dorado et al., 1987). Coffee also induced mutations in Chinese hamster lung cells in vitro (Nakasato et al., 1984). Direct-acting mutagenic activity of coffee in *S. typhimurium* strains TA100 and TA102 was confirmed by Friederich et al. (1985). This mutagenic activity was decreased by adding 10% rat liver S9 microsomal fraction, by adding reduced glutathione, and by increasing temperatures to 50°C; this observation led the authors to postulate that the reduction in mutagenic activity could be due to the mammalian enzyme methylglyoxalase, which exhibits similar inactivation properties in vitro (Friederich et al., 1985).

Although caffeine has been reported to be mutagenic to bacteria (Clarke and Wade, 1975; Demerec et al., 1948, 1951; Gezelius and Fries, 1952; Glass and Novick, 1959; Johnson and Bach, 1965; Kubitschek and Bendigkeit, 1958, 1964; Novick, 1956), it could not have been responsible for the mutagenicity observed in these studies of coffee, since decaffeinated coffee was as mutagenic as regular coffee and caffeine itself was not detected as a mutagen under the test conditions (Aeschbacher et al., 1980b; Nagao et al., 1979).

Caffeine was shown to induce gene mutations in bacteria and fungi, but its ability to induce point mutations in higher organisms is not well documented (Haynes and Collins, 1984). At higher concentrations, approximately 0.01 M, it produces chromosome aberrations in plant and animal cells

(Kihlman and Sturelid, 1975; Weinstein et al., 1972). Caffeine can enhance the genotoxic effects of other agents, including radiation and chemicals, presumably because of its ability to inhibit repair of DNA damage induced by these agents (Frei and Venitt, 1975; Haynes and Collins, 1984; Jenssen and Ramel, 1978).

Black tea, green tea, and roasted tea behaved as direct-acting mutagens in *S. typhimurium* strain TA100 (Nagao et al., 1979). The flavonoids quercetin, kaempferol, and myricetin were responsible for most of the mutagenic activity of an acid hydrolysate of green tea (Uyeta et al., 1981).

In summary, caffeine causes mutations in microorganisms. Its ability to induce mutations in higher organisms is not certain. Tea was shown to be mutagenic in the Ames *Salmonella* assay.

Coronary Heart Disease (CHD)

Epidemiologic Studies

Several recent studies suggest an association between coffee intake and increased levels of serum cholesterol. Some of these studies indicate positive associations in men and women (Green and Jucha, 1986; Haffner et al., 1985; Kark et al., 1985; Thelle et al., 1983); one in women only (Mathias et al., 1985); but in some, no relationship between coffee intake and increased serum cholesterol level was apparent (Dawber et al., 1974; Hofman et al., 1983; Kannel, 1977; Kovar et al., 1983; Shekelle et al., 1983; Yano et al., 1977). Overall, the evidence suggests that coffee intake may be positively associated with serum total cholesterol levels, especially low-density-lipoprotein (LDL) cholesterol. In a study of the association of coffee, tea, and whole eggs with serum lipids in 658 male workers from six factories in Israel, tea consumption was negatively associated with serum cholesterol, whereas coffee was positively associated and egg consumption appeared to have no association (Green and Jucha, 1986).

The epidemiologic evidence for a direct association between coffee drinking and CHD is inconsistent. For example, in a cohort study of 16,911 people followed for 11.5 years in the United States, Murray et al. (1981) failed to find any relationship between reported coffee intake and death from ischemic heart disease. However, in a cohort study of 1,130 college students followed for 19 to 35 years, La Croix et al. (1986) found a relative risk of 2.5 (95% confidence interval, range 1.1 to 5.8) for men drinking five cups of coffee or more a day compared to those drinking none, after adjusting for other factors, including smoking. In a study conducted during 1957–1958 to assess 19-year mortality in 1,191 white men ages 40 to 56 years employed by the Chicago Western Electric Company, higher mortality from CHD and from noncoronary causes, such as cancer and cardiovascular diseases other than chronic heart disease, was found among those consuming six or more cups per day than among those consuming one cup per day (LeGrady et al., 1987).

In two early case-control studies (Boston Collaborative Drug Surveillance Program, 1972; Jick et al., 1973), associations were found between coffee drinking and risk of heart disease, but several later case-control studies (Hennekens et al., 1976; Hrubec, 1973; Klatsky et al., 1973; Rosenberg et al., 1980) did not substantiate these findings. Methodological problems, especially the use of hospital controls, may have contributed to these discrepancies. Several studies have also shown that caffeine from such other sources as tea or colas has no association (Curb et al., 1986).

In summary, there is evidence that coffee drinking is associated with increased levels of LDL cholesterol, and in view of the established association between LDL cholesterol and the risk of ischemic heart disease, there is a plausible basis for an association between coffee intake and such risk. The failure to observe this in some epidemiologic studies could be due to the relatively small change in risk produced by the typical differences in coffee drinking in North America as compared to Europe. However, the cause of the association between coffee and serum cholesterol remains to be definitively established for the level and type of coffee drinking practiced in North America; it is possible that confounding by dietary factors such as fats could produce the changes in cholesterol level reported. Tea drinking, on the other hand, appears to have no association or a negative association with total serum cholesterol and coronary artery disease.

Reproductive Effects

Epidemiologic Studies

Contradictory results have been found in pregnant women who had consumed caffeine. Mau and Netter (1974) reported an increased risk of low birth-weight infants for women with high coffee intake after controlling for maternal age, parity, father's occupation, maternal weight, and smoking. No attempt was made in this study to determine the quantity or type of coffee consumed. In another study, an association of coffee with prematurity was attributed to smoking

(Van den Berg, 1977). However, when the data were reanalyzed after controlling for smoking and gestational age, a statistically significant relative risk of 1.24 for low birth weight was reported for heavy coffee drinkers (Hogue, 1981). In a retrospective survey, Mormon women with high caffeine consumption had higher rates of spontaneous abortion, stillbirth, and preterm deliveries than did women who consumed no caffeine (Weathersbee et al., 1977). The study, however, is biased in sampling (sampling method and number of women sampled in the population was unspecified) and there was a possible bias in reporting of abnormal pregnancies. In a case-control study, Berkowitz et al. (1982) found no association between preterm delivery and consumption of coffee or tea. Linn et al. (1982) reported no association between low birth weight, preterm delivery, or congenital malformation and heavy coffee consumption after controlling for smoking and other confounders. In a prospective study, Martin and Bracken (1987) reported that the consumption of caffeine in coffee, tea, colas, and drugs appears to cause growth retardation in full-term newborns. In a recent review, Leviton (1988) reported that moderate consumption of caffeine by pregnant women has no adverse effects on their fetuses.

Animal Studies

A great decrease in fertility was observed in fowls fed caffeine in a standard ration (Ax et al., 1976). Friedman et al. (1979) reported that caffeine fed to Osborne-Mendel rats for 3 to 16 months produced severe testicular atrophy and aspermatogenesis. Caffeine was shown to produce many underweight offspring when given to ICR (hereafter called CD/1) mice at doses up to 39 mg/kg body weight (bw) per day through four generations (Thayer and Kensler, 1973). When given as pellets to mice at 150 mg/kg bw per day, it reduced food intake and produced fetuses with cleft lip or palate (Elmazar et al., 1982), whereas in drinking water at the same dosage, it reduced both food and water intake and decreased ossification of the supraoccipital, sternebral, and xiphisternum bones (Sullivan, 1981). When fed throughout gestation to Sprague-Dawley rats, caffeine produced offspring with underdeveloped pelvises, decreased humerus density, statistically significant decreased organ-to-body-weight ratios for the brain, lungs, and liver at 30 mg/kg bw per day (equivalent to a woman consuming approximately 10 strong cups of coffee a day) (Palm et al., 1978), and delayed ossification of sternebrae at 80 mg/kg bw per day (Nolen, 1981). Offspring of rats given coffee to drink during gestation had reduced body, liver, and brain weight at birth and behavioral variations 30 days after birth (Groisser et al., 1982). Caffeine given in feed to rats at 1,000 mg/kg bw per day produced offspring with low birth weights (Aeschbacher et al., 1980a). Caffeine given in drinking water ad libitum to pregnant Osborne-Mendel rats at doses of 160.9 and 204.5 mg/kg bw per day decreased implantation efficiency, increased resorptions, and decreased the number of viable fetuses. Furthermore, fetal body weight and length were decreased and sternebral ossification deficiencies were increased, but no dose-related gross anomalies were observed (Collins et al., 1983).

In summary, caffeine at high dose causes reproductive defects in rodents. Some studies suggest that it may also lead to low birth weight in humans. The evidence, however, is neither uniform nor conclusive.

NONNUTRITIVE SWEETENERS

Occurrence and Exposure

The first artificial sweetener, saccharin, was introduced in the late nineteenth century, primarily in diets requiring restriction of natural and simple sugars and in times of sugar shortage, such as during the two world wars. The introduction of cyclamates coincided with a marked increase in the exposure of the general population to artificial sweeteners in the early 1960s, primarily in diet soft drinks and low-calorie foods. Aspartame, the dipeptide L-aspartyl-L-phenylalanine methyl ester, is approximately 180 times sweeter than sugar (Mazur, 1976). Its use as a sweetener or flavoring agent in foods was first approved by the FDA in 1981 (FDA, 1981). Later, in 1983 and 1984, it was approved for use in soft drinks and vitamin pills (FDA, 1983, 1984). A number of other sugar substitutes are likely to be introduced in the near future. In 1977, an estimated 2.2 million kg of saccharin and sodium saccharin were produced in the United States, and an additional 1.3 million kg were imported (NRC, 1978). At that time, approximately 2.9 million kg ($\approx$83% of the total) were used in foods (USDA, 1987b). A survey conducted in 1986 by the USDA showed that the amounts of saccharin and aspartame consumed per capita were equivalent to 5.5 and 13 pounds of sugar, respectively (USDA, 1987b).

Evidence Associating Nonnutritive Sweeteners with Chronic Diseases

To date, most evidence associating saccharin and cyclamate with chronic diseases relates to bladder cancer. Data from animal studies on saccharin, cyclamate, and aspartame, together with epidemiologic evidence relating saccharin and cyclamate to bladder cancer risk, are reviewed below. Both sweeteners are the only ones on the market long enough to make epidemiologic assessment possible in view of the long latency period needed for the development of bladder cancer. Since cyclamate and saccharin were used as a 10:1 mixture in most studies, it is difficult to distinguish the effect of one or the other on bladder-induced tumorigenesis in epidemiologic studies.

Saccharin: Studies of Cancer

Epidemiologic Studies

In view of the substantial increase in the use of saccharin from 1950 on, any major effect of saccharin on bladder cancer risk should be evident by an increase in bladder cancer rates; however, there is no evidence for any increase in rates of this cancer over the past 30 years and, if anything, there is a decrease among females (Burbank and Fraumeni, 1970). The possibility that a long latency period could mask any secular effect could explain the lack of any trend in the earlier data (Armstrong and Doll, 1974; Kessler, 1970), but one would expect to see some increase in bladder cancer rates within the past decade if saccharin were a bladder carcinogen.

People with diabetes use artificial sweeteners extensively. Therefore, any increased bladder cancer risk associated with the use of these products should be observable in this population. Two large-scale studies have evaluated this possibility. Armstrong and Doll (1974) conducted a case-control study in England and Wales using as cases 18,733 deaths from bladder cancer recorded between 1966 and 1972. Controls consisted of a random sample of deaths from other causes. No increased risk was found for diabetes as recorded on the death certificate. In a cohort study of 21,447 diabetics in the United States, Kessler (1970) also found no evidence of any excess risk of bladder cancer. Neither of these studies was able to relate the use of artificial sweeteners by a particular individual to bladder cancer in that same person.

A number of case-control studies have been conducted on saccharin and cancer. Kessler (1976) and Kessler and Clark (1978) found no evidence of any increased risk associated with the use of artificial sweeteners per se, dietetic beverages, or low-calorie foods. In contrast, a case-control study conducted in Canada showed a statistically significant association in males using artificial sweeteners (Howe et al., 1977, 1980). The data also showed a significant dose–response relationship. In contrast, no effect was found in females. Subsequently, a much larger case-control study involving almost 9,000 subjects (3,010 cases and 5,783 controls) (Hoover and Strasser, 1980) showed no overall increased risk associated with use of artificial sweeteners. However, small but statistically significant increases of about 50% were found among subjects who reported using tabletop artificial sweeteners and diet drinks, as well as the heavy use of one of these. Other case-control studies of bladder cancer and artificial sweetener use have been reported (Cartwright et al., 1981; Møller-Jensen et al., 1983; Morrison and Buring, 1980; Morrison et al., 1982a; Najem et al., 1982; Risch et al., 1988; Silverman et al., 1983; Wynder and Stellman, 1980). Most results from these studies were negative. Others indicated an increased risk in some subgroups (e.g., Cartwright et al., 1981; Morrison et al., 1982a; Risch et al., 1988), but these findings were not consistent among themselves or with the findings of Hoover and Strasser (1980). Thus, overall the epidemiologic evidence does not suggest that consumption of saccharin materially increases the risk of bladder cancer.

Animal Studies

No evidence of saccharin-induced carcinogenesis was provided in single-generation studies in which various doses of saccharin were fed to several strains of mice and rats (Furuya et al., 1975; Homburger, 1978; National Institute of Hygienic Sciences, 1973; Roe et al., 1970; Schmähl, 1973) and to hamsters and rhesus monkeys (Althoff et al., 1975; McChesney et al., 1977). Other single-generation feeding studies in rats showed that a high incidence of neoplasia occurred at high doses of saccharin (Arnold et al., 1977, 1980; Chowaniec and Hicks, 1979).

In a two-generation study, there was no difference in the incidence of tumors in treated or control Swiss specific-pathogen-free mice in either generation (Kroes et al., 1977). In three two-generation studies with Charles River and Sprague-Dawley rats (Arnold et al., 1977, 1980; DHEW, 1973a,b; Taylor and Friedman, 1974; Tisdel et al., 1974), the incidence of bladder tumors in treated male rats of the F_1 generation given the highest dose was significantly higher than that in controls in all three studies and in the F_0 males in one study (Arnold et al., 1977, 1980). In another two-generation study in which male rats were fed dietary levels of sodium

saccharin ranging from 1 to 7.5%, a clear dose–response for urinary bladder tumors was observed in the second-generation male rats; the 1% dietary level was considered to be a no-effect level (Schoenig et al., 1985).

Saccharin was shown to have tumor-promoting and cocarcinogenic potential in the bladder of rats, as shown by either increased incidence of, or decreased latency period for, tumor development in animals treated with *N*-methyl-*N*-nitrosourea (MNU) (Chowaniec and Hicks, 1979; Hicks et al., 1978) or with *N*-[4-(5-nitro-2-furyl)-2-thiazolyl] formamide (Cohen, 1985; Cohen et al., 1979; Fukushima et al., 1981).

Short-Term Tests

In several in vitro systems, saccharin produced effects associated with tumor-promoting properties (Brennessel and Keyes, 1985; Milo et al., 1983; Trosko et al., 1980). Sodium saccharin was not reactive to DNA (Ashby, 1985) and is not a gene mutagen in vitro (Clive et al., 1979). At high levels, it has intermittent activity as a very weak germ-cell mutagen (Rao and Qureshi, 1972), is a somatic-cell mutagen in vivo (Fahrig, 1982; Mahon and Dawson, 1982), causes chromosome aberrations in mammalian cells (Abe and Sasaki, 1977; McCann, 1977; S. Yoshida et al., 1978), and leads to sister chromatid exchanges in human cells (Wolff and Rodin, 1978). Its mode of action in these respects may be related to its ability to promote bladder tumors in rats at elevated doses, which defines it as a significant contributor to the biologic medium (solvent) rather than as a trace xenobiotic toxin (solute) (Ashby, 1985).

Cyclamate: Studies of Cancer

Epidemiologic Studies

Since cyclamate is usually formulated as a 10-to-1 cyclamate–saccharin mixture, it has rarely been possible to separate the effects of the two substances in studies in the United States. Thus, most epidemiologic studies focused either on saccharin alone or on the mixture, until cyclamate was banned in the United States in 1969.

In Canada, however, saccharin was banned as a food and soft-drink additive in 1978 but cyclamate was not. Thus, in a recent Canadian case-control study, it was possible to separate saccharin and cyclamate use (Risch et al., 1988). No consistent increase in risk was found for either males or females.

Animal Studies

In 1985, a National Research Council (NRC) committee conducted a comprehensive review of 22 long-term bioassays in which cyclamate alone was fed to rats or mice or given in drinking water (NRC, 1985). In mice, there were several equivocal findings of carcinogenicity at sites known to have a high incidence of spontaneous tumors (Muranyi-Kovacs et al., 1975, 1976; Rudali et al., 1969). None of these findings were confirmed in later, more extensive tests (Brantom et al., 1973; Homburger et al., 1973; Roe et al., 1970). Multigeneration studies designed specifically to evaluate the production of tumors of the urinary bladder provided no evidence for carcinogenicity (NRC, 1985).

In studies of the metabolite cyclohexylamine, no evidence for carcinogenicity has been obtained in rats or mice (Gaunt et al., 1974; Schmähl, 1973). Studies of cyclamate–saccharin mixtures have also been conducted. One study showed an increased incidence of bladder tumors in rats (Price et al., 1970), but in two more detailed studies, investigators failed to find an increase in bladder tumors (Ikeda et al., 1975; Schmähl and Habs, 1984). Overall, studies do not provide convincing evidence that cyclamate–saccharin mixtures are carcinogenic in rats.

Two studies, one in rats and one in mice, suggest that cyclamate may enhance the carcinogenic effect of other substances in the urinary bladder. In one of the studies, cyclamate was incorporated into a cholesterol pellet and implanted into the bladders of mice (Bryan and Ertürk, 1970); in the other, it was fed to rats after a carcinogen, N-methyl-N-nitrosourea, had been instilled into the bladder (Hicks et al., 1975). In both experiments, more bladder cancers formed in animals receiving cyclamate in combination with other agents than in those receiving the other agent alone, suggesting that cyclamate has cocarcinogenic as well as tumor-promoting activities.

Short-Term Tests

Positive cytogenetic effects by themselves were of uncertain significance with regard to carcinogenicity, but they were consistent with the possibility of a neoplasm-promoting action. Likewise, results of five in vitro studies conducted to explore effects associated with tumor-promoting properties were positive for cyclamate (Boyland and Mohiuddin, 1981; Ishii, 1982; Knowles et al., 1986; Lee, 1981; Malcolm et al., 1983).

Cyclamate and its major metabolite cyclohexylamine have been extensively subjected to a variety of short-term tests for DNA damage, gene mutations, and chromosome aberrations and have been evaluated by an NRC committee (NRC, 1985). Tests for gene mutations in bacteria have been uniformly negative for cyclamate and cyclohexylamine. A notable deficiency in the data, however, is the absence of assays for mammalian-cell DNA damage and gene mutation for cyclamate and a gene mutation assay for cyclohexylamine. Positive results have been obtained in mammalian cytogenetic tests and in some tests for recessive lethals and chromosome abnormalities in the fruit fly (Drosophila melanogaster). Many of these cytogenetic tests had limitations (e.g., lack of appropriate controls and use of cytotoxic concentrations of cyclamate), indicating a need for more refined studies. The combined evidence from short-term tests, as evaluated by two different techniques (the decision point approach and the carcinogenicity prediction and battery selection method), indicates that neither cyclamate nor cyclohexylamine is likely to be a DNA-reactive carcinogen.

Reproductive Effects of Cyclamate

At high doses, cyclamate and its metabolite cyclohexylamine appear to induce testicular atrophy. For example, testicular reduction was seen in rats fed a 10-to-1 cyclamate–saccharin mixture at 2,500 mg per kg of body weight per day (Oser et al., 1975), in rats fed calcium cyclamate at 5 to 10% of total diet weight (Nees and Derse, 1967), and in rats fed sodium cyclamate at 5% of total diet (Ikeda et al., 1975). Experiments with cyclohexylamine showed that testicular weight decreases at doses of approximately 5,000 ppm in rats or 250 mg per kg of body weight per day (Gaunt et al., 1974; Mason and Thompson, 1977; Oser et al., 1976). This effect raises concern because of its implication for humans, since microorganisms in the human gut have been shown to convert cyclamate to cyclohexylamine (NRC, 1985).

Aspartame: Studies of Cancer

Epidemiologic Studies

Since aspartame has been on the market only a short time, no relevant epidemiologic studies have been completed.

Animal Studies and Short-Term Tests

A number of long-term feeding studies have been conducted in laboratory animals. Charles

River mice fed aspartame at 1, 2, or 4 g/kg body weight per day in their diet for 2 years did not develop any tumors (Searle and Company, 1974b). Mice whose bladders were implanted for 6 weeks with cholesterol pellets containing aspartame or diketopiperazine (DKP), its breakdown product, had no bladder tumors (Searle and Company, 1973b).

In a long-term feeding study, male and female Sprague-Dawley rats were fed aspartame at various levels for 2 years and were observed for the development of brain tumors (Searle and Company, 1973c). An independent board of inquiry appointed by the FDA concluded that aspartame may lead to an increase in brain neoplasms (FDA, 1980a). Investigators at G. D. Searle and Company (the manufacturer of aspartame) disagreed. They used current instead of historic controls in their statistical analysis and contended that the FDA board of inquiry made errors regarding the time of death of certain rats (FDA, 1980a).

In a follow-up study by the Searle group, the difference in tumor incidence in rats exposed to aspartame in utero for their lifetime at 2 or 4 g/kg body weight per day and controls was not statistically significant (Searle and Company, 1974a). Ishii et al. (1981) reported no evidence that aspartame or DKP was carcinogenic in a chronic feeding study in Wistar rats. No evidence of neoplasia was found in beagle dogs fed aspartame at 1, 2, or 4 g/kg body weight per day in their diet for more than 106 weeks (Searle and Company, 1973a).

Other Health Effects of Aspartame

Six hundred twenty-three consumer complaints about side effects of aspartame were submitted to the FDA, to Searle, and to several private scientists. In February 1984, the FDA asked the Centers for Disease Control (CDC) to help analyze these complaints. Because of time constraints, CDC made in-depth review of only 231 cases that were received and coded by June 1984. The data did not provide evidence for the existence of serious, widespread, adverse health consequences associated with aspartame use, but some of the symptoms reported could be due to an as yet unconfirmed sensitivity to aspartame in these people. For a more thorough evaluation, focused clinical studies have been recommended (Bradstock et al., 1986); these are under way.

Waggoner (1984) and the Council on Scientific Affairs (1985) reviewed the data and concluded that when consumed in amounts two to three times higher than the maximum daily intake—34 mg/kg per day, which is substantially below the acceptable daily intake (ADI) of 50 mg/kg/of body weight set by the FDA (1981)—aspartame is not associated with any harmful effects in the general population. However, in individuals afflicted with phenylketonuria, a genetic disorder in which phenylalanine metabolism is blocked and progressive mental retardation may occur, intake should be strictly limited. Because phenylalanine is one product of the hydrolysis of aspartame in the gut (Waggoner, 1984), it should not be included in the diet of these individuals; hence, the FDA (1983) requires labeling of all foods or soft drinks containing aspartame.

Although questions are being raised as to whether nonnutritive sweeteners can contribute to weight reduction, a study of obese subjects by Porikos et al. (1977) showed that covert substitution of aspartame-sweetened products for their sucrose counterparts resulted in an immediate 25% reduction in spontaneous energy intake.

PRESERVATIVES, ANTIOXIDANTS, FOOD COLORS, AND OTHER INTENTIONALLY ADDED SUBSTANCES

Nitrites, Nitrates, and *N*-Nitroso Compounds

Occurrence and Exposure

Nitrites and to a lesser extent nitrates are used as preservatives in many foods and can be converted to *N*-nitroso compounds under a variety of conditions (NRC, 1981; Olsen et al., 1984). They can also occur naturally in foods, and because many *N*-nitroso compounds are strongly carcinogenic in many species (Magee and Barnes, 1967; Rao et al., 1984), there has been much concern during the past two decades about their role in the etiology of cancer in humans. Nitrites are present in saliva and in the urine of people with bladder infections. *N*-nitroso compounds can be formed in the stomach and bladder from action of the nitrite on ingested amines, which can be naturally present in food, from residues of agricultural chemicals in food, and from drugs and medicines (Lijinsky, 1986).

The concentrations of nitrates and nitrites in foods depend on many factors, including agricultural practices and storage conditions. An NRC committee estimated that the average U.S. diet provides approximately 75 mg of nitrates and 0.8 mg of nitrites daily (NRC, 1981). Vegetables contribute the largest proportion of nitrates, followed by nitrate-rich drinking water and fruit juices. The largest dietary source of nitrites, however, is cured meats, which provide more than one-third of the total dietary nitrites. Baked goods and cereals provide another third of total nitrites, whereas vegetables contribute approximately one-fifth.

Preformed nitrosamines may also be present in the diet, chiefly in foods cured with nitrate or nitrite. Beer was the largest single dietary source of nitrosamines until recently, when the malting process was modified. Currently, the most important dietary sources are cured meats, especially bacon, which may provide an average of 0.17 μg of nitropyrrolidine per person daily (NRC, 1981). This amount may be considerably lower if bacon is treated with antioxidants such as ascorbic acid. In the United States, the daily intake of nitrosamines from all dietary sources is estimated to be 1.1 μg/person (NRC, 1981). Residual nitrites in cured meats and fish are an important source of nitrosating agents in the stomach, since they provide concentrations of nitrites much higher than those in saliva. Many N-nitroso compounds can be formed in vivo from these sources, and the carcinogenic effects of many of them are unknown. All organs are potential targets (Lijinsky, 1986).

Evidence Associating Nitrites, Nitrates, and N-Nitroso Compounds with Chronic Diseases

Epidemiologic Studies

Findings from epidemiologic studies conducted in Colombia, Chile, Japan, Iran, China, England, and Hawaii show an association between increased incidence of cancers of the stomach and the esophagus and exposure to high levels of nitrate or nitrite in the diet or drinking water (Armijo and Coulson, 1975; Armijo et al., 1981; Correa et al., 1975; Cuello et al., 1976; Haenszel et al., 1972; Higginson, 1966; Meinsma, 1964). However, the NRC Committee on Nitrite and Alternative Curing Agents in Food concluded that those studies do not provide conclusive evidence for a causal relationship between exposure to nitrates and nitrites and the occurrence of cancers in humans at those sites (NRC, 1981).

Although bladder cancer has been correlated with nitrates in the water supply and with urinary tract infections (Howe et al., 1980; Wynder et al.,

1963), no difference in consumption of nitrite-preserved meats such as ham or pork sausages was observed between cases and controls (Howe et al., 1980). Nitrosamines have been found in the urine of patients with urinary tract infections, suggesting that the formation of these compounds may be responsible for bladder carcinogenesis (Radomski et al., 1978).

In China, an increased risk of esophageal cancer was associated with the ingestion of moldy food containing N-nitroso compounds, possibly produced by fungal contaminants (Yang, 1980). More recent studies showed a correlation between lesions of the esophageal epithelium and the amount of nitrosamines present in inhabitants of Linxian Province in China (Lu et al., 1986). Earlier studies in Iran, however, showed no differences in nitrosamine levels in foods consumed in regions of high and low risk for esophageal cancer (Joint Iran–International Agency for Research on Cancer Study Group, 1977).

Several studies in different parts of the world have shown an association between stomach cancer and frequent consumption of cured pickles or smoked foods (Choi et al., 1971; Joint Iran–International Agency for Research on Cancer Study Group, 1977; Kriebel and Jowett, 1979; Lijinsky and Shubik, 1964). In southern Louisiana, consumption of smoked foods and homemade or home-cured meats was found to increase the risk of gastric cancer in higher-risk blacks but not in lower-risk whites (Correa et al., 1985). In Canada, consumption of nitrites, smoked meats, and smoked fish was found to be a risk factor for gastric cancer (Risch et al., 1985). However, it was estimated that the major contributor to risk was consumption of nitrites; each milligram of nitrites increased the odds of cancer by 2.6 (95% confidence intervals, range 1.6–4.2). Thus, although salt, nitrates, nitrites, N-nitroso compounds, and PAHs have all been considered as potential causative agents, it seems most likely that consumption of nitrites and subsequent endogenous production of nitrosamines make a major contribution to the risk of stomach cancer.

Animal Studies

The few experiments conducted in animals have provided no conclusive evidence that nitrates are carcinogenic (Flamm, 1985; NRC, 1981). There is also no evidence of direct nitrite carcinogenicity in animals (NRC, 1981). However, nitrites may interact with specific components of diets consumed by humans and animals or with endogenous metabolites to produce N-nitroso compounds that induce cancer (NRC, 1981).

N-nitroso compounds comprise a large group of carcinogens and mutagens that have been examined in a number of test systems. There are large differences between species in response to N-nitroso compounds. For example, nitrosoalkylamides induce tumors at many sites in rats, but only in the spleen and forestomach of hamsters (Lijinsky, 1985).

Nitrosamines require metabolic activation to be mutagenic or carcinogenic (Lijinsky, 1985). The carcinogenic action of several N-nitroso compounds can be inhibited in systems where the formation of N-nitroso compounds has been prevented by such agents as ascorbic acid, and its isomers, sorbic acids, some phenols, and α-tocopherol (Mirvish, 1981). Formation of N-nitroso compounds can also be enhanced by a variety of ions that are normally present in foods, especially thiocyanate and iodide, which may catalyze the nitrosation reaction in the stomach (Mirvish et al., 1975).

Short-Term Tests

Nitrates do not appear to be directly mutagenic (Konetzka, 1974). In microbial systems, nitrites may be mutagenic by three different mechanisms (Zimmermann, 1977): deamination of DNA bases in single-strand DNA; formation of 2-nitroinosine and intrastrand or interstrand lesions leading to helix distortions in double-stranded DNA; and formation of mutagenic N-nitroso compounds by combining with nitrosatable substrates. Nitrites were positive in the Ames Salmonella assay and produced chromosome aberrations (Ishidate et al., 1984; Törnquist et al., 1983).

Many N-nitroso compounds have been found to be mutagenic in a variety of test systems, including bacterial assays, mammalian cells in culture, and Drosophila melanogaster under a variety of conditions (Mochizuki et al., 1984; Montesano and Bartsch, 1976) and to induce malignant transformations of human fetal lung fibroblasts in vitro (Huang et al., 1986).

Phenolic Antioxidants—Butylated Hydroxyanisole and Butylated Hydroxytoluene

Occurrence and Exposure

The phenolic compounds butylated hydroxyanisole (BHA) and butylated hydroxytoluene (BHT) are widely used as food additives, mainly because of their preservative and antioxidant properties. They are used extensively at levels ranging from 10 to 200 ppm in dry cereals and shortenings as well as in potato sprouts, granules, and flakes. BHA is also permitted as a food additive in active dry yeasts, in dry beverage and dessert mixes, and in beverages made from such mixes. Both BHA and BHT are limited in foods by a total antioxidant content of not more than 0.02% of the fat or oil content of foods. They are also permitted in food packaging materials subject to a migration limit of 0.005% in foods. In 1976, approximately 9 million pounds of BHT were produced for use in foods in the United States (Roberts, 1981). The total average daily intakes of BHA and BHT are 5.6 mg/person and 1.8 mg/person, respectively (D.L. Houston, Food and Drug Administration, personal communication, 1987).

Evidence Associating Phenolic Antioxidants with Chronic Diseases

BHA: Studies of Cancer

EPIDEMIOLOGIC STUDIES There is no epidemiologic evidence that relates risk of developing cancer to consumption of BHA.

ANIMAL STUDIES Repeated intraperitoneal injections of BHA at high doses produced a slight, although not statistically significant, increase in lung tumors in male A/J mice (Witschi et al., 1981). The addition of BHA to the diet of Fischer 344 rats induced a high incidence of papilloma and squamous cell carcinoma of the forestomach in both sexes (Ito et al., 1985). Male hamsters given BHA for 24 weeks also developed papillomas with a downward growth into the submucosa of the forestomach (Hirose et al., 1986). The 3-*tert* isomer—3-*tert*-butyl-4-hydroxyanisole—seemed to be responsible for the carcinogenicity of crude BHA in the forestomach of rats and hamsters. In two-stage carcinogenesis in rats, after appropriate initiations BHA enhanced carcinogenesis in the forestomach, kidney, and urinary bladder of rats, but inhibited carcinogenesis in the liver (Ito et al., 1985; Tsuda et al., 1984).

However, a diet containing BHA did not enhance the development of lung tumors in A/J mice when fed for 8 weeks after administration of the carcinogens urethane, benzo[a]pyrene, or dimethylnitrosamine (Witschi and Doherty, 1984). BHA was shown to decrease the incidence and density of large-bowel neoplasms in female CF/1 mice given 24 weekly doses of the carcinogen 1,2-dimethylhydrazine (Jones et al., 1984) and to decrease colon tumor incidence and multiplicity in animals given the carcinogen methylazoxymethanol acetate (Reddy and Maeura, 1984). BHA has been shown to inhibit the activity of a variety of carcinogens, such as benzo[a]pyrene, dimethylbenz[a]anthracene, 4-nitroquinoline-N-oxide, and urethane (NRC, 1982).

Evidence suggests that exposure to BHA before administration of a carcinogen often has a protective effect, whereas exposure to BHA after an exposure to a carcinogen has sometimes been protective and sometimes has no influence (Witschi, 1984).

SHORT-TERM TESTS There is no evidence that BHA is genotoxic. It does not increase the frequency of sister chromatid exchanges, induce mutations to 6-thioguanine resistance in V79 Chinese hamster lung cells activated by rat or hamster hepatocytes (Rogers et al., 1985), or produce chromosome aberrations in Chinese hamster cells (Abe and Sasaki, 1977). BHA has also been shown to inhibit host-mediated mutagenesis resulting from exposure to hycanthone, mitrifonate, praziquantel, and metronidazole (Batzinger et al., 1978).

MECHANISMS OF ACTION Data suggest that two factors may be of importance in carcinogenesis induced by the 3-tert isomer (3-BHA): (1) thiol depletion resulting from direct binding of quinone metabolites of 3-BHA to tissue thiols or (2) an attack on tissue constitutents by reactive metabolites of 3-BHA and possibly also by oxygen radicals produced as a result of redox cycling of quinone and hydroxyquinone metabolites of 3-BHA (deStafney et al., 1986).

BHT: Studies of Cancer

EPIDEMIOLOGIC EVIDENCE There is no epidemiologic evidence that relates risk of developing cancer to consumption of BHT.

ANIMAL STUDIES Female B6C3F$_1$ mice fed a diet containing 0, 0.3, or 0.6% BHT for approximately 2 years developed alveolar/bronchiolar adenomas or carcinomas only at the low dose (NCI, 1979), whereas male C3H mice fed a diet containing BHT had a significant increase in incidence of liver tumors (Lindenschmidt et al., 1986). However, BHT was not found to be carcinogenic in the forestomach of rats, mice, or Syrian hamsters (Hirose et al., 1986; Ito et al., 1985).

In a two-generation study in which Wistar rats were exposed in utero to BHT up to 250 mg/kg per day, a dose-related statistical increase in the number of hepatocellular adenomas and carcinomas was detected in the F$_1$ male rats, whereas in treated F$_1$ female rats, a statistical increase was observed only for adenomas. Hepatocellular tumors were detected in all F$_1$ rats more than 2 years old (Olsen et al., 1986). A diet containing 0.75% BHT enhanced the development of lung tumors in A/J mice when fed for 2 weeks after administration of the carcinogen urethane and for 8 weeks after exposure to 3-methylcholanthrene, benzo[a]pyrene, or N-nitrosodimethylamine (Witschi and Morse, 1983).

Male BALB/c mice treated subcutaneously with the carcinogen dimethylhydrazine and fed a diet containing BHT had a significant increase in the incidence of colon tumors, but male BALB/c mice exposed to the carcinogen N-methyl-N-nitrosourea intrarectally then fed BHT in the diet did not. This observation leads to the conclusion that the effect of BHT on tumor development depends on the exposure route and the carcinogens used (Lindenschmidt et al., 1986).

In studies of the enhancement of hepatocarcinogenesis by BHT, Maeura and Williams (1984) found that BHT fed to rats slightly enhanced hepatocellular foci produced by feeding them N-2-fluorenylacetamide for 8 weeks. In rats simultaneously fed N-2-fluorenylacetamide and BHA, hepatocarcinogenesis was inhibited but bladder carcinogenesis was enhanced (Williams et al., 1983). In a two-stage carcinogenesis study on rats, BHT enhanced the induction of urinary bladder tumors, inhibited the induction of liver tumors, and was believed to promote thyroid carcinogenesis (Ito et al., 1985).

The evidence suggests that in certain tissues, exposure first to BHT and then to a carcinogen has no effect on tumorigenesis (Witschi, 1984), whereas in others, it may suppress tumorigenesis, depending on the level of BHT in the diet, the type of diet in which BHT is administered, and the dosage of the carcinogen administered (Cohen et al., 1984, 1986).

SHORT-TERM TESTS BHT was negative in a sister chromatid exchange assay and did not induce chromosome aberrations (Abe and Sasaki, 1977). BHT can either enhance or inhibit mutagenic potency, depending on the substance tested; for example, in the Ames Salmonella assay, BHT is antimutagenic toward benzo[a]pyrene, but increases the numbers of *Salmonella* revertants induced by aflatoxin B_1 (Malkinson, 1983). BHT inhibited cell-to-cell communication between mammalian cells in vitro, an indication of possible promoting activity (Trosko et al., 1982).

MECHANISMS OF ACTION   BHT is one of the few compounds to have both tumor-prophylactic and tumor-promoting capabilities. The temporal sequence in which BHT and a carcinogen are administered to test animals seems to determine how BHT affects the response to these carcinogens. In common with other antioxidants, BHT inhibits the ability of carcinogens to induce tumors in various rodent organs when the animal is given BHT prior to treatment with a carcinogen. Unlike other antioxidants, however, the number of tumors increases when BHT is administered after exposure to a carcinogen (Malkinson, 1983). The anticarcinogenic activity of BHT may be due, in part, to preferential enhancement of hepatic detoxifying mechanisms, with the result that intracellular concentrations of reactive metabolites are reduced and fewer covalently bound products are formed (Salocks et al., 1984).

Food Colors

Occurrence and Exposure

Approximately 10% of the food consumed in the United States contains added certified colors. In 1982, approximately 2 million pounds of food colors were added to food products (NRC, 1984), amounting to a per-capita exposure of approximately 100 mg/day. The major categories of foods containing added colors are cereals and baked goods, candies, desserts, ice creams and sherbets, sausages, beverages, snack foods, and miscellaneous foods such as salad dressings, jams, and jellies (NRC, 1971). The concentration of colors in these foods ranges from 5 to 600 ppm; the average is approximately 150 ppm. The soft-drink industry is the single largest user of certified colors. The question of whether these colors pose a significant cancer risk has been debated since 1960, when the current regulatory system of toxicologic review was enacted (U.S. Congress, 1960). Food colors that have been examined most carefully for their toxic properties are FD&C Blue No. 2, FD&C Red No. 3 (erythrosine), FD&C Yellow No. 5 (tartrazine), and FD&C Yellow No. 6 (sunset yellow FCF). Only

the most recent long-term studies using toxicologic protocols adopted by the FDA are mentioned here (Rulis et al., 1984). There are no relevant epidemiologic studies on food colors.

Evidence Associating Food Colors with Chronic Diseases

Animal Studies and Short-Term Tests

FD&C BLUE NO. 2   In a chronic feeding study in mice and in a companion multigeneration feeding study in rats, no statistically significant compound-related adverse effects, including tumors, were observed (Borzelleca and Hogan, 1985; Borzelleca et al., 1985).

FD&C RED NO. 3 (ERYTHROSINE)   In a multigeneration study, Charles River CD rats exposed in utero to 4% erythrosine mixed in diet for 24 months exhibited a significant increase in incidence of follicular thyroid adenomas and carcinomas (Goldenthal, 1982). However, such effects may result from a thyroid hormone imbalance induced by the high concentrations of colorant used (DHHS, 1985).

Erythrosine was tested for its ability to induce mutations in the *Bacillus subtilis rec* assay; results were negative in one assay (Kada et al., 1972) and positive in another (Fujita et al., 1976). In *E. coli*, a slight but statistically significant mutagenic effect was observed by some investigators (Lück et al., 1963); no effects were found by others (Fujita et al., 1976). Erythrosine was negative in the Ames *Salmonella* assay but produced chromosome aberrations in vitro in the Chinese hamster fibroblast cell line (Ishidate et al., 1984).

FD&C YELLOW NO. 5 (TARTRAZINE)   FD&C Yellow No. 5 has been approved for general use in foods since 1969. It is not considered to be carcinogenic (Hesser, 1984). However, it exerted dose-dependent mutagenic activities in the Ames *Salmonella* assay with *S. typhimurium* TA98 after metabolic activation with rat liver S9 mix (Henschler and Wild, 1985); it induced chromosome aberrations in vitro in Chinese hamster fibroblasts (Ishidate et al., 1984) and in barking deer (*Muntiacus mantjak*) fibroblasts (Patterson and Butler, 1982); and it has been associated with allergic reactions such as itching, hives, and headaches in humans (Hesser, 1984). In recent analyses, the FDA determined that FD&C Yellow No. 5 contains the carcinogenic impurities 4-aminoazobenzene, 4-aminobiphenyl, aniline, azobenzene, benzidine, and 1,3-diphenyltriazine (DHHS, 1985). A risk evaluation by FDA revealed that the normal use of this colorant would not result in high exposures to the carcinogenic contaminants, provided that the current low level of contamination is not exceeded (DHHS, 1985).

FD&C Yellow No. 6 (Sunset Yellow FCF)
FD&C Yellow No. 6 remains provisionally approved for food use, because the most recent chronic feeding studies have not been completely evaluated. It appears to be noncarcinogenic in mice, but studies in rats require further review (DHHS, 1985).

Fat Substitute (Sucrose Polyester)

Sucrose polyester (SPE)—a nonabsorbable mixture of hexa-, hepta-, and octa-fatty-acid esters of sucrose with physical and organoleptic properties very similar to those of conventional fats—is now under investigation by the FDA as a potential food substitute that could help people to lose weight while lowering serum levels of cholesterol, LDLs, and triglycerides (Fallat et al., 1976; Mellies et al., 1985). SPE is not absorbed by the gut, which lacks the enzymes to break it down. Among the safety questions being addressed is whether any amount of SPE, however minute, will be absorbed by the body, since if even very minute amounts are absorbed, safety issues become more complex. Another concern is the possibility that SPE decreases the levels of some fat-soluble vitamins in the plasma, especially vitamin E. Mellies et al. (1985) reported a 17% decrease in the mean vitamin E baseline value in SPE-treated subjects, but attributed this decrease to a concomitant reduction in the LDL.

INDIRECT ADDITIVES, CONTAMINANTS, AND BY-PRODUCTS OF FOOD PROCESSING

Polychlorinated Biphenyls (PCBs)

Occurrence and Exposure

PCBs are highly persistent in the environment and have been detected in human tissues (Kutz and Strassman, 1976). In the United States, the general population may be exposed to small amounts of PCBs through food, water, and air. High exposures may occur among sports fishermen who consume freshwater fish from contaminated steams and lakes. Since fish is also a source of food for domesticated animals, PCBs may be found in milk, eggs, and poultry. In one survey, approximately

20% of all fish were contaminated with PCBs, although only a small percentage exceeded the tolerance level of 5 ppm established by the FDA (McNally, 1978). Recently, the tolerance levels have been lowered for several classes of foods—to 1.5 ppm in milk and dairy products and to 3 ppm in poultry. Other dietary exposures to PCBs can result from contamination of the food supply through industrial accidents and migration of PCBs to foods from packaging materials contaminated with PCBs.

Jelinck and Corneliussen (1975) reported a great reduction of PCB contamination from 1969 to 1975 in all foods except fish, in which no trend was observed. The average daily intake of PCBs per person in the United States from 1980 to 1982 was estimated to be 0.19 μg (Gartrell et al., 1986).

Evidence Associating PCBs with Chronic Diseases

Epidemiologic Studies

In Japan, more than 1,200 cases of Yusho disease (a disorder involving ocular, dermatologic, and nervous symptoms) were reported over a 9-year period (1968 to 1975) in humans who accidentally consumed rice oil contaminated with PCBs (Higuchi, 1976; Kuratsune, 1976). Nine out of 22 (41%) of the deaths reported as long as 5.5 years after the initial exposure were due to malignant neoplasia (Kuratsune, 1976; Urabe, 1974); however, the investigators did not compare this incidence with the rate of expected deaths from various cancers in the population (NRC, 1982).

Occupational exposure studies have also linked PCBs to cancer. In a retrospective study of 2,567 workers employed for at least 3 months in a plant using PCBs, Brown and Jones (1981) reported more liver cancers than expected (3 versus 1.07), even though total mortality and mortality from cancers were lower than expected. In a follow-up report on this study, two additional deaths from cancer of the liver and biliary passages were found. These resulted in a standard mortality ratio (SMR) for the combined sites of 2.1. However, one of the liver cancers originally reported was found to have metastasized from another site (Brown, 1987).

Bahn et al. (1976, 1977) reported two malignant melanomas among 31 workers heavily exposed to PCBs (20 times the expected incidence) and one melanoma among 41 less heavily exposed workers; however, these workers were also exposed to other chemicals. In an electrical capacitor manufacturing facility in Italy, 26 malignancies were observed compared to 12.9 expected (Bertazzi et al., 1987). Among males, the excess cancers were in the digestive tract (including one liver cancer); among females, excess cancers were in the lymphatic hematopoietic system. In a study of a small cohort of similar workers in Sweden, no significant excess of cancer deaths was noted (Gustavsson et al., 1986).

The International Agency for Research on Cancer (IARC, 1987) concluded that there is *limited* evidence for the carcinogenicity of PCBs in humans.

Animal Studies and Short-Term Tests

Laboratory experiments indicate that some PCBs produce liver tumors in rodents, but mostly at doses much higher than those generally present in the average U.S. diet (NRC, 1982). Evidence indicates that some PCBs may act primarily as tumor-promoting agents (Preston et al., 1981).

The PCBs Aroclor 1221 and 1268 have been shown to induce microsomal activation in the Ames *Salmonella* assay (Wyndham et al., 1976). Other PCBs (e.g., Aroclor 1254) are negative in the dominant lethal assay in rats and do not induce chromosome aberrations in human lymphocytes (Hoopingarner et al., 1972). Aroclor 1242 did not induce chromosome aberrations in bone marrow (Green et al., 1973).

Polybrominated Biphenyls (PBBs)

Occurrence and Exposure

PBBs, which are chemically related to PCBs, were used at one time as flame retardants in industrial processes, but their use has been prohibited because of their toxicity and because, like PCBs, they persist in the environment and can accumulate in body fat.

Evidence Associating PBBs with Chronic Diseases

Epidemiologic Studies

In Michigan in 1973, PBBs were accidently added to animal feed. As a consequence, cattle, poultry, and humans in surrounding areas were widely exposed (Kay, 1977). Because of the short interval between time of exposure and the measurement of effects, no definitive epidemiologic information linking PBBs to cancer were established.

Animal Studies and Short-Term Tests

Sherman rats given a single oral dose of PBBs by gavage developed neoplastic liver nodules after 6 months (Kimbrough et al., 1978). In a follow-up study, Sherman rats were given a single large dose of PBBs or 12 divided doses by gavage. Both treatments resulted in a high incidence of hepatocellular carcinomas. In the rats given multiple high doses, the incidence of tumors was higher and some of the liver carcinomas were less differentiated than in rats given the single dose (Kimbrough et al., 1981).

PBBs did not induce mutations either in the Ames *Salmonella* assay or in Chinese hamster uterine cells. When administered orally to mice, they did not induce chromosome aberrations in bone marrow cells (Wertz and Ficsor, 1978).

Polyvinyl Chloride (PVC)

Occurrence and Exposure

PVC is classified as an indirect food additive by the FDA, whereas the monomer, which may be present at low levels as a residue in PVC, is regarded as a contaminant (CPSC, 1974). PVC is the parent compound for a series of copolymers used in food packaging materials. The monomer may migrate into foods, and PVC has been detected in a variety of alcoholic drinks (0.2 to 1.0 mg/liter) (Williams, 1976a,b), in vinegars (~9 mg/liter) (Williams and Miles, 1975), and in products packaged and stored in PVC containers, for example, edible oils (0.05 to 14.8 mg/liter) (Rösli et al., 1975), margarine and butter (0.5 mg/kg) (Fuchs et al., 1975), and finished drinking water in the United States (10.0 µg/liter) (EPA, 1975a). There are no estimates of average daily dietary exposure to PVC.

Evidence Associating PVC with Chronic Diseases

Epidemiologic Studies

No epidemiologic studies on exposure to PVC as a food contaminant have been reported, but serveral studies of occupational exposure have linked PVC exposure to cancer. Creech and Johnson (1974) associated inhalation of PVC with the occurrence of hepatic angiosarcomas. Tabershaw and Gaffey (1974) observed increases in cancer of the alimentary tract, liver, respiratory tract, and lymphomas in male workers exposed to PVC for 1 year. Several other studies showed associations between exposure to PVC and increased mortality from cancer at various sites (e.g., Duck and Carter, 1976; Fox and Collier, 1977; Monson et al., 1974; Nicholson et al., 1975; Sweeney et al., 1986; Thériault and Allard, 1981; Waxweiler et al., 1976, 1981). Male workers occupationally exposed to PVC were reported to have more chromosome aberrations than were observed in unexposed cohorts (Funes-Cravioto et al., 1975; Heath and Dumont, 1977; Purchase et al., 1975).

IARC (1987) concluded that there is *sufficient* evidence that PVC is carcinogenic in humans.

Animal Studies and Short-Term Tests

Animal studies showed that PVC induces tumors in rats and hamsters (Feron et al., 1975, 1981; Maltoni, 1977; Maltoni et al., 1974, 1975). In short-term tests, PVC vapors induced mutations in Ames *Salmonella* strains (Andrews et al., 1976; Bartsch et al., 1979), *Escherichia coli* (Greim et al., 1975), *Schizosaccharomyces pombé* (Loprieno et al., 1976), *Drosophila melanogaster* (Verburgt and Vogel, 1977), and mammalian cells (Huberman et al., 1975) and produced gene conversions in yeast (Eckardt et al., 1981). Chromosome aberrations have been observed among workers exposed to PVC vapors (Poncelet et al., 1984).

Polycyclic Aromatic Hydrocarbons (PAHs)

Occurrence and Exposure

Low levels of approximately 100 PAHs have been identified as contaminants in a variety of foods. Major contributors to this contamination are smoking and broiling of foods and the use of curing smokes. The two major sources of PAH contamination of foods are pyrolysis and contact with petroleum and coal-tar products. Charbroiling of meats and fish over an open flame, in which fat drippings can be pyrolyzed, contributes substantially to dietary PAH exposure. Benzo[*a*]pyrene constitutes a significant portion of the total amount of carcinogenic PAHs in the environment; levels as high as 50 μg/kg have been detected in charcoal-broiled steaks. In contrast, data on dietary exposure to other carcinogenic PAHs are fragmentary (NRC, 1982). There have been no comprehensive surveys of the benzo[*a*]pyrene content of smoked foods in the United States. In Canada, smoked foods have been reported to contain benzo[*a*]pyrene at levels ranging from 0.2 to 15 μg/kg (Panalaks, 1976). Foods smoked at

home may contain higher levels of benzo[*a*]pyrene than commercial foods treated with liquid smoke. Edible marine species may contribute substantially to PAH intake. Food packaging materials contaminated with PAHs are also a major dietary source.

PAHs are not monitored by the FDA, and no acceptable daily intake of PAHs has been established. The total daily intake of PAHs in the United States is estimated to range from 1.6 to 16.0 μg (Santodonato et al., 1981).

Evidence Associating PAHs with Chronic Diseases

Of the more than 100 PAHs found in the environment, approximately 20 are carcinogenic in several species of laboratory animals (EPA, 1975b; Lo and Sandi, 1978) and many are potent mutagens (NRC, 1982). The PAHs exert their toxic, carcinogenic, and mutagenic effects only after metabolic activation (Freudenthal and Jones, 1976). Their carcinogenic activity varies from very weak to potent. Of the five PAHs found to be carcinogenic in animals when administered orally and mutagenic in several short-term tests, three— benzo[*a*]pyrene, dibenz[*a,h*]-anthracene, and benzanthrazene—occur in the average U.S. diet (NRC, 1982). Although occupational studies show an association between PAHs and the incidence of skin and lung cancer, there are no epidemiologic studies linking consumption of food contaminated with low levels of PAHs and the occurrence of cancer in humans (NRC, 1982).

Acrylonitrile

The appearance of acrylonitrile in foods as an indirect additive or contaminant may be attributed to its use in food packaging and the migratory quality of the monomer, which is present in small amounts in the polymer. It has been detected in Great Britain in margarine tubs and in food packaging films. In the United States, acrylonitrile has been detected in margarine (13 to 45 μg/kg) and olive oil (38 to 50 μg/liter), and in minute quantities in nuts (C.V. Breder, Food and Drug Administration, personal communication, 1980).

There are no estimates of average daily exposure to acrylonitrile in the United States. The effects of human exposure to acrylonitrile from food packaging or drinking water have not been completely evaluated. However, a retrospective study of male employees exposed to acrylonitrile at a textile plant indicated a trend toward increased risk of cancer at all sites, especially the lung (O'Berg,

1980). This limited evidence, plus the findings that acrylonitrile is carcinogenic in rats upon ingestion or inhalation (Norris, 1977) and mutagenic in three *Salmonella* strains (Milvy, 1978; Milvy and Wolff, 1977) and in *E. coli* (Venitt et al., 1977), suggests that acrylonitrile, under certain circumstances, might increase cancer risks in humans.

Diethylstilbestrol (DES)

Among the approximately 20 growth hormones commonly used in animal feed, attention has focused mainly on DES. Residues of this compound have been monitored for many years following reports that it was carcinogenic in animals (Fitzhugh, 1964; Jukes, 1974). The use of DES in humans for various preventive and therapeutic applications terminated in 1978. Until 1979, DES was permitted as a growth promoter for cattle and sheep under certain conditions delineated by the FDA (1979a).

There are no epidemiologic reports on the health effects of DES residues in food. There is, however, sufficient evidence that therapeutic doses of DES during pregnancy produces vaginal and cervical cancer in the female offspring of treated women (Herbst and Cole, 1978). In animals, it produced mainly mammary tumors in mice (Gass et al., 1974), rats (Gibson et al., 1967; Sumi et al., 1985), and Syrian hamsters (Rustia, 1979). In a host of short-term tests, it also induced positive results such as chromosome aberrations in Chinese hamster fibroblasts (Ishidate and Odashima, 1977) and in murine bone marrow cells in vivo (Ivett and Tice, 1981), mutations in mouse lymphoma cells (Clive, 1977), unscheduled DNA synthesis in HeLa cells (Martin et al., 1978), aneuploidy in mice in vivo (Chrisman, 1974), and morphological and neoplastic transformation of Syrian hamster embryo cells in the absence of cell proliferation (McLachlan et al., 1982).

Pesticides

Occurrence and Exposure

Residues of pesticides often remain on agricultural commodities after they have been harvested and prepared for consumer purchase. They are also found in processed foods derived from these commodities. The use of several organochlorine pesticides (e.g., DDT, dieldrin, heptaclor, ke-

pone, chlordane) has been gradually suspended by the Environmental Protection Agency (EPA) because they have a propensity to persist in the environment; to accumulate in fat-containing foods, such as meat, fish, poultry, and dairy products (DHEW, 1969; FDA, 1980b); and to concentrate in body tissues (IARC, 1979). Organophosphate pesticides (e.g., parathion and diazinon) are generally more common in cereal products (FDA, 1980a).

The Market Basket Surveys conducted by the FDA since the 1960s indicate that the levels of pesticides in foods are generally very low and tend to vary only slightly from region to region (Gartrell et al., 1986). In these surveys, pesticides were found most frequently in oils from fats and meat, fish, and poultry. The fewest residues were found in legumes and vegetables. The greatest variety of chemicals was found in the fruit and the oil–fat groups. Of the pesticides measured, only the intake of dieldrin and malathion have approached the ADI in recent years. However, any assessment of the health effects of exposure to pesticide residues must take into account the potential synergistic interactions and the limited nature of the toxicity data on several compounds. In one large-scale survey, Murphy et al. (1983) reported wide-scale contamination of body tissues and detected organochlorine pesticides in 4 to 14% of the serum and 93 to 97% of the adipose tissue samples examined.

There has been considerable concern recently about the use of the halogenated hydrocarbon pesticide ethylene dibromide (EDB) in food products. EDB was used as a soil fumigant to protect agricultural crops from attack by nematodes (root worms), until its emergency suspension by the EPA in September 1983. At the same time, the EPA announced cancellation and phaseout of all other major pesticide uses of EDB such as the postharvest fumigation of fruits and grains to prevent the spread of insects, spot fumigation of vaults, beehives, and timbers, and termite control (U.S. Senate, 1984).

Under its EDB compliance program in 1984, the FDA detected EDB in 462 out of 1,776 samples of grains at trace amounts to 150 ppb, at 150 to 500 ppb in 80 samples, at 500 to 900 ppb in 23 samples, and >900 ppb in 12 samples. No EDB was detected in 1,199 samples. Of 292 ready-to-eat food products analyzed, 277 contained no EDB, 10 contained a trace, and 5 contained 2 to 30 ppb (C. Carnevale, FDA, personal communication, 1988).

Evidence Associating Pesticides with Chronic Diseases

Cancer

EPIDEMIOLOGIC STUDIES Few epidemiologic studies have examined cancer risk following exposure to pesticides. Several industrial cohort mortality studies of exposure to dioxin or phenoxyacetic acid herbicides did not show an increase in the frequency of death from soft-tissue sarcomas (STS), Hodgkin's disease (HD), or non-Hodgkin's lymphoma (NHL) (Cook et al., 1980; Ott et al., 1980a; Riihimaki et al., 1982; Zack and Suskind, 1980). However, the total number of workers exposed was only 2,705. In the Ranch Hand Study—a cohort study conducted by the U.S. Air Force on exposure of 1,247 people to Agent Orange (dioxin) in Vietnam—no increase in incidence of or mortality from these cancers was detected as of December 1982, but less than one such death was expected in this small cohort (U.S. Air Force, 1983). In a case-control study based on 217 cases of STS from the files of the Armed Forces Institute of Pathology and 599 controls from the logs of referring pathologists, no evidence was found of increased risk of STS associated with military service in Vietnam (Kang et al., 1987).

In a series of case-control studies conducted in rural Sweden in the 1970s, investigators found highly significant relative risks—five- and sixfold in magnitude—for all three cancers (STS, HD, and NLH) following exposure to the phenoxyacetic acid herbicides and chlorophenols, regardless of whether or not exposures involved contamination by polychlorinated dibenzodioxins or polychlorinated dibenzofurans (Erickson et al., 1981; Hardell and Sandstrom, 1979; Hardell et al., 1981). A case-control study conducted in New Zealand yielded a negative result for STS (Smith et al., 1984).

In several studies, increased incidence of STS and NHL was observed among workers producing phenoxyacetic acid herbicides (Cook, 1981; Honchar and Halperin, 1981; Johnson et al., 1981; Moses and Selikoff, 1981) and among farmers (Buesching and Wollstadt, 1984; Cantor, 1982; Pearce et al., 1985; Stubbs et al., 1984). More recently, a population-based case-control study in rural Kansas (Hoar et al., 1986) indicated that the use of herbicides not likely to be contaminated by dioxins, especially the phenoxyacetic herbicides such as 2,4-dichlorophenoxyacetic acid (2,4-D) and 2,4,5-trichlorophenoxyacetic acid (2,4,5-T) (Cochrane et al., 1981), was associated with a sixfold increase of NHL among farmers exposed to

herbicides more than 20 days per year. The positive association was with phenoxyacetic acid herbicide and not insecticide use. Negative findings were reported for STS and HD.

In a population-based case-control study of exposure to phenoxyherbicides conducted in the western part of Washington State (Woods et al., 1987), no excess risk was found for STS. However, excess risk for NHL was found for farmers, forestry herbicide applicators, and others exposed for at least 15 or more years before NHL was diagnosed.

When the analyses were restricted to workers of Scandinavian descent, there was a suggestion of an increase in risk of STS following exposure to phenoxyherbicides. An additional explanation for the differences in findings in Sweden and the United States is the estimation by Woods et al. (1987) that their exposed workers had approximately half the exposure of Swedish workers. Since more than 42 million pounds of phenoxyacetic acid herbicides were applied to U.S. farmlands in 1976 (Eichers et al., 1978), the potential carcinogenic effects from exposure to these herbicides is of concern.

Occupational studies of workers exposed to EDB were not conclusive; the studies had small cohorts, exposure data were incomplete or missing, and exposure periods were short (Ott et al., 1980b; Haar, 1980; Wong et al., 1979).

ANIMAL STUDIES AND SHORT-TERM TESTS The general population is exposed to several common organochlorine pesticides (e.g., toxaphene and chlordane) that cause cancer in mice and in some other animal species (IARC, 1974; NRC, 1982). However, with the exception of parathion, organophosphate pesticides (e.g., malathion and diazinon) have not been found to be carcinogenic in laboratory animals (NRC, 1982). Of the two carbamates currently used, aldicarb does not appear to be carcinogenic in rats or mice, and data on the carcinogenicity of carbaryl are inconclusive. Carbaryl is capable of reacting with nitrites under mildly acidic conditions to produce carcinogenic N-nitroso compounds (Lijinsky and Taylor, 1976). The results of mutagenicity and related short-term tests for some organochlorine pesticides did not coincide with data from carcinogenicity tests in animals (NRC, 1982).

On the basis of studies in animals, and in the absence of adequate data from epidemiologic studies, the NRC Committee on Diet, Nutrition, and Cancer concluded that kepone (chlordecone), toxaphene, hexachlorobenzene, and perhaps heptachlor (with chlordane) and lindane present a carcinogenic risk to humans (NRC, 1982).

EDB was found to produce squamous cell carcinomas of the forestomach in Osborne-Mendel rats and to a lesser extent in B6C3F$_1$ mice when administered by gavage (NCI, 1978b). Van Duuren et al. (1979) reported an increased incidence of skin papillomas, skin carcinomas, and lung tumors in Swiss mice receiving EDB by skin application. In an inhalation study sponsored by the National Toxicology Program and National Cancer Institute, EDB was found to cause tumors of the nasal cavity in Fischer 344 rats and B6C3F$_1$ mice (NCI, 1982). An inhalation study sponsored by the National Institute for Occupational Safety and Health showed EDB to be carcinogenic to Sprague-Dawley rats (Wong et al., 1982). EDB was reported to induce large numbers of sex-linked recessive lethal mutations in *Drosophila melanogaster* males (Kale and Baum, 1979).

Broad-spectrum fungicides—benomyl, ethylene-bisdithiocarbamates (EBDCs), captan, captafol, folpet, chlorothalonil—are now being studied by the EPA because of their oncogenic potential (NRC, 1987). Their use in agriculture is concentrated in humid regions of the United States, particularly in the East and the Southeast. Fungicides from this group that are widely used and thus may pose considerable health hazards as discussed below.

Benomyl (benlate) and its metabolite methyl-2-benzimidazole carbamate have been characterized as "moderately severe oncogens" in mice (NRC, 1987). Studies have been conduced on EBDCs, whose major product trade names include Maneb, Zineb, Nabam, Mancozeb, and Metiram, and their conversion product ethylenethiourea (ETU), which is produced during cooking or processing of foods treated with these fungicides. Findings include increased lung adenomas in mice fed EBDCs, increased liver and lung tumors and lymphomas in mice fed ETU, and thyroid carcinomas in rats fed ETU (NRC, 1987).

Captan (Merpan) induces adenocarcinomas and mucosal hyperplasia in both sexes of mice and causes an increase in malignant and benign kidney tumors in rats (Innes et al., 1969; NCI, 1977).

Reproductive Effects in Laboratory Animals

Teratogenesis resulting from exposure to the herbicides 2,4,5-trichlorophenoxyacetic acid and 2,4-dichlorophenoxyacetic acid was found to occur only in mouse strains with a tendency to have a high rate of spontaneous congenital abnormalities

and is limited to cleft palate, renal lesions, some other soft-tissue histological changes, and abnormalities in the frontal bones and vertebrae (Pearn, 1985). In contrast, 2,3,7,8-tetrachlorodibenzo-*p*-dioxin (2,3,7,8-TCDD) is an unusually potent teratogen in mice, rats, and hamsters (Collins and Williams, 1971; Courtney and Moore, 1971; Khera and Ruddick, 1973). TCDD is transplacentally toxic to embryos and fetuses in rodents and primates, resulting in low fetal weight and reduced litter size (Pearn, 1985).

The herbicide dimethoate, at doses causing toxicity in pregnant female Wistar rats, produced rib abnormalities in embryos and reduced fetal weight (Pearn, 1985). The herbicide diuron was teratogenic in mice at high doses (250 to 500 mg/kg of body weight) and could cause skull abnormalities (Khera and Ruddick, 1973). With the exception of dioxin, it is unlikely that in a real-life situation, humans would experience the massive exposure to herbicides that is sufficient to be teratogenic in a large susceptible mammal (Pearn, 1985).

Among the organochlorine insecticides, DDT was shown to prevent embryotoxic or teratogenic effects of several compounds such as sodium salicylate, benomyl, and chlordane in rats when given during the first 10 to 12 days of pregnancy (Shentberg and Torchinskii, 1976). Moreover, DDT at 200 ppm in diet was shown to prolong the reproductive life of rats to 14 months, as compared to 9 months in control rats (Ottoboni, 1972).

Aldrin produced alterations in the estrous cycle of rats (Ball et al., 1952) and of beagle dogs (Deichmann et al., 1971); dieldrin produced the same phenomenon in mice (Guthrie et al., 1971) and resulted in a reduction in pregnancies in rats (Treon and Cleveland, 1955) and in dogs (Deichmann et al., 1971). High doses of aldrin, dieldrin, and endrin (half the LD$_{50}$ given as a single oral dose in corn oil) produced teratogenic effects, including cleft palate, open eyes, and webbed feet in hamsters and mice (Ottolenghi et al., 1974).

Kepone adversely affected reproduction in mice, reduced hatchability in chickens at relatively high doses (Naber and Ware, 1965), and produced testicular atrophy in quail (McFarland and Lacy, 1969). Mirex at high doses (6 to 12 mg/kg of body weight) caused a reduction in pregnancies, decreased fetal weight, a significant increase in visceral anomalies, and death (Khera et al., 1976).

Among the organophosphorous insecticides, malathion and related compounds were not shown to be teratogenic. At high doses, however, they may decrease survival and growth of the progeny of treated animals (IARC, 1983). EDB was shown to induce testicular atrophy at low doses in rats (NRC, 1986).

Mutagens and Carcinogens Produced in Cooked Food

Beef grilled over a gas or charcoal fire was reported to contain a variety of PAHs (Lijinsky and Shubik, 1964; see also above section on PAHs). The source of the PAHs was the smoke generated when pyrolyzed fat dripped from meat onto hot coals (Lijinsky and Ross, 1967). When meat was cooked in a manner that prevented exposure to smoke generated by the dripping fat, contamination was either reduced or eliminated (Lijinsky and Ross, 1967).

The following mutagenic heterocyclic amines are formed from pyrolyzed proteins and amino acids:

- 3-amino-1,4-dimethyl-5H-pyrido[4,3-b]indole (Trp-P-1) and 3-amino-1-methyl-5H-pyrido[4,3-b]indole (Trp-P-2) from a tryptophan pyrolysate (Sugimura et al., 1977);
- 2-amino-6-methyldipyrido[1,2-a:3'2'-d]imidazole (Glu-P-1) and 2-aminodipyrido[1,2-a:3',2'-d]imidazole (Glu-P-2) from a glutamic acid pyrolysate (Yamamoto et al., 1978);
- 3,4-cyclopentenopyrido[3,2-a]carbazole (Lys-P-1) from pyrolyzed lysine (Wakabayashi et al., 1983);
- 2-amino-5-phenylpyridine (Phe-P-1) from phenylalanine pyrolysate (Sugimura et al., 1977); and
- amino-α-carboline (AαC) and methylamino-α-carboline (MeAαC) from a pyrolysate of soybean globulin (D. Yoshida et al., 1978).

Mutagenic aminoimidazoquinoline (IQ) and aminomethylimidazoquinoline (MeIQ) were isolated from broiled sun-dried sardines (Kasai et al., 1980), and aminomethylimidazoquinoline (MeIQx) from fried beef (Kasai et al., 1981). All these heterocyclic amines were highly mutagenic toward *Salmonella typhimurium* TA98 treated with S9 mix (Sugimura et al., 1986). Four of the mutagenic pyrolysates—Trp-P-1, Trp-P-2, Glu-P-1, and AαC—induced sister chromatid exchanges in a permanent line of human lymphoblastoid cells (Tohda et al., 1980), and the basic fraction extracted from pyrolyzed tryptophan caused mutation resulting in resistance to ouabain or 8-azaguanine in cultured Chinese hamster lung cells (Inui et al., 1980). Trp-P-1, Trp-P-2, and Glu-P-1 transformed primary Syrian golden hamster embryo cells (Takayama et al., 1979). Several of these mutagenic pyrolysates were tested for carcinogenicity in rodents.

CD$_2$F$_1$ (BALB)/c AnNCrj × DBA/2NCrjF$_1$, Charles River, Japan, Atsugi, Kanagawa) mice given IQ at 0.03% in the diet produced hepatocellular carcinomas and adenomas, squamous cell carcinomas of the forestomach, and lung tumors (Ohgaki et al., 1984). Hepatocellular carcinomas, adenocarcinomas in the large intestine, squamous cell carcinomas in the skin, Zymbal gland, and clitoral gland, and mammary tumors were induced in Fischer 344 rats given 0.03% IQ (Takayama et al., 1984; Tanaka et al., 1985). Ishikawa et al. (1985) observed that IQ activates *Ha-ras* and *raf* oncogenes in rat hepatomas. MeIQ at 0.04% induced a high incidence of squamous cell carcinomas, hepatocellular carcinomas and adenomas, and intestinal adenocarcinomas and adenomas in the forestomach of mice (Ohgaki et al., 1985).

Liver tumors (hepatocellular carcinomas or adenomas) were induced in CDF$_1$ mice fed Trp-P-1 and Trp-P-2 at 0.02% (Matsukura et al., 1981). Hepatocellular carcinomas were induced in Fischer 344 rats given Glu-P-1, Glu-P-2, and MeAαC; AαC induced blood vessel tumors (mainly hemangioendothelial sarcomas) as well as liver tumors (mostly hepatocellular carcinomas and adenomas) when given to CDF$_2$ mice at 0.05 and 0.08% (Ohgaki et al., 1984). In Fischer 344 rats, Glu-P-1 and Glu-P-2 at 0.05% induced hepatocellular carcinomas, adenocarcinomas in the small and large intestine, and squamous cell carcinomas in the Zymbal and clitoral glands. Glu-P-2 activated the *N-ras* oncogene in the small intestine of a rat (Sugimura et al., 1986). MeAαC induced severe atrophy of the salivary glands and cancer cells in pancreas of rats (Takayama et al., 1985).

The presence of a carcinogenic chemical in a pyrolyzed amino acid or protein mixture does not necessarily imply that the carcinogen will also be present in normally cooked, uncharred food (NRC, 1982). Data on the quantities in food indicate that intakes of heterocyclic amines are negligible (one five-thousandths of the dose needed to develop cancers in 50% of animals fed carcinogens over their lifetime). Thus, these compounds may not pose a serious risk for cancer in humans (Sugimura et al., 1986).

Ohnishi et al. (1985) observed the formation of the highly mutagenic and carcinogenic compounds 1-nitropyrene and dinitropyrenes in grilled chicken. An activated *Ki-ras* gene was found in a rat fibrosarcoma induced by repeated subcutaneous injections of 1,8-dinitropyrene, and activation of the *Ha-ras* gene was reported in a tumor induced in a rat by 1,6-dinitropyrene (Ochiai et al., 1985).

Browning of food results from the reaction of amines with sugars and produces substances that are mutagenic; the increase in mutagenic activity over time parallels the increase in browning (Shinohara et al., 1980). Pyrazine and four of its alkyl products formed by heating mixtures of sugars and amino acids were nonmutagenic in *S. typhimurium* but induced chromosome aberrations in cultured Chinese hamster ovary cells (Stich et al., 1980). Commercial caramel and caramelized samples of several sugars prepared by heating sugar solutions also caused chromosome aberrations in Chinese hamster ovary cells (Stich et al., 1981a). Furan and six of its derivatives, which can be produced in foods by heating carbohydrates (Maga, 1979), also caused chromosome aberrations in Chinese hamster ovary cells, but they were not mutagenic in bacteria (Stich et al., 1981b).

Cooking accelerates the rancidity reaction of cooking oils and fat in meat (Shorland et al., 1981), thereby leading to increased consumption of mutagens and carcinogens (Ames, 1983).

Metabolites of Animal Origin

Tryptophan and Its Metabolites

Tryptophan is one of the essential amino acids and is present in most proteins. Proteins of animal origin contain $\simeq 1.4\%$ tryptophan. Most vegetable proteins contain $\simeq 1\%$, but corn products have only 0.6% (Orr and Watt, 1957). Average intake of tryptophan in the United States is estimated to be 1.2 g daily, representing about 1.2% of dietary protein (Munro and Crim, 1980).

Animal studies show that tryptophan is carcinogenic in dogs and exerts a promoting effect on the formation of urinary bladder tumors in rats. In addition, four of its metabolites (3-hydroxykynurenine, 3-hydroxyanthranilic acid, 2-amino-3-hydroxyacetophenone, and xanthurenic acid-8-methyl ether) induced bladder tumors when implanted as pellets in the urinary bladders of mice (Clayson and Garner, 1976). However, attempts to relate the development of tumors in the urinary bladder of humans to abnormalities in the metabolism of tryptophan have not been definitive (Clayson and Garner, 1976). Tryptophan and its metabolites were not mutagenic in the Ames *Salmonella* assay (Bowden et al., 1976).

Ethyl Carbamate (Urethane)

Ethyl carbamate, or urethane, is a product of fermentation in foods and beverages (e.g., wines, bread, beers, and yogurt). It has been detected in a wide range of alcoholic beverages at levels up to several thousand ppb (Mitchell and Jacobson, 1987).

Ethyl carbamate was shown to induce tumors in rodents when administered orally, by inhalation, or by subcutaneous or intraperitoneal injection. The susceptible tissues include the lungs, lymphoid tissue, skin, liver, mammary gland, and Zymbal gland (Iversen, 1984).

The role of naturally occurring ethyl carbamate in foods in the development of cancer in humans is unknown, but the levels found in foods are very low in comparison to those used to induce tumors in laboratory animals (NRC, 1982). Ethyl carbamate was not mutagenic in the Ames *Salmonella* assay (Simmon, 1979) or in the host-mediated assay (Simmon et al., 1979); however, it induced cell transformations (Pienta, 1981) and sister chromatid exchanges (Goon and Conner, 1984; Neft et al., 1985).

NATURALLY OCCURRING TOXICANTS IN FOODS

Mycotoxins

Occurrence and Exposure

Mycotoxins are toxic secondary products produced by the metabolism of molds. At least 45 mycotoxins have been identified as eliciting some type of carcinogenic or mutagenic response; only 17 of them have been reported to occur naturally in food (Stoloff, 1982).

The most thoroughly studied of this group are the aflatoxins, which are generally restricted to crops invaded by the molds *Aspergillus flavus* and *A. parasiticus* before harvest. In the United States, humans are unavoidably exposed to aflatoxins mostly in corn and peanuts (FDA, 1979b); cottonseed is also frequently attacked. Other direct dietary sources, such as tree nuts (including almonds, walnuts, pecans, and pistachios), are of minor significance, either because contamination is infrequent or because only small quantities are consumed. It is unlikely that significant exposures result from the ingestion of aflatoxin residues in tissues of animals fed aflatoxin-contaminated feed (Stoloff, 1979). In the United States, the maximum allowable limit for total aflatoxins in peanuts is 20 μg/kg (20 ppb).

Evidence Associating Mycotoxins with Chronic Diseases

Epidemiologic Studies

Various studies conducted in Africa and Asia have shown strong correlations between estimated levels of ingested aflatoxins and liver cancer incidence (Linsell and Peers, 1977). Two such studies were conducted in different areas of Swaziland (Keen and Martin, 1971) and Uganda (Alpert et al., 1971). Later studies from Swaziland (Peers et al., 1976, 1987), from the Murang'a district of Kenya (Peers and Linsell, 1973), and from Mozambique, which has perhaps the highest rates of liver cancer in the world (van Rensburg et al., 1974, 1985), have confirmed strong associations between liver cancer incidence and estimated levels of aflatoxins. Oettlé (1965) suggested that the geographic distribution of liver cancer in Africa could be due to differential exposures to aflatoxins in the diet.

In Asia, an overall correlation between estimated aflatoxin intake and liver cancer incidence was found in two regions of Thailand (Shank et al., 1972a,b; Wogan, 1975). In Guangxi Province in China and in Taiwan, the frequency of food contamination with aflatoxins has been correlated with liver cancer mortality (Armstrong, 1980; Tung and Ling, 1968). In several areas of China, Yen and Shen (1986) found that food contamination with aflatoxin B_1 is a high-risk factor for primary liver cancer. In a case-control study in the Philippines, Bulatao-Jayme et al. (1982), utilizing data on mean aflatoxin contamination levels in dietary items and relating them to individual consumption, reported an increased risk of hepatocellular cancer for those with high intakes of aflatoxins, suggesting a dose–response relationship.

Several studies have shown a high correlation between exposure to hepatitis B virus and primary hepatocellular carcinoma (Ayoola, 1984; Beasley et al., 1981; Chien et al., 1981; Prince et al., 1975; Simons et al., 1972; Stoloff, 1983; Stora and Dvorackova, 1987; Tong et al., 1971; Vogel et al., 1970). Van Rensburg (1977) and van Rensburg et al. (1985) concluded that preexisting viral infection may be necessary for malignant transformation by aflatoxins.

In three studies, an attempt was made to take serological evidence of chronic hepatitis B infection into account while evaluating elevated aflatoxin ingestion. In China, aflatoxin levels in both diet and urine were found to be related to the incidence of hepatocellular cancer, but corresponding differences in the prevalence of hepatitis B carriers were not found (Sun and Chu, 1984; Yeh et al., 1985). In Swaziland, liver cancer incidence was strongly associated with estimated levels of aflatoxins in food. In this study, exposure to aflatoxins was a more important determinant of

liver cancer incidence than was the prevalence of hepatitis B infection in a multivariate analysis (Peers et al., 1987).

Animal Studies and Short-Term Tests

Aflatoxin B_1, the most potent hepatocarcinogen known, was reported to induce tumors in many animal species, including ducks, hamsters, mice, rats, and trout. The male Fischer 344 rat was most sensitive (NRC, 1982).

Aflatoxin B_1 was also shown to be mutagenic to microbial and mammalian cells (Mangold et al., 1986; Ueno and Kubota, 1976; Ueno et al., 1978; Umeda et al., 1977) and to enhance transformation of metabolically activated C3H/10T½ cells in culture (Billings et al., 1985). Aflatoxin M_1, the metabolite of aflatoxin B_1, was mutagenic in the Ames *Salmonella* assay (Wong and Hsieh, 1976) but was inactive in the *Bacillus subtilis rec* assay (Ueno and Kubota, 1976).

Several mycotoxins other than aflatoxins that may be found in food (e.g., sterigmatocystin, ochratoxin A, zearalenone, patulin, griseofulvin, luteoskyrin, and cyclochlorotine) were shown to be mutagenic in bacterial systems and other short-term tests, had promoting activities, or were carcinogenic in laboratory animals (Bendele et al., 1985; Creppy et al., 1985; Curry et al., 1984; NRC, 1982); however, there are no epidemiologic studies on their role in human neoplasia.

Hydrazines in Mushrooms

Several hydrazines and hydrazones known to be carcinogenic in mice and mutagenic in *Salmonella typhimurium* have been isolated from two commonly eaten mushrooms, *Agaricus bisphorus* (the commonly eaten mushroom) and *Gyromitra esculenta* (false morel) (Toth, 1984; Toth and Patil, 1981). The uncooked mushroom *A. bisphorus* was shown to induce tumors in the bone, forestomach, liver, and lung of mice (Toth and Erickson, 1986). The precise contribution of exposure to these carcinogens to cancers in humans is difficult to determine due to the lack of epidemiologic studies (Palmer and Mathews, 1986). However, Prival (1984) estimated that the consumption of 4-hydroxymethylbenzonium from raw mushrooms in the United States is 0.058 mg/kg or about 1/7,000th of the dose that produced tumors in 31% of mice tested. If only 1% of the mushrooms sold in the United States are eaten raw, the cancer risk is estimated to be less than one per million per lifetime in the U.S. population.

Plant Constituents and Metabolites

Occurrence and Exposure

Flavonoid glycosides, especially quercetin and kaempferol glycosides, are found in the edible portion of most food plants, including citrus fruits, berries, leafy vegetables, roots, tubers, spices, cereal grains, tea, and cocoa. Many of these flavonoid glycosides are known to be mutagenic (NRC, 1982). Brown (1980) estimated that the intake of all mutagenic glycosides in the United States was 50 mg/day, i.e., about 1/70th of the dose of quercetin that produced tumors in rats in one study (Pamukcu et al., 1980).

Several alkyl benzene compounds are found in herbs and spices. For example, estragole is found in sweet basil and tarragon, and its daily intake is estimated to be 1 μg/kg. On the basis of the results of a carcinogenesis bioassay in female CD/1 mice fed a 0.23% estragole diet for 12 months, the estimated lifetime carcinogenic risk would be one cancer in 420,000 people (Prival, 1984). Other alkylbenzene derivatives found in herbs include safrole, methyleugenol, β-asarone, and isosafrole. Plants in nature as well as those in the diet of humans synthesize a large amount of toxic chemicals, apparently as a primary defense against varieties of bacteria, fungi, insects, or animal predators (Ames, 1983). Some of these toxins are discussed below.

Evidence Associating Plant Constituents with Chronic Disease

A number of epidemiologic studies have focused on the consumption of fruits and vegetables in the human diet. In several of them, intake of fiber-containing foods was found to have a protective effect against colorectal cancer (see Chapter 10). In other studies, intake of foods containing vitamin A or β-carotene was found to have a protective effect against lung cancer (see Chapter 11). In still others (see Chapter 12), the contribution of vitamin C made by fruit and vegetable consumption was found to have a protective effect against stomach cancer. In one study of colorectal cancer, Macquart-Moulin et al. (1986) found the protective effect of vegetable intake to be strongest for vegetables lowest in fiber, suggesting that some factors other than fiber in vegetables were responsible for the protective effect.

Other epidemiologic studies on the association of fruit or vegetable consumption with cancer risk did not focus specifically on fiber, vitamin A, β-carotene, or vitamin C intake. For example, in a case-control study of colorectal cancer, Graham et al. (1978) found evidence that a protective effect was provided by cabbage and other vegetables of the *Brassica* genus. The protective effects were particularly related to the frequent ingestion of raw vegetables, especially cabbage, Brussels sprouts, and broccoli. Haenszel et al. (1980) also found an inverse association between cabbage consumption and colorectal cancer in a case-control study in Japan. These associations may be due to the inhibition of the microsomal monooxygenase system, which in turn will inhibit the activation of chemical carcinogens (Wattenberg, 1981). In a subsequent case-control study of colorectal cancer, Miller et al. (1983) found only weak evidence of a protective effect of such vegetables only in females, after taking into account saturated fatty acid intake.

In several epidemiologic studies, evidence that vegetable consumption had a protective effect against lung cancer was found (Hirayama, 1986; MacLennan et al., 1977; Ziegler et al., 1986). These studies have generally been interpreted as providing further evidence for a protective effect of β-carotene. It is possible, however, that other factors in the vegetables may have been responsible for some of the protective effect. Indeed, in the cohort study by Hirayama (1986), a protective effect of green and yellow vegetable consumption was found for several cancer sites, including the stomach, colon, and lung (see Chapters 11 and 12).

In summary, there is consistent evidence that fruit and vegetable consumption is protective against several cancers. Although much of this effect could be due to components of dietary fiber (for colorectal cancer), vitamin C (for stomach cancer), and β-carotene (for lung cancer), the possibility remains that other protective factors in foods may be responsible for at least part of the effects. Therefore, in considering appropriate preventive measures, consumption of the relevant foods—not the putative protective components of those foods—should be encouraged.

Pyrrolizidine Alkaloids

Pyrrolizidine alkaloids are found in many inedible plant species, including the genera *Senecio* (ragworts), *Cortalaria* (rattleboxes), and *Heliotropium* (heliotropes), in amounts ranging from traces to as much as 5% of the dry weight of the plant. Alkaloids that are derivatives of 1-hydroxymethyl-1,2-dehydropyrrolizine have been shown to induce liver tumors in animals (Hirono et al., 1981; Schoental, 1968). Such lesions have been found in female rats fed these alkaloids during pregnancy

(Newberne, 1968; Schoental, 1959)—a phenomenon with a counterpart in some African tribes that prescribe alkaloid-containing herbal mixtures to pregnant women. Several of these alkaloids induce DNA repair synthesis and sister chromatoid exchanges (Bruggeman and van der Hoeven, 1985; Griffin and Segall, 1986; Mori et al., 1985b). Recent studies suggest that the hepatocarcinogenicity of pyrrolizidine alkaloids may be due to their promoting effects on initiated hepatocytes rather than to their very weak initiating activity (Hayes et al., 1985). No epidemiologic studies are available on these compounds.

Bracken Fern Toxins

Bracken fern (*Pteridium aquilinum*) grows widely in nature and is consumed by humans in several parts of the world, especially in Japan (Hirono, 1981). For at least 30 years, it has been known that consumption of this plant damages the bone marrow and intestinal mucosa of cattle, but the harmful component of this plant has not been identified (Pamukcu et al., 1980). In a cohort study in Japan, high risk of esophageal cancer was associated with daily intake of bracken fern (Hirayama, 1979). On the other hand, in a case-control study in Canada, no association between bladder cancer and consumption of fiddlehead greens (related to bracken fern) was found (Howe et al., 1980). Indirect evidence for carcinogenicity is derived from observations that milk from cows fed high levels of bracken fern contained compounds shown to be carcinogenic in rats (Pamukcu et al., 1980). Carcinomas of the intestine, urinary bladder, and kidney were observed in rats fed high levels of fresh or powdered milk from cows that had consumed 1 g of bracken fern per kilogram of body weight daily for approximately 2 years, but not in rats fed milk from control cows (Pamukcu et al., 1980). In another laboratory, however, dietary administration of quercetin (which occurs as a conjugate in the fern) did not result in a high incidence of tumors in ACI rats (Hirono et al., 1981). Mutagenic components of bracken fern (aquilide A and quercetin) and one that is carcinogenic and mutagenic (ptaquiloside) with a structure similar to aquilide have reportedly been isolated and identified (Hirono, 1986; Mori et al., 1985a; Umezawa et al., 1977; van der Hoeven et al., 1983).

Cycasin

Cycasin (methylazoxymethanol-α-glucoside) is one of the most potent carcinogens found in plants (IARC, 1976; Magee et al., 1976). This compound and at least one related glucoside (macrozamin) are present in the palm-like cycad trees of the family Cycadaceae. These trees have provided food for humans and their livestock in tropical and subtropical regions. The crude flour prepared from the unwashed nuts of these trees induced kidney and liver tumors in rats when fed at 2% of the diet (Zedeck, 1984). When administered orally, cycasin was highly carcinogenic in the liver, kidney, and colon of rats, and induced tumors in other species (Laqueur and Spatz, 1968).

Cycasin was not mutagenic in the standard Ames *Salmonella* assay (Ames et al., 1975), but it became mutagenic when preincubated with almond α-glucosidase (Matsushima et al., 1979). In Guam and Okinawa, the ingestion of cycasin in cycad nuts has been proposed as an etiologic factor in the development of liver cancer in humans, which occurs at high rates in those countries. However, in a descriptive study conducted in the Miyako Islands of Okinawa, no correlation between mortality from hepatoma and the ingestion of cycad nuts was found (Hirono et al., 1970).

OTHER SUBSTANCES   Safrole, estragole, methyleugenol, and related compounds are present in many edible plants and are carcinogenic in rodents; several of their metabolites have mutagenic potential (Miller et al., 1979). Black pepper contains a small amount of safrole and approximately 10% of the closely related compound piperine (Concon et al., 1979). Extracts of black pepper produce tumors in mice at various sites (Concon et al., 1979).

Linear furocoumarins (e.g., psoralen derivatives) are potent light-activated carcinogens and mutagens that are widespread in the Umbelliferae, such as celery, parsnip, figs, and parsley (Ivie et al., 1981). Psoralens are activated by sunlight and then damage DNA, induce tumors (Ashwood-Smith and Poulton, 1981), and produce oxygen radicals (Potapenko et al., 1982).

The glycoalkaloids solanine and chaconine, which are present in potatoes, are strong cholinesterase inhibitors and potential teratogens (Hall, 1979; Jadhav et al., 1981). Quinones and their phenolic precursors act as electrophiles producing semiquinone radicals that either react directly with DNA (Morimoto et al., 1983) or produce superoxide radicals (Kappus and Sies, 1981), which oxidize fat in cell membranes by a peroxidation chain reaction that generates mutagens and carcinogens (Brown, 1980; Levine et al., 1982). Plants such as rhubarb contain mutagenic quinone derivatives (Brown, 1980). Some dietary phenols (e.g., catechol derivatives) spontaneously autooxidize to quinones, producing hydrogen peroxides (Stich et al., 1981c). Catechol is a strong promotor and induces DNA damage (Carmella et al., 1982).

Allyl isothiocyanate, a major flavor ingredient in oil of mustard and horseradish, is a toxin that causes chromosome aberrations in hamster cells (Kasamaki et al., 1982) and is carcinogenic in rats (Dunnick et al., 1982). Gossypol, a major toxin in cottonseed oil, accounting for approximately 1% of its dry weight, was reported to be a potent initiator and promotor of carcinogens in mouse skin (Haroz and Thomasson, 1980). It also caused dominant lethal mutations (Ames, 1983), produced genetic damage in embryos sired by treated male rats, and caused pathological changes in the testes of rats and humans, leading to abnormal sperm and male sterility (Ames, 1983), probably through production of oxygen radicals (Coburn et al., 1980).

Cyclopropenoid fatty acids present in oils from seed plants of *Malvacealidae* (e.g., cotton, okra) are carcinogenic in trout and enhance the carcinogenicity of aflatoxins in trout. They are also mitogenic in rats, have a variety of toxic effects in farm animals, and cause atherosclerosis in rabbits, probably through the formation of peroxides and radicals (Hendricks et al., 1980).

Leguminous plants such as lupine contain potent teratogens. One such teratogen is anagyrine, which causes crooked calf abnormality in cows and goats foraging on these plants and passes to humans through milk (Ames, 1983).

Sesquiterpene lactone, a major toxin in the white sap of the poison lettuce *Lactuca virosa*, has been shown to be mutagenic (Manners et al., 1978). Canavanine, which accounts for 15% of the dry weight of alfalfa sprouts, appears to be the active ingredient causing a severe lupus erythematosus-like syndrome in monkeys. This condition is characterized by defects in the immune system, chromosome breaks, and other types of tissue injury (Malinow et al., 1982) believed to result from the production of oxygen radicals (Emerit et al., 1980).

The toxins vicine and convicine, which account for 2% of the dry weight of the broad bean *Vicia faba*, can lead to severe hemolytic anemia in some humans. This is caused by enzymatic hydrolysis of vicine to its aglycone—divicine—which forms a quinone that generates oxygen radicals in sensitive individuals ingesting the fava beans (Chevion and Navok, 1983).

Other plant constituents and metabolites, such as allylic propenylic benzene derivatives, estrogenic compounds, methylxanthines, thiourea, tannic acid and tannins, coumarin, and parasorbic acid, have been shown to be carcinogenic in animals or mutagenic in short-term tests. Many of these naturally occurring mutagens and carcinogens act by producing free radicals that damage DNA and thus may lead to cancer and mutations (Ames, 1983). Ames et al. (1987) suggested that the hazards from several man-made chemicals are much less severe than those of natural substances, but he did not conclude whether the natural exposure is of major or minor importance. Epstein and Swartz (1988) and Perera and Boffetta (1988) have argued against the conclusions of Ames.

SUMMARY

There is no convincing epidemiologic evidence relating coffee or tea to any type of cancer. Results of mutagenicity and carcinogenicity studies show that caffeine is mutagenic in microorganisms, but its ability to induce mutations in higher organisms or to produce tumors in animals is not certain. There are no adequate carcinogenicity studies on tea or tannins. A few short-term tests in microorganisms showed that tea is mutagenic. The strongest evidence for a possible deleterious health effect of coffee drinking is its association with increased LDL cholesterol levels. However, there is no convincing evidence from epidemiologic studies that the level of coffee consumed in North America increases risk of death from cardiovascular diseases. Caffeine, however, has been shown to cause reproductive defects, to be teratogenic in rodents, and, possibly, to lead to spontaneous abortion, stillbirth, preterm deliveries, and low birth weight in humans.

Nearly 3,000 substances are intentionally added to foods during processing in the United States. Another estimated 12,000 chemicals, such as polyvinyl chloride and acrylonitrile, which are used in food packaging, are classified as indirect additives. However, the annual per-capita exposure to most of these substances is very small. Except for the studies on nonnutritive sweeteners and on nitrates, nitrites, and N-nitroso compounds, very few epidemiologic studies have been conducted to examine the effect of food additives on cancer incidence.

Of the few direct food additives that have been tested and found to be carcinogenic in animals, all except saccharin have been banned from use in the food supply. The major deleterious health effect of artificial sweetener use, for which animal data provide evidence, is increased risk of bladder cancer. The substantial amount of epidemiologic evidence collected to date, however, indicates that the levels of saccharin and cyclamate in most diets do not confer an increased risk of bladder cancer in humans. Animal studies and short-term tests indicate that saccharin and possibly cyclamate have tumor-promoting potential. Cyclamate and its conversion metabolite cyclohexylamine have been shown to cause testicular atrophy in rodents. The nonnutritive sweetener aspartame does not appear to be carcinogenic.

Nitrates appear to be neither carcinogenic nor mutagenic. Nitrites are probably not direct carcinogens, but they are mutagenic in microbial systems. There is some epidemiologic evidence that nitrites and N-nitroso compounds play a role in the development of gastric and esophageal cancer.

There are no epidemiologic data on the relationship between the antioxidants BHA and BHT and human health. Animal studies showed that BHA induces carcinogenesis in the forestomach of rats and hamsters. The isomer 3-tert-butyl-4-hydroxyanisole seems responsible for this effect. It also has an inhibitory effect on the development of tumors, depending on the time of administration. It is not genotoxic, i.e., it does not damage DNA. Animal studies show that BHT enhances liver tumors and has a tumor-promoting effect. It can inhibit neoplasia induced by a number of chemicals depending on its level in the diet, the type of diet in which it is administered, and the dosage of the carcinogen given. It does not appear to be genotoxic and can either enhance or inhibit the mutagenic potency of other chemicals.

In the absence of epidemiologic studies, experimental evidence to date would suggest that exposure to individual food colors is unlikely to increase the burden of cancer in humans. Minute residues of a few indirect contaminants from food packaging known to produce cancer in animals (e.g., polyvinyl chloride and acrylonitrile) or to be carcinogenic in humans (e.g., polyvinyl chloride) are occasionally detected in foods. There is no evidence suggesting that such contamination or the increasing use of other food additives has contributed significantly to the overall risk of cancer for humans. Indeed, the decreasing incidence of stomach cancer (see Chapter 5) suggests that they have had little or no adverse effect. However, the lack of a detectable effect could be due to the relatively recent use of some of these substances, to lack of

carcinogenicity, or to the inability of epidemiologic techniques to detect weak effects of contaminants against the background of common cancers from other causes.

The results of standard chronic toxicity tests indicate that a number of environmental contaminants in foods (e.g., some organochlorine pesticides, PCBs, and PAHs) cause cancer in laboratory animals. Some epidemiologic studies have shown a five- to sixfold increase in non-Hodgkin's lymphoma in workers exposed to phenoxyacetic acid herbicides. These herbicides were also found to be teratogenic in mice. Reproductive and teratogenic defects have been attributed to some of the phenoxyacetic acid herbicides and dioxin, as well as to some organochlorine insecticides (aldrin, dieldrin, endrin, kepone, and mirex).

Various mutagens and carcinogens are formed during broiling, charring, and grilling of meat and fish, and browning of foods. However, the amounts formed may be too small to pose a serious risk for the developement of cancer in humans.

Aflatoxins, mycotoxins that occur naturally in grains and other food commodities, are carcinogenic in several species of animals, including mice, rats, trout, ducks, and monkeys, and there is evidence of a dose–response. In addition, they have been shown to be mutagenic in bacterial and mammalian systems. Several other mycotoxins found in food are carcinogenic or mutagenic in laboratory tests. With the exception of aflatoxins, which have been implicated in liver cancer in some parts of the world, there is no epidemiologic evidence concerning other mycotoxins and neoplasia in humans. Because levels of aflatoxins in foods in the United States are generally controlled, the risk to human health is considered negligible.

Hydrazine derivatives of two mushrooms—Agaricus bisporus and Gyromitra esculenta—both of which are consumed throughout the world, appear to be carcinogenic in mice and, under certain conditions, in hamsters. They are also mutagenic in bacteria. The significance of these findings for risk to humans cannot be determined, since there are no epidemiologic data.

Several pyrrolizidine alkaloids are carcinogenic in animals or mutagenic in several test systems. Cycad nuts, which are eaten in some parts of the world, contain cycasin (methylazoxymethanol-β-glucoside), a compound known to be carcinogenic in animals. It is also mutagenic in the Ames Salmonella assay after addition of β-glucosidase. Long- and short-term tests showed that bracken fern is carcinogenic in animals and may also be mutagenic. No evidence has been presented for the carcinogenicity of pyrrolizidine alkaloids, bracken fern, and cycasin in humans. Other constituents of plants, such as methylxanthines, thiourea, tannins, coumarin, parasorbic acid, safrole, estragole and eugenol, furocoumarins, glycolalkaloids, quinones and their phenolic precursors, allyl isothiocyanate, gossypol, cyclopropenoid fatty acids, and plant estrogens such as zearalenone, are carcinogenic in laboratory animals or mutagenic in bacterial or mammalian cell systems.

Overall, there is shortage of data on the complete range of nonnutritive substances present in the diet. Thus, no reliable estimates can be made of the most significant exposures. Exposure to individual nonnutritive chemicals, in the minute quantities normally present in the average diet, is unlikely to contribute to the overall cancer risk to humans in the United States. The risk from simultaneous exposure to many such compounds cannot be quantified on the basis of current knowledge.

The life span of humans in Western countries is steadily increasing, and age-specific mortalities from most common cancers such as breast and colon cancer show, at most, small increases over the past generation and many were decreased. These facts suggest that our society as a whole is not facing a health crisis posed by environmental agents. Nevertheless, potentially teratogenic, carcinogenic, or mutagenic chemicals and other pollutants do exist. Therefore, various regulatory decisions regarding avoidance of exposure need to be made. These decisions are difficult to reach, since they must be based on studies conducted in other organisms and the resulting data are difficult to extrapolate to humans. In many cases human exposure standards are inaccurate; therefore a conservative stance not to allow the introduction of potentially noxious agents is mandatory. Factors affecting risk assessment include interspecies variation and human variability due to intraspecies genetic variation. Since the latency period between initiation and clinical cancer may last a generation, careful epidemiologic surveillance for various cancers needs to be continued.

DIRECTIONS FOR RESEARCH

There are two major limitations to drawing definitive conclusions about the association between nonnutritive dietary constituents and chronic diseases: a dearth of precise data on the range of these chemicals in the diet and the poorly understood potential for synergistic or antagonistic interactions among nutritive and nonnutritive dietary substances. The following directions for research are aimed at filling these gaps in knowledge. With the exception of coffee, which has been weakly linked to hypercholesterolemia and cardiovascular diseases, nonnutritive substances are generally associated primarily with cancer risk. Therefore, the majority of the recommendations apply only to cancer.

• Research is needed on the mechanisms by which coffee and its constituents affect serum cholesterol levels. Possible modifiers of such adverse effects—e.g., additives such as cream, milk, lemon, and sugar, and the temperature at which beverages are consumed—should also be investigated. Studies should also be undertaken to obtain accurate measures of the intake of these beverages and to examine the methods used to decaffeinate them.

• There is a need for better measurements of the average intake of food additives as well as the distribution of intake among population subgroups. Such studies should assess exposure to both direct and indirect additives. If populations with significantly different levels of exposure are identified, epidemiologic studies should be undertaken to examine the effect of major additives on health.

• Additional studies should be conducted to determine the relevance of the tumor-promoting effects of BHT and the tumor-inhibiting effects of both BHT and BHA.

• Data from the series of USDA's Nationwide Food Consumption Surveys and the National Center for Health Statistics' Health and Nutrition Examination Surveys should be examined to see what information they can provide about exposure to and the long-term health effects of additives. Future surveys might be designed to include such data after appropriate markers are identified.

• Studies are needed to determine the effect of diet on the endogenous formation of mutagens, such as nitrosamines and fecal and urinary mutagens, and to assess the carcinogenicity of such mutagens. Efforts to identify nitrosatable precursors and endogenously produced mutagens should be continued.

• Studies are needed to characterize the distribution of intake of such carcinogens and mutagens in foods as hydrazines in mushrooms, aflatoxins and other mycotoxins, polycyclic aromatic hydrocarbons, mutagenic flavonoids and glyoxals, and mutagens produced during cooking. The data should include the patterns and frequencies of household and commercial cooking practices, cooking temperatures, and the duration of cooking for various types of food in which mutagens or carcinogens are produced during heating.

- Epidemiologic studies, including intervention trials when appropriate, should be conducted to determine whether consumption of foods containing high concentrations of nonnutritive inhibitors of carcinogenesis results in a lower incidence of cancer.

- Additional techniques for assessing the mutagenic effects of chemicals on human cells in vivo should be developed. Such techniques should be applied to diets believed to present a high or low risk for cancer in humans.

REFERENCES

Abe, S., and M. Sasaki. 1977. Chromosome aberrations and sister chromatid exchanges in Chinese hamster cells exposed to various chemicals. J. Natl. Cancer Inst. 58:1635–1641.

Abrams, I.J. 1977. Frequency Distributions of Intake of Caffeine Expected Milligrams per Kilogram of Body Weight per Person—Based on a 14-Day Average for Six Food Categories by 5 Age Groups. Classified by Their Intake of Caffeine From All Foods and Beverages. Market Research Corporation of America, Northbrook, Ill. 1044 pp.

Aeschbacher, H.U., and H.P. Würzner. 1980. An evaluation of instant and regular coffee in the Ames mutagenicity test. Toxicol. Lett. 5:139–145.

Aeschbacher, H.U., H. Milon, A. Poot, and H.P. Würzner. 1980a. Effect of caffeine on rat offspring from treated dams. Toxicol. Lett. 7:71–77.

Aeschbacher, H.U., C. Chappuis, and H.P. Würzner. 1980b. Mutagenicity testing of coffee: a study of problems encountered with the Ames Salmonella test system. Food Cosmet. Toxicol. 18:605–613.

Alpert, M.E., M.S. Hutt, G.N. Wogan, and C.S. Davidson. 1971. Association between aflatoxin content of food and hepatoma frequency in Uganda. Cancer 28:253–260.

Althoff, J., A. Cardesa, P. Pour, and P. Shubik. 1975. A chronic study of artificial sweeteners in Syrian golden hamsters. Cancer Lett. 1:21–24.

Ames, B.N. 1983. Dietary carcinogens and anticarcinogens. Oxygen radicals and degenerative diseases. Science 221:1256–1264.

Ames, B.N., J. McCann, and E. Yamasaki. 1975. Methods for detecting carcinogens and mutagens with the Salmonella/mammalian-microsome mutagenicity test. Mutat. Res. 31:347–364.

Ames, B.N., R. Magaw, and L.S. Gold. 1987. Ranking possible carcinogenic hazards. Science 236:271–280.

Andrews, A.W., E.S. Zawistowski, and C.R. Valentine. 1976. A comparison of the mutagenic properties of vinyl chloride and methyl chloride. Mutat. Res. 40:273–276.

Armijo, R., and A.H. Coulson. 1975. Epidemiology of stomach cancer in Chile—the role of nitrogen fertilizers. Int. J. Epidemiol. 4:301–309.

Armijo, R., A. Gonzalez, M. Orellana, A.H. Coulson, J.W. Sayre, and R. Detels. 1981. Epidemiology of gastric cancer

in Chile. II. Nitrate exposures and stomach cancer frequency. Int. J. Epidemiol. 10:57–62.

Armstrong, B. 1980. The epidemiology of cancer in the People's Republic of China. Int. J. Epidemiol. 9:305–315.

Armstrong, B., and R. Doll. 1974. Bladder cancer mortality in England and Wales in relation to cigarette smoking and saccharin consumption. Br. J. Prev. Soc. Med. 28:233–240.

Arnold, D.L., C.A. Moodie, B. Stavric, D.R. Stoltz, H.C. Grice, and I.C. Munro. 1977. Canadian Saccharin Study. Science 197:320.

Arnold, D.L., C.A. Moodie, H.C. Grice, S.M. Charbonneau, B. Stavric, B.T. Collins, P.F. McGuire, Z.Z. Zawidzka, and I.C. Munro. 1980. Long-term toxicity of orthotoluenesulfonamide and sodium saccharin in the rat. Toxicol. Appl. Pharmacol. 52:113–152.

Ashby, J. 1985. The genotoxicity of sodium saccharin and sodium chloride in relation to their cancer-promoting properties. Food Chem. Toxicol. 23:507–519.

Ashwood-Smith, M.J., and G.A. Poulton. 1981. Inappropriate regulations governing the use of oil of bergamot in suntan preparations. Mutat. Res. 85:389–390.

Ax, R.L., R.J. Collier, and J.R. Lodge. 1976. Effects of dietary caffeine on the testis of the domestic fowl, Gallus domesticus. J. Reprod. Fertil. 47:235–238.

Ayoola, E.A. 1984. Synergism between hepatitis B virus and aflatoxin in hepatocellular carcinoma. IARC Sci. Publ. (63):167–179.

Bahn, A.K., I. Rosenwakie, N. Herrmann, P. Grover, J. Stellman, and K. O'Leary. 1976. Melanoma after exposure to PCBs. N. Engl. J. Med. 295:450.

Bahn, A.K., P. Grover, I. Rosenwaike, K. O'Leary, and J. Stellman. 1977. A reply to PCBs and melanoma. N. Engl. J. Med. 296:108.

Ball, W.L., K. Kay, and J.W. Sinclair. 1952. Observations on toxicity of aldrin. I. Growth and estrus in rats. Arch. Ind. Hyg. Occup. Med. 7:292–300.

Bartsch, H., C. Malaveille, A. Barbin, and G. Planche. 1979. Mutagenic and alkylating metabolites of halo-ethylenes, chlorobutadienes and dichlorobutenes produced by rodent or human liver tissues. Evidence for oxirane formation by P450-linked microsomal mono-oxygenases. Arch. Toxicol. 41:249–277.

Batzinger, R.P., S.Y. Ou, and E. Bueding. 1978. Antimutagenic effects of 2(3)-tert-butyl-4-hydroxyanisole and of antimicrobial agents. Cancer Res. 38:4478–4485.

Bauer, A.R., Jr., R.K. Rank, R. Kerr, R.L. Straley, and J.D. Mason. 1977. The effects of prolonged coffee intake on genetically identical mice. Life Sci. 21:63–70.

Beasley, R.P., L.Y. Hwang, C.C. Lin, and C.S. Chien. 1981. Hepatocellular carcinoma and hepatitis B virus. Lancet 2:1129–1133.

Bendele, A.M., W.W. Carlton, P. Krogh, and E.B. Lillehoj. 1985. Ochratoxin A carcinogenesis in the (C57BL/6J X C3H)F$_1$ mouse. J. Natl. Cancer Inst. 75:733–742.

Berkowitz, G.S., T.R. Holford, and R.L. Berkowitz. 1982. Effects of cigarette smoking, alcohol, coffee, and tea consumption on preterm delivery. Early Hum. Dev. 7:239–250.

Bertazzi, P.A., L. Riboldi, A. Pesatori, L. Radice, and C. Zocchetti. 1987. Cancer mortality of capacitor manufacturing workers. Am. J. Ind. Med. 11:165–176.

Bichel, J., and A. Bach. 1968. Investigation on the toxicity of small chronic doses of tannic acid with special reference to possible carcinogenicity. Acta Pharmacol. Toxicol. 26:41–45.

Billings, P.C., C. Heidelberger, and J.R. Landolph. 1985. S-9 metabolic activation enhances aflatoxin-mediated transformation of C3H/10T1/2 cells. Toxicol. Appl. Pharmacol. 77: 58–65.

Binstock, M., D. Krakow, J. Stamler, J. Reiff, V. Persky, K. Liu, and D. Moss. 1983. Coffee and pancreatic cancer: an analysis of international mortality data. Am. J. Epidemiol. 118:630–640.

Borzelleca, J.F., and G.K. Hogan. 1985. Chronic toxicity/carcinogenicity study of FD&C Blue No. 2 in mice. Food Chem. Toxicol. 23:719–722.

Borzelleca, J.F., G.K. Hogan, and A. Koestner. 1985. Chronic toxicity/carcinogenicity study of FD&C Blue No. 2 in rats. Food Chem. Toxicol. 23:551–558.

Boston Collaborative Drug Surveillance Program. 1972. Coffee drinking and acute myocardial infarction. Lancet 2: 1278–1281.

Bowden, J.P., K.T. Chung, and A.W. Andrews. 1976. Mutagenic activity of tryptophan metabolites produced by rat intestinal microflora. J. Natl. Cancer Inst. 57:921–924.

Boyland, E., and J. Mohiuddin. 1981. Surface activity of some tumour promoters. IRCS Med. Sci. 9:753–754.

Bradstock, M.K., M.K. Serdula, J.S. Marks, R.J. Barnard, N.T. Crane, P.L. Remington, and F.L. Trowbridge. 1986. Evaluation of reactions to food additives: the aspartame experience. Am. J. Clin. Nutr. 43:464–469.

Brantom, P.G., I.F. Gaunt, and P. Grasso. 1973. Long-term toxicity of sodium cyclamate in mice. Food Cosmet. Toxicol. 11:735–746.

Brennessel, B.A., and K.J. Keyes. 1985. Saccharin induces morphological changes and enhances prolactin production in GH4C1 cells. In Vitro Cell. Dev. Biol. 21:402–408.

Brown, D.P. 1987. Mortality of workers exposed to polychlorinated biphenyls—an update. Arch. Environ. Health 42: 333–339.

Brown, D.P., and M. Jones. 1981. Mortality and industrial hygiene study of workers exposed to polychlorinated biphenyls. Arch. Environ. Health 36:120–129.

Brown, J.P. 1980. A review of the genetic effects of naturally occurring flavonoids, anthraquinones and related compounds. Mutat. Res. 75:243–277.

Bruggeman, I.M., and J.C. van der Hoeven. 1985. Induction of SCE by some pyrrolizidine alkaloids in V79 Chinese hamster cells co-cultured with chick embryo hepatocytes. Mutat. Res. 142:209–212.

Bryan, G.T., and E. Ertürk. 1970. Production of mouse urinary bladder carcinomas by sodium cyclamate. Science 167:996–998.

Buesching, D.P., and L. Wollstadt. 1984. Cancer mortality among farmers. J. Natl. Cancer Inst. 72:503–504.

Bulatao-Jayme, J., E.M. Almero, M.C. Castro, M.T. Jardeleza, and L.A. Salamat. 1982. A case-control dietary study of primary liver cancer risk from aflatoxin exposure. Int. J. Epidemiol. 11:112–119.

Burbank, F., and J.F. Fraumeni, Jr. 1970. Synthetic sweetener consumption and bladder cancer trends in the United States. Nature 227:296–297.

Byers, T., J. Marshall, S. Graham, C. Mettlin, and M. Swanson. 1983. A case-control study of dietary and nondietary factors in ovarian cancer. J. Natl. Cancer Inst. 71: 681–686.

Cantor, K.P. 1982. Farming and mortality from non-Hodgkin's lymphoma: a case-control study. Int. J. Cancer 29:239–247.

Carmella, S.G., E.J. La Voie, and S.S. Hecht. 1982. Quantitative analysis of catechol and 4-methylcatechol in human urine. Food Chem. Toxicol. 20:587–590.

Cartwright, R.A., R. Adib, R. Glashan, and B.K. Gray. 1981. The epidemiology of bladder cancer in West Yorkshire. A preliminary report on non-occupational aetiologies. Carcinogenesis 2:343–347.

Challis, B.C., and C.D. Bartlett. 1975. Possible cocarcinogenic effects of coffee constituents. Nature 254:532–533.

Chevion, M., and T. Navok. 1983. A novel method for quantitation of favism-inducing agents in legumes. Anal. Biochem. 128:152–158.

Chien, M.C., M.J. Tong, K.J. Lo, J.K. Lee, D.R. Milich, G.N. Vyas, and B.L. Murphy. 1981. Hepatitis B viral markers in patients with primary hepatocellular carcinoma in Taiwan. J. Natl. Cancer Inst. 66:475–479.

Choi, N.W., D.W. Entwistle, W. Michaluk, and N. Nelson. 1971. Gastric cancer in Icelanders in Manitoba. Isr. J. Med. Sci. 7:1500–1508.

Chowaniec, J., and R.M. Hicks. 1979. Response of the rat to saccharin with particular reference to the urinary bladder. Br. J. Cancer 39:355–375.

Chrisman, C.L. 1974. Aneuploidy in mouse embryos induced by diethylstilbestrol diphosphate. Teratology 9:229–232.

Clarke, C.H., and M.J. Wade. 1975. Evidence that caffeine, 8-methoxypsoralen and steroidal diamines are frameshift mutagens for E. coli K-12. Mutat. Res. 28:123–125.

Clayson, D.B., and R.C. Garner. 1976. Carcinogenic aromatic amines and related compounds. Pp. 366–461 in C.E. Searle, ed. Chemical Carcinogens. ACS Monograph 173. American Chemical Society, Washington, D.C.

Clive, D. 1977. A linear relationship between tumorigenic potency in vivo and mutagenic potency at the heterozygous thymidine kinase (TK$^{+/-}$) locus of L5178Y mouse lymphoma cells coupled with mammalian metabolism. Pp. 241–247 in D. Scott, B.A. Bridges, and F.H. Sobels, eds. Progress in Genetic Toxicology: Developments in Toxicology and Environmental Science, Vol. 2. Proceedings of the Second International Conference on Environmental Mutagens, Edinburgh, July 11–15, 1977. Elsevier/North-Holland, Amsterdam.

Clive, D., K.O. Johnson, J.F. Spector, A.G. Batson, and M.M. Brown. 1979. Validation and characterization of the L5178Y/TK$^{+/-}$ mouse lymphoma mutagen assay system. Mutat. Res. 59:61–108.

Coburn, M., P. Sinsheimer, S. Segal, M. Burgos, and W. Troll. 1980. Oxygen free radical generation by gossypol: a possible mechanism of antifertility action in sea urchin sperm. Biol. Bull. 159:468.

Cochrane, W.P., J. Singh, W. Miles, and B. Wakeford. 1981. Determination of chlorinated dibenzo-p-dioxin contaminants in 2,4-D products by gas chromatography-mass spectrometric techniques. J. Chromatogr. 217:289–299.

Cohen, L.A., M. Polansky, K. Furuya, M. Reddy, B. Berke, and J.H. Weisburger. 1984. Inhibition of chemically induced mammary carcinogenesis in rats by short-term exposure to butylated hydroxytoluene (BHT): interrelationships among BHT concentration, carcinogen dose, and diet. J. Natl. Cancer Inst. 72:165–174.

Cohen, L.A., K. Choi, S. Numoto, M. Reddy, B. Berke, and J.H. Weisberger. 1986. Inhibition of chemically induced mammary carcinogenesis in rats by long-term exposure to butylated hydroxytoluene (BHT): interrelations among BHT concentration, carcinogen dose, and diet. J. Natl. Cancer Inst. 76:721–730.

Cohen, S.M. 1985. Multi-stage carcinogenesis in the urinary bladder. Food Chem. Toxicol. 23:521–528.

Cohen, S.M., M. Arai, J.B. Jacobs, and G.H. Friedell. 1979. Promoting effect of saccharin and DL-tryptophan in urinary bladder carcinogenesis. Cancer Res. 39:1207–1217.

Cole, P. 1971. Coffee-drinking and cancer of the lower urinary tract. Lancet 1:1335–1337.

Collins, T.F., and C.H. Williams. 1971. Teratogenic studies with 2,4,5-T and 2,4-D in the hamster. Bull. Environ. Contam. Toxicol. 6:559–567.

Collins, T.F., J.J. Welsh, T.N. Black, and D.I. Ruggles. 1983. A study of the teratogenic potential of caffeine ingested in drinking-water. Food Chem. Toxicol. 21:763–777.

Concon, J.M., D.S. Newburg, and T.W. Swerczek. 1979. Black pepper [Piper nigrum]: evidence of carcinogenicity. Nutr. Cancer 1:22–25.

Cook, R.R. 1981. Dioxin, chloracne, and soft tissue sarcoma. Lancet 1:618–619.

Cook, R.R., J.C. Townsend, M.G. Ott, and L.G. Silverstein. 1980. Mortality experience of employees exposed to 2,3,7,8-tetrachlorodibenzo-p-dioxin (TCDD). J. Occup. Med. 22:530–532.

Correa, P., W. Haenszel, C. Cuello, S. Tannenbaum, and M. Archer. 1975. A model for gastric cancer epidemiology. Lancet 2:58–60.

Correa, P., E. Fontham, L.W. Pickle, V. Chen, Y.P. Lin, and W. Haenszel. 1985. Dietary determinants of gastric cancer in south Louisiana inhabitants. J. Natl. Cancer Inst. 75:645–654.

Council on Scientific Affairs. 1985. Aspartame. Review of safety issues. J. Am. Med. Assoc. 254:400–402.

Courtney, K.D., and J.A. Moore. 1971. Teratology studies with 2,4,5-trichlorophenoxyacetic acid and 2,3,7,8-tetrachlorodibenzo-p-dioxin. Toxicol. Appl. Pharmacol. 20:396–403.

CPSC (U.S. Consumer Product Safety Commission). 1974. Self-pressurized household substances containing vinyl chloride monomer; classification as a banned hazardous substance. Fed. Reg. 39:30112–30114.

Creech, J.L., Jr., and M.N. Johnson. 1974. Angiosarcoma of liver in the manufacture of polyvinyl chloride. J. Occup. Med. 16:150–151.

Creppy, E.E., A. Kane, G. Dirheimer, C. Lafarge-Frayssinet, S. Mousset, and C. Frayssinet. 1985. Genotoxicity of ochratoxin A in mice: DNA single-strand break evaluation in spleen, liver and kidney. Toxicol. Lett. 28:29–35.

Cuello, C., P. Correa, W. Haenszel, G. Gordillo, C. Brown, M. Archer, and S. Tannenbaum. 1976. Gastric cancer in Colombia. I. Cancer risk and suspect environmental agents. J. Natl. Cancer Inst. 57:1015–1020.

Curb, J.D., D.M. Reed, J.A. Kautz, and K. Yano. 1986. Coffee, caffeine, and serum cholesterol in Japanese men in Hawaii. Am. J. Epidemiol. 123:648–655.

Curry, P.T., R.N. Reed, R.M. Martino, and R.M. Kitchin. 1984. Induction of sister-chromatid exchanges in vivo in mice by the mycotoxins sterigmatocystin and griseofulvin. Mutat. Res. 137:111–115.

Dawber, T.R., W.B. Kannel, and T. Gordon. 1974. Coffee and cardiovascular disease. Observations from the Framingham Study. N. Engl. J. Med. 291:871–874.

Deichmann, W.B, W.E. MacDonald, A.G. Beasley, and D. Cubit. 1971. Subnormal reproduction in beagle dogs induced by DDT and aldrin. Ind. Med. Surg. 40:10–20.

Demerec, M., B. Wallace, and E.M. Witkin. 1948. The gene. Carnegie Inst. Washington Yearb. 47:169–176.

Demerec, M., G. Bertani, and J. Flint. 1951. A survey of chemicals for mutagenic action on E. coli. Am. Nat. 85:119–136.

deStafney, C.M., U.D. Prabhu, V.L. Sparnins, and L.W. Wattenberg. 1986. Studies related to the mechanism of 3-BHA-induced neoplasia of the rat forestomach. Food Chem. Toxicol. 24:1149–1157.

Dews, P., H.C. Grice, A. Neims, J. Wilson, and R. Wurtman. 1984. Report of Fourth International Caffeine Workshop, Athens, 1982. Food Chem. Toxicol. 22:163–169.

DHEW (Department of Health, Education, and Welfare). 1969. Report of the Secretary's Commission on Pesticides and Their Relationship to Environmental Health, Parts I and II. U.S. Government Printing Office, Washington, D.C. 677 pp.

DHEW (Department of Health, Education, and Welfare). 1973a. Histopathologic Evaluation of Tissues from Rats Following Continuous Dietary Intake of Sodium Saccharin and Calcium Cyclamate for a Maximum Period of Two Years. Final Report, December 21, 1973. Project P-169-170. Division of Pathology, Food and Drug Administration, U.S. Department of Health, Education, and Welfare. Washington, D.C.

DHEW (Department of Health, Education, and Welfare). 1973b. Subacute and Chronic Toxicity and Carcinogenicity of Various Dose Levels of Sodium Saccharin. Final Report. Project P-169-170. Division of Pathology, Food and Drug Administration, U.S. Department of Health, Education, and Welfare. Washington, D.C.

DHHS (Department of Health and Human Services). 1985. Provisional Listing of Certain Color Additives, Proposal to Extend Closing Dates. Fed. Reg. 50:2637–2638.

Dorado, G., M. Barbancho, and C. Pueyo. 1987. Coffee is highly mutagenic in the L-arabinose resistance test in Salmonella typhimurium. Environ. Mutagen. 9:251–260.

Duck, B.W., and J.T. Carter. 1976. Response to letter (vinyl chloride and mortality). Lancet 2:195.

Dunnick, J.K., J.D. Prejean, J. Haseman, R.B. Thompson, H.D. Giles, and E.E. McConnell. 1982. Carcinogenesis bioassay of allyl isothiocyanate. Fundam. Appl. Toxicol. 2:114–120.

Eckardt, F., H. Muliawan, N. de Ruiter, and H. Kappus. 1981. Rat hepatic vinyl chloride metabolites induce gene conversion in the yeast strain D7RAD in vitro and in vivo. Mutat. Res. 91:381–390.

Eichers, T.R., P.A. Andrilenas, and T.W. Anderson. 1978. Farmer's Use of Pesticides in 1976. Agricultural Economic Report 418. National Economic Analysis Division, Economics, Statistics, and Cooperative Service. U.S. Department of Agriculture, Washington, D.C. 58 pp.

Elmazar, M.M., P.R. McElhatton, and F.M. Sullivan. 1982. Studies on the teratogenic effects of different oral preparations of caffeine in mice. Toxicology 23:57–71.

Emerit, I., A.M. Michelson, A. Levy, J.P. Camus, and J. Emerit. 1980. Chromosome-breaking agent of low molecular weight in human systemic lupus erythematosus: protector effect of superoxide dismutase. Hum. Genet. 55:341–344.

EPA (Environmental Protection Agency). 1975a. Preliminary Assessment of Suspected Carcinogens in Drinking Water. Report to Congress. EPA-560/4-75-005. PB-25096. Office of Toxic Substances, U.S. Environmental Protection Agency, Washington, D.C. 55 pp.

EPA (Environmental Protection Agency). 1975b. Scientific and Technical Assessment Report on Particulate Polycyclic Organic Matter (PPOM), EPA-600/6-75-001. March 1975. Office of Research and Development, U.S. Environmental Protection Agency, Washington, D.C. 95 pp.

Epstein S.S., and J.B. Swartz. 1988. Carcinogenic risk estimation. Science 240:1043–1045.

Erickson, M., L. Hardell, N.O. Berg, T. Moller, and O. Axelson. 1981. Soft tissue sarcomas and exposure to chemical substances: a case-referent study. Br. J. Ind. Med. 38:27–33.

Fahrig, R. 1982. Effects in the mammalian spot test: cyclamate versus saccharin. Mutat. Res. 103:43–47.

Fallat, R.W., C.J. Glueck, R. Lutmer, and F.H. Mattson. 1976. Short term study of sucrose polyester, a nonabsorbable fat-like material as a dietary agent for lowering plasma cholesterol. Am. J. Clin. Nutr. 29:1204–1215.

FDA (Food and Drug Administration). 1979a. Assessment of Estimated Risk Resulting from Aflatoxins in Consumer Peanut Products and Other Food Commodities. Bureau of Foods, Food and Drug Administration, U.S. Department of Health, Education, and Welfare. Washington, D.C. 29 pp.

FDA (Food and Drug Administration). 1979b. Diethylstilbestrol; withdrawal of approval of new animal drug applications; Commissioner's decision. Fed. Regist. 44:54852–54900.

FDA (Food and Drug Administration). 1980a. Aspartame: Decision of the Public Board of Inquiry, Department of Health and Human Services. Docket No. 75F-0355. Food and Drug Administration, U.S. Department of Health, Education, and Welfare, Washington, D.C. 51 pp.

FDA (Food and Drug Administration). 1980b. FDA Compliance Program Report of Findings, FY 77 Total Diet Studies—Adult (7320.73). Bureau of Foods, Food and Drug Administration, U.S. Department of Health, Education, and Welfare, Washington, D.C. 33 pp.

FDA (Food and Drug Administration). 1981. Aspartame; Commissioner's Final Decision. Fed. Regist. 46:38283–38308.

FDA (Food and Drug Administration). 1983. Food Additives Permitted for Direct Addition to Food for Human Consumption, Aspartame. Fed. Regist. 48:31376–31382.

FDA (Food and Drug Administration). 1984. Food Additives Permitted for Direct Addition to Food for Human Consumption, Aspartame. Fed. Regist. 49:22468–22469.

Feron, V.J., A.J. Speek, M.E. Willems, D. van Battum, and A.P. de Groot. 1975. Observations on the oral administration and toxicity of vinyl chloride in rats. Food Cosmet. Toxicol. 13:633–638.

Feron, V.J., C.F. Hendriksen, A.J. Speek, H.P. Til, and B.J. Spit. 1981. Lifespan oral toxicity study of vinyl chloride in rats. Food Cosmet. Toxicol. 19:317–333.

Fitzhugh, O.G. 1964. Appraisal of the safety of residues of veterinary drugs and their metabolites in edible animal tissues. Ann. N.Y. Acad. Sci. 111:665–670.

Flamm, W.G. 1985. Nitrites: laboratory evidence. IARC Sci. Publ. (65):181–182.

Fox, A.J., and P.F. Collier. 1977. Mortality experience of workers exposed to vinyl chloride monomer in the manufacture of polyvinyl chloride in Great Britain. Br. J. Ind. Med. 34:1–10.

Fraumeni, J.F., Jr., J. Scotto, and L.J. Dunham. 1971. Coffee-drinking and bladder cancer. Lancet 2:1204.

Frei, J.V., and S. Venitt. 1975. Chromosome damage in the bone marrow of mice treated with the methylating agents methyl methanesulphonate and N-methyl-N-nitrosourea in the presence or absence of caffeine, and its relationship with thymoma induction. Mutat. Res. 30:89–96.

Freudenthal, R.I., and P.W. Jones, eds. 1976. Carcinogenesis—A Comprehensive Survey, Vol. 1. Polynuclear Aromatic Hydrocarbons: Chemistry, Metabolism, and Carcinogenesis. Raven Press, New York. 450 pp.

Friederich, U., D. Hann, S. Albertini, C. Schlatter, and F.E. Wurgler. 1985. Mutagenicity studies on coffee. The influence of different factors on the mutagenic activity in the Salmonella/mammalian microsome assay. Mutat. Res. 156:39–52.

Friedman, L., M.A. Weinberger, T.M. Farber, F.M. Moreland, E.L. Peters, C.E. Gilmore, and M.A. Khan. 1979. Testicular atrophy and impaired spermatogenesis in rats fed high levels of the methylxanthines caffeine, theobromine, or theophylline. J. Environ. Pathol. Toxicol. 2:687–706.

Fuchs, G., B.M. Gawell, L. Albanus, and S. Slorach. 1975. Vinyl chloride monomer levels in edible fats. Var Foeda 17:134–145.

Fujita, H., A. Mizuo, and H. Kogo. 1976. Mutagenetics of dyes in the microbial system. Tokyo Toritsu Eisei Kenkyusho Kenkyu Hokoku 27:153.

Fukushima, S., G.H. Friedell, J.B. Jacobs, and S.M. Cohen. 1981. Effect of L-tryptophan and sodium saccharin on urinary tract carcinogenesis initiated by N-[4-(5-nitro-2-furyl)-2-thiazolyl]formamide. Cancer Res. 41:3100–3103.

Funes-Cravioto, F., B. Lambert, J. Lindsten, L. Ehrenberg, A.T. Natarajan, and S. Osterman-Golkar. 1975. Chromosome aberrations in workers exposed to vinyl chloride. Lancet 1:459.

Furuya, T., K. Kawamata, T. Kaneko, O. Uchida, S. Horiuchi, and Y. Ikeda. 1975. Long-term toxicity study of sodium cyclamate and saccharin sodium in rats. Jpn. J. Pharmacol. 25:55P–56P.

Gartrell, M.J., J.C. Craun, D.S. Podrebarac, and E.L. Gunderson. 1986. Pesticides, selected elements, and other chemicals in adult total diet samples, October 1980-March 1982. J. Assoc. Off. Anal. Chem. 69:146–161.

Gass, G.H., J. Brown, and A.B. Okey. 1974. Carcinogenic effects of oral diethylstilbestrol on C3H mice with and without the mammary tumor virus. J. Natl. Cancer Inst. 53:1369–1370.

Gaunt, I.F., J. Hardy, P. Grasso, S.D. Gangolli, and K.R. Butterworth. 1974. Long-term toxicity of cyclohexylamine hydrochloride in the rat. Food Cosmet. Toxicol. 14:255–267.

Gezelius, K., and N. Fries. 1952. Phage resistant mutants induced in Escherichia coli by caffeine. Hereditas 38:112–114.

Gibson, J.P., J.W. Newberne, W.L. Kuhn, and J.R. Elsen. 1967. Comparative chronic toxicity of three oral estrogens in rats. Toxicol. Appl. Pharmacol. 11:489–510.

Gilbert, R.M. 1981. Caffeine: overview and anthology. Pp. 145–166 in S.A. Miller, ed. Nutrition & Behavior. Franklin Institute Press, Philadelphia.

Glass, E.A., and A. Novick. 1959. Induction of mutation in chloramphenicol-inhibited bacteria. J. Bacteriol. 77:10–16.

Gold, E.B., L. Gordis, M.D. Diener, R. Seltser, J.K. Boitnott, T.E. Bynum, and D.F. Hutcheon. 1985. Diet and other risk factors for cancer of the pancreas. Cancer 55:460–467.

Goldenthal, E.I. 1982. Long-Term Dietary Toxicity/Carcinogenicity Study in Rats. IRDC Report 410–011. International Research and Development Corporation, Mattawan, Mich.

Goon, D., and M.K. Conner. 1984. Simultaneous assessment of ethyl carbamate-induced SCE in murine lymphocytes, bone marrow and alveolar macrophage cells. Carcinogenesis 5:399–402.

Graham, D.M. 1978. Caffeine—its identity, dietary sources, intake, and biological effects. Nutr. Rev. 36:97–102.

Graham, S., H. Dayal, M. Swanson, A. Mittelman, and G. Wilkinson. 1978. Diet in the epidemiology of cancer of the colon and rectum. J. Natl. Cancer Inst. 61:709–714.

Green, M.S., and E. Jucha. 1986. Association of serum lipids with coffee, tea, and egg consumption in free-living subjects. J. Epidemiol. Community Health 40:324–329.

Green, S., K.A. Palmer, and E.J. Oswald. 1973. Cytogenic effects of the polychlorinated biphenyls (Aroclor 1242) on rat bone marrow and spermatogonial cells. Toxicol. Appl. Pharmacol. 25:482.

Greim, H., G. Bonse, Z. Radwan, D. Reichert, and D. Henschler. 1975. Mutagenicity in vitro and potential carcinogenicity of chlorinated ethylenes as a function of metabolic oxiran formation. Biochem. Pharmacol. 24:2013–2017.

Griffin, D.S., and H.J. Segall. 1986. Genotoxicity and cytotoxicity of selected pyrrolizidine alkaloids, a possible alkenal metabolite of the alkaloids, and related alkenals. Toxicol. Appl. Pharmacol. 86:227–234.

Groisser, D.S., P. Rosso, and M. Winick. 1982. Coffee consumption during pregnancy: subsequent behavioral abnormalities of the offspring. J. Nutr. 112:829–832.

Gustavsson, P., C. Hogstedt, and C. Rappe. 1986. Short-term mortality and cancer incidence in capacitor manufacturing workers exposed to polychlorinated biphenyls (PCBs). Am. J. Ind. Med. 10:341–344.

Guthrie, F.E., R.J. Monroe, and C.O. Abernathy. 1971. Response of the laboratory mouse to selection for resistance to insecticides. Toxicol. Appl. Pharmacol. 18:92–101.

Haar, G.T. 1980. An investigation of possible sterility and health effects from exposure to ethylene dibromide. Pp. 167–188 in B. Ames, P. Infante, and R. Reitz, eds. Banbury Report 5. Ethylene Dichloride: A Potential Health Risk? Cold Spring Harbor Laboratory, New York.

Haenszel, W., M. Kurihara, M. Segi, and R.K. Lee. 1972. Stomach cancer among Japanese in Hawaii. J. Natl. Cancer Inst. 49:969–988.

Haenszel, W., F.B. Locke, and M. Segi. 1980. A case-control study of large bowel cancer in Japan. J. Natl. Cancer Inst. 64:17–22.

Haffner, S.M., J.A. Knapp, M.P. Stern, H.P. Hazuda, M. Rosenthal, and L.J. Franco. 1985. Coffee consumption, diet, and lipids. Am. J. Epidemiol. 122:1–12.

Hall, R.L. 1979. Naturally occurring toxicants and food additives: our perception and management of risks. Nutr. Cancer 1:27–36.

Hardell, L., and A. Sandstrom. 1979. Case-control study: soft-tissue sarcomas and exposure to phenoxyacetic acids or chlorophenols. Br. J. Cancer 39:711–717.

Hardell, L., M. Eriksson, P. Lenner, and E. Lundgren. 1981. Malignant lymphoma and exposure to chemicals, especially organic solvents, chlorophenols and phenoxy acid: a case-control study. Br. J. Cancer 43:169–176.

Haroz, R.K., and J. Thomasson. 1980. Tumor initiating and promoting activity of gossypol. Toxicol. Lett. (sp. iss.) 6:72.

Hartge, P., R. Hoover, D.W. West, and J.L. Lyon. 1983.

Coffee drinking and risk of bladder cancer. J. Natl. Cancer Inst. 70:1021–1026.

Hayes, M.A., E. Roberts, and E. Farber. 1985. Initiation and selection of resistant hepatocyte nodules in rats given the pyrrolizidine alkaloids lasiocarpine and senecionine. Cancer Res. 45:3726–3734.

Haynes, R.H., and J.D.B. Collins. 1984. The mutagenic potential of caffiene. Pp. 221–238 in P.B. Dews, ed. Caffeine: Perspectives from Recent Research. Springer-Verlag, Berlin.

Heath, C.W., Jr., and C.R. Dumont. 1977. Chromosomal damage in men occupationally exposed to vinyl chloride monomer and other chemicals. Environ. Res. 14:68–72.

Heilbrun, L.K., A. Nomura, and G.N. Stemmermann. 1986. Black tea consumption and cancer risk: a prospective study. Br. J. Cancer 54:677–683.

Hendricks, J.D., R.O. Sinnhuber, P.M. Loveland, N.E. Pawlowski, and J.E. Nixon. 1980. Hepatocarcinogenicity of glandless cottonseeds and cottonseed oil to rainbow trout (Salmo gairdneri). Science 208:309–311.

Hennekens, C.H., M.E. Drolette, M.J. Jesse, J.E. Davies, and G.B. Hutchinson. 1976. Coffee drinking and death due to coronary heart disease. N. Engl. J. Med. 294:633–636.

Henschler, D., and D. Wild. 1985. Mutagenic activity in rat urine after feeding with the azo dye tartrazine. Arch. Toxicol. 57:214–215.

Herbst, A.L., and P. Cole. 1978. Epidemiologic and clinical aspects of clear cell adenocarcinoma in young women. Pp. 2–7 in A.L. Herbst, ed. Intrauterine Exposure to Diethylstilbestrol in the Human. Proceeding of Symposium on DES, 1977. American College of Obstetricians and Gynecologists, Chicago.

Hesser, L. 1984. Tartrazine on trial. Food Chem. Toxicol. 22: 1019–1024.

Heuch, I., G. Kvale, B.K. Jacobsen, and E. Bjelke. 1983. Use of alcohol, tobacco and coffee, can increase risk of pancreatic cancer. Br. J. Cancer 48:637–643.

Hicks, R.M., J. Wakefield, and J. Chowaniec. 1975. Evaluation of new model to detect bladder carcinogens or cocarcinogens; results obtained with saccharin, cyclamate and cyclophosphamide. Chem. Biol. Interact. 11:225–233.

Hicks, R.M., J. Chowaniec, and J.S.J. Wakefield. 1978. Experimental induction of bladder tumors by a two-stage system. Pp. 475–489 in T.J. Slaga, A. Sivak, and R.K. Boutwell, eds. Carcinogenesis: A Comprehensive Survey, Vol. 2. Mechanisms of Tumor Promotion and Cocarcinogenesis. Raven Press, New York.

Higginson, J. 1966. Etiological factors in gastrointestinal cancer in man. J. Natl. Cancer Inst. 37:527–545.

Higuchi, K. 1976. Outline. Pp. 3–7 in K. Higuchi, ed. PCB Poisoning and Pollution. Kodansha Ltd., Tokyo.

Hirayama, T. 1979. Epidemiological evaluation of the role of naturally occurring carcinogens and modulators of carcinogenesis. Pp. 359–380 in E.C. Miller, J.A. Millar, I. Hirono, T. Sugimura, and S. Takayama, eds. Naturally Occurring Carcinogens-Mutagens and Modulators of Carcinogenesis. Japan Scientific Societies Press, Tokyo.

Hirayama, T. 1986. Nutrition and cancer—a large scale cohort study. Pp. 299–311 in I. Knudsen, ed. Genetic Toxicology of the Diet: Progress in Clinical and Biological Research, Vol. 206. Alan R. Liss, New York.

Hirono, I. 1981. Natural carcinogenic products of plant origin. CRC Crit. Rev. Toxicol. 8:235–277.

Hirono, I. 1986. Carcinogenicity of plant constituents: pyrrolizidine alkaloids, flavonoids, bracken fern. Pp. 45–53 in I. Knudsen, ed. Genetic Toxicology of the Diet: Progress in Clinical and Biological Research, Vol. 206. Alan R. Liss, New York.

Hirono, I., H. Kachi, and T. Kato. 1970. A survey of acute toxicity of cycads and mortality rate from cancer in the Miyako Islands, Okinawa. Acta Pathol. Jpn. 20:327–337.

Hirono, I., I. Ueno, S. Hosaka, H. Takanashi, T. Matsushima, T. Sugimura, and S. Natori. 1981. Carcinogenicity examination of quercetin and rutin in ACI rats. Cancer Lett. 13:15–21.

Hirose, M., A. Masuda, Y. Kurata, E. Ikawa, Y. Mera, and N. Ito. 1986. Histologic and autoradiographic studies on the forestomach of hamsters treated with 2-tert-butylated hydroxyanisole, 3-tert-butylated hydroxyanisole, crude butylated hydroxyanisole, or butylated hydroxytoluene. J. Natl. Cancer Inst. 76:143–149.

Hoar, S.K., A. Blair, F.F. Holmes, C.D. Boysen, R.J. Robel, R. Hoover, and J.F. Fraumeni. 1986. Agricultural herbicide use and risk of lymphoma and soft-tissue sarcoma. J. Am. Med. Assoc. 256:1141–1147.

Hofman, A., A. van Laar, F. Klein, and H.A. Valkenburg. 1983. Coffee and cholesterol. N. Engl. J. Med. 309:1248–1249.

Hogue, C.J. 1981. Coffee in pregnancy. Lancet 1:554.

Homburger, F. 1978. Negative lifetime carcinogen studies in rats and mice fed 50,000 ppm saccharin. Pp. 359–373 in C.L. Galli, R. Paoletti, and G. Vettorazzi, eds. Chemical Toxicology of Food. Elsevier/North-Holland Biomedical Press, Amsterdam.

Homburger, F., A.B. Russfield, E.K. Weisburger, and J.H. Weisburger. 1973. Final Report: Studies on Saccharin and Cyclamate. Bio-Research Consultants, Cambridge, Mass.

Honchar, P.A., and W.E. Halperin. 1981. 2,4,5-T, trichlorophenol, and soft tissue sarcoma. Lancet 1:268–269.

Hoopingarner, R., A. Samuel, and D. Krause. 1972. Polychlorinated biphenyl interactions with tissue culture cells. Environ. Health Perspect. 1:155–158.

Hoover, R.N., and P.H. Strasser. 1980. Artificial sweeteners and human bladder cancer. Preliminary Results. Lancet 1:837–840.

Howe, G.R., J.D. Burch, A.B. Miller, B. Morrison, P. Gordon, L. Weldon, L.W. Chambers, G. Fodor, and G.M. Winsor. 1977. Artificial sweeteners and human bladder cancer. Lancet 2:578–581.

Howe, G.R., J.D. Burch, A.B. Miller, G.M. Cook, J. Esteve, B. Morrison, P. Gordon, L.W. Chambers, G. Fodor, and G.M. Winsor. 1980. Tobacco use, occupation, coffee, various nutrients, and bladder cancer. J. Natl. Cancer Inst. 64:701–713.

Hrubec, Z. 1973. Coffee drinking and ischaemic heart disease. Lancet 1:548.

Hsieh, C.C., B. MacMahon, S. Yen, D. Trichopoulos, K. Warren, and G. Nardi. 1986. Coffee and pancreatic cancer (Chapter 2). N. Engl. J. Med. 315:587–589.

Huang, M., Z.H. Wang, X.Q. Wang, and M. Wu. 1986. Malignant transformation of human fetal lung fibroblasts induced by nitrosamine compounds in vitro. Sci. Sin. 29:1192–1200.

Huberman, E., H. Bartsch, and L. Sachs. 1975. Mutation induction in Chinese hamster V79 cells by two vinyl chloride metabolites, chloroethylene oxide and 2-chloroacetaldehyde. Int. J. Cancer 16:639–644.

IARC (International Agency for Research on Cancer). 1974. Thiourea. Pp. 95–109 in IARC Monographs on the Evaluation of Carcinogenic Risk of Chemicals to Man, Vol. 7.

Some Anti-Thyroid and Related Substances, Nitrofurans and Industrial Chemicals. IARC, Lyon, France.

IARC (International Agency for Research on Cancer). 1976. IARC Monographs on the Evaluation of Carcinogenic Risk of Chemicals to Man, Vol. 10. Some Naturally-Occurring Substances. IARC, Lyon, France. 353 pp.

IARC (International Agency for Research on Cancer). 1979. IARC Monographs on the Evaluation of the Carcinogenic Risk of Chemicals to Humans, Vol. 20. Some Halogenated Hydrocarbons. IARC, Lyon, France. 609 pp.

IARC (International Agency for Research on Cancer). 1983. IARC Monographs on the Evaluation of the Carcinogenic Risk of Chemicals to Humans, Vol. 30. Miscellaneous Pesticides. IARC, Lyon, France. 424 pp.

IARC (International Agency for Research on Cancer). 1987. IARC Monographs on the Evaluation of the Carcinogenic Risk of Chemicals to Humans, Suppl. 7. Overall Evaluations of Carcinogenicity: An Updating of IARC Monographs, Vols. 1 to 42. IARC, Lyon, France. 440 pp.

ICO (International Coffee Organization). 1986. United States of America: Coffee Drinking Study, Winter, 1986. International Coffee Organization, London. 15 pp.

Ikeda, Y., S. Horiuchi, T. Furuya, K. Kawamata, T. Kaneko, and O. Uchida. 1975. Long-Term Toxicity Study of Sodium Cyclamate and Saccharin Sodium in Rats. Department of Toxicology, National Institute of Hygienic Sciences, Tokyo, Japan.

Innes, J.R.M., B.M. Ulland, M.G. Valerio, L. Petrucelli, L. Fishbein, E.R. Hart, A.J. Pallotta, R.R. Bates, H.L. Falk, J.J. Gart, M. Klein, I. Mitchell, and J. Peters. 1969. Bioassay of pesticides and industrial chemicals for tumorigenicity in mice: a preliminary note. J. Natl. Cancer Inst. 42:1101–1114.

Inui, N., Y. Nishi, M.M. Hasegawa, and T. Kawachi. 1980. Induction of 8-azaguanine or ouabain resistant somatic mutation of Chinese hamster lung cells by treatment with tryptophan products. Cancer Lett. 9:185–189.

Ishidate, M., Jr., and S. Odashima. 1977. Chromosome tests with 134 compounds on Chinese hamster cells in vitro—a screening for chemical carcinogens. Mutat. Res. 48:337–353.

Ishidate, M., Jr., T. Sofuni, K. Yoshikawa, M. Hayashi, T. Nohmi, M. Sawada, and A. Matsuoka. 1984. Primary mutagenicity screening of food additives currently used in Japan. Food Chem. Toxicol. 22:623–636.

Ishii, H., T. Koshimizu, S. Usami, and T. Fujimoto. 1981. Toxicity of aspartame and its diketopiperazine for Wistar rats by dietary administration for 104 weeks. Toxicology 21:91–94.

Ishii, D.N. 1982. Inhibition of iodinated nerve growth factor binding by the suspected tumor promoters saccharin and cyclamate. J. Natl. Cancer Inst. 68:299–303.

Ishikawa, F., F. Takaku, M. Nagao, M. Ochiai, K. Hayashi, S. Takayama, and T. Sugimura. 1985. Activated oncogenes in a rat hepatocellular carcinoma induced by 2-amino-3-methylimidazo[4,5-f]quinoline. Jpn. J. Cancer Res. 76:425–428.

Ito, N., S. Fukushima, and H. Tsuda. 1985. Carcinogenicity and modifications of the carcinogenic response by BHA, BHT and other antioxidants. CRC Crit. Rev. Toxicol. 15:109–150.

Iversen, O.H. 1984. Urethan (ethyl carbamate) alone is carcinogenic for mouse skin. Carcinogenesis 5:911–915.

Ivett, J.L., and R.R. Tice. 1981. Diethylstilbestrol-diphosphate induces chromosomal aberrations but not sister chromatid exchanges in murine bone marrow cells in vivo. Environ. Mutagen. 3:445–452.

Ivie, G.W., D.L. Holt, and M.C. Ivey. 1981. Natural toxicants in human foods: psoralens in raw and cooked parsnip root. Science 213:909–910.

Jadhav, S.J., R.P. Sharma, and D.K. Salunkhe. 1981. Naturally occurring toxic alkaloids in foods. CRC Crit. Rev. Toxicol. 9:21–104.

Jacobsen, B.K., E. Bjelke, G. Kvale, and I. Heuch. 1986. Coffee drinking, mortality, and cancer incidence: results from a Norwegian prospective study. J. Natl. Cancer Inst. 76:823–831.

Jelinck, C.F., and P.E. Corneliussen. 1975. Levels of PCB's in the U.S. food supply. Pp. 147–154 in National Conference on Polychlorinated Biphenyls, November, 1975, Chicago, Illinois. EPA-560/6–75–004. Office of Toxic Substances, U.S. Environmental Protection Agency, Washington, D.C.

Jensen, O.M., J. Wahrendorf, J.B. Knudsen, and B.L. Sorensen. 1986. The Copenhagen case-control study of bladder cancer. II. Effect of coffee and other beverages. Int. J. Cancer 37:651–657.

Jenssen, D., and C. Ramel. 1978. Factors affecting the induction of micronuclei at low doses of X-rays, MMS and dimethylnitrosamine in mouse erythroblasts. Mutat. Res. 58:51–65.

Jick, H., O.S. Miettinen, R.K. Neff, S. Shapiro, O.P. Heinonen, and D. Slone. 1973. Coffee and myocardial infarction. N. Engl. J. Med. 289:63–67.

Johnson, F.E., M.A. Kugler, and S.M. Brown. 1981. Soft tissue sarcomas and chlorinated phenols. Lancet 2:40.

Johnson, H.G., and M.K. Bach. 1965. Apparent suppression of mutation rates in bacteria by spermine. Nature 208:408–409.

Joint Iran–International Agency for Research on Cancer Study Group. 1977. Esophageal cancer studies in the Caspian Littoral of Iran: results of population studies—a prodrome. J. Natl. Cancer Inst. 59:1127–1138.

Jones, F.E., R.A. Komorowski, and R.E. Condon. 1984. The effects of ascorbic acid and butylated hydroxyanisole in the chemoprevention of 1,2-dimethylhydrazine-induced large bowel neoplasms. J. Surg. Oncol. 25:54–60.

Jukes, T.H. 1974. Estrogens in beefsteaks. J. Am. Med. Assoc. 229:1920–1921.

Kabat, G.C., G.S. Dieck, and E.L. Wynder. 1986. Bladder cancer in nonsmokers. Cancer 57:362–367.

Kada, T., K. Tutikawa, and Y. Sadaie. 1972. In vitro and host-mediated "rec-assay" procedures for screening chemical mutagens; and phloxine, a mutagenic red dye detected. Mutat. Res. 16:165–174.

Kaiser, H.E. 1967. Cancer-promoting effects of phenols in tea. Cancer 20:614–616.

Kale, P.G., and J.W. Baum. 1979. Sensitivity of Drosophila melanogaster to low concentrations of gaseous mutagens. II. Chronic Exposures. Mutat. Res. 68:59–68.

Kang, H., F.M. Enzinger, P. Breslin, M. Feil, Y. Lee, and B. Shepard. 1987. Soft tissue sarcoma and military service in Vietnam: a case-control study. J. Natl. Cancer Inst. 79:693–699.

Kannel, W.B. 1977. Coffee, cocktails and coronary candidates. N. Engl. J. Med. 297:443–444.

Kapadia, G.J., B.D. Paul, E.B. Chung, B. Ghosh, and S.N. Pradhan. 1976. Carcinogenicity of Camellia sinensis (tea) and some tannin-containing folk medicinal herbs adminis-

tered subcutaneously in rats. J. Natl. Cancer Inst. 57:207–209.

Kappus, H., and H. Sies. 1981. Toxic drug effects associated with oxygen metabolism: redox cycling and lipid peroxidation. Experientia 37:1233–1241.

Kark, J.D., Y. Friedlander, N.A. Kaufmann, and Y. Stein. 1985. Coffee, tea, and plasma cholesterol: the Jerusalem Lipid Research Clinic prevalence study. Br. Med. J. 291:699–704.

Kasai, H., Z. Yamaizumi, K. Wakabayashi, M. Nagao, T. Sugimura, S. Yokoyama, T. Miyazawa, N.E. Spingarn, J.H. Weisburger, and S. Nishimura. 1980. Potent novel mutagens produced by broiling fish under normal conditions. Proc. Jpn. Acad. 56B:278–283.

Kasai, H., Z. Yamaizumi, T. Shiomi, S. Yokoyama, T. Miyazawa, K. Wakabayashi, M. Nagao, T. Sugimura, and S. Nishimura. 1981. Structure of a potent mutagen isolated from fried beef. Chem. Lett. 4:485–488.

Kasai, H., K. Kumeno, Z. Yamaizumi, S. Nishimura, M. Nagao, Y. Fujita, T. Sugimura, H. Nukaya, and T. Kosuge. 1982. Mutagenicity of methylglyoxal in coffee. Gann 73:681–683.

Kasamaki, A., H. Takahashi, K. Tsumura, J. Niwa, T. Fujita, and S. Urasawa. 1982. Genotoxicity of flavoring agents. Mutat. Res. 105:387–392.

Kay, K. 1977. Polybrominated biphenyls (PBB) environmental contamination in Michigan, 1973–1976. Environ. Res. 13:74–93.

Keen, P., and P. Martin. 1971. The toxicity and fungal infestation of foodstuffs in Swaziland in relation to harvesting and storage. Trop. Geogr. Med. 23:35–43.

Kessler, I.I. 1970. Cancer mortality among diabetics. J. Natl. Cancer Inst. 44:673–686.

Kessler, I.I. 1976. Non-nutritive sweeteners and human bladder cancer: preliminary findings. J. Urol. 115:143–146.

Kessler, I.I., and J. P. Clark. 1978. Saccharin, cyclamate, and human bladder cancer. No evidence of an association. J. Am. Med. Assoc. 240:349–355.

Khera, K.S., and J.A. Ruddick. 1973. Polychlorodibenzo-p-dioxins: perinatal effects and the dominant lethal test in Wistar rats. Pp. 70–84 in E.H. Blair, ed. Chlorodioxins—Origin and Fate. Advances in Chemistry Series 120. American Chemical Society, Washington, D.C.

Khera, K.S., D.C. Villeneuve, G. Terry, L. Panopio, L. Nash, and G. Trivett. 1976. Mirex: a teratogenicity, dominant lethal and tissue distribution study in rats. Food Cosmet. Toxicol. 14:25–29.

Kihlman, B.A., and S. Sturelid. 1975. Enhancement by methylated oxypurines of the frequency of induced chromosomal aberrations. III. The effect in combination with x-rays on root tips of Vicia faba. Hereditas 80:247–254.

Kimbrough, R.D., V.W. Burse, and J.A. Liddle. 1978. Persistent liver lesions in rats after a single oral dose of polybrominated biphenyls (firemaster FF-1) and concomitant PBB tissue levels. Environ. Health Perspect. 23:265–273.

Kimbrough, R.D., D.F. Groce, M.P. Korver, and V.W. Burse. 1981. Induction of liver tumors in female Sherman strain rats by polybrominated biphenyls. J. Natl. Cancer Inst. 66:535–542.

Kinlen, L.J., and K. McPherson. 1984. Pancreas cancer and coffee and tea consumption: a case-control study. Br. J. Cancer 49:93–96.

Kirby, K.S. 1960. Induction of tumors by tannic extracts. Br.

J. Cancer 14:147–150.

Klatsky, A.L., G.D. Friedman, and A.B. Siegelaub. 1973. Coffee drinking prior to acute myocardial infarction. Results from the Kaiser-Permanente Epidemiologic Study of Myocardial Infarction. J. Am. Med. Assoc. 226:540–543.

Knowles, M.A., I.C. Summerhayes, and R.M. Hicks. 1986. Carcinogenesis studies using cultured rat and mouse bladder epithelium. Pp. 127–167 in M.M. Webber and L.I. Sekesy, eds. In Vitro Models for Cancer Research, Vol. IV. Carcinomas of the Urinary Bladder and Kidney. CRC Press, Boca Raton, Fla.

Konetzka, W.A. 1974. Mutagenesis by nitrate reduction in Eschericia coli. P. 37 in Abstracts of the Annual Meeting of the American Society for Microbiology 1974, May 12–17, 1974, Chicago, Illinois. American Society for Microbiology, Washington, D.C.

Korpássy, B., and M. Mosonyi. 1950. The carcinogenic activity of tannic acid; liver tumors induced in rats by prolonged subcutaneous administration of tannic acid solutions. Br. J. Cancer 4:411–420.

Kosugi, A., M. Nagao, Y. Suwa, K. Wakabayashi, and T. Sugimura. 1983. Roasting coffee beans produces compounds that induce prophage lambda in E. coli and are mutagenic in E. coli and S. typhimurium. Mutat. Res. 116:179–184.

Kovar, M.G., R. Fulwood, and M. Feinleib. 1983. Coffee and cholesterol. N. Engl. J. Med. 309:1248–1250.

Kriebel, D., and D. Jowett. 1979. Stomach cancer mortality in the north central states: high risk is not limited to the foreign-born. Nutr. Cancer 1:8–12.

Kroes, R., P.W. Peters, J.M. Berkvens, H.G. Verschuuren, T. de Vries, and G.J. van Esch. 1977. Long term toxicity and reproduction study (including a teratogenicity study) with cyclamate, saccharin and cyclohexylamine. Toxicology 8: 285–300.

Kubitschek, H.E., and H.E. Bendigkeit. 1958. Delay in the appearance of caffeine-induced T5 resistance in Escherichia coli. Genetics 43:647–661.

Kubitschek, H.E., and H.E. Bendigkeit. 1964. Mutation in continuous cultures. I. Dependence of mutational response upon growth-limiting factors. Mutat. Res. 1:113–120.

Kuenzig, W., J. Chau, E. Norkus, H. Holowaschenko, H. Newmark, W. Mergens, and A.H. Conney. 1984. Caffeic and ferulic acid as blockers of nitrosamine formation. Carcinogenesis 5:309–313.

Kuratsune, M. 1976. Epidemiologic studies on Yusho. Pp. 9–23 in K. Higuchi, ed. PCB Poisoning and Pollution. Kodansha Ltd., Tokyo.

Kutz, F.W., and S.C. Strassman. 1976. Residues of polychlorinated biphenyls in the general population of the United States. Pp. 139–143 in National Conference on Polychlorinated Biphenyls, November 1975, Chicago, Illinois. EPA-560/6–75–004, Office of Toxic Substances, U.S. Environmental Protection Agency, Washington, D.C.

La Croix, A.Z., L.A. Mead, K.Y. Liang, C.B. Thomas, and T.A. Pearson. 1986. Coffee consumption and the incidence of coronary heart disease. N. Engl. J. Med. 315:977–982.

Lam, L.K., V.L. Sparnins, and L.W. Wattenberg. 1982. Isolation and identification of kahweol palmitate and cafestol palmitate as active constituents of green coffee beans that enhance glutathione S-transferase activity in the mouse. Cancer Res. 42:1193–1198.

Laqueur, G.L., and M. Spatz. 1968. Toxicology of cycasin. Cancer Res. 28:2262–2267.

La Vecchia, C., S. Franceschi, A. Decarli, A. Gentile, P.

Liati, M. Regallo, and G. Tognoni. 1984. Coffee drinking and the risk of epithelial ovarian cancer. Int. J. Cancer 33: 559–562.

Lê, M.G. 1985. Coffee consumption, benign breast disease, and breast cancer. Am. J. Epidemiol. 122:721.

Lee, L.S. 1981. Saccharin and cyclamate inhibit binding of epidermal growth factor. Proc. Natl. Acad. Sci. U.S.A. 78: 1042–1046.

LeGrady, D., A.R. Dyer, R.B. Shekelle, J. Stamler, K. Liu, O. Paul, M. Lepper, and A.M. Shryock. 1987. Coffee consumption and mortality in the Chicago Western Electric Company Study. Am. J. Epidemiol. 126:803–812.

Levine, D.E., M. Hollstein, M.F. Christman, F.A. Schwiers, and B.N. Ames. 1982. A new Salmonella tester strain (TA102) with AT base pairs at the site of mutation detects oxidative mutagens. Proc. Natl. Acad. Sci. U.S.A. 79: 7445–7449.

Leviton, A. 1988. Caffeine consumption and the risk of reproductive hazards. J. Reprod. Med. 33:175–178.

Lijinsky, W. 1985. Carcinogenicity and mutagenicity of N-nitroso compounds. American Chemical Society Central Regional Meeting, June 5–7, 1985, University of Akron, Akron, Ohio. 44 pp.

Lijinsky, W. 1986. The significance of N-nitroso compounds as environmental carcinogens. J. Env. Sci. Health 4:1–45.

Lijinsky, W., and A.E. Ross. 1967. Production of carcinogenic polynuclear hydrocarbons in the cooking of food. Food Cosmet. Toxicol. 5:343–347.

Lijinsky, W., and P. Shubik. 1964. Benzo(a)pyrene and other polynuclear hydrocarbons in charcoal-broiled meat. Science 145:53–55.

Lijinsky, W., and H.W. Taylor. 1976. Carcinogenesis in Sprague-Dawley rats of N-nitroso-N-alkylcarbamate esters. Cancer Lett. 1:275–279.

Lindenschmidt, R.C., A.F. Tryka, M.E. Goad, and H.P. Witschi. 1986. The effects of dietary butylated hydroxytoluene on liver and colon tumor development in mice. Toxicology 38:151–160.

Linn, S., S.C. Schoenbaum, R.R. Monson, B. Rosner, P.G. Stubblefield, and K.J. Ryan. 1982. No association between coffee consumption and adverse outcomes of pregnancy. N. Engl. J. Med. 306:141–145.

Linsell, C.A., and F.G. Peers. 1977. Aflatoxin and liver cell cancer. Trans. R. Soc. Trop. Med. Hyg. 71:471–473.

Lo, M.T., and E. Sandi. 1978. Polycyclic aromatic hydrocarbons (polynuclears) in foods. Residue Rev. 69:35–86.

Loprieno, N., R. Barale, S. Baroncelli, C. Bauer, G. Bronzetti, A. Cammellini, G. Cercignani, C. Corsi, G. Gervasi, C. Leporini, R. Nieri, A.M. Rossi, G. Stretti, and G. Turchi. 1976. Evaluation of the genetic effects induced by vinyl chloride monomer (VCM) under mammalian metabolic activation: studies in vitro and in vivo. Mutat. Res. 40:89–96.

Lu, S.H., R. Montesano, M.S. Zhang, L. Feng, F.J. Luo, S.X. Chui, D. Umbenhauer, R. Saffhill, and M.F. Rajewsky. 1986. Relevance of N-nitrosamines to esophageal cancer in China. J. Cell. Physiol. Suppl. 4:51–58.

Lubin, F., E. Ron, Y. Wax, and B. Modan. 1985. Coffee and methylxanthines and breast cancer: a case-control study. J. Natl. Cancer Inst. 74:569–573.

Lück, H., P. Wallnöfer, and H. Bach. 1963. Lebensmittelzusatzstoffe und mutagene Wirkung. VII. Mitteilung Prüfung einiger Xanthen-Farbstoffe auf mutagene Wirkung an Escherichia coli. Pathol. Microbiol. 26:206–224.

Mack, T.M., M.C. Yu, R. Hanisch, and B.E. Henderson.

1986. Pancreas cancer and smoking, beverage consumption, and past medical history. J. Natl. Cancer Inst. 76:49–60.

MacLennan, R., J. Da Costa, N.E. Day, C.H. Law, Y.K. Ng, and K. Shanmugaratnam. 1977. Risk factors for lung cancer in Singapore Chinese, a population with high female incidence rates. Int. J. Cancer 20:854–860.

MacMahon, B., S. Yen, D. Trichopoulos, K. Warren, and G. Nardi. 1981. Coffee and cancer of the pancreas. N. Engl. J. Med. 304:630–633.

Macquart-Moulin, G., E. Riboli, J. Cornee, B. Charnay, P. Berthezene, and N. Day. 1986. Case-control study on colo-rectal cancer and diet in Marseilles. Int. J. Cancer 38:183–191.

Maeura, Y., and G.M. Williams. 1984. Enhancing effect of butylated hydroxytoluene on the development of liver altered foci and neoplasms induced by N-2-fluorenylacetamide in rats. Food Chem. Toxicol. 22:191–198.

Maga, J.A. 1979. Furans in foods. CRC Crit. Rev. Food Sci. Nutr. 11:355–400.

Magee, P.N., and J.M. Barnes, 1967. Carcinogenic nitroso compounds. Adv. Cancer Res. 10:163–246.

Magee, P.N., R. Montesano, and R. Preussman. 1976. N-Nitroso compounds and related carcinogens. Pp. 491–625 in C.E. Searle, ed. Chemical Carcinogens. ACS Monograph 173. American Chemical Society, Washington, D.C.

Mahon, G.A., and G.W. Dawson. 1982. Saccharin and the induction of presumed somatic mutations in the mouse. Mutat. Res. 103:49–52.

Malcolm, A.R., L.J. Mills, and E.J. McKenna. 1983. Inhibition of metabolic cooperation between Chinese hamster V79 cells by tumor promoters and other chemicals. Ann. N.Y. Acad. Sci. 407:448–450.

Malinow, M.R., E.J. Bardana, Jr., B. Pirofsky, S. Craig, and P. McLaughlin. 1982. Systemic lupus erythematosus-like syndrome in monkeys fed alfalfa sprouts: role of a nonprotein amino acid. Science 216:415–417.

Malkinson, A.M. 1983. Review: putative mutagens and carcinogens in foods. III. Butylated hydroxytoluene (BHT). Environ. Mutagen. 5:353–362.

Maltoni, C. 1977. Vinyl chloride carcinogenicity: an experimental model for carcinogenesis studies. Pp. 119–146 in H.H. Hiatt, J.D. Watson, and J.A. Winsten, eds. Origins of Human Cancer, Book A: Incidence of Cancer in Humans. Cold Spring Harbor Laboratory, New York.

Maltoni, C., G. Lefemine, P. Chieco, and D. Carretti. 1974. Vinyl chloride carcinogenesis: current results and perspectives. Med. Lav. 65:421–444.

Maltoni, C., A. Ciliberti, L. Gianni, and P. Chieco. 1975. Gli effetti oncogeni del cloruro di vinile somministrato per via orale mel ratto. Gli Ospedali della Vita 2:102–104.

Mangold, K.A., G.S. Bailey, and G.H. Thorgaard. 1986. Sister chromatid exchange induction in rainbow trout leukocytes by in vivo exposure to ethyl methanesulfonate or aflatoxin B_1. Proc. Am. Assoc. Cancer Res. 27:36.

Manners, G.D., G.W. Ivie, and J.T. MacGregor. 1978. Mutagenic activity of hymenovin in Salmonella typhimurium: association with the bishemiacetal functional group. Toxicol. Appl. Pharmacol. 45:629–633.

Marrett, L.D., S.D. Walter, and J.W. Meigs. 1983. Coffee drinking and bladder cancer in Connecticut. Am. J. Epidemiol. 117:113–127.

Martin, C.N., A.C. McDermid, and R.C. Garner. 1978. Testing of known carcinogens and noncarcinogens for their ability to induce unscheduled DNA synthesis in HeLa cells.

Cancer Res. 38:2621–2627.

Martin, T.R., and M.B. Bracken. 1987. The association between low birth weight and caffeine consumption during pregnancy. Am. J. Epidemiol. 126:813–821.

Mason, P.L., and G.R. Thompson. 1977. Testicular effects of cyclohexylamine hydrochloride in the rat. Toxicology 8:143–156.

Mathias, S., C. Garland, E. Barrett-Connor, and D.L. Wingard. 1985. Coffee, plasma cholesterol, and lipoproteins. A population study in an adult community. Am. J. Epidemiol. 121:896–905.

Matsukura, N., T. Kawachi, K. Morino, H. Ohgaki, T. Sugimura, and S. Takayama. 1981. Carcinogenicity in mice of mutagenic compounds from a tryptophan pyrolyzate. Science 213:346–347.

Matsushima, T., H. Matsumoto, A. Shirai, M. Sawamura, and T. Sugimura. 1979. Mutagenicity of the naturally occurring carcinogen cycasin and synthetic methylazoxymethanol conjugates in Salmonella typhimurium. Cancer Res. 39:3780–3782.

Mau, G., and P. Netter. 1974. Are coffee and alcohol consumpton risk factors in pregnancy? Geburtshilfe Frauenheilkd. 34:1018–1022.

Mazur, R.H. 1976. Aspartame—a sweet surprise. J. Toxicol. Environ. Health 2:243–249.

McCann, J.C. 1977. Short-term tests. Pp. 91–108 in Cancer Testing Technology and Saccharin. Office of Technology Assessment, Congress of the United States, Washington, D.C.

McChesney, E.W., F. Coulston, and K.F. Benitz. 1977. Six-year study of saccharin in rhesus monkeys. Toxicol. Appl. Pharmacol. 41:164.

McCutcheon, R.S. 1975. Toxicology and the Law. Pp. 728–741 in Toxicology: The Basic Science of Poisons. L.J. Casarett and J. Doull, eds. Macmillian Publishing Co., New York.

McFarland, L.Z., and P.B. Lacy. 1969. Physiologic and endocrinologic effects of the insecticide kepone in the Japanese quail. Toxicol. Appl. Pharmacol. 15:441–450.

McLachlan, J.A., A. Wong., G.H. Degen, and J.C. Barrett. 1982. Morphologic and neoplastic transformation of Syrian hamster embryo fibroblasts by diethylstilbestrol and its analogs. Cancer Res. 42:3040–3045.

McNally, J. 1978. Polybrominated biphenyls: environmental contamination of food. Pp. CRS1–CRS42 in Environmental Contaminants in Food, Vol. II. Part A: Working Papers. Food and Renewable Resources Program, Health and Life Sciences Division, Office of Technology Assessment, Washington, D.C.

Meinsma, L. 1964. Voeding en Kanker. Voeding 25:357–365.

Mellies, M.J., C. Vitale, R.J. Jandacek, G.E. Lamkin, and C.J. Glueck. 1985. The substitution of sucrose polyester for dietary fat in obese, hypercholesterolemic outpatients. Am. J. Clin. Nutr. 41:1–12.

Mettlin, C., and S. Graham. 1979. Dietary risk factors in human bladder cancer. Am. J. Epidemiol. 110:255–263.

Miller, A.B., G.R. Howe, M. Jain, K.J. Craib, and L. Harrison. 1983. Food items and food groups as risk factors in a case-control study of diet and colo-rectal cancer. Int. J. Cancer 32:155–161.

Miller, D.R., L. Rosenberg, D.W. Kaufman, S.P. Helmrich, D. Schottenfeld, J. Lewis, P.D. Stolley, N. Rosenshein, and S. Shapiro. 1987. Epithelial ovarian cancer and coffee drinking. Int. J. Epidemiol. 16:13–17.

Miller, E.C., J.A. Miller, I. Hirono, T. Sugimura, and S. Takayama, eds. 1979. Naturally Occurring Carcinogens—Mutagens and Modulators of Carcinogenesis. Japan Scientific Societies Press, Tokyo. 399 pp.

Milo, G.E., I. Noyes, J.W. Oldham, R.W. West, and F.F. Kadlubar. 1983. Co-carcinogenicity of saccharin and N-methylnitrosourea in human diploid fibroblasts. Proc. Am. Assoc. Cancer Res. 24:102.

Milvy, P. 1978. Re: mutatgenic studies with acrylonitrile. Mutat. Res. 57:110–112.

Milvy, P., and M. Wolff. 1977. Mutagenic studies with acrylonitrile. Mutat. Res. 48:271–278.

Mirvish, S.S. 1981. Inhibition of the formation of carcinogenic N-nitroso compounds by ascorbic acid and other compounds. Pp. 557–587 in J.H. Burchenal and H.F. Oettgen, eds. Cancer: Achievements, Challenges, and Prospects for the 1980s, Vol. 1. Grune & Stratton, New York.

Mirvish, S.S., A. Cardesa, L. Wallcave, and P. Shubik. 1975. Induction of mouse lung adenomas by amines or ureas plus nitrite and by N-nitroso compounds: effect of ascorbate, gallic acid, thiocyanate, and caffeine. J. Natl. Cancer Inst. 55:633–636.

Mitchell, C.P., and M.F. Jacobson. 1987. Tainted Booze: The Consumer's Guide to Urethane in Alcoholic Beverages. Center for Science in the Public Interest, Washington, D.C. 71 pp.

Mochizuki, M., M. Osabe, T. Anjo, E. Suzuki, and M. Okada. 1984. Mutagenicity of alpha-hydroxy N-nitrosamines in V79 Chinese hamster cells. J. Cancer Res. Clin. Oncol. 108:290–295.

Møller-Jensen, O., J.B. Knudsen, B.L. Sorensen, and J. Clemmesen. 1983. Artificial sweeteners and absence of bladder cancer risk in Copenhagen. Int. J. Cancer 32:577–582.

Monson, R.R., J.M. Peters, and M.N. Johnson. 1974. Proportional mortality among vinyl-chloride workers. Lancet 2:397–398.

Montesano, R., and H. Bartsch. 1976. Mutagenic and carcinogenic N-nitroso compounds: possible environmental hazards. Mutat. Res. 32:179–228.

Morgan, R.W., and M.G. Jain. 1974. Bladder cancer: smoking, beverages and artificial sweeteners. Can. Med. Assoc. J. 111:1067–1170.

Mori, H., S. Sugie, I. Hirono, K. Yamada, H. Niwa, and M. Ojika. 1985a. Genotoxicity of ptaquiloside, a bracken carcinogen, in the hepatocyte primary culture/DNA-repair test. Mutat. Res. 143:75–78.

Mori, H., S. Sugie, N. Yoshimi, Y. Asada, T. Furuya, and G.M. Williams. 1985b. Genotoxicity of a variety of pyrrolizidine alkaloids in the hepatocyte primary culture-DNA repair test using rat, mouse, and hamster hepatocytes. Cancer Res. 45:3125–3129.

Morimoto, K., S. Wolff, and A. Koizumi. 1983. Induction of sister-chromatid exchanges in human lymphocytes by microsomal activation of benzene metabolites. Mutat. Res. 119:355–360.

Morrison, A.S., and J.E. Buring. 1980. Artificial sweeteners and cancer of the lower urinary tract. N. Engl. J. Med. 302:537–541.

Morrison, A.S., J.E. Buring, W.G. Verhoek, K. Aoki, I. Leck, Y. Ohno, and K Obata. 1982a. Coffee drinking and cancer of the lower urinary tract. J. Natl. Cancer Inst. 68:91–94.

Morrison, A.S., W.G. Verhoek, I. Leck, K. Aoki, Y. Ohno, and K. Obata. 1982b. Artificial sweeteners and bladder cancer in Manchester, U.K., and Nagoya, Japan. Br. J. Cancer 45:332–336.

Moses, M., and I.J. Selikoff. 1981. Soft tissue sarcomas, phenoxy herbicides, and chlorinated phenols. Lancet 1:1370.

Munro, H., and M.C. Crim. 1980. The proteins and amino acids. Pp. 51–98 in R.S. Goodhard and M.E. Shils, eds. Modern Nutrition in Health and Disease, 6th ed. Lea & Febiger, Philadelphia.

Muranyi-Kovacs, I., G. Rudali, and L. Aussepe. 1975. The Carcinogenicity of Sodium Cyclamate in Combination with Other Oncogenic Agents. Laboratorie de Genetique, Foundation Curie, Institut du Radium, Paris.

Muranyi-Kovacs, I., G. Rudali, and J. Imbert. 1976. Bioassay of 2,4,5-trichlorophenoxyacetic acid for the carcinogenicity in mice. Br. J. Cancer. 33:626–633.

Murphy, R.S., F.W. Kutz, and S.C. Strassman. 1983. Selected pesticide residues or metabolites in blood and urine specimens from a general population survey. Environ. Health Perspect. 48:81–86.

Murray, S.S., E. Bjelke, R.W. Gibson, and I.M. Schuman. 1981. Coffee consumption and mortality from ischemic heart disease and other causes: results from the Lutheran Brotherhood Study, 1966–1978. Am. J. Epidemiol. 113:661–667.

Naber, E.C., and G.W. Ware. 1965. Effect of kepone and mirex on reproductive performance in the laying hen. Poult. Sci. 44:875–880.

Nagao, M., Y. Takahashi, H. Yamanaka, and T. Sugimura. 1979. Mutagens in coffee and tea. Mutat. Res. 68:101–106.

Nagao, M., Y. Fujita, T. Sugimura, and T. Kosuge. 1986a. Methylglyoxal in beverages and foods: its mutagenicity and carcinogenicity. IARC Sci. Publ. (70):283–291.

Nagao, M., K. Wakabayashi, Y. Fujita, T. Tahira, M. Ochiai, and T. Sugimura. 1986b. Mutagenic compounds in soy sauce, Chinese cabbage, coffee and herbal teas. Pp. 55–62 in I. Knudsen, ed. Genetic Toxicology of the Diet. Progress in Clinical and Biological Research, Vol. 206. Alan R. Liss, New York.

Najem, G.R., D.B. Louria, J.J. Seebode, I.S. Thind, J.M. Prusakowski, R.B. Ambrose, and A.R. Fernicola. 1982. Life time occupation, smoking, caffeine, saccharine, hair dyes and bladder carcinogenesis. Int. J. Epidemiol. 11:212–217.

Nakasato, F., M. Nakayasu, Y. Fujita, M. Nagao, M. Terada, and T. Sugimura. 1984. Mutagenicity of instant coffee on cultured Chinese hamster lung cells. Mutat. Res. 141:109–112.

National Institute of Hygienic Sciences. 1973. Chronic Toxicity Study of Sodium Saccharin: 21 Months Feeding in Mice. National Institute of Hygienic Sciences, Tokyo.

NCI (National Cancer Institute). 1977. Bioassay of Captan for Possible Carcinogenicity. CAS No. 133-06-2, NCI-CG-TR-15. DHEW Publ. No. (NIH) 77-815. Carcinogenesis Program, National Institutes of Health, Public Health Service, U.S. Department of Health, Education, and Welfare, Bethesda, Md. 99 pp.

NCI (National Cancer Institute). 1978a. Bioassay of a Mixture of Aspirin, Phenacetin and Caffeine for Possible Carcinogenicity. DHEW Publ. No. (NIH) 78-1317. Carcinogenesis Testing Program, National Institutes of Health, U.S. Department of Health, Education, and Welfare, Bethesda, Md. 112 pp.

NCI (National Cancer Institute). 1978b. Bioassay of 1,2-Dibromomethane for Possible Carcinogenicity. CAS No. 106-93-4, NCI-CG-TR-86. DHEW Publ. No. (NIH) 78-1336. Carcinogenesis Testing Program. National Institutes of Health, Public Health Service, U.S. Department of Health, Education, and Welfare. Bethesda, Md. 64 pp.

NCI (National Cancer Institute). 1979. Bioassay of Butylated Hydroxytoluene (BHT) for Possible Carcinogenicity. CAS No. 128-37-0, NCI-CG-TR-150. NIH Publ. No. 79-1706. Carcinogenesis Testing Program. National Institutes of Health, Public Health Service, U.S. Department of Health, Education, and Welfare, Bethesda, Md. 114 pp.

NCI (National Cancer Institute). 1982. Carcinogenesis Bioassay of 1,2-Dibromoethane (CAS No. 106-93-4) in F344 Rats and B6C3F1 Mice (Inhalation Study). TR-210. NIH Publ. No. 81-1766. National Toxicology Program, National Institutes of Health, Public Health Service, U.S. Department of Health and Human Services, Bethesda, Md. 163 pp.

Nees, P.O., and P.H. Derse. 1967. Effect of feeding calcium cyclamate to rats. Nature 213:1191–1195.

Neft, R.E., M.K. Conner, and T. Takeshita. 1985. Long-term persistence of ethyl carbamate-induced sister chromatid exchanges in murine lymphocytes. Cancer Res. 45:4115–4121.

Newberne, P.M. 1968. The influence of a low lipotrope diet on response of maternal and fetal rats to lasiocarpine. Cancer Res. 28:2327–2337.

Nicholson, W.J., E.C. Hammond, H. Seidman, and I.J. Selikoff. 1975. Mortality experience of a cohort of vinyl chloride–polyvinyl chloride workers. Ann. N.Y. Acad. Sci. 246:225–230.

Nolen, G.A. 1981. The effect of brewed and instant coffee on reproduction and teratogenesis in the rat. Toxicol. Appl. Pharmacol. 58:171–183.

Nomura, A., L.K. Heilbrun, and G.N. Stemmermann. 1986. Prospective study of coffee consumption and the risk of bladder cancer. J. Natl. Cancer Inst. 76:587–590.

Norell, S.E., A. Ahlbom, R. Erwald, G. Jacobson, I. Lindberg-Navier, R. Olin, B. Törnberg, and K.L. Wiechel. 1986. Diet and pancreatic cancer: a case-control study. Am. J. Epidemiol. 124:894–902.

Norris, J.M. 1977. Status Report on the 2 Year Study Incorporating Acrylonitrile in the Drinking Water of Rats. Health and Environmental Research. The Dow Chemical Company, Midland, Mich. 14 pp.

Novick, A. 1956. Mutagens and antimutagens. Brookhaven Symp. Biol. 8:201–215.

NRC (National Research Council). 1971. Current usage of certified colors in foods. Pp. 10–16 in Food Colors. Report of the Committee on Food Protection, Food and Nutrition Board, Division of Biology and Agriculture. National Academy of Sciences, Washington, D.C. 46 pp.

NRC (National Research Council). 1978. Saccharin: Technical Assessment of Risks and Benefits, Part I. Report of the Committee for a Study on Saccharin and Food Safety Policy, Assembly of Life Sciences. National Academy of Sciences, Washington, D.C. (various pagings)

NRC (National Research Council). 1981. The Health Effects of Nitrate, Nitrite, and N-Nitroso Compounds. Report of the Committee on Nitrite and Alternative Curing Agents in Food, Assembly of Life Sciences. National Academy Press, Washington, D.C. (various pagings)

NRC (National Research Council). 1982. Diet, Nutrition, and Cancer. Report of the Committee on Diet, Nutrition, and Cancer, Assembly of Life Sciences. National Academy Press, Washington, D.C. 478 pp.

NRC (National Research Council). 1984. 1982 Poundage Update of Food Chemicals. Report of the Committee on Food Additives Survey Data, Food and Nutrition Board, Commission on Life Sciences. National Academy Press, Washington, D.C. 564 pp.

NRC (National Research Council). 1985. Evaluation of Cyclamate for Carcinogenicity. Report of Committee on the Evaluation of Cyclamate for Carcinogenicity, Commission on Life Sciences. National Academy Press, Washington, D.C. 196 pp.

NRC (National Research Council). 1986. Drinking Water and Health, Vol. 6. Board on Toxicology and Environmental Health Hazards, Commission on Life Sciences. National Academy Press, Washington, D.C. 457 pp.

NRC (National Research Council). 1987. Regulating Pesticides in Food: The Delaney Paradox. Report of the Committee on Scientific and Regulatory Issues Underlying Pesticide Use Patterns and Agricultural Innovation, Board on Agriculture. National Academy Press, Washington, D.C. 272 pp.

O'Berg, M.T. 1980. Epidemiologic study of workers exposed to acrylonitrile. J. Occup. Med. 22:245–252.

Ochiai, M., M. Nagao, T. Tahira, F. Ishikawa, K. Hayashi, H. Ohgaki, M. Terada, N. Tsuchida, and T. Sugimura. 1985. Activation of K-ras and oncogenes other than ras family in rat fibrosarcomas induced by 1,8-dinitropyrene. Cancer Lett. 29:119–125.

Oettlé, A.G. 1965. The etiology of primary carcinoma of the liver in Africa: a critical appraisal of previous ideas with an outline of the mycotoxin hypothesis. S. Afr. Med. J. 39:817–825.

Ohgaki, H., K. Kusama, N. Matsukura, K. Morino, H. Hasegawa, S. Sato, S. Takayama, and T. Sugimura. 1984. Carcinogenicity in mice of a mutagenic compound, 2-amino-3-methylimidazo[4,5-f]quinoline, from broiled sardine, cooked beef and beef extract. Carcinogenesis 5:921–924.

Ohgaki, H., H. Hasegawa, T. Kato, M. Suenaga, M. Ubukata, S. Sato, S. Takayama, and T. Sugimura. 1985. Induction of tumors in the forestomach and liver of mice by feeding 2-amino-3,4-dimethylimidazo[4,5-f]quinoline (MeIQ). Proc. Jpn. Acad. 61B:137–139.

Ohnishi, Y., T. Kinouchi, Y. Manabe, H. Tsutsui, H. Otsuka, H. Tokiwa, and T. Otofuji. 1985. Nitro compounds in environmental mixtures and foods. Pp. 195–204 in M.D. Waters, S.S. Sandhu, J. Lewtas, L. Claxton, G. Strauss, and S. Nesnow, eds. Short-Term Bioassays in the Analysis of Complex Environmental Mixtures IV.

Ohno, Y., K. Aoki, K. Obata, and A.S. Morrison. 1985. Case-control study of urinary bladder cancer in metropolitan Nagoya. Natl. Cancer Inst. Monogr. 69:229–234.

Olsen, P., J. Gry, I. Knudsen, O. Meyer, and E. Poulsen. 1984. Animal feeding study with nitrite-treated meat. IARC Sci. Publ. 57:667–675.

Olsen, P., O. Meyer, N. Bille, and G. Wurtzen. 1986. Carcinogenicity study on butylated hydroxytoluene (BHT) in Wistar rats exposed in utero. Food Chem. Toxicol. 24:1–12.

Orr, M.L., and B.K. Watt. 1957. Amino Acid Content of Foods. Home Economics Research Report No. 4. U.S. Government Printing Office, Washington, D.C. 82 pp.

Oser, B.L., and R.A. Ford. 1981. Caffeine: an update. Drug

Chem. Toxicol. 4:311–329.

Oser, B.L., S. Carson, G.E. Cox, E.E. Vogin, and S.S. Sternberg. 1975. Chronic toxicity study of cyclamate:saccharin (10:1) in rat. Toxicology 4:315–330.

Oser, B.L., S. Carson, G.E. Cox, E.E. Vogin, and S.S. Sternberg. 1976. Long-term and multigeneration toxicity studies with cyclohexylamine hydrochloride. Toxicology 6:47–65.

Ott, M.G., B.B. Holder, and R.D. Olson. 1980a. A mortality analysis of employees engaged in the manufacture of 2,4,5-trichlorophenoxyacetic acid. J. Occup. Med. 22:47–50.

Ott, M.G., H.C. Scharnweber, and R.R. Langner. 1980b. Mortality experience of 161 employees exposed to ethylene dibromide in two production units. Br. J. Ind. Med. 37:163–168.

Ottoboni, A. 1972. Effect of DDT on the reproductive life-span in the female rat. Toxicol. Appl. Pharmacol. 22:497–502.

Ottolenghi, A.D., J.K. Haseman, and F. Suggs. 1974. Teratogenic effects of aldrin, dieldrin, and endrin in hamsters and mice. Teratology 9:11–16.

Palm, P.E., E.P. Arnold, P.C. Rachwall, J.C. Leyczek, K.W. Teague, and C.J. Kensler. 1978. Evaluation of the teratogenic potential of fresh-brewed coffee and caffeine in the rat. Toxicol. Appl. Pharmacol. 44:1–16.

Palm, P.E., E.P. Arnold, M.S. Nick, J.R. Valentine, and T.E. Doerfler. 1984. Two-year toxicity/carcinogenicity study of fresh-brewed coffee in rats initially exposed in utero. Toxicol. Appl. Pharmacol. 74:364–382.

Palmer, S., and R.A. Mathews. 1986. The role of nonnutritive dietary constituents in carcinogenesis. Surg. Clin. North Am. 66:891–915.

Pamukcu, A.M., S. Yalçiner, J.F. Hatcher, and G.T. Bryan. 1980. Quercetin, a rat intestinal and bladder carcinogen present in bracken fern (Pteridium aquilinum). Cancer Res. 40:3468–3472.

Panalaks, T. 1976. Determination and identification of polycyclic aromatic hydrocarbons in smoked and charcoal-broiled food products by high pressure liquid chromatography and gas chromatography. J. Environ. Sci. Health 11:299–315.

Pao, E.M., K.H. Fleming, P.M. Guenther, and S.J. Mickle. 1982. Foods Commonly Eaten by Individuals: Amount Per Day and Per Eating Occasion. Home Economics Research Report No. 44. Human Nutrition Information Service, U.S. Department of Agriculture, Hyattsville, Md. 431 pp.

Patterson, R.M., and J.S. Butler. 1982. Tartrazine-induced chromosomal aberrations in mammalian cells. Food Chem. Toxicol. 20:461–465.

Pearce, N.E., A.H. Smith, and D.O. Fisher. 1985. Malignant lymphoma and multiple myeloma linked with agricultural occupations in a New Zealand Cancer Registry-based study. Am. J. Epidemiol. 121:225–237.

Pearn, J.H. 1985. Herbicides and congenital malformations: a review for the pediatrician. Aust. Pediatr. J. 21:237–242.

Peers, F.G., and C.A. Linsell. 1973. Dietary aflatoxins and liver cancer—a population-based study in Kenya. Br. J. Cancer 27:473–484.

Peers, F.G., G.A. Gilman, and C.A. Linsell. 1976. Dietary aflatoxins and human liver cancer. A study in Swaziland. Int. J. Cancer 17:167–176.

Peers, F., X. Bosch, J. Kaldor, A. Linsell, and M. Pluijmen. 1987. Aflatoxin exposure, hepatitus B virus infection and liver cancer in Swaziland. Int. J. Cancer 39:545–553.

Perera, F., and P. Boffetta. 1988. Perspectives on comparing risks of environmental carcinogens. J. Natl. Cancer Inst. 80:1282–1293.

Phillips, R.L., and D.A. Snowdon. 1985. Dietary relationship with fatal colorectal cancer among Seven-Day Adventists. J. Natl. Cancer Inst. 74:307–317.

Pienta, R.J. 1981. Transformation of Syrian hamster embryo cells by diverse chemicals and correlation with their reported carcinogenic and mutagenic activities. Chem. Mutagens 6:175–202.

Poncelet, F., M. Duverger-van Bogaert, M. Lambotte-Vandepaer, and C. de Meester. 1984. Mutagenicity, carcinogenicity, and teratogenicity of industrially important monomers. Pp. 205–279 in M. Kirsch-Volders, ed. Mutagenicity, Carcinogenicity, and Teratogenicity of Industrial Pollutants. Plenum Press, New York.

Porikos, K.P., G. Booth, and T.B. Van Itallie. 1977. Effect of covert nutritive dilution on the spontaneous food intake of obese individuals: a pilot study. Am. J. Clin. Nutr. 30:1638–1644.

Potapenko, A.Y., M.V. Moshnin, A.A. Kranovsky, Jr., and V.L. Sukhorukov. 1982. Dark oxidation of unsaturated lipids by the photo-oxidized 8-methoxypsoralen. Z. Naturforsch. 37:70–74.

Preston, B.D., J.P. Van Miller, R.W. Moore, and J.R. Allen. 1981. Promoting effects of polychlorinated biphenyls (Aroclor 1254) and polychlorinated dibenzofuran-free Aroclor 1254 on diethylnitrosamine-induced tumorigenesis in the rat. J. Natl. Cancer Inst. 66:509–515.

Price, J.M., C.G. Biava, B.L. Oser, E.E. Vogin, J. Steinfeld, and H.L. Ley. 1970. Bladder tumors in rats fed cyclohexylamine or high doses of a mixture of cyclamate and saccharin. Science 167:1131–1132.

Prince, A.M., W. Szmuness, J. Michon, J. Demaille, G. Diebolt, J. Linhard, C. Quenum, and M. Sankale. 1975. A case/control study of the association between primary liver cancer and hepatitis B infection in Senegal. Int. J. Cancer 16:376–383.

Prival, M.J. 1984. Carcinogens and mutagens present as natural components of food or induced by cooking. Nutr. Cancer 6:236–253.

Purchase, I.F.H., C.R. Richardson, and D. Anderson. 1975. Chromosomal and dominant lethal effects of vinyl chloride. Lancet 2:410–411.

Radomski, J.L., D. Greenwald, W.L. Hearn, N.L. Block, and F.M. Woods. 1978. Nitrosamine formation in bladder infections and its role in the etiology of bladder cancer. J. Urol. 120:48–50.

Rao, M.S., and A.B. Qureshi. 1972. Induction of dominant lethals in mice by sodium saccharin. Indian J. Med. Res. 60:599–603.

Rao, T.K., W. Lijinsky, and J.L. Epler, eds. 1984. Genotoxicicology of N-Nitroso Compounds. Plenum Press, New York. 271 pp.

Rebelakos, A., E. Trichopoulos, A. Tzonou, X. Zavitsanos, E. Velonakis, and A. Trichopoulos. 1985. Tobacco smoking, coffee drinking, and occupation as risk factors for bladder cancer in Greece. J. Natl. Cancer. Inst. 75:455–461.

Reddy, B.S., and Y. Maeura. 1984. Dose–response studies of the effect of dietary butylated hydroxyanisole on colon carcinogenesis induced by methylazoxymethanol acetate in female CF1 mice. J. Natl. Cancer Inst. 72:1181–1187.

Riihimaki, V., S. Asp, and S. Hernberg. 1982. Mortality of 2,4,-dichlorophenoxyacetic acid and 2,4,5-trichlorophenoxyacetic acid herbicide applicators in Finland: first report of an ongoing prospective cohort study. Scand. J. Work Environ. Health 8:37–42.

Risch, H.A., M. Jain, N.W. Choi, J.G. Fodor, C.J. Pfeiffer, G.R. Howe, L.W. Harrison, K.J. Craib, and A.B. Miller. 1985. Dietary factors and the incidence of cancer of the stomach. Am. J. Epidemiol. 122:947–959.

Risch, H.A., J.D. Burch, A.B. Miller, G.B. Hill, R. Steele, and G.R. Howe. 1988. Dietary factors and the incidence of cancer of the urinary bladder. Am. J. Epidemiol. 127:1179–1191.

Roberts, H.R., ed. 1981. Food Safety. Wiley, New York. 339 pp.

Roe, F.J., L.S. Levy, and R.L. Carter. 1970. Feeding studies on sodium cyclamate, saccharin and sucrose for carcinogenic and tumour-promoting activity. Food Cosmet. Toxicol. 8: 135–145.

Rogers, C.G., B.N. Nayak, and C. Héroux-Metcalf. 1985. Lack of induction of sister chromatid exchanges and of mutation to 6-thioguanine resistance in V79 cells by buty-lated hydroxyanisole with and without activation by rat or hamster hepatocytes. Cancer Lett. 27:61–69.

Rosenberg, L., D. Slone, S. Shapiro, D.W. Kaufman, P.D. Stolley, and O.S. Miettinen. 1980. Coffee drinking and myocardial infarction in young women. Am. J. Epidemiol. 111:675–681.

Rosenberg, L., D.R. Miller, S.P. Helmrich, D.W. Kaufman, D. Schottenfeld, P.D. Stolley, and S. Shapiro. 1985. Breast cancer and the consumption of coffee. Am. J. Epidemiol. 122:391–399.

Rösli, M., B. Zimmerli, and B. Marek. 1975. Ruckstände von Vinylchlorid—Monomer in Speiseölen. Mitt. Lebensmitte. Hyg. 66:507–511.

Rudali, G., E. Coezy, and I. Muranyi-Kovacs. 1969. Carcino-genic activity of sodium cyclamates in mice. C.R. Acad. Sci. 269:1910–1912.

Rulis, A.M., D.G. Hattan, and V.H. Morgenroth III. 1984. FDA's priority-based assessment of food additives. I. Prelim-inary results. Regul. Toxicol. Pharmacol. 4:37–56.

Rustia, M. 1979. Role of hormone imbalance in transplacental carcinogenesis induced in Syrian golden hamsters by sex hormones. Natl. Cancer Inst. Monogr. 51:77–87.

Salocks, C.B., D.P. Hsieh, and J.L. Byard. 1984. Effects of butylated hydroxytoluene pretreatment on the metabolism and genotoxicity of aflatoxin B$_1$ in primary cultures of adult rat hepatocytes: selective reduction of nucleic acid binding. Toxicol. Appl. Pharmacol. 76:498–509.

Santodonato, J., P. Howard, and D. Basu. 1981. Health and ecological assessment of polynuclear aromatic hydrocarbons. J. Environ. Pathol. Toxicol. 5:1–364.

Schmähl, D. 1973. Absence of carcinogenic activity of cycla-mate, cyclohexylamine and saccharin in rats. Arzneim.-Forsch. 23:1466–1470.

Schmähl, D., and M. Habs. 1984. Investigations on the carcinogenicity of the artificial sweeteners sodium cyclamate and sodium saccharin in rats in a two-generation experi-ment. Arzneim.-Forsch. 34:604–606.

Schoenig, G.P., E.I. Goldenthal, R.G. Geil, C.H. Frith, W.R. Richter, and F.W. Carlborg. 1985. Evaluation of the dose response and in utero exposure to saccharin in the rat. Food Chem. Toxicol. 23:475–490.

Schoental, R. 1959. Liver lesions in young rats suckled by mothers treated with the pyrrolizidine (senecio) alkaloids, lasiocarpine and retrorsine. J. Pathol. Bacteriol. 77:485–495.

Schoental, R. 1968. Toxicology and carcinogenic action of pyrrolizidine alkaloids. Cancer Res. 28:2237–2246.

Searle, G.D., and Company. 1973a. 106 week oral toxicity study in the dogs. P-T No. 855S270. G.D. Searle and Co., Skokie, Ill.

Searle, G.D., and Company. 1973b. A 26-Week Urinary Bladder Tumorigenicity Study in the Mouse by the Intra-vesical Pellet Implant Technique. P-T No. 1031OT72. Final Report. G.D. Searle and Co., Skokie, Ill.

Searle, G.D., and Company. 1973c. Two Year Toxicity Study in the Rat. P-T No. 838H71. Final Report. G.D. Searle and Co., Skokie, Ill. 104 pp.

Searle, G.D., and Company. 1974a. Lifetime toxicity study in the rat. P-T No. 892H72. Final Report. G.D. Searle and Co., Skokie, Ill. 255 pp.

Searle, G.D., and Company. 1974b. 104-Week Toxicity Study in the Mouse. P-T No. 984H73. Final Report. G.D. Searle and Co., Skokie, Ill. 295 pp.

Shank, R.C., J.E. Gordon, G.N. Wogan, A.Nondasuta, and B. Sabhamani. 1972a. Dietary aflatoxins and human liver cancer. III. Field survey of rural Thai families for ingested aflatoxins. Food Cosmet. Toxicol. 10:71–84.

Shank, R.C., N. Bhamarapravati, J.E. Gordon, and G.N. Wogan. 1972b. Dietary aflatoxins and human liver cancer. IV. Incidence of primary liver cancer in two municipal populations of Thailand. Food Cosmet. Toxicol. 10:171–179.

Shekelle, R.B., M. Gale, O. Paul, and J. Stamler. 1983. Letter to the editor re: coffee and cholesterol. N. Engl. J. Med. 309:1249–1250.

Shinohara, K., R.T. Wu, N. Jahan, M. Tanaka, N. Mori-naga, H. Murakami, and H. Omura. 1980. Mutagenicity of the browing mixtures by amino-carbonyl reactions on Sal-monella typhimurium TA 100. Agric. Biol. Chem. 44:671–672.

Shorland, F.B., J.O. Igene, A.M. Pearson, J.W. Thomas, R.K. McGuffey, and A.E. Aldridge. 1981. Effects of dietary fat and vitamin E on the lipid composition and stability of veal during frozen storage. J. Agric. Food. Chem. 29:863–871.

Shentberg, A.I., and A.M. Torchinskii. 1976. Evaluation of experimental data on teratogenic properties of substances foreign to the body in their combined effect. Gig. Sanit. 12:32–35.

Silverman, D.T., R.N. Hoover, and G.M. Swanson. 1983. Artificial sweeteners and lower urinary tract cancer: hospital vs. population controls. Am. J. Epidemiol. 117:326–334.

Simmon, V.F. 1979. In vitro assays for recombinogenic activ-ity of chemical carcinogens and related compounds with Saccharomyces cerevisiae D3. J. Natl. Cancer Inst. 62:901–909.

Simmon, V.F., H.S. Rosenkranz, E. Zeiger, and L.A. Poirier. 1979. Mutagenic activity of chemical carcinogens and re-lated compounds in the intraperitoneal host-mediated assay. J. Natl. Cancer Inst. 62:911–918.

Simon, D., S. Yen, and P. Cole. 1975. Coffee drinking and cancer of the lower urinary tract. J. Natl. Cancer Inst. 54:587–591.

Simons, M.J., E.H. Yap, and K. Shanmugaratnam. 1972. Australia antigen in Singapore Chinese patients with hep-atocellular carcinoma and comparison groups: influence of technique sensitivity on differential frequencies. Int. J. Cancer 10:320–325.

Smith, A.H., N.E. Pearce, D.O. Fisher, H.J. Giles, C.A.

Teague, and J.K. Howard. 1984. Soft tissue sarcoma and exposure to phenoxyherbicides and chlorophenols in New Zealand. J. Natl. Cancer Inst. 73:1111–1117.

Snowdon, D.A., and R.L. Phillips. 1984. Coffee consumption and risk of fatal cancers. Am. J. Publ. Health 74:820–823.

Stich, H.F., W. Stich, M.P. Rosin, and W.D. Powrie. 1980. Mutagenic activity of pyrazine derivatives: a comparative study with *Salmonella typhimurium, Saccharomyces cerevisiae*, and Chinese hamster ovary cells. Food. Cosmet. Toxicol. 18:581–584.

Stich, H.F., W. Stich, M.P. Rosin, and W.D. Powrie. 1981a. Clastogenic activity of caramel and caramelized sugars. Mutat. Res. 91:129–136.

Stich, H.F., M.P. Rosin, C.H. Wu, and W.D. Powrie. 1981b. Clastogenicity of furans found in food. Cancer Lett. 13:89–95.

Stich, H.F., M.P. Rosin, C.H. Wu, and W.D. Powrie. 1981c. A comparative genotoxicity study of chlorogenic acid (3-0-caffeoylquinic acid). Mutat. Res. 90:201–212.

Stocks, P. 1970. Cancer mortality in relation to national consumption of cigarettes, solid fuel, tea and coffee. Br. J. Cancer 24:215–225.

Stoloff, L. 1979. Mycotoxin residues in edible animal tissues. Pp. 157–166 in Interactions of Mycotoxins in Animal Production. Proceedings of a Symposium. National Academy of Sciences, Washington, D.C.

Stoloff, L. 1982. Mycotoxins as potential environmental carcinogens. Pp. 97–120 in H.F. Stich, ed. Carcinogens and Mutagens in the Environment, Vol. 1. Food Products. CRC Press, Boca Raton, Fla.

Stoloff, L. 1983. Aflatoxin as a cause of primary-call cancer in the United States: a probability study. Nutr. Cancer 5:165–186.

Stora, C., and I. Dvorackova. 1987. Aflatoxin, viral hepatitis and primary liver cancer. J. Med. 18:23–41.

Stubbs, H.A., J. Harris, and R.C. Spear. 1984. A proportionate mortality analysis of California agricultural workers, 1978–1979. Am. J. Ind. Med. 6:305–320.

Sugimura, T., M. Nagao, T. Kawachi, M. Honda, T. Yahagi, Y. Seino, S. Sato, N. Matsukura, T. Matsushima, A. Shirai, M. Sawamura, and H. Matsumoto. 1977. Mutagen-carcinogens in food, with special reference to highly mutagenic pyrolytic products in broiled foods. Pp. 1561–1577 in H.H. Hiatt, J.D. Watson, and J.A. Winsten, eds. Origin of Human Cancers Book C: Human Risk Assessment. Cold Spring Harbor Laboratory, New York.

Sugimura, T., S. Sato, H. Ohgaki, S. Takayama, M. Nagao, and K. Wakabayashi. 1986. Mutagens and carcinogens in cooked food. Pp. 85–107 in I. Knudsen, ed. Genetic Toxicity of the Diet. Progress in Clinical and Biological Research, Vol. 206. Alan R. Liss, New York.

Sullivan, F. 1981. Third International Caffeine Workshop: special report. Nutr. Rev. 39:183–191.

Sullivan, J.W. 1982. Epidemiologic survey of bladder cancer in greater New Orleans. J. Urol. 128:281–283.

Sumi, C., M. Iseki, M. Kishikawa, I. Sekine, and I. Nishimori. 1985. Diethylstilbestrol (DES) metabolism and rat hepatic tumorigenesis. Jpn. J. Cancer Res. Suppl. 76:36.

Sun, T.T., and Y.Y.Chu. 1984. Carcinogenesis and prevention strategy of liver cancer in areas of prevalence. J. Cell Physiol. Suppl. 3:39–44.

Sweeney, M.H., J.J. Beaumont, R.J. Waxweiler, and W.E. Halperin. 1986. An investigation of mortality from cancer and other causes of death among workers employed at an East Texas chemical plant. Arch. Environ. Health 41:23–28.

Tabershaw, I.R., and W.F. Gaffey. 1974. Mortality study of workers in the manufacture of vinyl chloride and its polymers. J. Occup. Med. 16:509–518.

Tajima, K., and S. Tominaga. 1985. Dietary habits and gastro-intestinal cancers: a comparative case-control study of stomach and large intestinal cancers in Nagoya, Japan. Jpn. J. Cancer Res. 76:705–716.

Takayama, S. 1981. Studies on Carcinogenicity Testing of Food Additives in Japan. Food Chemical Technical Report Series No. 1. Japanese Ministry of Health and Welfare, Tokyo.

Takayama, S., T. Hirakawa, M. Tanaka, T. Kawachi, and T. Sugimura. 1979. In vitro transformation of hamster embryo cells with a glutamic acid pyrolysis product. Toxicol. Lett. 4:281–284.

Takayama, S., M. Masuda, M. Mogami, H. Ohgaki, S. Sato, and T. Sugimura. 1984. Induction of cancers in the intestine, liver and various other organs of rats by feeding mutagens from glutamic acid pyrolysate. Gann 75:207–213.

Takayama, S., Y. Nakatsura, H. Ohgaki, S. Sato, and T. Sugimura. 1985. Carcinogenicity in rats of a mutagenic compound, 3-amino-1,4-dimethyl-5H-pyrido[4,3-b]indole, from tryptophan pyrolysate. Jpn. J. Cancer Res. 76:815–817.

Tanaka, T., W.S. Barnes, G.M. Williams, and J.H. Weisburger. 1985. Multipotential carcinogenicity of the fried food mutagen 2-amino-3-methylimidazo[4,5-f]quinoline in rats. Jpn. J. Cancer Res. 76:570–576.

Taylor, J.M., and L. Friedman. 1974. Combined chronic feeding and three generation reproduction study of sodium saccharin in the rat. Toxicol. Appl. Pharmacol. 29:154.

Thayer, P.S., and C.J. Kensler. 1973. Exposure of four generations of mice to caffeine in drinking water. Toxicol. Appl. Pharmacol. 25:169–179.

Thelle, D.S., E. Arnesen, and O.H. Forde. 1983. The Tromso Heart Study. Does coffee raise serum cholesterol? N. Engl. J. Med. 308:1454–1457.

Thériault, G., and P. Allard. 1981. Cancer mortality of a group of Canadian workers exposed to vinyl chloride monomer. J. Occup. Med. 23:671–676.

Tisdel, M.O., P.O. Nees, D.L. Harris, and P.H. Derse. 1974. Long-term feeding of saccharin in rats. Pp. 145–158 in G.E. Inglett, ed. Symposium: Sweeteners. AVI Publishing Co., Westport, Conn.

Tohda, H., A. Oikawa, T. Kawachi, and T. Sugimura. 1980. Induction of sister-chromatid exchanges by mutagens from amino acid and protein pyrolysates. Mutat. Res. 77:65–69.

Tong, M.J., S.C. Sun, B.T. Schaeffer, N.K. Chang, K.J. Lo, and R.L. Peters. 1971. Hepatitis-associated antigen and hepatocellular carcinoma in Taiwan. Ann. Intern. Med. 75:687–691.

Törnquist, M., U. Rannug, A. Jonsson, and L. Ehrenberg. 1983. Mutagenicity of methyl nitrite in *Salmonella typhimurium*. Mutat. Res. 117:47–54.

Toth, B. 1984. Carcinogens in edible mushrooms. Pp. 99–108 in H.F. Stich, ed. Carcinogens and Mutagens in the Environment, Vol. III. Naturally Occurring Compounds: Epidemiology and Distribution. CRC Press, Boca Raton, Fla.

Toth, B., and J. Erickson. 1986. Cancer induction in mice by feeding of the uncooked cultivated mushroom of commerce *Agaricus bisporus*. Cancer Res. 46:4007–4011.

Toth, B., and K. Patil. 1981. Gyromitrin as a tumor inducer.

Neoplasma 28:559–564.

Treon, J.F., and F.P. Cleveland. 1955. Toxicity of certain chlorinated hydrocarbon insecticides for laboratory animals, with special reference to aldrin and dieldrin. J. Agric. Food Chem. 3:402–408.

Trichopoulos, D., M. Papapostolou, and A. Polychronopoulou. 1981. Coffee and ovarian cancer. Int. J. Cancer 28:691–693.

Trosko, J.E., B. Dawson, L.P. Yotti, and C.C. Chang. 1980. Saccharin may act as a tumour promoter by inhibiting metabolic cooperation between cells. Nature 285:109–110.

Trosko, J.E., L.P. Yotti, S.T. Warren, G. Tsushimoto, and C.C. Chang. 1982. Inhibition of cell–cell communication by tumor promoters. Pp. 565–585 in E. Hecker, N.E. Fusenig, W. Kunz, F. Marx, and H.W. Thielmann, eds. Carcinogenesis—A Comprehensive Survey, Vol. 7. Carcinogenesis and Biological Effects of Tumor Promoters. Raven Press, New York.

Tsuda, H., T. Sakata, T. Masui, K. Imaida, and N. Ito. 1984. Modifying effects of butylated hydroxyanisole, ethoxyquin and acetaminophen on induction of neoplastic lesions in rat liver and kidney initiated by N-ethyl-N-hydroxyethylnitrosamine. Carcinogenesis 5:525–531.

Tung, T.C., and K.H. Ling. 1968. Study on aflatoxin of foodstuffs in Taiwan. J. Vitaminol. 14:48–52.

Ueno, Y., and K. Kubota. 1976. DNA-attacking ability of carcinogenic mycotoxins in recombination-deficient mutant cells of *Bacillus subtilis*. Cancer Res. 36:445–451.

Ueno, Y., K. Kubota, T. Ito, and Y. Nakamura. 1978. Mutagenicity of carcinogenic mycotoxins in *Salmonella typhimurium*. Cancer Res. 38:536–542.

Umeda, M., T. Tsutsui, and M. Saito. 1977. Mutagenicity and inducibility of DNA single-strand breaks and chromosome aberrations by various mycotoxins. Gann 68:619–625.

Umezawa, K., T. Matsushima, T. Sugimura, T. Hirakawa, M. Tanaka, Y. Katoh, and S. Takayama. 1977. In vitro transformation of hamster embryo cells by quercetin. Toxicol. Lett. 1:175–178.

Urabe, H. 1974. The fourth reports of the study on "Yusho" and PCB. Foreword. Fukuoka Igaku Zasshi 65:1–4.

USDA (U.S. Department of Agriculture). 1986. Nationwide Food Consumption Survey. Continuing Survey of Food Intakes of Individuals. Men 19–50 Years, 1 Day, 1985. Report No. 85-3. Nutrition Monitoring Division, Human Nutrition Information Service, Hyattsville, Md. 94 pp.

USDA (U.S. Department of Agriculture). 1987a. Nationwide Food Consumption Survey. Continuing Survey of Food Intakes of Individuals. Women 19–50 Years and Their Children 1–5 Years, 4 Days, 1985. Report No. 85-4. Nutrition Monitoring Division, Human Nutrition Information Service, Hyattsville, Md. 182 pp.

USDA (U.S. Department of Agriculture) 1987b. Sugar and Sweetener. Situation and Outlook Report, September 1987. SSRV 12N3. Economic Research Service, U.S. Department of Agriculture, Washington, D.C. 43 pp.

U.S. Air Force. 1983. Air Force Health Study (Project Ranch Hand II). An Epidemiologic Investigation of Health Effects in Air Force Personnel Following Exposure to Herbicides, Baseline Mortality Study Results. Epidemiology Division, Data Science Division, U.S. Air Force School of Aerospace Medicine, Brooks Air Force Base, San Antonio, Tex. 61 pp.

U.S. Congress. 1938. Federal Food, Drug, and Cosmetic Act of 1938. 21 U.S.C. § 301 et seq. June 25, 1938, c. 675, 52. Stat. 1040. Washington, D.C.

U.S. Congress. 1948. Miller Amendment. 21 U.S.C. § 331 Subsection K. June 24, 1948, c. 613, 62. Stat. 582. Washington, D.C.

U.S. Congress. 1958. Food Additives Amendment of 1978. 21 U.S.C. § 348 et. seq. September 6, 1958, P.L. 85–929, 72. Stat. 1784. Washington, D.C.

U.S. Congress. 1960. Color Additive Amendments of 1960. 21 U.S.C. § 321 et seq. July 12, 1960, P.L. 86–618, 74. Stat. 397. Washington, D.C.

U.S. Senate. 1984. Contamination from Ethylene Dibromide. Hearing (January 27, 1984) of the Subcommittee on Toxic Substances and Environmental Oversight, Committee on Environment and Public Works. Washington, D.C.

Uyeta, M., S. Taue, and M. Mazaki. 1981. Mutagenicity of hydrolysates of tea infusions. Mutat. Res. 88:223–240.

Van den Berg, B.J. 1977. Epidemiologic observations of prematurity: effects of tobacco, coffee, and alcohol. Pp. 157–177 in D.M. Reed and F.J. Stanley, eds. The Epidemiology of Prematurity. Urban & Schwarzenberg, Baltimore.

van der Hoeven, J.C., W.J. Langerweij, and M.A. Posthumus. 1983. Aquilide A, a new mutagenic compound isolated from bracken fern (*Pteridium aquilinum* (L.) Kuhn). Carcinogenesis 4:1587–1590.

Van Duuren, B.L., B.M. Goldschmidt, G. Loewengart, A.C. Smith, S. Melchionne, I. Seidman, and D. Roth. 1979. Carcinogenicity of halogenated olefinic and aliphatic hydrocarbons in mice. J. Natl. Cancer Inst. 63:1433–1439.

van Rensburg, S.J. 1977. Role of epidemiology in the elucidation of mycotoxin health risks. Pp. 699–711 in J.V. Rodricks, C.W. Hesseltine, and M.A. Mehlman, eds. Mycotoxins in Human and Animal Health. Pathotox Publ., Park Forest South, Ill.

van Rensburg, S.J., J.J. van der Watt, I.F. Purchase, L. Pereira-Coutinho, and R. Markham. 1974. Primary liver cancer rate and aflatoxin intake in a high cancer area. S. Afr. Med. J. 48:2508A–2508D.

van Rensburg, S.J., P. Cook-Mozaffari, D.J. van Schalkwyk, J.J. van der Watt, T.J. Vincent, and I.F. Purchase. 1985. Hepatocellular carcinoma and dietary aflatoxin in Mozambique and Transkei. Br. J. Cancer 51:713–726.

Venitt, S., C.T. Bushell, and M. Osborne. 1977. Mutagenicity of acrylonitrile (cyanoethylene) in *Escherichia coli*. Mutat. Res. 45:283–288.

Verburgt, F.G., and E. Vogel. 1977. Vinyl chloride mutagenesis in *Drosophila melanogaster*. Mutat. Res. 48:327–336.

Vogel, C.L., P.P. Anthony, N. Mody, and L.F. Barker. 1970. Hepatitis-associated antigen in Ugandan patients with hepatocellular carcinoma. Lancet 2:621–624.

Waggoner, W.F. 1984. Aspartame—a review. Pediatr. Dent. 6:153–158.

Wakabayashi, K., M. Ochiai, H. Sait, M. Tsuda, Y. Suwa, M. Nagao, and T. Sugimura. 1983. Presence of 1-methyl-1,2,3,4-tetrahydro-β-carboline-3-carboxylic acid, a precursor of a mutagenic nitroso compound, in soy sauce. Proc. Natl. Acad. Sci. U.S.A. 80:2912–2916.

Wattenberg, L.W. 1981. Inhibitors of chemical carcinogens. Pp. 517–539 in J.H. Burchenal and H.F. Oettgen, eds. Cancer: Achievements, Challenges and Prospects for the 1980s, Vol. 1. Grune & Stratton, New York.

Waxweiler, R.J., W. Stringer, J.K. Wagoner, J. Jones, H. Falk, and C. Carter. 1976. Neoplastic risk among workers exposed to vinyl chloride. Ann. N.Y. Acad. Sci. 271:40–48.

Waxweiler, R.J., A.H. Smith, H. Falk, and H.A. Tyroler. 1981. Excess lung cancer risk in a synthetic chemicals plant. Environ. Health Perspect. 41:159–165.

Weathersbee, P.S., L.K. Olsen, and J.R. Lodge. 1977. Caffeine and pregnancy: a retrospective study. Postgrad. Med. 62:64–69.

Weinstein, D., I. Mauer, and H.M. Solomon. 1972. The effects of caffeine on chromosomes of human lymphocytes. In vivo and in vitro studies. Mutat. Res. 16:391–399.

Wertz, G.F., and G. Ficsor. 1978. Cytogenetic and teratogenic test of polybrominated biphenyls in rodents. Environ. Health Perspect. 23:129–132.

Whittemore, A.S., R.S. Paffenbarger, Jr., K. Anderson, and J. Halpern. 1983. Early precursors of pancreatic cancer in college men. J. Chronic Dis. 36:251–256.

Williams, D.T. 1976a. Confirmation of vinyl chloride in foods by conversion to 1-chloro-1,2-dibromoethane. J. Assoc. Off. Anal. Chem. 59:32–34.

Williams, D.T. 1976b. Gas-liquid chromatographic headspace method for vinyl chloride in vinegars and alcoholic beverages. J. Assoc. Off. Anal. Chem. 59:30–31.

Williams, D.T., and W.F. Miles. 1975. Gas-liquid chromatographic determination of vinyl chloride in alcoholic beverages, vegetable oils, and vinegars. J. Assoc. Off. Anal. Chem. 58:272–277.

Williams, G.M., Y. Maeura, and J.H. Weisburger. 1983. Simultaneous inhibition of liver carcinogenicity and enhancement of bladder carcinogenicity of N-2-fluorenylacetamide by butylated hydroxytoluene. Cancer Lett. 19:55–60.

Witschi, H. 1984. The role of toxicological interactions in chemical carcinogens. Toxicol. Pathol. 12:84–88.

Witschi, H.R., and D.G. Doherty. 1984. Butylated hydroxyanisole and lung tumor development in A/J mice. Fundam. Appl. Toxicol. 4:795–801.

Witschi, H.R., and C.C. Morse. 1983. Enhancement of lung tumor formation in mice by dietary butylated hydroxytoluene: dose-time relationships and cell kinetics. J. Natl. Cancer Inst. 71:859–866.

Witschi, H.P., P.J. Hakkinen, and J.P. Kehrer. 1981. Modification of lung tumor development in A/J mice. Toxicology 21:37–45.

Wogan, G.N. 1975. Dietary factors and special epidemiological situations of liver cancer in Thailand and Africa. Cancer Res. 35:3499–3502.

Wolff, S., and B. Rodin. 1978. Saccharin-induced sister chromatid exchanges in Chinese hamster and human cells. Science 200:543–545.

Wong, J.J., and D.P. Hsieh. 1976. Mutagenicity of aflatoxins related to their metabolism and carcinogenic potential. Proc. Natl. Acad. Sci. U.S.A. 73:2241–2244.

Wong, L.C.K., J.M. Winston, C.B. Hong, and H. Plotnick. 1982. Carcinogenicity and toxicity of 1,2-dibromoethane in the rat. Toxicol. Appl. Pharmacol. 63:155–165.

Wong, O., H.M. Utidjian, and V.S. Karten. 1979. Retrospective evaluation of reproductive performance of workers exposed to ethylene dibromide (EDB). J. Occup. Med. 21:98–102.

Woods, J.A., L. Polissar, R.K. Severson, L.S. Heuser, and B.G. Kulander. 1987. Soft tissue sarcoma and non-Hodgkin's lymphoma in relation to phenoxyherbicide and chlorinated phenol exposure in western Washington. J.

Natl. Cancer Inst. 78:899–910.

Würzner, H.P., E. Lindström, L. Vuataz, and H. Lunginbühl. 1977. A 2-year feeding study of instant coffees in rats. II. Incidence and types of neoplasms. Food Cosmet. Toxicol. 15:289–296.

Wynder, E.L., and S.D. Stellman. 1980. Artificial sweetener use and bladder cancer: a case control study. Science 207:1214–1216.

Wynder, E.L., J. Onderdonk, and N. Mantel. 1963. An epidemiological investigation of cancer of the bladder. Cancer 16:1388–1407.

Wynder, E.L., N.E. Hall, and M. Polansky. 1983. Epidemiology of coffee and pancreatic cancer. Cancer Res. 43:3900–3906.

Wyndham, C., J. Devenish, and S. Safe. 1976. The in vitro metabolism, macromolecular binding and bacterial mutagenicity of 4-chloribiphenyl, a model PCB substrate. Res. Commun. Chem. Pathol. Pharmacol. 15:563–570.

Yamamoto, T., K. Tsuji, T. Kosuge, T. Okamoto, K. Shudo, K. Takeda, Y. Iitaka, K. Yamaguchi, Y. Seino, T. Yahagi, M. Nagao, and T. Sugimura. 1978. Isolation and structure determination of mutagenic substances in L-glutamic acid pyrolysate. Proc. Jpn. Acad. 54B:248–250.

Yang, C.S. 1980. Research on esophageal cancer in China: a review. Cancer Res. 40:2633–2644.

Yano, K., G.G. Rhoads, and A. Kagan. 1977. Coffee, alcohol and risk of coronary heart disease among Japanese men living in Hawaii. N. Engl. J. Med. 297:405–409.

Yeh, F.S., C.C. Mo, and R.C. Yen. 1985. Risk factors for hepatocellular carcinoma in Guangxi, People's Republic of China. Natl. Cancer Inst. Monogr. 69:47–48.

Yen, F.S., and K.N. Shen. 1986. Epidemiology and early diagnosis of primary liver cancer in China. Adv. Cancer Res. 47:297–329.

Yoshida, D., T. Matsumoto, R. Yoshimura, and T. Matsuzaki. 1978. Mutagenicity of amino-alpha-carbolines in pyrolysis products of soybean globulin. Biochem. Biophys. Res. Commun. 83:915–920.

Yoshida, S., M. Masubuchi, and K. Hiraga. 1978. Induced chromosome aberrations by artificial sweeteners in CHO-K1 cells. Mutat. Res. 54:262.

Zack, J.A., and R.R. Suskind. 1980. The mortality experience of workers exposed to tetrachlorodibenzodioxin in a trichlorophenol process accident. J. Occup. Med. 22:11–14.

Zedeck, M.S. 1984. Hydrazine derivatives, azo and azoxy compounds, and methylazoxymethanol and cycasin. Pp. 915–944 in C.E. Searle, ed. Chemical Carcinogens, 2nd ed., Revised and Expanded. ACS Monograph 182. American Chemical Society, Washington, D.C.

Zeitlin, B.R. 1972. Coffee and bladder cancer. Lancet 1:1066.

Ziegler, R.G., T.J. Mason, A. Stemhagen, R. Hoover, J.B. Schoenberg, G. Gridley P.W. Virgo, and J.F. Fraumeni, Jr. 1986. Carotenoid intake, vegetables, and the risk of lung cancer among white men in New Jersey. Am. J. Epidemiol. 123:1080–1093.

Zimmermann, F.K. 1977. Genetic effects of nitrous acid. Mutat Res. 39:127–147.

18

Dietary Supplements

The use of dietary or nutritional supplements in the United States is extensive and noticeably increasing (Miller, 1987b). People supplement their diets for several reasons, including uncertainty about the nutrient adequacy of their diets, a desire for a more positive standard of health than they perceive to be obtainable from medical consultation, and decisions to treat themselves for an illness. The use of dietary supplements is probably fostered by their wide availability, aggressive marketing, and media reports on studies suggesting that supplements may help to prevent or treat common health problems (Gussow and Thomas, 1986; McDonald, 1986).

Sales of dietary supplements increased sixfold in 15 years—from $500 million in 1972 (Anonymous, 1981) to $3 billion in 1987 (Dickinson, 1987). Industry data show the market share for various supplements in 1986 as follows: multivitamins, 37%; vitamin C, 13%; calcium, 12%; B complex, 10%; and vitamin E, 9% (Dickinson, 1987). Guthrie (1986) calculated that Americans who supplement their diets spend an average of $32 per person annually, whereas for less than $10 per year, consumers can purchase a one-a-day multiple vitamin/mineral product that supplies approximately 100% of the Recommended Dietary Allowances (RDAs) for most nutrients.

In the U.S. population, dietary supplement use varies widely according to age, lifestyle, socioeco-nomic status, geographic location, and other characteristics. Variation in survey-based estimates of supplement use can be attributed to the population sampled; the season of the year the survey is conducted; definition of the term dietary supplement (e.g., in some studies only vitamin- and mineral-containing products are defined as supplements, but in others, products such as bee pollen, lecithin, and alfalfa tablets are included); and definition of the frequency of supplement use (e.g., daily use versus irregular use) (Kurinij et al., 1986; Looker et al., 1987; McDonald, 1986; Stewart et al., 1985). The use of dietary supplements among adults, children, the elderly, and health professionals is described in the following four sections.

USE OF DIETARY SUPPLEMENTS

Adults

The most current data on dietary supplement use in the United States have been collected by the U.S. Department of Agriculture (USDA) in the Continuing Survey of Food Intakes by Individuals (CSFII)—a component of its Nationwide Food Consumption Survey (NFCS). In 1985, 45% of the men 19 to 50 years of age reported taking a dietary supplement either regularly or occasionally—up from 26% in 1977 (USDA, 1986). In 1986, 55% of the women 19 to 50 years of age took supplements regularly or occasionally—up from 39% in 1977 (USDA, 1987b). Of the survey's low-income women 19 to 50 years of age, 45% took supplements during 1986 (USDA, 1987a).

The most comprehensive survey of dietary supplement use in the United States was conducted by the Food and Drug Administration (FDA) in 1980 through telephone interviews with 2,991 representative Americans over 15 years of age (Stewart et al., 1985). The FDA found that 35.9% of the men and 43.8% of the nonpregnant, nonlactating women consumed supplements daily. The supplement users were grouped into four categories: light users (who on average consumed the equivalent of 70% of the RDA for each nutrient), moderate users (168% of the RDA), heavy users (400% of the RDA), and very heavy users (777% of the RDA) (Levy and Schucker, 1987). The majority of the users took only one nutrient or combination product, although 10.9% of the sample consumed from 5 to 14 separate products (Stewart et al., 1985). Dietary supplement use was most prevalent in the western United States and among Caucasian people with relatively high incomes and at least a high school education.

The FDA investigators also noted that specialized vitamin and mineral preparations were most commonly taken by the heavy and very heavy users (28% and 14% of all users, respectively). The light and moderate users (42% and 16% of all users, respectively) favored the broad-spectrum, multinutrient products (Levy and Schucker, 1987). Compared to light and moderate users of dietary supplements, heavy and very heavy users were more likely to shop in health food stores, buy supplements through the mail, read specialized health literature, believe they had personal control over their health, engage in daily exercise, avoid involving their physicians in their decisions about supplements, and perceive specific rather than general health benefits from their supplements. The FDA investigators described the light and moderate users as people who consume supplements as insurance against dietary deficiencies. They described heavy and very heavy users as those who take supplements as part of an active effort to achieve better health.

Fairly high rates of dietary supplement use were also found in earlier national surveys conducted for the FDA. In 1969, 27% of the adults surveyed had taken a supplement on the day of the interview, and 57% of the sample said they had taken supplements at some time (National Analysts, Inc., 1972). Subjects most commonly took supple-

ments to improve health, to obtain "more pep and energy," to prevent colds, to reduce their risk of becoming ill, and to remain healthy while dieting. In 54% of the households contacted in 1973, at least one family member took supplements. The most frequent user was the homemaker (usually female), followed by the spouse and preteen child (FDA, 1974). In a similar study conducted in 1975, 47% of the households contained at least one member who took supplements. Again, the most frequent user was the female homemaker (FDA, 1976). The extent of dietary supplement use in the United States during the late 1970s was determined by Koplan et al. (1986), who evaluated data from the National Health and Nutrition Examination Survey (NHANES II). They found that 21.4% of adults in the United States took supplements daily and that another 13.5% took them at least once a week. Higher rates of supplement use were associated with women, whites, older age (ages 51 to 74 compared to ages 18 to 50), higher incomes, higher educational levels, and higher nutrient intakes from food.

Schutz et al. (1982) found that 67% of 2,451 randomly selected adults surveyed in seven western states took supplements over a 2-year period. Multiple vitamins with or without iron, vitamins C and E, and the B complex vitamins were most commonly taken. The most frequently given reasons for taking supplements, selected from a list provided by the investigators, were "to prevent colds and other illnesses," "to give me energy," and "to make up for what is not in food." Factors found to be significantly associated with supplement use included age (higher use at younger ages), education (greater use at higher educational levels), sex (women were heavier users), and the perception that the nutritional quality of food had decreased over the past decade. When a subsample of 689 people was questioned further, 59% of the users reported that their supplements were of "some benefit" to their health, and another 34% found them to be of "great benefit" (Read et al., 1985). In a study of a subsample of 1,673 people, differences were found between those who took multivitamins/minerals and those who took individual supplements of either vitamins A, C, or E in the importance placed on the need for supplementation and where nutrition information was obtained (Read et al., 1987). Users of one of these nutrients were significantly more likely than users of multivitamins/minerals to have a lower opinion of today's food quality, to classify their diets as being either poor or very poor, to believe in the value of unproven uses of nutrients as therapeutic agents, to rely on health food stores for nutrition information, and to feel that they would experience serious health problems if they were forced to discontinue their use of supplements.

Investigators have frequently studied or surveyed dietary supplement use among various population subgroups and small samples of adults (see, for example, Bootman and Wertheimer, 1980; Bowerman and Harrill, 1983; English and Carl, 1981; Read and Thomas, 1983; Rhee and Stubbs, 1976; Saegert and Saegert, 1976). The evidence accumulated over the past 20 years from these studies, as well as those mentioned above, conclusively demonstrates that dietary supplement use is popular in the United States. Today it is entirely possible that the majority of adults in the United States supplement their diets at least occasionally with extra vitamins and minerals.

The Elderly

The elderly might be expected to take dietary supplements in an attempt to prevent or cure chronic disease, to treat the symptoms of aging, or to prolong life. In fact, studies conducted more than 20 years ago indicate that between one-fourth and one-half of the elderly consumed supplements (Davidson et al., 1962; Le Bovit, 1965; Steinkamp et al., 1965).

In a more recent study, Hale et al. (1982) reported that among 3,192 ambulatory elderly participants, more than 46% of the women and 34% of the men took supplements. All were at least 65 years of age and enrolled in a health screening program. The participants typically consumed multivitamins or minerals, usually daily, as well as vitamins E and C. The users gave the following reasons for taking vitamin C (from most to least frequent): to treat deficiency states, to prevent coughs and colds, and to treat ophthalmic disorders, urinary tract infections, and rheumatic conditions. They used vitamin E primarily to treat or prevent deficiency states and leg cramps and as a vasodilator. In a study of 11,888 residents of a southern California retirement community, 62% of the men and 69% of the women were found to consume supplemental vitamins and minerals (Gray et al., 1986).

One of the most recent studies on dietary supplement use in the elderly involved 236 upper-class people from a retirement community in rural Maryland (Sobal et al., 1986). Fifty-three percent reported that they had taken supplements within the past 6 months, usually on a daily basis. A single multivitamin pill was usually consumed, but products containing vitamin C, potassium, calcium, B complex, vitamin E, and iron were popular as well. Participants most commonly justified their supplement use to combat tiredness (44% of users), to ensure good nutrition (30%), to increase energy (28%), and as treatment for illness (22%). Physicians were said to be most influential in the subjects' decision to consume these products. The investigators reported that the frequency and duration of supplement use was not significantly related to age, sex, level of education, reported health status, or frequency of worrying about health.

The studies described above as well as several others (see, for example, Garry et al., 1982; Gray et al., 1983; Kellett et al., 1984; McGandy et al., 1986; Ranno et al., 1988; Read and Graney, 1982; Yearick et al., 1980) over the past several decades demonstrate that many elderly people in the United States consume dietary supplements. In addition, the data indicate, as might be expected, that the elderly often take supplements to feel better and to treat the illnesses that afflict them as they age.

Children

There is relatively little information on dietary supplement use by children. The most current data on supplement use among U.S. children 1 to 5 years of age comes from USDA's CSFII. The proportion of children taking supplements in 1985 and 1986 was 60 and 59%, respectively, up from 47% in 1977 (USDA, 1987b). Forty-four percent of the children from low-income families receiving food stamps were reported to take supplements in 1986; 47% of the children in similar families not receiving food stamps also took supplements (USDA, 1987a).

Two surveys provide data on the extent of dietary supplement use among children of all ages. Bowering and Clancy (1986) examined data from NHANES II and found that dietary supplement use among children decreased with age—from 39% for 2-year-olds to slightly more than 10% for teenagers. No sex differences in supplement use were noted until the age of 13, when usage by boys plateaued at about 10% but began to increase among girls. Children were more likely to receive supplements if the head of the household was white and better educated. Also in NHANES II, supplements, generally multivitamins, were found to be commonly consumed daily from the ages of 1 to 10; from 11 to 19 years, supplement use was more likely to be irregular (Looker et al., 1987). Kovar (1985) reported that approximately 36% of more than 15,000 children under 18 years of age who had participated in the National Health Interview Survey in 1981 took supplements during the 2 weeks before the interview. Supplement use was most common among children under 7 years of age.

In a more limited study, Farris et al. (1985) examined supplement use among 10- and 13-year-old children randomly selected from the biracial community of Bogalusa, Louisiana, between 1973 and 1977. Sixteen to 18% of the 10-year-olds and 12% of the 13-year-olds were found to consume supplements daily, typically multivitamins with or without iron. There were no race or sex differences in supplement use. Similarly, Sharpe and Smith (1985) reported supplement use to be 11% among the 1,616 children in northern Mississippi households that participated in the Aid to Families with Dependent Children program administered by the U.S. Department of Health and Human Services.

Thomsen et al. (1987), in their 1985 survey of 163 adolescents from rural-based Iowa high schools, provided data on the reasons for dietary supplement use among that group. The 86 subjects who took supplements most commonly agreed with the following statements for their use: "they made me healthy"; "my doctor tells me to take them"; and "they help give me energy." Fifty-six percent of the sample agreed that "most teenagers need vitamin and mineral supplements."

In summary, dietary supplement use among children is not as extensive as it is among adults. Studies suggest that supplement use is highest at early ages, and then steadily declines until adolescence, when it may increase. Since most studies of supplement use focus on adults and the elderly, less information is available regarding the types of supplements children take, the nutrient doses involved, and the rationale for their use.

Health Professionals

Several studies suggest that supplement use is common among health professionals—a group likely to argue that nutrient needs can and should be met from foods. Worthington-Roberts and Breskin (1984) discovered that nearly 60% of the 665 Washington State dietitians who responded to a mail questionnaire admitted that they regularly took supplements—usually multivitamins/minerals, vitamin C, and iron—for personal health. The investigators hypothesized that these dietitians took supplements to ensure an adequate intake of nutrients in light of their occasional dietary indiscretions and calorie restrictions to regulate weight.

Willett et al. (1981) found that 38% of 1,742 registered nurses surveyed in 10 states consumed multiple vitamins, 23% took vitamin C, 15% took vitamin E, and 4% took vitamin A. The use of supplements of vitamins A, C, and E increased progressively with age. Use of any of the four supplements was strongly associated with use of the other three.

Several surveys demonstrate that supplement use among physicians and medical students is not infrequent. Nine out of 36 family practice residents surveyed in one study said they "usually" supplemented their diets (Pally et al., 1984). In another, 14% of 595 faculty members from Harvard Medical School admitted to taking multivitamins daily. In addition, 14% said they took extra vitamin C to protect against colds (Goldfinger, 1982). Among new medical students at the University of Maryland School of Medicine, more than 60% said they "regularly," "usually," or "sometimes" took dietary supplements (Sobal and Muncie, 1985).

Several studies indicate that physicians exert the most influence on the public (their patients) in making decisions to take supplements (Kellett et al., 1984; National Analysts, Inc., 1972; Pally et al., 1984; Read and Graney, 1982; Sobal et al., 1986, 1987; Yearick et al., 1980). A 1983 survey revealed that 27% of 1,419 primary care physicians (representing family/general practice, internal medicine, and obstetrics/gynecology) in Maryland believed that supplementation was either "very" or "somewhat" important in contrast to 97% who believed that a balanced diet was important (Sobal et al., 1987). Dietary supplementation was considered important primarily among obstetricians/gynecologists, female physicians, and those who said they were more likely to take continuing medical education courses in nutrition.

One study suggests that physicians need to become more knowledgeable about the appropriate use of supplements. After reviewing the medical charts of 433 elderly patients admitted to several health-care facilities in New York State, Sorensen et al. (1979) concluded that physicians prescribed specific vitamins and minerals for 43 patients in the absence of a diagnosis of deficiency. For five patients, however, vitamin and mineral supplements were not prescribed even though the medical diagnosis indicated that they should have been.

Pharmacists may also be involved in the inappropriate promotion of supplements. *Consumer Reports* magazine reported that of 30 pharmacists visited in three states by reporters who pretended to suffer from fatigue, tension, or nervousness, 17 of them recommended vitamin supplements and one recommended an amino acid preparation (Anonymous, 1986).

NUTRIENT ADEQUACY AND SUPPLEMENT USE

The above review of survey data and other studies indicate that dietary supplementation is usually related to subjective perceptions of health, well-being, and balanced diets and to beliefs about food, vitamins, and minerals (Worsley, 1986). But by more objective measures, are supplements being used appropriately? The effect of supplementation on nutritional status has occasionally been compared among users and nonusers by measuring dietary intake and biological indices. In general, the studies show little correlation between nutrient needs and nutrient supplementation (Guthrie, 1986).

Adults

Bowerman and Harrill (1983) analyzed the 3-day dietary records of 150 adults living in Colorado and found no major differences in mean dietary intake among users and nonusers. Dietary intakes of protein, phosphorus, vitamin A, riboflavin, niacin, and vitamin C were above RDA levels for men as well as women. Women 19 to 50 years of age, however, consumed less than two-thirds of the RDA for both iron and zinc. In an analysis of NHANES I data obtained from 3,227 nonpregnant women 15 to 41 years of age, Kurinij et al. (1986) found that dietary supplement users consumed more nutrient-dense diets than did nonusers. Although intakes of calcium, iron, and vitamins A and C were less than 50% of the RDA for many subjects in both groups, a greater proportion of nonusers had low intakes of these four nutrients. Using data on adults from NHANES II, Looker et al. (1988) failed to find an association between daily use of dietary supplements (which in most cases contained iron) and either improved iron status or a lower prevalence of impaired iron status. In addition, daily supplement users were found to consume more vitamin C from foods and to eat more fruits and vegetables compared to nonusers. Read and Thomas (1983) discovered that 41 of 49 adult lacto-ovovegetarians ingested dietary supplements, but an analysis of their diets revealed that

with the exception of iron (especially for females less than 51 years of age), they all met or surpassed the established RDAs for nine nutrients from food alone.

The Elderly

Several studies of elderly populations indicated that dietary supplement users consumed more nutrients from food than did nonusers (Garry et al., 1982; McGandy et al., 1986). In one study of 51 elderly people, dietary supplement use was found to be unrelated to dietary intake (Gray et al., 1983). Several studies show, however, that the diets of many elderly people fail to meet the RDAs for several nutrients—including calcium, zinc, vitamins B_6, B_{12}, D, E, and folate (Garry et al., 1982; McGandy et al., 1986). Yearick et al. (1980) reported that the majority of people they surveyed consumed diets low in calcium, vitamin A, thiamin, and iron and did not take supplements of these nutrients. Kirsch and Bidlack (1987) noted that many elderly people are at risk of nutrient deficiencies for reasons that include physiological decline, poor economic status, inadequate food intake, disease processes, and medical treatments. In addition, Ranno et al. (1988) found that the use or nonuse of supplements by 60 elderly volunteers was unrelated to the perceived adequacy of their diets.

Children

Using data from NHANES II for children from 1 to 19 years of age, Bowering and Clancy (1986) and Looker et al. (1987) found no differences in iron status indicators (e.g., hemoglobin, transferrin saturation, serum ferritin) between dietary supplement users and nonusers. In addition, both sets of investigators found that supplement users consumed more vitamin C from food. Looker and colleagues also noted that the users consumed more fruits and vegetables. Breskin et al. (1985) studied the dietary intakes and related biochemical indices of several B vitamins and vitamin C among 30 children aged $3\frac{1}{3}$ to 9 years and found that mean intakes of most of these nutrients from food alone met the subjects' needs. Furthermore, there were no major differences in the nutrient content of the diets of supplement users and nonusers. Since no nutrient deficiencies in either group were evident from the biochemical measures, the investigators concluded that improvements in biochemical indices resulting from supplement use were only relative and did not suggest that supplements were beneficial. Sharpe and Smith (1985) reported that low-income children in Mississippi who took supplements usually used preparations lacking in iron—one of the nutrients most likely to be poorly supplied in their diets.

EVIDENCE ASSOCIATING DIETARY SUPPLEMENTS WITH CHRONIC DISEASES

Supplements are often taken in high doses with the aim of preventing or treating various health problems or promoting longevity. However, there are relatively few controlled studies concerning the effects of dietary supplements on the risk of specific chronic diseases. Therefore, very little is known about the health effects of chronic use of high-potency dietary supplements (Miller, 1987b). In one prospective study of 479 elderly people, investigators found no clear reduction in mortality from the use of dietary supplements over a 6-year period (Enstrom and Pauling, 1982). Similarly, no association was noted between the use of vitamin C supplements and subsequent mortality among 3,119 adults in California followed for 10 years (Enstrom et al., 1986).

Cancer

Vitamin A

In one case-comparison study, low doses of vitamin A supplements were found to be associated with a lowered risk of cancer (Smith and Jick, 1978). Gregor et al. (1980) reported an inverse association between vitamin A intake and lung cancer risk primarily due to the intake of liver (which is high in vitamin A) and vitamin A preparations. Another study has shown that dietary supplementation with both retinol and β-carotene reversed micronucleus formation (a marker for cellular genetic damage) in buccal mucosal cells among Filipino chewers of betel nut and tobacco (Stitch et al., 1984). As discussed in Chapter 11, however, the weight of the evidence does not show that vitamin A from foods or supplements has a protective effect against cancer (La Vecchia et al., 1988; Samet et al., 1985; Shekelle et al., 1981; Ziegler et al., 1984). However, several studies have shown an inverse relationship between the consumption of fruits and vegetables rich in β-carotene and a reduced risk of cancer at various sites. Several prospective studies are in progress to determine whether supplements of β-carotene (with and without other nutrients) have the same protective

effect, but results are not expected before 1990 (DHHS, 1988; Greenwald, 1988).

Calcium

Lipkin and Newmark (1985) conducted a pilot study of the effect of calcium supplements on proliferation of colonic cells in patients considered to be at increased risk for colon cancer. They reported that the administration of 1.2 g/day of calcium led to the reduction of colonic crypt labeling with tritiated thymidine, in vitro, that approximated the pattern seen in a low-risk control population.

Zinc

Zinc intake from food and supplements was assessed in one case-control study of cancer. Kolonel et al. (1988) found that patients with prostate cancer who were 70 years old and older ingested *more* zinc (from supplements, but not from food) than did matched population controls prior to the onset of cancer.

Vitamin C

Cameron and Pauling (1976, 1978) reported that 100 patients with terminal cancer at various sites who were given vitamin C at 10 g/day had a mean survival time more than 4.1 times greater than that of a group of matched controls who did not receive the vitamin. None of the patients in these studies had received chemotherapy. In two subsequent controlled studies, investigators failed to find differences in survival time among 127 patients with advanced cancer at various sites (Creagan et al., 1979) and 100 patients with advanced colorectal cancer who had not received chemotherapy (Moertel et al., 1985) and who were randomly assigned to treatment with either 10 g of vitamin C per day or a placebo. Because the focus of this report is the prevention of chronic diseases rather than their treatment, the committee has not included the literature on nutritional supplements as therapy for cancer or other diseases.

Coronary Heart Disease

Vitamin E

An initial report (Vogelsang and Shute, 1946) of dramatic improvement in angina pectoris patients taking large doses of vitamin E was not confirmed in four placebo-controlled clinical trials (Anderson and Reid, 1974; Donegan et al., 1949; Makinson et al., 1948; Rinzler et al., 1950) and two double-blind trials (Anderson and Reid, 1974; Rinzler et al., 1950). Preliminary reports that vitamin E might raise the concentration of HDL cholesterol (Barboriak et al., 1982; Hermann et al., 1979) were not confirmed in a randomized, double-blind, placebo-controlled study (Stampfer et al., 1983).

Vitamin C

Spittle (1972) found that in healthy people under 25 years of age, cholesterol levels tended to fall with the addition of 1 g of vitamin C to their normal diets. Placebo-controlled studies, however, fail to show that vitamin C supplements lower serum cholesterol levels (Aro et al., 1988). For example, in a double-blind crossover study with 26 elderly female subjects, vitamin C in amounts as high as 2 g/day had no effect on serum cholesterol levels as compared to a placebo (Aro et al., 1988).

Calcium

Most intervention studies in which calcium supplements were used demonstrate a mild short-term reduction in blood pressure in certain normotensive and hypertensive subjects (Belizan et al., 1983; Grobbee and Hofman, 1986; McCarron and Morris, 1985; Resnick et al., 1984; Singer et al., 1985). However, in some patients with hypertension and increased concentrations of plasma renin, blood pressure may actually rise in response to calcium supplementation (Resnick et al., 1984).

Zinc

Supplementation of the diet of 12 adult men with more than 10 times the RDA of zinc in the presence of normal levels of copper for 5 weeks led to a significant decrease in HDL cholesterol but no change in total cholesterol (Hooper et al., 1980). Other studies have confirmed that zinc supplements suppress HDL levels (Chandra, 1984; Goodwin et al., 1985).

Chromium

The evidence is contradictory as to whether chromium supplementation affects blood lipoproteins in a favorable manner. As the trivalent ion in chromium chloride or glucose tolerance factor (GTF), chromium lowered serum total cholesterol and raised the HDL fraction in healthy participants in supplementation trials (Anderson, 1986; Riales and Albrink, 1981; Simonoff, 1984). Other trials have not shown an effect from chromium supplementation on serum lipoprotein levels (Anderson et al., 1983; Rabinowitz et al., 1983; Uusitupa et al., 1983).

Osteoporosis

It is not known whether calcium supplements, commonly consumed by women in the United States, are useful in the prevention and treatment of osteoporosis. The results of short-term investigations (2 years or less) are mixed. In general, they show a slowing of cortical but not trabecular bone loss. All studies in which estrogen treatment was also used show that calcium supplementation is inferior to estrogen in slowing cortical bone loss and that estrogen completely prevents trabecular bone loss (Cann et al., 1980; Ettinger et al., 1987; Horsman et al., 1977; Lamke et al., 1978; Nilas et al., 1984; Recker and Heaney, 1985; Recker et al., 1977; Riis et al., 1987; Smith et al., 1981). (See Chapter 13 for further details.) The evidence relating calcium supplementation to fracture prevalence is scanty. The only relevant study was a nonrandomized, prospective assessment of the effect of various treatments on the occurrence of future vertebral fractures in patients with generalized osteopenia (Riggs et al., 1982). Eighteen women receiving calcium carbonate (1,500–2,500 mg/day) and 19 patients given a combination of calcium plus vitamin D (50,000 units once or twice a week) had 50% fewer vertebral fractures than did 18 untreated women and 27 patients given a placebo ($p < .001$). This decrease in fracture rate is impressive and suggests that a long-term, randomized, blind study of fracture rates among placebo- and calcium-treated postmenopausal and elderly women might provide information crucial to the formulation of recommendations for calcium intakes in the elderly.

Other Diseases

Vitamin C is widely purported to help prevent or treat the common cold, as originally hypothesized by Linus Pauling (1986). However, the several studies conducted to test this hypothesis generally indicate that vitamin C taken even in gram quantities does not prevent colds and at best only reduces the frequency and severity of symptoms in cold sufferers (Anderson et al., 1972, 1974; Coulehan et al., 1974; Karlowski et al., 1975).

NUTRIENT TOXICITIES

Excess vitamin and mineral consumption is associated with numerous acute adverse health effects. Most reported vitamin intoxications have resulted from the consumption of supplements, not foods, although one notable exception is vitamin A poisoning among Arctic explorers who consumed polar bear liver (Greger, 1987; McLaren, 1984). There are laboratory animal data on the toxicity of single vitamins and minerals and clinical data on adverse health effects from high intakes of nutrients by individuals. Most of the data pertain to acute rather than chronic use.

Many case reports of human injury presumed to result from vitamin and mineral overdoses lack data on the actual dosages of nutrients consumed, formulation of the supplements, and periods of exposure. In addition, those reports rarely relate intake of the supplement to the levels of nutrients in a person's diet. It is difficult to determine the levels at which nutrient toxicities are likely to occur. Size, age, genetic disposition, and overall health, as well as the duration of supplementation and the quantity and form of nutrients consumed, greatly affect responses to nutrient overconsumption (Greger, 1987).

There are several comprehensive reviews of nutrient toxicity (see, e.g., Campbell et al., 1980; Rechcigl, 1978). The following paragraphs summarize some of the potential adverse health effects of excessive supplementation.

Vitamin A

Toxicity has been observed in people who have either chronically or acutely consumed more than 10 times the RDA. Acute hypervitaminosis A occurs following a single massive dose of retinol (e.g., from ingestion of polar bear or seal liver). Chronic hypervitaminosis A results from continued ingestion of high doses (e.g., supplements). Symptoms of hypervitaminosis A include dryness of the skin, headache, anorexia, weakness, hair loss, joint pain, vomiting, irritability, enlarged liver and spleen, and in babies, a bulging fontanelle and increased intracranial pressure (Olson, 1988). The clinical manifestations and the published literature on hypervitaminosis A have been reviewed in detail by Bauernfeind (1980) and Kamm et al. (1984). Hypervitaminosis A has not been reported to be a public health problem in any population. Vitamin A toxicity is unlikely to occur from food, unless very large amounts of liver are ingested. However, the widespread availability of vitamin A preparations in very large doses, publicity about the use of vitamin A in treating acne and preventing cancer, and the increasing prevalence of food supplementation are causes for concern that hypervitaminosis A may become com-

mon (Goodman, 1984). Uses of vitamin A supplements that exceed the RDA pose a potential for toxicity.

Of special note, consumption of excessive amounts of vitamin A during early pregnancy is potentially teratogenic. A related retinoid, 13-cis-retinoic acid, is a known teratogen (Costas et al., 1987). Yet, according to a study by the New York State Department of Health, 16 of 492 women who delivered live-born infants without birth defects over an 11-month period took supplements containing high doses of vitamin A during their pregnancy. Three of the 16 took 25,000 IU or more per day; the other 13 took from 15,000 to 24,999 IU/day. The Centers for Disease Control consider this finding to be of public health concern (Costas et al., 1987).

Vitamin B₆

In 1983, Schaumburg and colleagues reported on seven people who developed ataxia and sensory neuropathy after taking 2 to 6 g of pyridoxine daily for 2 to 40 months. When the supplement was discontinued, all patients noted an improvement in their neurological disability and gait and suffered less discomfort in their extremities. Subsequently, Berger and Schaumburg (1984) observed sensory neuropathy and symptoms resembling multiple sclerosis in a patient taking as little as 500 mg of pyridoxine daily for several years. Even smaller doses may cause problems. Pyridoxine toxicity was the apparent cause of neurological symptoms (including paraesthesia, bone pain, muscle weakness, and numbness) among 103 women attending a private clinic who were given supplements of this nutrient to treat premenstrual syndrome, depression, and other disorders (Dalton and Dalton, 1987). The women took an average of 117 ± 92 mg of this nutrient over a period ranging from more than 6 months to more than 5 years, and all developed high serum vitamin B₆ levels. Within 3 months after discontinuing pyridoxine supplementation, 55% reported partial or complete recovery from their neurological symptoms; by 6 months, all had recovered completely.

Vitamin E

No side effects were reported by 28 adults who had consumed vitamin E supplements in doses ranging from 100 to 800 IU/day for an average of 3 years (Farrell and Bieri, 1975). In a double-blind study of 202 adults given 600 IU of vitamin E per day for 4 weeks, subjects experienced a considerable reduction in serum thyroid hormone levels (Tsai et al., 1978). In the female subjects, serum triglyceride levels became elevated. Neither development, however, was associated with clinical symptoms. Bendich and Machlin (1988), in their recent review of the literature concerning the safety of vitamin E, concluded that few side effects have been observed in humans at intakes as high as 3,200 IU/day. They concluded that the majority of reported side effects have been based on individual case reports or uncontrolled studies and on reports in letters to the editors of journals. These side effects have not been seen in large, well-controlled studies.

Calcium

No adverse effects have been seen in healthy persons consuming up to 2,500 mg of calcium per day (Avioli, 1988). There is concern, however, that people with undiagnosed abnormalities of calcium metabolism could develop hypercalcemia with excessive calcium intake. High calcium intakes also appear to suppress bone remodeling, which could prevent repair of microfractures and eventually result in bone fragility (Meuleman, 1987). Calcium intakes greater than 1,500 mg/day may promote the development of urinary stones in some people (NIH, 1984).

Zinc

People consuming more than 25 mg/day have developed nausea, epigastric distress, and a metallic taste in the mouth (Solomons, 1988). Larger doses of zinc are sometimes used as an emetic. Zinc deficiency as well as zinc excess impair immune system function. In one study, 11 healthy men given 300 mg of zinc for 6 weeks developed impaired lymphocyte and polymorphonuclear (PMN) leukocyte function. T cells exhibited reduced response to antigens; chemotactic migration and phagocytosis of PMN leukocytes were also impaired (Chandra, 1984). Large doses of zinc promote the loss of copper from the body, leading to copper deficiency anemia (Solomons, 1988).

Summary

In summary, to date there is no evidence that low levels of dietary supplements adversely affect the general population. The FDA's most recent national survey of dietary supplement use (Stewart et al., 1985) shows that the use of various nutrients among men and women in the 95th percentile was in most cases well below the toxic levels reported by Hathcock (1985) (see Table 18–1). However, several surveys show that *some* people ingest supplements in potentially harmful amounts (Bowerman and Harrill, 1983; Gray et al., 1983, 1986; Levy and Schucker, 1987; Read et al., 1981; Willett et al., 1981).

In 1986, the FDA and the American Dietetic Association asked physicians nationwide to document their patients' use of dietary supplements, as is currently done with drugs, and to report any harmful effects to FDA's Adverse Reaction Monitoring System. FDA plans to use such data to determine the extent to which these products pose risks to health and to determine the most effective course of action (ADA, 1986; Miller, 1987b).

ADDITIONAL CONCERNS

Health professionals are also concerned about the public's use of dietary supplements for reasons other than the potential risks to health from nutrient overdoses. One reason is the complications attributable to supplementation that may occur in the diagnosis and treatment of certain diseases among people taking large doses of vitamins and minerals. Vitamin B_6, for example, acts as an antagonist to L-dopa, which is used to treat Parkinson's disease (Dreyfus, 1988). Large vitamin C intakes may interfere with the results of clinical laboratory tests used to detect the presence of fecal and urinary occult blood (Levine, 1983).

Nutrients interact in the human body, so that relatively large intakes of one nutrient may affect the absorption, metabolism, or excretion of others and, therefore, affect their requirements. Ascorbic acid, for example, increases the absorption of nonheme iron in food and decreases the intestinal absorption of copper (Hornig et al., 1988). Copper bioavailability is also depressed by extra zinc (Solomons, 1988). Calcium excretion is increased by diets rich in protein and magnesium (Avioli, 1988). In fact, absorption of nutrients from supplements containing many vitamins and minerals at levels exceeding the RDAs may be low because of multiple nutritional interactions that undoubtedly occur after the product is ingested (Weight et al., 1988).

On several occasions, supplements have been found to be contaminated. In 1982, for example, the FDA warned physicians that some samples of two popular calcium supplements—bone meal and dolomite—could contain substantial amounts of

TABLE 18–1 Vitamin and Mineral Safety Indexes[a]

Nutrient	Highest Recommended Adult Intake[b]	Source of Recommended Intake	Estimated Daily Adult Oral Minimum Toxic Dose	References
Vitamin A	5,000 IU	USRDA	25,000 to 50,000 IU	Miller and Hayes, 1982
Vitamin D	400 IU	USRDA	50,000 IU	Miller and Hayes, 1982
Vitamin E	30 IU	USRDA	1,200 IU	Miller and Hayes, 1982
Vitamin C	60 mg	RDA	1,000 to 5,000 mg	Miller and Hayes, 1982
Thiamin	1.5 mg	USRDA	300 mg	Itokawa, 1978; Miller and Hayes, 1982
Riboflavin	1.7 mg	USRDA	1,000 mg[c]	Miller and Hayes, 1982; Rivlin, 1978
Niacin (nicotinamide)	20 mg	USRDA	1,000 mg	Miller and Hayes, 1982; Waterman, 1978
Pyridoxine	2.2 mg	RDA	2,000 mg[d]	Schaumburg et al., 1983
Folacin	0.4 mg	USRDA	400 mg	Miller and Hayes, 1982
Biotin	0.3 mg	USRDA	50 mg	Miller and Hayes, 1982
Pantothenic acid	10 mg	USRDA	1,000 mg	Miller and Hayes, 1982
Calcium	1,200 mg	RDA	12,000 mg	Goto, 1978
Phosphorus	1,200 mg	RDA	12,000 mg	Draper and Bell, 1978
Magnesium	400 mg	USRDA	6,000 mg	Lipsitz, 1978
Iron	18 mg	USRDA	100 mg	Crosby, 1978
Zinc	15 mg	USRDA	500 mg	Lantzsch and Schenkel, 1978
Copper	3 mg	ESAADDI	100 mg	Moffitt, 1978
Fluoride	4 mg	ESAADDI	4 to 20 mg	Miller and Hayes, 1982
Iodine	0.15 mg	USRDA	2 mg	Vidor, 1978
Selenium	0.2 mg	ESAADDI	1 mg	Miller and Hayes, 1982

[a]Adapted from Hathcock, 1985.
[b]Figures represent the highest published value for each nutrient, either the Recommended Dietary Allowances (RDA) (except those for pregnancy and lactation) or Estimated Safe and Adequate Daily Dietary Intakes (ESAADDI) (NRC, 1980), or the U.S. Recommended Daily Allowances (USRDA).
[c]However, only ~25 mg of riboflavin can be absorbed in a single oral dose given to an adult.
[d]More recent data suggest that the toxic dose of pyridoxine for some individuals is much lower. See text.

lead. The agency recommended that infants, young children, and pregnant and lactating women avoid these products (Miller, 1987a). Several commercial samples of spirulina, an alga available as a dietary supplement, were found to contain mercury at concentrations exceeding limits set by the FDA (Johnson and Shubert, 1986). Four major brands of fish oil capsules were found to be free of mercury, but they contained trace amounts of DDT metabolites and polychlorinated biphenyls. Frequently these pollutants appeared at levels lower than those considered to be a health hazard (Ebel et al., 1987). In the United States, 13 people developed selenium intoxication as a result of taking an improperly manufactured dietary supplement that contained 27.3 mg of selenium per tablet—more than 180 times the amount labelled and considered safe (Helzlsouer et al., 1985). Symptoms included nausea, abdominal pain, diarrhea, nail and hair changes, peripheral neuropathy, fatigue, and irritability. The woman who consumed the most selenium (2,387 mg over a 2.5 month period) experienced hair loss, fingernail tenderness and loss, nausea and vomiting, a sour-milk breath odor, and increasing fatigue (Jensen et al., 1984).

In other cases, supplements have failed to meet advertised claims. Carr and Shangraw (1987), for example, found that the majority of 35 commercial brands of calcium carbonate supplements failed to meet U.S. Pharmacopoeia (USP) standards for disintegration or dissolution of calcium carbonate-containing drugs. Studies by Shangraw (in press) confirmed that more than half the calcium carbonate supplements tested failed to meet the USP standard. These incidents raise questions about the bioavailability of nutrients obtained from supplements. Dietary supplements are considered to be foods and not drugs and are therefore exempt from USP standards. In general, the absorption of nutrients from soft elastic gelatin capsules appears to be more efficient than absorption from tablets (Thakker et al., 1987). Factors that influence the bioavailability of nutrients from a supplement include the hardness of the tablet, the nature of its excipients, and substances used to coat the tablet (Shangraw, in press).

Only 19% of the 257 multivitamin and vitamin/mineral products evaluated by Bell and Fairchild (1987) were found to contain "appropriate" levels of nutrients (defined by the authors as no nutrient present in amounts greater than 50 to 200% of the U.S. RDA or 50 to 100% of the Estimated Safe and Adequate Daily Dietary Intakes proposed by the Food and Nutrition Board). The authors noted that most of the supplements they evaluated contained some vitamins in amounts two or more times the U.S. RDA for adults. In contrast, half the supplements targeted for children and for pregnant and lactating women were deemed appropriate by the authors' definition.

LEGAL STATUS

Because supplements are considered to be foods and not drugs, there are few regulations governing their availability and sale in the United States. In 1973, the FDA attempted to establish definitions, standards of identity, and labeling requirements for supplements and proposed specifications for the minimum and maximum quantities of allowable nutrients in supplement preparations (Hile, 1979). FDA's attempts to implement these and subsequent regulations were defeated, however, by public opinion, lawsuits by affected parties, and congressional action. At present, the FDA is prohibited by law from (1) limiting nutrients in supplements to levels considered nutritionally useful, (2) classifying a dietary supplement as a drug because one or more of the nutrients it contains is present at a level beyond that considered nutritionally rational or useful, and (3) requiring the presence of only essential nutrients in supplements and prohibiting the inclusion of ingredients considered useless or as having no nutritional value (Malbin, 1976).

COMMITTEE CONCLUSIONS

In the United States, dietary supplement use is widespread, especially among adults whose diets more closely meet the RDAs, women, and educated, higher-income whites. A large percentage of U.S. adults supplement their diets at least occasionally with vitamins and minerals; however, there appears to be little relationship between documented nutrient needs and the use of nutrient supplements. Furthermore, very few controlled studies have been conducted to examine the long-term health effects of supplement use and to assess their purported benefits in preventing or treating various chronic diseases. Several vitamins and minerals if consumed in excess can be toxic and cause numerous adverse health effects, but there is no evidence that the public is harming itself by the use of low levels of supplements.

Professional medical and nutrition societies agree that healthy people can and should obtain essential nutrients by eating a wide variety of foods. The following statement was issued jointly by the American Dietetic Association, American Institute of Nutrition, American Society for Clinical Nutrition, and the National Council Against Health Fraud (ADA, 1987):

> Healthy children and adults should obtain adequate nutrient intakes from dietary sources. Meeting nutrient needs by choosing a variety of foods in moderation, rather than by supplementation, reduces the potential risk for both nutrient deficiencies and nutrient excesses. Individual recommendations regarding supplements and diets should come from physicians and registered dietitians.
>
> Supplement usage may be indicated in some circumstances including:
>
> Women with excessive menstrual bleeding may need to take iron supplements.
>
> Women who are pregnant or breastfeeding need more of certain nutrients, especially iron, folic acid, and calcium.
>
> People with very low calorie intakes frequently consume diets that do not meet their needs for all nutrients.
>
> Some vegetarians may not be receiving adequate calcium, iron, zinc, and vitamin B_{12}.
>
> Newborns are commonly given, under the direction of a physician, a single dose of vitamin K to prevent abnormal bleeding.
>
> Certain disorders or diseases and some medications may interfere with nutrient intake, digestion, absorption, metabolism, or excretion and thus change requirements.
>
> Nutrients are potentially toxic when ingested in sufficiently large amounts. Safe intake levels vary widely from nutrient to nutrient and may vary with the age and health of the individual. In addition, high-dosage vitamin and mineral supplements can interfere with the normal metabolism of other nutrients and with the therapeutic effects of certain drugs.
>
> The Recommended Dietary Allowances represent the best currently available assessment of safe and adequate intakes and serve as the basis for the U.S. Recommended Daily Allowances shown on many product labels. There are no demonstrated benefits of self supplementation beyond these allowances (ADA, 1987, p. 1342).

The American Medical Association (Council on Scientific Affairs, 1987), the American Heart Association (AHA, 1987), the National Institute on Aging (NIA, 1983), the U.S. Departments of

Agriculture and Health and Human Services (USDA/DHHS, 1985) in their report *Dietary Guidelines for Americans*, and the *Surgeon General's Report on Nutrition and Health* (DHHS, 1988) essentially agree with this statement. In addition, the American Academy of Pediatrics has stated that dietary supplements are not necessary for properly nourished and healthy children (AAP, 1980).

This committee agrees with the positions these organizations have taken on dietary supplements. It also agrees with Dodds (1987) that professionally trained nutritionists from accredited institutions of higher education, along with physicians and registered dietitians, should offer the public responsible recommendations on supplement use.

DIRECTIONS FOR RESEARCH

• Investigators should continue to document the extent of dietary supplement use in the U.S. population and characterize the practice by various demographic and socioeconomic categories (e.g., sex, age, household income, region of country). Such studies should also describe the types and dosages of supplemental nutrients consumed and the reasons people give for using these products.

• Rigorous criteria need to be developed to enable the scientific community to document, in a more systematic and comprehensive manner, potential benefits as well as toxicities from the use of dietary supplements.

• An optimal system to monitor the use of dietary supplements should be developed. Its application would enable the scientific community, regulatory agencies, and the nutrient supplement industry to more effectively study, identify trends in, and evaluate this increasingly common practice.

• Most attention needs to be focused on further research to answer questions related to the potential benefits and risks from long-term dietary supplement use: Does supplement use affect mortality or general health status? Does supplement use help to prevent or treat health problems or chronic diseases in the general population or in particular population subgroups? By objective measures of need (e.g., inadequate nutrient intake from food, biochemical evidence of inadequacies), are supplements being used appropriately? What groups might be particularly vulnerable to health risks from the use of supplements? It is important to monitor the health effects from chronic high-dose levels of supplementation.

• More studies are needed to determine the quality of dietary supplement formulations, e.g., their potency, nutrient balance, nutrient bioavailability, and possible contamination with undesirable substances.

REFERENCES

AAP (American Academy of Pediatrics). 1980. Vitamin and mineral supplement needs in normal children in the United States. Pediatrics 66:1015–1021.

ADA (American Dietetic Association). 1986. Pills Versus Food: An Emerging Controversy. Scientific Panel Alarmed Over Supplement Use; Calls on Physicians to Report Harmful Effects. Press release, May 5. Marketing and Communications Department, American Dietetic Association, Chicago. 4 pp.

ADA (American Dietetic Association). 1987. Recommendations concerning supplement usage: ADA statement. J. Am. Diet. Assoc. 46:1342–1343.

AHA (American Heart Association). 1987. Vitamin and Mineral Supplements: Position Statement. Report of the Nutrition Committee, American Heart Association, Dallas. 1 p.

Anderson, R.A. 1986. Chromium metabolism and its role in disease processes in man. Clin. Physiol. Biochem. 4:31–41.

Anderson, R.A., M.M. Polansky, N.A. Bryden, E.E. Roginski, W. Mertz, and W. Glinsmann. 1983. Chromium supplementation of human subjects: effects on glucose, insulin, and lipid variables. Metabolism 32:894–899.

Anderson, T.W., and D.B.W. Reid. 1974. A double-blind trial of vitamin E in angina pectoris. Am. J. Clin. Nutr. 27: 1174–1178.

Anderson, T.W., D.B. Reid, and G.H. Beaton. 1972. Vitamin C and the common cold: a double-blind trial. Can. Med. Assoc. J. 107:503–508.

Anderson, T.W., G. Suranyi, and G.H. Beaton. 1974. The effect on winter illness of large doses of vitamin C. Can. Med. Assoc. J. 111:31–36.

Anonymous. 1981. The booming U.S. vitamins and minerals business—changes and challenges. Nutr. Today 16:26.

Anonymous. 1985. Calcium: how much is too much? Nutr. Rev. 43:345–346.

Anonymous. 1986. The vitamin pushers. Consum. Rep. 51: 170–175.

Aro, A., M. Kyllästinen, E. Kostiainen, C.G. Gref, S. Elfving, and U. Uusitalo. 1988. No effect on serum lipids by moderate and high doses of vitamin C in elderly subjects with low plasma ascorbic acid levels. Ann. Nutr. Metabol. 32:133–137.

Avioli, L.V. 1988. Calcium and phosphorus. Pp. 142–158 in M.E. Shils and V.R. Young, eds. Modern Nutrition in Health and Disease, 7th ed. Lea & Febiger, Philadelphia.

Barboriak, J.J., A.Z. el Ghatit, K.R. Shetty, and J.H. Kalbfleisch. 1982. Vitamin E supplements and plasma high-density lipoprotein cholesterol. Am. J. Clin. Pathol. 77: 371–372.

Bauernfeind, J.C. 1980. The safe use of vitamin A: A report of the International Vitamin A Consultive Group (IVACG). The Nutrition Foundation, New York. 44 pp.

Belizan, J.M., J. Villar, O. Pineda, A.E. Gonzalez, E. Sainz, G. Garrera, and R Sibrian. 1983. Reduction of blood pressure with calcium supplementation in young adults. J. Am. Med. Assoc. 249:1161–1165.

Bell, L.S., and M. Fairchild. 1987. Evaluation of commercial multivitamin supplements. J. Am. Diet. Assoc. 87:341–343.

Bendich, A., and L.J. Machlin. 1988. Safety of oral intake of vitamin E. Am. J. Clin. Nutr. 48:612–619.

Berger, A., and H.H. Schaumburg. 1984. More on neuropathy from pyridoxine abuse. N. Engl. J. Med. 311:986–987.

Bootman, J.L., and A.I. Wertheimer. 1980. Patterns of vitamin usage in a sample of university students. J. Am. Diet. Assoc. 77:58–60.

Bowering, J., and K.L. Clancy. 1986. Nutritional status of children and teenagers in relation to vitamin and mineral use. J. Am. Diet. Assoc. 86:1033–1038.

Bowerman, S.J., and I. Harrill. 1983. Nutrient consumption of individuals taking or not taking nutrient supplements. J. Am. Diet. Assoc. 83:298–305.

Breskin, M.W., C.M. Trahms, B. Worthington-Roberts, R.F. Labbe, and B. Koslowski. 1985. Supplement use: vitamin intakes and biochemical indexes in 40- to 108-month-old children. J. Am. Diet. Assoc. 85:49–56.

Cameron, E., and L. Pauling. 1976. Supplemental ascorbate in the supportive treatment of cancer: prolongation of survival times in terminal human cancer. Proc. Natl. Acad. Sci. U.S.A. 73:3685–3689.

Cameron, E., and L. Pauling. 1978. Supplemental ascorbate in the supportive treatment of cancer: reevaluation of prolongation of survival times in terminal human cancer. Proc. Natl. Acad. Sci. U.S.A. 75:4538–4542.

Campbell, T.C., R.G. Allison, and C.J. Carr. 1980. Feasibility of Identifying Adverse Health Effects of Vitamins and Essential Minerals in Man. Life Sciences Research Office, Federation of American Societies for Experimental Biology, Bethesda, Md. 76 pp.

Cann, C.E., H.K. Genant, B. Ettinger, and G.S. Gordan. 1980. Spinal mineral loss in oophorectomized women. Determination by quantitative computed tomography. J. Am. Med. Assoc. 244:2056–2059.

Carr, C.J., and R.F. Shangraw. 1987. Nutritional and pharmaceutical aspects of calcium supplementation. Am. Pharm. NS27:49–57.

Chandra, R.K. 1984. Excessive intake of zinc impairs immune responses. J. Am. Med. Assoc. 252:1443–1446.

Costas, K., R. Davis, N. Kim, A.S. Stark, S. Thompson, H.L. Vallet, and D.L. Morse. 1987. Use of supplements containing high-dose vitamin A—New York State, 1983–1984. J. Am. Med. Assoc. 257:1292, 1297.

Coulehan, J.L., K.S. Reisinger, K.D. Rogers, and D.W. Bradley. 1974. Vitamin C prophylaxis in a boarding school. N. Engl. J. Med. 290:6–10.

Council on Scientific Affairs. 1987. Vitamin preparations as dietary supplements and as therapeutic agents. J. Am. Med. Assoc. 257:1929–1936.

Creagan, E.T., C.G. Moertel, J.R. O'Fallon, A.J. Schutt, M.J. O'Connell, J. Rubin, and S. Frytak. 1979. Failure of high-dose vitamin C (ascorbic acid) therapy to benefit patients with advanced cancer. A controlled trial. N. Engl. J. Med. 301:687–690.

Crosby, W.H. 1978. The effect of nutrient toxicities in animals and man: iron. Pp. 177–192 in M. Rechcigl, Jr., ed. CRC Handbook Series in Nutrition and Food. Section E: Nutritional Disorders, Vol. l. CRC Press, West Palm Beach, Fla.

Dalton, K., and M.J.T. Dalton. 1987. Characteristics of pyridoxine overdose neuropathy syndrome. Acta Neurol. Scand. 76:8–11.

Davidson, C.S., J. Livermore, P. Andersen, and S. Kaufman. 1962. The nutrition of a group of apparently healthy aging persons. Am. J. Clin. Nutr. 10:181–199.

DHHS (U.S. Department of Health and Human Services). 1988. The Surgeon General's Report on Nutrition and Health. DHHS (PHS) Publ. No. 88-50210. Public Health Service, U.S. Department of Health and Human Services. U.S. Government Printing Office, Washington, D.C. 712 pp.

Dickinson, A. 1987. Benefits of Nutritional Supplements. Council for Responsible Nutrition, Washington, D.C. 55 pp.

Dodds, J. 1987. Message from the president. J. Nutr. Educ. 19:153.

Donegan, C.K., A.L. Messer, E.S. Orgain, and J.M. Ruffin. 1949. Negative results of tocopherol therapy in cardiovascular disease. Am. J. Med. Sci. 217:294–299.

Draper, H.H., and R.R. Bell. 1978. Nutrient toxicities in animals and man: phosphorus. Pp. 109–112 in M. Rechcigl, Jr., ed. CRC Handbook Series in Nutrition and Food. Section E: Nutritional Disorders, Vol. 1. CRC Press, West Palm Beach, Fla.

Dreyfus, P.M. 1988. Diet and nutrition in neurologic disorders. Pp. 1458–1470 in M.E. Shils and V.R. Young, eds. Modern Nutrition in Health and Disease, 7th ed. Lea & Febiger, Philadelphia.

Ebel, J.G., Jr., R.H. Eckerlin, G.A. Maylin, W.H. Gutenmann, and D.J. Lisk. 1987. Polychlorinated biphenyls and p,p'-DDE in encapsulated fish oil supplements. Nutr. Rep. Int. 36:413–417.

English, E.C., and J.W. Carl. 1981. Use of nutritional supplements by family practice patients. J. Am. Med. Assoc. 246:2719–2721.

Enstrom, J.E., and L. Pauling. 1982. Mortality among health-conscious elderly Californians. Proc. Natl. Acad. Sci. U.S.A. 79:6023–6027.

Enstrom, J.E., L.E. Kanim, and L. Breslow. 1986. The relationship between vitamin C intake, general health practices, and mortality in Alameda County, California. Am. J. Public Health 76:1124–1130.

Ettinger, B., H.K. Genant, and C.E. Cann. 1987. Postmenopausal bone loss is prevented by treatment with low-dosage estrogen with calcium. Ann. Intern. Med. 106:40–45.

Farrell, P.M., and J.G. Bieri. 1975. Megavitamin E supplementation in man. Am. J. Clin. Nutr. 28:1381–1386.

Farris, R.P., J.L. Cresanta, L.S. Webber, G.C. Frank, and G.S. Berenson. 1985. Dietary studies of children from a biracial population: intakes of vitamins in 10- and 13-year-olds. J. Am. Coll. Nutr. 4:539–552.

FDA (U.S. Food and Drug Administration). 1974. Consumer Nutrition Knowledge Survey: Report I, 1973–74. DHEW Publ. No. (FDA) 76-2058. Division of Consumer Studies, Office of Nutrition and Consumer Sciences, Bureau of Foods, Public Health Service, U.S. Department of Health, Education, and Welfare, Washington, D.C. 109 pp.

FDA (U.S. Food and Drug Administration). 1976. Consumer Nutrition Knowledge Survey: Report II, 1975. DHEW Publ. No. (FDA) 76-2059. Division of Consumer Studies, Office of Nutrition and Consumer Sciences, Bureau of Foods, Public Health Service, U.S. Department of Health, Education, and Welfare, Washington, D.C. (various pagings).

Garry, P.J., J.S. Goodwin, W.C. Hunt, E.M. Hooper, and A.G. Leonard. 1982. Nutritional status in a healthy elderly population: dietary and supplemental intakes. Am. J. Clin. Nutr. 36:319–331.

Goldfinger, S. 1982. What do you do, doctor? Harv. Med.

Sch. Health Let. 7:3–6.

Goodman, D.S. 1984. Vitamin A and retinoids in health and disease. N. Engl. J. Med. 310:1023–1031.

Goodwin, J.S., W.C. Hunt, P. Hooper, and P.J. Garry. 1985. Relationship between zinc intake, physical activity, and blood levels of high-density lipoprotein cholesterol in a healthy elderly population. Metabolism 34:519–523.

Goto, S. 1978. Effect of nutrient toxicities in animals: calcium. Pp. 103–107 in M. Rechcigl, Jr., ed. CRC Handbook Series in Nutrition and Food. Section E: Nutritional Disorders, Vol. 1. CRC Press, West Palm Beach, Fla.

Gray, G.E., A. Paganini-Hill, and R.K. Ross. 1983. Dietary intake and nutrient supplement use in a Southern California retirement community. Am. J. Clin. Nutr. 38:122–128.

Gray, G.E., A. Paganini-Hill, R.K. Ross, and B.E. Henderson. 1986. Vitamin supplement use in a Southern California retirement community. J. Am. Diet. Assoc. 86:800–802.

Greenwald, P. 1988. Current status of chemoprevention in humans. Pp. 266–279 in J.G. Fortner and J.E. Rhoads, eds. General Motors Cancer Research Foundation's Accomplishments in Cancer Research 1987. J.B. Lippincott Co., Philadelphia.

Greger, J.L. 1987. Food, supplements, and fortified foods: scientific evaluations in regard to toxicology and nutrient bioavailability. J. Am. Diet. Assoc. 87:1369–1373.

Gregor, A., P.N. Lee, F.J.C. Roe, M.J. Wilson, and A. Melton. 1980. Comparison of dietary histories in lung cancer cases and controls with special reference to vitamin A. Nutr. Cancer 2:93–97.

Grobbee, D.E., and A. Hofman. 1986. Effect of calcium supplementation on diastolic blood pressure in young people with mild hypertension. Lancet 2:703–706.

Gussow, J.D., and P.R. Thomas. 1986. Nutritional supplements: to pill or not to pill, is that the question? Pp. 268–341 in The Nutrition Debate: Sorting Out Some Answers. Bull Publishing, Palo Alto, Calif.

Guthrie, H.A. 1986. Supplementation: a nutritionist's view. J. Nutr. Ed. 18:130–132.

Hale, W.E., R.B. Stewart, J.J. Cerda, R.G. Marks, and F.E. May. 1982. Use of nutritional supplements in an ambulatory elderly population. J. Am. Geriatr. Soc. 30:401–403.

Hathcock, J.N. 1985. Quantitative evaluation of vitamin safety. Pharm. Times 51:104–113.

Helzlsouer, K., R. Jacobs, and S. Morris. 1985. Acute selenium intoxication in the United States. Fed. Proc. 44:1670.

Hermann, W.J., Jr., K. Ward, and J. Faucett. 1979. The effect of tocopherol on high-density lipoprotein cholesterol. A clinical observation. Am. J. Clin. Pathol. 72:848–852.

Hile, J.P. 1979. Vitamin and mineral products; revocation of regulations. Fed. Reg. 44:16005-16006.

Hooper, P.L., L. Visconti, P.J. Garry, and G.E. Johnson. 1980. Zinc lowers high-density lipoprotein-cholesterol levels. J. Am. Med. Assoc. 244:1960–1961.

Hornig, D.H., U. Moser, and B.E. Glatthaar. 1988. Ascorbic acid. Pp. 417–435 in M.E. Shils and V.R. Young, eds. Modern Nutrition in Health and Disease, 7th ed. Lea & Febiger, Philadelphia.

Horsman, A., J.C. Gallagher, M. Simpson, and B.E. Nordin. 1977. Prospective trial of oestrogen and calcium in postmenopausal women. Br. Med. J. 2:789–792.

Itokawa, Y. 1978. Effect of nutrient toxicities in animals and man: thiamine. Pp. 3–23 in M. Rechcigl, Jr., ed. CRC Handbook Series in Nutrition and Food. Section E: Nutritional Disorders, Vol. 1. CRC Press, West Palm Beach, Fla.

Jensen, R., W. Closson, and R. Rothenberg. 1984. Selenium intoxication—New York. J. Am. Med. Assoc. 251:1938.

Johnson, P.E., and L.E. Shubert. 1986. Accumulation of mercury and other elements by Spirulina (Cyanophyceae). Nutr. Rep. Int. 34:1063–1070.

Kamm, J.J., C.W. Ehmann, and K.O. Ashenfelter. 1984. Preclinical and clinical toxicity of selected retinoids. Pp. 287–326 in M.B. Sporn, A.B. Roberts, and D.S. Goodman, eds. The Retinoids, Vol. 2. Academic Press, New York.

Karlowski, T.R., T.C. Chalmers, L.D. Frenkel, A.Z. Kapikian, T.L. Lewis, and J.M. Lynch. 1975. Ascorbic acid for the common cold. A prophylactic and therapeutic trial. J. Am. Med. Assoc. 231:1038–1042.

Kellett, M., E. Kelleher, J. Crutchfield, M. Dubes, S.C. Glasser, and G. Lazure. 1984. Vitamin and mineral supplement usage by retired citizens. J. Nutr. Elderly 3:7–19.

Kirsch, A., and W.R. Bidlack. 1987. Nutrition and the elderly: vitamin status and efficacy of supplementation. Nutrition 3:305–314.

Kolonel, L.N., C.N. Yoshizawa, and J.H. Hankin. 1988. Diet and prostatic cancer: a case-control study in Hawaii. Am. J. Epidemiol. 127:999–1012.

Koplan, J.P., J.L. Annest, P.M. Layde, and G.L. Rubin. 1986. Nutrient intake and supplementation in the United States (NHANES II). Am. J. Public Health 76:287–289.

Kovar, M.G. 1985. Use of medications and vitamin-mineral supplements by children and youths. Public Health Rep. 100:470–473.

Kurinij, N., M.A. Klebanoff, and B.I. Graubard. 1986. Dietary supplement and food intake in women of childbearing age. J. Am. Diet. Assoc. 86:1536–1540.

Lamke, B., H.E. Sjöberg, and M. Sylvén. 1978. Bone mineral content in women with Colles' fracture: effect of calcium supplementation. Acta Orthop. Scand. 49:143–146.

Lantzsch, H.J., and H. Schenkel. 1978. Effect of specific nutrient toxicities in animals and man: zinc. Pp. 291–307 in M. Rechcigl, Jr., ed. CRC Handbook Series in Nutrition and Food. Section E: Nutritional Disorders, Vol. 1. CRC Press, West Palm Beach, Fla.

La Vecchia, C., A. Decarli, M. Fasoli, F. Parazzini, S. Franceschi, A. Gentile, and E. Negri. 1988. Dietary vitamin A and the risk of intraepithelial and invasive cervical neoplasia. Gynecol. Oncol. 30:187–195.

Le Bovit, C. 1965. The food of older persons living at home. J. Am. Diet. Assoc. 46:285–289.

Levine, M. 1983. New concepts in the biology and biochemistry of ascorbic acid. N. Engl. J. Med. 314:892–902.

Levy, A.S., and R.E. Schucker. 1987. Patterns of nutrient intake among dietary supplement users: attitudinal and behavioral correlates. J. Am. Diet. Assoc. 87:754–760.

Lipkin, M., and H. Newmark. 1985. Effect of added dietary calcium on colonic epithelial-cell proliferation in subjects at high risk for familial colonic cancer. N. Engl. J. Med. 313:1381–1384.

Lipsitz, P.J. 1978. Nutrient toxicities in animals and man: magnesium. Pp. 113–117 in M. Rechcigl, Jr., ed. CRC Handbook Series in Nutrition and Food. Section E: Nutritional Disorders, Vol. 1. CRC Press, West Palm Beach, Fla.

Looker, A.C., C.T. Sempos, C.L. Johnson, and E.A. Yetley. 1987. Comparison of dietary intakes and iron status of vitamin-mineral supplement users and nonusers, aged 1–19 years. Am. J. Clin. Nutr. 46:665–672.

Looker, A.C., C.T. Sempos, C. Johnson, and E.A. Yetley.

1988. Vitamin-mineral supplement use: association with dietary intake and iron status of adults. J. Am. Diet. Assoc. 88:808–814.

Makinson, D.H., S. Oleesky, and R.V. Stone. 1948. Vitamin E in angina pectoris. Lancet 1:102.

Malbin, I. 1976. Vitamin-mineral legislation. FDA Talk Paper, April 27, T76-32. U.S. Food and Drug Administration Press Office, Public Health Service, U.S. Department of Health, Education, and Welfare, Washington, D.C. 2 pp.

McCarron, D.A., and C.D. Morris. 1985. Blood pressure response to oral calcium in persons with mild to moderate hypertension. Ann. Int. Med. 103:825–831.

McDonald, J.T. 1986. Vitamin and mineral supplement use in the United States. Clin. Nutr. 5:27–33.

McGandy, R.B., R.M. Russell, S.C. Hartz, R.A. Jacob, S. Tannenbaum, H. Peters, N. Sahyoun, and C.L. Otradovec. 1986. Nutritional status survey of healthy noninstitutionalized elderly: energy and nutrient intakes from three-day diet records and nutrient supplements. Nutr. Res. 6:785–798.

McLaren, D.S. 1984. Vitamin A deficiency and toxicity. Pp. 192–208 in R.E. Olson, H.P. Broquist, C.O. Chichester, W.J. Darby, A.C. Kolbye, Jr., and R.M. Stalvey, eds. Nutrition Reviews' Present Knowledge in Nutrition, 5th ed. The Nutrition Foundation, Washington, D.C.

Meuleman, J. 1987. Beliefs about osteoporosis. A critical appraisal. Arch. Intern. Med. 147:762–765.

Miller, D.R., and K.C. Hayes. 1982. Vitamin excess and toxicity. Pp. 81–133 in J.N. Hathcock, ed. Nutritional Toxicology, Vol. 1. Academic Press, New York.

Miller, S.A. 1987a. Lead in calcium supplements. J. Am. Med. Assoc. 257:1810.

Miller, S.A. 1987b. Women's health: nutrition. Introductory remarks. Public Health Rep., suppl. July/August:20–22.

Moertel, C.G., T.R. Fleming, E.T. Creagan, J. Rubin, M.J. O'Connell, and M.M. Ames. 1985. High-dose vitamin C versus placebo in the treatment of patients with advanced cancer who have had no prior chemotherapy. N. Engl. J. Med. 312:137–141.

Moffitt, A.E., Jr. 1978. Effect of nutrient toxicities in animals and man: copper. Pp. 195–202 in M. Rechcigl, Jr., ed. CRC Handbook Series in Nutrition and Food. Section E: Nutritional Disorders, Vol. 1. CRC Press, West Palm Beach, Fla.

National Analysts, Inc. 1972. A Study of Health Practices and Opinions; Final Report, June 12. Report No. PB-210–978, Survey Conducted for the U.S. Food and Drug Administration. National Technical Information Service, Springfield, Va. 343 pp.

NIA (National Institute on Aging). 1983. Dietary Supplements: More Is Not Always Better. Publ. No. 1986-491-280/40002. National Institutes of Health, Public Health Service, U.S. Department of Health and Human Services. U.S. Government Printing Office, Washington, D.C. 2 pp.

NIH (National Institutes of Health). 1984. Osteoporosis: NIH Consensus Development Conference. National Institute of Arthritis, Diabetes, and Digestive and Kidney Diseases and the Office of Medical Applications of Research, Bethesda, Md. 87 pp.

Nilas, L., C. Christiansen, and P. Rodbro. 1984. Calcium supplementation and postmenopausal bone loss. Br. Med. J. 289:1103–1106.

NRC (National Research Council). 1980. Recommended Dietary Allowances, 9th ed. Report of the Committee on Dietary Allowances, Food and Nutrition Board, Division of Biological Sciences, Assembly of Life Sciences. National Academy Press, Washington, D.C. 185 pp.

Olson, J.A. 1988. Vitamin A, retinoids, and carotenoids. Pp. 292–312 in M.E. Shils and V.R. Young, eds. Modern Nutrition in Health and Disease, 7th ed. Lea & Febiger, Philadelphia.

Pally, A., J. Sobal, and H.L. Muncie, Jr. 1984. Nutritional supplement utilization in an urban family practice center. J. Fam. Prac. 18:249–253.

Pauling, L. 1986. How to Live Longer and Feel Better. Avon Books, New York. 413 pp.

Rabinowitz, M.B., H.C. Gonick, S.R. Levin, and M.B. Davidson. 1983. Effects of chromium and yeast supplements on carbohydrate and lipid metabolism in diabetic men. Diabetes Care 6:319–327.

Ranno, B.S., G.M. Wardlaw, and C.J. Geiger. 1988. What characterizes elderly women who overuse vitamin and mineral supplements? J. Am. Diet. Assoc. 88:347–348.

Read, M.H., and A.S. Graney. 1982. Food supplement usage by the elderly. J. Am. Diet. Assoc. 80:250–253.

Read, M.H., and D.C. Thomas. 1983. Nutrient and food supplement practices of lacto-ovo vegetarians. J. Am. Diet. Assoc. 82:401–404.

Read, M.H., V. Bhalla, I. Harrill, R. Bendel, J.E. Monagle, H.G. Schutz, E.T. Sheehan, and B.R. Standal. 1981. Potentially toxic vitamin supplementation practices among adults in seven Western states. Nutr. Rep. Int. 24:1133–1138.

Read, M., H.G. Schutz, R. Bendel, V. Bhalla, I. Harrill, M.E. Mitchell, E.T. Sheehan, and B.R. Standal. 1985. Attitudinal and demographic correlates of food supplementation practices. J. Am. Diet. Assoc. 85:855–857.

Read, M.H., M.A. Bock, R. Bendel, M. Mitchell, V. Bhallia, I. Harrill, H. Schutz, E. Sheehan, and B. Standal. 1987. Vitamin supplement users subgroup comparisons. Nutr. Rep. Int. 36:751–755.

Rechcigl, M., Jr., ed. 1978. CRC Handbook Series in Nutrition and Food. Section E: Nutritional Disorders, Vol. 1. CRC Press, West Palm Beach, Fla. 518 pp.

Recker, R.R., and R.P. Heaney. 1985. The effect of milk supplements on calcium metabolism, bone metabolism, and calcium balance. Am. J. Clin. Nutr. 41:254–263.

Recker, R.R., P.D. Saville, and R.P. Heaney. 1977. Effect of estrogens and calcium carbonate on bone loss in postmenopausal women. Ann. Intern. Med. 87:649–655.

Resnick, L.M., J.P. Nicholson, and J.H. Laragh. 1984. Outpatient therapy of essential hypertension with dietary calcium supplementation. J. Am. Coll. Cardiol. 3:616.

Rhee, K., and A.C. Stubbs. 1976. Health food users in two Texas cities. Nutritional and socioeconomic implications. J. Am. Diet. Assoc. 68:542–545.

Riales, R., and M.J. Albrink. 1981. Effect of chromium chloride supplementation on glucose tolerance and serum lipids including high-density lipoprotein of adult men. Am. J. Clin. Nutr. 34:2670–2678.

Riggs, B.L., E. Seeman, S.F. Hodgson, D.R. Taves, and W.M. O'Fallon. 1982. Effect of the fluoride/calcium regimen on vertebral fracture occurrence in postmenopausal osteoporosis. Comparison with conventional therapy. N. Engl. J. Med. 306:446–450.

Riis, B., K. Thomsen, and C. Christiansen. 1987. Does calcium supplementation prevent postmenopausal bone loss? A double-blind, controlled clinical study. N. Engl. J. Med. 316:173–177.

Rinzler, S.H., H. Bakst, Z.H. Benjamin, A.L. Bobb, and J.

Travell. 1950. Failure of alpha tocopherol to influence chest pain in patients with heart disease. Circulation 1:288–293.

Rivlin, R.S. 1978. Effect of nutrient toxicities (excess) in animals and man: riboflavin. Pp. 25–27 in M. Rechcigl, Jr., ed. CRC Handbook Series in Nutrition and Food. Section E: Nutritional Disorders, Vol. 1. CRC Press, West Palm Beach, Fla.

Saegert, J., and M.M. Saegert. 1976. Consumer attitudes and food faddism: the case of vitamin E. J. Consum. Aff. 10:156–169.

Samet, J.M., B.J. Skipper, C.G. Humble, and D.R. Pathak. 1985. Lung cancer risk and vitamin A consumption in New Mexico. Am. Rev. Respir. Dis. 131:198–202.

Schaumburg, H., J. Kaplan, A. Windebank, N. Vick, S. Rasmus, D. Pleasure, and M.J. Brown. 1983. Sensory neuropathy from pyridoxine abuse. A new megavitamin syndrome. N. Engl. J. Med. 309:445–448.

Schutz, H.G., B. Read, R. Bendel, V.S. Bhalla, I. Harrill, J.E. Monagle, E.T. Sheehan, and B.R. Standal. 1982. Food supplement usage in seven Western states. Am. J. Clin. Nutr. 36:897–901.

Shangraw, R.F. In press. Factors to consider in the selection of a calcium supplement. Public Health Rep., suppl.

Sharpe, T.R., and M.C. Smith. 1985. Use of vitamin-mineral supplements by AFDC children. Public Health Rep. 100:321–324.

Shekelle, R.B., M. Lepper, S. Liu, C. Maliza, W.J. Raynor, Jr., A.H. Rossof, O. Paul, A.M. Shryock, and J. Stamler. 1981. Dietary vitamin A and risk of cancer in the Western Electric study. Lancet 2:1186–1190.

Simonoff, M. 1984. Chromium deficiency and cardiovascular risk. Cardiovasc. Res. 18:591–596.

Singer, D.R.J., N.D. Markandu, F.P. Cappuccio, G.W. Beynon, A.C. Shore, S.J. Smith, and G.A. MacGregor. 1985. Does oral calcium lower blood pressure: a double blind study. J. Hypertension 3:661.

Smith, E.L., Jr., W. Reddan, and P.E. Smith. 1981. Physical activity and calcium modalities for bone mineral increase in aged women. Med. Sci. Sports Exerc. 13:60–64.

Smith, P.G., and H. Jick. 1978. Cancers among users of preparations containing vitamin A: a case-control investigation. Cancer 42:808–811.

Sobal, J., and H.L. Muncie, Jr. 1985. Vitamin use and vitamin beliefs among students entering medical school. J. Nutr. Ed. 17:123–125.

Sobal, J., H.L. Muncie, Jr., and A.S. Baker. 1986. Use of nutritional supplements in a retirement community. Gerontologist 26:187–191.

Sobal, J., H.L. Muncie, Jr., C.M. Valente, B.R. DeForge, and D. Levine. 1987. Physicians' beliefs about vitamin supplements and a balanced diet. J. Nutr. Ed. 19:181–185.

Solomons, N.W. 1988. Zinc and copper. Pp. 238–262 in M.E. Shils and V.R. Young, eds. Modern Nutrition in Health and Disease, 7th ed. Lea & Febiger, Philadelphia.

Sorensen, A.A., D.I. Sorensen, and J.G. Zimmer. 1979. Appropriateness of vitamin and mineral prescription orders for residents of health-related facilities. J. Am. Geriatr. Soc. 27:425–430.

Spittle, C.R. 1972. Atherosclerosis and vitamin C. Lancet 1:798.

Stampfer, M.J., W. Willett, W.P. Castelli, J.O. Taylor, J. Fine, and C.H. Hennekens. 1983. Effect of vitamin E on lipids. Am. J. Clin. Pathol. 79:714–716.

Steinkamp, R.C., N.L. Cohen, and H.E. Walsh. 1965.

Resurvey of an aging population—fourteen-year follow-up. J. Am. Diet. Assoc. 46:103–110.

Stewart, M.L., J.T. McDonald, A.S. Levy, R.E. Schucker, and D.P. Henderson. 1985. Vitamin/mineral supplement use: a telephone survey of adults in the United States. J. Am. Diet. Assoc. 85:1585–1590.

Stich, H.F., M.P. Rosin, and M.O. Vallejera. 1984. Reduction with vitamin A and beta-carotene administration of proportion of micronucleated buccal mucosal cells in Asian betel nut and tobacco chewers. Lancet 1:1204–1206.

Thakker, K.M., H.S. Sitren, J.F. Gregory III, G.L. Schmidt, and T.G. Baumgartner. 1987. Dosage form and formulation effects on the bioavailability of vitamin E, riboflavin, and vitamin B_6 from multivitamin preparations. Am. J. Clin. Nutr. 45:1472–1479.

Thomsen, P.A., R.D. Terry, and R.J. Amos. 1987. Adolescents' beliefs about and reasons for using vitamin/mineral supplements. J. Am. Diet. Assoc. 87:1063–1065.

Tsai, A.C., J.J. Kelley, B. Peng, and N. Cook. 1978. Study on the effect of megavitamin E supplementation in man. Am. J. Clin. Nutr. 31:831–837.

USDA (U.S. Department of Agriculture). 1986. Nationwide Food Consumption Survey. Continuing Survey of Food Intakes of Individuals. Men 19–50 Years, 1 Day, 1985. Report No. 85-3. Nutrition Monitoring Division, Human Nutrition Information Service, Hyattsville, Md. 94 pp.

USDA (U.S. Department of Agriculture). 1987a. Nationwide Food Consumption Survey. Continuing Survey of Food Intakes of Individuals. Low-Income Women 19–50 Years and Their Children 1–5 Years, 1 Day, 1986. Report No. 86-2. Nutrition Monitoring Division, Human Nutrition Information Service, Hyattsville, Md. 166 pp.

USDA (U.S. Department of Agriculture). 1987b. Nationwide Food Consumption Survey. Continuing Survey of Food Intakes of Individuals. Women 19–50 Years and Their Children 1–5 Years, 1 Day, 1986. Report No. 86-1. Nutrition Monitoring Division, Human Nutrition Information Service, Hyattsville, Md. 98 pp.

USDA/DHHS (U.S. Department of Agriculture/Department of Health and Human Services). 1985. Nutrition and Your Health: Dietary Guidelines for Americans, 2nd ed. Home & Garden Bulletin No. 232. U.S. Government Printing Office, Washington, D.C. 24 pp.

Uusitupa, M.I.J., J.T. Kumpulainen, E. Voutilainen, K. Hersio, H. Sarlund, K.P. Pyörälä, P.E. Kovistoinen, and J.T. Lehto. 1983. Effect of inorganic chromium supplementation on glucose tolerance, insulin response, and serum lipids in noninsulin-dependent diabetics. Am. J. Clin. Nutr. 38:404–410.

Vidor, G.I. 1978. Iodine toxicity in man and animals. Pp. 219–282 in M. Rechcigl, Jr., ed. CRC Handbook Series in Nutrition and Food. Section E: Nutritional Disorders, Vol. 1. CRC Press, West Palm Beach, Fla.

Vogelsang, A., and E.V. Shute. 1946. Effect of vitamin E in coronary heart disease. Nature (London) 157:772.

Waterman, R.A. 1978. Nutrient toxicities in animals and man: niacin. Pp. 29–42 in M. Rechcigl, Jr., ed. CRC Handbook Series in Nutrition and Food. Section E: Nutritional Disorders, Vol. 1. CRC Press, West Palm Beach, Fla.

Weight, L.M., K.H. Myburgh, and T.D. Noakes. 1988. Vitamin and mineral supplementation: effect on the running performance of trained athletes. Am. J. Clin. Nutr. 47:192–195.

Willett, W., L. Sampson, C. Bain, B. Rosner, C.H. Hennekens, J. Witschie, and F.E. Speizer. 1981. Vitamin supplement use among registered nurses. Am. J. Clin. Nutr. 34:1121–1125.

Worsley, A. 1986. Health, wellbeing and dietary supplementation. Recent Adv. Clin. Nutr. 2:43–56.

Worthington-Roberts, B., and M. Breskin. 1984. Supplementation patterns of Washington State dietitians. J. Am. Diet. Assoc. 84:795–800.

Yearick, E.S., M.S. Wang, and S.J. Pisias. 1980. Nutritional status of the elderly: dietary and biochemical findings. J. Gerontol. 35:663–671.

Ziegler, R.G., T.J. Mason, A. Stemhagen, R. Hoover, J.B. Schoenberg, G. Gridley, P.W. Virgo, R. Altman, and J.F. Fraumeni, Jr. 1984. Dietary carotene and vitamin A and risk of lung cancer among white men in New Jersey. J. Natl. Cancer Inst. 73:1429–1435.

PART III

Impact of Dietary Patterns on Chronic Diseases

19

Atherosclerotic Cardiovascular Diseases

Atherosclerosis is the pathological process in the coronary arteries, cerebral arteries, iliac and femoral arteries, and aorta that is responsible for coronary heart disease (CHD), stroke, and peripheral arterial disease (PAD). It begins during childhood in the intima of the large elastic and muscular arteries with deposits of lipids, principally cholesterol and its esters, in macrophages and smooth muscle cells (Figure 19–1). The lesions, called *fatty streaks,* produce only minimal intimal thickening and cause no disturbances in blood flow during early childhood, but they rapidly become more extensive during adolescence. In young adults, more lipid is deposited at some sites, and a core of lipid and necrotic debris becomes covered by a cap of smooth muscle and fibrous tissue. These changes produce elevated lesions called *fibrous plaques* that project into the lumen and begin to disturb blood flow.

The relationship between fatty streaks and fibrous plaques has been one of the most controversial aspects of the pathogenesis of atherosclerosis. The coronary arteries differ from most other arteries by having a prominent intimal layer of longitudinal smooth muscle and fibrous tissue that is apparent even in childhood. By the age of 20, the thickness of this layer is about equal to that of the media, even when it does not contain abnormal lipid (Stary, 1987a,b). This fibromuscular intimal layer occurs in all populations, even in those not predisposed to coronary atherosclerosis in adulthood (Geer et al., 1968) and is considered to be a normal anatomic structure rather than an atherosclerotic lesion.

Some evidence suggests that fibrous plaques are created by cellular proliferation and subsequent fatty degeneration without prior lipid deposition (Benditt, 1974), and some observations are not consistent with the progression of fatty streaks to fibrous plaques. For example, fatty streaks are more extensive in the thoracic aortas of children, but fibrous plaques are more extensive in the abdominal aortas of adults. Young women have more extensive fatty streaks in their coronary arteries and aortas than do young men, but among adults this pattern is reversed. (McGill, 1968).

Overall, however, evidence supports the association of fatty streaks with fibrous plaques. Lesions in the arteries of young adults have many histological and chemical characteristics of fatty streaks as well as fibrous plaques—an observation suggesting a continuous progression from one type of lesion to the other (Geer et al., 1968; Katz, 1981; Stary, 1987a,b). Furthermore, in contrast to the differences in location of fatty streaks and fibrous plaques in the aorta, the sites of fatty streaks in the coronary arteries of children are the most common sites of fibrous plaques in adults (Montenegro and Eggen, 1968). The major risk factors, hypercholesterolemia and hypertension, are closely associ-

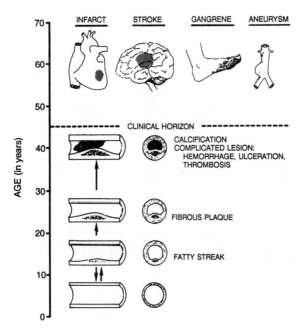

FIGURE 19–1   Natural history of atherosclerosis, showing progressive arterial occlusion and resultant health effects. From McGill et al. (1963).

ated with the extent of fibrous plaques in adults (Solberg and Strong, 1983). The few relevant data indicate that there is an association between serum cholesterol and low-density lipoprotein (LDL) cholesterol concentrations with fatty streaks in childhood (Freedman et al., 1988; Newman et al., 1986). Furthermore, it seems most likely that fatty streaks in children are labile, i.e., some may regress or remain as fatty streaks whereas others progress and evolve into fibrous plaques. This later process occurs particularly in the coronary arteries and abdominal aorta, where some fatty streaks are gradually converted to fibrous plaques by continued lipid deposition and reactive chronic inflammation and repair. For a review of this subject, see McGill (1988).

Regardless of their origin, fibrous plaques undergo a variety of qualitative changes in early middle age in the U.S. population, as illustrated in Figure 19–1. These changes result in fibrous plaques that vary in their content of lipids, smooth muscle cells, connective tissue, calcium, and vessels. The most serious complication is ulceration of the connective tissue and smooth muscle cap of fibrous plaque, a change that exposes blood to the lipid-rich necrotic debris of the core and is likely to precipitate thrombosis. Another serious complication is hemorrhage into the plaque. This causes sudden swelling of the plaque and may precipitate ulceration and thrombosis.

Thrombosis overlying an advanced atherosclerotic fibrous plaque is the most common event that occludes the lumen of the coronary artery and causes ischemia. At a point, determined by such factors as blood pressure, collateral circulation, and tissue oxygen demand, the blood supply is reduced below a critical level and ischemic necrosis occurs in the tissue supplied by the affected artery.

Lesions in the coronary arteries lead to CHD, which is the most common and most serious manifestation of atherosclerotic cardiovascular diseases in middle-aged adults. The atherosclerotic process that occurs in the cerebral and peripheral arteries is similar to that which occurs in the coronary arteries, but the lesions usually develop a decade or two later than those in the coronary arteries.

In approximately one-third of all CHD cases, coronary artery occlusion causes a fatal arrhythmia within a few minutes or hours (sudden cardiac death). If the patient survives the first few hours, ischemic necrosis of the myocardium occurs (myocardial infarction). Afterward, the necrotic tissue is removed and replaced by connective tissue. The subsequent clinical outcome is determined, for the most part, by the amount and location of cardiac muscle that is lost. A few days after infarction, and before much connective tissue has formed, the heart may rupture at the site of infarction (cardiac tamponade). The patient surviving this stage may recover cardiac function as the remaining heart hypertrophies to compensate for myocardium lost by infarction. At any stage, the patient may die from failure of the heart to pump sufficient blood (congestive heart failure) or from a disturbance in the conduction system controlling the distribution of the contractile impulse (arrhythmia). Stenosis of the coronary arteries sometimes is sufficient to cause ischemic pain, but not infarction, especially on exertion (angina pectoris). This condition indicates the presence of severe lesions and high risk of myocardial infarction. All these syndromes (angina pectoris, myocardial infarction, sudden cardiac death) are included in the term *coronary heart disease*.

If thrombosis forms over an atherosclerotic plaque in a cerebral artery, ischemic necrosis occurs in the brain (cerebral infarct). Cerebral infarction (one type of *stroke*) typically causes paralysis on the contralateral side due to lack of upper motor neuron function, and disturbances of speech, vision, hearing, and memory, depending on the anatomic location of the infarct. Death may occur due to involvement of the brain centers controlling respiration or to cerebral edema. The necrotic tissue is converted to a liquid-filled cavity. Function is usually recovered to some degree as edema subsides, but neurons do not regenerate. Neural control of muscles and sensory organs may be regained in part as other pathways are developed. If the arterial occlusion is partial or temporary, temporary functional cerebral impairment may occur for a few minutes to a few hours (transient ischemic attacks). These episodes, which are analogous to angina pectoris, indicate that the patient has a high risk of developing cerebral infarction.

Another type of stroke is cerebral hemorrhage, which includes intracerebral hemorrhage (bleeding into the brain) and subarachnoid hemorrhage (bleeding into the space between the arachnoid membrane and the surface of the brain). In an intracerebral hemorrhage, an artery within the brain ruptures and causes a large area of tissue destruction. Its clinical manifestations are similar to those of cerebral infarction, except that it is more rapid in onset and more likely to be fatal. This type of stroke is almost always associated with severe hypertension. Since hypertension augments cerebral atherosclerosis, it is a major risk factor for both cerebral infarction and intracerebral hemorrhage.

The rupture of an artery into the subarachnoid space is usually at the site of a developmental defect in the artery wall. Either the defect, or its rupture, or both may be enhanced by hypertension. The clinical manifestations of a subarachnoid hemorrhage are similar to those of other types of stroke.

Peripheral arterial disease (PAD) occurs when atherosclerosis and its complications in the abdominal aorta, iliac arteries, and femoral arteries produce temporary arterial insufficiency in the lower extremities upon exertion (intermittent claudication) or ischemic necrosis of the extremities (gangrene). In the abdominal aorta, weakening of the media underlying the atherosclerotic plaque leads to an aneurysm, which may become filled with a thrombus or rupture into the abdominal cavity.

The major risk factors associated with clinically manifest atherosclerotic diseases also are associated with the severity of atherosclerosis. In particular, LDL cholesterol levels are positively correlated with fibrous plaques and other advanced lesions, and high-density lipoprotein (HDL) cholesterol levels are inversely associated with advanced lesions (Solberg and Strong, 1983). Hypertension is more closely associated with advanced atherosclerosis in the cerebral arteries than in other arteries, a selective effect consistent with the identification

of hypertension as the dominant risk factor for stroke. Cigarette smoking is associated with advanced atherosclerosis of the abdominal aorta and iliac-femoral arteries, and consequently with PAD (DHHS, 1983). Smoking also is associated with advanced coronary atherosclerosis, but the increased coronary atherosclerosis in smokers is not sufficient to account for their much greater risk of CHD; other mechanisms, particularly thrombosis, are probably involved. Diabetes mellitus also is associated with severity of atherosclerosis in all arteries. Men have more severe coronary atherosclerosis than women, just as they have a higher frequency of CHD, but there is no sex difference in the severity of atherosclerosis of the aorta or cerebral arteries.

In populations with low serum cholesterol levels, atherosclerosis is less severe in those without hypertension and diabetes. However, among the latter, the severity of the disease is less than in populations where hyperlipidemia is prevalent (Robertson and Strong, 1968). Thus, hyperlipidemia, hypertension, and diabetes are additive in their effect on atherosclerosis, just as they are additive in their effect on risk of clinical disease. There is less information about the effects of cigarette smoking among different populations, but the evidence (Keys, 1980; Robertson et al., 1977) suggests that a similar relationship exists.

CHD risk factors for which no associations with severity of atherosclerosis have been found include physical activity and obesity (Solberg and Strong, 1983). The relationship of other putative risk factors to the severity of atherosclerosis has not been determined.

Results of animal experiments are consistent with observations in humans. LDL cholesterol and HDL cholesterol levels, and the ratio of the two lipoprotein cholesterol concentrations to one another are highly predictive of lesions in laboratory animals. High blood pressure combined with hyperlipidemia accelerates experimentally induced atherosclerosis. Despite several attempts, no effect of cigarette smoking on experimentally induced atherosclerosis has been demonstrated (Rogers et al., 1988).

CORONARY HEART DISEASE

Occurrence in the U.S. Population

By 1920, CHD had become a major cause of death and a public health issue in the United States. CHD mortality rates increased thereafter by 1 to 2% per year until the mid-1960s and reached a peak of greater than 300 deaths per year per 100,000 population (Stallones, 1980; Woolsey and Moriyama, 1948). In the 1960s, a healthy 40-year-old man had a 20% chance of developing CHD before age 60 (DHHS, 1987), and 30 to 35% of first heart attacks were fatal within the first 3 weeks (Kuller, 1969; Stamler, 1967). U.S. mortality from CHD began to decline about 1967. The decline began earlier on the West Coast (Rosenberg and Klebba, 1979). By 1983, the most recent year for which official statistics have been published, age-adjusted risk of CHD death had declined by 28% from 328.1 to 236.1 per 100,000 population (DHHS, 1987). Unofficial reports indicate that the decline has continued at least through 1986 at a slightly slower rate. The decline has also occurred in men and women, in blacks and other nonwhite people, and in the young and the elderly. The decline was proportionately greater in the younger compared to the older groups (Pell and Fayerweather, 1985) and in salaried workers compared to wage earners (Thom et al., 1985) (for further details, see Chapter 5). The decline has also occurred in out-of-hospital deaths, in sudden and unexpected deaths, in hospital case-fatality rates, and in acute nonfatal myocardial infarctions (Anastasiou-Nana et al., 1982; Folsom et al., 1987; Gillum et al., 1983; Gomez-Marin et al., 1987; Inter-Society Commission for Heart Disease Resources, 1984). Thus, improved medical care, better availability of medical care, and preventive measures in the population are probably all responsible for the decline. Despite the downward trend in mortality, CHD continues to be the leading cause of death in the United States. Of 2,091,200 deaths in the United States in 1983, 27% were attributed to CHD, 22% to malignant neoplasms, 21% to cardiovascular diseases other than CHD, 5% to accidents, and 25% to all other causes combined (DHHS, 1987).

Risk of CHD death is low during early adulthood but increases rapidly with age. The risk is higher for men than for women. Among men, risk is higher for whites than for blacks, but the reverse is found among women. Risk of CHD is inversely related to socioeconomic status now, but this association may have been positive earlier (Marmot et al., 1978).

Evidence Associating Dietary Factors with CHD

Animal Studies

The first animal model of atherosclerosis was discovered early in the twentieth century by Igna-

towski (1909) while investigating the effects of animal protein fed to rabbits. A few years later in 1913, Anitschkow (1967) demonstrated that cholesterol was the dietary component responsible for experimentally induced hypercholesterolemia and atherosclerosis in rabbits. Subsequently, a variety of animal species, including guinea pigs, swine, fowl, and nonhuman primates, were also found to be susceptible to the serum cholesterol raising effects of dietary cholesterol. The excess serum cholesterol was carried primarily in the LDL fraction (see Chapter 7).

Similar effects were found in laboratory animals after the effects of dietary saturated fatty acids (SFAs) on serum lipids were discovered in 1952. Dietary SFAs elevated both LDL and HDL cholesterol, as in humans, and augmented experimentally induced atherosclerosis (see Chapter 7). In a few studies, prolonged feeding of cholesterol- and fat-enriched diets to laboratory animals produced severe obstructive atherosclerotic lesions and myocardial infarction or PAD.

The responses of serum lipids and lipoproteins to dietary cholesterol and SFAs vary among animal species, but experimentally induced atherosclerosis is strongly and consistently associated with elevated serum cholesterol levels. In particular, LDL cholesterol concentrations are directly associated, and HDL cholesterol is inversely associated, with experimentally induced atherosclerosis. Rabbits, guinea pigs, swine, and rhesus and cynomolgus monkeys are among the most susceptible species, more so than humans, whereas rats and dogs are more resistant than humans. Baboons and vervet monkeys are moderately susceptible, within the same range of susceptability as humans. Within species, there is interindividual variation in responsiveness to dietary fat and cholesterol. Variability among and within species is due in part to genetically determined differences in lipid metabolism. Heritability of this characteristic has been demonstrated in several species (see Chapter 7).

Proteins, carbohydrates, fibers, metals, trace elements, and vitamins have been examined for their effects on serum lipid levels and experimentally induced atherosclerosis. Evidence regarding these components is reviewed in Chapters 8, 9, 10, 11, 12, and 14 of this report. Although there have been some reports that these dietary components affect serum lipids, lipoproteins, and atherosclerosis in one or more animal species, none of the components has emerged as a consistent and strong determinant of either the biochemical intervening variables associated with atherosclerosis or of atherosclerosis itself. Thus, the evidence in laboratory animals is consistent with the evidence in humans and indicates that cholesterol and fats are the major dietary determinants of atherosclerotic cardiovascular diseases.

Human Studies

Experimental Studies on Diet and Hyperlipidemia

More than three decades of experiments in humans have demonstrated that dietary saturated fatty acids and cholesterol are major determinants of serum cholesterol and lipoprotein concentrations (see Chapter 7). The average response of adults to changes in dietary fat and cholesterol intake was expressed in the following equation by Keys (1965):

$$\Delta Chol = 1.35 (2S - P) + 1.52 Z,$$

where $\Delta Chol$ is the change in serum cholesterol concentration in mg/dl; S and P are changes in percent of calories derived from saturated (S) and polyunsaturated (P) fatty acids; and Z is the difference between the square roots of the old and new cholesterol intakes expressed as mg/1,000 kcal.

This equation has been useful in predicting the effects of changes in dietary fat and cholesterol intakes, and its validity has been confirmed by subsequent experiments (Keys, 1984). However, not all SFAs raise serum cholesterol levels. The major cholesterol-raising SFAs are palmitic (C16) and myristic (C12) acids (see Chapter 7). In addition, individuals vary in their responses to SFAs (Grundy and Vega, 1988) and to cholesterol (Katan et al., 1986). Much of this variability is due to genetically controlled differences in lipid metabolism (see Chapters 4 and 7).

The Keys equation deals only with serum cholesterol concentrations. Dietary cholesterol leads predominantly to elevation of LDL cholesterol concentrations, whereas SFAs elevate both LDL and HDL cholesterol. When substituted for SFAs, polyunsaturated fatty acids (PUFAs) lead to both lower LDL and HDL cholesterol concentrations. Monounsaturated fatty acids (MUFAs) substituted for SFAs lead to decreased LDL cholesterol but have little or no effect on HDL cholesterol. Stearic acid has no effect on serum or lipoprotein cholesterol concentrations (see Chapter 7).

Most studies of PUFAs and plasma lipoproteins have used the more common ω-6 PUFAs, which are abundant in vegetable oils. ω-3 PUFAs derived from marine animals lower plasma triglyceride levels, but their effects on LDL cholesterol levels are not consistent. Their effects on lipid and lipoprotein metabolism are under investigation (see Chapter 7).

The effects of many other dietary components on serum lipids and lipoproteins are reviewed in detail in Chapters 6, 7, 8, 9, 10, 11, 12, 14, 16, and 17 of this report. Substitution of vegetable protein for animal protein reduces the serum cholesterol concentration slightly, although it probably is not an important factor within the usual ranges of intake (see Chapter 8). Dietary carbohydrates affect serum lipids and lipoproteins only when substituted for fats (see Chapter 9). Water-soluble, but not insoluble, dietary fiber lowers serum cholesterol levels (see Chapter 10). Alcohol consumption can elevate serum lipid levels, primarily by its elevating effect on serum triglyceride levels (see Chapter 16). Coffee consumption has been associated with slight elevations in serum cholesterol in some epidemiologic studies, but there is no consistent evidence that tea or other nonnutritive dietary components affect serum lipid concentrations (see Chapter 17).

Observational Studies on Diet, Serum Cholesterol Levels, and CHD

The percentage of calories derived from SFAs in the food supply is strongly associated with mean population cholesterol levels and CHD rates (Keys, 1970, 1980), whereas the percentage of calories derived from PUFAs and MUFAs is not strongly related. Mean per capita intakes of other dietary components, such as starches and fiber, and habitual physical activity, mean body mass index, cigarette smoking, and blood pressure have little or no independent association with CHD rates for populations (Keys, 1980).

Until recently, cross-sectional studies detected little or no association between the fatty acid composition of the diet and serum cholesterol concentrations (see Chapter 7). In at least two studies, inverse associations were observed between the intake of SFAs and serum cholesterol concentrations (Shekelle et al., 1982). However, methodological problems in cross-sectional studies include unreliability in assessment of dietary intake (Beaton et al., 1979; Keys, 1965; Liu et al., 1978) and in measurement of serum cholesterol concentrations (Jacobs et al., 1979; Keys, 1965) and dietary changes by people after learning of their high serum cholesterol levels (Shekelle et al.,

1982). Even after adjustment for these variables, cross-sectional studies have indicated that only a small proportion of the variation among individuals within a population can be attributed to the lipid composition of the diet.

In within-population studies carefully designed to reduce variation and in which the Keys equation was used, both SFAs alone and SFAs combined with PUFAs and cholesterol have been associated with serum cholesterol levels or CHD risk in individuals. Until recently, epidemiologic studies failed to show any association between a person's dietary cholesterol intake and serum cholesterol levels or CHD risk (see Chapter 7). However, these early studies did not adequately adjust for the confounding effect of caloric intake (Willet and Stampfer, 1986), were not accurate in measuring intake of dietary cholesterol (Beaton et al., 1979; Keys, 1965; Liu et al., 1978), or were biased due to systematic errors dietary change in people after learning of their hypercholesterolemia (Shekelle et al., 1981).

Since 1981, four prospective epidemiologic investigations—the Western Electric Study (Shekelle et al., 1981), the Ireland-Boston Diet-Heart Study (Kushi et al., 1985), the Zutphen Study (Kromhout and de Lezenne Coulander, 1984), and the Honolulu Heart Program (McGee et al., 1984)—have dealt adequately with these problems, and all found a positive association between the intake of dietary cholesterol and subsequent risk of CHD after adjustment for potentially confounding factors such as age, blood pressure, serum cholesterol concentration, and cigarette smoking.

Many studies have found that total energy intake is inversely associated with risk of CHD (see Chapter 6). This inverse association is probably due to a protective effect of physical activity on susceptibility to CHD and the positive correlation between physical activity and intake of energy.

Certain vegetable proteins (e.g., soy protein) and water-soluble dietary fiber can lower serum cholesterol in people with high cholesterol levels. The evidence for a protective role of these dietary constituents in CHD risk is, however, inconclusive (see Chapters 8 and 10).

Alcohol consumption in most cross-sectional epidemiologic studies is associated with an increased concentration of HDL cholesterol (Gordon et al., 1981), primarily of the HDL subclass, HDL_3 (William et al., 1985), as well as of apolipoproteins AI (apo AI) and AII (apo AII) (Camargo et al., 1985). Small intakes of alcohol (a range of 50–100 g distributed throughout the week) are associated in several studies with lower risk of CHD. A causal protective role for alcohol has not been established, however, and consumption of larger quantities of alcohol (e.g., >500 g/week) is associated with increased risk of CHD, stroke, and other diseases (see Chapter 16).

The association between coffee consumption and CHD risk is weak and inconsistent. Some cohort studies have found that habitual consumption of five to six cups or more per day is associated with increased risk (La Croix et al., 1986; LeGrady et al., 1987). No association between consumption of tea and risk of CHD has been observed (see Chapter 16).

Experimental Studies on Diet and CHD

Early experiments in humans to prevent CHD by modification of diet had promising results (Dayton et al., 1968; Miettinen et al., 1972). These findings were not conclusive, however, either because of the small number of subjects or the absence of appropriate control groups. Although the National Heart, Lung, and Blood Institute Task Force on Arteriosclerosis (NHLBI, 1971) concluded that a large-scale diet-heart trial was not feasible, it recommended an intervention trial on multiple coronary risk factors. The results of that trial (MRFIT Research Group, 1982) showed no effect of intervention on risk of coronary death after 7 years of follow-up, but this finding has been questioned because of the inadequate power of the study.

In contrast, a primary prevention trial conducted in Oslo, Norway, with normotensive hypercholesterolemic men achieved a reduction in CHD risk following dietary changes to lower serum cholesterol and a reduction in cigarette smoking (Hjermann et al., 1981). Other clinical trials (e.g., the Lipid Research Clinics Program, 1984), as summarized in Chapter 7, demonstrated that CHD incidence in middle-aged hypercholesterolemic men decreased in proportion to the reduction in plasma LDL cholesterol concentrations.

Clinical trials to lower serum cholesterol and CHD are reviewed in detail in Chapter 7. The combined results of all such trials in which diet or drugs were used indicate that a reduction in CHD risk is proportional to the degree and duration of serum cholesterol lowering achieved. Although a statistically nonsignificant but consistent excess of non-CHD deaths occurred in the aggregate experimental groups, this excess was not directly attributable either to the change in diet or to the lowering of total cholesterol; it was probably due to a combination of chance and the occurrence of deaths from causes that were previously masked by earlier death from CHD (Mann and Marr, 1981; Tyroler, 1985).

Evidence Associating Nondietary Factors with CHD

Cigarette Smoking

Cigarette smoking is an important risk factor for CHD in the United States and in other countries where the average diet is high in SFAs (i.e., >10% of total calories) and cholesterol and where serum cholesterol levels are high (Doll et al., 1980; Pooling Project Research Group, 1978). CHD risk within populations increases with the number of cigarettes smoked per day. A report by the Pooling Project Research Group (1978) indicated that the relative risk for men smoking more than one pack a day in comparison to nonsmokers was 3.2. In contrast, the association is weak in countries where intakes of SFAs and cholesterol and serum cholesterol concentrations are low. For example, cigarette smoking was not associated with the incidence of CHD in Japan, but was associated among men of Japanese descent living in Hawaii (Robertson et al., 1977). In the Seven Countries Study, cigarette smoking was strongly associated with risk of CHD death among U.S. and northern European men, but only weakly associated with risk in men from southern Europe where overall CHD risk was low (Keys, 1980).

Many observational studies have noted that former cigarette smokers have a substantially lower risk of CHD than current smokers (Doll and Hill, 1964; Friedman et al., 1981; Gordon et al., 1974). In high-risk men, randomized trials have shown a possible benefit of smoking cessation, even though the power of these studies to demonstrate an effect was only borderline (Holme, 1982; MRFIT Research Group, 1982; Rose et al., 1982).

High Blood Pressure

High blood pressure is a well-established major risk factor for CHD and stroke in the United States (Pooling Project Research Group, 1978) and other countries (Keys, 1980) (see Chapters 5 and 20). However, differences in prevalence of hypertension are less important than differences in serum cholesterol levels in accounting for population rates of CHD (Keys, 1980; Winkelstein et al., 1975).

Obesity

The precise role of obesity in the etiology of atherosclerosis and CHD is unclear. Cigarette smokers tend to be leaner than nonsmokers, and smokers who quit gain several pounds of body fat (Blitzer et al., 1977; Brozek and Keys, 1957; Goldbourt and Medalie, 1977; Gordon et al., 1975), but ex-smokers have lower risk of CHD. Adiposity is inversely correlated with HDL cholesterol concentration in some populations. Weight gain is associated with a decrease in HDL cholesterol levels (Garrison et al., 1980; Rhoads et al., 1976) and weight loss associated with moderate exercise with increased HDL cholesterol (Brownell et al., 1982). Adiposity is positively associated with the prevalence and incidence of hypertension (Kannel et al., 1967) and with the prevalence of glucose intolerance and hyperinsulinemia (Cahill, 1977) (see Chapter 21). Autopsy studies (Amad et al., 1965; Montenegro and Solberg, 1968) and angiographic studies (Anderson et al., 1978; Cramér et al., 1966) failed to show an association between obesity and severity of coronary artery disease.

Age-standardized 10-year incidence of nonfatal myocardial infarction and coronary death among 15 cohorts in the Seven Countries Study was not associated with mean body mass index or mean skinfold thickness (Keys, 1980). Within populations, however, prospective epidemiologic studies have generally shown an association between obesity and risk of coronary death at the upper range of body weight—e.g., ≥140% of ideal body weight or a body mass index ≥30 (see Chapter 21). For example, CHD incidence in the Honolulu Heart Study was positively associated with body mass index as well as subscapular skinfold thickness, even after controlling for other CHD risk factors (Donahue et al., 1987). Other studies (Lapidus et al., 1986; Larsson et al., 1984) support the hypothesis that the pattern of fat distribution (e.g., waist-to-hip ratio) may be an important risk factor for CHD; people with central fat distribution (typical in males) may be at increased risk of CHD in comparison to people with peripheral fat distribution (typical in females).

The evidence on body weight and CHD risk suggests that certain lifestyle variables, including diet, contribute to overweight and that obesity, especially severe obesity, increases CHD risk. Thus, maintaining moderate body weight is an important preventive measure to lower CHD risk in populations where obesity and high serum cholesterol levels are widespread.

Genetic Factors

CHD has long been known to cluster in families. Osler (1897) described a family in which three generations were affected. In a pioneering study of young men with myocardial infarction, Gertler and White (1954) found that a family history of CHD was 2.5 times as frequent among the affected cases as among the controls. First-degree relatives of people with CHD had a higher than average risk of the disease (Rose, 1964; Shanoff et al., 1961; Slack and Evans, 1966; Thomas, 1958). There was a high degree of concordance between twins of the same sex in incidence of CHD (Harvald and Hauge, 1970). Thus, a family history of premature CHD was established as a risk factor. This genetic predisposition is likely to involve multiple mechanisms, but attention has been focused on the genetic control of serum cholesterol and lipoprotein concentrations, knowledge of which accumulated rapidly after 1970.

Familial hypercholesterolemia first described by Müller (1938) is the most extreme example of genetic dyslipoproteinemia predisposing to premature CHD. It results from an autosomal dominant trait that occurs in the heterozygous form in about 1 in 500 people and in a severe homozygous form in about 1 in 1 million people. Affected people are deficient in the LDL receptor, which is essential for the cellular uptake and internalization of LDL. Heterozygous people have about half the normal LDL receptor activity and approximately double the normal LDL concentrations from birth and often develop CHD in their forties. Homozygous people have very little or no LDL receptor activity, LDL concentrations 6 to 10 times the normal, and CHD in childhood. The molecular defect involved in familial hypercholesterolemia and the structure of the LDL receptor and its gene were determined by Brown and Goldstein (1986). Animal models of this defect have been found in rabbits (Goldstein et al., 1983; Tanzawa et al., 1980; Watanabe et al., 1985) and rhesus monkeys (Scanu et al., 1988).

LDL cholesterol concentrations of people with familial hypercholesterolemia are not reduced to desirable levels when dietary cholesterol and SFA intakes are reduced, and treatment depends on pharmacological intervention with cholesterol-lowering drugs. Since people with familial hypercholesterolemia make up less than 1% of the population and only a small percentage of all people with hyperlipidemia, this genetic dyslipoproteinemia is not a major consideration in making dietary recommendations for a population.

Another genetic dyslipoproteinemia associated with increased incidence of CHD is familial combined hyperlipidemia, characterized by elevated fasting plasma cholesterol and triglyceride concentrations (Goldstein et al., 1972, 1973a,b). The metabolic disorders involved in this condition are not well delineated and are under investigation.

The wide variation in responsiveness within a population to the serum cholesterol raising effects of dietary cholesterol and SFAs suggests genetic control, which has been demonstrated in nonhuman primates (Clarkson et al., 1971, 1985; Flow et al., 1981; La Ville et al., 1987; McGill et al., 1988). There is less direct evidence in humans, because it is not possible to undertake comparable dietary intervention in families.

Apolipoprotein E (Apo E) isoforms (see Chapter 7 for definitions) are associated with variations in serum cholesterol levels and in CHD risk, and there is considerable evidence regarding the molecular mechanism by which these effects are produced (Davignon et al., 1988; Mahley, 1988). Apo B variants are associated with serum cholesterol concentrations (Kwiterovich et al., 1987; Young et al., 1987a,b, 1988). Apo AI variants are associated with abnormalities in HDL cholesterol levels (Franceschini et al., 1987). Genetic control of lipoprotein metabolism is an active topic of investigation. Investigators hope to find many new associations between genetic variants and serum lipoprotein levels as well as genetic markers for susceptibility to the serum cholesterol raising effect of dietary fat and cholesterol.

A family history of CHD is also a risk factor for the disease, even after adjusting for other known CHD risk factors (Barrett-Connor and Khaw, 1984; Colditz et al., 1986; Hammond et al., 1971; Sholtz et al., 1975; ten Kate et al., 1982; and reviewed by Goldbourt and Neufeld, 1986). These studies suggest that increased risk in men with a family history of CHD is about 1.5 to 2 times greater than in men without such a history, but is less in women. The physiological mechanism by which this independent effect is produced is not known. An intervening variable could theoretically be a genetically modulated risk factor such as dyslipoproteinemia, but evidence for this is still lacking.

Physical Activity

Physical inactivity (measured directly, or indirectly by caloric intake) is associated with an increased CHD risk and mortality in some cohort studies (Ekelund et al., 1988; Morris et al., 1977; Paffenbarger et al., 1978), but not in all. For example, variation in CHD mortality among cohorts in the Seven Countries Study was unrelated to habitual occupational activity; the two most active populations resided in areas with the highest (East Finland) and lowest (Japan) CHD rates (Keys, 1970, 1980).

Sustained physical activity is associated with an increased concentration of HDL cholesterol in humans (Hartung et al., 1980; Huttunen et al., 1979; Wood and Haskell, 1979) and with retardation in the development of coronary atherosclerosis in monkeys (Macaca fascicularis) receiving an atherogenic diet (Kramsch et al., 1981).

The evidence suggests an indirect and possibly direct role of physical activity in reducing risk of fatal CHD. Evidence on the level of physical activity required to reduce risk is conflicting.

Psychosocial Factors

Research completed in the 1970s supported the hypothesis that the Type A behavior pattern—a pattern composed primarily of competitiveness, excessive drive, and an enhanced sense of time urgency—was associated with increased risk of CHD independently of other known risk factors (Review Panel on Coronary-Prone Behavior and Coronary Heart Disease, 1981). Although some later studies in healthy populations also indicated an association between Type A behavior and increased risk of CHD (French–Belgium Collaborative Group, 1982; Haynes et al., 1983), most subsequent studies in the United States, particularly in high-risk groups, have been unable to repeat these early findings (Case et al., 1985; Ragland and Brand, 1988a,b; Shekelle et al., 1985a,b). Inconsistent findings have also been reported in studies on the association of Type A behavior and the presence and degree of angiographically determined coronary atherosclerosis (Williams et al., 1988). These inconsistent findings do not support a conclusion that Type A behavior is an established risk factor for CHD. Evidence regarding other aspects of emotional stress or other psychosocial factors is insufficient to justify firm conclusions about their role in the etiology of CHD in humans (Shepard and Weiss, 1987). Furthermore, Type A behavior did not modify the association of such other established risk factors as serum cholesterol concentration, cigarette smoking, or blood pressure with CHD (Rosenman et al., 1976), and there is no substan-

tial evidence to indicate that other psychosocial factors might do so.

Unstable social conditions were associated with coronary atherosclerosis in highly competitive male cynomolgus monkeys consuming an atherogenic diet (Kaplan et al., 1982), but there are no other laboratory data on this issue.

Summary

In summary, CHD is the most common clinical manifestation of atherosclerosis and it is the major cause of deaths among adults in the United States and many industrial societies. A large body of evidence indicates that the incidence of CHD is associated with three major risk factors: high serum cholesterol and low-density lipoprotein concentrations, high blood pressure, and cigarette smoking. Men are at much higher risk than are women. Other major risk factors include a low HDL–cholesterol concentration, diabetes mellitus, and a positive family history of early (premature) CHD. Other conditions (e.g., obesity, physical inactivity, personality type) also are associated with increased risk, but the associations are weaker and the evidence is less complete. There is a strong genetic component in risk of CHD in individuals and most of it is mediated through genetic/environmental interactions that determine the major risk factors. The predominant determinant of the average serum cholesterol and lipoprotein concentrations for populations is habitual diet, mainly the dietary intakes of cholesterol-raising SFAs and cholesterol. Individual CHD risk within populations is determined by genetic-environmental interactions affecting serum lipoproteins and blood pressure and by cigarette smoking. The observation that the established CHD risk factors account for about half the observed variation in CHD in multivariate analyses despite the lack of precision in measuring lifetime exposure to these variables underscores their importance as etiologic factors.

PERIPHERAL ARTERIAL DISEASE

Occurrence in the U.S. Population

PAD includes several clinical syndromes of arterial insufficiency in the extremities, characterized by pain, inflammation, and ischemic damage to soft tissues from partial or complete occlusion of major arteries. The most characteristic symptom of PAD is intermittent claudication, described as cramping, aching, and numbness of the extremities induced by exercise and resolved promptly by stopping the exercise. An advanced form of PAD is an aneurysm of the abdominal aorta, leading to occlusion of major aortic branches or to rupture and massive hemorrhage. PAD is caused by the obliteration of the arterial lumen due to thrombi overlying atherosclerotic plaques.

PAD is diagnosed by the clinical history of intermittent claudication, decreased arterial pulsations or pressure, and decreased blood flow. New ultrasound techniques promise effective noninvasive diagnosis, but x-ray angiography remains the definitive diagnostic method (Criqui et al., 1985c).

There are few systematic data pertaining to the frequency of PAD among or within populations. Mortality rates for PAD are unreliable because the disease occurs in a variety of syndromes and is not frequently a direct cause of death (Criqui et al., 1985a). Furthermore, there is no reliable information on trends in prevalence or deaths from PAD. In one U.S. study in which standardized diagnostic procedures were used, large-vessel PAD was found in 11.7% of the subjects, predominately whites with an average age of 66 years (Criqui et al., 1985b).

Evidence Associating Dietary Factors with PAD

Diet affects PAD through its effects on serum lipids and lipoproteins. The relationship of the serum cholesterol concentration to PAD risk or prevalence varies from strong in some studies to none in others. Where positive relationships occur, serum triglyceride and very-low-density lipoprotein (VLDL) cholesterol levels are more closely related to PAD than are HDL and LDL cholesterol levels (see Chapters 5 and 7).

No systematic studies have related dietary intakes to PAD risk; however, two diet-related conditions—diabetes and hypertension—are important PAD risk factors. Intermittent claudication (IC) is more common in diabetics than in nondiabetics in the Framingham study, and a substantial part of the risk for IC in that population was attributable to diabetes mellitus (Kannel and Mc-Gee, 1985). Risk ratios of 4 to 1 for IC were found with impaired glucose tolerance. PAD is a common late complication of diabetes; it was found in 45% of the diabetics studied in Rochester, Minnesota, for 20 years after diagnosis (Melton et al., 1980). Somewhat lower risk ratios are seen for

hypertension. In the Framingham study, a multiple factor (age, blood cholesterol, electrocardiogram reading, systolic blood pressure, relative weight, hemoglobin, and cigarette smoking) coronary risk index was strongly related to the incidence of IC; IC risk doubled in the upper quintile of the coronary risk score. The clustering of IC with other cardiovascular diseases was also pronounced in the Framingham study (Kannel and McGee, 1985).

Evidence Associating Nondietary Factors with PAD

PAD increases steadily and dramatically with age, rising more steeply after age 55. The clinical onset of PAD may be delayed beyond that of other atherosclerotic manifestations, because an extreme degree of obstructive disease is required to impair blood flow through the large arteries serving the lower extremities (Kannel and McGee, 1985).

Clinical and population-based studies suggest that PAD, expressed as intermittent claudication, is more frequent in men than in women up to age 65—occurring in 11.6% of men and 5.3% of women over 26 years of follow-up (Kannel and McGee, 1985)—after which incidence rates in both sexes are similar. There are no data on ethnic and racial differences or on associations with socioeconomic and psychosocial factors. There is no strong familial or genetic clustering of PAD other than the association with diabetes. Older clinical studies suggested that most patients with PAD were cigarette smokers. In more systematic follow-up studies, the frequency of intermittent claudication rose steadily and steeply according to number of cigarettes smoked, even beyond age 65 (see Chapter 5). This observation was confirmed by studies showing more severe atherosclerosis in the aortas of smokers than in those of nonsmokers (Solberg and Strong, 1983).

Multiple Risk Factors

Age, smoking, diabetes and fasting plasma glucose level, and systolic blood pressure were associated with PAD, whereas obesity and levels of LDL and HDL cholesterol were only marginally related to large-vessel PAD (Criqui et al., 1980). More important is the difference emerging in risk-factor configurations associated with each major atherosclerotic end point, i.e., CHD, stroke, and PAD. For example, diabetes, cigarette smoking, serum triglyceride level, and glucose tolerance predict PAD better than do serum lipid concentrations and blood pressure, whereas LDL and HDL cholesterol levels more strongly predict CHD, and blood pressure more strongly predicts stroke.

Summary

In summary, PAD is a large but poorly documented public health problem. There is little information on its prevalence or incidence or on population differences or trends. Evidence suggests a different combination of risk factors for PAD than for other atherosclerotic manifestations, with an emphasis on diabetes, glucose intolerance, smoking, and plasma triglyceride concentrations. Because CHD risk factors strongly predict PAD risk in the U.S. population, measures that would control CHD would also be expected to control PAD.

STROKE

Occurrence in the U.S. Population

Stroke is a clinical syndrome of neurological disabilities due to infarction of the brain by thrombosis over an atherosclerotic plaque or to destruction of brain tissue by hemorrhage from a ruptured artery. Transient ischemic attacks (TIAs) are episodes of temporary neurological disability due to insufficient arterial blood supply to the brain.

Most strokes are due to cerebral infarction. The next most frequent causes are the two major forms of cerebral hemorrhage: intracerebral and subarachnoid. Stroke has been recognized since antiquity and remains a major cause of death in adults worldwide. In many industrial countries, it is third among causes of death, following heart diseases and cancer. In the United States, strokes of all types were responsible for the deaths of approximately 182,000 people in 1977 (DHHS, 1987). The American Heart Association estimated that the 1981 prevalence of stroke was 1.87 million compared to 4.6 million cases of CHD (AHA, 1983). In the United States, the short-term case fatality from stroke is about 15%. Another 16% of the cases require institutional care, and 50% of survivors are permanently disabled (Kannel and Wolf, 1983).

Prevalence rates for stroke differ greatly among populations. For example, age-adjusted prevalence rates for stroke in 1970 were approximately 556 per 100,000 people in Rochester, Minnesota, compared to 363 in the United Kingdom (Kurtzke, 1976). Among countries, the distribution of and mortality rates from the different types of stroke, particularly cerebral infarct versus hemorrhage, also vary widely (Omae et al., 1976). Generally, the frequency of cerebral infarct deaths parallels that of CHD, whereas the frequency of intracerebral hemorrhage parallels that of hypertension. For example, stroke is the leading cause of death among adults in Japan, where hypertension is prevalent but CHD is uncommon (Komachi, 1977). Hypertension selectively augments atherosclerosis of the large cerebral arteries and thereby contributes to cerebral infarction. It also damages smaller cerebral arteries and contributes to cerebral hemorrhage.

Stroke deaths in the United States have declined for several decades, and the decline has accelerated since 1972 (Levy, 1979). Between 1968 and 1981, the age-adjusted stroke death rate fell by 46% (Inter-Society Commission for Heart Disease Resources, 1984). The incidence of cerebral infarction and intracerebral hemorrhage is also declining in Rochester, Minnesota, and the latter began to decline well before the wide availability of computerized brain tomography for diagnosis (Garraway and Whisnant, 1987).

In contrast, short-term fatality and survival rates for hospitalized stroke patients have not changed appreciably. This observation suggests that stroke incidence and deaths have declined as a result of preventive measures in the population, including hypertension control (Gillum et al., 1985), rather than as a result of improved treatment.

Evidence Associating Dietary Factors with Stroke

As reviewed in Chapter 7, a U-shaped relationship has been found in several studies between serum cholesterol level and incidence of stroke or cerebral infarct (i.e., the highest stroke rates are associated with both low and high levels of serum cholesterol, and the lowest rates with moderate levels) (Kannel and Wolf, 1983; Reed et al., 1986). Improved discrimination between hemorrhage and thrombosis suggests that the left side of the U-shaped curve is related to a higher frequency of cerebral hemorrhage in persons with hypertension at low cholesterol levels; the right side reflects a positive relationship between serum cholesterol level and cerebral infarct. Similarly, there is an inverse relationship between HDL cholesterol levels and stroke rates in subjects in the Honolulu Heart Program (Reed et al., 1986).

Hypertension is consistently, strongly, and independently related to individual risk of stroke (Dyken et al., 1984). Relative body weight was positively related to stroke incidence in the Framingham population under age 65, and inversely related at older ages (Kannel and Wolf, 1983). Abdominal obesity was positively related to stroke in Göteborg men (Welin et al., 1987). Age-adjusted stroke incidence rises steadily with alcohol intake in several populations (Gill et al., 1986) (see Chapters 5 and 16).

The paradoxical relationship of certain dietary components to stroke is discussed in Chapters 7 and 28. Animal fat, SFAs, and total fat were positively related to the risk of cerebral infarct (Reed et al., 1986). However, where hemorrhage occurs in the major proportion of stroke cases, as in Japan, animal protein and saturated fatty acid intake were inversely related to the incidence of cerebral hemorrhage and, therefore, to overall stroke incidence (Tanaka et al., 1982, 1985). Among omnivorous Seventh-Day Adventists in the United States, consumption of meats, eggs, milk, or cheese was unrelated to stroke risk (Snowdon, 1988).

Evidence Associating Nondietary Factors with Stroke

Fatal and nonfatal stroke are uncommon under age 45, after which stroke rates climb dramatically with age—rising from about 1/1,000 at ages 45 to 54, to 3.5/1,000 at ages 55 to 64, 9.0/1,000 at ages 65 to 74, 20/1,000 at ages 75 to 84, and 40/1,000 at ages 85 and over. Before age 65, rates are higher for men. After that, the rates are approximately the same for both sexes.

Downward trends in stroke deaths in the United States started earlier and have been greater in women, partly because of more effective hypertension control in women (Garraway and Whisnant, 1987). Stroke incidence and death are higher in blacks than in whites. However, migrant studies suggest that environment has a greater influence on stroke incidence than race or ethnicity. For example, stroke rates were substantially greater in people of Japanese extraction living in Japan than in those who migrated to Hawaii and California (Kagan et al., 1980), and greater in New Zealand migrants than in those who remained in their island homeland (Bonita and Beaglehole, 1982). Close relatives of stroke patients are at slightly greater risk of stroke than are unrelated people, and maternal history of stroke confers a slightly greater risk than does paternal history (Heyden et al., 1969; Welin et al., 1987).

Smoking was associated with cerebral infarct below age 65 in the Honolulu and Framingham studies (Abbott et al., 1986) but not in the Chicago Stroke Study (Ostfeld et al., 1974). Other cardiovascular diseases were strongly associated with the risk of stroke, particularly CHD, PAD, and hypertensive heart disease (Ostfeld et al., 1974).

Summary

In summary, stroke is the third most frequent cause of death among adults in many industrial countries. Risk rises steeply with age, and there are proportionately more deaths among blacks than among whites in the United States. The proportion of strokes due to infarction compared to strokes due to hemorrhage varies among countries. The frequency of cerebral infarction parallels that of CHD, and the frequency of hemorrhage parallels that of hypertension. Despite little change in hospital case-fatality and survival rates, stroke deaths in the United States have been declining for several decades. Blood pressure is the most consistent characteristic associated with the risk of stroke in populations and in individuals, but all the major risk factors for atherosclerosis, including diet, serum lipids, and smoking, contribute to the risk of stroke. Alcohol is also a strong risk factor for cerebral hemorrhage.

OVERALL SUMMARY

Atherosclerotic cardiovascular diseases make up the largest group of vascular diseases in the United States and have the greatest effect on morbidity and mortality. Comparisons of populations show large differences in incidence and mortality from the atherosclerotic cardiovascular diseases and in the underlying pathological process—atherosclerosis. The differences in population rates are strongly associated with average levels and distributions of the blood lipoproteins (for CHD) and with blood pressure (for stroke). The age-adjusted death rate from CHD in the United States declined 2 to 3% per year from 1968 to 1982 and has continued to fall since 1982 but at a slower rate. CHD deaths have increased at similar rates in some other countries. These trends in mortality and the rapid changes in risk factors and CHD risk observed among migrant populations indicate the potential for prevention. Despite the downward trend, CHD remains the major cause of deaths among U.S. adults.

CHD rates and population risk are most strongly related to the average serum cholesterol level (or, more specifically, to the average LDL cholesterol level). The mean cholesterol level in turn is strongly influenced by the composition of a population's habitual diet, chiefly its intake of saturated fatty acids and cholesterol. Within high-risk populations, the effect of diet on individual risk is strongly influenced by genetic differences in blood lipoprotein levels and by other factors such as arterial blood pressure and cigarette smoking. Within populations, the major risk factors—serum cholesterol concentration, blood pressure, and cigarette smoking—individually and combined are related to an individual's risk of clinical events in a continuously graded fashion.

Change in dietary composition, particularly in fatty acids (type and amount) and cholesterol, influences lipoprotein levels in small-group experiments. In randomized clinical trials, lowering of serum and LDL cholesterol, and possibly elevation of HDL cholesterol, has consistently demonstrated a reduction in CHD risk proportionate to the degree and duration of the reduced exposure. An excess of traumatic and other noncardiovascular deaths in the treated groups in these trials is not statistically significant and is not directly attributable to the lowering of serum cholesterol levels.

Hypertension, cigarette smoking, and diabetes mellitus are powerful influences on individual risk in populations with high CHD rates, but the role of overweight (except for severe obesity) and weight gain is variable, apparently determined more by dietary composition and lifestyle than by overweight itself. Genetic influences strongly affect an individual's susceptibility within high risk populations, but probably explain little of the large differences in rates among populations. Habitual physical activity has not been unequivocally related to population rates of CHD but may reduce individual risk as well as case-fatality rates in myocardial infarction. The evidence is inconclusive on the role of psychosocial factors.

PAD and cerebral infarction are influenced by the same risk factors as is CHD, but the relative importance of these risk factors is different. Smoking and diabetes are the most important risk factors for PAD, and hypertension is the most important risk factor for cerebral infarction and cerebral hemorrhage.

Congruence of evidence from laboratory, clinical, and population studies concerning the etiology and potential for prevention of atherosclerotic cardiovascular diseases provides a strong basis for public health recommendations. Furthermore, from the epidemiologic data, one can estimate the potential public health benefit of dietary modifications.

DIRECTIONS FOR RESEARCH

Animal Studies

• The physiological and molecular mechanisms by which hyperlipidemia causes atherosclerosis; identification and characterization of the specific lipoprotein subclasses or the modified lipoproteins that are directly involved in lipid deposition in the arterial wall and in progression of atherosclerosis.

• The mechanisms that control the responses to dietary fat and cholesterol or to other dietary components affecting serum lipoproteins, experimental atherosclerosis, or both.

• The basis for the differences in susceptibility to atherosclerosis among species and among different arterial beds within a species.

Human Studies

• The nature and the regulation (including the dietary regulation) of heterogeneity within each major class of lipoproteins and the roles of different lipoprotein subclasses in atherosclerosis and CHD, PAD, and stroke.

• The role of postprandial lipoproteins in atherosclerosis and in CHD, PAD, and stroke; the effects of diet on postprandial lipoproteins.

• The major dietary determinants of plasma HDL and the role of HDL and the mechanism whereby it protects against CHD.

• The extent and mechanism of individual variability in response to dietary saturated fatty acid intake.

• The extent and mechanism of individual variability in response to dietary cholesterol.

• The U-shaped relationship between serum cholesterol level and cerebral hemorrhage and atherothrombotic brain infarction and possible mechanisms of action.

• The effects of monounsaturated fatty acids and stearic acid on plasma lipid and lipoprotein levels and on atherosclerotic cardiovascular disease risk.

• The long-term consequences of the ingestion of different levels of ω-6 polyunsaturated vegetable oils on lipoproteins and atherosclerotic cardiovascular disease risk.

- The effects of ω-3 PUFAs (fish oils) on serum lipids and lipoproteins.
- The effects of total energy intake and expenditure on atherosclerotic cardiovascular disease risk factors and risk of atherosclerotic cardiovascular diseases, especially CHD.
- The effects of different types of protein (animal and vegetable) on serum lipid and lipoprotein levels and atherosclerotic cardiovascular disease risk.
- The long-term effects of increasing the proportion of dietary complex carbohydrates (starches and fibers) on serum lipid and lipoprotein levels and atherosclerotic cardiovascular disease risk.
- The metabolic mechanisms by which alcohol intake influences serum lipid and lipoprotein levels and risk of CHD and stroke.
- The influence of specific dietary components and dietary patterns compared to that of other environmental and genetic factors (and their interactions) on atherosclerotic cardiovascular disease risk.

REFERENCES

Abbott, R.D., Y. Yin, D.M. Reed, and K. Yano. 1986. Risk of stroke in male cigarette smokers. N. Engl. J. Med. 315:717–720.

AHA (American Heart Association). 1983. 1984 Heart Facts. Office of Communications, Dallas. 25 pp.

Amad, K.H., J.C. Brennan, and J.K. Alexander. 1965. The cardiac pathology of chronic exogenous obesity. Circulation 32:740–745.

Anastasiou-Nana, M., S. Nanas, J. Stamler, J. Marquardt, R. Stamler, H.A. Lindberg, D.M. Berkson, K. Liu, E. Stevens, M. Mansour, and T. Kokich. 1982. Changes in rates of sudden CHD death with first vs. recurrent events, Chicago Peoples Gas Company Study, 1960–1980. Circulation, Suppl. 66:II-236.

Anderson, A.J., J.J. Barboriak, and A.A. Rimm. 1978. Risk factors and angiographically determined coronary occlusion. Am. J. Epidemiol. 107:8–14.

Anitschkow, N.N. 1967. A history of experimentation on arterial atherosclerosis in animals. Pp. 21–44 in H.T. Blumenthal, ed. Cowdry's Arteriosclerosis: a Survey of the Problem, 2nd ed. C.C. Thomas, Springfield, Ill.

Barrett-Connor, E., and K.T. Khaw. 1984. Family history of heart attack as an independent predictor of death due to cardiovascular disease. Circulation 69:1065–1069.

Beaton, G.H., J. Milner, P. Corey, V. McGuire, M. Cousins, E. Stewart, M. de Ramos, D. Hewitt, P.V. Grambsch, N. Kassim, and J.A. Little. 1979. Sources of variance in 24-hour dietary recall data: implications for nutrition study design and interpretation. Am. J. Clin. Nutr. 32:2546–2549.

Benditt, E.P. 1974. Evidence for a monoclonal origin of human atherosclerotic plaques and some implications. Circulation 50:650–652.

Blitzer, P.H., A.A. Rimm, and E.E. Giefer. 1977. The effect of cessation of smoking on body weight in 57,032 women: cross-sectional and longitudinal analyses. J. Chron. Dis. 30:415–429.

Bonita, R., and R. Beaglehole. 1982. Trends in cerebrovascular disease mortality in New Zealand. N.Z. Med. J. 95:411–414.

Brown, M.S., and J.L. Goldstein. 1986. A receptor-mediated pathway for cholesterol homeostasis. Science 232:34–47.

Brownell, K.D., P.S. Bachorik, and R.S. Ayerle. 1982. Changes in plasma lipid and lipoprotein levels in men and women after a program of moderate exercise. Circulation 65:477–484.

Brozek, J., and A. Keys. 1957. Changes of body weight in normal men who stop smoking cigarettes. Science 125:1203.

Cahill, G.H., Jr. 1977. Obesity and diabetes. Pp. 101–110 in G. Bray, ed. Recent Advances in Obesity Research, Vol. II. John Libbey and Co., London.

Camargo, C.A., Jr., P.T. Williams, K.M. Vranizan, J.J. Albers, and P.D. Wood. 1985. The effect of moderate alcohol intake on serum apolipoproteins A-I and A-II. J. Am. Med. Assoc. 253:2854:2857.

Case, R.B., S.S. Heller, N.B. Case, A.J. Moss, and the Multicenter Post-Infarction Research Group. 1985. Type A behavior and survival after acute myocardial infarction. N. Engl. J. Med. 312:737–741.

Clarkson, T.B., H.B. Lofland, Jr., B.C. Bullock, and H.O. Goodman. 1971. Genetic control of plasma cholesterol: studies on squirrel monkeys. Arch. Pathol. 92:37–45.

Clarkson, T.B., J.R. Kaplan, and M.R. Adams. 1985. The role of individual differences in lipoprotein, artery wall, gender, and behavioral responses in the development of atherosclerosis. Ann. N.Y. Acad. Sci. 454:28–45.

Colditz, G.A., M.J. Stampfer, W.C. Willett, B. Rosner, F.E. Speizer, and C.H. Hennekens. 1986. A prospective study of parental history of myocardial infarction and coronary heart disease in women. Am. J. Epidemiol. 123:48–58

Cramér, K., S. Paulin, and L. Werkö. 1966. Coronary angiographic findings in correlation with age, body weight, blood pressure, serum lipids, and smoking habits. Circulation 33:888–900.

Criqui, M.H., E. Barrett-Connor, M.J. Holbrook, M. Austin, and J.D. Turner. 1980. Clustering of cardiovascular disease risk factors. Prev. Med. 9:525–533.

Criqui, M.H., S.S. Coughlin, and A. Fronek. 1985a. Noninvasively diagnosed peripheral arterial disease as a predictor of mortality: results from a prospective study. Circulation 72:768–773.

Criqui, M.H., A. Fronek, E. Barrett-Connor, M.R. Klauber, S. Gabriel, and D. Goodman. 1985b. The prevalence of peripheral arterial disease in a defined population. Circulation 71:510–515.

Criqui, M.H., A. Fronek, M.R. Klauber, E. Barrett-Connor, and S. Gabriel. 1985c. The sensitivity, specificity, and predictive value of traditional clinical evaluation of peripheral arterial disease: results from noninvasive testing in a defined population. Circulation 71:516–522.

Davignon, J., R.E. Gregg, and C.F. Sing. 1988. Apolipoprotein E polymorphism and atherosclerosis. Arteriosclerosis 8:1–21.

Dayton, S., M.L. Pearce, H. Goldman, A. Harnish, D. Plotkin, M. Shickman, M. Winfield, A. Zager, and W. Dixon. 1968. Controlled trial of a diet high in unsaturated fat for prevention of atherosclerotic complications. Lancet 2:1060–1062.

DHHS (U.S. Department of Health and Human Services).

1983. Arteriosclerosis. Pp. 13–62 in The Health Conse-
quences of Smoking: Cardiovascular Disease. DHHS (PHS)
Publ. No. 84–50204. A Report of the Surgeon General,
Office on Smoking and Health, Public Health Service, U.S.
Department of Health and Human Services, Rockville, Md.

DHHS (U.S. Department of Health and Human Services).
1987. Monthly Vital Statistics Report, Vol. 36: The Ad-
vance Report of Final Mortality Statistics, 1985. DHHS
Publ. No. (PHS) 87–1120. National Center for Health
Statistics, Public Health Service, U.S. Department of
Health and Human Services, Hyattsville, Md. 48 pp.

Doll, R., and A.B. Hill. 1964. Mortality in relation to
smoking: ten years' observations of British doctors. Br. Med.
J. 1:1399–1410.

Doll, R., R. Gray, B. Hafner, and R. Peto. 1980. Mortality in
relation to smoking: 22 years' observations on female British
doctors. Br. Med. J. 280:967–971.

Donahue, R.P., R.D. Abbott, E. Bloom, D.M. Reed, and K.
Yano. 1987. Central obesity and coronary heart disease in
men. Lancet 1:821–824.

Dyken, M.L., P.A. Wolf, H.J.M. Barnett, J.J. Bergan, W.K.
Hass, W.B. Kannel, L. Kuller, J.F. Kurtzke, and T.M.
Sundt. 1984. Risk factors in stroke: a statement for physicians by the Subcommittee on Risk Factors and Stroke of
the Stroke Council. Stroke 15:1105–1111.

Ekelund, L.G., W.L. Haskell, J.L. Johnson, F.S. Whaley,
M.H. Criqui, and D.S. Sheps. 1988. Physical fitness as a
predictor of cardiovascular mortality in asymptomatic North
American men: the Lipid Research Clinics Mortality Follow-up Study. N. Engl. J. Med. 319:1379–1384.

Flow, B.L., T.C. Cartwright, T.J. Kuehl, G.E. Mott, D.C.
Kraemer, A.W. Kruski, J.D. Williams, and H.C. McGill,
Jr. 1981. Genetic effects on serum cholesterol concentra-
tions in baboons. J. Hered. 72:97–103.

Folsom, A.R., O. Gomez-Marin, R.F. Gillum, T.E. Kottke,
W. Lohman, and D.R. Jacobs, Jr. 1987. Out-of-hospital
coronary death in an urban population—validation of death
certificate diagnosis: the Minnesota Heart Survey. Am. J.
Epidemiol. 125:1012–1018.

Franceschini, G., L. Calabresi, C. Tosi, C.R. Sirtori, C.
Fragiacomo, G. Noseda, E. Gong, P. Blanche, and A.V.
Nichols. 1987. Apolipoprotein A-IMilano. Correlation between high density lipoprotein subclass distribution and
triglyceridemia. Arteriosclerosis 7:426–435.

Freedman, D.S., W.P. Newman III, R.E. Tracy, A.E. Voors,
S.R. Srinivasan, L.S. Webber, C. Restrepo, J.P. Strong,
and G.S. Berenson. 1988. Black-white differences in aortic
fatty streaks in adolescence and early adulthood: the Bogalusa Heart Study. Circulation 77:856–864.

French-Belgian Collaborative Group. 1982. Ischemic heart
disease and psychological patterns: prevalence and incidence studies in Belgium and France. Adv. Cardiol. 29:25–
31.

Friedman, G.D., D.B. Petitti, R.D. Bawol, and A.B. Siegelaub. 1981. Mortality in cigarette smokers and quitters:
effect of base-line differences. N. Engl. J. Med. 304:1407–
1410.

Garraway, W.M., and J.P. Whisnant. 1987. The changing
pattern of hypertension and the declining incidence of
stroke. J. Am. Med. Assoc. 258:214–217.

Garrison, R.J., P.W. Wilson, W.P. Castelli, M. Feinleib,
W.B. Kannel, and P.M. McNamara. 1980. Obesity and
lipoprotein cholesterol in the Framingham Offspring Study.
Metabolism 29:1053–1060.

Geer, J.C., H.C. McGill, Jr., W.B. Robertson, and J.P.
Strong. 1968. Histologic characteristics of coronary artery
fatty streaks. Lab. Invest. 18:565–570.

Gertler, M.M., and P.D. White. 1954. Coronary Heart
Disease in Young Adults; a Multidisciplinary Study. Harvard
University Press, Cambridge, Mass. 218 pp.

Gill, J.S., A.V. Zezulka, M.J. Shipley, S.K. Gill, and D.G.
Beevers. 1986. Stroke and alcohol consumption. N. Engl. J.
Med. 315:1041–1046.

Gillum, R.F., A. Folsom, R.V. Luepker, D.R. Jacobs, Jr.,
T.E. Kottke, O. Gomez-Marin, R.J. Prineas, H.L. Taylor,
and H. Blackburn. 1983. Sudden death and acute myocardial infarction in a metropolitan area, 1970–1980: the
Minnesota Heart Survey. N. Engl. J. Med. 309:1353–1358.

Gillum, R.F., O. Gomez-Marin, T.E. Kottke, D.R. Jacobs,
Jr., R.J. Prineas, A.R. Folsom, R.V. Luepker, and H.
Blackburn. 1985. Acute stroke in a metropolitan area, 1970
and 1980: the Minnesota Heart Survey. J. Chron. Dis. 38:
891–898.

Goldbourt, U., and J.H. Medalie. 1977. Characteristics of
smokers, non-smokers and ex-smokers among 10,000 adult
males in Israel. Am. J. Epidemiol. 105:75–86.

Goldbourt, U., and H.N. Neufeld. 1986. Genetic aspects of
arteriosclerosis. Arteriosclerosis 6:357–377.

Goldstein, J.L., W.R. Hazzard, H.G. Schrott, E.L. Bierman,
and A.G. Motulsky. 1972. Genetics of hyperlipidemia in
coronary heart disease. Trans. Assoc. Am. Phys. 85:120–
138.

Goldstein, J.L., W.R. Hazzard, H.G. Schrott, E.L. Bierman,
and A.G. Motulsky. 1973a. Hyperlipidemia in coronary
heart disease. I. Lipid levels in 500 survivors of myocardial
infarction. J. Clin. Invest. 52:1533–1543.

Goldstein, J.L., H.G. Schrott, W.R. Hazzard, E.L. Bierman,
and A.G. Motulsky. 1973b. Hyperlipidemia in coronary
heart disease. II. Genetic analysis of lipid levels in 176
families and delineation of a new inherited disorder, combined hyperlipidemia. J. Clin. Invest. 52:1544–1568.

Goldstein, J.L., T. Kita, and M.S. Brown. 1983. Defective
lipoprotein receptors and atherosclerosis: lessons from an
animal counterpart of familial hypercholesterolemia. N.
Engl. J. Med. 309:288–296.

Gomez-Marin, O., A.R. Folsom, T.E. Kottke, S.C. Wu, D.R.
Jacobs Jr., R.F. Gillum, S.A. Edlavitch, and H. Blackburn.
1987. Improvement in long-term survival among patients
hospitalized with acute myocardial infarction, 1970 to 1980:
the Minnesota Heart Survey. N. Engl. J. Med. 316:1353–
1359.

Gordon, T., W.B. Kannel, D. McGee, and T.R. Dawber.
1974. Death and coronary attacks in men after giving up
cigarette smoking: a report from the Framingham Study.
Lancet 2:1345–1348.

Gordon, T., W.B. Kannel, T.R. Dawber, and D. McGee.
1975. Changes associated with quitting cigarette smoking:
the Framingham Study. Am. Heart. J. 90:322–328.

Gordon, T., N. Ernst, M. Fisher, and B.M. Rifkind. 1981.
Alcohol and high-density lipoprotein cholesterol. Circulation, Suppl. 64:III63–III67.

Grundy, S.M., and G.L. Vega. 1988. Plasma cholesterol
responsiveness to saturated fatty acids. Am. J. Clin. Nutr.
47:822–824.

Hammond, E.C., L. Garfinkel, and H. Seidmann. 1971.
Longevity of parents and grandparents in relation to coronary heart disease and associated variables. Circulation 43:
31–44.

Hartung, G.H., J.P. Foreyt, R.E. Mitchell, I. Vlasek, and A.M. Gotto, Jr. 1980. Relation of diet to high-density-lipoprotein cholesterol in middle-aged marathon runners, joggers, and inactive men. N. Engl. J. Med. 302:357–361.

Harvald, B., and M. Hauge. 1970. Coronary occlusion in twins. Acta Genet. Med. Gemellol. 19:248–250.

Haynes, S.G., M. Feinleib, and E.D. Eaker. 1983. Type A behaviour and the 10-year incidence of coronary heart disease in the Framingham Heart Study. Pp. 80–92 in R.H. Rosenman, ed. Psychosomatic Risk Factors and Coronary Heart Disease: Indications for Specific Preventive Therapy. Hans Huber Publishers, Bern, Switzerland.

Heyden, S., A. Heyman, and L. Camplong. 1969. Mortality patterns among parents of patients with atherosclerotic cerebrovascular disease. J. Chron. Dis. 22:105–110.

Hjermann, I., K.V. Byre, I. Holme, and P. Leren. 1981. Effect of diet and smoking intervention on the incidence of coronary heart disease. Lancet 2:1303–1310.

Holme, I. 1982. On the separation of the intervention effects of diet and antismoking advice on the incidence of major coronary events in coronary high risk men. The Oslo Study. J. Oslo City Hosp. 32:31–54.

Huttunen, J.K., E. Länsimies, E. Voutilainen, C. Ehnholm, E. Hietanen, I. Pentillä, O. Siitonen, and R. Rauramaa. 1979. Effect of moderate physical exercise on serum lipoproteins: a controlled clinical trial with special reference to serum high-density lipoproteins. Circulation 60:1220–1229.

Ignatowski, A. 1909. Über die Wirkung des tierischen Eiweisses auf die Aorta und die parenchymatösen Organe der Kaninchen. Virchows Arch. Pathol. 198:248–270.

Inter-Society Commission for Heart Disease Resources. 1984. Optimal resources for primary prevention of atherosclerotic diseases. Circulation 70:157A–205A.

Jacobs, D.R., Jr., J.T. Anderson, and H. Blackburn. 1979. Diet and serum cholesterol: do zero correlations negate the relationship? Am. J. Epidemiol. 110:77–87.

Kagan, A., J.S. Popper, and G.C. Rhoads. 1980. Factors related to stroke incidence in Hawaii Japanese men: the Honolulu Heart Study. Stroke 11:14–21.

Kannel, W.B., and D.L. McGee. 1985. Update on some epidemiologic features of intermittent claudication: the Framingham Study. J. Am. Geriatr. Soc. 33:13–18.

Kannel, W.B., and P.A. Wolf. 1983. Epidemiology of cerebrovascular disease. Pp. 1–24 in R.W.R. Russell, ed. Vascular Disease of the Central Nervous System. Churchill Livingstone, Edinburgh.

Kannel, W.B., N. Brand, J.J. Skinner, Jr., T.R. Dawber, and P.M. McNamara. 1967. The relation of adiposity to blood pressure and development of hypertension: the Framingham Study. Ann. Intern. Med. 67:48–59.

Kaplan, J.R., S.B. Manuck, T.B. Clarkson, F.M. Lusso, and D.M. Taub. 1982. Social status, environment, and atherosclerosis in cynomolgus monkeys. Arteriosclerosis 2:359–368.

Katan, M.B., A.C. Beynen, J.H.M. De Vries, and A. Nobels. 1986. Existence of consistent hypo- and hyperresponders to dietary cholesterol in man. Am. J. Epidemiol. 123:221–234.

Katz, S.S. 1981. The lipids of grossly normal human aortic intima from birth to old age. J. Biol. Chem. 256:12275–12280.

Keys, A. 1965. Dietary survey methods in studies on cardiovascular epidemiology. Voeding 26:464–483.

Keys, A. 1970. Coronary heart disease in seven countries. Circulation, Suppl. 41:I1-I211.

Keys, A. 1980. Seven Countries: A Multivariate Analysis of Death and Coronary Heart Disease. Harvard University Press, Cambridge, Mass. 381 pp.

Keys, A. 1984. Serum cholesterol response to dietary cholesterol. Am. J. Clin. Nutr. 40:351–359.

Komachi, Y. 1977. Recent problems in cerebrovascular accidents: characteristics of stroke in Japan. Nippon Ronen Igakkai Zasshi 14:359–364.

Kramsch, D.M., A.J. Aspen, B.M. Abramowitz, T. Kreimendahl, and W.B. Hood, Jr. 1981. Reduction of coronary atherosclerosis by moderate conditioning exercise in monkeys on an atherogenic diet. N. Engl. J. Med. 305:1483–1489.

Kromhout, D., and C. de Lezenne Coulander. 1984. Diet, prevalence and 10-year mortality from coronary heart disease in 871 middle-aged men: the Zutphen Study. Am. J. Epidemiol. 119:733–741.

Kuller, L. 1969. Sudden death in arteriosclerotic heart disease: the case for preventive medicine. Am. J. Cardiol. 24:617–628.

Kurtzke, J.F. 1976. An introduction to the epidemiology of cerebrovascular disease. Pp. 239–253 in P. Scheinberg, ed. Cerebrovascular Diseases: Tenth Princeton Conference. Raven Press, New York.

Kushi, L.H., R.A. Lew, F.J. Stare, C.R. Ellison, M. el Lozy, G. Bourke, L. Daly, I. Graham, N. Hickey, R. Mulcahy, and J. Kevaney. 1985. Diet and 20-year mortality from coronary heart disease: the Ireland-Boston Diet-Heart Study. N. Engl. J. Med. 312:811–818.

Kwiterovich, P.O., Jr., S. White, T. Forte, P.S. Bachorik, H. Smith, and A. Sniderman. 1987. Hyperapobetalipoproteinemia in a kindred with familial combined hyperlipidemia and familial hypercholesterolemia. Arteriosclerosis 7:211–225.

La Croix, A.Z., L.A. Mead, K.Y. Liang, C.B. Thomas, and T.A. Pearson. 1986. Coffee consumption and the incidence of coronary heart disease. N. Engl. J. Med. 315:977–982.

Lapidus, L., H. Andersson, C. Bengtsson, and I. Bosaeus. 1986. Dietary habits in relation to incidence of cardiovascular disease and death in women: a 12-year follow-up of participants and the population study of women in Gothenburg, Sweden. Am. J. Clin. Nutr. 44:444–448.

Larsson, B., K. Svärdsudd, L. Welin, L. Wilhelmsen, P. Björntorp, and G. Tibblin. 1984. Abdominal adipose tissue distribution, obesity, and risk of cardiovascular disease and death: 13 year follow up of participants in the study of men born in 1913. Br. Med. J. 288:1401–1404.

La Ville, A., P.R. Turner, R.M. Pittilo, S. Martini, C.B. Marenah, P.M. Rowles, G. Morris, G.A. Thomson, N. Woolf, and B. Lewis. 1987. Hereditary hyperlipidemia in the rabbit due to overproduction of lipoproteins. I. Biochemical studies. Arteriosclerosis 7:105–112.

LeGrady, D., A.R. Dyer, R.B. Shekelle, J. Stamler, K. Liu, O. Paul, M. Lepper, and A.M. Shryock. 1987. Coffee consumption and mortality in the Chicago Western Electric Company Study. Am. J. Epidemiol. 126:803–812.

Levy, R.I. 1979. Stroke decline: implications and prospects. N. Engl. J. Med. 300:490–491.

Lipid Research Clinics Program. 1984. The Lipid Research Clinics Coronary Primary Prevention Trial Results. II. The relationship of reduction in incidence of coronary heart disease to cholesterol lowering. J. Am. Med. Assoc. 251:365–374.

Liu, K., J. Stamler, A. Dyer, J. McKeever, and P. McKeever.

1978. Statistical methods to assess and minimize the role of intra-individual variability in obscuring the relationship between dietary lipids and serum cholesterol. J. Chron. Dis. 31:399–418.

Mahley, R.W. 1988. Apolipoprotein E: cholesterol transport protein with expanding role in cell biology. Science 240: 622–630.

Mann, J.I., and J.W. Marr. 1981. Coronary heart disease prevention: trials of diets to control hyperlipidemia. Pp. 197–210 in N.E. Miller and B. Lewis, eds. Lipoproteins, Atherosclerosis and Coronary Heart Disease: Metabolic Aspects of Cardiovascular Disease, Vol. 1. Elsevier/North-Holland, Amsterdam.

Marmot, M.G., A.M. Adelstein, N. Robinson, and G.A. Rose. 1978. Changing social-class distribution of heart disease. Br. Med. J. 2:1109–1112.

McGee, D.L., D.M. Reed, K. Yano, A. Kagan, and J. Tillotson. 1984. Ten-year incidence of coronary heart disease in the Honolulu Heart Program: relationship to nutrient intake. Am. J. Epidemiol. 119:667–676.

McGill, H.C., Jr. 1968. Fatty streaks in the coronary arteries and aorta. Lab. Invest. 18:560–564.

McGill, H.C., Jr. 1988. The pathogenesis of atherosclerosis. Clin. Chem. 34:B33-B39.

McGill, H.C., Jr., J.C. Geer, and J.P. Strong. 1963. Natural history of human atherosclerotic lesions. Pp. 39–65 in M. Sandler and G.H. Bourne, eds. Atherosclerosis and Its Origin. Academic Press, New York.

McGill, H.C., Jr., C.A. McMahan, G.E. Mott, Y.N. Marinez, and T.J. Kuehl. 1988. Effects of selective breeding on the cholesterolemic responses to dietary saturated fat and cholesterol in baboons. Arteriosclerosis 8:33–39.

Melton, L.J., III, K.M. Macken, P.J. Palumbo, and L.R. Elveback. 1980. Incidence and prevalence of clinical peripheral vascular disease in a population-based cohort of diabetic patients. Diabetes Care 3:650–654.

Miettinen, M., O. Turpeinen, M. Karvonen, R. Elosuo, and E. Paavilainen. 1972. Effect of cholesterol-lowering diet on mortality from coronary heart-disease and other causes. Lancet 2:835–838.

Montenegro, M.R., and D.A. Eggen. 1968. Topography of atherosclerosis in the coronary arteries. Lab. Invest. 18:586–593.

Montenegro, M.R., and L.A. Solberg. 1968. Obesity, body weight, body length, and atherosclerosis. Lab. Invest. 18: 594–603.

Morris, J.N., J.W. Marr, and D.G. Clayton. 1977. Diet and heart: a postscript. Br. Med. J. 2:1307–1314.

MRFIT (Multiple Risk Factor Intervention Trial) Research Group. 1982. Multiple Risk Factor Intervention Trial: risk factor changes and mortality results. J. Am. Med. Assoc. 248:1465–1477.

Müller, C. 1938. Xanthomata, hypercholesterolemia, angina pectoris. Acta Med. Scand. Suppl. 89:75–84.

Newman, W.P., III, D.S. Freedman, A.W. Voors, P.D. Gard, S.R. Srinivasan, J.L. Cresanta, G.D. Williamson, L.S. Webber, and G.S. Berenson. 1986. Relation of serum lipoprotein levels and systolic blood pressure to early atherosclerosis. The Bogalusa Heart Study. N. Engl. J. Med. 314: 138–144.

NHLBI (National Heart, Lung, and Blood Institute). 1971. Arteriosclerosis: A Report by the National Heart, Lung and Blood Task Force on Arteriosclerosis, Vol. 1. DHEW Publ. No. (NIH) 72–219. National Institutes of Health, Public

Health Service, U.S. Department of Health, Education, and Welfare, Bethesda, Md. 365 pp.

Omae, T., M. Takeshita, and Y. Hirota. 1976. The Hisayama Study and Joint Study on cerebrovascular diseases in Japan. Pp. 255–265 in P. Scheinberg, ed. Cerebrovascular Diseases: Tenth Princeton Conference. Raven Press, New York.

Osler, W. 1897. Lectures on Angina Pectoris and Allied States. Appleton, New York. 160 pp.

Ostfeld, A.M., R.B. Shekelle, H. Klawans, and H.M. Tufo. 1974. Epidemiology of stroke in an elderly welfare population. Am. J. Public Health 64:450–458.

Paffenbarger, R.S., Jr., A.L. Wing, and R.T. Hyde. 1978. Physical activity as an index of heart attack risk in college alumni. Am. J. Epidemiol. 108:161–175.

Pell, S., and W.E. Fayerweather. 1985. Trends in the incidence of myocardial infarction and in associated mortality and morbidity in a large employed population, 1957–1983. N. Engl. J. Med. 312:1005–1011.

Pooling Project Research Group. 1978. Relationship of blood pressure, serum cholesterol, smoking habit, relative weight and ECG abnormalities to incidence of major coronary events: final report of the Pooling Project. J. Chron. Dis. 31: 201–306.

Ragland, D.R., and R.J. Brand. 1988a. Coronary heart disease mortality in the Western Collaborative Group Study: follow-up experience of 22 years. Am. J. Epidemiol. 127:462–475.

Ragland, D.R., and R.J. Brand. 1988b. Type A behavior and mortality from coronary heart disease. N. Engl. J. Med. 318: 65–69.

Reed, D., K. Yano, and A. Kagan. 1986. Lipids and lipoproteins as predictors of coronary heart disease, stroke, and cancer in the Honolulu Heart Program. Am. J. Med. 80: 871–878.

Review Panel on Coronary-Prone Behavior and Coronary Heart Disease. 1981. Coronary-prone behavior and coronary heart disease: a critical review. Circulation 63:1199–1215.

Rhoads, G.G., C.L. Gulbrandsen, and A. Kagan. 1976. Serum lipoproteins and coronary heart disease in a population study of Hawaii Japanese men. N. Engl. J. Med. 294: 293–298.

Robertson, W.B., and J.P. Strong. 1968. Atherosclerosis in persons with hypertension and diabetes mellitus. Lab. Invest. 18:538–551.

Robertson, T.L., H. Kato, T. Gordon, A. Kagan, G.G. Rhoads, C.E. Land, R.M. Worth, J.L. Belsky, D.S. Dock, M. Miyanishi, and S. Kawamoto. 1977. Epidemiologic studies of coronary heart disease and stroke in Japanese men living in Japan, Hawaii and California. Am. J. Cardiol. 39: 244–249.

Rogers, W.R., K.D. Cary, C.A. McMahan, M.M. Montiel, G.E. Mott, H.S. Wigodsky, and H.C. McGill, Jr. 1988. Cigarette smoking, dietary hyperlipidemia, and experimental atherosclerosis in the baboon. Exp. Mol. Pathol. 48:135–151.

Rose, G. 1964. Familial patterns in ischaemic heart disease. Br. J. Prev. Soc. Med. 18:75–80.

Rose, G., P.J.S. Hamilton, L. Colwell, and M.J. Shipley. 1982. A randomised controlled trial of anti-smoking advice: 10-year results. J. Epidemiol. Community Health 36:102–108.

Rosenberg, H.M., and A.J. Klebba. 1979. Trends in cardiovascular mortality with a focus on ischemic heart disease: United States, 1950–1976. Pp. 11–41 in R.J. Havlik, M. Feinlieb, T. Thom, B. Krames, A.R. Sharrett, and R. Garrison, eds. Proceedings of the Conference on the Decline in Coronary Heart Disease Mortality. NIH Publ. No. 79–1610. National Heart, Lung, and Blood Institute, National Institutes of Health, Public Health Service, U.S. Department of Health, Education, and Welfare, Bethesda, Md.

Rosenman, R.H., R.J. Brand, R.I. Sholtz, and M. Friedman. 1976. Multivariate prediction of coronary heart disease during 8.5 year follow-up in the Western Collaborative Group Study. Am. J. Cardiol. 37:903–910.

Scanu, A.M., A. Khalil, L. Neven, M. Tidore, G. Dawson, D. Pfaffinger, E. Jackson, K.D. Carey, H.C. McGill, and G.M Fless. 1988. Genetically determined hypercholesterolemia in a rhesus monkey family due to a deficiency of the LDL receptor. J. Lipid Res. 29:1671–1681.

Shanoff, H.M., A. Little, E.A. Murphy, and H.E. Rykert. 1961. Studies of male survivors of myocardial infarction due to "essential" atherosclerosis. I. Characteristics of the patients. Can. Med. Assoc. J. 84:519–530.

Shekelle, R.B., A.M. Shryock, O. Paul, M. Lepper, J. Stamler, S. Liu, and W.J. Raynor, Jr. 1981. Diet, serum cholesterol, and death from coronary heart disease: the Western Electric Study. N. Engl. J. Med. 304:65–70.

Shekelle, R.B., J. Stamler, O. Paul, A.M. Shryock, S. Liu, and M. Lepper. 1982. Dietary lipids and serum cholesterol level: change in diet confounds the cross-sectional association. Am. J. Epidemiol. 115:506–514.

Shekelle, R.B., S.B. Hulley, J.D. Neaton, J.H. Billings, N.O. Borhani, T.A. Gerace, D.R. Jacobs, N.L. Lasser, M.B. Mittlemark, and J. Stamler for the Multiple Risk Factor Intervention Trial Research Group. 1985a. The MRFIT Behavior Pattern Study. II. Type A behavior and incidence of coronary heart disease. Am. J. Epidemiol. 122:559–570.

Shekelle, R.B., M. Gale, and M. Norusis. 1985b. Type A score (Jenkins Activity Survey) and risk of recurrent coronary heart disease in the Aspirin Myocardial Infarction Study. Am. J. Cardiol. 56:221–225.

Shepard, J.T., and S.M. Weiss, eds. 1987. Conference on behavioral medicine and cardiovascular disease. Circulation, Suppl. 76:II–I227.

Sholtz, R.I., R.H. Rosenman, and R.J. Brand. 1975. The relationship of reported parental history to the incidence of coronary heart disease in the Western Collaborative Group Study. Am. J. Epidemiol. 102:350–356.

Slack, J., and K.A. Evans. 1966. The increased risk of death from ischaemic heart disease in first degree relatives of 121 men and 96 women with ischaemic heart disease. J. Med. Genet. 3:239–257.

Snowdon, D.A. 1988. Animal product consumption and mortality because of all causes combined, coronary heart disease, stroke, diabetes, and cancer in Seventh-Day Adventists. Am. J. Clin. Nutr. 48:739–748.

Solberg, L.A., and J.P. Strong. 1983. Risk factors and atherosclerotic lesions. A review of autopsy studies. Arteriosclerosis 3:187–198.

Stallones, R.A. 1980. The rise and fall of ischemic heart disease. Sci. Am. 243:53–59.

Stamler, J. 1967. Lectures on Preventive Cardiology. Grune & Stratton, New York. 434 pp.

Stary, H.C. 1987a. Evolution and progression of atherosclerosis in the coronary arteries of children and adults. Pp 20–

36 in S.R. Bates and E.C. Gangloff, eds. Atherogenesis and Aging. Springer-Verlag, New York.

Stary, H.C. 1987b. Macrophages, macrophage foam cells, and eccentric intimal thickening in the coronary arteries of young children. Atherosclerosis 64:91–108.

Tanaka, H., Y. Ueda, M. Hayashi, C. Date, T. Baba, H. Yamashita, H. Shoji, Y. Tanaka, K. Owada, and R. Detels. 1982. Risk factors for cerebral hemorrhage and cerebral infarction in a Japanese rural community. Stroke 13:62–73.

Tanaka, H., M. Hayashi, C. Date, K. Imai, M. Asada, H. Shoji, K. Okazaki, H. Yamamoto, K. Yoshikawa, T. Shimada, and S.I. Lee. 1985. Epidemiologic studies of stroke in Shibata, a Japanese provincial city: preliminary report on risk factors for cerebral infarction. Stroke 16:773–780.

Tanzawa, K., Y. Shimada, M. Kuroda, Y. Tsujita, M. Arai, and H. Watanabe. 1980. WHHL-rabbit: a low density lipoprotein receptor-deficient animal model for familial hypercholesterolemia. FEBS Lett. 118:81–84.

ten Kate, L.P., H. Boman, S.P. Daiger, and A.G. Motulsky. 1982. Familial aggregation of coronary heart disease and its relation to known genetic risk factors. Am. J. Cardiol. 50:945–953.

Thom, T.J., F.H. Epstein, J.J. Feldman, and P.E. Leaverton. 1985. Trends in total mortality and mortality from heart disease in 26 countries from 1950 to 1978. Int. J. Epidemiol. 14:510–520.

Thomas, C.B. 1958. Familial and epidemiologic aspects of coronary disease and hypertension. J. Chron. Dis. 7:198–208.

Tyroler, H.A. 1985. Total serum cholesterol and ischemic heart disease risk in clinical trials and observation studies. Am. J. Prev. Med. 1:18–24.

Watanabe, Y., T. Ito, and M. Shiomi. 1985. The effect of selective breeding on the development of coronary atherosclerosis in WHHL rabbits: an animal model for familial hypercholesterolemia. Atherosclerosis 56:71–79.

Welin, L., K. Svärdsudd, L. Wilhelmsen, B. Larsson, and G. Tibblin. 1987. Analysis of risk factors for stroke in a cohort of men born in 1913. N. Engl. J. Med. 317:521–526.

Willett, W., and M.J. Stampfer. 1986. Total energy intake: implications for epidemiologic analyses. Am. J. Epidemiol. 124:17–27.

William, P.T., R.M. Kraus, P.D. Wood, J.J. Albers, D. Dreon, and N. Ellsworth. 1985. Associations of diet and alcohol intake with high-density lipoprotein subclasses. Metab. Clin. Exp. 34:524–530.

Williams, R.B., Jr., J.C. Barefoot, T.L. Haney, F.E. Harrell, Jr., J.A. Blumenthal, D.B. Pryor, and B. Peterson. 1988. Type A behavior and angiographically documented coronary atherosclerosis in a sample of 2,289 patients. Psychosom. Med. 50:139–152.

Winkelstein, W., Jr., A. Kagan, H. Kato, and S.T. Sacks. 1975. Epidemiologic studies of coronary heart disease and stroke in Japanese men living in Japan, Hawaii and California: blood pressure distributions. Am. J. Epidemiol. 102:502–513.

Wood, P.D., and W.L. Haskell. 1979. The effect of exercise on plasma high density lipoproteins. Lipids 14:417–427.

Woolsey, T.D., and I.M. Moriyama. 1948. Statistical studies of heart diseases. II. Important factors in heart disease mortality trends. Public Health Rep. 63:1247–1273.

Young, S.G., S.J. Bertics, T.M. Scott, B.W. Dubois, W.F. Beltz, L.K. Curtiss, and J.L. Witztum. 1987a. Apolipoprotein B allotypes MB19(1) and MB19(2) in subjects with coronary artery disease and hypercholesterolemia. Arteriosclerosis 7:61–65.

Young, S.G., S.J. Bertics, L.K. Curtiss, B.W. Dubois, and J.L. Witztum. 1987b. Genetic analysis of a kindred with familial hypobetalipoproteinemia. Evidence for two separate gene defects: one associated with an abnormal apolipoprotein B species, apolipoprotein B-37; and a second associated with low plasma concentrations of apolipoprotein B-100. J. Clin. Invest. 79:1842–1851.

Young, S.G., S.T. Northey, and B.J. McCarthy. 1988. Low plasma cholesterol levels caused by a short deletion in the apolipoprotein B gene. Science 241:591–593.

20

Hypertension

Hypertension is defined herein as sustained elevated arterial blood pressure measured indirectly by an inflatable cuff and pressure manometer. Hypertension can involve many organ systems, including the heart, endocrine organs, kidneys, and central and autonomic nervous systems. It has been clearly shown to increase the risk of developing stroke, coronary heart disease, congestive heart failure, peripheral vascular disease, and nephrosclerosis (Gordon and Kannel, 1972; Johansen, 1983; Stamler et al., 1980). Blood pressure is a continuously distributed variable in human populations, and the degree of cardiovascular risk is quantitatively related to the level of both systolic blood pressure (SBP) and diastolic blood pressure (DBP) throughout the entire range from highest to lowest (Kannel and Sorlie, 1975; Society of Actuaries, 1959). Thus, definitions of hypertension are arbitrary and serve only to classify people into risk categories and to analyze the effects of interventions designed to reduce blood pressure.

An individual's blood pressure usually is not constant but varies to a certain extent from day to day. Many people with elevated blood pressure on one occasion will have lower levels at a second visit. Ordinarily, blood pressure must be measured on two or more separate visits before a diagnosis of hypertension is made. As a result, cross-sectional surveys in which blood pressure is measured on only one visit will usually result in an overestimate

of the prevalence of sustained hypertension (JNC, 1984; Working Group on Risk and High Blood Pressure, 1985).

The classification of blood pressure most commonly used is that of the World Health Organization (WHO) Expert Committee published in 1978 (WHO, 1978):

- *Normotension*: SBP ≤ 140 mm Hg and DBP ≤ 90 mm Hg;
- *Borderline hypertension*: SBP 141–159 mm Hg and DBP 91–94 mm Hg;
- *Hypertension*: SBP ≥ 160 mm Hg or DBP ≥ 95 mm Hg.

Since borderline hypertension as well as isolated systolic hypertension (i.e., elevation of SBP without a concomitant increase in DBP) have been found to increase risk of cardiovascular diseases, a new classification has been promoted by the Third Joint National Committee (JNC III) for the Detection, Evaluation and Treatment of High Blood Pressure (JNC, 1984). JNC III classified adults with DBP between 85 and 89 mm Hg as "high normal" and reclassified some categories of patients into mild, moderate, and severe hypertension based on DBP criteria and into borderline and definite systolic hypertension based on SBP criteria. These definitions have been retained in the 1988 JNC report (JNC IV) and are given in Table 20–1 (JNC, 1988).

TABLE 20-1 Classification of Blood Pressure in Adults 18 Years and Older[a]

Blood Pressure Range (mm Hg)	Classification[b]
Diastolic	
<85	Normal blood pressure
85–89	High-normal blood pressure
90–104	Mild hypertension
105–114	Moderate hypertension
≥115	Severe hypertension
Systolic, when diastolic blood pressure is <90	
<140	Normal blood pressure
140–159	Borderline isolated systolic hypertension
≥160	Isolated systolic hypertension

[a]Adapted from JNC (1988). Blood pressures are based on the average of two or more readings on two or more occasions.
[b]A classification of borderline isolated systolic hypertension (SBP 140–159 mm Hg) or isolated systolic hypertension (SBP ≥ 160 mm Hg) takes precedence over a classification of normal diastolic blood pressure (DBP < 85 mm Hg) or high-normal diastolic blood pressure (DBP 85–89 mm Hg) when either occurs in the same person. A classification of high-normal diastolic blood pressure (DBP 85–89 mm Hg) takes precedence over a classification of normal systolic blood pressure (SBP < 140 mm Hg) when both occur in the same person.

Population comparisons indicate that there are substantial differences in mean blood pressure values and distributions and in the frequency of adult hypertension that cannot be explained solely by problems of standardization and reliability of measurement. Data derived from the 1976–1980 National Health and Nutrition Examination Survey (NHANES II) conducted by the National Center for Health Statistics (Carroll et al., 1983) indicate that approximately 25 million adults in the United States (17.7%) have definite hypertension according to WHO criteria and that an additional 17 million (12.0%) have borderline hypertension (DHHS, 1986). If the JNC IV criteria are used, 42 million adults (29.7%) are hypertensive. Average SBP is higher among blacks than among whites in most adult age groups. Mean DBP is generally higher in men than in women and higher in black adults than in white adults. Isolated systolic hypertension was found to be rare below age 55 (DHHS, 1986).

Comparison of NHANES II data (DHHS, 1986) with those from two previous surveys—one during 1960–1962 (DHEW, 1963) and one during 1971–1975 (DHEW, 1979)—indicates no significant trend in population mean or in distribution of

average blood pressure for any ages between the 1960–1962 and 1971–1975 surveys, but NHANES II (1976–1980) showed a lower average SBP at all ages above 30 and a lower overall prevalence of hypertension in people over 40, based on either the WHO or the JNC IV criteria. The relative contributions to this possible lowering of average blood pressure made by detection and control programs and by primary prevention could not be determined from the data. Although both factors have probably played a role, there is no direct evidence of a decline in mean population blood pressure that is independent of medical treatment. Similarly, there is no evidence that the decline in high blood pressure has resulted from a change in the average weight of the population, since this has risen in recent years in the United States.

Additional data on the distribution of hypertension in the population are given in Chapter 5.

EVIDENCE ASSOCIATING DIETARY FACTORS WITH HYPERTENSION

Human Studies

The relationships among body mass, obesity, and hypertension have been extensively examined in human populations (see Chapter 21). In virtually every epidemiologic study of blood pressure throughout the world, investigators have found strong correlations between body mass and blood pressure and between obesity and hypertension. Although problems of measurement occur when cuff size is not properly adjusted to arm circumference in obese people, the relationship between body mass and blood pressure remains highly significant, even when this source of error is controlled. Blood pressure and body mass are well correlated in both the hypertensive and the normal ranges.

Weight gain during adult life is associated with increased blood pressure levels. In the Framingham study, the risk of developing hypertension among those normotensive at entry was proportional to subsequent weight gain (Kannel et al., 1967). In general, risk appears greatest in people who gain weight during the third and fourth decades of life, after which the relationship weakens (Oberman et al., 1967; Stamler et al., 1975). Loss of weight by obese hypertensives is associated with a reduction in blood pressure, especially during active weight loss (Chiang et al., 1969; Reisin et al., 1978; Tuck et al., 1981; Tyroler et al., 1975). Little is known, however, about the effects of sustained weight loss on blood pressure. Moreover, the mechanisms by which body mass and obesity influence blood pressure are not well understood, and there are no established animal models for studying these relationships.

The strongest body of evidence for an effect of nutrients on hypertension concerns the electrolytes sodium and potassium (see Chapter 15). No optimal range of salt intake has been established, and human populations vary widely in habitual intake. In many unacculturated societies where salt intake is habitually low (<4 g of salt per day), blood pressure does not rise with age, and hypertension is rare or absent (Page, 1979). There are no well-documented examples of societies that habitually ingest a moderately high-salt diet (approximately 6 g of salt or more per day) and in which hypertension is absent (Denton, 1984; Prineas and Blackburn, 1985). Many interpopulation comparisons show a positive correlation of salt intake with SBP as well as DBP (Froment et al., 1979; Gleibermann, 1973; Simpson, 1985), but the evidence is not entirely consistent (Intersalt Cooperative Research Group, 1988) (see Chapter 15). Studies of blood pressure and sodium intake or excretion within populations have also yielded inconsistent results, showing either a positive association (Kesteloot et al., 1980; Khaw and Barrett-Connor, 1988; Page et al., 1981; Tao et al., 1984) or no association (Dawber et al., 1967; Holden et al., 1983; Karvonen and Punsar, 1977; Ljungman et al., 1981; McCarron et al., 1982; Schlierf et al., 1980).

The lack of association in many studies may reflect a high and relatively homogeneous salt intake within study populations; weaknesses in study design, including lack of control of potential confounding factors (e.g., obesity, sex, age, alcohol intake) (Prineas and Blackburn, 1985); or insufficient statistical power to detect a true association (Watt et al., 1983). Epidemiologic studies of populations with a high prevalence of hypertension (e.g., American blacks) have also demonstrated a positive correlation between salt intake and blood pressure level (Voors et al., 1983). In addition, studies of pressor responses to short-term changes in salt intake and salt depletion suggest that some people are more salt-responsive than others (Bittle et al., 1985; Fujita et al., 1980; Kawasaki et al., 1978; Luft et al., 1979a, 1982; Mark et al., 1975) and that responses are somewhat greater in hypertensives (Weinberger et al., 1986), in blacks of all ages, and in whites over the age of 40 (Luft et al., 1979b). Together, these data

suggest that a habitual high-salt intake may increase the risk of developing hypertension. There is as yet, however, no certain method for identifying susceptible people or for ascertaining how many of them become hypertensive as a result of excessive salt intake. Dietary salt modification can be more effectively targeted when reliable genetic markers for identifying salt-sensitive people at increased risk for hypertension are identified.

Low-potassium diets (e.g., 20 to 46 mEq/day) have been associated with increased risk of hypertension, stroke, and hypertension-related end-stage renal disease in several U.S. populations (Langford, 1985; Rostand et al., 1982; Walker et al., 1979) and elsewhere (Kromhout et al., 1985; Tobian, 1986). In addition, urinary sodium-to-potassium ratios have been positively correlated with DBP in several populations, even when no association with urinary sodium excretion was observed (Intersalt Cooperative Research Group, 1988; Langford, 1985; Page et al., 1981).

Clinical studies show that supplemental potassium given to hypertensives can reduce SBP as much as 6 mm Hg and DBP as much as 4 mm Hg (Kaplan et al., 1985; MacGregor et al., 1982; Morino et al., 1978; Svetkey et al., 1986). Diets rich in natural sources of potassium have been associated with decreased rates of hypertension and stroke (Khaw and Barrett-Connor, 1984; Khaw and Rose, 1982; Kromhout et al., 1985; Reed et al., 1985). In a 12-year cohort study in people over age 50 in the United States, potassium intake was negatively correlated with stroke-related mortality. The inverse association remained even after controlling for age, caloric intake, SBP or DBP, dietary fiber, magnesium, and calcium (Khaw and Barrett-Connor, 1987). Within the past decade, a considerable amount of new evidence has been obtained about the role of dietary calcium in blood pressure regulation (see Chapter 13). However, no clear conclusions can be reached, partly because the differences in study results are not fully explained. In some epidemiologic studies, for example, reduced calcium intake was found to be the best dietary predictor of hypertension (Ackley et al., 1983; Garcia-Palmieri et al., 1984; Kok et al., 1986; McCarron et al., 1984), whereas other studies demonstrated no association (Feinleib et al., 1984; Gruchow et al., 1985) or even a positive association between level of calcium intake and blood pressure (Harlan et al., 1984). These varied findings may have resulted in part from the high degree of collinearity among other dietary components associated with blood pressure (e.g., calcium, potassium, and protein) (Reed et al., 1985) and from limitations in the methods for assessing calcium intake in noninstitutionalized populations (Kaplan and Meese, 1986; Lau and Eby, 1985).

Clinical findings have been more consistent than epidemiologic findings, demonstrating a mild, short-term reduction in blood pressure from calcium supplementation in some normotensives and hypertensives (Belizan et al., 1983; Grobbee and Hofman, 1986; McCarron and Morris, 1985; Resnick et al., 1984; Singer et al., 1985). However, in certain patients with hypertension and high levels of renin, blood pressure may increase (Resnick et al., 1984). As yet, there has been no clinical trial of calcium that is adequate in size and design.

In population studies, consumption of more than two alcoholic drinks per day (>30 ml of alcohol per day) has generally been associated with a higher mean blood pressure and hypertension prevalence than found in those consuming lower levels of alcohol (Criqui, 1987) (see Chapter 16). Alcohol intake has also been associated with risk of hemorrhagic stroke and cerebral infarction in prospective studies (Donahue et al., 1986; Kagan et al., 1980, 1981) and case-control studies (Gill et al., 1986; Taylor et al., 1984; von Arbin et al., 1985). In the Framingham Offspring Study (Garrison et al., 1987), consumption of alcohol was associated with risk of hypertension after adjustment for adiposity and other variables in women but not in men. The reason for this difference is not clear, since the cross-sectional association between alcohol consumption and blood pressure level appears to be weaker in women than in men (Fortmann et al., 1983; Jackson et al., 1985; MacMahon and Leeder, 1984). In a randomized, crossover, single-blind study of alcohol restriction in mildly hypertensive Japanese office workers ages 30 to 59, Ueshima et al. (1987) found a modest reduction in SBP but not in DBP.

Observational, clinical, and community intervention studies in humans suggest that a high ratio of dietary polyunsaturated to saturated fat (P/S) in the presence of low total fat produces a modest reduction in blood pressure in normotensive and mildly hypertensive people. The modest hypotensive effect of the high P/S diet was not evident in people consuming a low-salt (77 mM/day) diet (Puska et al., 1983).

Studies on the relationship of protein intake to hypertension have yielded weak and inconsistent results (see Chapter 8). Chronically malnourished people exhibit low blood pressures (Viart, 1977), but the relative contribution of protein deficiency to this effect cannot be readily determined. Likewise, although epidemiologic studies have shown blood pressure levels (independent of age and weight) to be lower in populations consuming predominately vegetarian diets than in those consuming omnivorous diets (Armstrong et al., 1977; Ophir et al., 1983; Rouse and Beilin, 1984; Sacks et al., 1974), the findings cannot necessarily be ascribed to differences in plant and animal protein intakes, since it is likely that most types of vegetarians (complete vegetarians, lacto-ovovegetarians, and others) differ from omnivores in other dietary (e.g., lower fat and higher fiber intakes) and nondietary (e.g., lifestyle) factors that may confound the association between protein intake and blood pressure levels. Clinical findings are inconsistent, demonstrating either lower blood pressure levels in lacto-ovovegetarians than in omnivores (Rouse et al., 1983) or no difference in blood pressure (Brussaard et al., 1981).

Epidemiologic studies of dietary fiber and blood pressure, like those of protein (see Chapter 10), indicate that blood pressures are lower in vegetarian populations than in omnivorous populations (Armstrong et al., 1977; Rouse et al., 1982; Sacks et al., 1974; Trowell, 1981). Clinical studies also indicate a fairly consistent blood pressure-lowering effect of high-fiber diets in normal as well as hypertensive subjects (Anderson, 1986; Dodson et al., 1984; Lindahl et al., 1984). Although study findings are fairly consistent, the potential influence of other dietary factors associated with these high-fiber diets (e.g., lower fat and animal protein; varied sodium, potassium, and calcium content) cannot be dismissed, nor can the findings be ascribed solely to an effect of dietary fiber.

Other dietary factors have been studied in relation to hypertension. Lead, for example, has been associated with hypertension in several studies (Batuman et al., 1983; Beevers et al., 1980; Medeiros and Pellum, 1984), but there was no consistent relation to blood pressure in occupational studies and in studies of normotensives (see Chapter 14). This lack of consistency may in part reflect inadequate methods of measuring the body burden of lead (Batuman et al., 1983; Hansen and Pedersen, 1986). Pantothenic acid, magnesium, cadmium, chromium, and mercury have also been studied in relation to blood pressure levels, but again no consistent association in humans is apparent (see Chapters 12, 13, and 14).

Animal Studies

Experiments in animals provide strong evidence that salt intake plays a role in the causation of hypertension (see Chapter 15). The hypertensive effect of dietary salt is not observed in all animal models, but seems to operate most clearly when an underlying renal defect diminishes the ability to excrete salt rapidly (Tobian, 1983; Tobian et al., 1977). Studies indicate that Dahl S and Dahl R rats have blood pressures within the normal range when dietary salt is low, but the Dahl S rat has a slightly higher blood pressure than the Dahl R rat as well as some evidence of a defect in renal salt excretion. When both strains are fed a high-salt diet, the blood pressure of the Dahl R rat does not rise, whereas that of the Dahl S strain increases quickly and markedly (Dahl et al., 1962). The hypertensive effect of high-salt diets is also seen in other animal models with a diminished renal capacity to excrete salt, including the Kyoto spontaneously hypertensive rat (SHR) (Wilczynski and Leenen, 1987) and in animals given subtotal nephrectomy (Coleman and Guyton, 1969), injections of angiotensin (Muirhead et al., 1975), or doses of mineral corticoids sufficient to cause renal dysfunction and salt retention (Kaplan, 1982). These findings suggest that a combination of excessive dietary salt and reduced salt excretion may play a role in the development of hypertension in humans. This contention is consistent with epidemiologic evidence that populations with a lifelong low-salt diet seem to have no hypertension whatsoever and evidence from human genetics that susceptibility to hypertension may be related to a diminished capacity for rapid sodium excretion (Grim et al., 1979).

Supplemental potassium moderates the effects of hypertension in susceptible animals. Although the addition of potassium reduces blood pressure only modestly (Tobian et al., 1985), it appears to retard the gradual progressive changes in renal structure and function seen in hypertensive animals, including progressive destruction of the kidney tubules. High-potassium diets also prevent injury to the endothelial cells in many arteries. This may explain why such diets prevent much of the thickening of the intimal and medial layers of arteries in susceptible animals and preserve endothelium-dependent relaxation in their arteries (Tobian et al., 1984, 1987). The addition of potassium to high-salt diets also markedly decreases stroke incidence and overall mortality in stroke-prone spontaneously hypertensive rats and Dahl S rats (Tobian et al., 1985) as well as in Sprague-Dawley rats (Meneely and Ball, 1958). It also protects against the vascular lesions observed in arteries of hypertensive rabbits (Gordon and Drury, 1956) and rats (Goldby and Beilin, 1972; Tobian, 1986), which could explain the reduction in stroke mortality. The mechanism by which increased dietary potassium protects against endothelial and vascular injury is not known.

In most animal models (see Chapter 15), non-chloride salts failed to elevate blood pressure (Berghof and Geraci, 1929; Kurtz and Morris, 1985; Whitescarver et al., 1984). These data suggest that both sodium and chloride are necessary to produce hypertension in these animal models, but more studies on the effects of different salts are needed.

A number of animal studies indicate that calcium supplementation can lower blood pressure in the spontaneously hypertensive rat (Ayachi, 1979; Kageyama et al., 1986; Lau et al., 1984; McCarron et al., 1981, 1985), but that the effect is not produced consistently in normotensive control animals, such as the Wistar-Kyoto rat (see Chapter 13). There is insufficient experimental evidence to support an inverse association between dietary calcium and blood pressure level.

Studies of dietary fatty acids and blood pressure in animals suggest that diets deficient in linoleic acid increase blood pressure (see Chapter 7) and that the addition of linoleic acid to a low-fat, low-salt diet can decrease blood pressure (Düsing et al., 1983; MacDonald et al., 1981; Moritz et al., 1985).

Cadmium exposure has been linked to increased hypertension risk in animal studies, but the findings are inconsistent and possible mechanisms of action are not known (see Chapter 14). Cadmium doses insufficient to produce other signs of cadmium toxicity have induced hypertension in some studies, but in others, doses high enough to produce chronic toxicity had no effect (Eakin et al., 1980; Fingerle et al., 1982; Whanger, 1979). Perry and Kopp (1983) suggested that the presence of other trace elements such as selenium, copper, and zinc may counteract the hypertensive action of cadmium, but this has not been confirmed.

Other dietary factors, including protein, pantothenic acid, chromium, mercury, lead, and fluoride, have also been examined in relation to hypertension (see Chapters 8, 12, and 14). None of the laboratory studies has provided convincing evidence of a relationship between these factors and blood pressure levels.

EVIDENCE ASSOCIATING NONDIETARY FACTORS WITH HYPERTENSION

Heredity

A genetic predisposition to hypertension is generally acknowledged both for humans and laboratory animals (Folkow, 1982). Although it has not been determined whether a single gene (McManus, 1983; Platt, 1947) or polygenic inheritance (Folkow, 1982) is involved, the current consensus is that for humans, the predisposition is polygenic and permissive rather than determinative. Thus, the tendency to develop hypertension remains latent unless one or more environmental influences activate the mechanisms that raise blood pressure.

Primary hypertension in humans probably does not result from genetic influences alone. Because predisposition of humans to hypertension is polygenic, it is probable that different genes or gene products are activated or suppressed by single or multiple environmental influences, including sodium and potassium intake, psychosocial stress, and other environmental or nutritional influences. The resulting effect on blood pressure may in turn affect cardiovascular control mechanisms involving endocrine, renal, or cardiac factors, the central nervous system, or other systems. Thus, the factors triggering the onset, progression, and outcome of hypertension in genetically susceptible individuals are probably many and varied (Folkow, 1982).

Because of the complexity of genetic composition, it is unlikely that a single uniform cause of hypertension in humans will be found. It is nevertheless possible that some predisposing constellations of genetic factors may occur commonly in humans. Furthermore, one or more environmental factors may initiate a cascade of physiological events that lead to hypertension, even after the initiating factors are no longer operating.

There is considerable variety in the factors triggering hypertension among the various strains of genetically susceptible rodents. As described above, the Dahl S and R rat strains differ strikingly in their response to salt loading (Dahl et al., 1962). The SHR strain (Okamoto and Aoki, 1963) is sensitive to sodium loading as well as psychosocial stimuli, but will develop hypertension without either. The Milan hypertensive rat is also sensitive to salt loading but not to psychological stimuli (Folkow, 1982; Hallback et al., 1977).

The variety of precipitating factors is more complex in humans because of our greater genetic heterogeneity, far more complex environment, and longer lifespan. Strong evidence exists for interaction of genetic predisposition with electrolytes and obesity. Evidence for the role of other nutrients, psychosocial stress, and other influences is weaker and less consistent.

Studies in humans have provided strong evidence of similar blood pressures among twins, siblings, and other first-degree relatives (Feinleib et al., 1975; Miller and Grim, 1983; Zinner et al., 1971). However, efforts to identify genetic markers for susceptibility to hypertension or for sodium sensitivity have not been successful (see Chapter 15). Apart from relatively crude and qualitative indicators derived from knowledge of blood pressure in relatives, no valid method exists for predicting susceptibility to hypertension.

Racial Influences

Many studies demonstrate that blood pressure is higher and hypertension more prevalent among blacks of African origin than in Caucasians living in similar environments (Stamler et al., 1975). This has been borne out in three surveys of blood pressure by the National Center for Health Statistics (DHHS, 1986). It is possible that a variety of genetic, physiological, dietary, and psychosocial influences are important in producing these differences. Comparisons of black and white schoolchildren show differences in plasma renin activity, dopamine β-hydroxylase activity, glucose tolerance, and resting heart rate (Berenson, 1980). Several studies demonstrate marked differences between black and white Americans in dietary intake and excretion of sodium and potassium (Cushman and Langford, 1983; Grim et al., 1980) and in response to acute sodium loading (Luft et al., 1979b). Among black and white hypertensives, there may also be differences in sodium-lithium countertransport in blood cells (Canessa et al., 1984) and in response to different classes of antihypertensive medications (Cushman and Langford, 1983). Differences in blood pressure among other racial groups have also been reported (DHHS, 1985), but data are not sufficiently extensive or of high enough quality to permit firm conclusions to be drawn.

Psychosocial and Sociocultural Influences

Although many studies have related short-term changes in blood pressure to psychosocial and sociocultural factors, little is known about how these factors might interact with diet to increase risk of sustained hypertension. This is undoubtedly due in part to the heterogeneity of subjects, the complexity of blood pressure control mechanisms, and the complexity of the psychosocial environment.

Cross-sectional and longitudinal studies of populations undergoing a cultural change from traditional to more westernized or industrialized ways of life usually show an increase in both SBP and DBP (Cassel, 1975; Cruz-Coke et al., 1973; Maddocks, 1967; Page et al., 1974; Sever et al., 1980). Such increases have been observed in migrants and in populations undergoing rapid industrialization (Beaglehole et al., 1977; Page and Friedlaender, 1986; Poulter et al., 1985; Prior et al., 1977). When other factors, such as change in body weight or diet are controlled, however, variance in blood pressure due to such environmental factors as psychosocial stress appears to be small. For example, in a longitudinal study of Polynesians who migrated from the Tokelau Islands to / New Zealand, Beaglehole et al. (1977) found that the degree of social interactions with white New Zealanders accounted for only 2.1% of the blood pressure variance in males and 1.4% in females after controlling for dietary change. In a study of migrants who relocated from a rural tribal area in Kenya to Nairobi, Poulter et al. (1985) found that SBP and DBP were elevated within the first 60 days after migration and that intake of sodium, potassium, calcium, and other nutrients had also changed.

Exercise and Activity

Many studies have focused on the effects of activity and exercise in both hypertensive and normotensive people (Berkson et al., 1960; Bonanno and Lies, 1974; De Vries, 1970; Jennings et al., 1984; Urata et al., 1987), but the long-term hypotensive effects of activity and exercise have not been studied. Furthermore, most studies on this topic are poorly designed, lack appropriate control subjects (Leon and Blackburn, 1982), and have not demonstrated an association with dietary factors.

PEDIATRIC DIET AND ADULT HYPERTENSION

The relationship of blood pressure in childhood to adult hypertension has not been clearly estab-

lished. The inconsistency in study findings may relate in part to the difficulty of obtaining accurate blood pressure readings in children (Berenson, 1980; Lauer and Clarke, 1980). Two studies of cardiovascular risk factors in schoolchildren (Berenson et al., 1980; Lauer and Clarke, 1980) demonstrate a strong relationship between body size and blood pressure during growth but do not show a strong relationship of blood pressure to diet or to specific nutrients. Children tend to remain in the same percentile of SBP and DBP relative to their peers until adolescence (Lauer and Clarke, 1980). Differences between blacks and whites are small during infancy and early childhood (Berenson et al., 1980; Schacter et al., 1982) but become stronger during adolescence (Berenson et al., 1980).

Few intervention studies have been conducted in infants and children. In one randomized trial of sodium intake and blood pressure during the first 6 months of life, infants who consumed a low-salt formula approximating the salt content of human breast milk (365 mg of sodium chloride per liter) had an SBP slightly lower than in those on normal formula (1,100 mg of sodium chloride per liter) (Hofman et al., 1983). Growth rate and body size were the same in the two groups. After 1 year, there were no differences in blood pressure between the two groups. In a study conducted in China by Kangmim et al. (1987), no single nutrient was correlated with blood pressure in boys ages 7 and 8, although the ratios of sodium to potassium and potassium to calcium were correlated with SBP in multivariate analyses.

SUMMARY

Frequency of high blood pressure, average blood pressure, and population distributions of blood pressures vary widely among populations. Some populations are characterized by a rarity of adult hypertension and the absence of an increase in blood pressure with age. Others, such as the U.S. population, are characterized by an increase in blood pressure with age and a high prevalence of hypertension among adults. In such populations, where exposure to environmental factors affecting blood pressure is presumably widespread, familial and genetic factors appear to have a strong influence on individual blood pressure levels.

Obesity and habitual high-alcohol intake appear to be associated with an increased risk of hypertension. Habitual high-salt intake appears to have a major adverse effect on hypertension risk in some susceptible people, but there is no certain method for identifying such people or ascertaining how many of them will become hypertensive as a result of excessive salt intake. Potassium may modulate the blood pressure-raising effects of sodium and provide some protection against death from stroke, even when blood pressure is not reduced.

Some evidence suggests that reduced fat intake and a high P/S ratio also reduce blood pressure. Data on calcium are inconclusive. Psychosocial and sociocultural factors affecting risk of sustained hypertension are also inconclusive, and no linkage to diet has been reported. Some data suggest that increased physical activity and exercise have a long-term hypotensive effect, either independently or in association with diet.

DIRECTIONS FOR RESEARCH

- The mechanisms by which nutrients affect the development of hypertension. Such research should further examine the effects and interactions of sodium, potassium, calcium, alcohol, lipids, and proteins of different origin and composition.
- The combined action of diet and physical fitness on blood pressure.
- Nutrient consumption, with particular attention to foods and nutrients known to influence blood pressure.
- Racial differences in blood pressure level and risk of hypertension, particularly in respect to the higher risks of hypertension and hypertension-related mortality in blacks compared to whites.
- The pediatric antecedents, dietary and other, of adult hypertension through the continued application of longitudinal study.
- Identification of genetic markers of susceptability to dietary effects on blood pressure.

REFERENCES

Ackley, S., E. Barrett-Connor, and L. Suarez. 1983. Dairy products, calcium and blood pressure. Am. J. Clin. Nutr. 38:457–461.

Anderson, J.W. 1986. High-fiber, hypocaloric vs very-low-calorie diet effects on blood pressure of obese men. Am. J. Clin. Nutr. 43:695.

Armstrong, B., H. Coates, and A.J. van Merwyk. 1977. Blood pressure in Seventh-Day Adventist vegetarians. Am. J. Epidemiol. 105:444–449.

Ayachi, S. 1979. Increased dietary calcium lowers blood pressure in the spontaneously hypertensive rat. Metabolism 28:1234–1238.

Batuman, V., E. Landy, J.K. Maesaka, and R.P. Wedeen. 1983. Contribution of lead to hypertension with renal impairment. N. Engl. J. Med. 309:17–21.

Beaglehole, R., C.E. Salmond, A. Hooper, J. Huntsman, J.M. Stanhope, J.C. Cassel, and I.A. Prior. 1977. Blood pressure and social interaction in Tokelauan migrants in New Zealand. J. Chronic Dis. 30:803–812.

Beevers, D.G., J.K. Cruickshank, W.B. Yeoman, G.F. Carter, A. Goldberg, and M.R. Moore. 1980. Blood-lead and cadmium in human hypertension. J. Environ. Pathol. Toxicol. 4:251–260.

Belizan, J.M., J. Villar, O. Pineda, A.E. Gonzalez, E. Sainz, G. Garrera, and R. Sibrian. 1983. Reduction of blood pressure with calcium supplementation in young adults. J. Am. Med. Assoc. 249:1161–1165.

Berenson, G.S. 1980. Cardiovascular Risk Factors in Children. Oxford University Press, New York. 453 pp.

Berenson, G.S., A.W. Voors, and L.S. Webber. 1980. Importance of blood pressures in children. Pp. 71–97 in H. Kesteloot and J.V. Joossens, eds. Epidemiology of Arterial Blood Pressure: Developments in Cardiovascular Medicine, Vol. 8. Martinus Nijhoff, The Hague.

Berghoff, R.S., and A.S. Geraci. 1929. Influence of sodium chloride on blood pressure. Ill. Med. J. 56:395–397.

Berkson, D.M., J. Stamler, H.A. Lindberg, W. Miller, H. Mathies, H. Lasky, and Y. Hall. 1960. Socioeconomic correlates of atherosclerotic and hypertensive heart diseases. Ann. N.Y. Acad. Sci. 84:835–850.

Bittle, C.C., Jr., D.J. Molina, and F.C. Bartter. 1985. Salt sensitivity in essential hypertension as determined by the Cosinor method. Hypertension 7:989–994.

Bonanno, J.A., and J.E. Lies. 1974. Effects of physical training on coronary risk factors. Am. J. Cardiol. 33:760–764.

Brussaard, J.H., J.M. van Raaij, M. Stasse-Wolthuis, M.B. Katan, and J.G. Hautvast. 1981. Blood pressure and diet in normotensive volunteers: absence of an effect of dietary fiber, protein, or fat. Am. J. Clin. Nutr. 34:2023–2029.

Canessa, M., A. Spalvins, N. Adragna, and B. Falkner. 1984. Red cell sodium countertransport and cotransport in normotensive and hypertensive blacks. Hypertension 6:344–351.

Carroll, M.D., S. Abraham, and C.M. Dresser. 1983. Dietary Intake Source Data: United States, 1976–80. Vital and Health Statistics, Ser. 11, No. 231. DHHS Publ. No. (PHS) 83-1681. National Center for Health Statistics, Public Health Service, U.S. Department of Health and Human Services, Hyattsville, Md. 483 pp.

Cassel, J. 1975. Studies of hypertension in migrants. Pp. 41–58 in O. Paul, ed. Epidemiology and Control of Hypertension. Stratton Intercontinental Medical Book Co., New York.

Chiang, B.N., L.V. Perlman, and F.H. Epstein. 1969. Overweight and hypertension: a review. Circulation 39:403–421.

Coleman, T.G., and A.C. Guyton. 1969. Hypertension caused by salt loading in the dog. III. Onset transients of cardiac output and other circulatory variables. Circ. Res. 25:153–160.

Criqui, M.H. 1987. Alcohol and hypertension: new insights from population studies. Euro. Heart J. 8 Suppl. B:19–26.

Cruz-Coke, R., H. Donoso, and R. Berrera. 1973. Genetic ecology of hypertension. Clin. Sci. Mol. Med. 45:55s–65s.

Cushman, W.C., and H.G. Langford. 1983. Urinary electrolyte differences in black and white hypertensives: Veterans Administration Cooperative Study Group on antihypertensive agents. Clin. Res. 31:843A.

Dahl, L.K., M. Heine, and L. Tassinari. 1962. Effects of chronic excess salt ingestion. Evidence that genetic factors play an important role in susceptibility to experimental hypertension. J. Exp. Med. 115:1173–1190.

Dawber, T.R., W.B. Kannel, A. Kagan, R.K. Donabedian, P.M. McNamara, and G. Pearson. 1967. Environmental factors in hypertension. Pp. 255–288 in J. Stamler, R. Stamler, and T.N. Pullman, eds. The Epidemiology of Hypertension. Grune and Stratton, New York.

Denton, D. 1984. The Hunger for Salt: An Anthropological, Physiological and Medical Analysis. Springer-Verlag, Berlin. 650 pp.

De Vries, H.A. 1970. Physiological effects of an exercise training regimen upon men aged 52 to 88. J. Gerontol. 25:325–336.

DHEW (U.S. Department of Health, Education, and Welfare). 1963. Origin, Program, and Operation of the U.S. National Health Survey. Vital and Health Statistics, Ser. 1, No. 1. PHS Publ. No. 1000. National Center for Health Statistics, Public Health Service, U.S. Department of Health, Education, and Welfare, Washington, D.C. 41 pp.

DHEW (U.S. Department of Health, Education, and Welfare). 1979. Dietary Intake Source Data: United States, 1971–74. DHEW Publ. No. (PHS) 79-1221. National Center for Health Statistics, Public Health Service, U.S. Department of Health, Education, and Welfare, Hyattsville, Md. 421 pp.

DHHS (U.S. Department of Health and Human Services). 1985. Plan and Operation of the Hispanic Health and Nutrition Examination Survey 1982–84. Vital and Health Statistics, Ser. 1, No. 19. DHHS Publ. No. (PHS) 85-1321. National Center for Health Statistics, Public Health Service, U.S. Department of Health and Human Services, Hyattsville, Md. 429 pp.

DHHS (U.S. Department of Health and Human Services). 1986. Blood Pressure Levels in Persons 18–74 Years of Age in 1976–80, and Trends in Blood Pressure from 1960 to 1980 in the United States. Data from the National Health Survey, Ser. 11, No. 234. DHHS Publ. No. (PHS) 86-1684. National Center for Health Statistics, Public Health Service, U.S. Department of Health and Human Services, Hyattsville, Md. 68 pp.

Dodson, P.M., P.J. Pacy, P. Bal, A.J. Kubicki, R.F. Fletcher, and K.G. Taylor. 1984. A controlled trial of a high fibre, low fat and low sodium diet for mild hypertension in Type 2 (non-insulin-dependent) diabetic patients. Diabetologia 27:522–526.

Donahue, R.P., R.D. Abbott, D.M. Reed, and K. Yano. 1986. Alcohol and hemorrhagic stroke. J. Am. Med. Assoc. 255:2311–2314.

Düsing, R., R. Scherhag, K. Glänzer, U. Budde, and H.J. Kramer. 1983. Dietary linoleic acid deprivation: effects on blood pressure and PGI2 synthesis. Am. J. Physiol. 244:H228–H233.

Eakin, D.J., L.A. Schroeder, P.D. Whanger, and P.H. Weswig. 1980. Cadmium and nickel influence on blood pressure, plasma renin, and tissue mineral concentrations. Am. J. Physiol. 238:E53–E61.

Feinleib, M., C. Lenfant, and S.A. Miller. 1984. Hypertension and calcium. Science 226:384–389.

Feinleib, M., R. Garrison, N. Borhani, R. Rosenman, and J. Christian. 1975. Studies of hypertension in twins. Pp. 3–20 in O. Paul, ed. Epidemiology and Control of Hypertension. Stratton Intercontinental Medical Book Co., New York.

Fingerle, H., G. Fischer, and H.G. Classen. 1982. Failure to produce hypertension in rats by chronic exposure to cadmium. Food Chem. Toxicol. 20:301–306.

Folkow, B. 1982. Physiological aspects of primary hypertension. Physiol. Rev. 62:347–504.

Fortmann, S.P., W.L. Haskell, K. Vranizan, B.W. Brown, and J.W. Farquhar. 1983. The association of blood pressure and dietary alcohol: differences by age, sex, and estrogen use. Am. J. Epidemiol. 118:497–507.

Froment, A., H. Milon, and C. Gravier. 1979. Relationship of sodium intake and arterial hypertension: contribution of geographical epidemiology. Rev. Epidemiol. Sante Publique 27:437–454.

Fujita, T., W.L. Henry, F.C. Bartter, C.R. Lake, and L.S. Delea. 1980. Factors influencing blood pressure in salt-sensitive patients with hypertension. Am. J. Med. 69:334–344.

Garcia-Palmieri, M.R., R. Costas, Jr., M. Cruz-Vidal, P.D. Sorlie, J. Tillotson, and R.J. Havlik. 1984. Milk consumption, calcium intake, and decreased hypertension in Puerto Rico. Puerto Rico Heart Health Program study. Hypertension 6:322–328.

Garrison, R.J., W.B. Kannel, J. Stokes III, and W.P. Castelli. 1987. Incidence and precursors of hypertension in young adults: the Framingham Offspring Study. Prev. Med. 16:235–251.

Gill, J.S., A.V. Zezulka, M.J. Shipley, S.K. Gill, and G. Beevers. 1986. Stroke and alcohol consumption. N. Engl. J. Med. 315:1041–1046.

Gleibermann, L. 1973. Blood pressure and dietary salt in human populations. Ecol. Food Nutr. 2:143–156.

Goldby, F.S., and L.J. Beilin. 1972. Relationship between arterial pressure and the permeability of arterioles to carbon particles in acute hypertension in the rat. Cardiovasc. Res. 6:384–390.

Gordon, D.B., and D.R. Drury. 1956. Effect of potassium on occurrence of petechial hemorrhages in renal hypertensive rabbits. Circ. Res. 4:167–172.

Gordon, T., and W.B. Kannel. 1972. Predisposition to atherosclerosis in the head, heart, and legs. J. Am. Med. Assoc. 221:661–666.

Grim, C.E., F.C. Luft, J.Z. Miller, P.L. Brown, M.A. Gannon, and M.H. Weinberger. 1979. Sodium labeling and depletion in normotensive first degree relatives of essential hypertensives. J. Lab. Clin. Med. 94:764–771.

Grim, C.E., F.C. Luft, J.Z. Miller, G.R. Meneely, H.D. Battarbee, C.G. Hames, and L.K. Dahl. 1980. Racial difference in blood pressure in Evans County, Georgia: relationship to sodium and potassium intake and plasma renin activity. J. Chronic Dis. 33:87–94.

Grobbee, D.E., and A. Hofman. 1986. Effect of calcium supplementation on diastolic blood pressure in young people with mild hypertension. Lancet 2:703–707.

Gruchow, H.W., K.A. Sobocinski, and J.J. Barboriak. 1985. Alcohol, nutrient intake, and hypertension in U.S. adults. J. Am. Med. Assoc. 253:1567–1570.

Hallback, M., J.V. Jones, G. Bianchi, and B. Folkow. 1977. Cardiovascular control in the Milan strain of spontaneously hypertensive rat (MHS) at "rest" and during acute mental "stress." Acta Physiol. Scand. 99:208–216.

Hansen, J.C., and H.S. Pedersen. 1986. Environmental exposure to heavy metals in North Greenland. Arct. Med. Res. 41:21–34.

Harlan, W.R., A.L. Hull, R.L. Schmouder, J.R. Landis, F.E. Thompson, and F.A. Larkin. 1984. Blood pressure and nutrition in adults. The National Health and Nutrition Examination Survey. Am. J. Epidemiol. 120:17–18.

Hofman, A., A. Hazebroek, and H.A. Valkenburg. 1983. A randomized trial of sodium intake and blood pressure in newborn infants. J. Am. Med. Assoc. 250:370–373.

Holden, R.A., A.M. Ostfeld, D.H. Freeman, Jr., K.G. Hellenbrand, and D.A. D'Atri. 1983. Dietary salt intake and blood pressure. J. Am. Med. Assoc. 250:365–369.

Intersalt Cooperative Research Group. 1988. Intersalt: an international study of electrolyte excretion and blood pressure. Results for 24 hour urinary sodium and potassium excretion. Br. Med. J. 297:319–328.

Jackson, R., A. Stewart, R. Beaglehole, and R. Scragg. 1985. Alcohol consumption and blood pressure. Am. J. Epidemiol. 122:1037–1044.

Jennings, G.L., L. Nelson, M.D. Esler, P. Leonard, and P.I. Korner. 1984. Effects of changes in physical activity on blood pressure and sympathetic tone. J. Hypertens. 2 Suppl. 3:139–141.

Johansen, H.L. 1983. Hypertension in Canada: risk factor review and recommendations for further work. Can. J. Public Health 74:123–128.

JNC (Joint National Committee on Detection, Evaluation, and Treatment of High Blood Pressure). 1984. The 1984 report of the Joint National Committee on Detection, Evaluation, and Treatment of High Blood Pressure. Arch. Intern. Med. 144:1045–1057.

JNC (Joint National Committee on Detection, Evaluation, and Treatment of High Blood Pressure). 1988. The 1988 report of the Joint National Committee on Detection, Evaluation, and Treatment of High Blood Pressure. Arch. Intern. Med. 148:1023–1038.

Kagan, A., J.S. Popper, and G.G. Rhoads. 1980. Factors related to stroke incidence in Hawaii Japanese men. The Honolulu Heart Study. Stroke 11:14–21.

Kagan, A., K. Yano, G.G. Rhoads, and D.L. McGee. 1981. Alcohol and cardiovascular disease: the Hawaiian experience. Circulation 64:27–31.

Kageyama, Y., H. Suzuki, K. Hayashi, and T. Saruta. 1986. Effects of calcium loading on blood pressure in spontaneously hypertensive rats: attenuation of the vascular reactivity. Clin. Exp. Hypertens. 8:355–370.

Kangmim, Z., H. Shangpu, P. Xiaoqin, Z. Xianrong, and G. Yuan. 1987. The relation of urinary cations to blood pressure in boys aged seven to eight years. Am. J. Epidemiol. 126:658–663.

Kannel, W.B., and P. Sorlie. 1975. Hypertension in Framingham. Pp. 553–592 in O. Paul, ed. Epidemiology and Control of Hypertension. Stratton Intercontinental Medical Book Co., New York.

Kannel, W.B., N. Brand, J.J. Skinner, Jr., T.R. Dawber, and P. McNamara. 1967. The relation of adiposity to blood pressure and the development of hypertension. The Framingham Study. Ann. Intern. Med. 67:48–59.

Kaplan, N.M.. 1982. Clinical Hypertension, 3rd ed. Williams and Wilkins, Baltimore. 454 pp.

Kaplan, N.M., and R.B. Meese. 1986. The calcium deficiency hypothesis of hypertension: a critique. Ann. Intern. Med. 105:947–955.

Kaplan, N.M., A. Carnegie, P. Raskin, J.A. Heller, and M. Simmons. 1985. Potassium supplementation in hypertensive patients with diuretic-induced hypokalemia. N. Engl. J. Med. 312:746–749.

Karvonen, M.J., and S. Punsar. 1977. Sodium excretion and blood pressure of West and East Finns. Acta Med. Scand. 202:501–507.

Kawasaki, T., C.S. Delea, F.C. Bartter, and H. Smith. 1978. The effect of high-sodium and low-sodium intakes on blood pressure and other related variables in human subjects with idiopathic hypertension. Am. J. Med. 64:193–198.

Kesteloot, H., B.C. Park, C.S. Lee, E. Brems-Heyns, J. Claessens, and J.V. Joossens. 1980. A comparative study of blood pressure and sodium intake in Belgium and in Korea. Eur. J. Cardiol. 11:169–182.

Khaw, K.T., and E. Barrett-Connor. 1984. Dietary potassium and blood pressure in a population. Am. J. Clin. Nutr. 39: 963–968.

Khaw, K.T., and E. Barrett-Connor. 1987. Dietary potassium and stroke-associated mortality: a 12-year prospective population study. N. Engl. J. Med. 316:235–240.

Khaw, K.T., and E. Barrett-Connor. 1988. The association between blood pressure, age, and dietary sodium and potassium: a population study. Circulation 77:53–61.

Khaw, K.T., and G. Rose. 1982. Population study of blood pressure and associated factors in St. Lucia, West Indies. Int. J. Epidemiol. 11:372–377.

Kok, F.J., J.P. Vandenbroucke, C. van der Heide-Wessel, and R.M. van-der Heide. 1986. Dietary sodium, calcium, and potassium, and blood pressure. Am. J. Epidemiol. 123: 1043–1048.

Kromhout, D., E.B. Bosschieter, and C.D. Coulander. 1985. Potassium, calcium, alcohol intake and blood pressure: the Zutphen Study. Am. J. Clin. Nutr. 41:1299–1304.

Kurtz, T.W., and R.C. Morris, Jr. 1985. Dietary chloride as a determinant of disordered calcium metabolism in salt-dependent hypertension. Life Sci. 36:921–929.

Langford, H.G. 1985. Potassium and hypertension. Pp. 147–153 in M.J. Horan, M. Blaustein, J.B. Dunbar, W. Kachadorian, N.M. Kaplan, and A.P. Simopoulos, eds. NIH Workshop on Nutrition and Hypertension: Proceedings from a Symposium. Biomedical Information Corp., New York.

Lau, K., and B. Eby. 1985. The role of calcium in genetic hypertension. Hypertension 7:657–667.

Lau, K., D. Zikos, J. Spirnak, and B. Eby. 1984. Evidence for an intestinal mechanism in hypercalciuria of spontaneously hypertensive rats. Am. J. Physiol. 247:E625–E633.

Lauer, R.M., and W.R. Clarke. 1980. Immediate and long-term prognostic significance of childhood blood pressure levels. Pp. 281–290 in R.M. Lauer and R.B. Shekelle, eds. Childhood Prevention of Atherosclerosis and Hypertension. Raven Press, New York.

Leon, A.S. and H. Blackburn. 1982. Physical activity and hypertension. Pp. 14–36 in P. Sleight and E. Freis, eds. Hypertension: Cardiology, Vol. 1. Butterworth Scientific, London.

Lindahl, O., L. Lindwall, A. Spångberg, A. Stenram, and P.A. Ockerman. 1984. A vegan regimen with reduced medication in the treatment of hypertension. Br. J. Nutr. 52:11–20.

Ljungman, S., M. Aurell, M. Hartford, J. Wikstrand, L. Wilhelmsen, and G. Berglund. 1981. Sodium excretion and blood pressure. Hypertension 3:318–326.

Luft, F.C., L.I. Rankin, R. Bloch, A.E. Weyman, L.R. Willis, R.H. Murray, C.E. Grim, and M.H. Weinberger. 1979a. Cardiovascular and humoral responses to extremes of sodium intake in normal black and white men. Circulation 60:697–706.

Luft, F.C., C.E. Grim, N. Fineberg, and M.C. Weinberger. 1979b. Effects of volume expansion and contraction in normotensive whites, blacks, and subjects of different ages. Circulation 59:643–650.

Luft, F.C., M.H. Weinberger, and C.E. Grim. 1982. Sodium sensitivity and resistance in normotensive humans. Am. J. Med. 72:726–736.

MacDonald, M.C., R.L. Kline, and G.J. Mogenson. 1981. Dietary linoleic acid and salt-induced hypertension. Can. J. Physiol. Pharmacol. 59:872–875.

MacGregor, G.A., S.J. Smith, N.D. Markandu, R.A. Banks, and G.A. Sagnella. 1982. Moderate potassium supplementation in essential hypertension. Lancet 2:567–570.

MacMahon, S.W., and S.R. Leeder. 1984. Blood pressure levels and mortality from cerebrovascular disease in Australia and the United States. Am. J. Epidemiol. 120:865–875.

Maddocks, I. 1967. Blood pressure in Melanesians. Med. J. Aust. 1:1123–1126.

Mark, A.L., W.J. Lawton, F.M. Abboud, A.E. Fitz, W.E. Connor, and D.D. Heistad. 1975. Effects of high and low sodium intake on arterial pressure and forearm vascular resistance in borderline hypertension. A preliminary report. Circ. Res. 36 Suppl. 1:194–198.

McCarron, D.A., and C.D. Morris. 1985. Blood pressure response to oral calcium in persons with mild to moderate hypertension. A randomized, double-blind, placebo-controlled, crossover trial. Ann. Intern. Med. 103:825–831.

McCarron, D.A., N.N. Yung, B.A. Ugoretz, and S. Krutzik. 1981. Disturbances of calcium metabolism in the spontaneously hypertensive rat. Hypertension 3:I162–I167.

McCarron, D.A., H.J. Henry, and C.D. Morris. 1982. Human nutrition and blood pressure regulation: an integrated approach. Hypertension 4:III2–III13.

McCarron, D.A., C.D. Morris, H.J. Henry, and J.L. Stanton. 1984. Blood pressure and nutrient intake in the United States. Science 224:1392–1398.

McCarron, D.A., P.A. Lucas, R.J. Shneidman, B. LaCour, and R. Dräke. 1985. Blood pressure development of the spontaneously hypertensive rat after concurrent manipulations of dietary Ca^{2+} and Na^+. Relation to intestinal fluxes. J. Clin. Invest. 76:1147–1154.

McManus, I.C. 1983. Bimodality of blood pressure levels. Stat. Med. 2:253–258.

Medeiros, D.M., and L.K. Pellum. 1984. Elevation of cadmium, lead, and zinc in the hair of adult black female hypertensives. Bull. Environ. Contam. Toxicol. 32:525–532.

Meneely, G.R., and C.O. Ball. 1958. Experimental epidemiology of chronic sodium chloride toxicity and the protective effect of potassium chloride. Am. J. Med. 25:713–725.

Miller, J.Z., and C.E. Grim. 1983. Heritability of blood pressure. Pp. 79–90 in T.A. Kotchen and J.M. Kotchen, eds. Clinical Approaches to High Blood Pressure in the Young. John Wright, Boston.

Morino, T., R. McCaa, and H.G. Langford. 1978. Effect of potassium loading on blood pressure, sodium excretion and plasma renin activity in hypertensive patients. Clin. Res. 26:805a.

Moritz, V., P. Singer, D. Förster, I. Berger, and S. Massow. 1985. Changes of blood pressure in spontaneously hypertensive rats dependent on the quantity and quality of fat intake. Biomed. Biochim. Acta 44:1491–1505.

Muirhead, E.E., B.E. Leach, J.O. Davis, F.B. Armstrong, J.A. Pitcock, and W.L.S. Brosius. 1975. Pathophysiology of angiotensin-salt hypertension. J. Lab. Clin. Med. 85:734–745.

Oberman, A., N.E. Lane, W.R. Harlan, A. Graybiel, and R.E. Mitchell. 1967. Trends in systolic blood pressure in the thousand aviator cohort over a twenty-four-year period. Circulation 36:812–822.

Okamoto, K., and K. Aoki. 1963. Development of a strain of spontaneously hypertensive rats. Jpn. Circ. J. 27:282–293.

Ophir, O., G. Peer, J. Gilad, M. Blum, and A. Aviram. 1983. Low blood pressure in vegetarians: the possible role of potassium. Am. J. Clin. Nutr. 37:755–762.

Page, L.B. 1979. Hypertension and atherosclerosis in primitive and acculturating societies. Pp. 1–12 in J.C. Hunt, ed. Hypertension Update, Vol. 1. Health Learning Systems, Lyndhurst, N.J.

Page, L.B., and J. Friedlaender. 1986. Blood pressure, age and cultural change: a longitudinal study of Solomon Islands populations. Pp. 11–26 in M.J. Horan, G.M. Steinberg, J.B. Dunbar, and E.C. Hadley, eds. NIH Workshop on Blood Pressure Regulation and Aging: Proceedings from a Symposium. Biomedical Information Corp., New York.

Page, L.B., A. Damon, and R.C. Moellering, Jr. 1974. Antecedents of cardiovascular disease in six Solomon Islands societies. Circulation 49:1132–1146.

Page, L.B., D.E. Vandevert, K. Nader, N.K. Lubin, and J.R. Page. 1981. Blood pressure of Qash'qai pastoral nomads in Iran in relation to culture, diet, and body form. Am. J. Clin. Nutr. 34:527–538.

Perry, H.M., Jr., and S.J. Kopp. 1983. Does cadmium contribute to human hypertension? Sci. Total Environ. 26:223–232.

Platt, R. 1947. Heredity in hypertension. Q. J. Med. 16:111–133.

Poulter, N.R., K.T. Khaw, M. Mugambi, W.S. Peart, and P.S. Sever. 1985. Migration-induced changes in blood pressure: a controlled longitudinal study. Clin. Exp. Pharmacol. Physiol. 12:211–216.

Prineas, R.J., and H. Blackburn. 1985. Clinical and epidemiologic relationships between electrolytes and hypertension. Pp. 63–85 in M.J. Horan, M. Blaustein, J.B. Dunbar, W. Kachadorian, N.M. Kaplan, and A.P. Simopoulos, eds. NIH Workshop on Nutrition and Hypertension: Proceedings from a Symposium. Biomedical Information Corp., New York.

Prior, I.A.M., A. Hooper, J. Huntsman, J.M Stanhope, and C.E. Salmond. 1977. The Tokelau Island migrant study. Pp. 165–186 in G.A. Harrison, ed. Population Structure and Human Variation. Cambridge University Press, London.

Puska, P., J.M. Iacono, A. Nissinen, H.J. Korhonen, E. Vartiainen, P. Pietinen, R. Dougherty, U. Leino, M. Mutanen, S. Moisio, and J. Huttunen. 1983. Controlled randomised trial of the effect of dietary fat on blood pressure. Lancet 1:1–5.

Reed, D., D. McGee, K. Yano, and J. Hankin. 1985. Diet, blood pressure, and multicollinearity. Hypertension 7:405–410.

Reisin, E., R. Abel, M. Modan, D.S. Silverberg, H.E. Eliahou, and B. Modan. 1978. Effect of weight loss without salt restriction on the reduction of blood pressure in overweight hypertensive patients. N. Engl. J. Med. 298:1–6.

Resnick, L.M., J.P. Nicholson, and J.H. Laragh. 1984. Outpatient therapy of essential hypertension with dietary calcium supplementation. J. Am. Coll. Cardiol. 3:616.

Rostand, S.G., K.A. Kirk, E.A. Rutsky, and B.A. Pate. 1982. Racial differences in the incidence of treatment for end-stage renal disease. N. Engl. J. Med. 306:1276–1279.

Rouse, I.L., B.K. Armstrong, and L.J. Beilin. 1982. Vegetarian diet, lifestyle and blood pressure in two religious populations. Clin. Exp. Pharmacol. Physiol. 9:327–330.

Rouse, I.L., L.J. Beilin, B.K. Armstrong, and R. Vandongen. 1983. Blood-pressure-lowering effect of a vegetarian diet: controlled trial in normotensive subjects. Lancet 1:5–10.

Rouse, I.L., and L.J. Beilin. 1984. Vegetarian diet and blood pressure. J. Hypertens. 2:231–240.

Sacks, F.M., B. Rosner, and E.H. Kass. 1974. Blood pressure in vegetarians. Am. J. Epidemiol. 100:390–398.

Schacter, J., L.H. Kuller, and C. Perfetti. 1982. Blood pressure during the first two years of life. Am. J. Epidemiol. 116:29–41.

Schlierf, G., L. Arab, B. Schellenberg, P. Oster, R. Mordasini, H. Schmidt-Gayk, and G. Vogel. 1980. Salt and hypertension: data from the "Heidelberg Study." Am. J. Clin. Nutr. 33:872–875.

Sever, P.S., D. Gordon, W.S Peart, and P. Beighton. 1980. Blood-pressure and its correlates in urban and tribal Africa. Lancet 2:60–64.

Simpson, F.O. 1985. Blood pressure and sodium intake. Pp. 175–190 in C.J. Bulpitt, ed. Handbook of Hypertension, Vol. 6. The Epidemiology of Hypertension. Elsevier Science Publ., New York.

Singer, D.R.J., N.D. Markandu, F.P. Cappuccio, G.W. Beynon, A.C. Shore, S.J. Smith, and G.A. MacGregor. 1985. Does oral calcium lower blood pressure: a double-blind study. J. Hypertension 3:661.

Society of Actuaries. 1959. Build and Blood Pressure Study, Vol 1. Society of Actuaries, Chicago. 268 pp.

Stamler, J., D.M. Berkson, A. Dyer, M.H. Lepper, H.A. Lindberg, O. Paul, H. McKean, P. Rhomberg, J.A. Schoenberger, R.B. Shekelle, and R. Stamler. 1975. Relationship of multiple variables to blood pressure—findings from four Chicago epidemiologic studies. Pp. 307–356 in O. Paul, ed. Epidemiology and Control of Hypertension. Stratton Intercontinental Medical Book Co., New York.

Stamler, J., E. Farinaro, L.M. Mojonnier, Y. Hall, D. Moss, and R. Stamler. 1980. Prevention and control of hypertension by nutritional-hygienic means. Long-term experience of the Chicago Coronary Prevention Evaluation Program. J. Am. Med. Assoc. 243:1819–1823.

Svetkey, L.P., W.E. Yarger, J.R. Feussner, E. DeLong, and P.E. Klotman. 1986. Placebo-controlled trial of oral potassium in the treatment of mild hypertension. Clin. Res. 34:487a.

Tao, S.C., R.S. Tsai, Z.G. Hong, and J. Stamler. 1984. Timed overnight sodium and potassium excretion and blood pressure in steel workers in Peoples' Republic of China, (PRC)-North. CVD Epidemiol. Newsletter (AHA) 35:64.

Taylor, J.R., T. Combs-Orme, D. Anderson, D.A. Taylor, and C. Koppenol. 1984. Alcohol, hypertension, and stroke. Alcoholism 8:283–286.

Tobian, L. 1983. Human essential hypertension: implications of animal studies. Ann. Intern. Med. 98:729–734.

Tobian, L. 1986. High potassium diets markedly protect against stroke deaths and kidney disease in hypertensive rats, a possible legacy from prehistoric times. Can. J. Physiol. Pharmacol. 64:840–848.

Tobian, L., J. Lange, S. Azar, J. Iwai, D. Koop, and K. Coffee. 1977. Reduction of intrinsic natriuretic capacity in kidneys of Dahl hypertension-prone rats. Trans. Assoc. Am. Physicians 90:401–406.

Tobian, L., D. MacNeill, M.A. Johnson, M.C. Ganguli, and J. Iwai. 1984. Potassium protection against lesions of the renal tubules, arteries, and glomeruli and nephron loss in salt-loaded hypertensive Dahl S rats. Hypertension 6:I170–I176.

Tobian, L., J. Lange, K. Ulm, L. Wold, and J. Iwai. 1985. Potassium reduces cerebral hemorrhage and death rate in hypertensive rats, even when blood pressure is not lowered. Hypertension 7:I110–I114.

Tobian, L., T. Sugimoto, M.A. Johnson, and S. Hanlon. 1987. High K diets protect against hypertensive intimal lesions and endothelial injury in arteries of stroke-prone hypertensive rats. Trans. Assoc. Am. Physicians 100:300–304.

Trowell, H. 1981. Hypertension, obesity, diabetes mellitus and coronary heart disease. Pp. 3–32 in H.C. Trowell and D.P. Burkitt, eds. Western Diseases: Their Emergence and Prevention. Edward Arnold, London.

Tuck, M.L., J. Sowers, L. Dornfeld, G. Kledzik, and M. Maxwell. 1981. The effect of weight reduction on blood pressure, plasma renin activity, and plasma aldosterone levels in obese patients. N. Engl. J. Med. 304:930–933.

Tyroler, H.A., S. Heyden, and C.G. Hames. 1975. Weight and hypertension: Evans County studies of blacks and whites. Pp. 177–204 in O. Paul, ed. Epidemiology and Control of Hypertension. Stratton Intercontinental Medical Book Co., New York.

Ueshima, H., T. Ogihara, S. Baba, Y. Tabuchi, K. Mikawa, K. Hashizume, T. Mandai, H. Ozawa, Y. Kumahara, S. Asakura, and M. Hisanari. 1987. The effect of reduced alcohol consumption on blood pressure: a randomised, controlled, single blind study. J. Hum. Hypertens. 1:113–119.

Urata, H., Y. Tanabe, A. Kiyonaga, M. Ikeda, H. Tanaka, M. Shindo, and K. Arakawa. 1987. Antihypertensive and volume-depleting effects of mild exercise on essential hypertension. Hypertension 9:245–252.

Viart, P. 1977. Hemodynamic findings in severe protein-calorie malnutrition. Am. J. Clin. Nutr. 30:334–348.

von Arbin, M., M. Britton, U. de Faire, and A. Tisell. 1985. Circulatory manifestations and risk factors in patients with acute cerebrovascular disease and in matched controls. Acta Med. Scand. 218:373–380.

Voors, A.W., E.R. Dalferes, Jr., G.C. Frank, G.G. Aristimuno, and G.S. Berenson. 1983. Relation between ingested potassium and sodium balance in young blacks and whites. Am. J. Clin. Nutr. 37:583–594.

Walker, W.G., P.K. Whelton, H. Saito, R.P. Russell, and J. Hermann. 1979. Relation between blood pressure and renin, renin substrate, angiotensin II, aldosterone and urinary sodium and potassium in 574 ambulatory subjects. Hypertension 1:287–291.

Watt, G.C., C.J. Foy, and J.T. Hart. 1983. Comparison of blood pressure, sodium intake, and other variables in offspring with and without a family history of high blood pressure. Lancet 1:1245–1248.

Weinberger, M.H., J.Z. Miller, F.C. Luft, C.E. Grim, and N.S. Fineberg. 1986. Definitions and characteristics of sodium sensitivity and blood pressure resistance. Hypertension 8:II127–II134.

Whanger, P.D. 1979. Cadmium effects in rats on tissue iron, selenium, and blood pressure; blood and hair cadmium in some Oregon residents. Environ. Health Perspect. 28:115–121.

Whitescarver, S.A., C.E. Ott, B.A. Jackson, G.P. Guthrie, Jr., and T.A. Kotchen. 1984. Salt-sensitive hypertension:

contribution of chloride. Science 223:1430–1432.

Wilczynski, E.A., and F.H. Leenen. 1987. Dietary sodium intake and age in spontaneously hypertensive rats: effects on blood pressure and sympathetic activity. Life Sci. 41:707–715.

WHO (World Health Organization). 1978. Arterial Hypertension. Report of a WHO Expert Committee. Technical Report Series 628. World Health Organization, Geneva. 58 pp.

Working Group on Risk and High Blood Pressure. 1985. An epidemiological approach to describing risk associated with blood pressure levels. Hypertension 7:641–651.

Zinner, S.H., P.S. Levy, and E.H. Kass. 1971. Familial aggregation of blood pressure in childhood. N. Engl. J. Med. 284:401–404.

21

Obesity and Eating Disorders

For more than 50 years, the life insurance industry has pointed out that increased body weight is associated with excess mortality. This has been one stimulus for including measures of body weight, stature, and occasionally skinfolds in epidemiologic studies on the factors associated with the development of cardiovascular diseases and cancer. In recent years, fat distribution has also been included. It is now clear that two important factors associated with the risk of developing several chronic diseases are total body fat (most often estimated from ratios of body weight to height) and the distribution of that fat on the abdomen and trunk or peripherally on the arms and legs.

Overweight, obesity, and *adiposity* are commonly used terms. *Overweight* can be expressed as *relative weight* or *ratios of weight to height. Relative weight* is the ratio of actual to standard weight as determined from a table of reference body weights expressed relative to height, frequently as a percentage. *Weight-to-height ratios* can be expressed in several ways. The most widely used is the body mass index (BMI) or Quetelet index (QI), which is body weight (in kilograms) divided by the square of the height (in meters), i.e., weight/(height)^2. The BMI is more highly correlated with body fat than with other indices of height and weight (Benn, 1971). The nomogram in Figure 21–1 allows rapid determination of BMI for given levels of height and weight.

Obesity refers to an excess of total body fat, which can be assessed by a variety of techniques (see Chapter 6).

Adiposity refers to both the distribution and the size of the adipose tissue depots. Since half or more of the body fat is subcutaneous, measurement of skinfold thickness has been used frequently to estimate fat and its distribution. Other techniques involve the use of soft tissue x-rays, ultrasound, electrical conductivity, electrical impedance, computed tomographic scans, and magnetic resonance imaging scans. From a practical point of view, both the ratio of waist-to-hip (WHR) circumference and the ratio of triceps-to-subscapular skinfolds have proven useful.

Fat cells in specific depots can be measured by needle biopsies of adipose tissue followed by osmium fixation of the fat cell (Hirsch and Gallian, 1968) or separation of isolated fat cells and then measurement of their size under a microscope (Lavau et al., 1977).

WEIGHT STANDARDS

Body Weight

The generation of national weight standards requires information on a large group of subjects. For most of the twentieth century, the life insurance industry has provided the data base for the

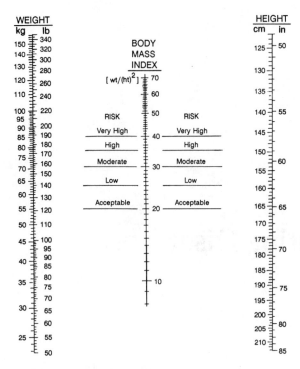

FIGURE 21–1 Nomogram for determining BMI. To use this nomogram, place a ruler or other straight edge between the body weight in kilograms or pounds (without clothes) located on the left-hand column and the height in centimeters or in inches (without shoes) located on the right-hand column. The BMI is read from the middle of the scale and is in metric units. Copyright 1978, George A. Bray. Used by permission.

TABLE 21–1 Desirable Body Mass Index in Relation to Age

Age Group (years)	BMI (kg/m^2)
19–24	19–24
25–34	20–25
35–44	21–26
45–54	22–27
55–65	23–28
>65	24–29

most widely used tables of desirable body weight. Both the 1959 and the 1983 Metropolitan Life Insurance tables were based on data obtained from the pooled experience of the life insurance industry in the United States (Society of Actuaries, 1959, 1980a,b). Although these surveys of weight and stature among insured individuals provide data on nearly 5 million people, they suffer from a self-selection bias, i.e., they provide data only on people who choose to take out life insurance. The insured tend to have a longer life expectancy, to be healthier, and, on average, to weigh less than the general population.

A second data base has been generated by the National Center for Health Statistics (NCHS), which in the past 20 years performed five surveys, including measurements of weight and stature of a representative sample of Americans from census tracts in the United States (Abraham et al., 1983). These surveys include approximately 20,000 people.

Appropriate weight standards can be determined in two ways. First, the normal distribution of weight in relation to height can be arbitrarily divided into overweight and severely overweight groups. This approach has been used by the NCHS, which defines overweight as those in the 85th percentile of weight for height using as reference the weights of 20- to 29-year-olds. With this technique, a BMI higher than 27.8 kg/m^2 for men and above 27.3 kg/m^2 for women is considered overweight, and the top 5th percentile is severely overweight. This approach was used in the *Surgeon General's Report on Nutrition and Health* (DHHS, 1988) but not by the National Institute on Aging. There are several drawbacks with this approach. First, the standards change as the weight distribution of the population changes. Second, the 85th percentile values of the BMI, 27.8 kg/m^2 and 27.3 kg/m^2 for men and women, respectively, will be very difficult for health professionals and the public to remember or understand. Third, and more important, is the underlying assumption that average weight is a healthy or preferred weight. Lastly, it is assumed in this approach that optimal weights remain constant at different ages—an assumption that may not be justified (Andres, 1985).

Weight standards can also be based on the BMI associated with the lowest overall risk to health. The minimal death rate in several prospective studies is associated with a BMI of 22 to 25 kg/m^2. Andres (1985) reanalyzed the Build and Blood Pressure Study of 1979 (Society of Actuaries, 1980a,b) and showed that the BMI associated with the lowest mortality increased with age. A similar increase in the BMI distribution curve with age is evident from a study conducted in Norway (Waaler, 1984). On the basis of these collated data, the ranges for BMI in relation to age proposed in Table 21–1 seem reasonable. Although the BMI is adjusted for age, the range overlaps. For example, the highest BMI for 19- to 24-year-olds is 24 kg/m^2, which is the lowest for those over 65. A BMI above 25 kg/m^2 was associated with increased risk of death in 78,612 young men followed for 32 years (Hoffmans et al., 1988). Alternatively, one might adopt the system used by the British and Australians, who define a normal BMI range as 20 to 25 kg/m², overweight as a BMI of 25 to 30 kg/m², severe overweight as a BMI above 30 kg/m², and massive overweight as a BMI above 40 kg/m².

Data from several longitudinal surveys in the United States might also provide sufficient information for preparing weight tables. Longitudinal data bases are also available from foreign countries. For example, Waaler (1984) reported the relationship of weight and height to morbidity and mortality for all 1.7 million Norwegians, except those living in Oslo and Bergen. The size of this sample and the 5-year follow-up provide a useful basis on which to determine relationships between weight and risks for cardiovascular diseases, hypertension, and diabetes (Waaler, 1984).

Fat Distribution

Fat distribution can be estimated by skinfolds, by waist-to-hip circumference ratios, or by such sophisticated techniques as ultrasound, computed tomography, or magnetic resonance imaging. The ratio of central (abdominal) to peripheral (gluteal) fat distribution can also be estimated from subscapular skinfold thickness (Donahue et al., 1987; Stokes et al., 1985). Skinfold measurements on the trunk and extremities can be used for principal component analysis (Ducimetiere et al., 1986; Mueller, 1983).

Data bases for circumferences may be developed from Swedish studies in Göteborg (Lapidus et al., 1984; Larsson et al., 1984), from studies in Milwaukee, Wisconsin (Hartz et al., 1984; Kissebah et al., 1982), and from the Canadian Fitness Survey (Fitness and Amateur Sport, 1986). A nomogram for determining the abdominal-to-gluteal circumference ratio (AGR), or WHR, is shown in Figure 21–2. The percentile distribution of these values for men and women in relation to age is plotted in Figure 21–3 from data obtained in the Canadian Fitness Surveys (Fitness and Amateur Sport, 1986).

ADIPOSITY STANDARDS

Height and weight data have been accumulated on millions of people. In contrast, quantitative estimates of total fat have been determined only from much smaller samples (Cheek, 1968; Cohn et al., 1984; Garrow, 1978; Segal et al.,

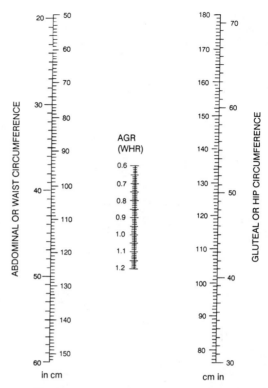

FIGURE 21–2 Nomogram for determining abdominal-to-gluteal circumference ratio (waist-to-hip ratio). Place a straight edge between the column for waist circumference and the column for hip circumference and read the ratio from the point where this straight edge crosses the AGR or WHR line. The waist, or abdominal, circumference is the smallest circumference below the rib cage and above the umbilicus, and the hip, or gluteal, circumference is the largest circumference at the posterior extension of the buttocks. From Bray and Gray (1988).

1985). Durnin and Womersley (1974) provided tables for estimating body fat from skinfolds measured at four different sites. No one as yet has tried to apply these Scottish standards to other populations. Steinkamp and colleagues (1965a,b) and several other groups have also provided useful equations for estimating body fat for men and women of various ages, using skinfolds from selected sites (Lohman, 1981; Lukaski, 1987; Steinkamp et al., 1965a,b). Triceps and subscapular skinfolds were measured in the surveys conducted by the NCHS (Abraham et al., 1979); however, these measurements cannot be used to establish standards for determining fatness because no data were collected on the relationship of these skinfolds to other measures of body fat. It is nonetheless possible to divide the population into percentiles of body fat by determining skinfold measurements from triceps and the subscapular region.

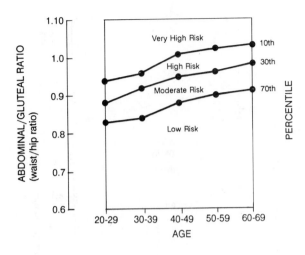

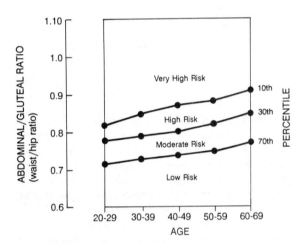

FIGURE 21–3 Percentiles of fat distribution. The percentiles of the ratio of abdominal-to-gluteal circumference (waist-to-hip ratio) are depicted for men and women by age groups along with relative risk. From Bray and Gray (1988). Plotted from tabular data in the Canadian Standardized Test of Fitness, 1986.

Fat Cell Size and Number

The number of fat cells can be estimated from measurements of total body fat and the average size of a fat cell. A reliable estimate of the total number of fat cells should be based on the average size of fat cells from more than one location, because fat cells differ in size from one region to another. Normally, there are no more than 60 billion fat cells. In general, cells proliferate most rapidly from birth to 2 years of age and during late childhood and puberty. In some types of obesity, they can increase 3 to 5 times more than the normal number. In *hypercellular* obesity, the number of fat cells are

increased. This type of obesity usually occurs in early or middle childhood but may also occur in adult life.

A higher-than-normal number of fat cells is usually present in people more than 75% above their desirable weight (Björntorp, 1985; Hirsch and Batchelor, 1976). When obesity begins during adult life, it often involves enlargement of adipose tissue cells. *Hypertrophic* obesity tends to correlate with an android or truncal fat distribution and is often associated with metabolic disorders such as glucose intolerance, hyperlipidemia, hypertension, and coronary artery disease (Feldman et al., 1969; Kissebah et al., 1982; Krotkiewski et al., 1983; Vague, 1956).

Stability of Total and Regional Fat

In several epidemiologic studies, investigators have examined the correlation between weights at two different ages (Borkan et al., 1986; Clarke et al., 1986; Noppa and Hällström, 1981; Zack et al., 1979). People in the lowest quintile for body weights at the end of childhood or adolescence may only have a small subsequent variation in body weight. For people in the middle or upper quintiles, however, there is considerable variability in weight; many individuals shift their weight one quintile up or down over a 5-year period. Mean body weights may show only a small upward trend during adult life, which camouflages considerable year-to-year fluctuations. In 1,302 women from Göteborg, Sweden, mean weight gain was 1.4 kg ± 5.1 kg SD over a 6-year period; 28 of the women lost more than 10 kg and 59 women gained more than 10 kg (Noppa and Hällström, 1981). In the normative aging study of 1,396 men, the weight of 168 of the subjects increased more than 10% and 75 men lost more than 10%. The baseline weight of those who lost weight was higher (84.1 kg) than that of those who gained weight (77.3 kg) (Borkan et al., 1986).

A prospective follow-up study over 36 years points to the variability in body weight with age (Bradden et al., 1986). At age 36, 3,322 people born in 1946 were divided into weight categories, based on BMI. In this cohort, 5.3% of the men and 8.4% of the women were severely overweight (BMI >30 kg/m²) and 38.0% of the men and 24.2% of women were overweight (BMI of 25 to 29.9 kg/m²). The correlation between BMI at ages 26 and 36 was $R = .64$ for men and $R = .66$ for women. The authors drew the following conclusions: First, approximately 25% of the men and women in the cohort were obese both as children and as adults. Second, the remaining 75% of this cohort became obese adults—an event that could not be predicted from weights before age 20. Those who became obese between the ages of 11 and 36 were often not the heaviest during childhood. On the basis of all socioeconomic, demographic, and weight data, only 50 to 60% of the men and women in the top decile for weight at age 36 could be correctly predicted at age 26 to attain that weight.

CAUSES OF OBESITY: INCREASED ENERGY INTAKE OR DECREASED ENERGY EXPENDITURE?

Energy Intake

There is little question that extreme changes in food intake produce corresponding changes in body weight (Bray, 1976; Forbes, 1987; Garrow, 1978). Short-term studies in men and one in women demonstrate that normal or overweight people who overeat on a metabolic ward gain considerable amounts of body fat. However, this is influenced by the genetic makeup of individuals (Poehlman et al., 1986) (see below). Total weight gain can be predicted for groups from the degree of excess caloric ingestion (Forbes, 1987). Early in this century, Gulick (1922) and Neumann (1902) suggested that overeating might not produce obesity. In a reanalysis of these two studies, Forbes (1984) showed a linear relationship for each subject between degree of increased food intake and change in body weight. On the other hand, previously obese individuals at normal or near-normal weight may require fewer calories to maintain this weight (Geissler et al., 1987; Leibel and Hirsch, 1984).

Keys and colleagues (1950), in their classic study of starvation in humans, demonstrated that reduced-calorie diets were associated with weight loss in normal, healthy volunteers. Kinsell et al. (1964) and others (e.g., Bray, 1976; Forbes, 1987; Garrow, 1978) reported that calorie restriction in obese subjects reduced body weight and fat stores. A vast literature collected primarily in developing countries also demonstrates a correlation between calorie restriction, body weight, and other indices of malnutrition.

In animals, there is also little question that increasing total caloric intake causes them to increase body weight. There are several ways of increasing voluntary food intake in animals, in-

cluding the provision of more palatable diets (Cruce et al., 1974; Sclafani and Springer, 1976), the administration of calorically dense drinking solutions (Faust et al., 1978), switching diets frequently (Collier, 1985), and increasing the fat content of the diet (Schemmel et al., 1970). In most of these cases, the ability to voluntarily increase intake is complicated by dietary composition. Thus, it is frequently difficult to separate the effects of caloric intake per se from the specific effects of dietary macronutrients, i.e., fats, carbohydrates, and proteins. In addition, such dietary manipulations have sometimes been confounded by the ingestion of diets whose protein-to-energy ratio is too low to support normal growth and maintenance.

There is no epidemologic evidence indicating that total fat intake per se, independent of total caloric intake, is associated with increased adiposity in the population. Obesity itself has not been found to be associated with dietary fat in either inter- or intrapopulation studies. A few clinical studies suggest that a high saturated fatty acid intake may be positively associated with obesity (see Chapter 7). Animal studies suggest that both the type and the amount of dietary fat, independent of total caloric intake, may contribute to obesity, possibly through more efficient metabolism of this nutrient relative to other nutrients (see Chapters 6 and 7).

Female rats fed isocaloric high-fat and high-carbohydrate diets spontaneously overingest the high-fat diet, compared to male rats, and become fatter (Hoyenga and Hoyenga, 1982; Sclafani and Gorman, 1977). In general, reduction in dietary fat leads to weight reduction, but this effect may be secondary to concomitant reductions in caloric intake. A more detailed discussion of the association of dietary fat with obesity can be found in Chapter 7.

Energy Intake and Energy Expenditure

As discussed in Chapter 6, epidemiologic studies of the relationship between body weight and energy intake have shown either no correlation or an inverse correlation (Baecke et al., 1983; Braitman et al., 1985; Keen et al., 1979; Kromhout, 1983; Lapidus et al., 1986; Romieu et al., 1988). In contrast, the direct measurements of energy expenditure for periods ranging from a few hours to 72 hours by indirect or direct calorimeters show a direct positive correlation between energy expenditure and body weight, body fat, fat-free mass, and body surface area (de Boer et al., 1986; Garrow, 1978; Jequier, 1984; Owen et al., 1986, 1987; Ravussin et al., 1986). This direct positive correlation between energy expenditure and fat-free mass has an important genetic component, since the variance among siblings is smaller than the variance among families (Bogardus et al., 1986; Bouchard et al., 1986). Thus, increases in adiposity in some cases must reflect decreases in energy expenditure or changing metabolic efficiency.

Metabolic Efficiency

Animal studies provide clear evidence that increased energy intake is not required to induce obesity (Bray and York, 1971, 1979). The most clear-cut examples are animals with recessively inherited forms of obesity, which, despite precise paired feeding, had greater weight gain and fat deposition than their lean littermates (Cleary et al., 1980; Coleman, 1979; Cox and Powley, 1981). These differences cannot be explained by differences in work-related energy expenditure.

Similar studies have been conducted in animals with hyperphagia and obesity resulting from damage to the hypothalamus (Bray and York, 1979; Cox and Powley, 1981). When such animals are pair-fed with lean animals, the animals with lesions become obese but the lean animals do not. These studies imply differences in metabolic efficiency.

Studies in animals indicate that increased energy intake usually results in obesity (Bray, 1987a) but is not essential for the development of modest levels of obesity. If this phenomenon exists among heterogeneous groups of obese humans, then some forms of obesity are probably associated with enhanced metabolic efficiency, whereas others may require increased energy intake or decreased energy expenditure. Recent prospective studies of Pima Indians (Ravussin et al., 1988) and infants born to overweight mothers (Roberts et al., 1988) further support the possibility that lower energy expenditure can predict the subsequent development of obesity.

GENETIC FACTORS IN OBESITY

It has been known for decades that obesity is a familial trait (Bray, 1976). Since members of a kindred share many dietary and other environmental exposures, the identification of genetic factors is complex. As discussed in Chapter 4, the most compelling evidence for a genetic component in

obesity comes from examinations of monozygotic and dizygotic twins (e.g., Börjeson, 1976; Bouchard, 1988; Fabsitz et al., 1980; Feinleib et al., 1977; Medlund et al., 1976; Stunkard et al., 1986). Börjeson (1976) studied 40 monozygotic and 61 same-sex dizygotic twin pairs and estimated heritability of obesity to be 88%. (Heritability may range from 0, i.e., no genetic factors, to 100%, indicating that a trait is entirely genetically determined.) A similar conclusion by Brook et al. (1975) was based on studies of monozygotic and dizygotic twins. Two large studies of twins confirmed the importance of genetic factors in obesity and the distribution of body fat (Bouchard, 1988; Stunkard et al., 1986). A strong interaction between genetic predisposition and environmental stimuli is suggested by the findings of Poehlman et al. (1986), who reported differential responses of twin pairs to overfeeding. Although weight gain was closely correlated within a pair of twins, there was wide scatter in values among pairs of twins. Studies of twins suggest that there is an important genetic component in the etiology of human obesity.

In addition to obesity per se, there is increasing evidence that patterns of fat distribution are inherited. This was indicated in a study of twins (Bouchard, 1988) and in several studies of ethnic groups (Mueller, 1988). These patterns may be apparent among children. For example, Mexican-American children have a pronounced upper-body distribution of fat, which is sometimes independent of adiposity per se (Mueller, 1988), whereas children of European origin seem to have a more peripheral fat distribution (Mueller, 1988).

The specific genes involved in obesity are still unknown. Such genes may have played an important evolutionary role by improving the survival of people who could store fat more efficiently during periods of prosperity and use it during caloric deprivation. If this is true, then one might expect to find some people who develop obesity more readily than others.

Obesity in mice and rats can be caused by several different single gene mutations (Bray and York, 1979). Some strains of pigs (Steele et al., 1974) and rats become obese, whereas control animals fed the same diet do not (Schemmel et al., 1970). The exact biochemical or metabolic defects leading to such observations have not yet been discovered. Intensive research is under way to clone relevant candidate genes.

Monogenic animal models of obesity will most probably not fully explain the genetic factors operative in human obesity, which do not appear to be monogenic; however, some genes involved in monogenic animal obesity may play some role in human obesity. Information on the genes involved in animal obesity will provide a basis for the direct testing of similar genes in humans with the techniques of molecular genetics.

EVIDENCE ASSOCIATING OVERWEIGHT OR OBESITY WITH CHRONIC DISEASES AND PHYSIOLOGIC FUNCTION

Epidemiologic data on the relationship between body weight and the risk of chronic diseases, or between body weight and mortality, indicate that the relationship is curvilinear and often J- or U-shaped. That is, mortality increases as body weight increases or decreases away from the mean. This J-shaped relationship applies to overall mortality as well as to cardiovascular diseases, cancer, diabetes, hypertension, gallbladder disease, and osteoporosis (Bray, 1985). For example, data from the Pooling Project show that the underweight group has the highest mortality (McGee and Gordon, 1976).

Cardiovascular Diseases

Epidemiologic Studies

Many epidemiologic studies have contributed to our current perspective on the relationship of overweight and adiposity to atherosclerotic cardiovascular diseases. These include retrospective as well as prospective studies.

Cardiovascular diseases are the major cause of death in the United States. This fact has provided the stimulus for many epidemiologic studies, which have attempted to identify the risk factors associated with these multifactorial diseases. In a review of many such studies, Manson et al. (1987) concluded that overweight generally increases the risk of death, especially sudden death, although it is not always an independent risk factor. Manson et al. (1987) also pointed out in a review of mortality statistics related to body weight indices that there are three major drawbacks to most studies in this area. First, the authors frequently do not separate smokers, who tend to have lower weights and higher mortality, from nonsmokers, who have lower mortality. Second, they fail to take into account the impact of early mortality on longer-range mortality trends. Third, they focus on the identification of obesity as an independent risk factor rather than on its relationship to intermediary complications such as diabetes, hypertension, or hyperlipidemia through which the effects of increased body weight on chronic diseases are likely to become manifest. Obesity must modify some intermediate mechanism, such as cardiac function or the metabolism of lipid or glucose, to produce its effects on risks that have not otherwise been controlled for or identified. Overweight and obesity are more likely to be identified as significant risk factors in studies with large numbers of subjects of all ages, with a large proportion of younger people, and with a follow-up longer than 15 years.

Obesity itself is not independently associated with the severity of atherosclerosis (Solberg and Strong, 1983), and the precise role of obesity in the etiology of atherosclerosis and CHD is unclear. However, some studies show that there is an association between obesity and risk of coronary death at the upper range of body weight, e.g. > 140% of ideal body weight or a BMI >30 (Donahue et al., 1987). Furthermore, the pattern of fat distribution, as discussed below, may be an important risk factor for CHD. In general, dietary composition (e.g., type of fat) and lifestyle are more closely associated with risk of CHD than is overweight, except for severe overweight.

Retrospective Life Insurance Studies

Applicants for individual life insurance policies usually undergo a medical examination. In the Build and Blood Pressure Study of 1979 (Society of Actuaries, 1980a,b), weights were measured for approximately 87% of the almost 4 million men and 600,000 women on whom policies were written (Society of Actuaries, 1980a,b).

The lowest death rate occurred at a body weight slightly lower than the average weight for the entire population. As body weight increased, there was a progressive increase in mortality. Life insurance data show that mortality is increased to 125% of expected levels in individuals who are 5 to 15% overweight and rises to more than 500% of the expected level in people who are 25% or more overweight. There was also an increase in excess mortality at very low body weights, but the causes were different from the causes of death for people with a high BMI.

The curvilinear relationship of excess mortality to excess body weight is evident for all age groups in the life insurance studies published in 1959 and 1980 (Society of Actuaries, 1959, 1980a,b). The lowest mortality occurred at high BMIs in this study as well as in a study conducted by Waaler (1984) in Norway.

Data on the association between BMI and mortality in the elderly are limited. Mattila et al. (1986) reported that survival over a 5-year observation period was related to the BMI of 674 people 65 years of age or older. Those with a BMI of 22 kg/m² or less had a lower survival rate compared to people with a BMI between 22 and 28 kg/m². These data are consistent with most population data, which show that increased risk is associated with underweight and that it also increases gradually with BMI above 25 kg/m².

Few morbidly obese people (greater than twice the ideal body weight) receive life insurance and, thus, are not represented in life insurance statistics. Drenick et al. (1980) have provided some insight into the effects of gross obesity on life expectancy. They reviewed medical records of 200 morbidly obese men (average weight, 143.5 kg), who were admitted to a Veterans Administration hospital for a weight control program and then followed for an average of 7.5 years. One hundred eighty-five of these men were followed until death or termination of the study. The mortality rate for these subjects was higher at all ages when compared with the mortality expected for the general population of U.S. males. In men ages 25 to 34, mortality increased 12-fold. In those ages 35 to 44, mortality increased fivefold. For the 55- to 64-year-old group, however, the mortality rate was only double that of the average U.S. population.

Prospective Studies

In the Pooling Project, data from five prospective studies of factors involved in the development of coronary heart disease (CHD) were pooled for analytical purposes. These studies included three occupation-based studies (Albany Civil Servants, Chicago Gas Company, Chicago Western Electric Company) and two community-based studies (Framingham, Massachusetts, and Tecumseh, Michigan). The subjects were 8,422 white men ages 40 to 64 years. The mean length of follow-up was 8.6 years. A high relative weight was associated with an increased risk of a first major coronary event only for men in their forties. For the older groups, there was no effect of age on the risk of developing CHD. Using quintiles of body weight at 5-year age intervals, the investigators found that the relative risk of developing heart disease was 2.1 among 40- to 44-year-old men and that the risk fell to 1.6 for men ages 45 to 49. This analysis means that men ages 40 to 44 in the highest quintile for

relative weight were 2.1 times as likely to develop a first coronary event within an average of 3.6 years than men in the lowest quintile. In the men over 55, the gradual increase in risk with increasing weight was negligible.

The Framingham Study included 2,252 men and 2,818 women living in Framingham, Massachusetts. Participants were initially examined between 1948 and 1950 and reexamined at 2-year intervals thereafter. The median body weights of these subjects were almost identical to the upper limits for large-frame people in life insurance tables published in 1959 by the Metropolitan Life Insurance Company. On the basis of these tables, 15% of the men and 19% of the women were 20% overweight, and 3% of the men and 9% of the women were more than 50% overweight. Weight gain was associated with an increase in serum cholesterol, blood pressure, uric acid, and blood glucose (Ashley and Kannel, 1974). Overweight was also associated with an increased risk of sudden death, presumably from CHD; however, the exact cause is unknown.

After 26 years, there were 870 deaths among the men and 688 among the women. Relative weight at entry into the study was an independent predictor for development of cardiovascular diseases, particularly in women (Hubert et al., 1983). The 26-year incidence of CHD (including angina pectoris), death from CHD, and the likelihood of developing congestive heart failure in men was predicted from the initial degree of overweight using multiple logistic regression analysis. The predictive power for the relative degree of overweight was independent of age, cholesterol levels, systolic blood pressure, cigarette smoking, or glucose intolerance.

Relative body weight of the women was also positively and independently predictive of the likelihood for developing cardiovascular diseases, stroke, congestive heart failure, and death from CHD. Weight gain after the young adult years increased the risk of cardiovascular diseases in both sexes. There was, however, either no effect or a small inverse relationship of body weight to the frequency of intermittent claudication (Kannel and McGee, 1985).

Although excess weight was shown to be predictive of developing CHD in the Framingham study, it is not predictive of the outcome. Survival and functional status after a myocardial infarct were not affected by weight status (Kannel and Schatzkin, 1984) (see Chapter 19).

The Seven Countries Study involved an international collaborative examination of risk factors for development of CHD in 16 cohorts of men in the United States, Europe, and Japan. Men at entry into this prospective study were between 40 and 59 years old. Overweight was defined as a BMI greater than 27 kg/m^2, and obesity as the sum of triceps and subscapular skinfolds greater than 37 mm. On the basis of these criteria, more than half (52%) of the U.S. participants were obese. This was a substantially higher prevalence of obesity compared to that of the northern European group, but it was comparable to the prevalence in the southern European group.

Among the men from the United States and southern Europe, few, if any, significant relationships were found between body weight, the risk of myocardial infarction, and CHD death, but overweight was found to be correlated with angina pectoris. Among the men from northern Europe, the findings were nearly reversed. There were statistically significant correlations between all measures of body weight and "hard" criteria (an actual occurrence) for coronary events, but no significant association was found between body weight and "soft" diagnostic criteria (e.g., elevated blood lipids) for CHD.

In the 15-year follow-up of these groups, there were 2,289 deaths—618 of which were from CHD. Relative body weight did not predict the risks of death from all causes or from CHD alone. These findings are contrary to the conclusions based on life insurance statistics.

The American Cancer Society studied the association of mortality with body weight in more than 750,000 people followed prospectively between 1959 and 1972 (Lew and Garfinkel, 1979). Relative death rates among subgroups that deviated above or below the average body weight were compared to the death rate for the group with weights that were 90 to 109% of the group mean. The overall mortality rate increased with increasing body weight.

This study also indicated that mortality for a smoker with a normal body weight (a BMI of 25 kg/m^2) is comparable to that of a nonsmoker with a BMI of 30 to 35 kg/m^2. Cardiovascular disease was a major factor in this increased mortality. No increase in mortality was observed until the BMI exceeded 25 kg/m^2, at which point the increase in relative mortality was almost linear for both sexes. These findings are similar to the increases observed both in the Build and Blood Pressure Study of 1979 (Society of Actuaries, 1980a,b) and in the Framingham study (Kannel and Schatzkin, 1984).

In the Norwegian prospective study, height and weight measurements were obtained for most of that country's population during the course of mass x-ray screenings conducted between 1963 and 1975 (Waaler, 1984). For more than 95% of the subjects, BMIs were calculated on the basis of body weights and heights measured without shoes and with the upper body undressed in preparation for the x-rays. Of the 1.7 million men and women ages 15 to 90 followed in this study, 176,574 deaths occurred from 1963 to 1979. A J-shaped relationship was found between mortality and BMI, with the lowest mortality rates for males and females occurring at a BMI of 23 kg/m^2, and increased rates observed for BMIs of less than 23 kg/m^2. Relative mortality increased only slightly when at BMIs between 23 and 27 kg/m^2. As the BMI increased above 27 kg/m^2, however, there was a curvilinear increase in excess mortality.

There was also a strong inverse association between mortality and height. That is, short people had a higher death rate. The principal causes of excess mortality in the shorter people were tuberculosis, obstructive lung diseases, and cancer of the stomach and lung. Among the overweight subjects, the principal causes of death were cerebrovascular diseases, cardiovascular diseases, diabetes mellitus, and cancer of the colon. From his analysis, Waaler (1984) concluded that at the optimal BMI, the total mortality would be reduced by an additional 15%.

Clinical Studies

Lipoprotein Metabolism

Associations of obesity with alterations in lipoprotein metabolism may be related to the risk of developing coronary atherosclerosis (Egusa et al., 1985; Grundy et al., 1979) (see Chapter 19). First, high-density-lipoprotein (HDL$_2$) cholesterol decreases in obese males and females (Gordon et al., 1977b). Second, serum total cholesterol in obesity is normal or only slightly elevated, although the transport of low-density-lipoprotein (LDL) cholesterol through the plasma compartment increases. This increased transport is consistent with the correlation between increased cholesterol production and obesity, which amounts to approximately 20 more milligrams of cholesterol for each extra kilogram of body fat (Miettinen, 1971; Nestel et al., 1973). Third, the production of very-low-density-lipoprotein (VLDL) triglyceride and the corresponding apoprotein (VLDL-B) tends to increase in relation to the degree of obesity in

Caucasians and Pima Indians (Bennion and Grundy, 1978). Whether or not triglyceride levels increase, as reported in many studies, depends on the rate at which triglycerides are cleared from the plasma. Fourth, the high rate of apoprotein B synthesis in LDL-B is probably related to the high rate of synthesis of apoprotein B for incorporation into VLDL. Fifth, lipoprotein lipase, the clearing-factor enzyme for lipoproteins, increases in obesity and may help prevent elevated triglyceride levels in some subjects. Finally, free fatty acid concentrations frequently increase in obesity, reflecting their higher rate of turnover.

Hypertension

It is widely believed that the indirect auscultatory method of obtaining blood pressure with an inflatable cuff produces higher readings in obese individuals than does direct intraarterial measurement. This may not occur, however, if the blood pressure cuff bladder is sufficiently long. With short cuffs, greater differences have been observed between systolic and diastolic pressures measured by direct intraarterial methods and indirect measurements. Despite this potential problem, there is clear evidence that increased body weight is associated with hypertension (Chaing et al., 1969; Havlik et al., 1983).

The increased blood pressure probably results from increased peripheral arteriolar resistance (Messerli, 1982), but the etiology of the increase in peripheral resistance is unknown. Tuck et al. (1981) suggested that it results from the increased secretion of catecholamines due to a hyperactive sympathetic nervous system.

Several associations emerge from a review of the relationship between body weight and hypertension. First, hypertension has a striking correlation not only with body weight but also with lateral body build. People with a large chest circumference relative to their height and weight have higher blood pressure than do slender individuals. In one study, hypertension was present in 37% of the broad-chested men but in only 3% of the narrow-chested men (Bray 1976). Body build was associated with an almost proportional effect on systolic and diastolic blood pressure. Second, when blood pressure was compared in groups with constant body build, there was no significant correlation between obesity and hypertension. The greatest correlation of blood pressure with obesity was observed in men with a slender build. A much smaller correlation was found in the broad-chested men. From these data, it appears that body build

may be more important than obesity per se in the positive correlation between blood pressure and body weight (Weinsier et al., 1985). Two recent epidemiologic studies suggest that the effect of hypertension may be less severe in obese subjects than in normal-weight subjects. Two different groups found that the risk of cardiovascular mortality associated with hypertension and obesity is less than the risk of hypertension in normal-weight people (Barrett-Connor and Khaw, 1985; Cambien et al., 1985).

Messerli (1982) compared the cardiovascular consequences of hypertension in subjects with and without obesity. Cardiac output is increased in obese people, but not in nonobese, hypertensive people. The preload (volume inside the heart before it contracts), which is increased in obese people with or without hypertension, is normal in nonobese, hypertensive individuals. The presence of hypertension and obesity increases abnormalities of most other cardiac parameters, including afterload (resistance against which heart has to beat), stroke work (volume that the heart ejects in one heart beat against resistant pressure), and left ventricular mass. On the other hand, the nonobese hypertensive subject has a smaller chamber volume but a larger relative thickness of the left ventricular wall. Total peripheral resistance is sharply elevated in nonobese hypertensives but may decrease in obese people and become only modestly elevated in those who are obese and hypertensive. These data suggest an interaction between obesity and hypertension with reduced morbidity in obese hypertensives. However, this does not imply that becoming obese is an effective approach to treatment of hypertension, but may suggest that type of obesity, distribution of body fat (Hartz et al., 1984), weight history, or other lifestyle factors may be more important.

A reduction in blood pressure usually follows weight loss. During periods of caloric deprivation, such as World War I or World War II, hypertension was almost nonexistent. A number of clinical studies correlating changes in blood pressure with weight reduction have shown that blood pressure drops in 50 to 70% of those who lose weight. One explanation might be the reduced intake of salt that is associated with reduced caloric intake. However, Reisin et al. (1978) and Tuck et al. (1981) showed that blood pressure decreased even when salt intake was not reduced. Weight reduction is more effective in lowering systolic than diastolic pressure. Because reduction in blood pressure takes place as soon as food restriction begins, and then levels off, it has been suggested that the lowering of blood pressure may be a direct result of caloric deprivation rather than the result of eliminating obesity (Ernsberger and Nelson, 1988; Nelson and Ernsberger, 1984). Whether the therapeutic effect of weight reduction is related to the magnitude of the decline in body weight or to other environmental factors is still not clear. However, weight reduction was observed to produce a significant reduction in blood pressure in more than half of the hypertensive patients studied by MacMahon et al. (1986).

Diabetes Mellitus

Epidemiologic Studies

A variety of epidemiologic data indicate that adiposity increases the risk of noninsulin-dependent (Type II) diabetes mellitus (NIDDM). The U.S. National Diabetes Commission (DHEW, 1976) reported that the chance of becoming diabetic more than doubles with every 20% excess in body weight. In an epidemiologic study of 10,000 Israeli civil servants, those destined to develop diabetes were found to be considerably fatter. In a study of Pima Indians, the incidence of NIDDM was strongly related to preexisting obesity. When BMI was below 20 kg/m^2, the incidence of diabetes was 0.8 cases per 1,000 person-years. The rate increased steadily as BMI increased, peaking at 72.2 cases per 1,000 person-years at a BMI over 40 kg/m^2. This effect remained when subjects were classified according to the diabetic status of their parents (Knowler et al., 1978, 1981).

Rimm et al. (1975) investigated the relationship between diabetes and obesity in a retrospective analysis of more than 73,000 responses to a questionnaire submitted to members of a voluntary weight-loss group. Increases in body weight and aging were associated with increases in the frequency of NIDDM. Less than 1% of normal-weight women ages 25 to 44 reported NIDDM, whereas 7% of those of the same age who were 100% overweight (twice the ideal weight) reported this disease. Data from the Framingham study (Gordon et al., 1977a) also show that obesity is significantly associated with diabetes. Only plasma glucose was a better predictor than body weight for the risk of developing glucose intolerance over a 14-year period. Moreover, fasting glucose level changed in the same direction as body weight (Ashley and Kannel, 1974).

The increase in percentage of body weight for males and females between the ages of 25 and 60 in four different countries is also related to the frequency of diabetes. The mortality from NIDDM was highest among females who had the greatest gain in weight between ages 25 and 60. Canadian and U.S. populations had the greatest percentage increases in body weight between these ages compared to other populations of countries and thus had the highest mortality from diabetes.

The epidemiologic data are buttressed by the cross-cultural studies of West and Kalbfeisch (1971), who examined the prevalence of diabetes in 12 age-matched populations from 11 countries. There was a positive correlation ($R = .89$) between the prevalence of diabetes and standard weight in these populations. Larsson et al. (1981) also demonstrated a positive correlation between obesity and the development of diabetes over a 10-year period in a longitudinal study of nearly 900 middle-aged men in Göteborg.

Clinical Studies

In a retrospective analysis of patient charts, Joslin et al. (1935) found that 51% of diabetic males and 59% of diabetic females were at least 20% overweight and that 17% of the males and 26% of the females were actually 40% or more above average weight. Patients who developed diabetes between the ages of 20 and 35—presumably a mixture of insulin-dependent diabetes mellitus (IDDM) and NIDDM—had appreciably less excess body weight compared to those in older age groups.

Pyke and Please (1957) extended these studies by comparing the body weights of 946 patients. Below age 30, there was little difference in weight distribution between subjects with and without diabetes. Among 30-year-olds, the percentage of overweight diabetics exceeded that of nondiabetics. Among the older diabetics, 43 to 55% of the men and 51 to 55% of the women exceeded 110% of normal weight. Among nondiabetics, only 21 to 27% were >110% of normal weight.

Early studies demonstrated that impaired glucose tolerance is related to the duration of obesity. The prevalence of glucose intolerance in grossly obese subjects has been repeatedly found to be around 50%, varying somewhat with age, sex, and genetics. Lillioja et al. (1987) demonstrated that obese Pima Indians are at high risk of developing NIDDM and that this phenomenon aggregates in families. The risk of developing diabetes was highest among those with the most resistance to the effects of insulin (lowest rate of glucose disposal), and this resistance ran in families. Why only half the obese develop glucose intolerance remains an unresolved question. Its answer may be related to the impact of regional fat distribution.

Vague (1956) suggested that increased central body fat is more likely to be associated with the onset of diabetes mellitus. The female (or gynoid) type of body fat distribution (i.e., fat deposited primarily on the hips and thighs) was found to have a lower association with diabetes than the male (or android) type of obesity (i.e., fat deposited predominantly on the abdomen and upper body). Subsequently, Feldman et al. (1969), Hartz et al. (1984), and Ohlson et al. (1985) confirmed this association by demonstrating that diabetic subjects showed a significant shift toward an android or abdominal distribution of fat after onset of diabetes. Kissebah and colleagues (1982), who were pioneers in this area of research, conducted glucose tolerance tests and found that glucose and insulin levels increased more in subjects with upper-body obesity (high WHR) than in those with lower-body obesity when both groups had comparable amounts of total body fat. Krotkiewski et al. (1983), who also conducted a glucose tolerance test, found that both high total body fat and upper-body fat distribution were associated with a greater rise in glucose and insulin.

Recent data from the San Antonio Heart Study have extended these observations to 2,217 randomly selected Mexican-American individuals ages 25 to 60 (Haffner et al., 1987). A high ratio of subscapular to tricep skinfold or high WHR in a medically examined subset of 736 subjects was associated with high rates of NIDDM. BMI, a high WHR, and the ratio of subscapular tricep skinfold measurements all were independent predictors for the risk of NIDDM onset in females but not in males.

Beginning with the work of Himsworth (1935) and Newburgh and Conn (1939), studies have consistently shown that weight loss in obese subjects could improve glucose tolerance and that weight gain could worsen it. Glucose levels rise when normal-weight subjects gain weight and decline when they lose weight (Ashley and Kannel, 1974). This relationship was demonstrated most elegantly by Drenick et al. (1972), who showed the marked amelioration in glucose tolerance and insulin secretion after weight loss. In five obese men with normal glucose tolerance, insulin levels rose less during a glucose tolerance test when weight fell from 270 to 196 lb (112.5 to 81.6 kg) than before weight loss. After a 10- to 20-pound (4.5- to 9.0-kg) weight gain, glucose tolerance deteriorated substantially, and insulin secretion

was inadequate. In another group of six men with abnormal glucose tolerance, there was improvement in insulin secretion and glucose tolerance after weight fell from 132.3 kg to 94.1 kg. After a modest regain of weight to 103.2 kg, glucose tolerance deteriorated significantly.

When normal-weight subjects voluntarily overeat to gain weight, not only is there a small but significant increase in plasma glucose but there is also a rise in the fasting insulin level (Sims et al., 1973). Basal levels of insulin increase linearly with the degree of overweight. This primarily represents increased insulin secretion associated with insulin resistance. Obese people also have a reduced response to the infusion of exogenous insulin, which indicates insulin resistance. This has been shown when the human forearm is perfused in vivo, when total glucose disposal is measured during the infusion of insulin, and when various tissues are studied in vitro (Olefsky et al., 1982; Rabinowitz, 1970). One mechanism for the resistance to insulin may be a reduction in the number of receptor sites on fat cells and other tissue cells (Olefsky et al., 1982). A second mechanism in some obese people is a postreceptor disturbance, in which genetic factors play an important role (Lillioja et al., 1987).

Animal Studies

Almost all forms of experimental obesity in animals are associated with hyperinsulinemia, and most of the animals have abnormalities in glucose tolerance. This is most prominent in obese (ob/ob) and diabetic (db/db) mice and obese (fa/fa) rats. This impairment in glucose tolerance can be mild, as in the fatty rat or the rat with hypothalamic obesity, or can be pronounced with associated ketoacidosis, as observed in the diabetic mouse (Bray and York, 1979) and the Wistar fatty rat (Ikeda et al., 1981; Kava et al., 1989). The impairment in glucose tolerance and the diabetic features of these animals have been shown to be improved by adrenalectomy (Bray, 1987a).

The mechanism for the hyperinsulinemia in obesity is only partly understood. Both humoral and neural mechanisms may play a role. The raised levels of several amino acids could act synergistically with glucose to enhance the secretion of insulin. Increased vagal tone or reduced sympathetic tone could also augment the release of insulin. The increased secretion of β-endorphin by the pituitary may stimulate insulin secretion, or alteration in fat storage enzymes such as lipoprotein lipase may lead to increased fat cell size and insulin resistance.

Gallbladder Disease

Epidemiologic Studies

According to the American Cancer Society study by Lew and Garfinkel (1979), digestive diseases, primarily gallbladder disease, are next to diabetes in demonstrating the detrimental curvilinear effect of excess and substandard body weight. In a cross-sectional study of 62,739 respondents to a questionnaire developed by a self-help group, Bernstein et al. (1977) found that the prevalence of gallbladder disease increases with age, body weight, and parity. Eighteen percent of women between 25 and 34 years of age whose weight was twice or more higher than the ideal weight had gallbladder disease compared to nearly 35% of the women at ages 45 to 55 who were in the same weight category. In this study, 88% of the variation in frequency of gallbladder disease was accounted for by weight, age, and parity; weight was the most important variable. Obese women between 20 and 30 years of age had a sixfold increase in the risk of developing gallbladder disease compared to normal-weight women. By age 60, nearly one-third of obese women can expect to develop gallbladder disease. In the Framingham study (Friedman et al., 1966), people at least 20% above the median weight for their height had about twice the risk of developing gallbladder disease as those who were less than 90% of the median weight for height.

In a case-control autopsy study, Sturdevant et al. (1973) found that the body weight of men without gallstones was considerably less than that of men with gallstones. The incidence of gallstones at autopsy was 16% (25/156) in men who were more than 9.1 kg overweight.

Clinical Studies

Increased cholesterol production and secretion provide one explanation for the increased risk of gallbladder disease in overweight people. Nestel et al. (1973) showed that cholesterol production rate was correlated with body weight and the number of fat cells. For each kilogram of excess body weight, cholesterol production increased 22 mg/day. Miettinen (1971) estimated that an additional 20 mg of cholesterol per day was produced for each additional kilogram of adipose tissue. Bennion and Grundy (1978) found that bile was more highly saturated with cholesterol in 23 obese subjects than in the 23 nonobese controls. The hepatic secretion of cholesterol was higher in 11 subjects before weight loss than afterward, but neither phospholipids nor bile salt secretion changed.

Cancers

Epidemiologic Studies

In the American Cancer Society cohort study conducted between 1959 and 1972, Lew and Garfinkel (1979) reported positive associations between excess weight and cancers of the gallbladder, biliary duct, endometrium, ovary, breast, and cervix in women and cancers of the colon and prostate in men. The finding of an increase in risk for endometrial cancer with increasing weight has been a consistent finding in the majority of case-control studies in northern Italy (La Vecchia et al., 1986), Denmark (Jensen, 1985), and the United States (Henderson et al., 1983), including the Framingham cohort study.

Studies of breast cancer have also provided evidence for an association between obesity and increased risk. The effect has primarily been observed in postmenopausal women in studies in the Netherlands (de Waard and Baanders-van Halewijn, 1975), northern Italy (Talamini et al., 1984), and Israel (Lubin et al., 1985). Associations have also been reported in premenopausal women (Kelsey et al., 1981), although less consistently. On the other hand, Willett et al. (1985) used BMI as a basis for examining the relationship between weight status and the development of premenopausal breast cancer among 121,964 U.S. women ages 30 to 55 who were enrolled in the Nurses Health Study. There was a significant inverse relationship between the BMI and age-adjusted relative risks for breast cancer. In the Israeli case-control study (Lubin et al., 1985), risk decreased in postmenopausal women past the age of 60 who had lost weight during their adult life. Several studies suggest that height rather than weight may be the better predictor of breast cancer risk (de Waard and Baanders-van Halewijn, 1974; Tulinius et al., 1985). If this is the case, nutritional status during adolescence may be a determinant of breast cancer risk.

In one case-control study of ovarian cancer, there was a weakly positive association with weight (Tzonou et al., 1984). In another, there was a weakly negative association (Byers et al., 1983). Several, but not all, studies have suggested that weight gain is associated with increased risk of prostate cancer (Kolonel et al., 1988; Snowdon et al., 1984; Talamini et al., 1986).

There have been isolated reports of increased risk of various cancers associated with decreases in weight, for example, cancers of the esophagus (Ziegler et al., 1981) and lung (Tulinius et al., 1985). It seems likely, however, that these are indicators of less-than-optimal nutritional status, which may reflect social factors or the use of tobacco or alcohol.

Clinical Studies

The incidence of endometrial cancer has been shown to increase in obese women, especially in postmenopausal obese women when endogenous estrogen levels fall. One explanation for this increased risk might be the increased production of estrogen in fat tissue. Urinary estrone production rates are increased in obese postmenopausal women; 50 to 120 μg/day are produced in obese women in contrast to 20 to 40 μg/day in nonobese women. In postmenopausal women, the increased estrogen appears to be produced by the conversion of the adrenal steroid androstenedione to estrogen by the stromal cells in adipose tissue.

Animal Studies

Most animal studies of diet and cancer have been designed to assess the effects of total caloric intake or the effects of specific nutrients on the induction or prevention of various cancers. Some of these are reviewed under the sections on total energy intake in this chapter and in more detail in Chapter 22. Thus, body weight gain or adiposity may affect cancer incidence, but most probably because of the effect of specific macronutrients rather than because of obesity per se.

Effects of Fluctuations in Body Weight

Epidemiologic Studies

Weight gain in adults (Ashley and Kannel, 1974; Borkan et al., 1986; Noppa, 1980) and in children (Clarke et al., 1986) has been associated with increased blood pressure and blood lipids, suggesting an increased risk of heart disease. Borkan et al. (1986) found that changes in weight status were long-term predictors of changes in blood pressure, triglycerides, serum cholesterol, glucose, and uric acid. Clarke et al. (1986) reported that changes in adiposity among children were also directly related to changes in blood pressure.

Dieting to reduce body weight has become a major phenomenon due to health and cosmetic concerns in the United States and many other industrialized societies. The Health Promotion and Disease Prevention Questionnaire, a part of the National Health Interview Survey (1985), indicated that the prevalence of dieting in 1974 and 1975 was 47% among 18- to 44-year-old women, 45% among 45- to 64-year-old women, and 24% and 30%, respectively, among men in the same age groups. A 1985 Gallup poll revealed that almost 90% of Americans believed that they weighed too much, 16% of the women questioned considered themselves perpetual dieters, and 31% reported dieting at least once monthly.

Most dieters eventually regain the weight they lose. Recidivism rates after weight loss have been estimated to range between 60 and 90%. Most people engage in many dieting attempts in their pursuit of thinness (Brownell, 1982; Jeffery et al., 1984; Stunkard, 1980).

Although adherence to weight reduction diets is traditionally viewed as a health-enhancing behavior, it is clear that some dieting practices, such as those associated with eating disorders, can seriously damage health. Furthermore, there is evidence that repeated cycles of weight loss and regain alone may enhance metabolic efficiency in animals (Brownell et al., 1986). Given the high prevalence of dieting, it is surprising that the long-term consequences of weight loss and weight gain are not well understood, especially in relation to the normal aging process, and that even less is known about the health consequences of repeated cycles of dieting. The few studies that have addressed these issues in humans are summarized below.

Weight Gain

In the Framingham study, weight gain was shown to be a risk factor for atherogenesis and total mortality (Ashley and Kannel, 1974; Hubert et al., 1983). These analyses indicate that even small weight gains carry incremental health risks. In contrast, an analysis of life insurance data suggests that the optimal BMI, or that associated with minimal mortality, increases slightly with age (Table 21–1) (Andres, 1985). This observation is consistent with the results of two longitudinal studies, which also suggest that moderate increments in body weight over a lifetime may be beneficial (Avons et al., 1983; Rhoads and Kagan, 1983). Some investigators have found positive associations between weight gain and cardiovascular diseases (Abraham et al., 1971; Noppa, 1980; Shapiro et al., 1969), whereas others have found no association (Barrett-Connor, 1985; Heyden et al., 1971; Hsu et al., 1977).

Weight Loss

Weight loss was associated with decreased relative risk of CHD in the Framingham study, which is consistent with the negative consequences of weight gain observed in the same group (Ashley and Kannel, 1974). In contrast, results of a study of Parisian civil servants associated weight loss with elevated mortality from all causes and from cancer, although the possibility that occult disease was present during the periods of weight loss makes it difficult to ascribe causality with certainty (Avons et al., 1983). Paradoxically, data from the Honolulu Heart Study indicate that weight loss is associated with a decrease in CHD risk but with an increase in CHD mortality (Bloom et al., 1987). One possible interpretation of this finding is that weight loss in the absence of disease is beneficial but that weight loss is also an indicator of antecedent disease.

Cycles of Weight Loss and Gain

In the Framingham study, a 30% increase in CHD was associated with a 10% weight gain, and a 20% decrease in CHD was associated with a 10% weight loss (Ashley and Kannel, 1974). Repeated cycles of weight loss and gain might exert a net negative effect; however, relatively few attempts have been made to address this question directly by studying subjects who lose and subsequently regain weight.

Data from the Chicago Gas and Electric Study indicate that one cycle of gain and loss is a risk factor for death from CHD independent of high BMI (Hamm et al., 1989). In that study, Hamm et al. (1989) examined the self-reported weights of Western Electric workers at ages 20, 25, 30, 35, and 40. They divided them into three groups: those who had a large gain in weight and no loss, those who gained little or no weight, and those who had both a large weight gain and a large weight loss. The gain-and-loss group had a significantly higher risk of CHD mortality when compared to the no-change group. The adjusted relative risk was 1.8 for the gain-and-loss group compared to the no-change group. No significant effects were observed in the gain-and-no-loss group.

Methodologic Considerations

The study of the temporal sequence of weight change in relation to chronic diseases is particularly challenging in humans. It is critical that epidemiologic studies of weight change and chronic diseases be long term and prospective in nature. Body weight should be measured repeatedly before the onset of disease. People who lose large amounts of weight immediately before diagnosis of CHD should be excluded from the analysis. In such studies, systematic trends in body weight need to be distinguished from random or periodic fluctuations. Such data are accumulating in several ongoing longitudinal studies. Thus, it may soon be possible to address this issue more thoroughly.

Clinical Studies

Keys et al. (1950) observed in clinical studies that healthy male volunteers who lost weight by food restriction and then regained it were fatter after regain than at the beginning of their weight reduction. Over time, the body weight and composition returned to preweight reduction levels. During studies of overfeeding, Sims and colleagues (1973) observed an increase in circulating cholesterol and triglycerides as well as a small increase in glucose and insulin. Weight loss has been associated with considerable reductions in blood pressure and levels of triglycerides, insulin, and glucose (Henry et al., 1985; Tuck et al., 1981). In another study of the loss–regain cycle, Drenick et al. (1964) and Johnson and Drenick (1977) placed approximately 200 obese men on total fasts, some for more than 2 months and the rest for 3 to 8 weeks. After refeeding, the men regained their lost weight, often exceeding their original weight. Eighty percent developed diabetes; one-half of these cases were severe.

Weight loss may be accompanied by changes in several chronic disease risk factors, e.g., lowered blood pressure or lowered triglycerides. If weight is regained, however, levels of these parameters return to preweight-loss level. (See section on Clinical Studies under Evidence Relating Total Energy Intake to Chronic Diseases: Atherosclerotic Cardiovascular Disease, Chapter 6.)

Animal Studies

Some animal studies of cycles of weight gain and weight loss and regain suggest that repeated cycles are associated with increases in metabolic efficiency, i.e., greater energy storage at a fixed energy intake (Brownell et al., 1986; Reed et al., 1988) and increases in abdominal fat depots (Reed et al., 1988), but others have not found an increase in energy efficiency (Gray et al., 1988; Hill et al., 1984).

Effects of Regional Fat Distribution

Prospective Epidemiologic Studies

The Göteborg Studies

In a prospective study of men living in Göteborg, Sweden, Larsson et al. (1984) showed that BMI and WHR (AGR) were positively correlated in those who developed strokes. That is, over a 13-year period, men in the highest tertile, both for WHR ratio and BMI, had 20.8% of the total number of strokes compared to 5.6% for men in the lowest tertile of BMI and WHRs. For cardiovascular diseases, there was a much different relationship. The highest risk was observed in the group with the highest tertile of WHR and the lowest tertile of BMI. Thus, carrying extra fat around the waist poses a particular risk, regardless of BMI.

A similar set of relationships apply to women (Lapidus et al., 1986). Among 14,462 women between 38 and 60 years of age, the 12-year age-specific incidence rates for myocardial infarction, stroke, and overall death were correlated with WHR. Among the highest quintile, the relative risk of myocardial infarction was 8.2 times higher than the risk for those in the lowest quintile. For stroke and overall death rate, the relative risk was increased 3.8 and 2.0 times, respectively, for those in the highest quintile for WHR compared to those in the lowest quintile. When women in the top 5% were compared to women in the lowest quintile, the risk of myocardial infarction was increased 14.8 times, the risk of having a stroke was increased 11.0 times, and the risk of death from all causes was increased 4.8 times. Increasing BMI along with a higher WHR enhanced the risk of developing CHD in women.

Framingham Study

At the fourth biennial examination in the Framingham study, several measures of regional fat distribution were taken, including waist, but not hip, circumference, plus measurements of subscapular, tricep, abdominal, and quadricep skinfolds. The 22-year incidence of CHD was significantly related to thickness of the subscapular skinfold. For men, only the relationship to CHD with serum total cholesterol was stronger than the relationship to subscapular skinfold thickness. For women, cholesterol and blood pressure coefficients were higher (.222 and .293, respectively) (Stokes et al., 1985).

Honolulu Heart Study

This study of 8,006 men of Japanese ancestry living in Hawaii provided data on the 12-year incidence of CHD in relation to BMI and subscapular skinfold thickness. The men in the highest tertile for subscapular skinfold experienced a more than twofold excess relative risk compared to those in the lowest tertile. There was a direct and significant relationship between the rate of CHD and subscapular skinfold within each tertile of BMI. Men in the middle tertile of subscapular skinfold thickness experienced a 70% excess of definite CHD. After adjustment for concomitant risk factors, those in the middle tertile still had a 40% excess risk of CHD and those in the highest tertile of subscapular skinfold thickness still had a 50% excess risk (Donahue et al., 1987).

Paris Study

In a prospective study conducted on 7,535 civil servants in Paris, investigators examined the relationship between body weight and fat distribution based on a principal-component analysis of several skinfolds in men ages 42 to 53. This analysis provides three parameters that correspond to total fatness, trunk versus extremity fatness, and upper extremity versus lower extremity fatness. The parameter corresponding to the trunk/extremity estimate of fatness had a linear relationship to the annual incidence of CHD, for which there was a nearly threefold increase in risk ratio between the lowest and highest quintiles (Ducimetiere et al., 1986).

All these studies indicate that regional fat distribution is a more important variable than BMI for predicting risks associated with adiposity.

Cardiac Function

Heart mass increases as body weight rises, whether assessed by postmortem examination or by echocardiographic measurements of the posterior wall and interventricular septal dimensions (Bray, 1987b). This increase involves left and right ventricles and is related not only to the degree of obesity but also to its duration.

The increased cardiac mass observed in obese people is associated with a number of functional changes. Blood volume increases along with intracellular and extracellular fluid volumes. Cardiac output and stroke volume are elevated and positively correlated with body weight and the degree of overweight. Left and right ventricular end-diastolic pressures are high as are the pulmonary artery and pulmonary capillary wedge pressures. In the most obese subjects, cardiac catheterization studies have revealed the presence of impaired left ventricular function, and a cardiomyopathy of obesity has been clearly identified (Bray, 1987b).

In contrast to most other cardiac indices, heart rate does not increase in very obese subjects. However, abnormalities can be detected on the electrocardiogram. Data from the second National Health and Nutrition Examination Survey (NHANES II) show that there is a leftward shift of the mean QRS complex with increasing fatness in both men and women (Zack et al., 1984). This effect is independent of age and blood pressure. However, this shift in the QRS complex is confined to the normal range, since left-axis deviation (QRS axis of $-30°$ or less) is not associated with body fatness. In a study of more than 1,000 electrocardiograms from obese people, the PR interval, QRS duration, QTc interval, and voltage increased with increasing obesity. ST and T wave abnormalities were present in 11% of the subjects and correlated better with increasing age and blood pressure than with the magnitude of the obesity. A prolonged QTc interval was present in 28.3% of those tested (Frank et al., 1986). Changes in the QTc interval have been considered a harbinger of potential cardiac dysrhythmia in obese individuals during prolonged starvation or when eating very low-calorie diets.

Pulmonary Function

Abnormalities of pulmonary function have been observed in obese subjects (Ray et al., 1983). At one extreme are patients with the Pickwickian syndrome, named after Joe, the overweight boy in Dickens's *Pickwick Papers*. This syndrome, also called the obesity–hypoventilation syndrome, is characterized by somnolence, obesity, and alveolar hypoventilation. At the other extreme are impairments in work capacity and pulmonary function that are due to obesity itself. In obese subjects, there is a fairly uniform decrease in expiratory reserve volume (i.e., the volume of air that can be exhaled after normal respiration) (Ray et al., 1983). There is also a low maximum rate of voluntary respiration as well as a tendency toward a general reduction in lung volumes. Lung compliance appears to be normal, but studies on the mechanics of breathing show increased oxygen consumption associated with breathing, since more work is required to move the mass of the

obese chest (Sharp et al., 1980). Finally, there appears to be some element of venous admixture: segments of the lung that are not well perfused but are ventilated and other regions that are perfused but not adequately ventilated, leading to the consistent but modest decrease in arterial oxygenation without a corresponding increase in arterial carbon dioxide content.

Extensive alterations in pulmonary function are observed primarily in massively obese subjects or in obese people with some other respiratory or cardiovascular problem. In a careful study of 29 obese women and 14 obese men, there was a progressive decrease in expiratory reserve volume as the weight-to-height (kg/cm) ratio increased. On the other hand, vital capacity, inspiratory capacity, residual volume, and diffusion capacity remained fairly constant over a range of weights, except in subjects who were massively obese (i.e., with a WHR above 1.0 kg/cm) (Ray et al., 1983).

In a study by Sharp et al. (1980), the higher metabolic rate of obese subjects at rest and during exercise resulted in an increased oxygen uptake and carbon dioxide output. This demand is met by increased minute ventilation. The extra weight on the chest and abdomen of subjects weighing 114 kg on average was associated with a two- to fourfold increase in the mechanical work required to passively ventilate the lungs. The compliance of the chest wall, however, was not related to BMI (Suratt et al., 1984).

Hematologic and Immunologic Consequences

Epidemiologic Studies

An increase in the hemoglobin levels in obese subjects was reported by Garn and Ryan (1982). Data from the NCHS show a difference of approximately 0.2 g/dl between the obese (the top 15% of the sample) and the lean (the lowest 15% by triceps skinfold). This increase in hemoglobin concentration in obese subjects was not associated with race.

Clinical Studies

Nutritional factors influence the immune response under many conditions, including obesity. For example, Krishnan et al. (1982) showed that when monocytes were incubated in vitro, the number that matured into macrophages was significantly less in obese people than in lean subjects. The generation of migration-inhibiting factor by lymphocytes from obese subjects with normal glucose levels was also significantly less in the presence of purified protein derivative than in normal controls. In obese and lean children, the levels of serum immunoglobulins, the complement components C3 and C4, as well as the numbers of T and B lymphocytes were similar. The obese children and adolescents had a variably impaired cell-mediated immune response and reduced intracellular bacterial killing by polymorphonuclear leukocytes. In the search for an explanation, Krishnan et al. (1982) examined serum copper and zinc levels, since it is well known that zinc deficiency can impair immune functions. They found a subclinical deficiency of both micronutrients. To test this further, the authors treated patients with zinc and copper for 4 weeks and found that immunologic function improved. These data suggest that immunologic responses may be impaired in obese subjects, in part because of other nutritional deficiencies.

Bone, Joint, and Skin Disorders

Epidemiologic Studies

Added body weight might be expected to increase trauma to the weight-carrying joints and thus accelerate the development of osteoarthritis. The literature on this issue is contradictory (Bray, 1985). The distribution of body weight in people with primary and secondary osteoarthritis of the hip is similar to that of people with normal hip joints. Surprisingly, one study of people with more than twice ideal body weight indicated that the incidence of osteoarthritis, determined by x-ray, was only 12%. Several authors reported an increased prevalence of osteoarthritis in obese subjects, and an increased mean weight for people with osteoarthritis has been reported in other studies. The knee joint seems to be the most frequently involved. The prevalence of osteoarthritis of the hands and the ankles increased with age among 2,548 people divided into four age groups in NHANES II (Engel, 1968). Within each age group, however, there was a clear increase in the prevalence of osteoarthritis in relation to body weight for all groups of women over 35 years of age. The slope of the increase with weight was sharpest below 90 kg (200 lbs), suggesting that body weight is only one factor.

Obesity is also associated with an increased risk of gout. Rimm et al. (1975), in a study of 73,532 weight-conscious women, found that the crude relative risks for gout and arthritis were 2.56 and 1.55, respectively. In women whose weights were 85% higher than desirable, the frequency of gout

was 1.56 times that of women who were less than 10% overweight. There was also a significant correlation between serum uric acid levels and body weight (Ashley and Kannel, 1974). This effect was particularly marked in the 35- to 44-year age group; somewhat lower correlation coefficients were found in the older age groups. The risk of osteoporosis is reduced in the obese (Dalen et al., 1975), possibly because of the increased bone mass accrued during the early years of bone formation.

Clinical Studies

In a study of obese and normal subjects, Bell et al. (1985) found that obese white people had an increase in serum immunoreactive parathyroid hormone, serum 1,25-dihydroxy vitamin D, and urinary cyclic adenosine monophosphate. There was a corresponding decrease in urinary calcium excretion comparable to that observed in obese menopausal women who were also found to have a lower ratio of urinary calcium to creatinine compared to nonobese postmenopausal controls.

Complications of Pregnancy

Body weight before pregnancy and weight gain during pregnancy both influence the course of labor and its outcome. Among heavy women (the top 10% in weight of 3,939 women), the frequency of toxemia and hypertension was greatly increased, and the duration of labor was longer (Peckham and Christianson, 1971). In more than 7% of the heavy women, labor lasted more than 24 hours. This occurred in only 0.8% of the light-weight women (the lowest 10%). Caesarean section was performed in 5.5% of the overweight patients but in only 0.7% of the light-weight ones, indicating that obese patients had more obstetrical complications than the nonobese ones. Gross et al. (1980) reviewed 2,746 consecutive deliveries, which included 279 obese women weighing more than 90 kg. The obese women were older, had a higher parity, and had an increased incidence of hypertension, diabetes mellitus, and twin gestation. The occurrence of abnormal labor, including oxytocin infusion and caesarean section, was also higher among the obese women.

Infants born to heavy women weigh more than the offspring of light women. There is also a direct relationship between placental weight and prepregnancy body weight. At the age of 7, approximately 50% of the incremental weight gain can be accounted for by the differences in placental weight at birth and the remaining 50% is attributable to postnatal environment. Naeye (1979) found that the fewest fetal and neonatal deaths occurred when mothers who were overweight at the beginning of the pregnancy gained an average of 7.3 kg (16 lb) or less. The optimal weight gain during pregnancy was 9.1 kg (20 lb) for normal-weight women and 13.6 kg (30 lb) for those under weight.

Endocrine Disorders

Epidemiologic Studies

There is a reduction in the concentration of total serum testosterone and sex-hormone binding globulin (SHBG) in obese males. The decline in testosterone is directly related to the degree of overweight. There is also a weight-related increase in estradiol and estrone in males. The low testosterone level sometimes found in obese men probably results from the reduced concentrations of SHBG, which transports testosterone in the serum. Although the mechanism for the SHBG reduction is presently unknown, the concentration of free testosterone remains essentially normal, except in massively obese men, in whom free testosterone is often low. Testicular size and the basal concentration of pituitary gonadotropins, follicle-stimulating hormones (FSH), and luteinizing hormones (LH), are normal. Similarly, the pituitary release of LH and FSH in response to an injection of luteinizing hormone-releasing hormone (LHRH) is normal, as is the concentration of these pituitary peptides during treatment with clomiphene.

Menarche occurs at younger ages among heavy women and is somewhat delayed among light women (Bray, 1976). Obese females often experience irregular menstrual cycles and an increased frequency of menstrual abnormalities. But obesity frequently occurs secondary to menstrual and other hormonal disorders, for example, abnormal steroid hormone metabolism. In these disorders, weight loss does not correct the hormonal imbalance. In one study (Bray, 1976), 43% of the 100 women with menstrual disorders, including amenorrhea, functional uterine bleeding, premature menopause, and infertility, were 20% above standard weight. In contrast, only 13% of 201 women with no menstrual abnormalities were overweight. Forty-eight percent of the women with amenorrhea were overweight, and 58% of the 19 patients with functional uterine bleeding were obese. Women with hirsutism and anovulatory cycles (i.e., irregular cycles of greater than 36 days) were on average

14 kg heavier than women with no menstrual abnormalities. There was also an increasing percentage of women with anovulatory cycles as the degree of excess weight increased. Among women less than 20% overweight, only 2.6% had anovulatory cycles compared to 8.4% of the women who were more than 74% overweight. Facial hair was associated with a longer duration of obesity.

Teenage-onset obesity was associated with a greater number of never-pregnant married women and with a higher likelihood of surgery for polycystic ovaries (Hartz et al., 1979). (The syndrome of polycystic ovaries, however, is associated with obesity, as discussed in the next section, and is not corrected by weight loss.) Thus, it appears that alterations in body weight can influence both the onset of menstruation as well as the subsequent initiation of menstruation in women who have developed secondary amenorrhea. Just as menarche occurs earlier in obese women, ovarian failure in menopause with its increased FSH production begins on average 4 years earlier in obese than in normal-weight women.

Clinical Studies

There are two abnormalities in the menstrual cycle of obese women (Sherman and Korenman, 1974). First, the rise in FSH production in the first half of the cycle is lower than in normal-weight women. Second, progesterone fails to rise normally in the second half of the menstrual cycle. The mechanism leading to these abnormalities in obese women is unknown, but it is clear that they are reversible with weight loss.

Function of the reproductive system in women is complicated by the metabolism of steroids in nonendocrine organs. Androstenedione, a product of the adrenal cortex, can be converted to estrone by nonsteroid-producing tissues. This conversion probably takes place in the stromal cells of adipose tissue. Muscle can also convert estrone to estradiol. Despite this enhanced rate of conversion of androstenedione to estrone, most studies do not demonstrate an increase in the circulating concentration of estrogens in premenopausal females (Zumoff, 1982); however, in the obese postmenopausal woman, the concentration of estrogen appears to be increased (Lobo et al., 1982). When bilaterally oophorectomized obese and nonobese women with estradiol implants were compared, the obese women had higher levels of androstenediol, androstenedione, and unbound testosterone.

The polycystic ovary syndrome is associated with obesity. This syndrome is defined clinically by the presence of oligomenorrhea, or amenorrhea, and obesity in 16 to 49% of the cases reported in various studies. Hirsutism, hyperandrogenism, elevated LH-to-FSH ratio, and polycystic ovaries are also present. In one study, SHBG was reduced in obese women with or without this syndrome, but levels of testosterone, albumin-bound testosterone, and androstenedione were higher than normal in those with polycystic ovaries (Pasquali et al., 1982). These alterations suggest that women with the polycystic ovary syndrome may have a defective control of hormone secretion.

Animal Studies

Many endocrine abnormalities accompany the obese condition in animals. Much of the pathology associated with obesity may in fact result from the accompanying endocrine dysfunction. Hyperinsulinemia is a prominent feature of virtually all experimentally induced or genetically determined obesities (Bray et al., in press). The hyperinsulinemia may precede, coincide with, or follow the development of hyperphagia in obese rodents (Berthaud and Jeanrenaud, 1979; Turkenkopf et al., 1982). Hyperinsulinemia contributes to the hypertriglyceridemia and glucose intolerance, further enhances adipose tissue lipoprotein lipase (LPL), and contributes to blood flow alterations in obese animals. In addition, the prevention of hyperinsulinemia in some experimentally, but not genetically, obese rodents can retard the development of obesity.

The role of sex hormones in the control of food intake has been extensively described (Wade and Gray, 1979). There is little question that sex hormones regulate certain aspects of food ingestion, fat distribution, and the redistribution of fat during pregnancy and lactation. In animals, much of the effect of the sex hormones on the distribution of fat is believed to be mediated through the action of the hormones on adipose tissue LPL activity.

There have been numerous reports of hypothalamus–pituitary dysfunction in obese rodents. These include altered levels of endorphin, adrenocorticotropic hormone (ACTH), LH, FSH, and somatomedin. Growth hormone abnormalities have also been observed in several strains and in experimentally produced obese animals. The removal of the pituitary reduces linear growth but does not prevent, and may enhance, the development of obesity (Han, 1967) in normally lean animals. In genetically obese rodents, hypophysectomy normalizes the growth curve but not the body

composition of treated animals (Cox and Powley, 1977); however, treatment with growth hormone does not reverse the development of the obesity. The role of glucocorticoids in the development of experimental and genetic obesities is somewhat unclear. There are few clear-cut examples of altered plasma glucocorticoids in experimental animals when conditions are carefully controlled. Nonetheless, the removal of the adrenal gland prevents the further development of obesity in genetically obese strains of rodents and reverses much of the associated pathology (Bray, 1987a). Overall, many of the endocrine abnormalities associated with obesity may cause certain aspects of the associated morbidity, but no single endocrine abnormality has been shown to be responsible for experimentally produced or genetically determined obesity.

MISCONCEPTIONS

Do Fat Children Become Fat Adults?

It is widely held that fat children become fat adults. Longitudinal studies show that the risk of a fat child becoming a fat adult is far less than many think. When a large sample of U.S. children were examined after an average of 3.5 years following the initial measurement of weight and height, considerable redistribution in relative weights was observed (Zack et al., 1984). Many children who are at the extreme end of the spectrum for weight relative to height at one age in childhood do not remain there in subsequent years. Of individuals who were overweight at age 26, less than 7% were overweight at age 7 (Bradden et al., 1986). The principal concern about obesity in childhood and adolescence should be focused on those whose proportion of body weight to height continues to deviate from the norm, especially in those with a family history of marked obesity.

For those with so-called progressive obesity, the risks of remaining obese in adult life appear to be substantially higher than for those in the upper 20% of weight for height but who remain in that category for several years. Current estimates suggest that more than 80% of obese adolescents remain obese into adulthood. The likelihood of remission decreases as severity increases. For example, 54% of 7-year-olds who are 130 to 145% of ideal body weight [50th percentile of the NHANES] will remit, whereas remission occurs in only 18% of 7-year-olds who are 157 to 165% over ideal body weight and in 0% among those who are

>165% of ideal body weight (Börjesson, 1962). Two factors influence whether or not an obese child becomes an obese adult: the time of onset and the degree of obesity. Obese adolescents who become obese adults may be fatter than obese adults whose obesity began in adulthood.

A variety of family variables are also associated with childhood and adolescent obesity. The association of obesity in children with parental obesity has been well described. This can be readily explained by environmental factors or family practices, although genetic factors may affect susceptibility (Dietz, 1987).

Do All Fat People Overeat?

Overweight individuals are popularly believed to be gluttons. Carefully controlled studies in animals indicate, however, that overeating is not a necessary requirement for the development of obesity (Bray and York, 1979; Bray et al., in press). The precise measurement of food intake by humans is difficult, but it is clear from several studies that normal as well as overweight individuals tend to underreport their dietary intake. Most studies comparing normal and overweight people suggest that those who are overweight eat fewer calories than those of normal weight (see Chapter 6). Yet, in-patient studies show that the energy required to maintain body weight in heavy people is greater than that required for lean subjects. In formerly obese people who have lost weight, energy requirements are lower than expected for their age (Leibel and Hirsch, 1984). If food intake, corrected for errors in reporting, is lower in overweight than in normal-weight people, this suggests that their energy expenditure may be proportionally lower or their metabolic efficiency may be greater. In the absence of techniques for modifying metabolic efficiency, people should be encouraged to increase their overall level of exercise and to moderate their food intake.

Do Fat Cells Increase in Number and Size During Adult Life?

Early studies on measurements of fat cell size and number indicated that most laboratory animals that became obese early in life had more fat cells than did lean controls. Development of obesity in older animals was initially believed to result entirely from an increase in the size of fat cells—not by an increase in the number. It has recently become clear, however, that the number of fat cells in laboratory animals eating a high-fat diet can increase at any age, although the increase is less than that seen in genetically obese animals (Faust et al., 1978; Lemonnier, 1972). Recent clinical data also suggest that the number of fat cells in the human body may increase in adult life (Sjöstrom and William-Olsson, 1981). When the number of fat cells in a group of 19 Swedish women were compared over 7 to 9 years, Sjöstrom and William-Olsson (1981) observed that the changes in the amount of body fat in women who gained weight or lost weight were related to the total number—not the size—of their fat cells. Data consistently indicate that very obese humans have an increased fat cell number and that this is not reversible.

Does Low Caloric Intake Increase Life Span?

For more than 40 years, studies in mice and rats have shown that reducing caloric intake below baseline levels prolongs life (Masoro, 1985; McCay et al., 1935). This reduction is also associated with slower rates of growth and smaller body sizes. The mechanism for these observations is not clear. In contrast to the substantial amount of data on animals, there are no convincing data that restricting energy intake in humans has any effect on life expectancy. Furthermore, there are no epidemiologic data regarding the timing of the imposition of the dietary restriction and its effect on life expectancy. Data from several natural famines indicate that the incidence of certain diseases was lowered following caloric restriction, but its effect on longevity is not known since caloric intake subsequently returned to normal.

EATING DISORDERS

Two major eating disorders, anorexia nervosa and bulimia, are becoming increasingly recognized as serious psychiatric disorders with physiological sequelae, especially among young white women in the middle and upper socioeconomic classes (Fadiman, 1982; Golden and Sacker, 1984; Levin, 1983). Anorexia nervosa is characterized by extreme weight loss, body-image disturbance, and an intense fear of becoming obese. Bulimia is characterized by binge-eating episodes in private followed by self-induced vomiting, fasting, or use of laxatives or diuretics (Herzog and Copeland, 1985). On college campuses, these disorders may affect as many as 20% of female students (Boskind-Lodahl and White, 1978; Cooper and Fairburn, 1983; Halmi et al., 1981; Kretchmar, 1984; Pyle et al., 1983). The term *epidemic* has been used in conjunction with eating disorders; however, there is disagreement over its applicability. For example, Williams and King (1987) suggest that this term is inappropriate because the statistics simply reflect a high hospital readmission rate and not necessarily new cases. They do note, however, that in the population they studied (patients admitted to psychiatric facilities in England between 1972 and 1981), although there was no increase in risk, there was an increase in the size of the population at risk for anorexia nervosa.

Anorexia Nervosa

Prevalence

Anorexia nervosa is found primarily among adolescent girls and young women; approximately 4 to 6% of the cases are male (Halmi, 1985). A recent British study estimates the incidence of anorexia nervosa at 3.82 per 100,000 per annum (Szmukler et al., 1986), while a Dutch study puts this figure at 5 per 100,000 per annum (Hoek and Brook, 1985). In a population-based study in Rochester, Minnesota, A. Lucas (Mayo Clinic, personal communication, 1989) reported that over a 45-year period (1935–1979) the overall rate for males and females was 7.3 per 100,000. Relentless pursuit of a thin body size despite emaciation is the central phenomenon that must always be present for a diagnosis of anorexia nervosa. Central to this weight phobia is a preoccupation with maintaining a low subpubertal body weight and avoiding any weight gain. Low body weight control may be sustained mainly by carbohydrate and fat avoidance—a form of starvation unique to anorexia nervosa (Crisp, 1977; Garfinkel and Garner, 1982).

Clinical Diagnosis

Several objective diagnostic clinical criteria have been developed (Feighner et al., 1972). According to the *Diagnostic and Statistical Manual DSM-III* (APA, 1987), onset usually occurs before 25 years of age. To be classified as anorectic, the subject must have lost at least 25% of original body weight or, if under 18 years of age, 9.25% of original body weight plus the amount of weight that would have been gained based on growth charts. Furthermore, there must be no other known medical or psychiatric illness accounting for the weight loss. The diagnostic criteria usually require evidence of a psychological disturbance in

addition to a morbid fear of becoming fat, e.g., a disturbance (misperception) of body image and a claim to feel fat even when emaciated (Dally, 1969; Morgan and Russell, 1975). The patient may resort to a variety of devices to lose weight (e.g., starvation, vomiting, laxatives). Patients with anorexia nervosa show a desperate need to control and manipulate their environments, and there is a refusal to maintain body weight over a minimal normal weight for age and height range. Despite severe weight loss, these people exhibit excessive activity. In the natural course of events, approximately 40% of anorectics recover within 6 years after initial diagnosis and about 5% die (Crisp, 1983).

A variety of endocrine abnormalities have been observed in anorectic patients. Among them are abnormal responses to exposure to heat and cold (Burman et al., 1977; Frankel and Jenkins, 1975), which suggest hypothalamic dysfunction. Amenorrhea, dry skin, constipation, bradycardia, and low basal metabolic rate have also been reported. Thyroid-stimulating hormone appears to be normal, but serum triiodothyronine (T_3) levels have been found to be low (Bhat and Cama, 1978; Burman et al., 1977; Curran-Celentano et al., 1985). Thyroxine (T_4) levels have also been found to be in the low-normal range, but not in all patients (Curran-Celentano et al., 1985; Schwabe et al., 1981). Since similar thyroid test results are found in other malnourished states, these findings cannot be considered specific to anorexia nervosa. All the endocrine abnormalities mentioned above are observed in other forms of starvation and are reversible with adequate refeeding and return of the resting metabolic rate to normal.

Hypercarotenemia is also associated with anorexia nervosa, but the mechanism for this has not been established (Curran-Celentano et al., 1985; Robboy et al., 1974). Other endocrine abnormalities include low basal plasma levels of FSH, LH, and estradiol (Russell, 1965; Vigersky et al., 1976). Resting levels of growth hormone can be greatly elevated (Frankel and Jenkins, 1975; Vigersky and Loriaux, 1977) as can basal plasma cortisol levels (Boyar et al., 1977).

Bulimia

Prevalence and Clinical Features

Bulimia is much more common than anorexia nervosa, especially during late adolescence and young adulthood (Halmi et al., 1981; Herzog, 1982). Halmi et al. (1981) found a prevalence of

13% in a population survey of 355 college students and a 7-to-1 ratio of females to males. Other studies show that the prevalence of bulimia may be as low as 3.2% among college women (Pyle et al., 1986). The wide range of results may be due to differences in methods of assessment and in the stringency with which the diagnostic criteria are applied. In addition to women of college age, other groups identified as being vulnerable to this disorder include jockeys, wrestlers, gymnasts, and ballet dancers.

Bulimia may exist concomitantly with anorexia nervosa or as an entirely separate disorder (Palmer and Guay, 1985). Bulimic patients are usually less cachectic than anorectics (Pyle et al., 1981) but are difficult to treat, since the pattern of binge eating and vomiting, or purging, is usually extremely difficult to interrupt (Smith, 1984).

Diagnostic criteria for bulimia include such behaviors as recurrent rapid consumption of a large amount of high-calorie, easily ingested food, such as carbohydrates, in a discrete period of time, usually less than 2 hours, and frequent weight fluctuations greater than 10 pounds due to alternating binges and fasts (APA, 1987). Body weight may, however, hover around normal or even be slightly higher. Other symptoms that may accompany bulimia include an increase in dental caries (possibly related to recurrent contact with acidic vomitus or excessive carbohydrate consumption during binging), hypoglycemia, parotid gland enlargement, and, in extreme cases, acute gastric dilation and rupture (Pyle et al., 1981).

SUMMARY

Overweight as defined by a BMI of 27 to 30 kg/m² afflicts more than 25% of the females and 31% of the males over 18 years of age in the U.S. population. Severe overweight—a BMI higher than 30 kg/m²—is present in 12%. For most adults, overweight results from the expenditure of fewer calories than are ingested. This may result from a sedentary lifestyle or increased metabolic efficiency. As BMI increases, there is an increased risk of chronic disease.

Obesity is an independent risk factor that modifies some intermediate mechanism, such as cardiac function or the metabolism of lipids or glucose, to produce its effects on risks that have not otherwise been identified or controlled for. For example, a high relative weight has been associated with an increased risk of a first major coronary event for men in their forties. As age increases, the relation-ship between weight and CHD decreases. In the Framingham study, relative body weight of women was positively and independently associated with developing CHD. In other studies, however, few significant relationships were found between body weight and the risk of myocardial infarction and CHD death. Associations of obesity with alterations in lipoprotein metabolism may be related to the risk of developing coronary atherosclerosis.

Although measuring blood pressure in obese patients is difficult, there is evidence that increased body weight is associated with hypertension. Hypertension also has a striking correlation with lateral body build, which may be more important than obesity in the positive correlation between blood pressure and body weight. Other researchers have reported that hypertension may be less severe in obese subjects than in normal-weight subjects. The relationship between hypertension and body size needs further exploration.

As adiposity increases, the risk of NIDDM also increases. Fasting glucose levels have also been reported to change in the same direction as body weight. It has been postulated that there is a genetic component that contributes to the risk of developing insulin resistance. In general, weight loss in obese subjects could improve glucose tolerance and weight gain could worsen it.

Certain cancers, such as cancers of the gallbladder, biliary duct, endometrium, ovary, breast, and cervix in women, and cancers of the colon and prostate in men, have been associated with excess weight. In particular, the incidence of endometrial cancer has been shown to increase among obese, postmenopausal women. The association of obesity with cancer is discussed further in Chapters 6 and 22.

Obesity is also associated with increased risk of gallbladder disease. Cholesterol production rate has been reported to correlate with body weight and the number of fat cells. Increased abdominal circumference relative to hip circumference is associated more strongly than BMI per se with early death and with the risk of developing heart disease, hypertension, stroke, diabetes mellitus, and in women, endometrial carcinoma.

Childhood obesity increases the likelihood of obesity in adult life, but only a minority of the overweight adults were overweight as children or adolescents. The degree and timing of obesity in childhood are the two most important factors that influence whether or not the obesity will carry over into adulthood. Weight gain in adult life usually results from a relative decrease in energy expenditure, which is on average greater than the decline in food intake. This conclusion arises from an epidemiologic study showing that energy intake by men decreased over 10 years during which body weight rose. Weight gain or gain-and-loss cycles in adults may carry greater risks for chronic disease than does stable body weight.

DIRECTIONS FOR RESEARCH

• It is now recognized that fat distribution, particularly the fat deposition in the abdominal and probably the intraabdominal region, is an important determinant of health risk; however, several important questions remain to be answered: Are intra- and extraabdominal subcutaneous fat equally important? Why does fat accumulate in one region as opposed to another? What are the relative risks of regional fat distribution? What are the feedback signals for regulation of fat stores? One possible clue to this last question is the observation that testosterone, estrogen, and adrenal steroids have powerful influences on the sites of fat deposition. The mechanisms by which these steroid hormones produce their effects on fat, and how this can be influenced, deserve high priority.

• Understanding food intake is a second area of importance. In most adults, body fat increases with age, even though average food intake declines (see Chapter 6). Research is needed to study why food intake does not decrease further to keep the stores of fat in balance, and why some humans and some animals are more susceptible to increasing body fat stores when eating a high-fat diet, whereas others are not responsive to this dietary shift. This implies that there are genetic or individual differences that are not understood and that deserve more research.

• Big eaters who are not obese tend to be more active. Research is needed to elucidate the relationship between physical activity and the ingestion and storage of fat and to understand the environmental and genetic interactions that regulate food intake as a function of physical activity. Better understanding of the mechanisms by which food intake and physical activity are related will provide new insights into the prevention and management of obesity.

REFERENCES

Abraham, S., G. Collins, and M. Nordsieck. 1971. Relationship of childhood weight status to morbidity in adults. HSMHA Health Rep. 86:273–284.

Abraham, S., C.L. Johnson, and M.F. Najjar. 1979. Weight and Height of Adults 18–74 Years of Age: United States, 1971–74. Vital and Health Statistics, Ser. 11, No. 211. DHEW Publ. No. PHS-79-1659. National Center for Health Statistics, Public Health Service, U.S. Department of Health, Education, and Welfare, Hyattsville, Md. 49 pp.

Abraham, S., M.D. Carroll, M.F. Najjar, and R. Fulwood. 1983. Obese and overweight adults in the United States. Vital and Health Statistics, Ser. 11, No. 230. DHHS Publ. No. (PHS) 83-1680. National Center for Health Statistics, Public Health Service, U.S. Department of Health and Human Services, Hyattsville, Md. 93 pp.

Andres, R. 1985. Mortality and obesity: the rationale for age-specific height-weight tables. Pp. 311–318 in R. Andres, E.L. Bierman, and W.R. Hazzard, eds. Principles of Geriatric Medicine. McGraw-Hill, New York.

APA (American Psychiatric Association). 1987. Diagnostic and Statistical Manual of Mental Disorders, 3rd ed. American Psychiatric Association, Washington, D.C. 567 pp.

Ashley, F.W., Jr., and W.B. Kannel. 1974. Relation of weight change to changes in atherogenic traits: the Framingham Study. J. Chronic Dis. 27:103–114.

Avons, P., P. Ducimetiere, and R. Rakotovao. 1983. Weight and mortality. Lancet 1:1104.

Baecke, J.A., W.A. van Staveren, and J. Burema. 1983. Food consumption, habitual physical activity, and body fatness in young Dutch adults. Am. J. Clin. Nutr. 37:278–286.

Barrett-Connor, E.L. 1985. Obesity, atherosclerosis, and coronary artery disease. Ann. Intern. Med. 103:1010–1019.

Barrett-Connor, E., and K.T. Khaw. 1985. Is hypertension more benign when associated with obesity? Circulation 72:53–60.

Bell, N.H., S. Epstein, A. Greene, J. Shary, M.J. Oexmann, and S. Shaw. 1985. Evidence for alteration of the vitamin D-endocrine system in obese subjects. J. Clin. Invest. 76:370–373.

Benn, R.T. 1971. Some mathematical properties of weight-for-height indices used as measures of adiposity. Br. J. Prev. Soc. Med. 25:42–50.

Bennion, L.J., and S.M. Grundy. 1978. Risk factors for the development of cholelithiasis in man (part 2). N. Engl. J. Med. 299:1221–1227.

Bernstein, R.A., E.E. Geifer, J.J. Vieira, L.H. Werner, and A.A. Rimm. 1977. Gallbladder disease. II. Utilization of the life table method in obtaining clinically useful information. A study of 62,739 weight-conscious women. J. Chronic Dis. 30:529–541.

Berthaud, H.R., and B. Jeanrenaud. 1979. Changes of insulinemia, glycemia and feeding behavior induced by VMH-procainization in the rat. Brain Res. 174:184–187.

Bhat, M.K., and H.R. Cama. 1978. Thyroidal control of hepatic release and metabolism of vitamin A. Biochim. Biophys. Acta 541:211–222.

Björntorp, P. 1985. Adipose tissue in obesity (Willendorf lecture). Pp. 163–170 in J. Hirsch and T.B. Van Itallie, eds. Recent Advances in Obesity Research, Vol. IV. John Libbey, London.

Bloom, E., K. Yano, J.D. Curb, D.M. Reed, and C.J. MacLean. 1987. Smoking cessation and incidence of coronary heart disease. CVD Epidemiol. Newsletter (AHA) 41:36.

Bogardus, C., S. Lillioja, E. Ravussin, W. Abbott, J.K. Zawadzki, A. Young, W.C. Knowler, R. Jacobowitz, and P.P. Moll. 1986. Familial dependence on the resting metabolic rate. N. Engl. J. Med. 315:96–100.

Börjeson, M. 1962. Overweight children. Acta Paediatr. 51 suppl. 132:1–76.

Börjeson, M. 1976. The aetiology of obesity in children. A study of 101 twin pairs. Acta Paediatr. Scand. 65:279–287.

Borkan, G.A., D. Sparrow, C. Wisniewski, and P.S. Vokonas. 1986. Body weight and coronary disease risk: patterns of risk factor change associated with long-term weight change. Am. J. Epidemiol. 124:410–419.

Boskind-Lodahl, M., and W.C. White, Jr. 1978. The definition and treatment of bulimarexia in college women—a pilot study. J. Am. Coll. Health Assoc. 27:84–86.

Bouchard, C. 1988. Inheritance of human fat distribution. Pp. 103–125 in C. Bouchard and F.E. Johnston, eds. Fat Distribution During Growth and Later Health Outcomes: Current Topics in Nutrition and Disease, Vol. 17. Alan R. Liss, New York.

Bouchard, C., R. Lesage, G. Lortie, J.A. Simoneau, P. Hamel, M.R. Boulay, L. Perusse, G. Theriault, and C. Leblanc. 1986. Aerobic performance in brothers, dizygotic and monozygotic twins. Med. Sci. Sports Exercise 18:639–646.

Boyar, R.M., L.D. Hellman, H. Roffwarg, J. Katz, B. Zumoff, J. O'Connor, H.L. Bradlow, and D.K. Fukushima. 1977. Cortisol secretion and metabolism in anorexia nervosa. N. Engl. J. Med. 296:190–193.

Bradden, F.E., B. Rodgers, M.E. Wadsworth, and J.M. Davies. 1986. Onset of obesity in a 36-year birth cohort study. Br. Med. J. 293:299–303.

Braitman, L.E., E.V. Adlin, and J.L. Stanton, Jr. 1985. Obesity and caloric intake: the National Health and Nutrition Examination Survey of 1971–1975 (HANES I). J. Chronic Dis. 38:727–732.

Bray, G.A. 1976. The Obese Patient: Major Problems in Internal Medicine, Vol. IX. W.B. Saunders, Philadelphia. 450 pp.

Bray, G.A. 1978. Definition, measurement, and classification of the syndromes of obesity. Int. J. Obes. 2:99–112.

Bray, G.A. 1985. Complications of obesity. Ann. Intern. Med. 103:1052–1062.

Bray, G.A. 1987a. Obesity—a disease of nutrient or energy balance? Nutr. Rev. 45:33–43.

Bray, G.A. 1987b. Obesity and the heart. Mod. Concepts Cardiovasc. Dis. 56:67–71.

Bray, G.A., and D.S. Gray. 1988. Obesity: Part I—Pathogenesis. West. J. Med. 149:429–441.

Bray, G.A., and D.A. York. 1971. Genetically transmitted obesity in rodents. Physiol. Rev. 51:598–646.

Bray, G.A., and D.A. York. 1979. Hypothalamic and genetic obesity in experimental animals: an autonomic and endocrine hypothesis. Physiol. Rev. 59:719–809.

Bray, G.A., D.A. York, and J.S. Fissler. In press. Experimental obesity: a homeostatic failure due to defective nutrient stimulation of the sympathetic nervous system. Vitam. Horm.

Brook, C.G., R.M. Huntley, and J. Slack. 1975. Influence of heredity and environment in determination of skinfold thickness in children. Br. Med. J. 2:719–721.

Brownell, K.D. 1982. Obesity: understanding and treating a serious, prevalent, and refractory disorder. J. Consult. Clin. Psychol. 50:820–824.

Brownell, K.D., M.R. Greenwood, E. Stellar, and E.E. Shrager. 1986. The effects of repeated cycles of weight loss and regain in rats. Physiol. Behav. 38:459–464.

Burman K.D., R.A. Vigersky, D.L. Loriaux, D. Strum, Y.Y. Djuh, F.D. Wright, and L. Wartofsky. 1977. Investigations concerning thyroxine deiodinative pathways in patients with anorexia nervosa. Pp. 255–261 in R.A. Vigersky, ed. Anorexia Nervosa. Raven Press, New York.

Byers, T., J. Marshall, S. Graham, C. Mettlin, and M. Swanson. 1983. A case-control study of dietary and non-dietary factors in ovarian cancer. J. Natl. Cancer Inst. 71: 681–686.

Cambien, F., J.M. Chretien, P. Ducimetiere, L. Guize, and J.L. Richard. 1985. Is the relationship between blood pressure and cardiovascular risk dependent on body mass index? Am. J. Epidemiol. 122:434–442.

Chaing, B.N., L.V. Perlman, and F.H. Epstein. 1969. Overweight and hypertension: a review. Circulation 39:403–421.

Cheek, D.B. 1968. Human Growth. Lea & Febiger, Philadelphia. 781 pp.

Clarke, W.R., R.F. Woolson, and R.M. Lauer. 1986. Changes in ponderosity and blood pressure in children: the Muscatine Study. Am. J. Epidemiol. 124:195–206.

Cleary, M.P., J.R. Vasselli, and M.R. Greenwood. 1980. Development of obesity in Zucker obese (fafa) rat in absence of hyperphagia. Am. J. Physiol. 238:E284-E292.

Cohn, S.H., A.N. Vaswani, S. Yasumura, K. Yuen, and K.J. Ellis. 1984. Improved models for determination of body fat by in vivo neutron activation. Am. J. Clin. Nutr. 40:255–259.

Coleman, D.L. 1979. Obesity genes: beneficial effects in heterozygous mice. Science 203:663–665.

Collier, G.H. 1985. Satiety: an ecological perspective. Brain Res. Bull. 14:693–700.

Cooper, P.J., and C.G. Fairburn. 1983. Binge-eating and self-induced vomiting in the community: a preliminary study. Br. J. Psychiatry 142:139–144.

Cox, J.E., and T.L. Powley. 1977. Development of obesity in diabetic mice pair-fed with lean siblings. J. Comp. Physiol. Psychol. 91:347–358.

Cox, J.E., and T.L. Powley. 1981. Prior vagotomy blocks VMH obesity in pair-fed rats. Am. J. Physiol. 240:E573-E583.

Crisp, A.H. 1977. Some psychobiological aspects of adolescent growth and their relevance for the fat/thin syndrome (anorexia nervosa). Int. J. Obes. 1:231–238.

Crisp, A.H. 1983. Treatment and outcome in anorexia nervosa. Pp. 91–104 in R.K. Goodstein, ed. Eating and Weight Disorders: Advances in Treatment and Research. Springer Publishing Co., New York.

Cruce, J.A., M.R. Greenwood, P.R. Johnson, and D. Quartermain. 1974. Genetic versus hypothalamic obesity: studies of intake and dietary manipulations in rats. J. Comp. Physiol. Psychol. 87:295–301.

Curran-Celentano, J., J.W. Erdman, Jr., R.A. Nelson, and S.J. Grater. 1985. Alterations in vitamin A and thyroid hormone status in anorexia nervosa and associated disorders. Am. J. Clin. Nutr. 42:1183–1191.

Dalen, N., D. Hallberg, and B. Lamke. 1975. Bone mass in obese subjects. Acta Med. Scand. 197:353–355.

Dally, P. 1969. Anorexia Nervosa. Grune & Stratton, New York. 137 pp.

de Boer, J.O., A.J. van Es, L.C. Roovers, J.M. van Raaij, and J.G. Hautvast. 1986. Adaptation of energy metabolism of overweight women to low-energy intake, studied with whole-body calorimeters. Am. J. Clin. Nutr. 44:585–595.

de Waard, F., and E.A. Baanders-van Halewijn. 1974. A prospective study in general practice on breast-cancer risk in postmenopausal women. Int. J. Cancer 14:153–160.

DHEW (Department of Health, Education, and Welfare). 1976. Report of the National Commission on Diabetes to the Congress of the United States, Vol. I: The Long Range Plan to Combat Diabetes. DHEW Publ. No. (NIH) 76-1018. National Institutes of Health, Public Health Service, U.S. Department of Health, Education, and Welfare, Washington, D.C. 97 pp.

DHHS (U.S. Department of Health and Human Services). 1988. The Surgeon General's Report on Nutrition and Health. DHHS (PHS) Publ. No. 88-50210. Public Health Service, U.S. Department of Health and Human Services. U.S. Government Printing Office, Washington, D.C. 712 pp.

Dietz, W.H. 1987. Pediatric obesity and the risk of obesity in adulthood. Presented at a workshop in La Jolla, California, on January 21, 1987, held by the Committee on Diet and Health, Food and Nutrition Board, Commission on Life Sciences, National Research Council, Washington, D.C. 7 pp.

Donahue, R.P., R.D. Abbott, E. Bloom, D.M. Reed, and K. Yano. 1987. Central obesity and coronary heart disease in men. Lancet 1:821–824.

Drenick, E.J., M.E. Swendseid, W.H. Blahd, and S.G. Tuttle. 1964. Prolonged starvation as treatment for severe obesity. J. Am. Med. Assoc. 187:100–105.

Drenick, E.J., A.S. Brickman, and E.M. Gold. 1972. Dissociation of the obesity-hyperinsulinism relationship following dietary restriction and hyperalimentation. Am. J. Clin. Nutr. 25:746–755.

Drenick, E.J., G.S. Bale, F. Seltzer, and D.G. Johnson. 1980. Excessive mortality and causes of death in morbidly obese men. J. Am. Med. Assoc. 243:443–445.

Ducimetiere, P., J. Richard, and F. Cambien. 1986. The pattern of subcutaneous fat distribution in middle-aged men and the risk of coronary heart disease: the Paris Prospective Study. Int. J. Obes. 10:229–240.

Durnin, J.V., and J. Womersley. 1974. Body fat assessed from total body density and its estimation from skinfold thickness: measurements on 481 men and women aged from 16 to 72 years. Br. J. Nutr. 32:77–97.

Egusa, G., W.F. Beltz, S.M. Grundy, and B.V. Howard. 1985. Influence of obesity on the metabolism of apolipoprotein B in humans. J. Clin. Invest. 76:596–603.

Engel, A. 1968. Osteoarthritis and body measurements. Vital Health Stat. 11:1–37.

Ernsberger, P., and D.O. Nelson. 1988. Refeeding hypertension in dietary obesity. Am. J. Physiol. 254:R47–R55.

Fabsitz, R., M. Feinleib, and Z. Hrubec. 1980. Weight changes in adult twins. Acta Genet. Med. Gemellol. 29:273–279.

Fadiman, A. 1982. The skeleton at the feast: a case study of anorexia nervosa. Life 5:62–76.

Faust, I.M., P.R. Johnson, J.S. Stern, and J. Hirsch. 1978. Diet-induced adipocyte number increase in adult rats: a new model of obesity. Am. J. Physiol. 235:E279–E286.

Feighner, J.P., E. Robins, S.B. Guze, R.A. Woodruff, Jr., G. Winokur, and R. Munoz. 1972. Diagnostic criteria for use in psychiatric research. Arch. Gen. Psychiatry 26:57–63.

Feinleib, M., R.J. Garrison, R. Fabsitz, J.C. Christian, Z. Hrubec, N.O. Borhani, W.B. Kannel, R. Rosenman, J.T. Schwartz, and J.O. Wagner. 1977. The NHLBI twin study of cardiovascular disease risk factors: methodology and summary of results. Am. J. Epidemiol. 106:284–285.

Feldman, R., A.J. Sender, and A.B. Sieglaub. 1969. Differ-ence in diabetic and non diabetic fat distribution patterns by skin fold measurements. Diabetics 18:478–486.

Fitness and Amateur Sport. 1986. Canadian Standardized Test of Fitness (for 15 to 69 Years of Age), 3rd ed. Operations Manual. FAS 7378. Minister of State, Fitness and Amateur Sport, Government of Canada, Ottawa, Ontario, Canada. 41 pp.

Forbes, G.B. 1984. Energy intake and body weight: a reexamination of two "classic" studies. Am. J. Clin. Nutr. 39:349–350.

Forbes, G.B. 1987. Lean body mass-body fat interrelationships in humans. Nutr. Rev. 45:225–231.

Frank, S., J.A. Colliver, and A. Frank. 1986. The electrocardiogram in obesity. Statistical analysis of 1,129 patients. J. Am. Coll. Cardiol. 7:295–299.

Frankel, R.J., and J.S. Jenkins. 1975. Hypothalamic-pituitary function in anorexia nervosa. Acta Endocrinol. 78:209–221.

Friedman, G.D., W.B. Kannel, and T.R. Dawber. 1966. The epidemiology of gallbladder disease: observations in the Framingham Study. J. Chronic Dis. 19:273–292.

Garfinkel, P.E., and D.M. Garner. 1982. Anorexia Nervosa: A Multidimensional Perspective. Brunner/Mazel, New York. 379 pp.

Garn, S.M., and A.S. Ryan. 1982. The effect of fatness on hemoglobin levels. Am. J. Clin. Nutr. 36:189–192.

Garrow, J.S. 1978. Energy Balance and Obesity in Man, 2nd ed. Elsevier/North Holland, New York. 243 pp.

Geissler, C.A., D.S. Miller, and M. Shah. 1987. The daily metabolic rate of the post-obese and the lean. Am. J. Clin. Nutr. 45:914–920.

Golden, N., and I.M. Sacker. 1984. An overview of the etiology, diagnosis, and management of anorexia nervosa. Clin. Pediatr. 4:209–214.

Gordon, T., W.B. Kannel, W.P. Castelli, M.C. Hjortland, W.B. Kannel, and T.R. Dawber. 1977a. Diabetes, blood lipids, and the role of obesity in coronary heart disease risk for women. The Framingham study. Ann. Intern. Med. 87:393–397.

Gordon, T., W.P. Castelli, M.C. Hjortland, W.B. Kannel, and T.R. Dawber. 1977b. High density lipoprotein as a protective factor against coronary heart disease. The Framingham Study. Am. J. Med. 62:707–714.

Gray, D.S., J.S. Fisler, and G.A. Bray. 1988. Effects of repeated weight loss and regain on body composition in obese rats. Am. J. Clin. Nutr. 47:393–399.

Gross, T., R.J. Sokol, and K.C. King. 1980. Obesity in pregnancy: risks and outcome. Obstet. Gynecol. 56:446–450.

Grundy, S.M., H.Y. Mok, L. Zech, D. Steinberg, and M. Berman. 1979. Transport of very low density lipoprotein triglycerides in varying degrees of obesity and hypertriglyceridemia. J. Clin. Invest. 63:1274–1283.

Gulick, A. 1922. A study of weight regulation in the adult human body during over-nutrition. Am. J. Physiol. 60:371–395.

Haffner, S.M., M.P. Stern, H.P. Hazuda, J. Pugh, and J.K. Patterson. 1987. Do upper-body and centralized adiposity measure different aspects of regional body-fat distribution? Relationship to non-insulin-dependent diabetes mellitus, lipids, and lipoproteins. Diabetes 36:43–51.

Halmi, K.A. 1985. Eating disorders. Pp. 1731–1736 in H.I. Kaplan and B.J. Sadock, eds. Comprehensive Textbook of Psychiatry IV, Vol. 2. Williams and Wilkins, Baltimore.

Halmi, K.A., J.R. Falk, and E. Schwartz. 1981. Binge-eating and vomiting: a survey of a college population. Psychol. Med. 11:697–706.

Hamm, P., R.B. Shekelle, and J. Stamler. 1989. Large fluctuations in body weight during young adulthood and twenty-five-year risk of coronary death in men. Am. J. Epidemiol. 129:312–318.

Han, P.W. 1967. Hypothalamic obesity in rats without hyperphagia. Trans. N.Y. Acad. Sci. 30:229–242.

Hartz, A.J., P.N. Barboriak, A. Wong, K.P. Katayama, and A.A. Rimm. 1979. The association of obesity with infertility and related menstrual abnormalities in women. Int. J. Obes. 3:57–73.

Hartz, A.J., D.C. Rupley, and A.A. Rimm. 1984. The association of girth measurements with disease in 32,856 women. Am. J. Epidemiol. 119:71–80.

Havlik, R.J., H.B. Hubert, R.R. Fabsitz, and M. Feinleib. 1983. Weight and hypertension. Ann. Intern. Med. 98:855–859.

Henderson, B.E., J.T. Casagrande, M.C. Pike, T. Mack, and I. Rosario. 1983. The epidemiology of endometrial cancer in young women. Br. J. Cancer 47:749–756.

Henry, R.R., L. Scheaffer, and J.M. Olefsky. 1985. Glycemic effects of intensive caloric restriction and isocaloric refeeding in noninsulin-dependent diabetes mellitus. J. Clin. Endocrinol. Metab. 61:917–925.

Herzog, D.B. 1982. Bulimia in the adolescent. Am. J. Dis. Child. 136:985–989.

Herzog, D.B., and P.M. Copeland. 1985. Eating disorders. N. Engl. J. Med. 313:295–303.

Heyden, S., C.G. Hames, A. Bartel, J.C. Cassel, H.A. Tyroler, and J.C. Cornoni. 1971. Weight and weight history in relation to cerebrovascular and ischemic heart disease. Arch. Intern. Med. 128:956–960.

Hill, J.O., S.K. Fried, and M. DiGirolamo. 1984. Effects of fasting and restricted refeeding on utilization of ingested energy in rats. Am. J. Physiol. 247:R318–R327.

Himsworth, H.P. 1935. Diet and incidence of diabetes mellitus. Clin. Sci. 2:117–148.

Hirsch, J., and B. Batchelor. 1976. Adipose tissue cellularity in human obesity. Clin. Endocrinol. Metab. 5:299–311.

Hirsch, J., and E. Gallian. 1968. Methods for the determination of adipose cell size in man and animals. J. Lipid Res. 9:110–119.

Hoek, W.H., and F.G. Brook. 1985. Patterns of care of anorexia nervosa. J. Psychiatr. Res. 19:155–160.

Hoffmans, M.D., D. Kromhout, and C. de Lezenne Coulander. 1988. The impact of body mass index of 78,612 18-year-old Dutch men on 32-year mortality from all causes. J. Clin. Epidemiol. 41:749–756.

Hoyenga, K.B., and K.T. Hoyenga. 1982. Gender and energy balance: sex differences in adaptations for feast and famine. Physiol. Behav. 28:545–563.

Hsu, P.H., F.A. Mathewson, H.A.Abu-Zeid, and S.W. Rabkin. 1977. Change in risk factor and the development of chronic disease. A methodological illustration. J. Chronic Dis. 30:567–584.

Hubert, H.B., M. Feinleib, P.M. McNamara, and W.P. Castelli. 1983. Obesity as an independent risk factor for cardiovascular disease: a 26-year follow-up of participants in the Framingham Heart Study. Circulation 67:968–977.

Ikeda, H., A. Shino, T. Matsuo, H. Iwatsuka, and Z. Suzuoki. 1981. A new genetically obese-hyperglycemic rat (Wistar fatty). Diabetes 30:1045–1050.

Jeffery, R.W., A.R. Folsom, R.V. Luepker, D.R. Jacobs, Jr., R.F. Gillum, H.L. Taylor, and H. Blackburn. 1984. Prevalence of overweight and weight loss behavior in a metropolitan adult population: the Minnesota Heart Survey experience. Am. J. Public Health 74:349–352.

Jensen, H. 1985. Endometrial carcinoma. A retrospective, epidemiological study. Dan. Med. Bull. 32:219–228.

Jequier, E. 1984. Energy expenditure in obesity. Clin. Endocrinol. Metab. 13:563–580.

Johnson, D., and E.J. Drenick. 1977. Therapeutic fasting in morbid obesity. Arch. Intern. Med. 137:1381–1382.

Joslin, E.P., L.I. Dublin, and H.H. Marks. 1935. Studies in diabetes mellitus; interpretations of variations in diabetes incidence. Am. J. Med. Sci. 189:163–192.

Kannel, W.B., and D.L. McGee. 1985. Update on some epidemiologic features of intermittent claudication: the Framingham Study. J. Am. Geriatr. Soc. 33:13–18.

Kannel, W.B., and A. Schatzkin. 1984. Risk factor analysis. Prog. Cardiovasc. Dis. 26:309–332.

Kava, R.A., D.B. West, V.A. Lukasik, and M.R.C. Greenwood. 1989. Sexual dimorphism of hyperglycemia and glucose tolerance in Wistar fatty rat. Diabetes 38:159–163.

Keen, H., B.J. Thomas, R.J. Jarrett, and J.H. Fuller. 1979. Nutrient intake, adiposity, and diabetes. Br. Med. J. 1:655–658.

Kelsey, J.L., D.B. Fischer, T.R. Holford, V.A. LiVoisi, E.D. Mostow, I.S. Goldenberg, and C. White. 1981. Exogenous estrogens and other factors in the epidemiology of breast cancer. J. Natl. Cancer Inst. 67:327–333.

Keys, A., J. Brozek, A. Henschel, O. Mickelsen, and H.L. Taylor. 1950. The Biology of Human Starvation, Vols. 1 and 2. University of Minnesota Press, Minneapolis. 1385 pp.

Kinsell, L.W., B. Gunning, G.D. Michaels, J. Richardson, S.E. Cox, and C. Lemon. 1964. Calories do count. Metabolism 13:195–204.

Kissebah, A.H., N. Vydelingum, R. Murray, D.J. Evans, A.J. Hartz, R.K. Kalkhoff, and P.W. Adams. 1982. Relation of body fat distribution to metabolic complications of obesity. J. Clin. Endocrinol. Metab. 54:254–260.

Knowler, W.C., P.H. Bennett, R.F. Hamman, and M. Miller. 1978. Diabetes incidence and prevalence in Pima Indians: a 19-fold greater incidence than in Rochester, Minnesota. Am. J. Epidemiol. 108:497–505.

Knowler, W.C., D.J. Pettitt, P.J. Savage, and P.H. Bennett. 1981. Diabetes incidence in Pima Indians: contributions of obesity and parental diabetes. Am. J. Epidemiol. 113:144–156.

Kolonel, L.N., C.N. Yoshizawa, and J.H. Hankin. 1988. Diet and prostatic cancer: a case-control study in Hawaii. Am. J. Epidemiol. 127:999–1012.

Kretchmar, L. 1984. A look at eating disorders on campus: feast and famine. Dartmouth Alumni Magazine 76:39–46.

Krishnan, E.C., L. Trost, S. Aarons, and W.R. Jewell. 1982. Study of function and maturation of monocytes in morbidly obese individuals. J. Surg. Res. 33:89–97.

Kromhout, D. 1983. Energy and macronutrient intake in lean and obese middle-aged men (the Zutphen study). Am. J. Clin. Nutr. 37:295–299.

Krotkiewski, M., P. Björntorp, L. Sjöström, and U. Smith. 1983. Impact of obesity on metabolism in men and women. Importance of regional adipose tissue distribution. J. Clin. Invest. 72:1150–1162.

Lapidus, L., C. Bengtsson, B. Larsson, K. Pennert, E. Rybo,

and L. Sjöström. 1984. Distribution of adipose tissue and risk of cardiovascular disease and death: a 12 year follow-up of participants in the population study of women in Gothenburg, Sweden. Br. Med. J. 289:1257–1261.

Lapidus, L., H. Andersson, C. Bengtsson, and I. Bosaeus. 1986. Dietary habits in relation to incidence of cardiovascular disease and death in women: a 12-year follow-up of participants in the population study of women in Gothenburg, Sweden. Am. J. Clin. Nutr. 44:444–448.

Larsson, B., P. Björntorp, and G. Tibblin. 1981. The health consequences of moderate obesity. Int. J. Obesity 5:97–116.

Larsson, B., K. Svärdsudd, L. Welin, L. Wilhelmsen, P. Björntorp, and G. Tibblin. 1984. Abdominal adipose tissue distribution, obesity, and risk of cardiovascular disease and death: 13 year follow-up of participants in the study of men born in 1913. Br. Med. J. 288:1401–1404.

Lavau, M., C. Susini, J. Knittle, S. Blanchet-Hirst, and M.R.C. Greenwood. 1977. A reliable photomicrographic method to determining fat cell size and number: application to dietary obesity. Proc. Soc. Exp. Biol. Med. 156:251–256.

La Vecchia, C., A. Decarli, M. Fasoli, and A. Gentile. 1986. Nutrition and diet in the etiology of endometrial cancer. Cancer 57:1248–1253.

Leibel, R.L., and J. Hirsch. 1984. Diminished energy requirements in reduced obese patients. Metabolism 33:164–170.

Lemonnier, D. 1972. Effect of age, sex, and site on the cellularity of the adipose tissue in mice and rats rendered obese by a high-fat diet. J. Clin. Inves. 51:2907–2915.

Levin, E. 1983. A sweet surface hid a troubled soul in the late Karen Carpenter, a victim of anorexia nervosa. People Weekly 19:52–59.

Lew, E.A., and L. Garfinkel. 1979. Variations in mortality by weight among 750,000 men and women. J. Chronic Dis. 32:563–576.

Lillioja, S., D.M. Mott, J.K. Zawadzki, A.A. Young, W.G. Abbott, W.C. Knowler, P.H. Bennett, P. Moll, and C. Bogardus. 1987. In vivo insulin action is familial characteristic in nondiabetic Pima Indians. Diabetes 36:1329–1335.

Lobo, R.A., C.M. March, U. Goebelsmann, and D.R. Mishell, Jr. 1982. The modulating role of obesity and 17 beta-estradiol (E_2) on bound and unbound E_2 and adrenal androgens in oophorectomized women. J. Clin. Endocrinol. Metab. 54:320–324.

Lohman, T.G. 1981. Skinfolds and body density and their relation to body fatness: a review. Hum. Biol. 53:181–225.

Lubin, F., A.M. Ruder, Y. Wax, and B. Modan. 1985. Overweight and changes in weight throughout adult life in breast cancer etiology. A case-control study. Am. J. Epidemiol. 122:579–588.

Lukaski, H.C. 1987. Methods for the assessment of human body composition: traditional and new. Am. J. Clin. Nutr. 46:537–556.

MacMahon, S.W., D.E. Wilcken, and G.J. Macdonald. 1986. The effect of weight reduction on left ventricular mass. A randomized controlled trial in young, overweight hypertensive patients. N. Engl. J. Med. 314:334–339.

Manson, J.E., M.J. Stampfer, C.H. Hennekens, and W.C. Willett. 1987. Body weight and longevity. A reassessment. J. Am. Med. Assoc. 257:353–358.

Masoro, E.J. 1985. Aging and nutrition—can diet affect life span? Trans. Assoc. Life Insur. Med. Dir. Am. 67:30–44.

Mattila, K., M. Haavisto, and S. Rajala. 1986. Body mass index and mortality in the elderly. Br. Med. J. 292:867–868.

McCay, C.M., M.F. Crowell, and L.A. Maynard. 1935. Effect of retarded growth upon length of life span and upon ultimate body size. J. Nutr. 10:63–79.

McGee, D., and T. Gordon. 1976. The results of the Framingham Study applied to four other U.S. based epidemiological studies of cardiovascular disease. Section 31 in W.B. Kannel and T. Gordon, eds. The Framingham Study: An Epidemiological Investigation of Cardiovascular Disease. DHEW Publ. No. (NIH) 76-1083. National Heart and Lung Institute, National Institutes of Health, Public Health Service, U.S. Department of Health, Education, and Welfare, Bethesda, Md.

Medlund, P., R. Cederlöf, B. Floderus-Myrhed, L. Friberg, and S. Sörensen. 1976. A new Swedish twin registry. Acta Med. Scand., Suppl. 600:1–111.

Messerli, F.H. 1982. Cardiovascular effects of obesity and hypertension. Lancet 1:1165–1168.

Miettinen, T.A. 1971. Cholesterol production in obesity. Circulation 44:842–850.

Morgan, H.G., and G.F. Russell. 1975. Value of family background and clinical features as predictors of long-term outcome in anorexia nervosa: four-year follow-up study of 41 patients. Psychol. Med. 5:355–371.

Mueller, W.H. 1983. The genetics of human fatness. Yearb. Phys. Anthropol. 26:215–230.

Mueller, W.H. 1988. Ethnic differences in fat distribution during growth. Pp. 127–145 in C. Bouchard and F.E. Johnston, eds. Current Topics in Nutrition and Disease, Vol. 17: Fat Distribution During Growth and Later Health Outcomes. Alan R. Liss, New York.

Naeye, R.L. 1979. Weight gain and the outcome of pregnancy. Am. J. Obstet. Gynecol. 135:3–9.

Nelson, D.O., and P. Ernsberger. 1984. Feed-starve cycling in dietary obesity induces moderate hypertension via alterations in the autonomic regulation of cardiovascular function. Soc. Neurosci. 10:716.

Nestel, P.J., P.H. Schreibman, and E.H. Ahrens, Jr. 1973. Cholesterol metabolism in human obesity. J. Clin. Invest. 52:2389–2397.

Neumann, R.O. 1902. Experimentelle Beiträge zur Lehre von dem täglichen Nahrungsbedarf des Menschen unter besonderer Berücksichtigung der notwendigen Eiweissmenge. Arch. Hyg. 45:1–87.

Newburgh, L.H., and J.W. Conn. 1939. New interpretation of hypergylcemia in obese middle-aged persons. J. Am. Med. Assoc. 112:7–11.

Noppa, H. 1980. Body weight change in relation to incidence of ischemic heart disease and change in risk factors for ischemic heart disease. Am. J. Epidemiol. 111:693–704.

Noppa, H., and T. Hällström. 1981. Weight gain in adulthood in relation to socioeconomic factors, mental illness and personality traits: a prospective study of middle-aged women. J. Psychosom. Res. 25:83–89.

Noppa, H., C. Bengtsson, H. Wedel, and L. Wilhelmsen. 1980. Obesity in relation to morbidity and mortality from cardiovascular disease. Am. J. Epidemiol. 111:682–692.

Ohlson, L.O., B. Larsson, K. Svärdsudd, L. Welin, H. Eriksson, L. Wilhelmsen, P. Björntorp, and G. Tibblin. 1985. The influence of body fat distribution on the incidence of diabetes mellitus. 13.5 years of follow-up of the participants in the study of men born in 1913. Diabetes 34:1055–1058.

Olefsky, J.M., O.G. Kolterman, and J.A. Scarlett. 1982. Insulin action and resistance in obesity and non insulin-dependent type II diabetes mellitus. Am. J. Physiol. 243: E15–E30.

Owen, O.E., E. Kavle, R.S. Owen, M. Polansky, S. Caprio, M.A. Mozzoli, Z.V. Kendrick, M.C. Bushman, and G. Boden. 1986. A reappraisal of caloric requirements in healthy women. Am. J. Clin. Nutr. 44:1–19.

Owen, O.E., J.L. Holup, D.A. D'Alessio, E.S. Craig, M. Polansky, K.J. Smalley, E.C. Kavle, M.C. Bushman, L.R. Owen, M.A. Mozzoli, Z.V. Kendrick, and G.H. Boden. 1987. A reappraisal of the caloric requirements of men. Am. J. Clin. Nutr. 46:875–885.

Palmer, E.P., and A.T. Guay. 1985. Reversible myopathy secondary to abuse of ipecac in patients with major eating disorders. N. Engl. J. Med. 313:1457–1459.

Pasquali, R., S. Venturoli, R. Paradis, M. Capelli, M. Parenti, and N. Melchionda. 1982. Insulin and C-peptide levels in obese patients with polycystic ovaries. Horm. Metab. Res. 14:284–287.

Peckham, C.H., and R.E. Christianson. 1971. The relationship between pre-pregnancy weight and certain obstetric factors. Am. J. Obstet. Gynecol. 111:1–7.

Poehlman, E.T., A. Tremblay, J.P. Deprés, E. Fontaine, L. Pérusse, G. Thériault, and C. Bouchard. 1986. Genotype-controlled changes in body composition and fat morphology following overfeeding in twins. Am. J. Clin. Nutr. 43:723–731.

Pyke, D.A., and N.W. Please. 1957. Obesity, parity and diabetes. J. Endocrinol. 15:xxvi–xxxiii.

Pyle, R.L., J.E. Mitchell, and E.D. Eckert. 1981. Bulimia: a report of 34 cases. J. Clin. Psychiatry 42:60–64.

Pyle, R.L., J.E. Mitchell, E. Eckert, P.A. Halvorson, P.A. Neuman, and G.M. Goff. 1983. The incidence of bulimia in freshman college students. Int. J. Eating Disorders 2:75–85.

Pyle, R.L., P.A. Halvorson, P.A. Neuman, and J.E. Mitchell. 1986. The increasing prevalence of bulimia in freshman college students. Int. J. Eating Disorders 5:631–636.

Rabinowitz, D. 1970. Some endocrine and metabolic aspects of obesity. Annu. Rev. Med. 21:241–258.

Ravussin, E., S. Lillioja, T.E. Anderson, L. Christin, and C. Bogardus. 1986. Determinants of 24-hour energy expenditure in man. Methods and results using a respiratory chamber. J. Clin. Invest. 78:1568–1578.

Ravussin, E., S. Lillioja, W.C. Knowler, L. Christin, D. Freymond, W.G. Abbott, V. Boyce, B.V. Howard, and C. Bogardus. 1988. Reduced rate of energy expenditure as a risk factor for body-weight gain. N. Engl. J. Med. 318:467–472.

Ray, C.S., D.Y. Sue, G. Bray, J.E. Hansen, and K. Wasserman. 1983. Effects of obesity on respiratory function. Am. Rev. Respir. Dis. 128:501–506.

Reed, D.R., R.J. Contreras, C. Maggio, and M.R. Greenwood, and J. Rodin. 1988. Weight cycling in female rats increases dietary fat selection and adiposity. Physiol. Behav. 42:389–395.

Reisin, E., R. Abel, M. Modan, D.S. Silverberg, H.E. Eliahou, and B. Modan. 1978. Effect of weight loss without salt restriction on the reduction of blood pressure in overweight hypertensive patients. N. Engl. J. Med. 298:1–6.

Rhoads, G.G., and A. Kagan. 1983. The relation of coronary disease, stroke, and mortality to weight in youth and in middle age. Lancet 1:492–495.

Rimm, A.A., L.H. Werner, B.V. Yserloo, and R.A. Bernstein. 1975. Relationship of obesity and disease in 73,532 weight-conscious women. Public Health Rep. 90:44–54.

Robboy, M.S., A.S. Sato, and A.D. Schwabe. 1974. The hypercarotenemia in anorexia nervosa: a comparison of vitamin A and carotene levels in various forms of menstrual dysfunction and cachexia. Am. J. Clin. Nutr. 27:362–367.

Roberts, S.B., J. Savage, W.A. Coward, B. Chew, and A. Lucas. 1988. Energy expenditure and intake in infants born to lean and overweight mothers. N. Engl. J. Med. 318:461–466.

Romieu, I., W.C. Willett, M.J. Stampfer, G.A. Colditz, L. Sampson, B. Rosner, C.H. Hennekens, and F.E. Speizer. 1988. Energy intake and other determinants of relative weight. Am. J. Clin. Nutr. 47:406–412.

Russell, G.F. 1965. Metabolic aspects of anorexia nervosa. Proc. R. Soc. Med. 58:811–814.

Schemmel, R., O. Mickelsen, and J.L. Gill. 1970. Dietary obesity in rats: body weight and body fat accretion in seven strains of rats. J. Nutr. 100:1041–1048.

Schwabe, A.D., B.M. Lippe, R.J. Chang, M.A. Pops, and J. Yager. 1981. Anorexia nervosa. Ann. Intern. Med. 94:371–381.

Sclafani, A., and A.N. Gorman. 1977. Effects of age, sex, and prior body weight on the development of dietary obesity in adult rats. Physiol. Behav. 18:1021–1026.

Sclafani, A., and D. Springer. 1976. Dietary obesity in adult rats: similarities to hypothalamic and human obesity syndromes. Physiol. Behav. 17:461–471.

Segal, K.R., B. Gutin, E. Presta, J. Wang, and T.B. Van Itallie. 1985. Estimation of human body composition by electrical impedance methods: a comparative study. J. Appl. Physiol. 58:1565–1571.

Shapiro, S., E. Weinblatt, C.W Frank, and R.V. Sager. 1969. Incidence of coronary heart disease in a population insured for medical care (HIP): myocardial infarction, angina pectoris, and possible myocardial infarction. Am. J. Public Health 59:1–101.

Sharp, J.T., M. Barrocas, and S. Chokroverty. 1980. The cardiorespiratory effects of obesity. Clin. Chest Med. 1:103–118.

Sherman, B.M., and S.G. Korenman. 1974. Measurement of serum LH, FSH, estradiol and progesterone in disorders of the human menstrual cycle: the inadequate luteal phase. J. Clin. Endocrinol. Metab. 39:145–149.

Sims, E.A., E. Danforth, Jr., E.S. Horton, G.A. Bray, J.A. Glennon, and L.B. Salans. 1973. Endocrine and metabolic effects of experimental obesity in man. Recent Prog. Horm. Res. 29:457–496.

Sjöström, L., and T. William-Olsson. 1981. Prospective studies on adipose tissue development in man. Int. J. Obes. 5:597–604.

Smith, M.S. 1984. Anorexia nervosa and bulimia. J. Fam. Practice 18:757–766.

Snowdon, D.A., R.L. Phillips, and W. Choi. 1984. Diet, obesity, and risk of fatal prostate cancer. Am. J. Epidemiol. 120:244–250.

Society of Actuaries. 1959. Build and Blood Pressure Study, Vol. 1. Society of Actuaries, Chicago. 268 pp.

Society of Actuaries. 1980a. Blood Pressure Study of 1979. Society of Actuaries/Association of Life Insurance Medical Directors of America, Chicago. 359 pp.

Society of Actuaries. 1980b. Build Study of 1979. Society of Actuaries/Association of Life Insurance Medical Directors of America, Chicago. 255 pp.

Solberg, L.A., and J.P. Strong. 1983. Risk factors and atherosclerotic lesions. A review of autopsy studies. Arteriosclerosis 3:187–198.

Steele, N.C., L.T. Frobish, and M. Keeney. 1974. Lipogenesis and cellularity of adipose tissue from genetically lean and obese swine. J. Anim. Sci. 39:712–719.

Steinkamp, R.C., N.L. Cohen, W.E. Siri, T.W. Sargent, and H.E. Walsh. 1965a. Measures of body fat and related factors in normal adults. I. Introduction and methodology. J. Chronic Dis. 18:1279–1291.

Steinkamp, R.C., N.L. Cohen, W.R. Gaffey, T. McKey, G. Bron, W.E. Siri, T.W. Sargent, and E. Isaacs. 1965b. Measures of body fat and related factors in normal adults. II. A simple clinical method to estimate body fat and lean body mass. J. Chronic Dis. 18:1291–1307.

Stokes, J., III, R.J. Garrison, and W.B. Kannel. 1985. The independent contributions of various indices of obesity to the 22-year incidence of coronary heart disease: the Framingham Heart Study. Pp. 49–57 in J. Vague, P. Björntorp, B. Guy-Grand, M. Rebuffé-Scrive, and P. Vague, eds. Metabolic Complications of Human Obesities. Excerpta Medica, Amsterdam.

Stunkard, A.J., ed. 1980. Obesity. W.B. Saunders, Philadelphia. 470 pp.

Stunkard, A.J., T.T. Foch, and Z. Hrubec. 1986. A twin study of human obesity. J. Am. Med. Assoc. 256:51–54.

Sturdevant, R.A., M.L. Pearce, and S. Dayton. 1973. Increased prevalence of cholelithiasis in men ingesting a serum-cholesterol-lowering diet. N. Engl. J. Med. 288:24–27.

Suratt, P.M., S.C. Wilhoit, H.S. Hsiao, R.L. Atkinson, and D.F. Rochester. 1984. Compliance of chest wall in obese subjects. J. Appl. Physiol. 57:403–407.

Szmukler, G., C. McCance, L. McCrone, and D. Hunter. 1986. Anorexia nervosia: a psychiatric case register study from Aberdeen. Psychol. Med. 16:49–58.

Talamini, R., C. La Vecchia, A. Decarli, S. Franceschi, E. Grattoni, E. Grigoletto, A. Liberati, and G. Tognoni. 1984. Social factors, diet and breast cancer in a northern Italian population. Br. J. Cancer 49:723–729.

Talamini, R., C. La Vecchia, A. Decarli, E. Negri, and S. Franceschi. 1986. Nutrition, social factors and prostatic cancer in a northern Italian population. Br. J. Cancer 53:817–821.

Tuck, M.L., J. Sowers, L. Dornfeld, G. Kledzik, and M. Maxwell. 1981. The effect of weight reduction on blood pressure, plasma renin activity, and plasma aldosterone levels in obese patients. N. Engl. J. Med. 304:930–933.

Tulinius, H., N. Sigfusson, H. Sigvaldason, and N.E. Day. 1985. Relative weight and human cancer risk. Int. Cong. Ser. (685):173–189.

Turkenkopf, I., P.R. Johnson, and M.R.C. Greenwood. 1982. Development of pancreatic and plasma insulin in prenatal and suckling Zucker rats. Am. J. Physiol. 242:E220–E229.

Tzonou, A., N.E. Day, D. Trichopoulos, A. Walker, M. Saliaraki, M. Papapostolou, and A. Polychronopoulou. 1984. The epidemiology of ovarian cancer in Greece: a case-control study. Eur. J. Cancer Clin. Oncol. 20:1045–1052.

Vague, J. 1956. Degree of masculine differentiation of obesities: factor determining predisposition to diabetes, atherosclerosis, gout, and uric calculous disease. Am. J. Clin. Nutr. 4:20–34.

Vigersky, R.A., and D.L. Loriaux. 1977. Anorexia nervosa as a model of hypothalamic dysfunction. Pp. 109–21 in R.A. Vigersky, ed. Anorexia Nervosa. Raven Press, New York.

Vigersky, R.A., D.L. Loriaux, A.E. Andersen, R.S. Mecklenburg, and J.L. Vaitukaitis. 1976. Delayed pituitary hormone response to LRF and TRF in patients with anorexia nervosa and with secondary amenorrhea associated with simple weight loss. J. Clin. Endocrinol. Metab. 43:893–900.

Waaler, H.T. 1984. Height, weight and mortality: the Norwegian experience. Acta Med. Scand., Suppl. 679:1–56.

Wade, G.N., and J.M. Gray. 1979. Gonadal effects on food intake and adiposity: a metabolic hypothesis. Physiol. Behav. 22:583–593.

Weinsier, R.L., D.J. Norris, R. Birch, R.S. Bernstein, J. Wang, M.U. Yang, R.N. Pierson, Jr., and T.B. Van Itallie. 1985. The relative contribution of body fat and fat pattern to blood pressure level. Hypertension 7:578–585.

West, K.M., and J.M. Kalbfleisch. 1971. Influence of nutritional factors on prevalence of diabetes. Diabetes 20:289–296.

Willett, W.C., M.L. Browne, C. Bain, R.J. Lipnick, M.J. Stampfer, B. Rosner, G.A. Colditz, C.H. Hennekens, and F.E. Speizer. 1985. Relative weight and risk of breast cancer among premenopausal women. Am. J. Epidemiol. 122:731–740.

Williams, P., and M. King. 1987. The "epidemic" of anorexia nervosa: another medical myth? Lancet 1:205–207.

Zack, P.M., W.R. Harlan, P.E. Leaverton, and J. Cornoni-Huntley. 1979. A longitudinal study of body fatness in childhood and adolescence. J. Pediatr. 95:126–130.

Zack, P.M., R.D. Wiens, and H.L. Kennedy. 1984. Left-axis deviation and adiposity: the United States Health and Nutrition Examination Survey. Am. J. Cardiol. 53:1129–1134.

Ziegler, R.G., L.E. Morris, W.J. Blot, L.M. Pottern, R. Hoover, and J.F. Fraumeni, Jr. 1981. Esophageal cancer among black men in Washington, D.C. II. Role of nutrition. J. Natl. Cancer Inst. 67:1199–1206.

Zumoff, B. 1982. Relationship of obesity to blood estrogens. Cancer Res. 42:3289s–3292s.

22

Cancer

In this chapter, the committee summarizes the role of dietary factors as they relate to the risks of various forms of cancer. Since the evidence regarding specific dietary constituents is discussed in detail in earlier chapters, it is only briefly summarized here. Some discussion of other risk factors for these cancers is included to put the role of diet in perspective. Epidemiologic data as well as supportive evidence from animal studies and from research on mechanisms of carcinogenesis are reviewed. Although the results of experiments in animals cannot be quantitatively extrapolated to humans, they provide evidence on the biologic plausibility of observed correlations between specific dietary constituents and cancer incidence or mortality in epidemiologic studies.

TRENDS IN CANCER INCIDENCE IN THE UNITED STATES AND THE ROLE OF DIET

Devesa et al. (1987) reviewed trends in the incidence of and mortality from specific forms of cancer in the white populations of five areas of the United States from 1947 to 1984. Overall trends were dominated by the well-known rise in lung cancer, clearly a direct result of exposure to tobacco smoke. The authors suggested that lung cancer rates in people with little or no exposure to tobacco smoke may also have increased, but the

evidence is not conclusive. Large increases in incidence were also found for melanoma of the skin, cancer of the prostate and testis, and non-Hodgkin's lymphoma. Smaller increases were found for cancers of the liver, kidney, colon, urinary bladder, and breast. Major decreases in incidence were observed for cancer of the stomach and for invasive cancer of the cervix. The combined impact of improved detection standards, diagnostic ability, and reporting on the published cancer incidence rates could not be precisely measured. It is unlikely that these factors were of major importance, however, except possibly for cancers of the cervix and breast.

Some investigators have estimated the overall impact of diet on total cancer incidence and mortality. Such estimates are based on a combination of evidence regarding established relationships between dietary factors and cancer risk, the dramatic shifts in site-specific cancer rates among migrants to the United States, secular trends in cancer for which a dietary etiology is likely, supportive evidence from animal experiments, and lack of more persuasive alternative hypotheses. Doll and Peto (1981) estimated that approximately 35% (range, 10 to 70%) of all cancer *mortality* in the United States is related to diet, whereas Wynder and Gori (1977) estimated that 40% of cancer *incidence* among men and nearly 60% among women is related to diet. Because few relationships between specific dietary components and cancer risk are well established, it is not possible to quantify the contribution of diet to individual cancers (and thus to total cancer rates) more precisely. Nevertheless, these estimates help to emphasize the importance of diet in the etiology and prevention of cancer in the United States today.

EVIDENCE ASSOCIATING DIETARY FACTORS WITH CANCER AT SPECIFIC SITES

Epidemiologic Studies

The discussion in this section is presented by specific cancer sites because the dietary associations are not the same for all cancer types. See Chapters 6 through 17 for more detailed review of evidence by dietary components.

Esophageal Cancer

Correlation analyses have shown direct associations between consumption of alcoholic beverages and esophageal cancer in Western countries (Breslow and Enstrom, 1974; Chilvers et al., 1979; Hinds et al., 1980; Kolonel et al., 1980; Lyon et al., 1980; Schoenberg et al., 1971). Case-control and cohort studies have also provided consistent evidence of an association between alcohol consumption and risk of esophageal cancer (Hakulinen et al., 1974; Pottern et al., 1981; Williams and Horn, 1977). Alcohol consumption appears to act synergistically with cigarette smoking to increase the risk. Wynder and Bross (1961) found that increases in the use of alcohol and tobacco were associated with an increased risk of squamous cell carcinoma of the esophagus and that alcohol and tobacco exert a multiplicative effect. Similar effects have been observed in Paris (Schwartz et al., 1962), Puerto Rico (Martinez, 1969), Brittany (Tuyns et al., 1977), and Normandy (Tuyns, 1983). Alcohol also seems to have an independent effect on cancer risk in the absence of smoking (Keller, 1980).

In correlation studies conducted in different parts of the world, investigators have found positive associations between esophageal cancer and several dietary factors, including (1) low intakes of lentils, green vegetables, fresh fruits, animal protein, vitamins A and C, riboflavin, nicotinic acid, magnesium, calcium, zinc, and molybdenum; (2) high intakes of pickles, pickled vegetables, and moldy foods containing N-nitroso compounds; and

(3) consumption of very hot foods and beverages (de Jong et al., 1974; Hormozdiari et al., 1975; Joint Iran–IARC Study Group, 1977; Thurnham et al., 1982; van Rensburg, 1981; Yang, 1980; Zaridze et al., 1985). Many of these findings have been supported by the results of case-control studies (Cook-Mozaffari, 1979; de Jong et al., 1974; Mettlin et al., 1981). The reported associations are consistent with the general hypothesis that certain nutrient deficiencies, such as found in many high-risk populations, including heavy alcohol drinkers, might increase the susceptibility of the esophageal epithelium to neoplastic transformation (van Rensburg, 1981). In the esophageal epithelium of humans, for example, riboflavin deficiency causes lesions that may be precursors of cancer (Foy and Mbaya, 1977), although an intervention trial with riboflavin (and zinc and retinol) in a high-risk Chinese population failed to show any effect of these nutrients (Muñoz et al., 1985).

In summary, esophageal cancer is associated with the use of tobacco and alcohol individually, but especially with their combined use. Studies suggest that consumption of certain types of preserved foods increases risk and that several vitamins and minerals are protective against esophageal cancer, but the reasons for these relationships are not yet clearly established.

Stomach Cancer

A high incidence of stomach cancer is found in South America, Japan, and other parts of Asia, but not in North America or Western Europe where the rates are low and still decreasing (Stukonis, 1978; Waterhouse et al., 1976). In the United States, stomach cancer rates are now among the lowest in the world, whereas in 1930, this was the leading cause of cancer death for men and the second leading cause in women (Page and Asire, 1985). Gastric cancer incidence has recently begun to decrease in Japan, and a gradual decline in incidence over several generations has been noted among Japanese migrants to Hawaii (Kolonel et al., 1980). It seems most likely that these trends are related to changes in food consumption patterns, since several dietary factors have been implicated in gastric cancer risk.

Several correlation and case-control studies have shown positive associations between gastric cancer and the consumption of dried, salted fish, smoked fish, or pickled vegetables (e.g., Dungal, 1966; Haenszel et al., 1976; Hirayama, 1967; Joossens and Geboers, 1987; Risch et al., 1985). These foods contain high concentrations of salt, nitrates, and nitrites. Other investigators have reported associations between gastric cancer and nitrate levels in the drinking water supplies of populations in such settings as Chile (Armijo and Coulson, 1975; Zaldivar, 1977), Colombia (Correa et al., 1976; Tannenbaum et al., 1979), and England (Hill et al., 1973). In a case-control study in Canada, Risch et al. (1985) found a significant association between nitrite consumption and stomach cancer risk. The above findings support a hypothesis that gastric cancer is related to the reduction of nitrates to nitrites in the stomach and the subsequent formation of N-nitroso compounds (NRC, 1981). A high intake of salt might facilitate this process either by irritating the gastric mucosa, which is then more susceptible to carcinogenic transformation, or by inducing atrophic gastritis, leading to colonization of the stomach with bacteria that can nitrosate dietary precursors to form nitrosamines (Correa et al., 1976). Chronic gastritis has been associated with gastric cancer risk in Japan (Imai et al., 1971).

A second major dietary association with stomach cancer has been a protective effect of fresh fruits, vegetables, and vitamins, especially vitamin C. Several case-control and correlation studies have shown this inverse relationship (Bjelke, 1978; Correa et al., 1985; Graham et al., 1972; Haenszel and Correa, 1975; Higginson, 1966; Kolonel et al., 1981; Risch et al., 1985), which is consistent with the ability of ascorbic acid to inhibit the formation of carcinogenic N-nitroso compounds (Mirvish et al., 1972).

Evidence relating certain other dietary components to stomach cancer risk is uncertain because of an inadequate replication of results. This evidence includes a direct association with carbohydrates and high-starch foods in two studies (Modan et al., 1974; Risch et al., 1985), a direct association with fried foods (Higginson, 1966), an inverse association with milk (Hirayama, 1977), and an inverse association with dietary fiber (Modan et al., 1974; Risch et al., 1985). Some studies suggest that stomach cancer risk is increased by alcoholic beverage consumption (Correa et al., 1985; Hoey et al., 1981), but others do not suggest it (Acheson and Doll, 1964; Graham et al., 1972; Haenszel et al., 1972; Tuyns et al., 1982).

In summary, stomach cancer is associated with diets comprising large amounts of salt-preserved foods (that possibly contain precursors of nitrosamines) and low levels of fresh fruits and vegetables (acting as possible inhibitors of nitrosamine formation). Dietary shifts away from this pattern could explain the great decline in stomach cancer mortality in the United States over the past 50 years, but the evidence is not conclusive.

Colorectal Cancer

International data show a strong correlation between the incidence of colorectal cancer and cancers of the breast, endometrium, ovary, and, to a lesser extent, prostate. Within the United States, mortality from colorectal cancer is higher in the north and in urban areas than in other parts of the country (Haenszel and Dawson, 1965). Although the incidence of and mortality from this cancer have been relatively stable over the past 30 to 40 years, there has been a recent decline in mortality among females and possibly the beginning of a decline among males. In epidemiologic studies, the risk of colorectal cancer has been associated with the fat and fiber content of the diet, but other dietary constituents have also been implicated.

Several correlation and case-control studies demonstrate positive associations between the risk for colorectal (primarily colon) cancer and dietary fat (Armstrong and Doll, 1975; Carroll and Khor, 1975; Dales et al., 1979; Drasar and Irving, 1973; Graham et al., 1988; Howe et al., 1986; McKeown-Eyssen and Bright-See, 1984; Miller et al., 1983; Pickle et al., 1984; Wynder, 1975). In several other studies, positive associations have been found between meat consumption and this cancer (Haenszel et al., 1973; Hirayama, 1979; Howell, 1975; Knox, 1977; Manousos et al., 1983; Pickle et al., 1984). Conversely, many other studies have shown no relationship between fat or meat intake and colorectal cancer (e.g., Enstrom, 1975; Graham et al., 1978; Haenszel et al., 1980; Kinlen, 1982; Lyon and Sorenson, 1978; Modan et al., 1975). The studies not showing a positive correlation usually included narrow ranges of fat intake. In general, the data suggest that if this association is real, saturated rather than unsaturated fatty acids are responsible.

Two other major dietary components—protein and calories—have been positively associated with colorectal cancer risk in some studies (Armstrong and Doll, 1975; Carroll and Khor, 1975; Gregor et al., 1969; Jain et al., 1980; Kune et al., 1987; Lyon et al., 1987; Macquart-Moulin et al., 1986; Potter and McMichael, 1986; Thind, 1986) but not in all (Bingham et al., 1979; International Agency for Research on Cancer Intestinal Microecology Group, 1977; Jensen et al., 1982; Tuyns et al., 1987). Since it is not possible to separate clearly the effects of these variables in epidemiologic analyses, it remains possible that dietary fats are not the only relevant factor. Two recent case-control studies in Europe suggest that monounsaturated fatty acids may actually have a protective effect against colorectal cancer (Macquart-Moulin et al., 1986; Tuyns et al., 1987), but this finding needs further confirmation.

Few studies have examined the relationship between *dietary* cholesterol and colorectal cancer, but one correlation study (Liu et al., 1979) and one case-control study (Jain et al., 1980) did show a positive effect. Furthermore, the correlation of high levels of meat consumption with colorectal cancer implies a positive association with dietary cholesterol. Reports that very low *serum* cholesterol levels are associated with an increased risk of colon cancer in some male cohorts have not been reproduced in a substantial number of similar cohorts; in some of these studies, the association has appeared to be due to undiagnosed colon cancer in the early years of observation (McMichael et al., 1984). A relationship of diet to these low levels of serum cholesterol has not been established, and present evidence does not support a causal relationship between low serum cholesterol and colon cancer.

The data relating dietary fiber to colorectal cancer are equivocal. Although several case-control and correlation studies have shown inverse relationships between the intake of high-fiber foods and colon cancer risk (Bjelke, 1978; Dales et al., 1979; Modan et al., 1975; Phillips, 1975), these foods (vegetables to a large extent) are rich sources of other nutritive and nonnutritive constituents with potential cancer-inhibiting properties. Thus, the observed effects cannot be attributed to fiber per se. The results of the few studies that attempted to assess the intake of fiber itself have also not been consistent. Some correlation and case-control studies (Bingham et al., 1985; Bjelke, 1978; Jensen et al., 1982; Kune et al., 1987; MacLennan et al., 1978; Malhotra, 1977; McKeown-Eyssen and Bright-See, 1984) support the hypothesis of a protective effect from dietary fiber, whereas other studies (Howe et al., 1986; Potter and McMichael, 1986; Smith et al., 1985) do not. The study by Potter and McMichael (1986) even suggests a direct association among females.

Certain other dietary components have been associated with colorectal cancer in some studies. A few investigators reported inverse relationships with the intake of vitamin A or with the consumption of vegetables that were not necessarily high in fiber content (Bjelke, 1978; Macquart-Moulin et al., 1986; Phillips, 1975). Although some studies show protective effects of vitamin C and calcium (Garland et al., 1985; Macquart-Moulin et al., 1986; Potter and McMichael, 1986), others do not (Heilbrun et al., 1986; Jain et al., 1980; Tuyns et al., 1987).

Several case-control and cohort studies suggest an association between alcohol intake and colorectal cancer, especially with rectal cancer (Bjelke, 1978; Dean et al., 1979; Kabat et al., 1986; Kune et al., 1987; Pollack et al., 1984; Tuyns et al., 1982). In some studies, colorectal cancer was associated with the consumption of alcoholic beverages in general. In others, there was an association with beer consumption specifically. Other studies did not find this relationship with alcohol (Dales et al., 1979; Graham et al., 1978; Jensen, 1979; Miller et al., 1983; Modan et al., 1975).

In summary, the data on diet and colorectal cancer are inconsistent, perhaps because of differences in the populations studied or in the dietary methodology used to assess intake. In general, increased risk of colorectal cancer appears to be associated with a dietary pattern consisting of a high fat intake (particularly saturated fats) and low vegetable intake. It is not clear whether dietary fiber per se is protective or whether the apparent protective effects in some studies are due to other food constituents such as vitamin C or calcium. Colorectal cancer risk may be increased by the consumption of alcoholic beverages, especially beer.

Liver Cancer

Primary liver cancer is relatively rare in the United States and most Western countries, but it is common in sub-Saharan Africa and Southeast Asia, where it is associated primarily with exposure to hepatitis B virus infection in early life and with consumption of foods contaminated with aflatoxins. Limited evidence links liver cancer to other possible dietary risk factors, including pyrrolizidine alkaloids, safrole, and cycasin (Anthony, 1977).

In Africa, liver cancer incidence and mortality by geographic area or among different population groups have been correlated with aflatoxin contamination of foodstuffs (Alpert et al., 1971; Peers et al., 1976; van Rensburg et al., 1974). Similar geographic correlations have been found in China (Armstrong, 1980), Thailand (Shank et al., 1972a,b; Wogan, 1975), Taiwan (Tung and Ling, 1968), and in a case-control study in the Philippines (Bulatao-Jayme et al., 1982).

Numerous reports have documented a high correlation between primary liver cancer and infection with hepatitis B virus, which has a worldwide distribution similar to that of aflatoxins (Chien et al., 1981). This association was confirmed in a large prospective cohort in Taiwan (Beasley et al., 1981).

Alcohol has been suggested as an etiologic agent for liver cancer in Western countries. Although liver cancer is associated with cirrhosis of the liver, which is in turn associated with heavy alcohol consumption, direct epidemiologic evidence linking alcohol to primary liver cancer is limited. Some studies show an association (Hakulinen et al., 1974; Inaba et al., 1984; Jensen, 1979; Yu et al., 1983), and others do not (Monson and Lyon, 1975; Nicholls et al., 1974; Pell and D'Alonzo, 1973; Robinette et al., 1979; Schmidt and de Lint, 1972; Trichopoulos et al., 1987).

In summary, liver cancer risk is most clearly associated with early-life infection with hepatitis B virus. Aflatoxins are also an etiologic factor, possibly in association with hepatitis B virus infection, in the high-risk areas of Africa and Southeast Asia. In Western countries, some studies show an association between heavy alcohol consumption and this cancer.

Pancreatic Cancer

An increasing trend in the incidence of pancreatic cancer in the United States over the past 20 to 30 years now appears to be stabilizing. In general, pancreatic cancer occurs more commonly in higher socioeconomic groups and is most clearly associated with cigarette smoking as a risk factor (DHEW, 1979). Pancreatic cancer has been associated with meat consumption in some studies (Hirayama, 1977; Ishii et al., 1968; Mack et al., 1986) but not in others (Gold et al., 1985; Norell et al., 1986). In a case-control study conducted in Boston, MacMahon et al. (1981) found a dose–response relationship between pancreatic cancer and coffee consumption, but in a subsequent study by some of the same authors (Hsieh et al., 1986), other case-control studies (Gold et al., 1985; Mack et al., 1986; Norell et al., 1986; Wynder et al., 1983), and large cohort studies in the United States (Whittemore et al., 1983) and Norway (Heuch et al., 1983), no consistent evidence was found to support this association. Some studies have related cancer of the pancreas to alcohol consumption (Blot et al., 1978; Burch and Ansari, 1968; Cubilla and Fitzgerald, 1978; Dørken, 1964), but most have not—even among alcoholics (Hakulinen et al., 1974; MacMahon et al., 1981;

Monson and Lyon, 1975; Tuyns et al., 1982; Williams and Horm, 1977; Wynder et al., 1973).

In summary, only cigarette smoking has been clearly established as a major risk factor for pancreatic cancer.

Lung Cancer

In most technologically advanced countries, lung cancer is the leading cause of death from cancer among men, and it is rapidly approaching this status among women (Miller, 1980). The most important causal factor is cigarette smoking (DHEW, 1979). Lung cancer risk in males is clearly increased by certain occupational exposures (e.g., to asbestos, nickel, chromate, gamma-radiation), several of which have been shown to interact synergistically with smoking (Fraumeni, 1975). In females, cigarette smoking appears to be the only major contributor to lung cancer incidence in most Western countries. Although most studies of dietary factors and lung cancer have controlled for cigarette smoking, possible interactions between tobacco and dietary factors have received little attention.

A prospective study in Norway showed that dietary vitamin A was inversely associated with lung cancer (Bjelke, 1975; Kvale et al., 1983). This result was supported by hospital-based studies in the United States (Mettlin and Graham, 1979) and in the United Kingdom (Gregor et al., 1980). Other studies (Byers et al., 1987; Hinds et al., 1984; Samet et al., 1985; Shekelle et al., 1981; Ziegler et al., 1984) suggest that the relevant dietary constituent may be β-carotene rather than retinol. This is consistent with several reports of an inverse association between lung cancer and the frequency of eating green or yellow vegetables (Hirayama, 1979; MacLennan et al., 1977). In prospective studies (Menkes et al., 1986; Nomura et al., 1985), the concentration of β-carotene in serum was inversely associated with the risk of lung cancer. Early reports of a similar inverse association for serum retinol were not confirmed by subsequent studies (Friedman et al., 1986; Kark et al., 1981; Menkes et al., 1986; Peleg et al., 1984; Salonen et al., 1985; Wald et al., 1980, 1986). No effect of dietary vitamin C on lung cancer risk has been found (Byers et al., 1987; Hinds et al., 1984; Kvale et al., 1983; Mettlin et al., 1981). Dietary fats (Byers et al., 1987; Wynder et al., 1987) and dietary cholesterol (Hinds et al., 1983) have been positively associated with lung cancer risk.

In summary, the main causal factor for lung cancer is cigarette smoke. Occupational exposures to asbestos, nickel, radiation, and other agents also increase risk, and some of these have been shown to interact synergistically with smoking. Frequent consumption of green and yellow vegetables (leading to a high intake of β-carotene and other constituents in such foods) appears to be protective against lung cancer.

Breast Cancer

Breast cancer is a common cause of death among U.S. women. This cancer is more common in Caucasians than in other racial groups, although rates have been rising among blacks, Hispanics, and women of Asian origin. Descriptive epidemiologic studies suggest that some aspects of lifestyle are related to the incidence of breast cancer. For example, breast cancer incidence among Japanese migrant women in Hawaii is much higher than that in Japan and is even higher in their daughters born in Hawaii (Kolonel et al., 1980).

Breast cancer risks are closely correlated with hormonal activity, and diet might be a major contributing factor through its effects on hormonal pathways and levels (MacMahon et al., 1973). A role of dietary factors is supported by descriptive epidemiologic studies, correlation studies, case-control and cohort studies, and evaluations of nutrition-mediated risk factors.

Correlation studies provide evidence of a direct association between breast cancer mortality and the intake of calories, fats, and specific sources of dietary fats, such as milk and beef (Armstrong and Doll, 1975; Carroll and Khor, 1975; Gaskill et al., 1979). Some studies show an inverse correlation between the intake of carbohydrates or fiber and the risk of breast cancer (Adelcreutz et al., 1982; Lubin et al., 1986).

Several case-control studies associate breast cancer risk with dietary constituents, especially fats. Lubin et al. (1981) and Phillips (1975) reported an association between the frequency of consumption of high-fat foods and breast cancer. Miller et al. (1978) found a positive association with total fat consumption in pre- and postmenopausal women and weaker associations with saturated fats and cholesterol in the premenopausal women, the strongest association relating to saturated fat intake (Howe, 1985). A similar association with dietary saturated fats was found by Hirohata et al. (1987). Lubin et al. (1986) reported an increased risk of breast cancer among women who consumed a diet containing high levels of fats and animal protein and low levels of fiber; Hislop et al. (1986) found a positive association with intake of fat-

containing foods, especially whole milk and beef; and Talamini et al. (1984) associated moderately increased risks with indices of fat intake. However, not all studies show these relationships (Graham et al., 1982; Hirohata et al., 1985; Willett et al., 1987a).

Several studies relate alcohol consumption to the risk of breast cancer in women (Begg et al., 1983; Byers and Funch, 1982; Hiatt and Bawol, 1984; Lê et al., 1986; Schatzkin et al., 1987; Willett et al., 1987b). However, it is unlikely that this association, even if established as causal, could account for a substantial fraction of the female breast cancer incidence in most populations.

Certain nutrition-mediated factors, notably body weight, height, and obesity (as reflected by body mass indices), have also been associated with breast cancer risk, primarily among postmenopausal women (de Waard et al., 1977; Lubin et al., 1985; Paffenbarger et al., 1980; Talamini et al., 1984). Height may be the best of these measures for predicting breast cancer risk (de Waard et al., 1977), but most studies show that the strongest association is with body mass index. However, these anthropometric measures have not been associated with risk in all populations (Kolonel et al., 1986).

In summary, breast cancer risk has been associated with the high-calorie Western diet, and dietary fat is the nutrient for which the data are strongest. However, the evidence is not conclusive, and other dietary factors may also be involved. Alcohol consumption may also be a risk factor for this cancer.

Endometrial Cancer

Endometrial cancer has been correlated with cancers of the breast, ovary, colon, and rectum (Miller, 1978). It tends to be more common in the United States than in other parts of the world and is more frequent in Caucasian women of higher socioeconomic status. The only well-established cause for this cancer is the use of exogenous estrogens at the high dosages commonly prescribed some years ago. Both noninsulin-dependent diabetes mellitus (NIDDM) and hypertension have been associated with this cancer (Elwood et al., 1977; La Vecchia et al., 1986). An association between endometrial cancer risk and excess weight was reported in several studies (Elwood et al., 1977; Henderson et al., 1983; Jensen, 1986; La Vecchia et al., 1986; Lew and Garfinkel, 1979; Wynder et al., 1966), and a hormonal mechanism has been postulated for this association (Henderson et al.,

1982). A protective effect of fiber has been reported (La Vecchia et al., 1986) but not confirmed.

In summary, endometrial cancer can be caused by exogenous estrogen hormones and is associated with obesity, hypertension, and NIDDM. Possible dietary risk factors for this cancer have not been established.

Ovarian Cancer

Ovarian cancer is more common in the United States and other Western countries than in Asia, and it occurs more frequently in countries where breast, colon, and endometrial cancers tend to occur. It tends to be more common in higher socioeconomic groups and less frequent in women who use oral contraceptives (Casagrande et al., 1979; Cramer et al., 1982; Nasca et al., 1984; Weiss et al., 1981).

Cramer et al. (1984) found that women with ovarian cancer consumed much greater amounts of animal fat and considerably less vegetable fat than did control subjects, whereas Byers et al. (1983) found no association. Weight and height, which in part reflect diet, were weakly but positively associated with ovarian cancer in one case-control study (Tzonou et al., 1984), but not in others (Annegers et al., 1979; Byers et al., 1983; Hildreth et al., 1981). Two case-control studies showed an association between coffee drinking and increased risk of ovarian cancer (La Vecchia et al., 1984; Trichopoulos et al., 1981), but a third study failed to detect this association (Byers et al., 1983); this matter remains unresolved.

In summary, ovarian cancer has been inversely related to oral contraceptive use, but no dietary associations have been established.

Bladder Cancer

Bladder cancer is more common in the United States than in many other parts of the world. It occurs more frequently in men than in women and in people of lower socioeconomic status. Bladder cancer risk is increased among cigarette smokers and among certain occupational groups exposed to certain chemicals, notably β-naphthylamine and benzidine.

One cohort study showed a statistically significant association between coffee drinking and death from bladder cancer (Snowdon and Phillips, 1984), and several case-control studies found that coffee was associated with elevated risks among males (Mettlin and Graham, 1979) and females (Cole, 1971; Fraumeni et al., 1971; Howe et al.,

1980; Simon et al., 1975). Other studies found only a weak association with coffee (Hartge et al., 1983; Marrett et al., 1983; Rebelakos et al., 1985), and several found no evidence of an association (Jacobson et al., 1986; Jensen et al., 1986; Morrison et al., 1982; Nomura et al., 1986; Ohno et al., 1985). Since the relative risks in most of the positive studies were low (<2.0) and few studies showed a dose–response relationship, this association is unlikely to be causal. Residual confounding by cigarette smoking may explain the apparent effect.

Conflicting findings have been reported for nonnutritive sweeteners and bladder cancer (see Chapter 17). Overall, however, it appears that use of such sweeteners does not measurably increase the risk of bladder cancer (Howe et al., in press).

There is limited epidemiologic evidence pertaining to the association of other dietary exposures with bladder cancer. Armstrong and Doll (1975) found a direct association of bladder cancer mortality with per-capita intake of fats and oils, particularly among women, but this association has not been confirmed in other studies. One case-control study (Mettlin and Graham, 1979) suggested an inverse association with carrots, milk, and an index of vitamin A intake, whereas another (Risch et al., 1988) showed no evidence of a protective effect of retinol or β-carotene, but an increased risk from consumption of dietary cholesterol. Although a direct association between beer intake and bladder cancer mortality in men was reported in a correlation study (Breslow and Enstrom, 1974), this finding has not been confirmed in case-control studies (Brownson et al., 1987; Thomas et al., 1983).

In summary, bladder cancer risk is clearly related to the use of cigarettes and to certain occupational exposures, such as benzidine and β-naphthylamine. Its relationship to dietary factors is less clear. Possible associations with coffee drinking, artificial sweetener use, and alcoholic beverage consumption have not been confirmed.

Prostate Cancer

Cancer of the prostate is common in the United States, and rates among black males are especially high. This cancer is relatively rare in males under 45 years. International incidence and mortality data generally show a positive correlation of prostate cancer with cancers of several other sites associated with diet, including cancers of the breast, corpus uteri, and colon (Berg, 1975; Howell, 1974; Wynder et al., 1971). Certain populations provide interesting exceptions, however: Mormons in Utah have high prostate but relatively low breast cancer incidence rates, whereas the native Polynesians of Hawaii have low prostate but high breast cancer incidence rates (Kolonel, 1980; Lyon et al., 1976).

Although male hormones appear to contribute to the risk for this disease, little is known about the etiology of prostate cancer. Some investigators have suggested a causal relationship to aspects of sexual behavior or to a venereally transmitted virus, but no convincing evidence supports these hypotheses (Mandel and Schuman, 1980; Ross et al., 1983).

Three dietary components appear to be related to this disease: fats, vitamin A, and the trace element cadmium. Several inter- and intracountry analyses show positive correlations between mortality from prostate cancer and per-capita intake of total fat (Armstrong and Doll, 1975; Blair and Fraumeni, 1978; Howell, 1974). These findings have been confirmed in several analytical studies showing an association of prostate cancer with the intake of high-fat foods (Rotkin, 1977; Schuman et al., 1982; Snowdon et al., 1984), as well as intake of fats per se (Graham et al., 1983; Heshmat et al., 1985; Kolonel et al., 1988).

Although studies of certain other cancers suggest that vitamin A (particularly β-carotene) may be a protective factor, case-control studies of prostate cancer have tended to identify vitamin A as a risk factor, especially among men age 70 years and older (Graham et al., 1983; Heshmat et al., 1985; Kolonel et al., 1987). In the study by Kolonel et al. (1987), the effect was specific for carotenes, not for retinol. A few studies based on food frequency data suggest inverse associations with the intake of some carotene-containing vegetables (Ross et al., 1983; Schuman et al., 1982).

Occupational exposure to cadmium has been associated with an increased risk for prostate cancer, but the evidence is not consistent (Friberg et al., 1986). The evidence regarding dietary cadmium is also equivocal. Some geographic analyses of estimated per-capita intakes or levels in drinking water or soil showed positive associations (Bako et al., 1982; Berg and Burbank, 1972; Schrauzer et al., 1977), whereas others did not (Inskip et al., 1982; Shigematsu, 1984). In one case-control study, Kolonel and Winkelstein (1977) found no effect of cadmium from dietary sources. Cadmium levels in prostate tissue of men with prostate cancer were higher than in men with benign prostatic hypertrophy or

normal prostate glands (Feustel and Wennrich, 1986; Feustel et al., 1982).

Increased weight or obesity has been positively associated with prostate cancer (Lew and Garfinkel, 1979; Snowdon et al., 1984; Talamini et al., 1986), but not in all studies (Kolonel et al., 1988).

In summary, prostate cancer risk appears to be higher in men consuming high-fat diets. A possible direct association with dietary vitamin A (notably carotenes) needs further confirmation. The effect of exposure to cadmium, either occupational or dietary, is not established.

Animal Studies

Animal models have been used extensively to study the effects of different dietary components on carcinogens. By using defined diets in such studies, it is possible to distinguish among the effects of different dietary constituents and to study mechanisms of action—both of which are difficult to accomplish in studies of humans. For this reason, and because there are no animal models for some cancer sites of importance in humans, this section is organized by dietary constituent rather than by cancer site.

Fats

Animal studies relating diet to carcinogenesis have been largely concerned with effects of dietary fats (Ip et al., 1986a; NRC, 1982). Tumors of the skin, mammary gland, colon, and pancreas develop more readily in animals fed high-fat diets than in those fed low-fat diets. Recent studies of treatment with carcinogens have been conducted in rats and, to a lesser extent, in mice and a few other species. Dietary fats appear to act primarily during the promotion stage of carcinogenesis, but the exact mechanism of action is not known and may depend on the tumor site (see Chapter 7).

Polyunsaturated vegetable oils promote tumorigenesis more effectively than saturated fats, apparently because of a requirement for ω-6 essential fatty acids, but a high level of dietary fats is also required for maximum effect (Ip, 1987). Fish oils, whose polyunsaturated fatty acids belong mainly to the ω-3 family, do not promote and may inhibit tumorigenesis at high levels of intake. However, a relatively large amount of fish oil is required to counteract the promoting effect of polyunsaturated vegetable oils (Cave and Jurkowski, 1987; O'Connor et al., 1987). Other types of fatty acids, including monounsaturated, medium-chain saturated, and *trans* fatty acids, do not appear to have specific promoting effects on carcinogenesis in animals (Cohen et al., 1986a,b; Ip et al., 1986b).

The fact that high-fat diets promote carcinogenesis in animals more effectively than low-fat diets supports the positive correlation between dietary fats and cancer incidence and mortality shown by epidemiologic data for different countries (Armstrong and Doll, 1975; Carroll and Khor, 1975) and in several case-control studies and suggests a causal relationship (see Chapter 7 for a detailed discussion). The consumption of monounsaturated fats in the form of olive oil has been suggested as a reason for the relatively low cancer rates in Mediterranean countries where fat intake is nevertheless quite high (Cohen, 1987).

The mechanism of action of dietary fats has been studied most extensively as it relates to mammary cancer (Welsch, 1987). This is reviewed in Chapter 7 and is summarized only briefly here. Although hormonal mechanisms are clearly important for breast cancer development, early suggestions that dietary fats might work through a hormonal mechanism now seem unlikely. Several other putative mechanisms relate to the requirement for ω-6 essential fatty acids. Evidence that the promoting effect can be prevented by prostaglandin synthesis inhibitors and that fish oils containing ω-3 fatty acids do not promote carcinogenesis suggest that prostaglandins may be involved. However, not all prostaglandin synthesis inhibitors counteract the promoting effect (Carter et al., 1987), and the extreme susceptibility of the ω-3 fatty acids in fish oil to oxidation may give rise to products other than prostaglandins that act as inhibitors of carcinogenesis (Carroll, in press).

Polyunsaturated fatty acids are characteristic components of the phospholipids of cellular membranes and are supplied entirely by the diet. Thus, dietary fats have the potential to alter the fatty acid composition of membrane phospholipids, thereby changing the fluidity of cell membranes and affecting other properties that could influence the potential for cellular growth, for example, immune responses, intercellular communication mediated by gap junctions, and responsiveness to growth factors such as protein kinase C (Welsch, 1987).

As indicated in Chapter 7, cancer mortality is positively correlated with total dietary fats but not with polyunsaturated fats. Why, then, is a high level of total dietary fat necessary for cancer promotion in animals in addition to the requirement for polyunsaturated fats? The promotional effect may result from the increased intake of

energy from high-fat, high-calorie diets. Recent studies indicate that caloric restriction may inhibit carcinogenesis in animals even when the diet is high in fats (Klurfeld et al., 1987; Pariza and Boutwell, 1987), but it has not been demonstrated conclusively that excessive energy intake per se promotes carcinogenesis (see Chapter 6).

Different mechanisms may be involved in the promotion of carcinogenesis at specific sites. For example, dietary fats may enhance colon cancer by increasing the colonic concentration of secondary bile acids that act as tumor promoters (see Chapter 7).

Protein

Dietary animal protein tends to be associated with dietary fat. In humans, therefore, animal protein and fats are correlated similarly with cancer incidence and mortality. The greater emphasis on dietary fat is due in part to the consistency of the evidence that high-fat diets are associated with increased tumor incidence and tumor yield in animal models; however, effects of dietary protein have also been investigated in a substantial number of experiments in animals (NRC, 1982; see also Chapter 8).

Diets with a low protein content have usually been found to suppress carcinogenesis, and a tumor-enhancing effect is generally observed at protein levels of 20 to 25%. Higher levels produce no further enhancement and may be inhibitory, possibly because of decreased food intake (NRC, 1982; Visek, 1986). Dietary protein appears to enhance tumorigenesis only when there is amino acid balance. Thus, the effect is not due to specific amino acids or to amino acid imbalance (NRC, 1982). It was at first suggested that the effects of dietary protein on hepatomas were due to a modification in aflatoxin B metabolism, but later studies suggest that effects occurring after initiation may be important (Appleton and Campbell, 1983; Campbell, 1983). Other studies show that the effect of dietary protein is so marked that the development of preneoplastic lesions is chiefly determined by protein intake, regardless of the level of aflatoxins consumed (Dunaif and Campbell, 1987). Low-protein diets are associated with inhibition of the growth of transplanted tumors, perhaps in conjunction with cellular immune function (see Chapter 8).

Carbohydrates

There have been relatively few studies of dietary carbohydrates in relation to carcinogenesis, but there is some evidence that rats fed sucrose or dextrose develop mammary tumors more readily than those fed lactose, starches, or dextrin (NRC, 1982; see also Chapter 9). This is of interest in connection with epidemiologic data suggesting a weak correlation between dietary sugar and breast cancer incidence and mortality.

Fiber

The role of dietary fiber has been investigated in animals primarily in relation to colon cancer. The original hypothesis was that dietary fiber inhibits colon carcinogenesis by adsorption or dilution of potential carcinogens or promoters in the colon or by decreasing colonic transit time, thereby reducing the length of exposure. Experimental studies have given variable results, however. Some types of fiber inhibit carcinogenesis, whereas others actually increase the yield of colon cancers (NRC, 1982; see also Chapter 10).

Fat-Soluble Vitamins

Extensive studies in animals show that retinoids can prevent cancer at such sites as the skin, mammary gland, and bladder, although no effect or even increased susceptibility has been reported in several instances. There is also some evidence that carotenoids can decrease the incidence of tumors in laboratory animals (see Chapter 11). Retinoids induce cell differentiation and may act directly on nonneoplastic cells to suppress malignant transformation. They also counteract the effects of phorbol esters and inhibit the proliferative effects of growth factors. Investigators have sought novel synthetic retinoids because the naturally occurring compounds are quite toxic at doses that inhibit carcinogenesis.

The antioxidant properties of vitamin E have stimulated interest in its possible anticarcinogenic properties, but experiments have yielded largely negative results. These studies, and research showing that vitamin K may have some effects on tumorigenesis in animals, are discussed in Chapter 11.

Water-Soluble Vitamins

Most of the water-soluble vitamins have been investigated in relation to cancer in animals (see Chapter 12). Vitamin C may prevent carcinogenesis by preventing the formation of N-nitroso compounds or by enhancing cellular immunity, but experiments to test its effects in tumor models have produced variable results (Glatthaar et al., 1986). Esophageal cancer has been associated with riboflavin deficiency in humans, and experiments

in animals have provided some supporting evidence (Rivlin, 1986). Rats fed diets deficient in lipotropes (choline, methionine, folate) are prone to develop liver tumors (Ghoshal et al., 1986; Newberne, 1986), perhaps because the deficient diet increases the initiating potency of carcinogens or serves as a promoter. Possible mechanisms include hypomethylation of DNA and alterations in membrane phospholipids, leading to structural and functional changes in membranes and increased peroxidation of membrane lipids (Shinozuka et al., 1986).

Trace Elements

Selenium inhibits virally and chemically induced tumors as well as transplanted tumors in animals and is effective during both initiation and proliferative phases of tumorigenesis (Ip, 1985, 1986; Milner, 1985, 1986). Various mechanisms for this inhibitory effect have been proposed. Selenium may prevent the activation of carcinogens such as dimethylbenzanthracene (DMBA) and may modify RNA transcription or translation (Milner, 1986). Its effect on the in vivo activation of aflatoxin B_1 to form covalent DNA adducts is equivocal (Chen et al., 1982a,b). The main function of selenium is to induce and maintain the enzyme glutathione peroxidase, which prevents cellular damage by catabolizing organic peroxides, but this function does not seem to be responsible for its chemopreventive effects (Medina, 1986). Other possible mechanisms of action include inhibition of DNA synthesis and enhancement of immune responses (Ip, 1985).

Dietary zinc deficiency has not been associated with an increased incidence of esophageal carcinoma in humans (see Chapter 14). In animals, zinc deficiency increases the incidence of esophageal carcinoma induced by methylbenzylnitrosamine (MBN), which requires metabolic activation. Zinc acts as a noncompetitive inhibitor of cytochrome P450 activity, and zinc deficiency activates the cytochrome P450-dependent metabolism of MBN, which may explain how zinc deficiency enhances the carcinogenic potential of this compound (Barch and Iannaccone, 1986). On the other hand, zinc is required for growth of both normal and neoplastic tissues, and zinc deficiency reduces the incidence of tumors induced in animals by 3-methylcholanthrene and 4-nitroquinoline-N-oxide (Barch and Iannaccone, 1986). Zinc deficiency affects immunocompetence and influences many other aspects of metabolism, including nucleic acid and protein synthesis.

Testicular tumors have been induced by direct injection of zinc. Excessive dietary zinc can sometimes enhance carcinogenesis, perhaps because it is required for synthesis of DNA, but in other animal models, excess zinc inhibits tumor formation. Other studies reviewed in Chapter 14 also demonstrate that zinc deficiency can either enhance or inhibit tumor growth, indicating that different mechanisms are involved. The role of zinc in carcinogenesis is complex and poorly defined (Kasprzak and Waalkes, 1986).

In rats fed an iodine-deficient diet, follicular adenomas of the thyroid develop by 12 months and follicular carcinomas by 18 months, probably because the iodine deficiency causes chronic hypersecretion of thyroid-stimulating hormone. Iodine deficiency, goitrogenic compounds, and thyroid toxins all act as potent tumor promoters in animals. These findings are not consistent with the weight of epidemiologic evidence, which does not show increased risk of thyroid cancer associated with goiter or living in iodine-deficient areas (see Chapter 14).

Some elements, such as iron and molybdenum, have been shown to enhance or inhibit cancer in different experiments. Others, such as chromium, manganese, and cadmium, were found to be mutagenic in short-term assays. In general, the relevance of these trace element studies to cancer in humans is not clear (see also Chapter 14).

Minerals

Salt has been implicated as a promoter of gastric cancer (Joossens and Geboers, 1987). Some experiments in animals indicate that dietary salt facilitates both initiation and promotion of gastric cancer (Takahashi, 1986; Takahashi et al., 1983). It may act by irritating and possibly damaging the gastric mucosa. (See Chapter 15 for further discussion of salt.)

Dietary calcium has been reported to increase the incidence of tumors in some animals (Kasprzak and Waalkes, 1986), whereas other studies focused on its possible protective effects in colon carcinogenesis (Bruce, 1987; Newmark et al., 1984). Calcium may bind bile acids and fatty acids, thereby preventing them from acting as tumor promoters, but in experiments on azoxymethane-induced colon tumors, rats fed a high-calcium diet developed more tumors than did those fed a low-calcium diet (Bull et al., 1987). On the other hand, Appleton et al. (1987) reported that calcium supplementation reduces colonic crypt-cell production rates and prevents the increase in intestinal tumor yields produced by enterectomy in

rats treated with azoxymethane. Pence and Buddingh (1987) also reported that supplemental calcium or vitamin D_3 inhibits the promotion by dietary fats of intestinal cancer induced in rats by 1,2-dimethylhydrazine. Furthermore, there is evidence that dietary calcium can reduce the yield of mammary tumors induced in rats by DMBA (Jacobson et al., 1987).

Nonnutritive Dietary Components

Animal studies of some of the constituents of coffee and tea, such as caffeine, phenolic compounds, and tannic acid, have yielded mixed results about the ability of these constituents to produce tumorigenesis (see Chapter 17). Nonnutritive sweeteners have been the subject of several long-term studies in animal cancer models. Two-generation studies have provided evidence of a positive association between dietary saccharin and bladder cancer in rats, and saccharin was also shown to have tumor-promoting and cocarcinogenic potential for bladder cancer induced in rats by other chemicals. Cyclamate does not appear to be carcinogenic in rats (NRC, 1985), but it may enhance the carcinogenic effect of other substances on the bladder. Aspartame has not been implicated as a bladder carcinogen, and there is conflicting evidence with regard to its effects on brain neoplasms in animals (see Chapter 17).

There is no conclusive evidence that nitrates or nitrites are carcinogenic in animals, but nitrites may interact with other dietary components to produce N-nitroso compounds (NRC, 1981). These compounds require metabolic activation to be mutagenic or carcinogenic, but can then induce a variety of tumors; however, there are large differences in the susceptibility of different species and different tissues (Lijinsky, 1986). The formation of N-nitroso compounds can be enhanced by a variety of ions present in food, especially thiocyanate and iodine, but can be prevented by other dietary components, including ascorbic acid and α-tocopherol.

Butylated hydroxyanisole (BHA) and butylated hydroxytoluene (BHT)—food additives that are widely used as preservatives and antioxidants—have been studied extensively in animal cancer models. BHA can induce tumors of the forestomach, but can also inhibit the activity of a variety of carcinogens (see Chapter 17), perhaps by preferential enhancement of hepatic detoxifying mechanisms. Unlike other antioxidants, however, BHT administered after carcinogens may increase the number of tumors.

Other nonnutritive components of foods studied for their cancer potential in animals are polychlorinated biphenyls, polybrominated biphenyls, polycyclic aromatic hydrocarbons, diethylstilbestrol, and various food colors (see Chapter 17). In addition to studies involving feeding trials of animals, many of these compounds have been investigated in short-term tests for genotoxicity and mutagenesis (Chapter 17). Positive results are frequently obtained, but Ames et al. (1987) emphasize that naturally occurring components of the diet often have mutagenic properties. Because these components may be associated with protective substances, it is difficult to assess the relative risks of these various mutagenic compounds in the overall context of human cancer.

SUMMARY

Although the contribution of diet to the total incidence of and mortality from cancer in the United States cannot be determined with certainty, it seems reasonable that approximately one-third of all cancer mortality may be related to diet. Over the past 30 years, the incidence of cancer at some sites associated with diet (e.g., breast, colon, prostate) has increased modestly, whereas for other sites (most notably the stomach), it has decreased substantially.

Cancers of the gastrointestinal tract have been positively associated in epidemiologic studies with a variety of dietary exposures, e.g., esophageal cancer with alcohol consumption (particularly combined with tobacco use), stomach cancer with a high intake of foods preserved with salt, colorectal cancer with dietary fats and alcoholic beverages (particularly beer), and liver cancer with aflatoxin-contaminated foods and possibly heavy alcohol consumption (but most strongly with hepatitis B virus infection). Inverse associations with some of these cancers have been noted for other dietary components, e.g., fresh fruits and vegetables (possibly reflecting vitamin C intake) with stomach cancer, and a high intake of vegetables (possibly reflecting intake of certain vitamins, components of fiber, or nonnutritive constituents) with colorectal cancer.

Cancers of the lung and bladder are most clearly associated with exposure to cigarette tobacco and certain industrial chemicals. Foods of plant origin, especially fruits, and green and yellow vegetables, rich in β-carotene (and other carotenoids) appear to exert a protective effect against lung cancer, but this effect could be due to some other constituent of these foods.

Cancers of the breast and prostate have been positively associated with dietary fats. Animal experiments support this positive association, but the epidemiologic evidence is not totally consistent. Alcohol consumption may also be a risk factor for breast cancer. Cancer of the endometrium is clearly associated with obesity, but no specific dietary risk factors for this cancer have been established.

Many of these epidemiologic associations are supported by evidence from experiments in animals. For example, high-fat diets clearly promote mammary and colon carcinogenesis in animals, whereas retinoids and selenium can inhibit experimentally induced tumors at several sites. Nitrites have been shown to interact with other dietary components to produce carcinogenic N-nitroso compounds. However, data on the carcinogenicity of most components of the human diet are quite limited. Although one or more mechanisms have been proposed for the carcinogenic effects of specific dietary factors, the exact mechanisms of carcinogenesis in humans are not yet established for any diet-related cancer.

DIRECTIONS FOR RESEARCH

• *Methodology* Although a considerable amount of research is being focused on the relationship of dietary constituents to cancer, few associations have been established with certainty. Progress in this field could be greatly facilitated by methodological improvements in several areas. For example, innovative methods for dietary assessment in population samples, including the identification of meaningful and practical biologic markers of exposure, might yield more reliable estimates of intake and less inconsistency among studies. Improvement is also needed in the quality and comprehensiveness of the food composition data bases used in this research, for example, those used to estimate the vitamin A and fiber content of foods.

• *Intervention Trials* To date, epidemiologic studies on diet and cancer in humans have been largely observational, i.e., intercountry comparisons, studies on migrants, or case-control and cohort studies. Although some findings are supported by animal studies, the results of such studies cannot be quantitatively extrapolated to humans. Furthermore, there are not always suitable animal models. Thus, to obtain definitive information on the role of diet and cancer in humans, it would be desirable to conduct intervention trials in which diets are modified in specific ways and the subjects are monitored for sufficient time to determine the impact on the incidence of cancer in a number of different sites. Such trials should be planned carefully on the basis of epidemiologic and experimental evidence; efforts should be made to identify the best study populations and the modifications in dietary patterns that most warrant investigation. Although intervention trials are likely to be very expensive, the magnitude of the health problem and the lack of satisfactory treatments for many major types of cancer warrant such an investment of human and financial resources.

• *Genetic Determinants* The role of genetic factors, particularly as they modify individual responses to environmental (dietary) exposures, has not been studied much. Research in this area might clarify some of the poorly understood relationships between dietary components and cancer.

• *Quantitative Relationships* The quantitative nature of the relationship between food constituents and cancer risk is as yet little understood. Such information will be necessary if the public is to be given more precise dietary recommendations than are currently possible.

• *Mechanisms of Action* Mechanisms of action for most dietary factors that affect cancer risk in humans are not completely understood. Elucidation of these mechanisms would help to establish the causal nature of some diet–cancer associations, but this information is not essential to the formulation of policy.

REFERENCES

Acheson, E.D., and R. Doll. 1964. Dietary factors in carcinoma of the stomach: a study of 100 cases and 200 controls. Gut 5:126–131.

Adelcreutz, H., T. Fotsis, R. Heikkinea, J.T. Dwyer, M. Woods, B.R. Goldin, and S.L. Gorbach. 1982. Excretion of the lignans enterolactone and enterodiol and of equol in omnivorous and vegetarian postmenopausal women and in women with breast cancer. Lancet 2:1295–1299.

Alpert, M.E., M.S. Hutt, G.N. Wogan, and C.S. Davidson. 1971. Association between aflatoxin content of food and hepatoma frequency in Uganda. Cancer 28:253–260.

Ames, B.N., R. Magaw, and L.S. Gold. 1987. Ranking possible carcinogenic hazards. Science 236:271–280.

Annegers, J.F., H. Strom, D.G. Decker, M.B. Dockerty, and W.M. O'Fallon. 1979. Ovarian cancer: incidence and case-control study. Cancer 43:723–729.

Anthony, P.P. 1977. Cancer of the liver: pathogenesis and recent aetiological factors. Trans. R. Soc. Trop. Med. Hyg. 71:466–470.

Appleton, B.S., and T.C. Campbell. 1983. Dietary protein intervention during the postdosing phase of aflatoxin B_1-induced hepatic preneoplastic lesion development. J. Natl. Cancer Inst. 70:547–549.

Appleton, G.V., P.W. Davies, J.B Bristol, and R.C. Williamson. 1987. Inhibition of intestinal carcinogenesis by dietary supplementation with calcium. Br. J. Surg. 74:523–525.

Armijo, R., and A.H. Coulson. 1975. Epidemiology of stomach cancer in Chile—the role of nitrogen fertilizers. Int. J. Epidemiol. 4:301–309.

Armstrong, B. 1980. The epidemiology of cancer in the People's Republic of China. Int. J. Epidemiol. 9:305–315.

Armstrong, B., and R. Doll. 1975. Environmental factors and cancer incidence and mortality in different countries, with specific reference to dietary practices. Int. J. Cancer 15:617–631.

Bako, G., E.S. Smith, J. Hanson, and R. Dewar. 1982. The geographical distribution of high cadmium concentrations in the environment and prostate cancer in Alberta. Can. J. Public Health 73:92–94.

Barch, D.H., and P.M. Iannaccone. 1986. Role of zinc deficiency in carcinogenesis. Pp. 517–527 in L.A. Poirier, P.M. Newberne, and M.W. Pariza, eds. Essential Nutrients in Carcinogenesis. Advances in Experimental Biology and Medicine, Vol. 206. Plenum Press, New York.

Beasley, R.P., L.Y. Hwang, C.C. Lin, and C.S. Chien. 1981. Hepatocellular carcinoma and hepatitis B virus: a prospective study of 22,707 men in Taiwan. Lancet 2:1129–1133.

Begg, C.B., A.M. Walker, B. Wessen, and M. Zelen. 1983. Alcohol consumption and breast cancer. Lancet 1:293–294.

Berg, J.W. 1975. Can nutrition explain the pattern of international epidemiology of hormone-dependent cancers? Cancer Res. 35:3345–3350.

Berg, J.W., and F. Burbank. 1972. Correlations between carcinogenic trace metals in water supplies and cancer mortality. Ann. N.Y. Acad. Sci. 199:249–264.

Bingham, S., D.R. Williams, T.J. Cole, and W.P. James. 1979. Dietary fibre and regional large-bowel cancer mortality in Britain. Br. J. Cancer 40:456–463.

Bingham, S.A., D.R. Williams, and J.H. Cummings. 1985. Dietary fibre consumption in Britain: new estimates and their relation to large bowel cancer mortality. Br. J. Cancer 52:399–402.

Bjelke, E. 1975. Dietary vitamin A and human lung cancer. Int. J. Cancer 15:561–565.

Bjelke, E. 1978. Dietary factors and the epidemiology of cancer of the stomach and large bowel. Aktuel. Ernaehrungsmed. Klin. Prax. Suppl. 2:10–17.

Blair, A., and J.F. Fraumeni, Jr. 1978. Geographic patterns of prostate cancer in the United States. J. Natl. Cancer Inst. 61:1379–1384.

Blot, W.J., J.F. Fraumeni, Jr., and B.J. Stone. 1978. Geographic correlates of pancreas cancer in the United States. Cancer 42:373–380.

Breslow, N.E., and J.E. Engstrom. 1974. Geographic correlations between cancer mortality rates and alcohol-tobacco consumption in the United States. J. Natl. Cancer Inst. 53: 631–639.

Brownson, R.C., J.C. Chang, and J.R. Davis. 1987. Occupation, smoking, and alcohol in the epidemiology of bladder cancer. Am. J. Public Health 77:1298–1300.

Bruce, W.R. 1987. Recent hypotheses for the origin of colon cancer. Cancer Res. 47:4237–4242.

Bulatao-Jayme, J., E.M. Almero, M.C.A. Castro, M.T. Jardeleza, and L.A. Salamat. 1982. A case-control dietary study of primary liver cancer risk from aflatoxin exposure. Int. J. Epidemiol. 11:112–119.

Bull, A., R.P. Bird, W.R. Bruce, N. Nigro, and A. Medine.

1987. Effect of calcium on azoxymethane induced intestinal tumors in rats. Gastroenterology 92:1332.

Burch, G.E., and A. Ansari. 1968. Chronic alcoholism and carcinoma of the pancreas: a correlative hypothesis. Arch. Intern. Med. 122:273–275.

Byers, T., and D.P. Funch. 1982. Alcohol and breast cancer. Lancet 1:799–800.

Byers, T., J. Marshall, S. Graham, C. Mettlin, and M. Swanson. 1983. A case-control study of dietary and nondietary factors in ovarian cancer. J. Natl. Cancer Inst. 71:681–686.

Byers, T.E., S. Graham, B.P. Haughey, J.R. Marshall, and M.K. Swanson. 1987. Diet and lung cancer risk: findings from the Western New York Diet Study. Am. J. Epidemiol. 125:351–363.

Campbell, T.C. 1983. Mycotoxins. Pp. 187–197 in E.L. Wynder, G.A. Leveille, J.H. Weisburger, and G.E. Livingston, eds. Environmental Aspects of Cancer: The Role of Macro and Micro Components of Foods. Food and Nutrition Press, Inc., Westport, Conn.

Carroll, K.K. In press. Experimental and epidemiological evidence on marine lipids and carcinogenesis. Health Effects of Omega-3 Fatty Acids. Proceedings of MIT Sea Grant College Program Lecture Seminar Series. Marcel Dekker, Inc.

Carroll, K.K., and H.T. Khor. 1975. Dietary fat in relation to tumorigenesis. Prog. Biochem. Pharmacol. 10:308–353.

Carter, C.A., M.M. Ip, and C. Ip. 1987. Response of mammary carcinogenesis to dietary linoleate and fat levels and its modulation by prostaglandin synthesis inhibitors. Pp. 253–260 in W.E.M. Lands, ed. Proceedings of the AOCS Short Course on Polyunsaturated Fatty Acids and Eicosanoids. American Oil Chemists' Society, Champaign, Ill.

Casagrande, J.T., E.W. Louie, M.C. Pike, S. Roy, R.K. Ross, and B.E. Henderson. 1979. "Incessant ovulation" and ovarian cancer. Lancet 2:170–173.

Cave, W.T., Jr., and J.J. Jurkowski. 1987. Comparative effects of omega-3 and omega-6 dietary lipids on rat mammary tumor development. Pp. 261–266 in W.E.M. Lands, ed. Proceedings of the AOCS Short Course on Polyunsaturated Fatty Acids and Eicosanoids. American Oil Chemists' Society, Champaign, Ill.

Chen, J., M.P. Goetchius, G.F. Combs, Jr., and T.C. Campbell. 1982a. Effects of dietary selenium and vitamin E on covalent binding of aflatoxin to chick liver cell macromolecules. J. Nutr. 112:350–355.

Chen, J., M.P. Goetchius, T.C. Campbell, and G.F. Combs, Jr. 1982b. Effects of dietary selenium and vitamin E on hepatic mixed-function oxidase activities and *in vivo* covalent binding of aflatoxin B_1 in rats. J. Nutr. 112:324–331.

Chien, M.C., M.J. Tong, K.J. Lo, J.K. Lee, D.R. Milich, G.N. Vyas, and B.L. Murphy. 1981. Hepatitis B viral markers in patients with primary hepatocellular carcinoma in Taiwan. J. Natl. Cancer Inst. 66:475–479.

Chilvers, C., P. Fraser, and V. Beral. 1979. Alcohol and oesophageal cancer: an assessment of the evidence from routinely collected data. J. Epidemiol. Community Health 33:127–133.

Cohen, L.A. 1987. Differing effects of high-fat diets rich in polyunsaturated, monounsaturated, or medium chain saturated fatty acids on rat mammary tumor promotion. Pp. 241–247 in W.E.M. Lands, ed. Proceedings of the AOCS Short Course on Polyunsaturated Fatty Acids and Ei-

cosanoids. American Oil Chemists' Society, Champaign, Ill.

Cohen, L.A., D.O. Thompson, Y. Maeura, K. Choi, M.E. Blank, and D.P. Rose. 1986a. Dietary fat and mammary cancer. I. Promoting effects of different dietary fats on N-nitrosomethylurea-induced rat mammary tumorigenesis. J. Natl. Cancer Inst. 77:33–42.

Cohen, L.A., D.O. Thompson, K. Choi, R.A. Karmali, and D.P. Rose. 1986b. Dietary fat and mammary cancer. II. Modulation of serum and tumor lipid composition and tumor prostaglandins by different dietary fats: association with tumor incidence patterns. J. Natl. Cancer Inst. 77:43–51.

Cole, P. 1971. Coffee-drinking and cancer of the lower urinary tract. Lancet 1:1335–1337.

Cook-Mozaffari, P. 1979. The epidemiology of cancer of the oesophagus. Nutr. Cancer 1:51–60.

Correa, P., C. Cuello, E. Duque, L.C. Burbano, F.T. Garcia, O. Bolanos, C. Brown, and W. Haenszel. 1976. Gastric cancer in Colombia. III. Natural history of precursor lesions. J. Natl. Cancer. Inst. 57:1027–1035.

Correa, P., E. Fontham, L.W. Pickle, V. Chen, Y.P. Lin, and W. Haenszel. 1985. Dietary determinants of gastric cancer in south Louisiana inhabitants. J. Natl. Cancer. Inst. 75:645–654.

Cramer, D.W., G.B. Hutchison, W.R. Welch, R.E. Scully, and R.C. Knapp. 1982. Factors affecting the association of oral contraceptives and ovarian cancer. N. Engl. J. Med. 307:1047–1051.

Cramer, D.W., W.R. Welch, G.B. Hutchinson, W. Willett, and R.E. Scully. 1984. Dietary animal fat in relation to ovarian cancer risk. Obstet. Gynecol. 63:833–838.

Cubilla, A.L., and P.J. Fitzgerald. 1978. Pancreas cancer (non-endocrine): a review—part II. Clin. Bull. 8:143–155.

Dales, L.G., G.D. Friedman, H.K. Ury, S. Grossman, and S.R. Williams. 1979. A case-control study of relationships of diet and other traits to colorectal cancer in American blacks. Am. J. Epidemiol. 109:132–144.

Dean, G., R. MacLennan, H. McLoughlin, and E. Shelley. 1979. Causes of death of blue-collar workers at a Dublin brewery, 1954–1973. Br. J. Cancer 40:581–589.

de Jong, U.W., N. Breslow, J.G. Hong, M. Sridharan, and K. Shanmugaratnam. 1974. Aetiological factors in oesophageal cancer in Singapore Chinese. Int. J. Cancer 13:291–303.

Devesa, S.S., D.T. Silverman, J.L. Young, Jr., E.S. Pollack, C.C. Brown, J.W. Horm, C.L. Percy, M.H. Myers, F.W. McKay, and J.F. Fraumeni, Jr. 1987. Cancer incidence and mortality trends among whites in the United States, 1947–1984. J. Natl. Cancer Inst. 79:701–770.

de Waard, F., J.P. Cornelis, K. Aoki, and M. Yoshida. 1977. Breast cancer incidence according to weight and height in two cities of the Netherlands and in Aichi prefecture, Japan. Cancer 40:1269–1275.

DHEW (Department of Health, Education, and Welfare). 1979. Smoking and Health: A Report of the Surgeon General. DHEW Publ. No. (PHS) 79-50066. Office on Smoking and Health, Office of the Assistant Secretary for Health, Public Health Service, U.S. Department of Health, Education, and Welfare, Rockville, Md. 1164 pp.

Doll, R., and R. Peto. 1981. The causes of cancer: quantitative estimates of avoidable risks of cancer in the United States today. J. Natl. Cancer Inst. 66:1191–1308.

Dörken, H. 1964. Einige Daten bei 280 Patienten mit Pankreaskrebs. Häufigkeit, Vor- und Begleitkrankheiten, exogene Faktoren. Gastroenterologia 102:46–77.

Drasar, B.S., and D. Irving. 1973. Environmental factors and cancer of the colon and breast. Br. J. Cancer 27:167–172.

Dunaif, G.E., and T.C. Campbell. 1987. Relative contribution of dietary protein level and aflatoxin B_1 dose in generation of presumptive preneoplastic foci in rat liver. J. Natl. Cancer Inst. 78:365–369.

Dungal, N. 1966. Stomach cancer in Iceland. Can. Cancer Conf. 6:441–450.

Elwood, J.M., P. Cole, K.J. Rothman, and S.D. Kaplan. 1977. Epidemiology of endometrial cancer. J. Natl. Cancer Inst. 59:1055–1060.

Enstrom, J.E. 1975. Colorectal cancer and consumption of beef and fat. Br. J. Cancer 32:432–439.

Feustel, A., and R. Wennrich. 1986. Zinc and cadmium plasma and erythrocyte levels in prostatic carcinoma, BPH, urological malignancies, and inflammations. Prostate 8:75–79.

Feustel, A., R. Wennrich, D. Steiniger, and P. Klauss. 1982. Zinc and cadmium concentration in prostatic carcinoma of different histological grading in comparison to normal prostate tissue and adenofibromyomatosis (BPH). Urol. Res. 10:301–303.

Foy, H., and V. Mbaya. 1977. Riboflavin. Prog. Food Nutr. Sci. 2:357–394.

Fraumeni, J.F., Jr. 1975. Respiratory carcinogenesis: an epidemiologic appraisal. J. Natl. Cancer Inst. 55:1039–1046.

Fraumeni, J.F., Jr., J. Scotto, and L.J. Dunham. 1971. Coffee-drinking and bladder cancer. Lancet 2:1204.

Friberg, L., C.G. Elinder, T. Kjellström, and G.F. Nordberg. 1986. Cadmium and Health: A Toxicological and Epidemiological Appraisal, Vol. II. Effects and Response. CRC Press, Boca Raton, Fla. 307 pp.

Friedman, G.D., W.S. Blaner, D.S. Goodman, J.H. Vogelman, J.L. Brind, R. Hoover, B.H. Fireman, and N. Orentreich. 1986. Serum retinol and retinol-binding protein levels do not predict subsequent lung cancer. Am. J. Epidemiol. 123:781–789.

Garland, C., R.B. Shekelle, E. Barrett-Connor, M.H. Criqui, A.H. Rossof, and O. Paul. 1985. Dietary vitamin D and calcium and risk of colorectal cancer: a 19-year prospective study in men. Lancet 1:307–308.

Gaskill, S.P., W.L. McGuire, C.K. Osborne, and M.P. Stern. 1979. Breast cancer mortality and diet in the United States. Cancer Res. 39:3628–3637.

Ghoshal, A.K., D.S.R. Sarma, and E. Farber. 1986. Ethionine in the analysis of the possible separate roles of methionine and choline deficiencies in carcinogenesis. Pp. 283–292 in L.A. Poirier, P.M. Newberne, and M.W. Pariza, eds. Essential Nutrients in Carcinogenesis. Advances in Experimental Biology and Medicine, Vol. 206. Plenum Press, New York.

Glatthaar, B.E., D.H. Hornig, and U. Moser. 1986. The role of ascorbic acid in carcinogenesis. Pp. 357–377 in L.A. Poirier, P.M. Newberne, and M.W. Pariza, eds. Essential Nutrients in Carcinogenesis. Advances in Experimental Biology and Medicine, Vol. 206. Plenum Press, New York.

Gold, E.B., L. Gordis, M.D. Diener, R. Seltser, J.K. Boitnott, T.E. Bynum, and D.F. Hutcheon. 1985. Diet and other risk factors for cancer of the pancreas. Cancer 55:460–467.

Graham, S., W. Schotz, and P. Martino. 1972. Alimentary factors in the epidemiology of gastric cancer. Cancer 30:927–938.

Graham, S., H. Dayal, M. Swanson, A. Mittelman, and G. Wilkinson. 1978. Diet in the epidemiology of cancer of the colon and rectum. J. Natl. Cancer Inst. 61:709–714.

Graham, S., J. Marshall, C. Mettlin, T. Rzepka, T. Nemoto, and T. Byers. 1982. Diet in the epidemiology of breast cancer. Am. J. Epidemiol. 116:68–75.

Graham, S., B. Haughey, J. Marshall, R. Priore, T. Byers, T. Rzepka, C. Mettlin, and J.E. Pontes. 1983. Diet in the epidemiology of carcinoma of the prostate gland. J. Natl. Cancer Inst. 70:687–692.

Graham, S., J. Marshall, B. Haughey, A. Mittelman, M. Swanson, M. Zielezny, T. Byers, G. Wilkinson, and D. West. 1988. Dietary epidemiology of cancer of the colon in western New York. Am. J. Epidemiol. 128:490–503.

Gregor, O., R. Toman, and F. Prusova. 1969. Gastrointestinal cancer and nutrition. Gut 10:1031–1034.

Gregor, A., P.N. Lee, F.J.C. Roe, M.J. Wilson, and A. Melton. 1980. Comparison of dietary histories in lung cancer cases and controls with special reference to vitamin A. Nutr. Cancer 2:93–97.

Haenszel, W., and P. Correa. 1975. Developments in the epidemiology of stomach cancer over the past decade. Cancer Res. 35:3452–3459.

Haenszel, W., and E.A. Dawson. 1965. A note on mortality from cancer of the colon and rectum in the United States. Cancer 18:265–272.

Haenszel, W., M. Kurihara, M. Segi, and R.K. Lee. 1972. Stomach cancer among Japanese in Hawaii. J. Natl. Cancer Inst. 49:969–988.

Haenszel, W., J.W. Berg, M. Segi, M. Kurihara, and F.B. Locke. 1973. Large-bowel cancer in Hawaiian Japanese. J. Natl. Cancer Inst. 51:1765–1779.

Haenszel, W., M. Kurihara, F.B. Locke, K. Shimuzu, and M. Segi. 1976. Stomach cancer in Japan. J. Natl. Cancer Inst. 56:265–274.

Haenszel, W., F.B. Locke, and M. Segi. 1980. A case-control study of large bowel cancer in Japan. J. Natl. Cancer Inst. 64:17–22.

Hakulinen, T., L. Lehtimaki, M. Lehtonen, and L. Teppo. 1974. Cancer morbidity among two male cohorts with increased alcohol consumption in Finland. J. Natl. Cancer Inst. 52:1711–1714.

Hartge, P., R. Hoover, D.W. West, and J.L. Lyon. 1983. Coffee drinking and risk of bladder cancer. J. Natl. Cancer Inst. 70:1021–1026.

Heilbrun, L.K., J.H. Hankin, A.M.Y. Nomura, and G.N. Stemmermann. 1986. Colon cancer and dietary fat, phosphorus, and calcium in Hawaiian-Japanese men. Am. J. Clin. Nutr. 43:306–309.

Henderson, B.E., R.K. Ross, M.C. Pike, and J.T. Casagrande. 1982. Endogenous hormones as a major factor in human cancer. Cancer Res. 42:3232–3239.

Henderson, B.E., J.T. Casagrande, M.C. Pike, T. Mack, and I. Rosario. 1983. The epidemiology of endometrial cancer in young women. Br. J. Cancer 47:749–756.

Heshmat, M.Y., L. Kaul, J. Kovi, M.A. Jackson, A.G. Jackson, G.W. Jones, M. Edson, J.P. Enterline, R.G. Worrell, and S.L. Perry. 1985. Nutrition and prostate cancer: a case-control study. Prostate 6:7–17.

Heuch, I., G. Kvale, B.K. Jacobsen, and E. Bjelke. 1983. Use of alcohol, tobacco and coffee, and risk of pancreatic cancer. Br. J. Cancer 48:637–643.

Hiatt, R.A., and R.D. Bawol. 1984. Alcoholic beverage consumption and breast cancer incidence. Am. J. Epidemiol. 120:676–683.

Higginson, J. 1966. Etiological factors in gastrointestinal cancer in man. J. Natl. Cancer Inst. 37:527–545.

Hildreth, N.G., J.L. Kelsey, V.A. LiVolsi, D.B. Fischer, T.R. Holford, E.D. Mostow, P.E. Schwartz, and C. White. 1981. An epidemiologic study of epithelial carcinoma of the ovary. Am. J. Epidemiol. 114:398–405.

Hill, M.J., G. Hawksworth, and G. Tattersall. 1973. Bacteria, nitrosamines, and cancer of the stomach. Br. J. Cancer 28: 562–567.

Hinds, M.W., L.N. Kolonel, J. Lee, and T. Hirohata. 1980. Associations between cancer incidence and alcohol/cigarette consumption among five ethnic groups in Hawaii. Br. J. Cancer 41:929–940.

Hinds, M.W., L.N. Kolonel, J.H. Hankin, and J. Lee. 1983. Dietary cholesterol and lung cancer risk in a multiethnic population in Hawaii. Int. J. Cancer 32:727–732.

Hinds, M.W., L.N. Kolonel, J.H. Hankin, and J. Lee. 1984. Dietary vitamin A, carotene, vitamin C and risk of lung cancer in Hawaii. Am. J. Epidemiol. 119:227–237.

Hirayama, T. 1967. The epidemiology of cancer of the stomach in Japan with special reference to the role of diet. Pp. 37–49 in R.J.C. Harris, ed. Proceedings of the 9th International Cancer Congress. UICC Monograph Series, Vol. 10. Springer-Verlag, Berlin.

Hirayama, T. 1977. Changing patterns of cancer in Japan with special reference to the decrease in stomach cancer mortality. Pp. 55–75 in H.H. Hiatt, J.D. Watson, and J.A. Winsten, eds. Origins of Human Cancer. Book A, Incidence of Cancer in Humans. Cold Spring Harbor Laboratory, New York.

Hirayama, T. 1979. Diet and cancer. Nutr. Cancer 1:67–81.

Hirohata, T., T. Shigematsu, A.M. Nomura, Y. Nomura, A. Horie, and I. Hirohata. 1985. Occurrence of breast cancer in relation to diet and reproductive history: a case-control study in Fukuoka, Japan. Natl. Cancer Inst. Monogr. 69: 187–190.

Hirohata, T., A.M. Nomura, J.H. Hankin, L.N. Kolonel, and J. Lee. 1987. An epidemiologic study on the association between diet and breast cancer. J. Natl. Cancer Inst. 78: 595–600.

Hislop, T.G., A.J. Coldman, J.M. Elwood, G. Brauer, and L. Kan. 1986. Childhood and recent eating patterns and risk of breast cancer. Cancer Detect. Prev. 9:47–58.

Hoey, J., C. Montvernay, and R. Lambert. 1981. Wine and tobacco: risk factors for gastric cancer in France. Am. J. Epidemiol. 113:668–674.

Hormozdiari, H., N.E. Day, B. Aramesh, and E. Mahboubi. 1975. Dietary factors and esophageal cancer in the Caspian Littoral of Iran. Cancer Res. 35:3493–3498.

Howe, G.R. 1985. The use of polytomous dual response data to increase power in case-control studies: an application to the association between dietary fat and breast cancer. J. Chronic Dis. 38:663–670.

Howe, G.R., J.D. Burch, A.B. Miller, G.M. Cook, J. Esteve, B. Morrison, P. Gordon, L.W. Chambers, G. Fodor, and G.M. Winsor. 1980. Tobacco use, occupation, coffee, various nutrients, and bladder cancer. J. Natl. Cancer Inst. 64:701–713.

Howe, G.R., A.B. Miller, and M. Jain. 1986. Re: "Total energy intake: implications for epidemiologic analyses." Am. J. Epidemiol. 124:157–159.

Howe, G.R., J.D. Burch, and H.A. Risch. In press. Artificial sweeteners, caloric intake and cancer: the epidemiologic evidence. Prev. Med.

Howell, M.A. 1974. Factor analysis of international cancer mortality data and per capita food consumption. Br. J. Cancer 29:328–336.

Howell, M.A. 1975. Diet as an etiological factor in the development of cancers of the colon and rectum. J. Chronic Dis. 28:67–80.

Hsieh, C.C., B. MacMahon, S. Yen, D. Trichopoulos, K. Warren, and G. Nardi. 1986. Coffee and pancreatic cancer (chapter 2). N. Engl. J. Med. 315:587–589.

Imai, T., T. Kubo, and H. Watanabe. 1971. Chronic gastritis in Japanese with reference to high incidence of gastric carcinoma. J. Natl. Cancer Inst. 47:179–195.

Inaba, Y., N. Maruchi, M. Matsuda, N. Yoshihara, and S.I. Yamamoto. 1984. A case-control study on liver cancer with special emphasis on the possible aetiological role of schistosomiasis. Int. J. Epidemiol. 13:408–412.

Inskip, H., V. Beral, and M. McDowall. 1982. Mortality of Shipham residents: 40-year follow-up. Lancet 1:896–899.

International Agency for Research on Cancer Intestinal Microecology Group. 1977. Dietary fibre, transit-time, faecal bacteria, steroids, and colon cancer in two Scandinavian populations. Lancet 2:207–211.

Ip, C. 1985. Selenium inhibition of chemical carcinogenesis. Fed. Proc. 44:2573–2578.

Ip, C. 1986. The chemopreventive role of selenium in carcinogenesis. Pp. 431–447 in L.A. Poirier, P.M. Newberne, and M.W. Pariza, eds. Essential Nutrients in Carcinogenesis. Advances in Experimental Biology and Medicine, Vol. 206. Plenum Press, New York.

Ip, C. 1987. Fat and essential fatty acids in mammary carcinogenesis. Am. J. Clin. Nutr. 45 suppl. 1:218–224.

Ip, C., D.F. Birt, A.E. Rogers, and C. Mettlin, eds. 1986a. Progress in Clinical and Biological Research, Vol. 222. Dietary Fat and Cancer. Alan R. Liss, New York. 885 pp.

Ip, C., M.M. Ip, and P. Sylvester. 1986b. Relevance of trans fatty acids and fish oil in animal tumorigenesis studies. Pp. 283–294 in C. Ip, D.F. Birt, A.E. Rogers, and C. Mettlin, eds. Progress in Clinical and Biological Research, Vol. 222. Dietary Fat and Cancer. Alan R. Liss, New York.

Ishii, K., K. Nakamura, H. Ozaki, N. Yamada, and T. Takeuchi. 1968. Epidemiological problems of pancreas cancer. Jpn. J. Clin. Med. 26:1839–1842.

Jacobsen, B.K., E. Bjelke, G. Kvale, and I. Heuch. 1986. Coffee drinking, mortality and cancer incidence: results from a Norwegian prospective study. J. Natl. Cancer Inst. 76:823–831.

Jacobson, E.A., R. Russell, H.L. Newmark, M.A. Amer, and K.K. Carroll. 1987. Fat, calcium and tumor development in dimethylbenz[a]anthracene (DMBA)-treated rats. Proc. Can. Fed. Biol. Sci. 30:112.

Jain, M., G.M. Cook, F.G. Davis, M.G. Grace, G.R. Howe, and A.B. Miller. 1980. A case-control study of diet and colo-rectal cancer. Int. J. Cancer. 26:757–768.

Jensen, H. 1986. Relationship of premorbid state of nutrition to endometrial carcinoma. Acta Obstet. Gynecol. Scand. 65:301–306.

Jensen, O.M. 1979. Cancer morbidity and causes of death among Danish brewery workers. Int. J. Cancer 23:454–463.

Jensen, O.M., R. MacLennan, and J. Wahrendorf. 1982. Diet, bowel function, fecal characteristics, and large bowel cancer in Denmark and Finland. Nutr. Cancer 4:5–19.

Jensen, O.M., J. Wahrendorf, J.B. Knudsen, and B.L. Sorenson. 1986. The Copenhagen case-control study of bladder cancer. II. The effect of coffee and other beverages. Int. J. Cancer 37:651–657.

Joint Iran-International Agency for Research on Cancer Study Group. 1977. Esophageal cancer studies in the Caspian

Littoral of Iran: results of population studies—a prodrome. J. Natl. Cancer Inst. 59:1127–1138.

Joossens, J.V., and J. Geboers. 1987. Dietary salt and risks to health. Am. J. Clin. Nutr. 45:1277–1288.

Kabat, G.C., C.P. Howson, and E.L. Wynder. 1986. Beer consumption and rectal cancer. Int. J. Epidemiol. 15:494–501.

Kark, J.D., A.H. Smith, B.R. Switzer, and C.G. Hames. 1981. Serum vitamin A (retinol) and cancer incidence in Evans County, Georgia. J. Natl. Cancer Inst. 66:7–16.

Kasprzak, K.S., and M.P. Waalkes. 1986. The role of calcium, magnesium, and zinc in carcinogenesis. Pp. 497–515 in L.A. Poirier, P.M. Newberne, and M.W. Pariza, eds. Essential Nutrients in Carcinogenesis. Advances in Experimental Biology and Medicine, Vol. 206. Plenum Press, New York.

Keller, A.Z. 1980. The epidemiology of esophageal cancer in the West. Prev. Med. 9:607–612.

Kinlen, L.J. 1982. Meat and fat consumption and cancer mortality: a study of strict religious orders in Britain. Lancet 1:946–949.

Klurfeld, D.M., M.M. Weber, and D. Kritchevsky. 1987. Inhibition of chemically induced mammary and colon tumor promotion by caloric restriction in rats fed increased dietary fat. Cancer Res. 47:2759–2762.

Knox, E.G. 1977. Foods and diseases. Br. J. Prev. Soc. Med. 31:71–80.

Kolonel, L.N. 1980. Cancer patterns of four ethnic groups in Hawaii. J. Natl. Cancer Inst. 65:1127–1139.

Kolonel, L.N., and W. Winkelstein, Jr. 1977. Cadmium and prostatic carcinoma. Lancet 2:566–567.

Kolonel, L.N., M.W. Hinds, and J.H. Hankin. 1980. Cancer patterns among migrant and native-born Japanese in Hawaii in relation to smoking, drinking, and dietary habits. Pp. 327–340 in H.V. Gelboin, M. MacMahon, T. Matsushima, T. Sugimura, S. Takayama, and H. Takebe, eds. Genetic and Environmental Factors in Experimental and Human Cancer. Japan Scientific Societies Press, Tokyo.

Kolonel, L.N., A.M. Nomura, T. Hirohata, J.H. Hankin, and M.W. Hinds. 1981. Association of diet and place of birth with stomach cancer incidence in Hawaii Japanese and Caucasians. Am. J. Clin. Nutr. 34:2478–2485.

Kolonel, L.N., A.M. Nomura, J. Lee, and T. Hirohata. 1986. Anthropometric indicators of breast cancer risk in postmenopausal women in Hawaii. Nutr. Cancer 8:247–256.

Kolonel, L.N., J.H. Hankin, and C.N. Yoshizawa. 1987. Vitamin A and prostate cancer in elderly men: enhancement of risk. Cancer Res. 47:2982–2985.

Kolonel, L.N., C.N. Yoshizawa, and J.H. Hankin. 1988. Diet and prostatic cancer: a case-control study in Hawaii. Am. J. Epidemiol. 127:999–1012.

Kune, S., G.A. Kune, and L.F. Watson. 1987. Case-control study of dietary etiological factors: the Melbourne Colorectal Cancer Study. Nutr. Cancer 9:21–42.

Kvale, G., E. Bjelke, and J.J. Gart. 1983. Dietary habits and lung cancer risk. Int. J. Cancer 31:397–405.

La Vecchia, C., S. Franceschi, A. Decarli, A. Gentile, P. Liati, M. Regello, and G. Tognoni. 1984. Coffee drinking and risk of epithelial ovarian cancer. Int. J. Cancer 33:559–562.

La Vecchia, C., A. Decarli, M. Fasoli, and A. Gentile. 1986. Nutrition and diet in the etiology of endometrial cancer. Cancer 57:1248–1253.

Lê, M.G., L.H. Moulton, C. Hill, and A. Kramar. 1986. Consumption of dairy produce and alcohol in a case-control study of breast cancer. J. Natl. Cancer Inst. 77:633–636.

Lew, E.A., and L. Garfinkel. 1979. Variations in mortality by weight among 750,000 men and women. J. Chronic Dis. 32:563–576.

Lijinsky, W. 1986. The significance of N-nitroso compounds as environmental carcinogens. J. Environ. Sci. Health C4:1–45.

Liu, K., J. Stamler, D. Moss, D. Garside, V. Persky, and I. Soltero. 1979. Dietary cholesterol, fat, and fibre, and colon-cancer mortality. An analysis of international data. Lancet 2:782–785.

Lubin, J.H., P.E. Burns, W.J. Blot, R.G. Ziegler, A.W. Lees, and J.F. Fraumeni, Jr. 1981. Dietary factors and breast cancer risk. Int. J. Cancer 28:685–689.

Lubin, F., A.M. Ruder, Y. Wax, and B. Modan. 1985. Overweight and changes in weight throughout adult life in breast cancer etiology. A case-control study. Am. J. Epidemiol. 122:579–588.

Lubin, F., Y. Wax, and B. Modan. 1986. Role of fat, animal protein, and dietary fiber in breast cancer etiology: a case-control study. J. Natl. Cancer Inst. 77:605–612.

Lyon, J.L., and A.W. Sorenson. 1978. Colon cancer in a low-risk population. Am. J. Clin. Nutr. 31 suppl. 10:S227–S230.

Lyon, J.L., M.R. Klauber, J.W. Gardner, and C.R. Smart. 1976. Cancer incidence in Mormons and non-Mormons in Utah, 1966–1970. N. Engl. J. Med. 294:129–133.

Lyon, J.L., J.W. Gardner, and D.W. West. 1980. Cancer risk and lifestyle: cancer among Mormons (1967–1975). Pp. 273–290 in H.V. Gelboin, B. MacMahon, T. Matsushima, T. Sugimura, S. Takayama, and H. Takebe, eds. Genetic and Environmental Factors in Experimental and Human Cancer. Japan Scientific Societies Press, Tokyo.

Lyon, J.L., A.W. Mahoney, D.W. West, J.W. Gardner, K.R. Smith, A.W. Sorenson, and W. Stanish. 1987. Energy intake: its relationship to colon cancer risk. J. Natl. Cancer Inst. 78:853–861.

Mack, T.M., M.C. Yu, R. Hanisch, and B.E. Henderson. 1986. Pancreas cancer and smoking, beverage consumption, and past medical history. J. Natl. Cancer Inst. 76:49–60.

MacLennan, R., J. Da Costa, N.E. Day, C.H. Law, Y.K. Ng, and K. Shanmugaratnam. 1977. Risk factors for lung cancer in Singapore Chinese, a population with high female incidence rates. Int. J. Cancer 20:854–860.

MacLennan, R., O.M. Jensen, J. Mosbech, and H. Vuori. 1978. Diet, transit time, stool weight, and colon cancer in two Scandinavian populations. Am. J. Clin. Nutr. 31 suppl. 10:S239–S242.

MacMahon, B., P. Cole, and J. Brown. 1973. Etiology of human breast cancer: a review. J. Natl. Cancer Inst. 50:21–42.

MacMahon, B., S. Yen, D. Trichopoulos, K. Warren, and G. Nardi. 1981. Coffee and cancer of the pancreas. N. Engl. J. Med. 304:630–633.

Macquart-Moulin, G., E. Riboli, J. Cornee, B. Charnay, P. Berthezene, and N. Day. 1986. Case-control study on colorectal cancer and diet in Marseilles. Int. J. Cancer 38:183–191.

Malhotra, S.L. 1977. Dietary factors in a study of colon cancer from cancer registry, with special reference to the role of saliva, milk and fermented milk products and vegetable fibre. Med. Hypotheses 3:122–126.

Mandel, J.S., and L.M. Schuman. 1980. Epidemiology of cancer of the prostate. Pp. 1–83 in A.M. Lilienfeld, ed.

Reviews in Cancer Epidemiology, Vol. 1. Elsevier/North-Holland, New York.

Manousos, O., N.E. Day, D. Trichopoulos, F. Gerovassilis, A. Tzonou, and A. Polychronopoulou. 1983. Diet and colorectal cancer: a case-control study in Greece. Int. J. Cancer 32:1–5.

Marrett, L.D., S.D. Walter, and J.W. Meigs. 1983. Coffee drinking and bladder cancer in Connecticut. Am. J. Epidemiol. 117:113–127.

Martinez, I. 1969. Factors associated with cancer of the esophagus, mouth, and pharynx in Puerto Rico. J. Natl. Cancer Inst. 42:1069–1094.

McKeown-Eyssen, G.E., and E. Bright-See. 1984. Dietary factors in colon cancer: international relationships. Nutr. Cancer 6:160–170.

McMichael, A.J., O.M. Jensen, D.M. Parkin, and D.G. Zaridze. 1984. Dietary and endogenous cholesterol and human cancer. Epidemiol. Rev. 6:192–216.

Medina, D. 1986. Mechanisms of selenium inhibition of tumorigenesis. Pp. 465–472 in L.A. Poirier, P.M. Newberne, and M.W. Pariza, eds. Essential Nutrients in Carcinogenesis. Advances in Experimental Biology and Medicine, Vol. 206. Plenum Press, New York.

Menkes, M.S., G.W. Comstock, J.P. Vuilleumier, K.J. Helsing, A.A. Rider, and R. Brookmeyer. 1986. Serum beta-carotene, vitamins A and E, selenium, and the risk of lung cancer. N. Engl. J. Med. 315:1250–1254.

Mettlin, C., and S. Graham. 1979. Dietary risk factors in human bladder cancer. Am. J. Epidemiol. 110:255–263.

Mettlin, C., S. Graham, R. Priore, J. Marshall, and M. Swanson. 1981. Diet and cancer of the esophagus. Nutr. Cancer 2:143–147.

Miller, A.B. 1978. An overview of hormone-associated cancer. Cancer Res. 38:3985–3990.

Miller, A.B. 1980. Epidemiology and etiology of lung cancer. Pp. 9–26 in H.H. Hansen and M. Roth, eds. Lung Cancer 1980. Excerpta Medica, Amsterdam.

Miller, A.B., A. Kelly, N.W. Choi, V. Matthews, R.W. Morgan, L. Munan, J.D. Burch, J. Feather, G.R. Howe, and M. Jain. 1978. A study of diet and breast cancer. Am. J. Epidemiol. 107:499–509.

Miller, A.B., G.R. Howe, M. Jain, K.J.P. Craib, and. L. Harrison. 1983. Food items and food groups as risk factors in a case-control study of diet and colo-rectal cancer. Int. J. Cancer 32:155–161.

Milner, J.A. 1985. Effect of selenium on virally induced and transplantable tumor models. Fed. Proc. 44:2568–2572.

Milner, J.A. 1986. Inhibition of chemical carcinogenesis and tumorigenesis by selenium. Pp. 449–463 in L.A. Poirier, P.M. Newberne, and M.W. Pariza, eds. Essential Nutrients in Carcinogenesis. Advances in Experimental Medicine and Biology, Vol. 206. Plenum Press, New York.

Mirvish, S.S., L. Wallcave, M. Eagen, and P. Shubik. 1972. Ascorbate-nitrite reaction: possible means of blocking the formation of carcinogenic N-nitroso compounds. Science 177:65–68.

Modan, B., F. Lubin, V. Barell, R.A. Greenberg, M. Modan, and S. Graham. 1974. The role of starches in the etiology of gastric cancer. Cancer 34:2087–2092.

Modan, B., V. Barell, F. Lubin, M. Modan, R.A. Greenberg, and S. Graham. 1975. Low-fiber intake as an etiologic factor in cancer of the colon. J. Natl. Cancer Inst. 55:15–18.

Monson, R.R., and J.L. Lyon. 1975. Proportional mortality among alcoholics. Cancer 36:1077–1079.

Morrison, A.S., J.E. Buring, W.G. Verhoek, K. Aoki, I. Leck, Y. Ohno, and K. Obata. 1982. Coffee drinking and cancer of the lower urinary tract. J. Natl. Cancer Inst. 68: 91–94.

Muñoz, N., J. Wahrendorf, L.J. Bang, M. Crespi, D.I. Thurnham, N.E. Day, Z.H. Ji, A. Grassi, L.W. Yan, L.G. Lin, L.Y. Quan, Z.C. Yun, Z.S. Fang, L.J. Yao, P. Correa, G.T. O'Conor, and X. Bosch. 1985. No effect of riboflavine, retinol, and zinc on prevalence of precancerous lesions of oesophagus. Randomised double-blind intervention study in high-risk population of China. Lancet 2:111–114.

Nasca, P.C., P. Greenwald, S. Chorost, R. Richart, and T. Caputo. 1984. An epidemiologic case-control study of ovarian cancer and reproductive factors. Am. J. Epidemiol. 119:705–713.

Newberne, P.M. 1986. Lipotropic factors and oncogenesis. Pp. 223–251 in L.A. Poirier, P.M. Newberne, and M.W. Pariza, eds. Essential Nutrients in Carcinogenesis. Advances in Experimental Biology and Medicine, Vol. 206. Plenum Press, New York.

Newmark, H.L., M.J. Wargovich, and W.R. Bruce. 1984. Colon cancer and dietary fat, phosphate, and calcium: a hypothesis. J. Natl. Cancer Inst. 72:1323–1325.

Nicholls, P., G. Edwards, and E. Kyle. 1974. Alcoholics admitted to four hospitals in England. II. General and cause-specific mortality. Q. J. Stud. Alcohol 35:841–855.

Nomura, A.M., G.N. Stemmermann, L.K. Heilbrun, R.M. Salkeld, and J.P. Vuilleumier. 1985. Serum vitamin levels and the risk of cancer of specific sites to men of Japanese ancestry in Hawaii. Cancer Res. 45:2369–2372.

Nomura, A., L.K. Heilbrun, and G.N. Stemmermann. 1986. Prospective study of coffee consumption and the risk of cancer. J. Natl. Cancer Inst. 76:587–590.

Norell, S.E., A. Ahlbom, R. Erwald, G. Jacobson, I. Lindberg-Navier, R. Olin, B. Tornberg, and K.L. Wiechel. 1986. Diet and pancreatic cancer: a case-control study. Am. J. Epidemiol. 124:894–902.

NRC (National Research Council). 1981. The Health Effects of Nitrate, Nitrite, and N-Nitroso Compounds. Report of the Committee on Nitrite and Alternative Curing Agents in Food, Assembly of Life Sciences. National Academy Press, Washington, D.C. 544 pp.

NRC (National Research Council). 1982. Diet, Nutrition, and Cancer. Report of the Committee on Diet, Nutrition, and Cancer, Assembly of Life Sciences. National Academy Press, Washington, D.C. 478 pp.

NRC (National Research Council). 1985. Evaluation of Cyclamate for Carcinogenicity. Report of the Committee on the Evaluation of Cyclamate for Carcinogenicity, Commission on Life Sciences. National Academy Press, Washington, D.C. 196 pp.

O'Connor, T.P., B.C. Roebuck, and T.C. Campbell. 1987. Effect of varying dietary omega-3:omega-6 fatty acid ratio on L-azaserine induced preneoplastic development in rat pancrease. Pp. 238–240 in W.E.M. Lands, ed. Proceedings of the AOCS Short Course on Polyunsaturated Fatty Acids and Eicosanoids. American Oil Chemists' Society, Champaign, Ill.

Ohno, Y., K. Aoki, K. Obata, and A.S. Morrison. 1985. Case-control study of urinary bladder cancer in metropolitan Nagoya. Natl. Cancer Inst. Monogr. 69:229–234.

Paffenbarger, R.S., J.B. Kampert, and H.G. Chang. 1980. Characteristics that predict risk of breast cancer before and after the menopause. Am. J. Epidemiol. 112:258–268.

Page, H.S., and A.J. Asire. 1985. Cancer Rates and Risks, 3rd ed. DHHS Publ. No. (NIH) 85–691. National Institutes of Health, Public Health Service, U.S. Department of Health and Human Services, Bethesda, Md. 136 pp.

Pariza, M.W., and R.K. Boutwell. 1987. Historical perspective: calories and energy expenditure in carcinogenesis. Am. J. Clin. Nutr. 45 suppl. 1:151–156.

Peers, F.G., G.A. Gilman, and C.A. Linsell. 1976. Dietary aflatoxins and human liver cancer. A study in Swaziland. Int. J. Cancer 17:167–176.

Peleg, I., S. Heyden, M. Knowles, and C.G. Hames. 1984. Serum retinol and risk of subsequent cancer: extension of the Evans County, Georgia, study. J. Natl. Cancer Inst. 73: 1455–1458.

Pell, S., and A. D'Alonzo. 1973. A five-year mortality study of alcoholics. J. Occup. Med. 15:120–125.

Pence, B.C., and F. Buddingh. 1987. Inhibition of dietary fat promotion of colon carcinogenesis by supplemental calcium or vitamin D. Proc. Am. Assoc. Cancer Res. 28:154.

Phillips, R.L. 1975. Role of life-style and dietary habits in risk of cancer among Seventh-Day Adventists. Cancer Res. 35: 3513–3522.

Pickle, L.W., M.H. Greene, R.G. Ziegler, A. Toledo, R. Hoover, H.T. Lynch, and J.F. Fraumeni, Jr. 1984. Colorectal cancer in rural Nebraska. Cancer Res. 44:363–369.

Pollack, E.S., A.M. Nomura, L.K. Heilbrun, G.N. Stemmermann, and S.B. Green. 1984. Prospective study of alcohol consumption and cancer. N. Engl. J. Med. 310:617–621.

Potter, J.D., and A.J. McMichael. 1986. Diet and cancer of the colon and rectum: a case-control study. J. Natl. Cancer Inst. 76:557–569.

Pottern, L.M., L.E. Morris, W.J. Blot, R.G. Ziegler, and J.F. Fraumeni, Jr. 1981. Esophageal cancer among black men in Washington, D.C. I. Alcohol, tobacco, and other risk factors. J. Natl. Cancer Inst. 67:777–783.

Rebelakos, A., D. Trichopoulos, A. Tzonou, X. Zavitsanos, E. Velonakis, and A. Trichopoulos. 1985. Tobacco smoking, coffee drinking, and occupation as risk factors for bladder cancer in Greece. J. Natl. Cancer Inst. 75:455–461.

Risch, H.A., M. Jain, N.W. Choi, J.G. Fodor, C.J. Pfeiffer, G.R. Howe, L.W. Harrison, K.J. Craib, and A.B. Miller. 1985. Dietary factors and the incidence of cancer of the stomach. Am. J. Epidemiol. 122:947–959.

Risch, H.A., J.D. Burch, A.B. Miller, G.B. Hill, R. Steele, and G.R. Howe. 1988. Dietary factors and the incidence of cancer of the urinary bladder. Am. J. Epidemiol. 127:1179–1191.

Rivlin, R.S. 1986. Riboflavin. Pp. 349–355 in L.A. Poirier, P.M. Newberne, and M.W. Pariza, eds. Essential Nutrients in Carcinogenesis. Advances in Experimental Biology and Medicine, Vol. 206. Plenum Press, New York.

Robinette, C.D., Z. Hrubec, and J.F. Fraumeni. 1979. Chronic alcoholism and subsequent mortality in World War II veterans. Am. J. Epidemiol. 109:687–700.

Ross, R.K., A. Paganini-Hill, and B.E. Henderson. 1983. The etiology of prostate cancer: what does the epidemiology suggest? Prostate 4:333–344.

Rotkin, I.D. 1977. Studies in the epidemiology of prostatic cancer: expanded sampling. Cancer Treat. Rep. 61:173–180.

Salonen, J.T., R. Salonen, R. Lappetelainen, P.H. Maenpaa, G. Alfthan, and P. Puska. 1985. Risk of cancer in relation to serum concentrations of selenium and vitamins A and E: matched case-control analysis of prospective data. Br. Med. J. 290:417–420.

Samet, J.M., B.J. Skipper, C.G. Humble, and D.R. Pathak. 1985. Lung cancer risk and vitamin A consumption in New Mexico. Am. Rev. Respir. Dis. 131:198–202.

Schatzkin, A., D.Y. Jones, R.N. Hoover, P.R. Taylor, L.A. Brinton, R.G. Ziegler, E.B. Harvey, C.L. Carter, L.M. Licitra, M.C. Dufour, and D.B. Larson. 1987. Alcohol consumption and breast cancer in the epidemiologic follow-up study of the first National Health and Nutrition Examination Survey. N. Engl. J. Med. 316:1169–1173.

Schmidt, W., and J. de Lint. 1972. Causes of death of alcoholics. Q. J. Stud. Alcohol, Part A 33:171–185.

Schoenberg, B.S., J.C. Bailar III, and J.F. Fraumeni, Jr. 1971. Certain mortality patterns of esophageal cancer in the United States, 1930–67. J. Natl. Cancer Inst. 46:63–73.

Schrauzer, G.N., D.A. White, and C.J. Schneider. 1977. Cancer mortality correlation studies—IV: associations with dietary intakes and blood levels of certain trace elements, notably Se-antagonists. Bioinorg. Chem. 7:35–56.

Schuman, L.M., J.S. Mandel, A. Radke, U. Seal, and F. Halberg. 1982. Some selected features of the epidemiology of prostatic cancer: Minneapolis-St. Paul, Minnesota case-control study, 1976–1979. Pp. 345–354 in K. Magnus, ed. Trends in Cancer Incidence: Causes and Practical Implications. Hemisphere Publishing Corp., Washington, D.C.

Schwartz, D., J. Lellouch, R. Flamant, and P.F. Denoix. 1962. Alcohol and cancer. Results of a retrospective investigation. Rev. Franc. Etud. Clin. Biol. 7:590–604.

Shank, R.C., J.E. Gordon, G.N. Wogan, A. Nondasuta, and B. Subhamani. 1972a. Dietary aflatoxins and human liver cancer. III. Field survey of rural Thai families for ingested aflatoxins. Food Cosmet. Toxicol. 10:71–84.

Shank, R.C., N. Bhamarapravati, J.E. Gordon, and G.N. Wogan. 1972b. Dietary aflatoxins and human liver cancer. IV. Incidence of primary liver cancer in two municipal populations of Thailand. Food Cosmet. Toxicol. 10:171–179.

Shekelle, R.B., M. Lepper, S. Liu, C. Maliza, W.J. Raynor, Jr., A.H. Rossof, O. Paul, A.M. Shryock, and J. Stamler. 1981. Dietary vitamin A and risk of cancer in the Western Electric study. Lancet 2:1186–1190.

Shigematsu, I. 1984. The epidemiological approach to cadmium pollution in Japan. Ann. Acad. Med. Singapore 13: 231–236.

Shinozuka, H., S.L. Katyal, and M.I.R. Perera. 1986. Choline deficiency and chemical carcinogenesis. Pp. 253–267 in L.A. Poirier, P.M. Newberne, and M.W. Pariza, eds. Essential Nutrients in Carcinogenesis. Advances in Experimental Biology and Medicine, Vol. 206. Plenum Press, New York.

Simon, D., S. Yen, and P. Cole. 1975. Coffee drinking and cancer of the lower urinary tract. J. Natl. Cancer Inst. 54: 587–591.

Smith, A.H., N.E. Pearce, and J.G. Joseph. 1985. Major colorectal aetiological hypotheses do not explain mortality trends among Maori and non-Maori New Zealanders. Int. J. Epidemiol. 14:79–85.

Snowdon, D.A., and R.L. Phillips. 1984. Coffee consumption and risk of fatal cancers. Am. J. Public Health 74:820–823.

Snowdon, D.A., R.L. Phillips, and W. Choi. 1984. Diet, obesity and risk of fatal prostate cancer. Am. J. Epidemiol. 120:244–250.

Stukonis, M.K. 1978. Cancer Incidence Cumulative Rates—International Comparison Based on Data from "Cancer Incidence in Five Continents." IARC Technical Report

No. 78/002. International Agency for Research on Cancer, Lyon, France. 54 pp.

Takahashi, M. 1986. Enhancing effect of a high salt diet on gastrointestinal carcinogenesis. Gan No Rinsho 32:667–673.

Takahashi, M., T. Kokubo, F. Furukawa, Y. Kurokawa, M. Tatematsu, and Y. Hayashi. 1983. Effect of high salt diet on rat gastric carcinogenesis induced by N-methyl-N'-nitro-N-nitrosoguanidine. Gann 74:28–34.

Talamini, R., C. La Vecchia, A. Decarli, S. Francechi, E. Grattoni, E. Grigoletto, A. Liberati, and G. Tognoni. 1984. Social factors, diet and breast cancer in northern Italian population. Br. J. Cancer 49:723–729.

Talamini, R., C. La Vecchia, A. Decarli, E. Negri, and S. Francechi. 1986. Nutrition, social factors and prostatic cancer in Northern Italian population. Br. J. Cancer 53:817–821.

Tannenbaum, S.R., D. Moran, W. Rand, C. Cuello, and P. Correa. 1979. Gastric cancer in Colombia. IV. Nitrite and other ions in gastric contents of residents from a high-risk region. J. Natl. Cancer Inst. 62:9–12.

Thind, I.S. 1986. Diet and cancer—an international study. Int. J. Epidemiol. 15:160–163.

Thomas, D.B., C.N. Uhl, and P. Hartge. 1983. Bladder cancer and alcoholic beverage consumption. Am. J. Epidemiol. 118:720–727.

Thurnham, D.I., P. Rathakette, K.M. Hambidge, N. Muñoz, and M. Crespi. 1982. Riboflavin, vitamin A, and zinc status in Chinese subjects in a high-risk area for oesophageal cancer in China. Hum. Nutr. Clin. Nutr. 36:337–349.

Trichopoulos, D., M. Papapostolou, and A. Polychronopoulou. 1981. Coffee and ovarian cancer. Int. J. Cancer 28:691–693.

Trichopoulos, D., N.E. Day, E. Kaklamani, A. Tzonou, N. Munoz, X. Zavitsanos, Y. Koumantaki, and A. Trichopoulou. 1987. Hepatitis B virus, tobacco smoking, and ethanol consumption in the etiology of hepatocellular carcinoma. Int. J. Cancer 39:45–49.

Tung, T.C., and K.H. Ling. 1968. Study on aflatoxin in foodstuffs in Taiwan. J. Vitaminol. 14:48–52.

Tuyns, A.J. 1983. Oesophageal cancer in non-smoking drinkers and in non-drinking smokers. Int. J. Cancer 32:443–444.

Tuyns, A.J., G. Péquinot, and O.M. Jensen. 1977. Le cancer de l'oesophage en Ille-et-Vilaine en fonction des niveaux de consommation d'alcool et de tabac. Des risques qui se multiplient. Bull. Cancer 64:45–60.

Tuyns, A.J., G. Péquignot, M. Gignoux, and A. Valla. 1982. Cancers of the digestive tract, alcohol and tobacco. Int. J. Cancer. 30:9–11.

Tuyns, A.J., M. Haelterman, and R. Kaaks. 1987. Colorectal cancer and the intake of nutrients: oligosaccharides are a risk factor, fats are not. A case-control study in Belgium. Nutr. Cancer 10:181–196.

Tzonou, A., N.E. Day, D. Trichopoulos, A. Walker, M. Saliaraki, M. Papapostolou, and A. Polychronopoulou. 1984. The epidemiology of ovarian cancer in Greece: a case-control study. Eur. J. Cancer Clin. Oncol. 20:1045–1052.

van Rensburg, S.J. 1981. Epidemiologic and dietary evidence for a specific nutritional predisposition to esophageal cancer. J. Natl. Cancer Inst. 67:243–251.

van Rensburg, S.J., J.J. van der Watt, I.F.H. Purchase, L.P. Coutinho, and R. Markham. 1974. Primary liver cancer

rate and aflatoxin intake in a high cancer area. S. Afr. Med. J. 48:2508a–2508d.

Visek, W.J. 1986. Dietary protein and experimental carcinogenesis. Pp. 163–186 in L.A. Poirier, P.M. Newberne, and M.W. Pariza, eds. Essential Nutrients in Carcinogenesis. Advances in Experimental Medicine and Biology, Vol. 206. Plenum Press, New York.

Wald, N., M. Idle, J. Boreham, and A. Bailey. 1980. Low serum-vitamin-A and subsequent risk of cancer. Preliminary results of a prospective study. Lancet 2:813–815.

Wald, N., J. Boreham, and A. Bailey. 1986. Serum retinol and subsequent risk of cancer. Br. J. Cancer 54:957–961.

Waterhouse, J., C. Muir, P. Correa, and J. Powell, eds. 1976. Cancer Incidence in Five Continents: Vol. III—1976. IARC Scientific Publ. No. 15. International Agency for Research on Cancer, Lyon, France. 584 pp.

Weiss, N.S., J.L. Lyon, J.M. Liff, W.M. Vollmer, and J.R. Daling. 1981. Incidence of ovarian cancer in relation to the use of oral contraceptives. Int. J. Cancer. 28:669–671.

Welsch, C.W. 1987. Enhancement of mammary tumorigenesis by dietary fat: review of potential mechanisms. Am. J. Clin. Nutr. 45 suppl. 1:192–202.

Whittemore, A.S., R.S. Paffenbarger, Jr., K. Anderson, and J. Halpren. 1983. Early precursors of pancreatic cancer in college men. J. Chronic Dis. 36:251–256.

Willett, W.C., M.J. Stampfer, G.A. Colditz, B.A. Rosner, C.H. Hennekens, and F.E. Speizer. 1987a. Dietary fat and the risk of breast cancer. N. Engl. J. Med. 316:22–28.

Willett, W.C., M.J. Stampfer, G.A. Colditz, B.A. Rosner, C.H. Hennekens, and F.E. Speizer. 1987b. Moderate alcohol consumption and the risk of breast cancer. N. Engl. J. Med. 316:1174–1180.

Williams, R.R., and J.W. Horm. 1977. Association of cancer sites with tobacco and alcohol consumption and socioeconomic status of patients: interview study from the Third National Cancer Survey. J. Natl. Cancer Inst. 58:525–547.

Wogan, G.N. 1975. Dietary factors and special epidemiological situations of liver cancer in Thailand and Africa. Cancer Res. 35:3499–3502.

Wynder, E.L. 1975. The epidemiology of large bowel cancer. Cancer Res. 35:3388–3394.

Wynder, E.L., and I.J. Bross. 1961. A study of etiological factors in cancer of the esophagus. Cancer 14:389–413.

Wynder, E.L., and G.B. Gori. 1977. Contribution of the environment to cancer incidence: an epidemiologic exercise. J. Natl. Cancer Inst. 58:825–832.

Wynder, E.L., G.C. Escher, and N. Mantel. 1966. An epidemiological investigation of cancer of the endometrium. Cancer 19:489–520.

Wynder, E.L., K. Mabuchi, and W.F. Whitmore, Jr. 1971. Epidemiology of cancer of the prostate. Cancer 28:344–360.

Wynder, E.L., K. Mabuchi, N. Maruchi, and J.G. Fortner. 1973. Epidemiology of cancer of the pancreas. J. Natl. Cancer Inst. 50:645–667.

Wynder, E.L., N.E. Hall, and M. Polansky. 1983. Epidemiology of coffee and pancreatic cancer. Cancer Res. 43:3900–3906.

Wynder, E.L., J.R. Hebert, and G.C. Kabat. 1987. Association of dietary fat and lung cancer. J. Natl. Cancer Inst. 79:631–637.

Yang, C.S. 1980. Research on esophageal cancer in China: a review. Cancer Res. 40:2633–2644.

Yu, M.C., T. Mack, R. Hanisch, R.L. Peters, B.E. Henderson, and M.C. Pike. 1983. Hepatitis, alcohol consumption, cigarette smoking, and hepatocellular carcinoma in Los Angeles. Cancer Res. 43:6077–6079.

Zaldivar, R. 1977. Nitrate fertilizers as environmental pollutants: positive correlation between nitrates ($NaNO_3$ and KNO_3) used per unit area and stomach cancer mortality rates. Experientia 33:264–265.

Zaridze, D.G., M. Blettner, N.N. Trapeznikov, J.P. Kuvshinov, E.G. Matiakin, B.P. Poljakov, B.K. Poddubni, S.M. Parshikova, V.I. Rottenberg, F.S. Chamrakulov, M.M.

Chodjaeva, H.F. Stich, M.P. Rosin, D.I. Thurnham, D. Hoffmann, and K.D. Brunnemann. 1985. Survey of a population with a high incidence of oral and oesophageal cancer. Int. J. Cancer 36:153–158.

Ziegler, R.G., T.J. Mason, A. Stemhagen, R. Hoover, J.B. Schoenberg, G. Gridley, P.W. Virgo, R. Altman, and J.F. Fraumeni, Jr. 1984. Dietary carotene and vitamin A and risk of lung cancer among white men in New Jersey. J. Natl. Cancer Inst. 73:1429–1435.

23

Osteoporosis

Osteoporosis is a multifactorial, complex disorder characterized by an asymptomatic reduction in the quantity of bone mass per unit volume. When bone mass becomes too low, structural integrity and mechanical support are not maintained and fractures occur with minimal trauma. The most common sites of osteoporotic fracture are the proximal femur, distal radius (Colles' fracture), vertebrae, humerus, pelvis, and ribs. In clinical research, the diagnosis of osteoporosis is frequently applied only to patients in whom one or more fractures have already occurred (NIH, 1984), even though it can now be detected by measuring bone mass with single- or dual-photon absorptiometry (Mazess and Barden, 1987) or with quantitative computed tomography (Genant et al., 1987).

Osteoporosis occurs most frequently in postmenopausal white women and in the elderly of both sexes (Cummings et al., 1985). Approximately 20% of women in the United States suffer one or more osteoporotic fractures by age 65, and as many as 40% sustain fractures after age 65.

Osteoporosis is not frequently observed in men and black women until after age 60, after which fracture rates progressively increase in these groups. For additional information on the distribution and importance of osteoporosis in the population, see Chapter 5.

BONE AND MINERAL METABOLISM

Bone is composed primarily of calcium and phosphorus, in the form of hydroxyapatite crystals deposited in a collagen matrix (Veis and Sabsay, 1987). Adult humans have two types of bone—cortical and trabecular. Cortical bone provides rigidity and is the major component of tubular bones (the appendicular skeleton). Trabecular bone is spongy in appearance, provides strength and elasticity, and constitutes at least 50% of the vertebrae (the axial skeleton) (Arnaud and Kolb, 1986).

Bone is a metabolically active tissue that is constantly being replaced. This process is regulated by cellular activities that resorb (osteoclastic) and form (osteoblastic) bone (Baron et al., 1984). In normal adult bone, resorption and formation are in balance. When one of these activities increases or decreases, the other shifts in degree and direction so that there is no net change in the total amount of bone (Frost, 1964, 1977).

Since the driving force for changing net bone mass is intrinsic to the cellular processes that govern bone resorption and formation, functional uncoupling of these cellular processes is required to either increase or decrease bone mass. The major mineral ions of bone (calcium, phosphorus, and magnesium) must be present at physiological concentrations in extracellular fluids for bone mineralization (formation) to occur normally (Marel et al., 1986) and play a passive role in any mass changes that occur. They help to replace minerals lost by obligatory processes (in urine, feces, and sweat) or those normally distributed to bone and soft tissues (Heaney, 1986).

Maximum bone mass is achieved by about 25 to 30 years of age, is maintained without much change until 35 to 45 years of age, and is lost at a constant rate of 0.2 to 0.5% per year in men and women thereafter (Heaney, 1986; Marcus, 1982; Parfitt, 1983). About 8 to 10 years immediately before and after menopause, women lose bone at a rate of 2 to 5% per year. Subsequently, bone loss returns to the slower rate shared by the sexes. Those few men who also lose sex hormone function usually very late in life (>70 years) also lose bone mass at rates similar to postmenopausal women (Odell and Swerdloff, 1976).

EVIDENCE ASSOCIATING DIETARY FACTORS WITH OSTEOPOROSIS

Epidemiologic and Clinical Studies
Calcium

Absorption and Balance

Calcium balance generally reflects the degree to which bone formation is coupled with resorption (see Chapter 13). Thus, negative balances are recorded when bone resorption exceeds formation, and positive balances occur when bone formation exceeds bone resorption. Since 99% of the body's calcium is located in bone, it is not possible to build bone without positive calcium balance or to be in negative balance without losing bone. The metabolic technique used to determine calcium balance has important theoretical and practical limitations that can result in inaccuracies in determining the amount of dietary calcium needed to achieve zero balance—data that are key to determining nutritional requirements for calcium.

Calcium balance depends on such factors as the amount of calcium in the diet, the efficiency of calcium absorption by the intestine, and the losses of calcium in the urine, feces, and sweat. Intestinal absorption decreases with age (Gallagher et al., 1979; Ireland and Fordtran, 1973). This may be due to the age-related decrease in serum levels of 1,25-dihydroxy vitamin D [1,25(OH)$_2$D$_3$] (Tsai et al., 1984)—the biologically active metabolite of vitamin D produced by the kidney that regulates intestinal absorption of calcium (DeLuca, 1983; Norman, 1985). The age-related decrease in cal-

cium absorption may lead to secondary hyperparathyroidism. That this endocrine adaptive response occurs is supported by the observation that serum immunoreactive and bioactive parathyroid hormone increases with age (Forero et al., 1987). Whether this response to decreased calcium absorption contributes to the decreased skeletal mass and increased incidence of fractures in the elderly is not known.

Relationship of Dietary Calcium to Bone Mass, Osteoporosis, and Fracture

There are two major methodological problems involved in evaluating the evidence relating dietary calcium to bone mass (see Chapter 13). First are the inaccuracies inherent in determining dietary calcium by historical recall. Second are the different methods used to measure bone mass—some measure predominantly cortical bone and others measure predominantly trabecular bone.

Decreased skeletal mass is the most important risk factor for bone fracture without significant trauma (Heaney, 1986; Heaney et al., 1982; Parfitt, 1983; Riggs and Melton, 1986). It is important to achieve genetically programmed peak bone mass, because the greater the mass attained before age-related loss, the less likely bone loss will reach the level at which fracture will occur (Heaney, 1986; Marcus, 1982; Parfitt, 1983).

The quantity of dietary calcium required to achieve peak bone mass is greater than that required to replace obligatory losses of this ion in urine, feces, and sweat (approximately 200 to 300 mg/day). Thus, as described in Chapter 13, people under the age of 25 years need to ingest sufficient calcium to ensure that they absorb more calcium from their intestines than they excrete and thus achieve positive balance.

Many published reports have shown either no relationship or only a modest positive relationship between dietary calcium and cortical bone mass (see Chapter 13). The most widely cited of the papers showing a positive effect of calcium is that of Matkovic et al. (1979), who reported a 5 to 10% greater metacarpal cortical volume in the inhabitants of a Yugoslavian district with a high calcium intake as compared with the inhabitants of a Yugoslavian district with a low calcium intake. The population in the high-calcium district also consumed more calories, fats, and protein and fewer carbohydrates than did the population in the low-calcium district. People in the high-calcium district had a 50% lower incidence of hip fractures and a significantly greater metacarpal cortical bone volume than did the inhabitants of the low-calcium district. Because the differences in bone mass as a function of age were constant, it is possible that high life-long calcium intakes did not prevent bone loss in this population but, rather, increased peak cortical bone mass. Contrasting sharply with these results are those of Riggs et al. (1987), who found no relationship between the calcium intakes (range, 260 to 2,003 mg/day; mean, 922 mg/day) of 106 normal women ages 23 to 84 years and the rates at which changes occurred in bone mineral density at the midradius (determined by single-photon absorptiometry) and the lumbar spine (determined by dual-photon absorptiometry) over a mean period of 4.1 years.

Dietary calcium intake has been associated with bone fracture rates in two ecological studies. In a comparison of 12 countries, Nordin (1966) reported an inverse graded association between frequency of osteoporotic vertebral fracture, as determined by x-rays of the spine, and calcium intakes. Japanese women, whose calcium intake averaged 400 mg/day, had the highest frequency of fracture, whereas women in Finland, where calcium intake was highest (1,300 mg/day), had the lowest frequency of fracture. This relationship did not hold in The Gambia and Jamaica, where there were low rates of osteoporotic fractures despite relatively low calcium intakes (Nordin, 1966). In the study described above, Matkovic et al. (1979) found that the incidence of hip fracture in the Yugoslavian district with a high-calcium intake was 50% lower than that in the low-calcium district, but no difference was detected in the incidence of fractures around the wrist.

Most clinical studies show lower calcium intakes by osteoporotic patients than by age-matched control subjects (see Chapter 13). Dietary calcium was lower than 800 mg/day for patients and controls in all these investigations. In one study of subjects with intakes greater than 800 mg/day (Nordin et al., 1979), no differences in calcium intake were found between osteoporotic patients and controls. This finding supports the view by Heaney (1986) that low dietary calcium may play a permissive rather than a causative role in the development of osteoporosis and that this role can be demonstrated best when dietary calcium is below a "saturation" level.

Effects of Supplementation on Bone Mass and Fracture

There is no direct evidence that the impairment of intestinal calcium absorption observed during menopause and aging can be overcome by calcium supplementation. Moreover, the evidence that calcium supplementation prevents the trabecular bone loss associated with menopause is at best weak. There is strong evidence, however, that calcium supplementation has a modest influence on preventing cortical bone loss. The evidence relating calcium supplementation to fracture prevalence is scanty. In a nonrandomized prospective study of the effect of various treatments on reducing vertebral fractures in women with generalized osteopenia, Riggs et al. (1982) observed that eight subjects receiving calcium carbonate (1,500–2,500 mg/day) and 19 receiving calcium supplementation plus vitamin D (50,000 IU once or twice a week) had 50% fewer vertebral fractures than did 27 placebo-treated subjects and 18 untreated controls.

As discussed in Chapter 13, calcium supplementation should therefore not be used as a substitute for sex hormone replacement, which prevents postmenopausal bone loss in most patients and appears to restore intestinal calcium absorption toward normal (Gallagher et al., 1980a). There is little justification for increasing the calcium intake above the Recommended Dietary Allowance (RDA) for women on estrogen replacement therapy. However, it seems prudent to recommend a higher calcium intake ($\sim$1,200 mg/day) for menopausal and postmenopausal women considered to be at risk for osteoporosis, but who either refuse to take estrogen or cannot do so for medical reasons. This could delay loss of cortical bone and prevent chronic secondary hyperparathyroidism. Some men over age 60 could benefit from supplementation for the same reasons. Evidence suggests that calcium intakes up to 2,000 mg/day are safe for teenagers and adults (Heath and Callaway, 1985; Knapp, 1947).

Phosphorus

Increased levels of dietary phosphorus have been shown to promote fecal calcium loss while reducing urinary excretion of calcium with the usual net effect of maintaining calcium balance. This explains why calcium balance is maintained in most normal people on a high-phosphorus diet (see Chapter 13).

The mechanism by which increased dietary phosphorus decreases intestinal absorption of calcium has been investigated by Portale et al. (1986). These investigators showed that increasing dietary phosphorus from a low intake of <500 mg/day to 3,000 mg/day decreased the production rate of $1,25(OH)_2D_3$ to the extent that its serum concentrations fell from a level 80% higher than normal to the low-normal range. This observation strongly suggests that the ability to adapt to decreases or increases in dietary phosphorus depends on the ability of the kidney to respond by increasing or decreasing its production of $1,25(OH)_2D_3$.

There is therefore a question whether increases in dietary phosphorus might adversely influence calcium economy in people whose kidneys have a limited capacity to produce $1,25(OH)_2D_3$ or in people who need to be in positive calcium balance. Portale et al. (1984) reported that normal dietary phosphorus levels were sufficient to suppress plasma concentrations of $1,25(OH)_2D_3$ in children with moderate renal insufficiency. No studies of the influence of dietary phosphorus on calcium and bone metabolism have been reported in other populations that may be unduly sensitive to increments in dietary phosphorus above the RDA (e.g., young people who are building bone or those such as the elderly who have a decreased ability to absorb or conserve calcium), even though there has been concern (Bell et al., 1977; Lutwak, 1975) that high phosphorus intakes may contribute to age-related bone loss in humans.

Vitamin D

Numerous studies during the past two decades suggest that elderly people in the United States, Israel, Great Britain, and Europe are at increased risk for developing vitamin D deficiency (see Chapter 11). Prolonged and severe deficiency of vitamin D results in osteomalacia—a disorder characterized by an increased proportion of bone matrix that is not mineralized (Frame and Parfitt, 1978; Parfitt et al., 1982).

Many recent studies show a progressive decline in the serum concentrations of the major circulating form of vitamin D—25-hydroxy vitamin D— with aging, but there is no convincing evidence that the incidence of osteomalacia is increased in the elderly. Poskitt et al. (1979) speculated that these decreased serum levels of 25-hydroxy vitamin D result from the tendency for older people to remain indoors and thus to have less exposure to the sun. However true this might be, MacLaughlin and Holick (1985) have provided data supporting an alternative and possibly complementary explanation. They have found an age-dependent decrease in the epidermal concentrations of 7-dehydrocholesterol (provitamin D_3). Skin biopsies showed that elderly subjects had as much as a twofold lower capacity to produce vitamin D_3 than

did young adults. It is likely, therefore, that the elderly have a decreased capacity to synthesize vitamin D in the skin.

Protein

Few epidemiologic investigations have assessed whether high levels of protein in natural mixed diets are a risk factor for osteoporosis (Marsh et al., 1980; Mazess and Mather, 1974). Studies conducted over most of the past half century have established that purified protein, taken in increased quantities as an isolated nutrient, dramatically increases the renal excretion of calcium (see Chapter 8). However, protein is not normally ingested as an isolated and purified nutrient; most protein-rich foods contain many other nutrients that could aggravate or counteract the calciuric effect of protein per se. For example, if phosphorus intake increases with protein intake, as it does in typical U.S. diets, the calciuric effect of protein is minimized (Hegsted et al., 1981; Schuette and Linkswiler, 1982).

Heaney and Recker (1982) evaluated the influence of a 50% increase in the protein content of natural whole foods on urinary calcium and calcium balance in 170 perimenopausal women who were given diets containing their usual individual intakes of calcium, phosphorus, nitrogen, and caffeine. These investigators found that the calciuric effect of natural protein was much smaller than that produced by purified proteins. Using a series of regression equations generated from the dietary intake and calcium balance data recorded in their study, they calculated that a 50% increase in natural protein intake would lead to a negative calcium balance of 32 mg/day—an amount that approaches the 40 mg/day negative balance needed to account for the mean 1 to 1.5% loss in skeletal mass per year observed in postmenopausal women. It is thus possible that increases in dietary protein exceeding 66 g/day contribute to the negative calcium balance frequently observed in perimenopausal women. In the United States, many perimenopausal women consume diets containing considerably more protein than this (Christakis and Frankle, 1974). The effects of high-protein diets on the elderly have not been systematically studied.

Fiber

Investigations over the past five decades (Dobbs and Baird, 1977; Ismail-Beigi et al., 1977; McCance et al., 1942; Reinhold et al., 1976) show that fiber chelates calcium (and other minerals) in the gastrointestinal tract and is therefore a potential cause of mineral deficiency. High-fiber diets may increase osteoporosis risk in such countries as Iran, where Bazari bread provides as much as 50% of the caloric needs of children. Although this bread contains more calcium than does white bread, its high fiber and phytate content leads to decreased intestinal absorption of calcium, magnesium, zinc, and phosphorus (Reinhold et al., 1976). The effect of fiber on mineral status at the levels consumed in the United States is unclear (see Chapter 10).

Kelsay et al. (1979) provided 12 adult males two different diets for 26 days (a high-fiber diet containing fruit and vegetables and a low-fiber diet containing fruit and vegetable juice) to determine their effects on calcium balance. Balance was +72 mg/day in those on the low-fiber diet and −122 mg/day in those on the high-fiber diet. In a follow-up study in which oxalate was removed from the diet, those investigators found that calcium balance was positive and was not influenced by fiber. Sandstead et al. (1979) reported that fiber added to diets caused negative calcium balance, and they calculated that the requirement for dietary calcium is increased as much as 150 mg/day when dietary fiber is increased by 26 g. Cummings et al. (1979) showed that the addition of 31 g of wheat fiber to the diets of subjects already consuming a high-protein diet produced a greater negative balance than the high-protein diet alone, suggesting an interaction of protein and fiber that causes greater negative calcium balance than when either is given alone.

Fluoride

Mertz (1981) has argued that fluoride is an essential trace element responsible for growth and maintenance of bones and teeth (see Chapter 14). However, since the dietary intake of fluoride is only 0.3 to 0.5 mg/day (Jenkins, 1967) and an additional 1 to 2 mg/day provided in drinking water (1 ppm) appears to have no demonstrable effect on bone structure (Riggs, 1984), it seems unlikely that fluoride is an important factor in osteoporosis risk for most Americans.

By contrast, the incidence of osteosclerosis is high in areas where the fluoride concentration in the drinking water is moderately high (5 to 10 ppm) (Leone et al., 1955), and there is a lower prevalence of osteoporosis in these areas than in low-fluoride regions (Bernstein et al., 1966; Leone, 1960). In areas with even higher fluoride intakes, such as the Punjab region of India, there is some crippling fluorosis (characterized by dense bones, exostoses, neurological complications, osteoarthritis, and ligamentous calcification) and, more commonly, asymptomatic osteosclerosis (Singh et al., 1963). In a prospective but unrandomized study, Riggs et al. (1982) observed that treatment of osteoporotic patients with pharmacological doses of fluoride and calcium reduced the vertebral fracture rate to approximately one-quarter that of untreated patients—a lower rate than was observed in patients treated with calcium alone.

Alcohol

Bone formation is decreased in patients who abuse alcohol. This causes a dramatic decrease in bone mass as compared with that in normal subjects (Bikle et al., 1985; Nilsson and Westlin, 1973). Since the risk of falling is increased in alcoholics, these two factors are probably responsible for the increased risk of hip and vertebral fracture reported in alcoholic men and women (see Chapter 16).

Animal Studies

Nordin (1960) reviewed an extensive literature describing the many species that develop decreased bone mass as a result of calcium deficiency (see Chapter 13). In all these studies, the bone disease produced by calcium deficiency most resembles osteoporosis. Low-calcium diets cause a loss of trabecular bone in adult cats (Bauer et al., 1929) and a generalized thinning of bone in dogs (Jaffe et al., 1932). After feeding adult cats a low-calcium diet for 5 months, Jowsey and Gershon-Cohen (1964) found that the animals had decreased skeletal weight, decreased bone density as determined radiographically, and increased bone resorption as shown by microradiographic evidence. These changes were partially reversed by refeeding the animals a diet containing more calcium. At present, however, there is no completely satisfactory animal model of postmenopausal or age-related osteoporosis. This deficiency is a major impediment to future progress in osteoporosis research.

In contrast to the apparent inability of rather dramatic changes in dietary phosphorus to influence calcium balance in normal human subjects, there is considerable evidence in animals that diets containing relatively larger quantities of phosphorus than calcium cause hyperparathyroidism and bone loss. Almost all the reports concern young growing or aged animals and thus differ from investigations in humans, which in general focus on young or middle-aged adults (see Chapter 13).

The committee found no relevant studies in animals focusing on the effects of dietary protein, fiber, and vitamin D on bone mass and rate of bone fracture.

EVIDENCE ASSOCIATING NONDIETARY FACTORS WITH OSTEOPOROSIS

Age and Sex

Age is a major risk factor for fracture, because bone mass is lost progressively with aging and the strength of bone is highly correlated with its mass and mineral content (Carter and Hayes, 1976; Dalen et al., 1976; Horsman and Currey, 1983; Rockoff et al., 1969). In the United States, the incidence of hip fracture increases dramatically after age 70 in both sexes but is twice as high among white women as among white men (Farmer et al., 1984; Gallagher et al., 1980b). Gallagher et al. (1980b) estimated that an adult white woman in the United States who attains the average lifespan of 80 years has a 15% lifetime risk of suffering a hip fracture compared to 5% for a white male whose life expectancy is 75 years. The risk of Colles' fracture is 6 to 8 times greater among elderly white women than among white men. Fractures of the humerus and pelvis are also more common in the elderly; 70 to 80% of these fractures result from minimal trauma (Melton et al., 1981; Rose et al., 1982). Several investigators speculated that the lower incidence of osteoporotic fractures in men may be due to the greater bone mass in men than in women of all ages (Cummings et al., 1985; Garn, 1970). However, there are no reliable data on the influence of age, sex, or race on vertebral fractures.

Race

Blacks in the United States suffer fewer osteoporotic fractures than do whites, presumably because they have a higher bone mass, greater bone density, thicker bony cortex, and greater vertebral density (Cohn et al., 1977; Smith and Rizek, 1966; Trotter et al., 1960). Black women have about one-half the age-specific incidence rates of hip fractures as white women (Bollett et al., 1965; Engh et al., 1968; Iskrant, 1968), and hip fractures are unusual among blacks in Africa (Solomon, 1968).

Asian-Americans have less cortical bone mass than age-matched whites (Garn et al., 1964; Yano et al., 1984). However, incidence rates of hip and other fractures have not been reported for Asian or Hispanic populations in the United States.

Genetics and Familial Factors

The role of heredity and family history in determining bone mass and susceptibility to fracture have not been well studied. Garn (1970) found that metacarpal dimensions of siblings were somewhat more highly correlated ($R = .37$) than those of parents and children ($R = .23$). In a study of young male twins, Smith et al. (1973) reported that there was a slightly greater variance in cortical bone mass between pairs of dizygotic twins than between pairs of monozygotic twins.

Peri- and Postmenopausal Estrogens

Nilas and Christiansen (1987) assessed bone mass in relation to age, menopausal status, and serum concentrations of sex hormones in 178 healthy Danish women ages 29 to 78 years. They observed that the menopause has a greater influence on bone loss than does chronological age.

Physiological doses of estrogen prevent or retard the bone loss associated with oophorectomy or menopause (Christiansen et al., 1980; Genant et al., 1982; Horsman and Currey, 1983; Horsman et al., 1977; Lindsay et al., 1976; Nachtigall et al., 1979; Recker et al., 1977; Riis et al., 1987). When estrogen therapy is discontinued, loss of cortical bone mass resumes at a rate similar to that observed immediately after the menopause (Christiansen et al., 1981; Lindsay et al., 1978).

The risk of hip and vertebral fracture appears to be reduced by at least 50% as long as estrogen is taken (Paganini-Hill et al., 1981; Weiss et al., 1980). Long-term use of estrogen has been reported to reduce rates of new vertebral deformities and fractures (Ettinger et al., 1985; Gordan et al., 1973; Lindsay et al., 1980; Riggs et al., 1982). It is not clear, however, whether postmenopausal women not taking estrogen who lose cortical bone rapidly have lower serum concentrations of estrogen than those who lose cortical bone slowly (Aloia et al., 1983; Avioli, 1981; Riis et al., 1984). Treatment with estrogen unopposed by progestogen is associated with an increased risk of endometrial cancer (Hulka et al., 1980; Kelsey and Hildreth, 1983; Ziel and Finkle, 1975). Hypogonadal males develop an osteoporotic syndrome similar to oophorectomized or postmenopausal women (Odell and Swerdloff, 1976).

Cigarette Smoking

Most, but not all, studies show that smoking is associated with reduced bone mass as well as an increased risk of vertebral and hip fractures in women (Aloia et al., 1985; Cummings et al., 1985) and of vertebral fractures in men (Seeman et al., 1983). These effects may involve an alteration in the hepatic metabolism of estrogen (Michonovicz et al., 1986) and a reduction in the amount of adipose tissue in most smokers, both of which result in decreased concentrations of circulating estrogen.

Physical Inactivity

Lack of physical activity results in decreased bone mass (Dietrick et al., 1948; Donaldson et al., 1970; Whedon and Shorr, 1957). The osteoporosis produced can be localized (associated with fracture casting or painful limbs), generalized (associated with prolonged bed rest or space travel), or neurological (associated with paraplegia or quadriplegia). Its causes are unknown; the absence of stress and muscle pull on bone may be a common etiologic factor. Resumption of normal weight-bearing activity restores both trabecular and cortical bone (Mazess and Whedon, 1983; Whedon, 1984).

Studies of the influence of increased physical activity on bone mass have produced mixed results. Many studies have shown that exercise of sufficient intensity and duration to produce amenorrhea can result in marked decreases in bone mineral density (Cann et al., 1984; Drinkwater et al., 1984; Lindberg et al., 1987; Marcus et al., 1985; Nelson et al., 1986). Among women who have amenorrhea from diverse causes, however, those who exercise regularly have greater bone density than those who are more sedentary (Rigotti et al., 1984).

Most controlled trials suggest that moderate exercise may have a modest effect in preventing postmenopausal bone loss (Aloia et al., 1978; Krolner et al., 1983; White et al., 1984). Unfortunately, a randomized design was not used in these studies, and sample size and statistical power were inadeqate in most. The effectiveness of walking in preventing bone loss has not been well studied.

Adiposity

The major source of estrogen in postmenopausal women is provided by the conversion of an-

drostenedione to estrone in adipose tissue (Grodin et al., 1973). Obese women produce more estrone than do thin women (MacDonald et al., 1978; Schindler et al., 1972). This difference has been suggested as the reason for the twofold increase in the risk of hip and Colles' fracture in thin women as compared to obese women (Cummings et al., 1985).

Concentrations of sex hormone-binding globulin also tend to be lower in obese women, further increasing the availability of free estrogen (Davidson et al., 1982; Grodin et al., 1973; MacDonald et al., 1978; Schindler et al., 1972). These observations may explain why thin women have less cortical bone mass than obese women (Danielli, 1976; Saville and Nilsson, 1966; Smith et al., 1972).

Reproductive History

High parity and long lactation periods are generally associated with increased bone mass and decreased risk of fracture (Alderman et al., 1986). This may be due to the increased intestinal absorption of calcium during pregnancy and lactation. Limited data suggest that age at menarche has no effect on the later development of osteoporotic fractures (Kreiger et al., 1982).

Previous Fractures

The occurrence of Colles' fracture in women is associated with only a small increase in risk for hip fracture (Owen et al., 1982). However, women who have had a hip fracture have twice the risk of suffering a contralateral hip fracture (Melton et al., 1982). It has not been established that hip fracture risk is increased in patients who have suffered vertebral fractures.

Other Medical Conditions

Patients with noninsulin-dependent diabetes mellitus are not at increased risk for hip fracture (Heath et al., 1980); however, some people with insulin-dependent diabetes have less bone mass than expected for their age (Hui et al., 1985). Other medical conditions that may aggravate bone loss and increase the incidence of fracture associated with aging include primary hyperparathyroidism, hyperthyroidism (spontaneous or iatrogenic), Cushing's syndrome (spontaneous or iatrogenic), chronic renal failure, hemochromatosis, vitamin C deficiency, and severe protein deficiency (Arnaud, 1987). Hip fractures are also more frequent in patients with severe disability from rheumatoid arthritis (Hooyman et al., 1984) and neurological disorders.

SUMMARY

Osteoporosis is a reduction in bone mass that is not usually apparent until minimal trauma causes a fracture. By age 65, approximately 20% of U.S. women suffer one or more osteoporotic fractures. In the elderly, secondary hyperparathyroidism, a condition that is generally associated with bone demineralization, may be caused by defects in intestinal calcium absorption. The long-term effects of increased calcium intake on bone mass after the menopause are not well established. Increased calcium intake is inferior to estrogen in slowing cortical bone loss during the period of rapid bone loss after menopause, and it has even less or no effect on the loss of trabecular bone. In contrast, estrogen prevents trabecular bone loss almost completely in most patients.

Relatively small increments in dietary phosphorus could interfere significantly with intestinal calcium absorption under conditions of increased physiological need for calcium or in patients who for one reason or another have a decreased renal capacity to produce $1,25(OH)_2D_3$ (such as patients with various degrees of renal failure). The calciuric effect of a high-protein diet is at least partially offset by the hypocalciuric effect of inorganic phosphorus, which is present in abundant quantities in most natural sources of protein. Although it is known that dietary fiber can chelate minerals and increase the fecal excretion of minerals, the effect of high dietary fiber on calcium balance is not clear.

Studies in rats, mice, cats, dogs, and nonhuman primates have shown that a diet low in calcium or high in phosphorus leads to increased bone resorption typical of hyperparathyroidism as well as a generalized decrease in bone mass.

White women are 2 to 3 times more likely to suffer a hip fracture than black women and men of both races. Other factors influencing osteoporosis risk are estrogen-replacement therapy, reproductive history, adiposity, cigarette smoking, alcohol intake, physical activity, previous fractures, and other medical conditions.

The evidence relating dietary calcium to bone mass is at best weak. A daily intake of 800 mg is appropriate for women between the ages of 25 and 45. Intakes of 1,200 mg/day between the ages of 10 and 25 may be required to achieve peak bone mass. High calcium intakes may help to prevent loss of cortical bone in some women after age 45 and in some men after age 65. Such intakes can be acheived with a judicious diet. However, patterns of food and beverage consumption associated with low calcium intakes (e.g., diets low in milk products) may necessitate calcium supplementation in some individuals.

DIRECTIONS FOR RESEARCH

• The age at which peak bone mass is achieved in men and women and the influence of calcium supplementation and exercise on peak bone mass need to be determined in prospective studies.

• Dietary requirements for calcium during and immediately before menopause need to be determined in different population groups by using modern measurement techniques. If consensus on the requirements can be reached, investigations can then proceed to determine if therapeutic lowering of requirements by increasing the fraction of calcium absorbed from the diet influences the rate at which bone is lost in these subjects.

• Intestinal absorption of calcium is decreased in people 65 years old and older. It is presently not known if calcium deficiency in this age group contributes to the progressive decline in skeletal mass observed with aging. Long-term studies should be conducted to determine the effect of calcium supplementation on the rate at which bone mass is lost in this age group.

• Dietary phosphorus, protein, and fiber each have separate and potentially deleterious effects on calcium economy. Studies should be conducted to determine their individual and joint effects on calcium balance in people with a diminished ability to increase the renal production of $1,25$-$(OH)_2D_3$ (i.e., the elderly) and in those with a need to be in positive calcium balance (i.e., adolescents).

• There is a need for continued research to develop noninvasive, quantitative, analytical techniques that can accurately identify individuals at risk for osteoporotic fracture.

REFERENCES

Alderman, B.W., N.S. Weiss, J.R. Daling, C.L. Ure, and J.H. Ballard. 1986. Reproductive history and postmenopausal risk of hip and forearm fracture. Am. J. Epidemiol. 124:262–267.
Aloia, J.F., S.H. Cohn, J.A. Ostuni, R. Cane, and K. Ellis. 1978. Prevention of involutional bone loss by exercise. Ann. Intern. Med. 89:356–358.

Aloia, J.F., A.N. Vaswani, J.K. Yeh, P. Ross, K. Ellis, and S.H. Cohn. 1983. Determinants of bone mass in postmenopausal women. Arch. Int. Med. 143:1700–1704.

Aloia, J.F., S.H. Cohn, A. Vaswani, J.K. Yeh, K. Yuen, and K. Ellis. 1985. Risk factors for postmenopausal osteoporosis. Am. J. Med. 78:95–100.

Arnaud, C.D. 1987. Calcium homeostasis and the pathogenesis of osteoporosis. Pp. 13–17 in H.K. Genant ed. Osteoporosis Update 1987: Perspectives for Internists, Gynecologists, Orthopaedists, Radiologists, and Nuclear Physicians. University of California Printing Services, Berkeley, Calif.

Arnaud, C.D., and F.O. Kolb. 1986. The calciotropic hormones and metabolic bone disease. Pp. 202–271 in F.S. Greenspan, and P.H. Forsham eds. Basic and Clinical Endocrinology, 2nd ed. Lange Medical Publ., Los Altos, Calif.

Avioli, L.V. 1981. The endocrinology of involutional osteoporosis. Pp. 343–351 in H.F. DeLuca, H.M. Frost, W.S.S. Jee, C.G. Johnston, Jr. and A.M. Parfitt, eds. Osteoporosis: Recent Advances in Pathogenesis and Treatment. University Park Press, Baltimore.

Baron, R., A. Vignery, and M. Horowitz. 1984. Lymphocytes, macrophages and the regulation of bone remodeling. Pp. 175–243 in W.A. Peck, ed. Bone and Mineral Research, Annual/2: A Yearly Survey of Developments in the Field of Bone and Mineral Metabolism. Elsevier, Amsterdam.

Bauer W., J.C. Aub, and F. Albright. 1929. Studies of calcium and phosphorus metabolism. V. A study of the bone trabeculae as a readily available reserve supply of calcium. J. Exp. Med. 49:145–161.

Bell, R.R., H.H. Draper, D.Y.M. Tszeng, H.K. Shin, and G.R. Schmidt. 1977. Physiological responses of human adults to foods containing phosphate additives. J. Nutr. 107:42–50.

Bernstein, D.S., N. Sadowski, D.M. Hegsted, C.D. Guri, and F.J. Stare. 1966. Prevalence of osteoporosis in high- and low-fluoride areas in North Dakota. J. Am. Med. Assoc. 198:499–504.

Bikle, D.D., H.K. Genant, C. Cann, R.R. Recker, B.P. Halloran, and G.J. Strewler. 1985. Bone disease in alcohol abuse. Ann. Intern. Med. 103:42–48.

Bollett, A.J., G. Engh, and W. Parson. 1965. Epidemiology of osteoporosis: sex and race incidence of hip fractures. Arch. Intern. Med. 116:191–194.

Cann, C.E., M.C. Martin, H.K. Genant, and R.B. Jaffee. 1984. Decreased spinal mineral content in amenorrheic women. J. Am. Med. Assoc. 251:626–629.

Carter, D.R., and W.C. Hayes. 1976. Bone compressive strength: the influence of density and strain rate. Science 194:1174–1176.

Christakis, G., and R.T. Frankle. 1974. Expensive beef: a blessing in disguise? Ann. Intern. Med. 80:547–549.

Christiansen, C., M.S. Christensen, P. McNair, C. Hagen, K.E. Stocklund, and I. Transbol. 1980. Prevention of early postmenopausal bone loss: controlled 2-year study in 315 normal females. Eur. J. Clin. Invest. 10:273–279.

Christiansen, C., M.S. Christensen, and I. Transbol. 1981. Bone mass in postmenopausal women after withdrawal of oestrogen/gestagen replacement therapy. Lancet 1:459–461.

Cohn, S.H., C. Abesamis, S. Yasumura, J.F. Aloia, I. Zanzi, and K.J. Ellis. 1977. Comparative skeletal mass and radial bone mineral content in black and white women. Metabolism 26:171–178.

Cummings, J.H., M.J. Hill, T. Jivraj, H. Houston, W.J. Branch, and D.J.A. Jenkins. 1979. The effect of meat protein and dietary fiber on colonic function and metabolism. I. Changes in bowel habit, bile acid excretion, and calcium absorption. Am. J. Clin. Nutr. 32:2086–2093.

Cummings, S.R., J.L. Kelsey, M.C. Nevitt, and K.J. O'Dowd. 1985. Epidemiology of osteoporosis and osteoporotic fractures. Epidemiol. Rev. 7:178–208.

Dalén, N., L.G. Hellström, and B. Jacobson. 1976. Bone mineral content and mechanical strength of the femoral neck. Acta Orthop. Scand. 47:503–508.

Daniell, H.W. 1976. Osteoporosis of the slender smoker. Vertebral compression fractures and loss of metacarpal cortex in relation to postmenopausal cigarette smoking and lack of obesity. Arch. Intern. Med. 136:298–304.

Davidson, B.J., R.K. Ross, A. Paganini-Hill, G.D. Hammond, P.K. Siiteri, and H.L. Judd. 1982. Total and free estrogens and androgens in post menopausal women with hip fractures. J. Clin. Endocrinol. Metab. 54:115–120.

DeLuca, H.F. 1983. The vitamin D endocrine system in health and disease. Pp. 41–67 in E.W. Haller, and G.E. Cotton, eds. Nutrition in the Young and the Elderly: A Symposium Held at the School of Medicine, University of Minnesota, Duluth, June 28–30, 1982. The Collamore Press, Lexington, Mass.

Dietrick, J.E., G.D. Whedon, and E. Shorr. 1948. Effects of immobilization upon various metabolic and physiologic functions of normal men. Am. J. Med. 4:3–36.

Dobbs, R.J., and I.M. Baird. 1977. Effect of wholemeal and white bread on iron absorption in normal people. Br. Med. J. 1:1641–1642.

Donaldson, C.L., S.B. Hulley, J.M. Vogel, R.S. Hattner, J.H. Bayers, and D.E. McMillan. 1970. Effect of prolonged bed rest on bone mineral. Metabolism 19:1071–1084.

Drinkwater, B.L., K. Nilson, C.H. Chesnut III, W.J. Brenner, S. Shainholtz, and M.B. Southworth. 1984. Bone mineral content of amenorrheic and eumenorrheic athletes. N. Engl. J. Med. 311:277–281.

Engh, G., A.J. Bollet, G. Hardin, and W. Parson. 1968. Epidemiology of osteoporosis. II. Incidence of hip fractures in mental institutions. J. Bone Jt. Surg., Am. Vol. 50:557–562.

Ettinger, B., H.K. Genant, and C.E. Cann. 1985. Long-term estrogen replacement therapy prevents bone loss and fractures. Ann. Intern. Med. 102:319–324.

Farmer, M.E., L.R. White, J.A. Brody, and K.R. Bailey. 1984. Race and sex differences in hip fracture incidence. Am. J. Public Health 74:1374–1380.

Forero, M.S., R.F. Klein, R.A. Nissenson, K. Nelson, H. Heath III, C.D. Arnaud, and B.L. Riggs. 1987. Effect of age on circulating immunoreactive and bioactive parathyroid hormone levels in women. J. Bone Min. Res. 2:363–366.

Frame, B., and A.M. Parfitt. 1978. Osteomalacia: current concepts. Ann. Intern. Med. 89:966–982.

Frost, H.M. 1964. Mathematical Elements of Lamellar Bone Remodellng. C.C. Thomas, Springfield, Ill. 127 pp.

Frost, H.M. 1977. A method of analysis of trabecular bone dynamics. Pp. 445–476 in P.J. Meunier, ed. Bone Histomorphometry. Armour Montagu, Paris.

Gallagher, J.C., B.L. Riggs, J. Eisman, A. Hamstra, S.B. Arnaud, and H.F. DeLuca. 1979. Intestinal calcium absorption and serum vitamin D metabolites in normal subjects and osteoporotic patients: effect of age and dietary calcium. J. Clin. Invest. 64:729–736.

Gallagher, J.C., B.L. Riggs, and H.F. DeLuca. 1980a. Effect of estrogen on calcium absorption and serum vitamin D metabolites in postmenopausal osteoporosis. J. Clin. Endocrinol. Metab. 51:1359–1364.

Gallagher, J.C., J.L. Melton, B.L. Riggs, and E. Bergstrath. 1980b. Epidemiology of fractures of the proximal femur in Rochester, Minnesota. Clin. Orthop. 150:163–171.

Garn, S.M. 1970. The Earlier Gain and the Later Loss of Cortical Bone, in Nutritional Perspective. C.C. Thomas, Springfield, Ill. 146 pp.

Garn, S.M., E.M. Pao, and M.E. Rihl. 1964. Compact bone in Chinese and Japanese. Science 143:1439–1440.

Genant, H.K., C.E. Cann, B. Ettinger, and G.S. Gordan. 1982. Quantitative computed tomography of vetebral spongiosa: a sensitive method for detecting early bone loss after oophorectomy. Ann. Intern. Med. 97:699–705.

Genant, H.K., J.E. Block, P. Steiger, and C.C. Glüer. 1987. Quantitative computed tomography in the assessment of osteoporosis. Pp. 49–71 in H.K. Genant, ed. Osteoporosis Update 1987: Perspectives for Internists, Gynecologists, Orthopaedists, Radiologists, and Nuclear Physicians. University of California Printing Services, Berkeley, Calif.

Gordan, G.S., J. Picchi, and B.S. Roof. 1973. Antifracture efficacy of long-term estrogens for osteoporosis. Trans. Assoc. Am. Physicians 86:326–332.

Grodin, J.M., P.K. Siiteri, and P.C. MacDonald. 1973. Source of estrogen production in postmenopausal women. J. Clin. Endocrinol. Metab. 36:207–214.

Heaney, R.P. 1986. Calcium, bone health, and osteoporosis. Pp. 255–301 in W.A. Peck, ed. Bone and Mineral Research, Annual 4: A Yearly Survey of Developments in the Field of Bone and Mineral Metabolism. Elsevier, Amsterdam.

Heaney, R.P., and R.R. Recker. 1982. Effects of nitrogen, phosphorus, and caffeine on calcium balance in women. J. Lab. Clin. Med. 99:46–55.

Heaney, R.P., J.C. Gallagher, C.C. Johnston, R. Neer, A.M. Parfitt, and G.D. Whedon. 1982. Calcium nutrition and bone health in the elderly. Am. J. Clin. Nutr. 36:986-1013.

Heath, H., III, and C.W. Callaway. 1985. Calcium tablets for hypertension? Ann. Intern. Med. 103:946–947.

Heath, H., III, L.J. Melton III, and C.P. Chu. 1980. Diabetes mellitus and risk of skeletal fracture. N. Engl. J. Med. 303:567–570.

Hegsted, M., S.A. Schuette, M.B. Zemel, and H.M. Linkswiler. 1981. Urinary calcium and calcium balance in young men as affected by level of protein and phosphorus intake. J. Nutr. 111:553–562.

Hooyman, J.R., L.J. Melton III, A.M. Nelson, W.M. O'Fallon, and B.L. Riggs. 1984. Fractures after rheumatoid arthritis. A population-based study. Arthritis Rheum. 27:1353–1361.

Horsman, A., and J.D. Currey. 1983. Estimation of mechanical properties of the distal radius from bone mineral content and cortical width. Clin. Orthop. 176:298–304.

Horsman, A., J.C. Gallagher, M. Simpson, and B.E.C. Nordin. 1977. Prospective trial of oestrogen and calcium in postmenopausal women. Br. Med. J. 2:789–792.

Hui, S.L., S. Epstein, and C.C. Johnston, Jr. 1985. A prospective study of bone mass in patients with type I diabetes. J. Clin. Endocrin. Metab. 60:74–80.

Hulka, B.S., R.C. Grimson, B.G. Greenberg, D.G. Kaufman, W.C. Fowler, Jr., C.J.R. Hogue, G.S. Berger, and C.C. Pulliam. 1980. "Alternative" controls in a case-control study of endometrial cancer and exogenous estrogen. Am. J. Epidemiol. 112:376–387.

Ireland, P., and J.S. Fordtran. 1973. Effect of dietary calcium and age on jejunal calcium absorption in humans studied by intestinal perfusion. J. Clin. Invest. 52:2672–2681.

Iskrant, A.P. 1968. The etiology of fractured hips in females. Am. J. Public Health 58:485–490.

Ismail-Beigi, F., J.G. Reinhold, B. Faraji, and P. Abadi. 1977. Effects of cellulose added to diets of low and high fiber content upon the metabolism of calcium, magnesium, zinc and phosphorus in man. J. Nutr. 107:510–518.

Jaffe, H.L., A. Bodansky, and J.P. Chandler. 1932. Ammonium chloride decalcification, as modified by calcium intake: the relation between generalized osteoporosis and ostitis fibrosa. J. Exp. Med. 56:823–834.

Jenkins, G.N. 1967. Fluoride. World Rev. Nutr. Diet. 7:138–203.

Jowsey, J., and J. Gershon-Cohen. 1964. Effect of dietary calcium levels on production and reversal of experimental osteoporosis in cats. Proc. Soc. Exp. Biol. Med. 116:437–441.

Kelsay, J.L., K.M. Behall, and E.S. Prather. 1979. Effect of fiber from fruits and vegetables on metabolic responses on human subjects. II. Calcium, magnesium, iron and silicon balances. Am. J. Clin. Nutr. 32:1876–1880.

Kelsey, J.L., and N.G. Hildreth. 1983. Breast and Gynecologic Cancer Epidemiology. CRC Press, Boca Raton, Fla. 168 pp.

Knapp, E.L. 1947. Factors influencing the urinary excretion of calcium. I. In normal persons. J. Clin. Invest. 26:182–202.

Kreiger, N., J.L. Kelsey, T.R. Holford, and T. O'Connor. 1982. An epidemiologic study of hip fracture in postmenopausal women. Am. J. Epidemiol. 116:141–148.

Krolner, B., B. Toft, S.P. Nielsen, and E. Tondevold. 1983. Physical exercise as prophylaxis against involutional vertebral bone loss: a controlled trial. Clin. Sci. 64:541–546.

Leone, N.C. 1960. The effects of the absorption of fluoride. I. Outline and summary. Arch. Indust. Health 21:324–325.

Leone, N.C., C.A. Stevenson, T.F. Hilbish, and M.C. Sosman. 1955. A roentgenologic study of a human population exposed to high-fluoride domestic water: a ten year study. Am. J. Roentgenol Radium Ther. Nucl. Med. 74:874–885.

Lindsay, R., D.M. Hart, J.M. Aitken, E.B. MacDonald, J.B. Anderson, and A.C. Clarke. 1976. Long-term prevention of postmenopausal osteoporosis by oestrogen. Lancet 1:1038–1041.

Lindsay, R., D.M. Hart, A. MacLean, A.C. Clark, A. Kraszewski, and J. Garwood. 1978. Bone response to termination of oestrogen treatment. Lancet 1:1325–1327.

Lindsay, R., D.M. Hart, C. Forrest, and C. Baird. 1980. Prevention of spinal osteoporosis in oopherectomised women. Lancet 2:1151–1154.

Lindberg, J.S., M.R. Powell, M.M. Hunt, D.E. Ducey, and C.E. Wade. 1987. Increased vetebral bone mineral in response to reduced exercise in amenorrheic runners. West. J. Med. 146:39–42.

Lutwak, L. 1975. Metabolic and biochemical considerations of bone. Ann. Clin. Lab. Sci. 5:185–194.

MacDonald, P.C., C.D. Edman, D.L. Hemsell, J.C. Porter, and P.K. Siiteri. 1978. Effect of obesity on conversion of plasma androstenedione to estrone in postmenopausal women with and without endometrial cancer. Am. J. Obstet. Gynecol. 130:448–455.

MacLaughlin, J., and M.F. Holick. 1985. Aging decreases the capacity of huuman skin to produce vitamin D₃. J. Clin. Invest. 76:1536–1538.

Marcus, R. 1982. The relationship of dietary calcium to the maintenance of skeletal integrity in man—an interface of endocrinology and nutrition. Metabolism 31:93–102.

Marcus, R., C. Cann, P. Madvig, J. Minkoff, M. Goddard, M. Bayer, M. Martin, L. Gaudiani, W. Haskell, and H. Genant. 1985. Menstrual function and bone mass in elite women distance runners. Endocrine and metabolic features. Ann. Intern. Med. 102:158–163.

Marel, G.M., M.J. McKenna, and B. Frame. 1986. Osteomalacia. Pp. 335–412 in W.A. Peck, ed. Bone and Mineral Research, Annual 4: A Yearly Survey of Developments in the Field of Bone and Mineral Metabolism. Elsevier, Amsterdam.

Marsh, A.G., T.V. Sanchez, O. Midkelsen, J. Keiser, and G. Mayor. 1980. Cortical bone density of adult lacto-ovo-vegetarian and omnivorous women. J. Am. Diet. Assoc. 76:148–151.

Matkovic, V., K. Kostial, I. Simonovic, R. Buzina, A. Brodarec, and B.E.C. Nordin. 1979. Bone status and fracture rates in two regions of Yugoslavia. Am. J. Clin. Nutr. 32:540–549.

Mazess, R.B., and H.S. Barden. 1987. Single and dual-photon absorptiometry for bone measurement in osteoporosis. Pp. 73–80 in H.K. Genant, ed. Osteoporosis Update 1987: Perspectives for Internists, Gynecologists, Orthopaedists, Radiologists, and Nuclear Physicians. University of California Printing Services, Berkeley, Calif.

Mazess, R.B., and W. Mather. 1974. Bone mineral content of North Alaskan Eskimos. Am. J. Clin. Nutr. 27:916–925.

Mazess, R.B., and G.D. Whedon. 1983. Immobilization and bone. Calcif. Tissue Int. 35:265–267.

McCance, R.A., E.M. Widdowson, and H. Lehmann. 1942. The effect of protein intake on the absorption of calcium and magnesium. Biochem. J. 36:686–691.

Melton, L.J., III, J.M. Sampson, B.F. Morrey, and D.M. Ilstrup. 1981. Epidemiologic features of pelvic fractures. Clin. Orthop. 155:43–47.

Melton, L.J., III, D.M. Ilstrup, R.D. Beckenbaugh, and B.L. Riggs. 1982. Hip fracture recurrence: a population-based study. Clin. Orthop. 167:131–138.

Mertz, W. 1981. The essential trace elements. Science 213:1332–1338.

Michnovicz, J.J., R.J. Hershcopf, H. Naganuma, H.L. Bradlow, and J. Fishman. 1986. Increased 2-hydroxylation of estradiol as a possible mechanism for the anti-estrogenic effect of cigarette smoking. N. Engl. J. Med. 315:1305–1309.

Nachtigall, L.E., R.H. Nachtigall, R.D. Nachtigall, and E.M. Beckman. 1979. Estrogen replacement therapy. I. A 10-year prospective study in the relationship to osteoporosis. Obstet. Gynecol. 53:277–281.

Nelson, M.E., E.C. Fisher, P.D. Catsos, C.N. Meredith, R.N. Turksoy, and W.J. Evans. 1986. Diet and bone status in amenorrheic runners. Am. J. Clin. Nutr. 43:910–916.

NIH (National Institutes of Health). 1984. Osteoporosis: consensus conference. J. Am. Med. Assoc. 252:799–802.

Nilas, L., and C. Christiansen. 1987. Bone mass and its relationship to age and the menopause. J. Clin. Endocrinol. Metab. 65:697–702.

Nilsson, B.E., and N.E. Westlin. 1973. Changes in bone mass in alcoholics. Clin. Orthop. 90:229–232.

Nordin, B.E.C. 1960. Osteomalacia, osteoporosis and calcium deficiency. Clin. Orthop. 17:235–258.

Nordin, B.E.C. 1966. International patterns of osteoporosis. Clin. Orthop. 45:17–30.

Nordin, B.E.C., A. Horsman, D.H. Marshall, M. Simpson, and G.M. Waterhouse. 1979. Calcium requirement and calcium therapy. Clin. Orthop. 140:216–239.

Norman, A.W. 1985. The vitamin D endocrine system. Physiologist 28:219–232.

Odell, W.D., and R.S. Swerdloff. 1976. Male hypogonadism. West. J. Med. 124:446–475.

Owen, R.A., L.J. Melton III, K.A. Johnson, D.M. Ilstrup, and B.L. Riggs. 1982. Incidence of Colles' fracture in a North American community. Am. J. Public Health 72:605–607.

Paganini-Hill, A., R.K. Ross, V.R. Gerkins, B.E. Henderson, M. Arthur, and T.M. Mack. 1981. Menopausal estrogen therapy and hip fractures. Ann. Intern. Med. 95:28–31.

Parfitt, A.M. 1983. Dietary risk factors for age-related bone loss and fractures. Lancet 2:1181–1185.

Parfitt, A.M., J.C. Gallagher, R.P. Heaney, C.C. Johnson, R. Neer, and G.D. Whedon. 1982. Vitamin D and bone health in the elderly. Am. J. Clin. Nutr. 36 suppl. 5:1014–1031.

Portale, A.A., B.E. Booth, B.P. Halloran, and R.C. Morris, Jr. 1984. Effect of dietary phosphorus on circulation concentrations of 1,25-dihydroxyvitamin D and immunoreactive parathyroid hormone in children with moderated renal insufficiency. J. Clin. Invest. 73:1580–1589.

Portale, A.A., B.P. Halloran, M.M. Murphy, and R.C. Morris, Jr. 1986. Oral intake of phosphorus can determine the serum concentration of 1,25-dihydroxyvitamin D by determining its production rate in humans. J. Clin. Invest. 77:7–12.

Poskitt, E.M.E., T.J. Cole, and D.E.M. Lawson. 1979. Diet, sunlight, and 25-hydroxyvitamin D in healthy children and adults. Br. Med. J. 1:221–223.

Recker, R.R., P.D. Saville, and R.P. Heaney. 1977. Effect of estrogens and calcium carbonate on bone loss in postmenopausal women. Ann. Intern. Med. 87:649–655.

Reinhold, J.G., B. Faradji, P. Abadi, and F. Ismail-Beigi. 1976. Decreased absorption of calcium, magnesium, zinc and phosphorus by humans due to increased fiber and phosphorus consumption as wheat bread. J. Nutr. 106:493–503.

Riggs, B.L. 1984. Treatment of osteoporosis with sodium fluoride: an appraisal. Pp. 366–393 in W.A. Peck, ed. Bone and Mineral Research, Annual 2: A Yearly Survey of Developments in the Field of Bone and Mineral Metabolism. Elsevier, Amsterdam.

Riggs, B.L., and L.J. Melton III. 1986. Involutional osteoporosis. N. Engl. J. Med. 314:1676–1686.

Riggs, B.L., E. Seeman, S.F. Hodgson, D.R. Taves, and W.M. O'Fallon. 1982. Effect of the fluoride/calcium regimen on vertebral fracture occurrence in postmenopausal osteoporosis. N. Engl. J. Med. 306:446–450.

Riggs, B.L., H.W. Wahner, L.J. Melton III, L.S. Richelson, H.L. Judd, and W.M. O'Fallon. 1987. Dietary calcium intake and rates of bone loss in women. J. Clin. Invest. 80:979–982.

Rigotti, N.A., S.R. Nussbaum, D.B. Herzog, and R.M. Neer. 1984. Osteoporosis in women with anorexia nervosa. N. Engl. J. Med. 311:1601–1606.

Riis, B.J., C. Christiansen, L.J. Deftos, and B.D. Catherwood. 1984. The role of serum concentrations of estrogens on postmenopausal osteoporosis and bone turnover. 1984. Pp. 333–336 in C. Christiansen, C.D. Arnaud, B.E.C. Nordin, A.M. Parfitt, W.A. Peck, and B.L. Riggs, eds. Osteoporosis: Proceedings of the Copenhagen International Symposium on Osteoporosis. Department of Clinical Chemistry, Glostrop Hospital, Copenhagen.

Riis, B., K. Thomsen, and C. Christiansen. 1987. Does calcium supplementation prevent postmenopausal bone loss: a double-blind controlled clinical study. N. Engl. J. Med. 316:173–177.

Rockoff, S.D., E. Sweet, and J. Bleustein. 1969. The relative contribution of trabecular and cortical bone to the strength of human lumbar vertebrae. Calcif. Tissue Res. 3:163–175.

Rose, S.H., L.J. Melton III, B.F. Morrey, D.M. Ilstrup, and B.L. Riggs. 1982. Epidemiologic features of humeral fractures. Clin. Orthop. 168:24–30.

Sandstead, H.H., L.M. Klevay, R.A. Jacob, J.M. Munoz, G.M. Logan, Jr., S.L. Reck, F.R. Dintzis, G.E. Inglett, and W.C. Shuey. 1979. Effects of dietary fiber and protein level on mineral element metabolism. Pp. 147–156 in G.E. Inglett, and S.I. Falkehag, eds. Dietary Fibers: Chemistry and Nutrition. Academic Press, New York.

Saville, P.D., and B.E. Nilsson. 1966. Height and weight in symptomatic postmenopausal osteoporosis. Clin. Orthop. 45:49–54.

Schindler, A.E., A. Ebert, and E. Friedrich. 1972. Conversion of androstenedione to estrone by human tissue. J. Clin. Endocrinol. Metab. 35:627–630.

Schuette, S.A., and H.M. Linkswiler. 1982. Effects on Ca and P metabolism in humans by adding meat, meat plus milk, or purified proteins plus Ca and P to a low protein diet. J. Nutr. 112:338–349.

Seeman, E., L.J. Melton III, W.M. O'Fallon, and B.L. Riggs. 1983. Risk factors for spinal osteoporosis in men. Am. J. Med. 75:977–983.

Singh, A., S.S. Jolly, B.C. Bansal, and C.C. Mathur. 1963. Endemic fluorosis: epidemiologic, clinical and biochemical study of chronic fluorine intoxication in Panjab (India). Medicine 42:229–246.

Smith, D.M., C.C. Johnston, Jr., and P.L. Yu. 1972. In vivo measurement of bone mass. Its use in demineralized states such as osteoporosis. J. Am. Med. Assoc. 219:325–329.

Smith, D.M., W.E. Nance, K.W. Kang, J.C. Christian, and C.C. Johnston, Jr. 1973. Genetic factors in determining bone mass. J. Clin. Invest. 52:2800–2808.

Smith, R.W., Jr., and J. Rizek. 1966. Epidemiologic studies of osteoporosis in women of Puerto Rico and Southeastern Michigan with special reference to age, race, national origin and to other related or associated findings. Clin. Orthop. 45:31–48.

Solomon, L. 1968. Osteoporosis and fracture of the femoral neck in the South African Bantu. J. Bone Jt. Surg., Br. Vol. 50:2–13.

Trotter, M., G.E. Broman, and R.R. Peterson. 1960. Densities of bones of white and negro skeletons. J. Bone Jt. Surg., Am. Vol. 42:50–58.

Tsai, K.S., H. Heath III, R. Kumar, and B.L. Riggs. 1984. Impaired vitamin D metabolism with aging in women: possible role in pathogenesis of senile osteoporosis. J. Clin. Invest. 73:1668–1672.

Veis, A., and B. Sabsay. 1987. The collagen of mineralized matrices. Pp. 1–63 in W.A. Peck, ed. Bone and Mineral Research, Annual 5: A Yearly Survey of Developments in the Field of Bone and Mineral Metabolism. Elsevier, Amsterdam.

Weiss, N.S., C.L. Ure, J.H. Ballard, A.R. Williams, and J.R. Daling. 1980. Decreased risk of fractures of the hip and lower forearm with postmenopausal use of estrogen. N. Engl. J. Med. 303:1195–1198.

Whedon, G.D. 1984. Disuse osteoporosis: physiological aspects. Calcif. Tissue Int. 36:S146–150.

Whedon, G.D., and E. Shorr. 1957. Metabolic studies in paralytic acute anterior poliomyelitis. II. Alterations in calcium and phosphorus metabolism. J. Clin. Invest. 36:966–981.

White, M.K., R.B. Martin, R.A. Yeater, R.L. Butcher, and E.L. Radin. 1984. The effects of exercise on the bones of postmenopausal women. Int. Orthop. 7:209–214.

Yano, K., R.D. Wasnich, J.M. Vogel, and L.K. Heilbrun. 1984. Bone mineral measurements among middle-aged and elderly Japanese residents in Hawaii. Am. J. Epidemiol. 119:751–764.

Ziel, H.K., and W.D. Finkle. 1975. Increased risk of endometrial carcinoma among users of conjugated estrogens. N. Engl. J. Med. 293:1167–70.

24

Diabetes Mellitus

Diabetes mellitus is a metabolic disorder characterized by high blood glucose levels and defective carbohydrate utilization due to a relative or absolute deficiency of insulin. As described in Chapter 5, there are two distinct primary forms of diabetes mellitus: type I, or insulin-dependent diabetes mellitus (IDDM), and type II, or noninsulin-dependent diabetes mellitus (NIDDM). This classification replaces the older terminology—juvenile-onset and adult-onset diabetes. IDDM usually results from destruction of the insulin-secreting beta cells in the pancreatic islets of Langerhans. It is believed to be linked to the immune system, i.e., there is an increased risk of IDDM in subjects with certain genes associated with the histocompatibility immune response (HLA) genes. In the United States, approximately 5 to 10% of the people with diabetes have IDDM. NIDDM is much more common; it is associated with unknown genetic factors and aging and is closely linked to the insulin resistance associated with adiposity (see Chapter 21). The very high concordance of the incidence of NIDDM in many identical twin pairs (Barnett et al., 1981) suggests that genes play a very important role in this disease. Little is known about gene–environment interactions in the etiology of NIDDM.

Diabetes (IDDM and NIDDM) is diagnosed by the presence of classical symptoms and elevated glucose levels (Callaway and Rossini, 1987). The disease has been diagnosed in approximately 6 million people in the United States, and an additional 4 million to 5 million individuals are believed to have undiagnosed diabetes (National Diabetes Data Group, 1985). Each year, approximately 500,000 new cases are diagnosed. IDDM afflicts about 0.3% of the population after age 20. NIDDM has been diagnosed in approximately 2.4% of the total population; among those 65 and older, almost 9% of the population may have this disease (Callaway and Rossini, 1987).

In the general U.S. population, more women than men are afflicted with diabetes (both IDDM and NIDDM). However, when corrections are made for degree of adiposity in men and women, the prevalence of the disease is greater among men. This may be attributable to the regional distribution of fat, which is strongly determined by genetic factors (see Chapter 4).

Interpopulation variations in the prevalence of diabetes are large and frequently attributable to environmental differences. In general, the intercountry incidence rates are correlated to the level of socioeconomic development. For example, rates in Central American and Southeast Asian countries are generally lower than those in Westernized countries.

There is an increased incidence of NIDDM with increasing age. Within age groups, demographic characteristics of diabetics are very similar to those of the general U.S. population. These characteristics include region and location of residence, marital status, and living arrangements. However, people with NIDDM have fewer years of schooling, are less likely to be employed, and have lower family incomes than the general adult population. Rates of NIDDM in the United States tend to be higher in rural areas and among people with relatively low socioeconomic status.

Genetic, environmental, and lifestyle factors can place a person at increased risk for developing NIDDM. Rates of NIDDM among adults of Hispanic origin, blacks, and Asian-Americans appear to be higher than among whites. The rates of diagnosed NIDDM among some Native Americans (e.g., Pima Indians) are among the highest in the world. It is likely, however, that this high frequency reflects a genetic origin. The most important risk factors for NIDDM are increasing age, higher blood glucose concentration, family history of diabetes, and adiposity. Central distribution of body fat (i.e., high waist-to-hip ratio) is also strongly associated with a higher risk of NIDDM (see Chapters 5 and 21).

Advanced maternal age and the presence of islet cell or insulin antibodies are associated with increased IDDM risk. The incidence of IDDM is similar in males and females, but is 1.5 times higher in whites than in blacks. Although incidence rates vary widely internationally, the risk for siblings of IDDM cases is 7 to 18 times higher than the risk in the general population. Siblings with certain HLA genes are at increased risk for developing IDDM (National Diabetes Data Group, 1985).

EVIDENCE ASSOCIATING DIETARY FACTORS WITH DIABETES MELLITUS

Epidemiologic and Clinical Studies

The only factor that has been consistently related to the prevalence of diabetes mellitus is relative body weight (West, 1978). In several migrant populations (e.g., Japanese who moved to Hawaii and California and Yemenites who migrated to Israel), the prevalence of diabetes has increased along with Westernization of diet and lifestyle (West, 1978). The association of diabetes (presumably NIDDM) with adiposity persists in both inter- and intrapopulation analyses, despite wide variation in intake of individual nutrients.

The prevalence of diabetes among adults is positively associated with higher percentages of total caloric intake as fats and inversely related to the percentage of calories as carbohydrates. Specific carbohydrates, such as sugar or starch, have not been shown to influence the risk of diabetes.

In a study comparing two Micronesian populations—one at high risk and one at low risk of NIDDM—King et al. (1984) found that estimates of fiber intake had no predictive value in estimating risk of subsequent disease. Metabolic studies indicate that soluble forms of dietary fiber (e.g., guar and pectin) may curtail the glycemic response (glucose levels reached in response to ingestion of a particular food) in people with overt diabetes (Jenkins et al., 1976, 1978, 1979; Monnier et al., 1978; Morgan et al., 1979; LSRO, 1987; Poynard et al., 1980), but there are no data on the possible role of dietary fiber in reducing the risk for this disease.

In large population studies, alcohol intake has been correlated with hyperglycemia. There is no ready explanation for this, except for alcoholics who develop insulin deficiency as a result of chronic pancreatitis. It was suspected that ethanol per se impaired glucose tolerance (Gerard et al., 1977). Yki-Järvinen and Nikkilä (1985) reported that insulin resistance results from excessive alcohol intake by otherwise healthy adults in the United States.

Studies in animals indicate that a decrease in glucose tolerance is induced by chromium deficiency and is reversed by the administration of chromium (see Chapter 14). In hyperglycemic humans, chromium supplementation improved glucose tolerance and lowered insulin levels (Anderson, 1986; Riales and Albrink, 1981; Simonoff, 1984), suggesting that chromium deficiency may be a contributing factor to disease onset. However, no population data have been reported implicating chromium deficiency in humans with diabetes, and chromium supplementation does not improve blood glucose or insulin levels in those with the disease (Anderson, 1986; Rabinowitz et al., 1983). Chromium deficiency in people with diabetes could thus be a consequence rather than a cause of the disease (Simonoff, 1984). In summary, other than data on total caloric intake and NIDDM, there is no evidence that dietary composition influences the risk of diabetes mellitus.

There is a long-standing controversy concerning the macronutrient composition of the diet used for management of people with IDDM and NIDDM (Bierman, 1979; Wood and Bierman, 1986), especially with regard to the optimal proportion of carbohydrate-containing foods. The nutritional requirements of people with diabetes are essentially the same as those for the general population. Restriction of total caloric intake to achieve ideal body weight is the primary dietary intervention recommended for NIDDM (NIH, 1986). Restriction of fat intake to ≤30% calories is also advised, and reduced intake of saturated fatty acids and dietary cholesterol (see Chapter 7) is advisable because of the very high rate of mortality from atherosclerotic coronary diseases among those with IDDM and NIDDM (Krowlewski et al., 1987; National Diabetes Data Group, 1985; West 1978).

Carbohydrates from vegetables and fruits are usually substituted for fats in the diet of diabetic patients (American Diabetes Association, 1987). There is some recent evidence that simple sugars such as sucrose need not be restricted (Bantle et al., 1983; Chantelau et al., 1985; Jellish et al., 1984; Peterson et al., 1986; Slama et al., 1984). There is no clear consensus, however, on this issue as well as on the proportion of carbohydrate needed in the diet for the management of diabetes mellitus (Garg et al., 1988; Jarrett, 1981; Nuttall, 1983; Reaven, 1980; Wood and Bierman, 1986). Reaven and colleagues caution against using a high-carbohydrate diet for long-term management of NIDDM because it can increase levels of postprandial glucose, insulin, and basal triglycerides (Coulston et al., 1987; Reaven, 1988). Other studies show wide variation in the glucose response to simple sugars and to foods containing complex carbohydrates (Crapo, 1985; Crapo et al., 1981; Jenkins et al., 1981).

Soluble dietary fiber, including guar, pectin, and oat bran, lowers plasma glucose levels among people with diabetes (Anderson et al., 1984; see also Chapter 10). However, the use of purified fiber supplements is not recommended for diabetes therapy since evidence of long-term efficacy and safety is lacking (NIH, 1986).

People with diabetes mellitus appear to have no special requirements for protein. There is increasing concern, however, that high protein intakes may be associated with increased risk of renal disease (diabetic nephropathy) in IDDM and NIDDM. Ciavarella (1987) reported that a 4- to 5-month dietary protein restriction in the diet of seven IDDM patients with early clinical nephropathy reduced albuminuria. This subject needs further investigation.

Hypertension appears to accelerate the progression of nephropathy in diabetics. The role of reduced sodium intake in slowing progression of this disorder remains to be elucidated (see Chapter 20).

Animal Studies

In normal strains of animals, it has been difficult to prove a specific effect of total caloric intake or the intake of specific nutrients on the emergence of diabetes mellitus (Glinsmann et al., 1986). As discussed in Chapter 6, large increases in total food intake that lead to adiposity in animals also lead to an increased incidence of insulin resistance (see section on total caloric intake and obesity in Chapter 6) (Hallfrisch et al., 1981; Johnson et al., 1975; Romsos and Leveille, 1974; Stern et al., 1975; Susini and Lavau, 1978; Turkenkopf et al., 1982) and some other aspects of NIDDM seen in humans.

The metabolic responses to increased total caloric intake usually become apparent only over a relatively long period. Thus, many of the animal studies of putative dietary-induced diabetes are confounded not only by the adiposity resulting from overfeeding, but also by the effects of aging inherent in long-term dietary studies. In most cases, the effects of increased caloric intake on insulin resistance can be reversed by weight reduction and restoration of a more normal body weight. Thus, it is difficult to separate any specific effect of calories on the development of diabetes from their effects on overall adiposity.

There are several animal models for studying the genetics of NIDDM and IDDM, particularly among rodents (Salans and Graham, 1982). Although there is some evidence that excessive consumption of certain nutrients may enhance (Cohen, 1978; Leiter et al., 1983) or provoke (Coleman, 1982; Greenwood et al., 1988; Ikeda et al., 1981) the appearance of incipient diabetes and exacerbate some pathological conditions (see Chapter 9), there is little evidence that the diabetic condition depends upon hyperphagia or ingestion of certain nutrients. One exception to this is the sand rat, which normally remains lean and nondiabetic in the wild but when housed under laboratory conditions becomes hyperphagic and often diabetic (Kalderon et al., 1986; Rice and Robertson, 1980). There is some evidence that dietary fiber may modulate the expression of hyperglycemia in chemically induced and spontaneous diabetes in rodents (see Chapter 10).

Diabetes mellitus can be induced experimentally in several ways, e.g., by the injection of streptozotocin or alloxan (beta-cell toxins) or by the surgical extirpation of all or part of the pancreas. Hypoinsulinemia follows such treatment and usually precedes any increase in food intake (although polyphagia may occur with polydipsia). Marked changes in the dietary preferences of diabetic rodents occur later and are not etiologically implicated in the initiation of the diabetes syndrome; they may, in fact, be symptoms of adaptation (Friedman, 1978; Kanarek et al., 1980).

SUMMARY

Relative body weight seems to be the only factor that has been consistently related to the prevalence of NIDDM, which is associated directly with the mean percentage of calories from fats and inversely with the mean percentage of calories from carbohydrates. This finding is attributed to the greater caloric density of high-fat diets rather than to any specific action of the nutrient itself. Fiber intake does not appear to be associated with the risk of developing NIDDM. Alcohol intake has been correlated with hyperglycemia, and ethanol is believed to impair glucose tolerance. The possible role of chromium deficiency in the etiology of diabetes is unresolved. There is no evidence that dietary composition influences the risk of developing diabetes mellitus.

DIRECTIONS FOR RESEARCH

The following areas need further investigation:

- Basic mechanisms through which genetic and dietary factors interact in the etiology of diabetes mellitus.
- The role of high carbohydrate diets with varying amounts and types of carbohydrates and fats in the long-term management of diabetes mellitus and its complications.
- The role of gene–environment interaction in NIDDM.
- Methods for reducing obesity and maintaining normal body weight in alleviating diabetes and its complications, and the nutritional, environmental, behavioral, and genetic aspects of obesity in the etiology of NIDDM.
- The role of saturated fatty acids and dietary cholesterol in mortality from coronary heart disease in people with diabetes.
- The role of protein intake in chronic renal failure in people with diabetes.
- The role of dietary fiber in reducing the risk of diabetes.

REFERENCES

American Diabetes Association. 1987. Nutritional recommendations and principles for individuals with diabetes mellitus: 1986. Diabetes Care 10:126–132.

Anderson, J.W., L. Story, B. Sieling, W.J. Chen, M.S. Petro, and J. Story. 1984. Hypocholesterolemic effects of oat-bran or bean intake for hypercholesterolemic men. Am. J. Clin. Nutr. 40:1146–1155.

Anderson, R.A. 1986. Chromium metabolism and its role in disease processes in man. Chem. Physiol. Biochem. 4: 31–41.

Bantle J.P., D.C. Laine, J.W. Castle, J.W. Thomas, B.J. Hoogwerf, and F.C. Goetz. 1983. Postprandial glucose and insulin responses to meals containing different carbohydrates in normal and diabetic subjects. N. Engl. J. Med. 309:7–12.

Barnett, A.H., C. Eff, R.D.G. Leslie, and D.A. Pyke. 1981. Diabetes in identical twins. Diabetologia 70:87–93.

Bierman, E.L. 1979. Nutritional management of adult and juvenile diabetics. Pp. 107–117 in M. Winick, ed. Nutritional Management of Genetic Disorders. Wiley, New York.

Callaway, C.W., and A.A. Rossini. 1987. Diabetes mellitus. Pp. 764–793 in W.T. Branch, Jr., ed. Office Practice of Medicine, 2nd ed. W.B. Saunders, Philadelphia.

Chantelau, E.A., G. Gösseringer, G.E. Sonnenberg, and M. Berger. 1985. Moderate intake of sucrose does not impair metabolic control in pump-treated diabetic out-patients. Diabetologia 28:204–207.

Ciavarella, A., G. DiMizio, S. Stefoni, L.C. Borgnino, and P. Vannini. 1987. Reduced albuminuria after dietary protein restriction in insulin-dependent diabetic patients with clinical nephropathy. Diabetes Care 10:407–413.

Cohen, A.M. 1978. Genetically determined response to different ingested carbohydrates in the production of diabetes. Horm. Metab. Res. 10:86–92.

Coleman, D.L. 1982. Diabetes-obesity syndromes in mice: proceedings of a task force on animals appropriate for studying diabetes mellitus and its complications. Diabetes 31 suppl. 1:1–6.

Coulston, A.M., C.B. Hollenbeck, A.L.M. Swislock, Y.D.I. Chen, and G.M. Reaven. 1987. Deleterious metabolic effect of high carbohydrate, sucrose-containing diets in patients with non-insulin-dependent diabetes mellitus. Am. J. Med. 82:213–220.

Crapo, P.A. 1985. Simple vs. complex carbohydrate in the diabetic diet. Annu. Rev. Nutr. 5:95–114.

Crapo, P.A., J. Insel, M. Sperling, and O.G. Kolterman. 1981. Comparison of serum glucose, insulin, and glucagon responses to different types of complex carbohydrate in noninsulin-dependent diabetic patients. Am. J. Clin. Nutr. 34:184–190.

Friedman, M.I. 1978. Hyperphagia in rats with experimental diabetes mellitus: a response to decreased supply of utilizable fuels. J. Comp. Physiol. Psychol. 92:109–117.

Garg, A., A. Bonanome, S.M. Grundy, Z.J. Zhang, and R.H. Unger. 1988. Comparison of a high-carbohydrate diet with a high-monounsaturated-fat diet in patients with non-insulin-dependent diabetes mellitus. N. Engl. J. Med. 310:829–839.

Gerard, M.J., A.L. Klatsky, A.B. Siegelaub, G.B. Friedman, and R. Feldman. 1977. Serum glucose levels and alcohol-consumption habits in a large population. Diabetes 26:780–785.

Glinsmann, W.H., H. Irausquin, and Y.K. Park. 1986. Evaluation of health aspects of sugars contained in carbohydrate sweeteners: report of Sugars Task Force, 1986. J. Nutr. 116:S1–S216.

Greenwood, M.R.C., R. Kava, D.B. West, and V.A. Lukasik. 1988. Wistar fatty rat: a sexually dimorphic model of human noninsulin-dependent diabetes. Pp. 316–318 in E. Shafrir and A.E. Renold, eds. Frontiers in Diabetes Research: Lessons from Animal Diabetes II. John Libbey, London.

Hallfrisch, J., L. Cohen, and S. Reiser. 1981. Effects of feeding rats sucrose in a high fat diet. J. Nutr. 111:531–536.

Ikeda, H., A. Shino, T. Matsuo, H. Iwatsuka, and Z. Suzuoki. 1981. A new genetically obese-hyperglycemic rat (Wistar fatty). Diabetes 30:1045–1050.

Jarrett, R.J. 1981. More about carbohydrate. Diabetologia 21:427–429.

Jellish, W.S., M.A. Emanuele, and C. Abraira. 1984. Graded sucrose/carbohydrate diets in overtly hypertriglyceridaemic diabetic patients. Am. J. Med. 77:1015–1022.

Jenkins, D.J.A., D.V. Goff, A.R. Leeds, K.G.M.M. Alberti, T.M.S. Wolever, M.A. Gassull, and T.D.R. Hockaday. 1976. Unabsorbable carbohydrates and diabetes: decreased post-prandial hyperglycemia. Lancet 2:172–174.

Jenkins, D.J.A., T.M.S. Wolever, R. Nineham, R. Taylor, G.L. Metz, S. Bacon, and T.D.R. Hockaday. 1978. Guar crisp bread in the diabetic diet. Br. Med. J. 2:1744–1746.

Jenkins, D.J.A., R.H. Taylor, R. Nineham, D.V. Goff, S.R. Bloom, D. Sarson, and K.G.M.M. Alberti. 1979. Combined use of guar and acarbose in reduction of post prandial glycemia. Lancet 2:924–927.

Jenkins, D.J.A., T.M.S. Wolever, R.H. Taylor, H. Barker, H. Fielden, J.M. Baldwin, A.C. Bowling, H.C. Mewman, A.L. Jenkins, and D.V. Goff. 1981. Glycemic index of foods: a physiological basis for carbohydrate exchange. Am. J. Clin. Nutr. 34:362–366.

Johnson, P.R., J.S. Stern, M.R.C. Greenwood, and J. Hirsch. 1975. Adipose tissue hyperplasia and hyperinsulinemia in Zucker obese female rats: a developmental study. Metabolism 27:1841–1854.

Kalderon, B., A. Gutman, E. Levy, E. Shafrir, and J.H. Adler. 1986. Characterization of stages in development of obesity–diabetes syndrome in sand rat (Psammomys obesus). Diabetes 35:717–724.

Kanarek, R.B., R. Marks-Kaufman, and B.J. Lipeles. 1980. Increased carbohydrate intake as a function of insulin administration in rats. Physiol. Behav. 25:779–782.

King, H., P. Zimmet, K. Pargeter, L.R. Raper, and V. Collins. 1984. Ethnic differences in susceptibility to non-insulin-dependent diabetes. A comparative study of two urbanized Micronesian populations. Diabetes 33:1002–1007.

Krowlewski, A.S., E.J. Kosinski, J.H. Warran, O.S. Leland, E.J. Busick, A.C. Asmal, L.F. Rand, A.R. Christlieb, R.F. Bradley, and C.R. Kahn. 1987. Magnitude and determinants of coronary artery disease in juvenile-onset, insulin-dependent diabetes mellitus. Am. J. Cardiol. 59:750–755.

Leiter, E.H., D.L. Coleman, D.K. Ingram, and M.A. Reynolds. 1983. Influence of dietary carbohydrate on the induction of diabetes in C57BL/KsJ-db/db diabetic mice. J. Nutr. 113:184–195.

LSRO (Life Sciences Research Office). 1987. Physiological Effects and Health Consequences of Dietary Fiber. Federation of American Societies for Experimental Biology, Bethesda, Md. 236 pp.

Monnier, L., T.C. Pham, L. Aguirre, A. Orseffi, and J. Mirouze. 1978. Influence of indigestible fibers on glucose tolerance. Diabetes Care 1:83–88.

Morgan, L.M., T.J. Goulder, D. Tsiolakis, V. Marks, and K.G.M.M. Alberti. 1979. The effect of unabsorbable carbohydrate on gut hormones: modification of post-prandial GIP secretion by guar. Diabetologia 17:85–89.

National Diabetes Data Group. 1985. Diabetes in America: Diabetes Data Compiled 1984. NIH Publ. No. 85-1468. National Institute of Arthritis, Diabetes and Digestive and Kidney Diseases, National Institutes of Health. Public Health Service, U.S. Department of Health and Human Services, Bethesda, Md. (various pagings).

NIH (National Institutes of Health). 1986. Diet and exercise in noninsulin-dependent diabetes mellitus. National Institutes of Health Consensus Development Conference Statement, Vol. 6. National Institute of Arthritis, Diabetes and Digestive and Kidney Diseases and the Office of Medical Applications of Research. U.S. Department of Health and Human Services, Bethesda, Md. 21 pp.

Nuttall, F.Q. 1983. Diet and the diabetic patient. Diabetes Care 6:197–207.

Peterson, D.B., J. Lambert, S. Gerring, D.P. Darling, R.D. Carter, R. Jelfs, and J.I. Mann. 1986. Sucrose in the diet of diabetic patients—just another carbohydrate? Diabetologia 29:216–220.

Poynard, T., G. Slama, A. Delage, and G. Tchobroutsky. 1980. Pectin efficacy in insulin-treated diabetics assessed by the artificial pancreas. Lancet 1:158.

Rabinowitz, M.B., H.C. Gonick, S.R. Levin, and M.B. Davidson. 1983. Effects on chromium and yeast supplements on carbohydrates and lipid metabolism in diabetic men. Diabetes Care 6:319–327.

Reaven, G.M. 1980. How high the carbohydrate? Diabetologia 19:409–413.

Reaven, G.R. 1988. Dietary therapy for non-insulin dependent diabetes mellitus. N. Engl. J. Med. 319:862–864.

Riales, R.M., and J. Albrink. 1981. Effect of chromium chloride supplementation on glucose tolerance and serum lipids including high-density lipoprotein of adult men. Am. J. Clin. Nutr. 34:2670–2678.

Rice, M.C., and R.P. Robertson. 1980. Re-evaluation of the sand rat as a model of diabetes mellitus. Am. J. Physiol. 239:E340–E345.

Romsos, D.R., and G.A. Leveille. 1974. Effect of meal frequency and diet composition on glucose tolerance in the rat. J. Nutr. 104:1503–1512.

Salans, L., and B. Graham, eds. 1982. Proceedings of a task force on animals appropriate for studying diabetes mellitus and its complications. Diabetes 31 suppl. 1:1–102.

Simonoff, M. 1984. Chromium deficiency and cardiovascular risk. Cardiovasc. Res. 18:591–596.

Slama, G., M.J. Haarat, P. Jean-Joseph, D. Costagliola, I. Goicolea, F. Bornet, F. Elgrably, and G. Tchobroutsky. 1984. Sucrose taken during a mixed meal has no additional hyperglycaemic action over isocaloric amounts of starch in well-controlled diabetics. Lancet 2:122–125.

Stern, J.S., P.R. Johnson, B.R. Batchelor, L.M. Zucker, and J. Hirsch. 1975. Pancreatic insulin release and peripheral tissue resistance in Zucker obese rats fed high- and low-carbohydrate diets. Am. J. Physiol. 228:543–548.

Susini, C., and M. Lavau. 1978. In vitro and in vivo responsiveness of muscle and adipose tissue to insulin in rats rendered obese by a high-fat diet. Diabetes 27:114–120.

Turkenkopf, I., P.R. Johnson, and M.R.C. Greenwood. 1982. Development of pancreatic and plasma insulin in prenatal and suckling Zucker rats. Am. J. Physiol. 242:E220–E229.

West, K.N. 1978. Epidemiology of Diabetes and Its Vascular Lesions. Elsevier/North-Holland, New York. 579 pp.

Wood, F.C., Jr., and E.L. Bierman. 1986. Is diet the cornerstone of management of diabetes? N. Engl. J. Med. 315:1224–1227.

Yki-Järvinen, H., and E.A. Nikkilä. 1985. Ethanol decreases glucose utilization in healthy man. J. Clin. Endocrinol. Metab. 61:941–945.

25

Hepatobiliary Disease

Hepatobiliary disease includes a heterogeneous group of diseases of the liver and biliary system caused by viral, bacterial, and parasitic infections, neoplasia, toxic chemicals, alcohol consumption, poor nutrition, metabolic disorders, and cardiac failure. The two predominant diseases of the liver in the United States are viral hepatitis and cirrhosis; the predominant chronic disease of the biliary system is cholelithiasis.

CIRRHOSIS OF THE LIVER

Cirrhosis of the liver is a chronic and usually relentlessly progressive disease characterized by loss of normal liver structure, fibrosis, impairment of the blood supply, and regeneration of disorganized liver lobules. These changes eventually result in liver failure. This disease has ranked among the 10 leading causes of death in the United States since 1950, and in middle-aged adults, it has ranked even higher in some years. In 1983, cirrhosis was the cause of 28,000 deaths, making it the ninth leading cause of death in the United States (Grant et al., 1986).

Cirrhosis may be caused by viral hepatitis, hemochromatosis, obstructive lesions of the biliary system, congestive heart failure, and chronic alcoholism. Specific causes of liver cirrhosis cannot be determined from conventional vital statistics, particularly from mortality statistics based on death certificates, even in technically developed countries. Physicians frequently fail to attribute liver cirrhosis to alcohol because of the social stigma attached to alcoholism. Estimates of the proportion of deaths from cirrhosis due to alcohol consumption in the United States range from 50 to 95% (NIAAA, 1983). In this chapter, it is assumed that most cases of liver cirrhosis are due to alcohol consumption, and rates of prevalence, incidence, and mortality for liver cirrhosis are used as indicators of alcoholic cirrhosis.

Evidence Associating Dietary Factors with Cirrhosis of the Liver

Role of Alcohol

The evidence for alcohol as a cause of cirrhosis derives from more than a century of anecdotal clinical observations made after the disease syndrome was described and named by Laënnec (1819). Further evidence is provided by many clinical and epidemiologic studies and by studies in laboratory animals (see Chapter 16). National mortality rates for liver cirrhosis were closely associated with fluctuations in the availability and consumption of alcohol in several countries before, during, and after World War II (Terris, 1967). The association was so strong and consistent that a causal relationship has been widely accepted. Recent epidemiologic studies have focused on the social and economic factors that influence alcohol consumption and thus the rates of mortality from cirrhosis. Early stages of alcoholic liver injury are reversible, but advanced stages are usually relentlessly progressive. The only known prevention for alcoholic cirrhosis is to limit consumption of alcohol.

Interactions of Alcohol with Diet

For many years cirrhosis among alcoholics was attributed to nutritional deficiencies associated with alcoholism and not to the direct effects of alcohol on the liver. This belief was based on experiments in animals, principally in rats, in which cirrhosis could be produced by protein deficiency but not by alcohol alone (see Chapter 16) and on the frequent occurrence of nutritional deficiencies among alcoholics. However, more recent experiments have demonstrated that alcohol produces liver toxicity independently of the adverse effects of nutrient deficiencies, and cirrhosis has been reproduced in baboons by alcohol in the absence of nutrient deficiencies (Lieber et al., 1975; Popper and Lieber, 1980; see also Chapter 16).

Evidence Associating Nondietary Factors with Cirrhosis of the Liver

Genetic Factors

It has long been known that alcoholism clusters in families, and rapidly accumulating evidence indicates that certain genotypes are more susceptible (see Chapters 4 and 16). A number of genetic markers have been associated with chronic alcoholism.

Most of these observations have been concerned with alcoholism and not specifically with cirrhosis. Since the major determinants of the effects of alcohol on tissue are the duration and intensity of exposure to alcohol and its metabolites, the genetic control of susceptibility to cirrhosis is probably associated with the alcohol-metabolizing enzymes of the liver (see Chapter 16). Therefore, both alcoholism and alcoholic cirrhosis are probably the results of genetic–environmental interactions.

GALLSTONES

There are two major varieties of gallstones: those composed primarily of cholesterol and those composed of heme pigments. Approximately 80% of the gallstones found in the U.S. population are composed of cholesterol. Therefore, the following

discussion is limited to those. The prevalence of cholelithiasis in adults in industrialized countries, including the United States, is about 10%; the prevalence among women is about twice that among men (Strom and West, 1985). The prevalence of cholelithiasis is much higher in populations with American Indian ancestry, reaching up to 65% in some American Indian groups (Hesse, 1959). Cholelithiasis and associated cholecystitis are not frequent causes of death, but they are frequent causes of hospital admission and surgical intervention.

Evidence Associating Dietary Factors with Gallstones

The physiological abnormality underlying the formation of gallstones is the accumulation of bile supersaturated with cholesterol. Supersaturation occurs when there is a high rate of cholesterol secretion, a low rate of bile acid secretion, a reduced bile acid pool, and low secretion of phospholipids.

Obesity increases risk of gallstones by increasing cholesterol secretion into bile. It seems logical that a high cholesterol intake would increase cholesterol secretion into the bile and increase the risk of gallstones, but there is no firm evidence from studies in humans that bile cholesterol saturation is increased by high intakes of cholesterol. Gastrointestinal disorders that impair the reabsorption of bile acids also may increase the risk of gallstone formation (reviewed by Bennion and Grundy, 1978a,b).

In general, dietary factors in gallstone formation—except for those involved in obesity—have not been conclusively identified. There is conflicting and inconsistent evidence regarding the effects of polyunsaturated fats on bile cholesterol saturation and cholelithiasis (see Chapter 7). In some experiments in humans, very high intakes of polyunsaturated fatty acids increase the cholesterol saturation of bile and increase its lithogenicity. There is no evidence that PUFA intakes of up to 10% of total calories affect the lithogenicity of bile.

Several species of rodents are highly susceptible to the induction of gallstones when fed diets enriched with cholesterol and fats and are thus useful in studying the pathogenesis of gallstones. However, this susceptibility appears to be due to a genetic variation in their ability to metabolize cholesterol and bile salts, and their existence does not establish a causal relationship with dietary fats or cholesterol in humans (see Chapter 7).

Evidence Associating Nondietary Factors with Gallstones

Genetic Factors

The predominant cause of gallstones and their accompanying complications—cholecystitis and bile duct obstruction—appears to be a genetically determined metabolic trait causing some people to secrete lithogenic bile. The strong predisposition to cholelithiasis among American Indians (Hesse, 1959) and people with American Indian ancestry supports the concept of genetic susceptibility. However, no specific genetic marker for this trait has been identified.

SUMMARY

Alcoholic cirrhosis and cholesterol gallstones are the major diseases of the liver and biliary system in the United States. Alcoholic cirrhosis results from prolonged and excessive consumption of alcoholic beverages. As with most diet-related diseases, there is a genetic basis for susceptibility both to alcohol abuse and to liver cirrhosis.

Cholesterol gallstones occur in approximately 10% of the U.S. population and are much more frequent among those with admixtures of American Indian blood. They are the major cause of chronic gallbladder disease and are responsible for a substantial number of surgical interventions, particularly in women. The only firmly established nutrition-related condition predisposing to gallstones is obesity, which causes excessive secretion of cholesterol into bile. Experiments in humans and animals suggest that polyunsaturated fat and cholesterol intake may contribute to cholesterol gallstones, but the evidence does not support a causal relationship for these dietary components in the general population. A subset of the population may be genetically susceptible to gallstone formation despite only average intakes of polyunsaturated fats and cholesterol.

DIRECTIONS FOR RESEARCH

Alcoholic Cirrhosis

- Major efforts are under way at the national level to control the abuse of alcoholic beverages (NIAAA, 1987). Efforts to develop effective educational and treatment regimens for alcohol de-

pendence should be continued. Research aimed at discovering the genetic basis of alcohol dependence is needed for designing more effective alcoholism prevention strategies.

Cholelithiasis and Cholecystitis

- The genetic–environmental (nutritional) interactions responsible for the formation of gallstones and lithogenic bile are poorly understood. Recent progress in the molecular biology of lipid and lipoprotein metabolism and in the genetic control of lipid metabolism should provide an opportunity for new studies on these diseases.

REFERENCES

Bennion, L.J., and S.M. Grundy. 1978a. Risk factors for the development of cholelithiasis in man (first of two parts). N. Engl. J. Med. 229:1161–1167.

Bennion, L.J., and S.M. Grundy. 1978b. Risk factors for the development of cholelithiasis in man (second of two parts). N. Engl. J. Med. 229:1221–1227.

Grant, B.F., J. Noble, and H. Malin. 1986. Decline in liver cirrhosis mortality and components of change: United States, 1973–1983. Alcohol Health Res. World 10:66–69.

Hesse, F.G. 1959. Incidence of cholecystitis and other diseases among Pima Indians of southern Arizona. J. Am. Med. Assoc. 170:1789–1790.

Laënnec, R.T.H. 1819. Traité de l'auscultation médiate et des maladies des poumons et du coeur. Brosson et Chaudé, Paris. 196 pp.

Lieber, C.S., L.M. DeCarli, and E. Rubin. 1975. Sequential production of fatty liver, hepatitis, and cirrhosis in subhuman primates fed ethanol with adequate diets. Proc. Natl. Acad. Sci. U.S.A. 72:437–441.

NIAAA (National Institute on Alcohol Abuse and Alcoholism). 1983. Fifth Special Report to the U.S. Congress on Alcohol and Health from the Secretary of Health and Human Services. DHHS Publ. No. (ADM) 84-1291. Public Health Service, U.S. Department of Health and Human Services, Rockville, Md. 146 pp.

NIAAA (National Institute on Alcohol Abuse and Alcoholism). 1987. Sixth Special Report to the U.S. Congress on Alcohol and Health from the Secretary of Health and Human Services. DHHS Publ. No. (ADM) 87-1519. Public Health Service, U.S. Department of Health and Human Services, Rockville, Md. 147 pp.

Popper, H., and C.S. Lieber. 1980. Histogenesis of alcoholic fibrosis and cirrhosis in the baboon. Am. J. Pathol. 98:695–716.

Strom, B.L., and S.L. West. 1985. The epidemiology of gallstone disease. Pp. 1–26 in S. Cohen and R.D. Soloway, eds. Contemporary Issues in Gastroenterology. Churchill Livingstone, New York.

Terris, M. 1967. Epidemiology of cirrhosis of the liver: national mortality data. Am. J. Public Health 57:2076–2088.

26

Dental Caries

Dental caries is the localized demineralization of the tooth surface caused by organic acid metabolites of oral microorganisms such as *Streptococcus mutans*. The disease leads to a chronic, progressive destruction of the teeth.

The prevalence of dental caries is most often expressed as *dmft* (decayed, missing, and filled teeth) for primary dentition and *DMFT* for permanent teeth (Barmes and Sardo-Infirri, 1977). Internationally, prevalence rates of dmft in 6-year-olds and DMFT in 12-year-olds range from a high of 9.3 per child in Japan and 10.6 per child in Switzerland, respectively, to a low of 0.9 per child in Cameroon and 0.1 in Zambia, respectively. U.S. prevalence rates are intermediate; dmft in 6-year-olds is 3.4 per child and DMFT in 12-year-olds is 4.0 per child (Sreebny, 1982a).

Caries prevalence in the United States has declined in the past 30 years. During 1971–1974, children from 5 to 17 years of age had decay or fillings in an average of 7.06 teeth. By 1981 this number had dropped to 4.77, a 32% decrease (NIDR, 1981). Caries of the tooth crown is still predominantly a disease of children and adolescents, although caries of the root surface of the teeth, secondary to exposure of the root by recession of the gingivae, is becoming more prevalent among older adults (Miller et al., 1987). Less is known about the causes of root caries than about caries of the tooth crown, but possible risk factors include increased longevity of the population and longer retention of teeth in adults (Carlos, 1984).

Although declining in prevalence, dental caries in the United States remains a significant health problem. Rates are highest in the Northeast, lowest in the Southwest, and at intermediate levels elsewhere (NIDR, 1981). Prevalence rates are highest in females of every age group (NIDR, 1981) and in people of both sexes in the lower socioeconomic groups (Ismail et al., 1987). The estimated costs of dental care in the United States amounted to $25.1 billion in 1984, or 6.5% of total health care costs (Levit et al., 1985). In 1990, the costs are projected to be as high as $42 billion (Arnett et al., 1986).

EVIDENCE ASSOCIATING DIETARY FACTORS WITH DENTAL CARIES

The relationship of diet to dental caries risk was suspected as early as the fourth century B.C., when Aristotle hypothesized that dental caries was caused by consumption of sweet figs, which stuck to the tooth (Forster, 1927). Current evidence from studies in humans and animals indeed indicates that dental caries does not develop in the absence of fermentable carbohydrates in the diet (Brown, 1975). Evidence also suggests that the cariogenic effect of fermentable carbohydrates can be amplified or attenuated by other dietary factors

637

as well as by oral microflora and host factors (e.g., genetic susceptibility and the composition and flow of saliva). However, as McDonald (1985a) points out, even after 23 centuries we know only a little more than Aristotle about the relative cariogenicity of foods.

Epidemiologic and Clinical Studies

Carbohydrates

Among the major carbohydrates in the diet—complex carbohydrates (e.g., starches) and simple sugars (e.g., sucrose and lactose)—sucrose appears to have the greatest cariogenic potential. Using data collected by the World Health Organization, Sreebny (1982a) reported a correlation coefficient of .72 between sugar availability in grams per person per day and DMFT in 12-year-old children in 47 countries. However, the correlation coefficient for dmft in 6-year-old children in 23 countries was only .31. Takeuchi (1961) provided time-trend data supportive of Sreebny's cross-sectional findings and reported that the prevalence of dental caries in Japanese children decreased precipitously during the late 1940s in association with the severe reduction in sugar supplies during World War II. Similar observations were made in Europe (Sognnaes, 1948; Toverud, 1957). In the United States, correlation analyses of time-trend data on per-capita sugar consumption and caries incidence suggest (1) that caries incidence increases when per-capita sugar consumption exceeds 40 g/day in the absence of fluoride use and 50 g/day when fluoride is used and (2) that the increase in caries incidence reaches a plateau when the per-capita consumption reaches approximately 130 g/day (Lehner, 1980; Newbrun, 1982; Sheiham, 1983, 1984; Sreebny, 1982b). As Glinsmann et al. (1986) noted, these data suggest that the current mean intake of added and total sugars in the United States (53 and 95 g/day, respectively) contributes substantially to overall caries risk and that reduction in sugar intake could be expected to reduce that risk. However, findings of other studies indicate that the correlation between sugar intake and caries occurrence is not entirely consistent. For example, caries incidence in Great Britain did not change appreciably from 1940 to 1977, despite an apparent doubling of sugar intake (Jackson, 1979). Likewise, the 32% decline in caries prevalence in the United States in the 1970s appears to have occurred despite a continued high intake of sugars. A similar observation was made in a study by DePaola et al. (1982), who noted that caries incidence in Massachusetts schoolchildren dropped markedly during a period in which total sugar consumption increased and then leveled out. Although total sugar consumption increased during the study period, however, the amount of sucrose consumed actually decreased.

Sucrose in solution stimulates the formation of plaque (Geddes et al., 1978)—a substance comprising microbial colonies embedded in a matrix of salivary proteins and extracellular polymers, which may serve as a medium for growth of caries-promoting bacteria. It also increases the mineral content of plaque and saliva, suggesting increased mineral resorption from the teeth (Tenovuo et al., 1984). Frequent rinsing with a sucrose solution over 2 months produced changes characteristic of early demineralization of tooth surfaces (Geddes et al., 1978). Small slabs of bovine enamel attached to human teeth for short periods also underwent demineralization when frequently exposed to sucrose (Pearce and Gallagher, 1979; Tehrani et al., 1983).

Sucrose in foods is also cariogenic. In a clinical trial at the University of Turku in Finland (Scheinin et al., 1975a,b), three groups consuming diets containing sucrose, fructose, and xylitol, respectively, were followed for 2 years. By the study's end, the average number of decayed, missing, or filled tooth surfaces (DMFS) was twice as high in the group consuming sucrose than in the fructose group. The xylitol group had virtually no DMFS. The lower cariogenicity of fructose relative to sucrose may explain in part the inability of some studies to demonstrate a cariogenic potential of presweetened foods such as cereals (Finn and Jamison, 1980; Glass and Fleisch, 1974), which differ considerably in their content of specific sugars (Glinsmann et al., 1986). The decline in caries prevalence in the United States since the 1970s, despite a continued high consumption of total sugars, may be partially due to the nation's increasing consumption of corn-derived sweeteners such as fructose and the declining use of sucrose (Glinsmann et al., 1986).

The composition of dietary carbohydrate also appears to influence cariogenicity. Early enamel erosion, a risk factor for caries, was noted in 12 children ages 9 to 15 years who had consumed large quantities of soft drinks (Asher and Read, 1987). The authors concluded that a major contributing factor was the high citric acid content and resulting low pH of the drinks. Consumption of canned pears and apples has also been noted to lower plaque pH—a factor believed to promote tooth demineralization (Shaw, 1987)—to a greater degree than sugar alone (Abelson and Pergola, 1984; Imfeld et al., 1978; Jensen and Schachtele, 1983). Likewise, comparisons of snack foods commonly consumed in the United States and in the United Kingdom demonstrate a wide variability in their ability to increase plaque and salivary acidity (Bibby et al., 1986; Edgar et al., 1975). In these studies, the sugar-to-starch ratio of the snack foods appears to be important, since some items low in sugar but high in starch caused a more severe and prolonged increase in plaque and saliva acidity than snacks high in sugar alone (Bibby et al., 1986; Mörmann and Mühlemann, 1981). The degree of plaque and salivary acidification does not necessarily correlate with the amount of enamel destruction that follows or with the extent of subsequent caries (McDonald, 1985a).

The sequence in which carbohydrate-containing foods are eaten also appears to influence cariogenesis. For example, a sharp decrease in the pH of saliva and plaque has been noted after use of a sugar rinse. The pH returns to baseline after approximately 30 minutes. However, when cheese is consumed 5 minutes after a sugar rinse, the sharp increase in acidity is blunted and the pH returns quickly to baseline (Edgar, 1981; Edgar et al., 1982; Schachtele and Jensen, 1983).

The frequency of carbohydrate consumption also appears to influence caries formation. In a classic cohort study conducted in a mental institution in Vipeholm, Sweden, the frequency of dental caries activity in adult patients was monitored over several years while their diet and eating schedule were controlled. Two important findings were noted. First, dental caries appeared to be influenced more by frequency of sucrose intake than by total amount consumed. Second, solid forms of sugar, which are more easily retained in teeth, appear to be more cariogenic than liquid forms of sucrose (Gustafsson et al., 1952).

In general, epidemiologic and clinical findings support the notion that all dietary carbohydrates are cariogenic to some degree and that cariogenesis is influenced not only by the composition of carbohydrate-containing foods but also by the sequence and frequency with which they are consumed. Beyond this, there are two basic reasons why little is known about the cariogenic potential of specific carbohydrate-containing foods: (1) because of cost and ethical considerations, few studies of specific foods and caries in humans have been or will be conducted and (2) findings from such studies are difficult to generalize to noninstitution-

alized humans. Furthermore, it is probably not possible to develop a valid cariogenic index for individual foods, since studies of caries incidence comparing groups consuming and not consuming various food items show little effect due to the strong cariogenic challenge from the rest of the diet (McDonald, 1985a).

Certain foods appear to be protective. As noted previously, consumption of cheese blunts the drop in pH characteristically seen after a sugar rinse (Edgar, 1981). Regular milk consumption by 14-year-old Danish schoolchildren was associated with a lower incidence of caries, but regular milk consumption was a marker of a better diet and could also have been an indicator of better preventive dental care (Hölund, 1987). Consumption of salted peanuts and cheddar cheese increases oral alkalinity (Geddes et al., 1977; Imfeld et al., 1978; Jensen and Schachtele, 1983)—a factor believed to protect against caries formation. Cocoa also contains substances that inhibit oral acidification (Paolino, 1982). Starchy fibrous foods require increased mastication and may inhibit cariogenesis by stimulating saliva and maintaining neutral plaque pH (Krasse, 1982). Studies suggest that polyols (sugar alcohols, including the 6-carbon sorbitol and 5-carbon xylitol) are noncariogenic and possibly even anticariogenic. Sorbitol-containing chewing gum, unlike sugar-containing gum, does not appear to promote tooth decay in children (Glass, 1983). Also, as noted earlier, the group on the xylitol diet in the University of Turku study had no DMFS. That finding was attributed to the fact that xylitol is not metabolized by oral microbes (Scheinin, 1976; Scheinin et al., 1975a,b). Substitution of xylitol for sucrose in many Finnish food products has been associated with a dramatic decrease in caries incidence over a 2-year period (Scheinin et al., 1975b). Similarly, the use of xylitol-containing chewing gum was associated in one study with low caries incidence, even in subjects who did not otherwise modify their diets. This led the authors to hypothesize that xylitol is actively anticariogenic rather than noncariogenic (Scheinin et al., 1975c).

With the exception of data on fluoride, there are few data relating dietary components to caries risk in humans. Several investigators have found a beneficial effect of supplemental vitamin D in children up to the age of 10 (McDonald, 1985b) and have suggested that the optimal daily intake is approximately 400 IU (Shaw, 1952). However, other studies have produced conflicting findings (Navia, 1970). As a result, the relationship of vitamin D to caries risk remains unresolved (McDonald, 1985b).

Fluoride

Of all dietary components exhibiting a protective effect against caries, the most effective is fluoride. In the 1930s, large-scale epidemiologic trials conducted in several suburban Chicago communities and later in 21 cities in four states demonstrated a strong inverse association between natural fluoride concentrations in community water supplies and DMFT prevalence in children ages 12 to 14 years (Dean et al., 1941, 1942). In these studies, DMFT prevalence was found to be approximately 60% lower in populations drinking water with natural flouride concentrations of 1 part per million (ppm) during tooth development than in populations consuming little or no fluoride. Once it was determined that the 1 ppm concentration of fluoride in drinking water is both optimal and safe and that the benefit of fluoride ingestion persists into middle age, a decision was made to undertake a large community trial in which water was fluoridated in three communities in North America (Grand Rapids, Michigan; Newburgh, New York; and Brantford, Ontario). A 50 to 60% reduction in caries prevalence was observed in all three communities, and no major adverse effects were noted in residents of any age (McClure, 1970). The findings from these and subsequent large-scale community trials led the American Dental Association and the U.S. Public Health Service in 1950 to endorse widespread fluoridation of the water supply as a preventive measure against dental caries (Schrotenboer, 1981). At present, approximately 130.8 million people in the United States are drinking water from public supplies with either natural fluoride at optimal levels (i.e., 0.7 to 1.2 ppm, depending on ambient temperature) or with fluoride added to meet optimal levels (T. Reeves, Centers for Disease Control, personal communication, 1987).

Ingestion of fluoride at such levels reduces caries risk in people of all ages. For example, consumption of optimally fluoridated water has been associated with an almost 50% reduction in caries incidence in children (Burt et al., 1986; Driscoll et al., 1981) as well as a reduced risk of root caries in adults (Anonymous, 1987; Stamm and Banting, 1980). Consumption of fluoridated water before the emergence of permanent molars appears most effective—producing an average risk reduction of 50 to 60%, which continues for the lifetime of the teeth as long as fluoride intake is maintained (Deatherage, 1943). If fluoride intake is discontinued, caries become more prevalent, but not to the degree that would be expected if there had been no previous exposure to fluoride (Lemke et al., 1970; Weatherell et al., 1977).

Although fluoridated water has been shown to be an effective, safe, and low-cost means of reducing caries risk in the general population, more than 45% of the U.S. population continues to drink water with less than optimal levels of fluoride (T. Reeves, Centers for Disease Control, personal communication, 1987). To address this need, the American Dental Association, the American Academy of Pediatrics, and the American Academy of Pediatric Dentistry have issued guidelines on fluoride supplementation for children receiving less than adequate levels of fluoride in their drinking water (see Table 26–1).

The extent of dietary fluoride supplementation in the United States is not known. In a 1982 survey of 4,000 dentists and 2,000 pediatricians, only 60% of the dentists and 70% of the pediatricians who responded reported prescribing dietary fluoride supplements (Gift and Hoerman, 1985). These figures are comparable with those of an earlier survey in which 81% of pediatricians and 63% of family physicians reported prescribing supplements (Margolis et al., 1980). The lower proportion of prescribers among dentists in both surveys may reflect a smaller number of children under age 2 in dentists' practices or a bias resulting from the survey's relatively low response rates, e.g., 75% and 49% among dentists and physicians,

TABLE 26–1 Recommended Daily Fluoride Supplements for Children in Three Age Categories, Based on Fluoride Concentration in the Water Supply[a]

Age of Child (years)[b]	Supplementation (ppm) Corresponding to Three Levels of Fluoride in the Water Supply (ppm)		
	<0.3	0.3 to 0.7	>0.7
0 to 2	0.25	0.00	0.00
2 to 3	0.50	0.25	0.00
3 to 13	1.00	0.50	0.00

[a]Adapted from Levy (1986). Recommended by the Council on Dental Therapeutics of the American Dental Association, by the Committee on Nutrition of the American Academy of Pediatrics, and by the American Academy of Pediatric Dentistry.
[b]The American Academy of Pediatrics recommends providing tablets from 2 weeks of age through at least 16 years of age.

respectively, in the 1982 survey (Gift and Hoerman, 1985).

The mechanism by which fluoride protects against root and surface caries is not well understood (Brown and König, 1977; Seichter, 1987). Since fluoride is found in enamel as well as in dentin, it is believed to inhibit caries formation primarily by promoting remineralization of early demineralized areas of the tooth (Driscoll, 1985; Silverstone, 1984) and by exerting an antimicrobial effect, thus suppressing cariogenic oral microflora (Shaw, 1987).

Fluoride is absorbed both systemically and topically (Brown et al., 1977; Ericsson, 1977; Weatherell et al., 1977). During tooth development, systemic fluoride appears to be incorporated into the tooth structure (Sognnaes, 1965; Weatherell et al., 1977). After tooth formation, fluoride is incorporated into the surface crystalline structure of the tooth, primarily through topical agents such as fluoridated water and dentifrices (Weatherell et al., 1977).

Overconsumption of fluoride during tooth development can lead to dental fluorosis characterized by mottling of the tooth surfaces. Consumption of water fluoridated at 1 ppm rarely results in clinical fluorosis of either the teeth or skeleton (Carr et al., 1985); however, other fluoride sources can add to overall fluoride load. For example, fluoride in the food chain is believed to contribute on average 0.2 to 0.6 mg of fluoride per person per day. Foods especially rich in fluoride include chicken, seafoods, and brewed tea (tea can contain as much as 1 to 4 mg of fluoride per cup) (Levy, 1986; McClure, 1970; Newbrun, 1975; Richmond, 1985). Fluoride can also be unintentionally ingested from fluoridated dentifrices, which can provide an average daily fluoride intake of as much as 0.3 mg for children under age 5 (Barnhart et al., 1974). Concern has also been expressed about the elevated fluoride levels in some baby formulas and foods (Adair and Wei, 1978; Singer and Ophaug, 1979). Because fluoride levels can vary considerably with the type of formula or food and where it is processed, manufacturers of infant formulas have reduced levels in their products (American Dental Association Council on Dental Therapeutics, 1984).

Overall, however, as noted in a review by Richmond (1985), the amount of fluoride ingested from foods and from the supervised use of fluoridated dentifrices is small, and when combined with levels in optimally fluoridated drinking water, is well within the margin of safety defined by the American Dental Association Council on Dental Therapeutics (1984). The large data base on fluoride indicates that consumption of optimal levels of fluoride substantially reduces caries incidence with little risk of side effects (e.g., dental fluorosis) and that the growing availability of fluoridated water is probably responsible for much of the decline in caries incidence in the United States over the past 15 to 20 years (Dunning, 1979).

Animal Studies

Results of animal studies on dietary carbohydrate and cariogenesis are consistent with those of studies in humans. In rats, for example, the incidence of caries increases with increases in the amounts of sucrose added to the diet; a cariogenic effect is seen at levels as low as 0.1% by weight of diet (Michalek et al., 1977). An increase in caries incidence with increasing sucrose dose has been observed at levels ranging from 8% (Kreitzman and Klein, 1976) to 40% of dietary sucrose (Hefti and Schmid, 1979). The cariogenic potential of sucrose is greater than that of equivalent amounts of glucose, fructose, or invert sugars (a mixture of dextrose and fructose obtained by hydrolyzing sucrose) (Birkhed et al., 1981; Horton et al., 1985).

As in humans, the cariogenicity of dietary carbohydrates in animal models appears to be influenced by the frequency, form, and composition of the diet. For example, frequent consumption of carbohydrates markedly accelerates caries formation in rats (Firestone et al., 1982; Skinner et al., 1982). Studies of the cariogenic potential of various forms of dietary carbohydrates in rats indicate that certain carbohydrate-containing foods, such as bananas, are much more cariogenic than sucrose alone or even sucrose-topped chocolate fed frequently in meals (Shrestha and Kreutler, 1983). Consumption of a cereal base with added sugar caused fewer caries in rats than did consumption of presweetened cereals with equal sucrose levels (McDonald and Stookey, 1977). Likewise, carbohydrates in the form of maize or wheat starch had virtually no cariogenic activity when consumed by gnotobiotic rats and macaques, respectively (Beighton and Hayday, 1984; Horton et al., 1985).

Studies of dietary composition in rats indicate that addition of certain cheeses (e.g., cheddar cheese) to a cariogenic diet protects against buccal (cheek side) decay both alone (Edgar et al., 1982; Harper et al., 1986) and with sulcal caries (toward the linear depression in the occlusal surface of the tooth) (Rosen et al., 1984). Other dietary substances inhibiting sucrose cariogenicity in animal models include mineral concentrates containing protein, calcium, and phosphate (Harper et al., 1987); cocoa (Paolino, 1982); and xylitol (Leach and Green, 1981; Shyu and Hsu, 1980) in rats; and saccharin in inbred hamsters (Linke, 1980). The mechanisms by which these items inhibit sucrose cariogenicity in animal models are not clearly understood, but may include enzyme inhibition in oral bacteria (Paolino, 1982); stimulation of saliva, which helps to maintain plaque pH in a neutral range (Krasse, 1982); and the influence of the texture and casein or calcium–phosphate content of cheeses (Harper et al., 1986).

The cariogenicity of other dietary components, including protein, vitamin D, niacin, pyridoxine, calcium, phosphorus, and certain trace elements, has also been investigated in animal studies. Offspring of rats fed marginal protein diets during pregnancy and lactation developed molars that were much more prone to caries than offspring of rats fed adequate protein diets (Shaw and Griffiths, 1963). Shaw (1987) hypothesized that the decreased amount and altered protein content of saliva in the protein-depleted rats may account for part of their increased caries susceptibility. Other studies have shown that children with protein–calorie malnutrition have not only a high rate of caries but also reduced salivary levels of immunoglobulin A (IgA), the predominant immunoglobulin in body secretions (McMurray et al., 1977; Reddy et al., 1976). McDonald (1985b) hypothesized that protein malnutrition disturbs IgA salivary concentration, thereby increasing caries risk.

In one early study in puppies, vitamin D deficiency was shown to disturb the rate of tooth eruption, tooth position, and calcification of enamel on permanent teeth (Mellanby, 1918). The B-complex vitamins niacin and pyridoxine were also shown in early studies to modify cariogenesis in animals; however, unlike vitamin D, their effect did not appear to be systemic. Niacin was believed to promote caries formation in the Syrian hamster by stimulating oral microflora (Orland et al., 1950). Unlike niacin, pyridoxine seemed to suppress caries formation in animals (Strean et al., 1956) and in humans (Strean, 1958). The paucity of more recent evidence on these vitamins suggests that neither plays a major role in cariogenesis.

The roles of calcium and phosphorus, both major constituents of teeth, were also the subject of early research (McDonald, 1985b). Reduction of dietary calcium in rats was shown to increase caries risk (Constant et al., 1954; Gustafson et al., 1963), whereas the addition of calcium chloride, calcium gluconate, or phosphorus decreased risk (Gustafson et al., 1964; Stanmeyer, 1963). There has been no confirmation of these findings, however. A number of trace elements, including aluminum, barium, boron, cadmium, copper, lead, and selenium, have also been examined for cariostatic potential, but again, no definitive data have been obtained (Losee and Ludwig, 1970).

Animal studies support findings in humans that dietary carbohydrates, especially sucrose, are a major risk factor for caries and that the frequency and sequence of carbohydrate consumption as well as the composition of the carbohydrates can also influence cariogenicity. Interpretation of the results from such studies must be tempered, however, by the knowledge that most of them are derived from a single animal species—the rat. The rat has been favored because of the rapidity with which it develops dental caries in the laboratory and the similarity of its sulcal and smooth-surface carious lesions to those of humans (Glinsmann et al., 1986); however, its feeding patterns and oral physiology (e.g., microbial composition, oral pH, salivary composition, flow rate, and buffering capacity) differ greatly from those of humans (McDonald, 1985a). For example, rats nibble throughout the day, and it is known that meal frequency correlates positively and strongly with caries formation in animals (Firestone et al., 1982; Skinner et al., 1982) and in humans (Gustafsson et al., 1952). Furthermore, foods must be given to rats in powdered form—not in the physical form usually consumed by humans. This can complicate attempts to assess cariogenicity of specific foods (Krasse, 1985). Differences in oral physiology may also influence findings. For example, although most types of phosphates effectively reduce caries in rats when added to sucrose-containing diets, phosphate supplementation in the human diet has been markedly unsuccessful in reducing caries incidence (Nizel and Harris, 1964).

EVIDENCE ASSOCIATING NONDIETARY FACTORS WITH DENTAL CARIES

Studies suggest that fermentable carbohydrates in the diet contribute to caries formation but are not sufficient by themselves to cause dental caries. Oral microflora and appropriate host factors must also be present and must interact with diet if caries are to form and progress (Navia, 1977).

Oral Microflora

The oral cavity is host to a variety of microbial flora that thrive in the moist nutrient-rich environment. At birth, the mouth is usually sterile; soon afterward, colonization occurs (Gibbons and van Houte, 1978). The cariogenic role of oral microflora was first noted in studies of rats delivered by Caesarean section and maintained under sterile conditions. The germ-free rats were caries-free from birth and remained so, even when fed a cariogenic diet (Orland et al., 1954).

Streptococcus mutans is most commonly associated with cariogenesis. *S. mutans* has been found in all human populations and is concentrated in plaque over the most active carious lesions (Kristofferson et al., 1985). Bacteriocin typing of *S. mutans* demonstrates that the mother is the major source of oral infection in the infant (Berkowitz and Jordan, 1975; Rogers, 1981). The mother also determines the extent of infection, since highly infected mothers tend to have children with higher counts of *S. mutans* than mothers with low infection rates (Köhler and Bratthall, 1978).

Both the presence and the extent of *S. mutans* infection in children are associated with caries risk. Köhler et al. (1986) reported that in children infected with *S. mutans* before age 2, caries prevalence is 8 times greater than in children not infected until age 4. Similarly, children who are more heavily infected tend to develop more caries than children with lower counts (Köhler et al., 1984).

Monoinoculation of germ-free rats with various isolates of human oral microflora has demonstrated that most strains of *S. mutans* can cause caries in the fissures and smooth surfaces of the teeth, although strains vary in virulence. Other microorganisms associated to various degrees with caries formation include *Streptococcus salivarius*, *S. sanguis*, *Lactobacillus casei*, and several strains of *Actinomyces* (Miller, 1981). However, generalizing these findings to humans should be approached with caution, since monoinfection in gnotobiotic rats does not mimic the process that occurs in the oral environment of humans where various microflora compete for available niches (Shaw, 1987).

The mechanisms by which *S. mutans*, *S. sanguis*, and other microorganisms promote caries are not well understood. *S. sanguis* is believed to help establish colonization of the tooth surface by *S. mutans* and other oral microflora (van Houte, 1976). If unimpeded, progressive colonization of the tooth surface results in plaque (Hardie and Bowden, 1976). Plaque holds acidic microbial metabolic by-products close to the tooth surface, protecting them from the buffering effect of saliva. These by-products are believed to demineralize the tooth surface and promote decay. The microbial content of plaque can vary considerably, however, both across a single tooth surface and over time. This limits our ability to identify specific causative agents. Furthermore, *S. mutans* is often not detectable in plaque over apparently active carious lesions (Shaw, 1987). Whether this results from an inability to measure small microbial concentrations, from mistaken sampling of inactive lesions, or from a true lack of effect is not known. However, the association of *S. mutans* infection with caries incidence in children and the fact that plaque concentrations over active lesions are reduced when sugar consumption is curtailed suggests that *S. mutans* is a major etiologic agent for caries of the tooth crown.

Host Factors

The role of genetic susceptibility in caries causation appears to be minor. Although monozygotic twins in one longitudinal twin study were found to have a more concordant incidence rate of caries than dizygotic twins (Kent and Moorrees, 1979), corroborative evidence is lacking.

The composition and the rate of flow of saliva appear to influence cariogenesis in several ways, although there is no evidence for genetic determination of these factors (Shaw, 1987). Saliva can act as a buffer, neutralizing acid by-products of oral microflora found on tooth surfaces and in carious lesions. The high concentrations of calcium and phosphorus and the low levels of fluoride found in saliva may facilitate remineralization of early carious lesions and form caries-resistant surface enamel (Silverstone, 1984). Saliva may also inhibit the metabolism and growth of cariogenic microflora, since it contains several potentially bacteriostatic agents, including lysozyme, lactoferrin, and secretory immunoglobulins (Cole et al., 1976; Evans et al., 1976; Pollock et al., 1976).

Decreasing saliva flow in rodents through removal or ligation of some or all the major salivary glands substantially increases caries incidence (Muhler and Shafer, 1957; Schwartz and Shaw, 1955; Schwartz and Weisberger, 1955). Destruction or absence of salivary glands in humans results in a marked increase in caries incidence (Bertram, 1967).

SUMMARY

Dental caries is a multifactorial disease. Diet and oral microflora are implicated in caries causation along with such host factors as salivary composition and flow. Genetic susceptibility does not appear to be a major risk factor for caries.

Fermentable carbohydrates appear to be the only component of the diet capable of inducing caries. All fermentable dietary carbohydrates, especially sucrose, are potentially cariogenic, but sucrose is generally accepted as the most cariogenic dietary factor. Sucrose consumption has been associated most strongly by and consistently with the frequency of dental caries in humans. Other sugars such as glucose and fructose have also been shown to be potentially cariogenic in human and laboratory studies, although they appear to be less cariogenic than sucrose. The cariogenic potential of carbohydrate-containing foods depends on their characteristics (e.g., stickiness), and the frequency and sequence of their consumption. The addition of certain foods and nonnutritive sweeteners, such as cheddar cheese, cocoa, and xylitol, to the diet appears to reduce the cariogenic potential of a sucrose-containing meal.

Caries will neither form nor progress in the absence of a suitable substrate (e.g., oral microflora). Of the oral microflora that have been implicated in caries causation, S. mutans has been the most consistently and strongly associated.

Consumption of fluoride in optimal amounts reduces caries incidence in people of all ages. Fluoride is strongly anticariogenic if consumed in optimal amounts before eruption of permanent teeth. Widespread fluoridation of water supplies and the use of topical fluorides (e.g., fluoridated dentifrices), combined with changing trends in sugar consumption (e.g., decreasing sucrose consumption), are probably the two factors most responsible for the recent decline in caries prevalence rates in the United States.

DIRECTIONS FOR RESEARCH

• Research should be continued on plaque and its specific role in cariogenesis and on dietary factors and food intake patterns that can modify plaque ecology or prevent plaque accumulation.

• More research should be undertaken on the environmental and genetic factors that influence risk of tooth and root cavities.

REFERENCES

Abelson, D.C., and G. Pergola. 1984. The effect of sucrose concentration on plaque pH in vivo. Clin. Prevent. Dent. 6:23–26.

Adair, S.M., and S.H.Y. Wei. 1978. Supplemental fluoride recommendations for infants based on dietary fluoride intake. Caries Res. 12:76–82.

American Dental Association Council on Dental Therapeutics. 1984. Fluoride compounds. Pp. 395–420 in Accepted Dental Therapeutics, 40th ed. American Dental Association, Chicago.

Anonymous. 1987. Fluoride and root surface caries. Nutr. Rev. 45:103–105.

Arnett, R.H., III, D.R. McKusick, S.R. Sonnefield, and C.S. Cowell. 1986. Projections of health care spending to 1990. Health Care Finan. Rev. 7:1–36.

Asher, C., and M.J.F. Read. 1987. Early enamel erosion in children associated with the excessive consumption of citric acid. Pediatr. Dent. 162:384–387.

Barmes, D.E., and J. Sardo-Infirri. 1977. World Health Organization activities in oral epidemiology. Community Dent. Oral Epidemiol. 5:22–29.

Barnhart, W.E., L.K. Hiller, G.J. Leonard, and E. Michaels. 1974. Dentifrice usage and ingestion among four age groups. J. Dent. Res. 53:1317–1322.

Beighton, D., and H. Hayday. 1984. The establishment of the bacterium Streptococcus mutans in dental plaque and the induction of caries in macaque monkeys (Macaca fascicularis) fed a diet containing cooked wheat flour. Arch. Oral Biol. 29:369–372.

Berkowitz, R.J., and H.V. Jordan. 1975. Similarity of bacteriocins of Streptococcus mutans from mother and infant. Arch. Oral Biol. 20:725–730.

Bertram, U. 1967. Xerostomia. Clinical aspects, pathology and pathogenesis. Acta Odont. Scand. 25 suppl. 49:1–126.

Bibby, B.G., S.A. Mundorff, D.T. Zero, and K.J. Almekinder. 1986. Oral food clearance and the pH of plaque and saliva. J. Am. Dent. Assoc. 112:333–337.

Birkhed, D., V. Topitsoglou, S. Edwardsson, and G. Frostell. 1981. Cariogenicity of invert sugar in long-term rat experiments. Caries Res. 15:302–307.

Brown, A.T. 1975. The role of dietary carbohydrates in plaque formation and oral disease. Nutr. Rev. 33:353–361.

Brown, W.E., and K.G. König, eds. 1977. Cariostatic mechanisms of fluorides. Caries Res. 11 suppl. 1:1–327.

Brown, W.E., T.M. Gregory, and L.C. Chow. 1977. Effects of fluoride on enamel solubility and cariostasis. Caries Res. 11 suppl. 1:118–141.

Burt, B.A., S.A. Eklund, and W.J. Loesche. 1986. Dental benefits of limited exposure to fluoridated water in childhood. J. Dent. Res. 65:1322–1325.

Carlos, J.P. 1984. Epidemiologic trends in caries: impact on adults and the aged. Pp. 131–148 in B. Guggenheim, ed. Cariology Today. S. Karger, Basel.

Carr, L.M., G.G. Craig, R. MacLennan, T.J. Martin, N.H. Stacey, and R. Woods. 1985. Fluorides in the control of dental caries. J. Food Nutr. 42:178–188.

Cole, M.F., R.R. Arnold, J. Mestecky, S. Prince, R. Kulhavy, and J.R. McGhee. 1976. Studies with human lactoferrin and Streptococcus mutans. Pp. 359–373 in H.M. Stiles, W.J. Loesche, and T.C. O'Brien, eds. Microbial Aspects of Dental Caries, Vol. 2. Information Retrieval, Inc., Washington, D.C.

Constant, M.A., H.W. Sievert, P.H. Phillips, and C.A.

Elvehjem. 1954. Dental caries in cotton rat: effect of tooth maturity and minerals on caries production by semi-synthetic diets. J. Nutr. 53:29–41.

Dean, H.T., P. Jay, F.A. Arnold, Jr., and E. Elvove. 1941. Domestic water and dental caries: study of 2,832 white children, aged 12–14 years, of 8 suburban Chicago communities, including *Lactobacillus acidophilus* studies of 1,761 children. Public Health Rep. 56:761–792.

Dean, H.T., F.A. Arnold, Jr., and E. Elvove. 1942. Domestic water and dental caries: additional studies of relation of fluoride domestic waters to dental caries experience in 4,425 white children aged 12 to 14 years, of 13 cities in 4 states. Public Health Rep. 57:1155–1179.

Deatherage, C.F. 1943. Fluoride domestic waters and dental caries experience in 2,026 white Illinois selective service men. J. Dent. Res. 22:129–137.

DePaola, P.F., P.M. Soparkar, M. Tavares, M. Allukian, Jr., and H. Peterson. 1982. A dental survey of Massachusetts school children. J. Dent. Res. (sp. iss.) 61:1356–1360.

Driscoll, W.S. 1985. What we know and don't know about dietary fluoride supplements—the research basis. J. Dent. Child. 52:259–264.

Driscoll, W.S., S.B. Heifetz, and J.A. Brunelle. 1981. Caries-preventive effects of fluoride tablets in schoolchildren four years after discontinuation of treatments. J. Am. Dent. Assoc. 103:878–881.

Dunning, J.M. 1979. Water fluoridation. Pp. 377–414 in Principles of Dental Public Health, 3rd ed. Harvard University Press, Cambridge, Mass.

Edgar, W.M. 1981. Effect of sequence in food intake on plaque pH. Pp. 279–287 in J.J. Hefferren and H.M. Koehler, eds. Foods, Nutrition and Dental Health, Vol. 1. Pathotox Publ., Park Forest South, Ill.

Edgar, W.M., B.G. Bibby, S. Mundorff, and J. Rowley. 1975. Acid production in plaques after eating snacks: modifying factors in foods. J. Am. Dent. Assoc. 90:148–425.

Edgar, W.M., W.H. Bowen, S. Amsbaugh, E. Monell-Torrens, and J. Brunelle. 1982. Effects of different eating patterns on dental caries in the rat. Caries Res. 16:384–389.

Ericsson, S.Y. 1977. Cariostatic mechanisms of fluorides: clinical observations. Caries Res. 11 suppl. 1:2–41.

Evans, R.T., R.J. Genco, F.G. Emmings, and R. Linzer. 1976. Antibody in the prevention of adherence: measurement of antibody to purified carbohydrates of *Streptococcus mutans* with an enzyme linked immunosorbent assay. Pp. 375–386 in H.M. Stiles, W.J. Loesche, and T.C. O'Brien, eds. Microbial Aspects of Dental Caries, Vol. 2. Information Retrieval, Inc., Washington, D.C.

Finn, S.B., and H.C. Jamison. 1980. The relative effects of three dietary supplements on dental caries. J. Dent. Child. 47:109–113.

Firestone, A.R., R. Schmid, and H.R. Mühlemann. 1982. Cariogenic effects of cooked wheat starch alone or with sucrose and frequency controlled feedings in rats. Arch. Oral Biol. 27:759–763.

Forster, E.S. 1927. The works of Aristotle, Vol. VII. Problemata. Oxford University Press, London. 931 pp.

Geddes, D.A., W.M. Edgar, G.N. Jenkins, and A.M. Rugg-Gunn. 1977. Apples, salted peanuts and plaque pH. Br. Dent. J. 142:317–319.

Geddes, D.A., J.A. Cooke, W.M. Edgar, and G.N. Jenkins. 1978. The effect of frequent sucrose mouthrinsing on the induction *in vivo* of caries-like changes in human dental enamel. Arch. Oral Biol. 23:663–665.

Gibbons, R.J., and J. van Houte. 1978. Oral bacterial ecology. Pp. 684–705 in J.H. Shaw, E.A. Sweeney, C.C. Cappuccino, and S.M. Meller, eds. Textbook of Oral Biology. W.B. Saunders, Philadelphia.

Gift, H.C., and K.C. Hoerman. 1985. Attitudes of dentists and physicians toward the use of dietary fluoride supplements. J. Dent. Child. 52:265–268.

Glass, R.L. 1983. A two-year clinical trial of sorbitol chewing gum. Caries Res. 17:365–368.

Glass, R.L., and S. Fleisch. 1974. Diet and dental caries: dental caries incidence and the consumption of ready-to-eat cereals. J. Am. Dent. Assoc. 88:807–813.

Glinsmann, W.H., H. Irausquin, and Y.K. Park. 1986. Evaluation of health aspects of sugars contained in carbohydrate sweeteners: report of Sugars Task Force, 1986. J. Nutr. 116:S1-S216.

Gustafson, G., E. Stelling, and E. Brunius. 1963. Cariogenic effect of variations in the salt mixture in a synthetic cariogenic diet. Experimental dental caries in golden hamsters, XI. Acta Odont. Scand. 21:297–308.

Gustafson, G., E. Stelling, and E. Brunius. 1964. Dietary calcium and caries. Experimental dental caries in golden hamsters. Acta Odont. Scand. 22:477–485.

Gustafsson, B.E., C.E. Quensel, L.S. Lanke, C. Lundqvist, H. Grahnen, B.E. Bonow, and B. Krasse. 1952. Vipeholm Dental Caries Study: the effect of different levels of carbohydrate intake on caries activity in 436 individuals observed for five years (Sweden). Acta Ondont. Scand. 11:232–364.

Hardie, J.M., and G.H. Bowden. 1976. The microbial flora in dental plaque: bacterial succession and isolation considerations. Pp. 63–86 in H.M. Stiles, W.J. Loesche, and T.C. O'Brien, eds. Microbial Aspects of Dental Caries, Vol. 1. Information Retrieval, Inc., Washington, D.C.

Harper, D.S., J.C. Osborn, J.J. Hefferren, and R. Clayton. 1986. Cariostatic evaluation of cheeses with diverse physical and compositional characteristics. Caries Res. 20:123–130.

Harper, D.S., J.C. Osborn, R. Clayton, and J.J. Hefferren. 1987. Modification of food cariogenicity in rats by mineral-rich concentrates from milk. J. Dent. Res. 66:42–45.

Hefti, A., and R. Schmid. 1979. Effect on caries incidence in rats of increasing dietary sucrose levels. Caries Res. 13:298–300.

Hölund, U. 1987. Relationship between diet-related behavior and caries in a group of 14-year-old Danish children. Community Dent. Oral Epidemiol. 15:184–187.

Horton, W.A., A.E. Jacobs, R.M. Green, V.F. Hillier, and D.B. Drucker. 1985. The cariogenicity of sucrose, glucose and maize starch in gnotobiotic rats mono-infected with strains of the bacteria *Streptococcus mutans*, *Streptococcus salivarius*, and *Streptococcus milleri*. Arch. Oral Biol. 30:777–780.

Imfeld, T., R.S. Hirsch, and H.R. Mühlemann. 1978. Telemetric recordings of interdental plaque pH during different meal patterns. Br. Dent. J. 144:40–45.

Ismail, A.L., B.A. Burt, and J.A. Brunelle. 1987. Prevalence of dental caries and periodontal disease in Mexican American children aged 5 to 17 years: results from southwestern HHANES, 1982–83. Am. J. Public Health 77:967–970.

Jackson, D. 1979. Caries experience in deciduous teeth of five-year-old English children: 1974–1977. Probe 20:404–406.

Jensen, M.E., and C.F. Schachtele. 1983. The acidogenic potential of reference foods and snacks at interproximal sites in the human dentition. J. Dent. Res. 62:889–892.

Kent, R.L., Jr., and C.F.A. Moorrees. 1979. Associations in interproximal caries prevalence from a longitudinal twin study. J. Dent. Res. (sp. iss.) 58:225.

Köhler, B., and D. Bratthall. 1978. Intrafamilial levels of Streptococcus mutans and some aspects of the bacterial transmission. Scand. J. Dent. Res. 86:35–42.

Köhler, B., I. Andréen, and B. Jonsson. 1984. The effect of caries-preventive measures in mothers on dental caries and the oral presence of the bacteria Streptococcus mutans and lactobacilli in their children. Arch. Oral Biol. 29:879–883.

Köhler, B., I. Andreen, and B. Jonsson. 1986. Streptococcus mutans infection and dental caries in young children—a longitudinal study. Caries Res. 20:171.

Krasse, B. 1982. Oral effect of other carbohydrates. Int. Dent. J. 32:24–32.

Krasse, B. 1985. The cariogenic potential of foods—a critical review of current methods. Int. Dent. J. 35:36–42.

Kreitzman, S.N., and R.M. Klein. 1976. Non-linear relationship between dietary sucrose and dental caries. J. Dent. Res. (sp. iss.) 55:B175.

Kristofferson, K., H.G. Grödahl, and D. Bratthall. 1985. The more Streptococcus mutans, the more caries on approximal surfaces. J. Dent. Res. 64:58–61.

Leach, S.A., and R.M. Green. 1981. Reversal of fissure caries in the albino rat by sweetening agents. Caries Res. 15:508–511.

Lehner, T. 1980. Future possibilities for the prevention of caries and periodontal disease. Br. Dent. J. 149:318–325.

Lemke, C.W., J.M. Doherty, and M.C. Arra. 1970. Controlled fluoridation: the dental effects of discontinuation in Antigo, Wisconsin. J. Am. Dent. Assoc. 80:782–786.

Levit, K.R., H. Lazenby, D.R. Waldo, and L.M. Davidoff. 1985. National health expenditures, 1984. Health Care Finan. Rev. 7:1–35.

Levy, S.M. 1986. Expansion of the proper use of systemic fluoride supplements. J. Am. Dent. Assoc. 112:30–34.

Linke, H.A. 1980. Inhibition of dental caries in the inbred hamster by saccharin. Ann. Dent. 39:71–74.

Losee, F.L., and T.G. Ludwig. 1970. Trace elements and caries. J. Dent. Res. 49:1229–1236.

Margolis, F.J., B.A. Burt, M.A. Schork, R.L. Bashshur, B.A. Whittaker, and T.L. Burns. 1980. Fluoride supplements for children: a survey of physicians' prescription practices. Am. J. Dis. Child. 134:865–868.

McClure, F.J. 1970. Water fluoridation: the search and the victory. National Institute of Dental Research, National Institutes of Health, Public Health Service, U.S. Department of Health, Education, and Welfare, Bethesda, Md. 302 pp.

McDonald, J.L., Jr. 1985a. Cariogenicity of foods. Pp. 320–345 in R.L. Pollack and E. Kravitz, eds. Nutrition in Oral Health and Disease. Lea & Febiger, Philadelphia.

McDonald, J.L., Jr. 1985b. Dietary and nutritional influences on caries. Pp. 151–160 in R.L. Pollack and E. Kravitz, eds. Nutrition in Oral Health and Disease. Lea & Febiger, Philadelphia.

McDonald, J.L., Jr., and G.K. Stookey. 1977. Animal studies concerning the cariogenicity of dry breakfast cereals. J. Dent. Res. 56:1001–1006.

McMurray, D.N., H. Rey, L.J. Casazza, and R.R. Watson. 1977. Effect of moderate malnutrition on concentrations of immunoglobulins and enzymes in tears and saliva of young Colombian children. Am. J. Clin. Nutr. 30:1944–1948.

Mellanby, M. 1918. The influence of diet on tooth formation. Lancet 2:767–770.

Michalek, S.M., J.R. McGhee, T. Shiota, and D. Devenyns. 1977. Low sucrose levels promote extensive Streptococcus mutans-induced dental caries. Infect. Immun. 16:712–714.

Miller, A.J., J.A. Brunelle, J.P. Carlos, L.J. Brown, and H. Löe. 1987. Oral Health of United States Adults. The National Survey of Oral Health in U.S. Employed Adults and Seniors: 1985–1986, National Findings. NIH Publ. No. 87-2868. Epidemiology and Oral Disease Prevention, National Institute of Dental Research, National Institutes of Health, Public Health Service, U.S. Department of Health and Human Services, Bethesda, Md. 168 pp.

Miller, C.H. 1981. Dental caries. Pp. 340–363 in G.I. Roth and R. Calmes, eds. Oral Biology. C.V. Mosby, St. Louis.

Mörmann, J.E., and H.R. Mühlemann. 1981. Oral starch degradation and its influence on acid production in human dental plaque. Caries Res. 15:166–175.

Muhler, J.C., and W.G. Shafer. 1957. Comparison between salivary gland extirpation and duct ligation on dental caries in rats. J. Dent. Res. 36:886–888.

Navia, J.M. 1970. Evaluation of nutritional and dietary factors that modify animal caries. J. Dent. Res. 49:1213–1228.

Navia, J.M. 1977. Experimental dental caries. Pp. 257–297 in Animal Models in Dental Research. University of Alabama Press, Tuscaloosa, Ala.

Newbrun, E., ed. 1975. Fluorides and Dental Caries, 2nd ed. C.C. Thomas, Springfield, Ill. 208 pp.

Newbrun, E. 1982. Sugar and dental caries: a review of human studies. Science 217:418–423.

NIDR (National Institute of Dental Research). 1981. The Prevalence of Dental Caries in United States Children: 1979–1980. NIH Publ. No. 82-2245. National Caries Program, National Institutes of Health, Public Health Service, U.S. Department of Health and Human Services, Bethesda, Md. 159 pp.

Nizel, A.E., and R.S. Harris. 1964. Effects of phosphates on experimental dental caries: a literature review. J. Dent. Res. 43:1123–1136.

Orland, F.J., E.S. Hemmens, and R.W. Harrison. 1950. Effect of partly synthetic diets on the dental caries incidence in Syrian hamsters. J. Dent. Res. 29:512–528.

Orland, F.J., R. Blayney, R.W. Harrison, J.A. Reyniers, P.C. Trexler, M. Wagner, H.A. Gordon, and T.D. Luckey. 1954. Use of the germfree animal technic in the study of experimental dental caries. I. Basic observations on rats reared free of all microorganisms. J. Dent. Res. 33:147–174.

Paolino, V. 1982. Anti-plaque activity of cocoa. Pp. 43–58 in J.J. Hefferren and H.M. Koehler, eds. Foods, Nutrition and Dental Health, Vol. 2: Third Annual Conference. American Dental Association, Chicago.

Pearce, E.I., and I.H. Gallagher. 1979. The behaviour of sucrose and xylitol in an intro-oral caries test. N.Z. Dent. J. 75:8–14.

Pollock, J.J., V.J. Iacono, H.G. Bicker, B.J. MacKay, L.I. Katona, L.B. Taichman, and E. Thomas. 1976. The binding, aggregation and lytic properties of lysozyme. Pp. 325–352 in H.M. Stiles, W.J. Loesche, and T.C. O'Brien, eds. Microbial Aspects of Dental Caries, Vol. 2. Information Retrieval, Inc., Washington, D.C.

Reddy, V., N. Raghuramulu, and C. Bhaskaram. 1976. Secretory IgA in protein-calorie malnutrition. Arch. Dis. Child. 51:871–874.

Richmond, V.L. 1985. Thirty years of fluoridation: a review. Am. J. Clin. Nutr. 41:129–138.

Rogers, A.H. 1981. The source of infection in the intrafamilial transfer of Streptococcus mutans. Caries Res. 15:26–31.

Rosen, S., D.B. Min, D.S. Harper, W.J. Harper, W.X. Beck, and F.M. Beck. 1984. Effect of cheese, with and without sucrose, on dental caries and recovery of *Streptococcus mutans* in rats. J. Dent. Res. 63:894–896.

Schachtele, C.F., and M.E. Jensen. 1983. Can foods be ranked according to their cariogenic potential? Pp. 136–146 in B. Guggenheim, ed. Cariology Today. S. Karger, Basel.

Scheinin, A. 1976. Caries control through the use of sugar substitutes. Int. Dent. J. 26:4–13.

Scheinin, A., K.K. Mäkinen, and K. Ylitalo. 1975a. Turku sugar studies. I. An intermediate report on the effect of sucrose, fructose and xylitol diets on the caries incidence in man. Acta Ondont. Scand. 32:383–412.

Scheinin, A., K.K. Makinen, and K. Ylitalo. 1975b. Turku sugar studies. V. Final report on the effect of sucrose, fructose and xylitol diets on the caries incidence in man. Acta Odont. Scand. 33:67–104.

Scheinin, A., K.K. Mäkinen, E. Tammisalo, and M. Rekola. 1975c. Turku sugar studies. XVIII. Incidence of dental caries in relation to 1-year consumption of xylitol chewing gum. Acta Odont. Scand. 33:307–316.

Schrotenboer, G.H. 1981. Fluoride benefits—after 36 years. J. Am. Dent. Assoc. 102:473–474.

Schwartz, A., and J.H. Shaw. 1955. Studies on the effect of selective desalivation on the dental caries incidence of albino rats. J. Dent. Res. 34:239–247.

Schwartz, A., and D. Weisberger. 1955. Salivary factors in experimental animal caries. Pp. 125–136 in R.F. Sognnaes, ed. Advances in Experimental Caries Research. American Association for the Advancement of Science, Washington, D.C.

Seichter, U. 1987. Root surface caries: a critical literature review. J. Am. Dent. Assoc. 115:305–310.

Shaw, J.H. 1952. Nutrition and dental caries. Pp. 415–507 in G. Toverud, S.B. Finn, G.J. Cox, C.F. Bodecker, and J.H. Shaw, eds. A Survey of the Literature of Dental Caries. A Report of the Committee on Dental Health, Food and Nutrition Board, National Research Council. National Academy of Sciences, Washington, D.C.

Shaw, J.H. 1987. Causes and control of dental caries. New Engl. J. Med. 317:996–1004.

Shaw, J.H., and D. Griffiths. 1963. Dental abnormalities in rats attributable to protein deficiency during reproduction. J. Nutr. 80:123–141.

Sheiham, A. 1983. Sugars and dental decay. Lancet 1:282–284.

Sheiham, A. 1984. Changing trends in dental caries. Int. J. Epidemiol. 13:142–147.

Shrestha, B.M., and P.A. Kreutler. 1983. A comparative rat caries study on cariogenicity of foods using the intubation and gel methods. J. Dent. Res. (sp. iss.) 62:685.

Shyu, K.W., and M.Y. Hsu. 1980. The cariogenicity of xylitol, mannitol, sorbitol and sucrose. Proc. Natl. Sci. Counc., Repub. China 4:21–26.

Silverstone, L.M. 1984. The significance of remineralization in caries prevention. Can. Dent. Assoc. J. 50:157–167.

Singer, L., and R. Ophaug. 1979. Total fluoride intake of infants. Pediatrics 63:460–466.

Skinner, A., P. Connolly, and M.N. Naylor. 1982. Influence of the replacement of dietary sucrose by maltose in solid and in solution on rat caries. Caries Res. 16:443–452.

Sognnaes, R.F. 1948. Analysis of wartime reduction of dental caries in European children. Am. J. Dis. Child. 75:792–821.

Sognnaes, R.F. 1965. Fluoride protection of bones and teeth. Science 150:989–993.

Sreebny, L.M. 1982a. Sugar availability, sugar consumption and dental caries. Community Dent. Oral Epidemiol. 10:1–7.

Sreebny, L.M. 1982b. The sugar–caries axis. Int. Dent. J. 32:1–12.

Stamm, J.W., and D.W. Banting. 1980. Comparison of root caries prevalence in adults with life-long residence in fluoridated and non-fluoridated communities. J. Dent. Res. 59:552.

Stanmeyer, W.R. 1963. The problem of dental caries in military dentistry: proceedings of the Conference on Phosphates and Dental Caries. J. Dent. Res. 43:997–998.

Strean, L.P. 1958. The importance of pyridoxine in the suppression of dental caries in school children and hamsters. N.Y. State Dent. J. 24:133–137.

Strean, L.P., E.W. Gilfillan, and G.A. Emerson. 1956. Suppressive effect of pyridoxine as dietary supplement on dental caries in Syrian hamster. N.Y. J. Dent. 22:325.

Takeuchi, M. 1961. Epidemiological study on dental caries in Japanese children, before, during and after World War II. Int. Dent. J. 11:443–457.

Tehrani, A., F. Brudevold, F. Attarzadeh, J. Van Houte, and J. Russo. 1983. Enamel demineralization by mouth rinses containing different concentrations of sucrose. J. Dent. Res. 62:1216–1217.

Tenovuo, J., K.K. Makinen, and K. Paunio. 1984. Effects on oral health of mouthrinses containing xylitol, sodium cyclamate and sucrose sweeteners in the absence of oral hygiene. IV. Analysis of whole saliva. Proc. Finn. Dent. Soc. 80:28–34.

Toverud, G. 1957. The influence of war and post-war conditions on the teeth of Norwegian school children. Milbank Mem. Fund Q. 35:373–459.

van Houte, J. 1976. Oral bacterial colonization: mechanisms and implications. Pp. 3–32 in H.M. Stiles, W.J. Loesche, and T.C. O'Brien, eds. Microbial Aspects of Dental Caries, Vol. 1. Information Retrieval, Inc., Washington, D.C.

Weatherell, J.A., D. Deutsch, C. Robinson, and A.S. Hallsworth. 1977. Assimilation of fluoride by enamel throughout the life of the tooth. Caries Res. 11 suppl. 1:85–115.

PART IV

Overall Assessment, Conclusions, and Recommendations

27

Overall Assessment and Major Conclusions

This chapter describes the committee's process for integrating the evidence relating dietary components to chronic diseases and presents its major conclusions concerning the role of diet in health. It is prefaced by a brief description of the special features of this study.

SPECIAL CHARACTERISTICS OF THE STUDY

Over the past half century, extensive epidemiologic, clinical, and experimental research has shown that diet is one of many factors that play an important role in the etiology and pathogenesis of major chronic diseases (AHA, 1988; Ahrens et al., 1979; DHEW, 1979; NRC, 1982; Page et al., 1961; U.S. Senate, 1977). In recent decades, scientists have identified many dietary factors that influence the incidence and course of specific chronic diseases and have attempted to define the pathophysiological mechanisms (AHA, 1982; Ahrens et al., 1979; Goldstein and Brown, 1984; Levy et al., 1979; NRC, 1980, 1982). Simultaneously, scientists, public health policymakers, the food industry, consumer groups, and others have been engaged in a debate about how much and what kind of evidence justifies giving dietary advice to the public and how best to control risk factors on which there is general agreement among scientists (Ahrens, 1985; Council on Scientific

Affairs, 1979; Blackburn, 1979; CAST, 1977; Connor, 1979; Habicht et al., 1979; Grobstein, 1983; Gussow and Thomas, 1986; Harper, 1978; Hegsted, 1978; NRC, 1980, 1982; O'Connor and Campbell, 1986; Olson, 1979; Palmer, 1983; U.S. Senate, 1977).

The present study was launched in an attempt to address the critical scientific issues that have been under debate, many of which are fundamental to nutrition policy on reducing the risk of chronic diseases. The committee recognized at the outset that the absence of consensus on certain diet–disease interrelationships derives partly from a lack of knowledge and partly from the absence of generally accepted criteria for interpretation and acceptability of the abundant though incomplete evidence on diet and chronic diseases. Several reports have addressed the importance of dietary factors in public health. With the exception of the recent *Surgeon General's Report on Nutrition and Health* (DHHS, 1988), however, they have focused primarily on identifying dietary risk factors for single diseases (e.g., American Diabetes Association, 1987; AHA, 1986, 1988; NIH, 1984a,b, 1985; NRC, 1982). With the exception of Ahrens et al. (1979), very few reports dealing with general health maintenance have documented in detail the criteria for acceptability of the evidence or provided a detailed basis for their conclusions. This report attempts to cross the boundary between identifying dietary risk factors for single diseases and determining how these risk factors influence the spectrum of chronic diseases and conditions, including atherosclerotic cardiovascular diseases, hypertension, obesity, cancer, osteoporosis, diabetes mellitus, hepatobiliary disease, and dental caries. The report complements and extends past efforts of government agencies and voluntary health and other scientific organizations by presenting an in-depth analysis of the overall relationship between diet and the major chronic diseases (e.g., AHA, 1988; DHHS, 1988; NRC, 1982; USDA, 1985; USDA/DHHS, 1980).

In the foregoing chapters, the committee reviews the evidence on all major public health conditions in which diet is believed to play an important role. In this chapter, it presents its overall conclusions about the effect of nutrients, foods and food groups, and dietary patterns on chronic diseases.

In Chapter 2, the committee presents criteria for assessing the data from single studies and explains the process for evaluating the cumulative evidence. The committee first considers the special strengths and weaknesses of each kind of epidemiologic and laboratory study on diet and chronic diseases and then evaluates the total evidence against the commonly used criteria for assessing causality, i.e., strength of association, dose–response relationship, temporally correct association, consistency of association, specificity of association, and biologic plausibility. It emphasizes, however, that these criteria alone do not define acceptability of the evidence.

Special attention is given to dietary interactions and competing risks, which are important considerations both for arriving at conclusions and for formulating dietary recommendations. For example, although diets containing high levels of plant foods have been associated with a lower risk of certain cancers, such diets, because of their high fiber content, could in principle initially inhibit the absorption of essential minerals such as calcium, thereby possibly enhancing other risks. Such potential competing risks and dietary interactions were considered in drawing the conclusions presented in this chapter.

The committee recognizes that genetically dependent variability among individuals and variability due to age, sex, and physiological status may affect physiological requirements for nutrients as well as responses to dietary exposures and, thus, the risk of chronic diseases. Therefore, to the extent possible, it addresses not only the risk to the general population, but also the feasibility of defining risks to subpopulations and individuals that may differ in susceptibility. Recognizing the limitations of the data on diet–disease relationships, the committee wishes to emphasize the necessarily interim nature of its conclusions.

CRITERIA AND PROCESS FOR INTERPRETING AND INTEGRATING EVIDENCE

Chapter 2 explains the many limitations to drawing conclusions about the association between dietary factors and chronic diseases. The term *insufficient data* could perhaps be applied to most issues concerning nutrition and health. In particular, it characterizes many of the relationships between diet and certain chronic diseases. The lack of certainty about causal associations and mechanisms of action is common and stems in part from attempts to relate a complex mixture such as diet to complex, multifactorial chronic diseases for which the pathophysiological, environmental, and genetic predisposing factors are imprecisely understood. Although this is a cause for concern, and therefore warrants further research (see Directions for Research in Chapter 28), it is not unusual in questions pertaining to human health.

In some cases, there is conclusive evidence that a particular dietary factor plays a role in the etiology of a particular chronic disease, but that is the exception rather than the rule. Despite such limitations, a large body of evidence has emerged in the past four decades concerning chronic diseases and their relationship to general dietary patterns or specific dietary components.

Studies in Humans

The strengths and limitations of different types of studies in humans and the methods of assessing dietary intake in such studies are described in Chapter 2. In general, the accuracy of assessing dietary intake is limited by the need to rely on the subjects' memories, the potential for misclassification, the bias of the subject or the investigator, the difficulty of precisely quantifying dietary exposure in years past (which would reflect the long latency period of most chronic diseases), the difficulty of standardizing the methodology of data collection, variation in accuracy of recall between subjects and controls, the likelihood of dietary modification by subjects over time, and the limitations of food composition data.

The committee recognizes that ecological correlations of dietary factors and chronic diseases among populations cannot be used alone to estimate the strength of the association between diet and disease. In general, due to the limitations summarized above, correlations among individuals in a population, including analyses of case-control and cohort studies, are likely to underestimate the strength of the association. Many prospective studies, such as the Framingham (Dawber et al., 1982) and Tecumseh (Nichols et al., 1976) studies, in which dietary practices of individuals were related to disease precursors or outcome (e.g., serum lipid levels or heart attacks), have failed to demonstrate the hypothesized relationship between the diet of an individual and the risk of disease. The absence of established relationships in such studies is probably due to a limited capacity to characterize the diet of an individual, the difficulty of taking into account the large day-to-day variability in dietary intake, and the variability in response (e.g., in serum total cholesterol levels) among people with similar dietary intakes. In contrast, the effect of diet has been more consistently demonstrated in comparisons of population groups with substantially different dietary practices (e.g., vegetarians and nonvegetarians, or Mediterraneans and northern Europeans). In the committee's judgment, when findings from studies within populations differ from those between populations, the latter assume greater importance because of the odds against identifying correlations between dietary factors and chronic disease within a population whose diet is fairly homogeneous.

Results of intervention studies that randomly allocate people to different diets are often considered ideal for assessing causal associations. These received special attention. The committee recognizes that rigid criteria for selecting participants in such studies lead to greater homogeneity in the study samples. In general, long exposures are required for the effects of dietary factors on disease risk to become manifest, and it is difficult to control the diets of noninstitutionalized populations for extended periods. The results of small-scale, short-term clinical investigations conducted under controlled conditions may have limited applicability to the general population or to chronic diseases with long latency periods.

Despite these limitations, in the committee's judgment, repeated and consistent findings of associations between certain dietary factors and certain diseases evaluated against the criteria described in Chapter 2 indicate that such associations are likely to be real and indicative of cause-and-effect relationships.

Studies in Animals

Animal experiments are an important counterpart to epidemiologic and clinical research on nutrition and chronic diseases. As described in Chapter 2, such studies can control genetic variability as well as dietary exposure and permit more intensive observation. However, in assessing the results of animal experiments, one must consider variability among species in diet and nutrient requirements, in absorption and metabolic phenomena, and thus in the comparability of their exposure and disease outcomes to humans.

The committee placed more confidence in data derived from studies on more than one animal species or test system, on results that have been reproduced in different laboratories, and on data that indicate a dose–response relationship.

Integrating the Overall Evidence

The committee recognizes that an a priori weighting scheme could be helpful in evaluating the many types of health-related data but concluded that its application to studies on diet and chronic diseases is not feasible in view of the limitations mentioned above. Thus, in addition to the criteria summarized above and discussed in more detail in Chapter 2, the committee based its conclusions on the totality of the evidence. It took the general view that the strength of the evidence should be evaluated on a continuum from highly likely to very inconclusive. The strength, consistency, and preponderance of the data and the degree of concordance in epidemiologic, clinical, and laboratory experiments determined the strength of the conclusions in the report.

In Section II of this report (Evidence on Dietary Components and Chronic Diseases), the criteria described in Chapter 2 provide the basis of a review of the evidence by *nutrients*. The 13 chapters in that section (6 through 18) summarize the relevant epidemiologic, clinical, and laboratory data pertaining to each nutrient or dietary factor and specific chronic diseases, including cardiovascular diseases, specific cancers, diabetes, hypertension, obesity, osteoporosis, hepatobiliary disease, and dental caries. Nutrient interactions and mechanisms of action are discussed where applicable.

Section III (Impact of Dietary Patterns on Chronic Diseases) briefly reassembles the evidence relating nutrients to specific chronic diseases or conditions and presents conclusions about the role of dietary components and patterns in the etiology of those diseases. Where data permit, the potential for reducing the risk of each disease by changes in dietary patterns is also discussed. This section goes beyond examining data on individual nutrients to consider the evidence on foods, food groups, and dietary patterns. Some of the evidence was obtained directly and some was obtained by extrapolation from data on nutrients or other dietary components. For example, much of the epidemiologic evidence on diet and colon cancer pertains to consumption of vegetables and diets with a high plant-fiber content or low levels of fat. Thus, it is possible to draw direct conclusions about dietary patterns rather than just about individual nutrients or nonnutritive components in these foods. In contrast, many metabolic studies on diet and osteoporosis have involved the measurement of calcium intake rather than the consumption of dairy products or other calcium-containing foods. Thus, extrapolation of the data from such studies is necessary to arrive at conclusions about dairy foods.

MAJOR CONCLUSIONS AND THEIR BASES

Following are the general conclusions drawn from the committee's in-depth review followed by specific conclusions pertaining to the major dietary components and specific chronic diseases. Each section begins with a brief discussion of the findings that served as a basis for the conclusions.

General Considerations

In the United States during this century, there have been noticeable changes in per capita availability of foods, in eating patterns, and in chronic disease trends (see Chapters 3 and 5). Although average per capita availability of calories does not appear to have varied substantially since 1909, the percentage of total calories from fat in this period increased by 11%, while calories from carbohydrates decreased. Since the 1960s, the per capita supply of fat has steadily increased, but remarkable changes have occurred in the sources and therefore the types of fat available. Use of whole milk has declined, whereas consumption of low-fat milk and whole-milk cheeses has increased. Beginning in the 1940s, the use of butter and lard greatly decreased, while the use of margarine and salad

and cooking oils dramatically increased. Most of these changes have resulted in increased per capita availability of polyunsaturated and monounsaturated fatty acids and a decreased supply of saturated fatty acids. Currently, the percentages of calories from fat by specific groups of fatty acids in the U.S. food supply are: approximately 17% monounsaturated (mainly oleic acid), 15% saturated, and 7% polyunsaturated (mainly linoleic acid) (see Chapter 3).

The use of eggs has also declined since 1947, resulting in lower average supplies of cholesterol. The use of poultry has increased steadily and markedly, while that of beef has declined slightly since the mid-1970s.

Complex carbohydrates in the food supply declined from 1909 to 1967, because of the decreased use of grain products and potatoes, but have increased by 9% since 1967. The proportion of carbohydrates from sugars in the food supply increased from approximately 33% in 1909 to slightly more than 50% in 1980. Use of sucrose declined remarkably since its peak use in 1971. Since then it has been partially replaced with corn syrups, including high-fructose corn syrup.

The average availability of protein in the U.S. population has remained at 11% of calories since 1909, but the proportion of protein from animal sources increased 16% by 1982 as a result of decreased use of flour, cereal products, and potatoes and increased use of meat, poultry, fish, and dairy products.

Per capita consumption of vegetables increased by 5% between 1970 and 1983. This includes a notable increase in the per capita intake of broccoli and cauliflower. An increased per capita availability of vitamin A since 1967 resulted from higher amounts of carotenoids in newer varieties of carrots and sweet potatoes. Growing supplies of citrus fruits since 1967 and increasing fortification of foods with vitamin C led to an increased availability of vitamin C in the food supply, and the large increase in the use of salad and cooking oils greatly increased the availability of vitamin E.

Estimates of nutrient availability in the food supply are higher than amounts actually consumed by the population, since food supply data are measured at the wholesale/retail level and do not take into account food wastage or nutrient losses that occur during food processing, marketing, and food preparation. Also, changes in the food supply over time are difficult to compare with data from national surveys that measure actual consumption of foods because of differences in survey methods.

Nevertheless, as described in Chapter 3, both food supply data and the national food consumption surveys have provided useful insights into food and nutrient availability and intake, as well as eating patterns.

The cross-sectional data on food consumption patterns in the national surveys do not permit simple correlations to be made between trends in eating patterns and trends in chronic disease incidence and mortality. The latter are reviewed in Chapter 5. Age- and sex-adjusted mortality from coronary heart disease in the United States has declined more than one-third in the last two decades. Even larger declines have been observed in mortality from stroke and other hypertension-related causes of death. On the other hand, recent surveys in the United States report increases in the prevalence of overweight both in men and women, especially in the younger age groups.

Cancers are responsible for approximately 22% of all deaths in the United States, and total cancer mortality has remained essentially unchanged in recent years in this country. However, the incidence and the mortality rates for specific cancers have shown noticeable changes with time. For example, the rates for lung cancer, one of the major causes of cancer mortality in the United States, have begun to decline for males following decades of increase; however, the incidence and mortality rates for lung cancer among females are increasing. The incidence of breast cancer in women has increased in the last 20 to 30 years, whereas mortality appears to have slightly decreased in premenopausal women and slightly increased in the postmenopausal group. In contrast, stomach cancer incidence and mortality have been declining sharply in both sexes for nearly half a century. Similarly, the incidence of (but not mortality from) endometrial cancer has risen in the past decade in the western part of the United States.

Approximately 15 to 20 million Americans are afflicted with osteoporosis in the United States, which has one of the highest rates of hip and other fractures in the world. These numbers are expected to increase steadily. The incidence of noninsulin-dependent diabetes mellitus (NIDDM), which is the seventh leading cause of mortality in the United States, is estimated to have increased sixfold in the past 50 years. By contrast, in the last 10 to 15 years, there has been a large and unprecedented decline in the prevalence of dental caries among U.S. children.

The committee analyzed these trends in the major chronic diseases as well as trends in eating patterns (Chapters 3 and 5). It reviewed the epidemiologic, clinical, and laboratory evidence pertaining to dietary factors and chronic diseases (Chapters 6 through 26) and attempted to put into perspective the role of diet versus the role of other environmental and genetic factors in the etiology of these diseases (Chapters 4 and 5).

Following are the general conclusions drawn from the committee's in-depth review as well as the specific conclusions pertaining to the major dietary components and specific chronic diseases.

General Conclusions

• A comprehensive review of the epidemiologic, clinical, and laboratory evidence indicates that diet influences the risk of several major chronic diseases. The evidence is very strong for atherosclerotic cardiovascular diseases and hypertension and is highly suggestive for certain forms of cancer (especially cancers of the esophagus, stomach, large bowel, breast, lung, and prostate). Furthermore, certain dietary patterns predispose to dental caries and chronic liver disease, and a positive energy balance produces obesity and increases the risk of NIDDM. However, the evidence is not sufficient for drawing conclusions about the influence of dietary patterns on osteoporosis and chronic renal disease.

• Most chronic diseases in which nutritional factors play a role also have genetic and other environmental determinants, but not all the environmental risk factors have been clearly characterized and susceptible genotypes usually have not been identified. Furthermore, the mechanisms of genetic and environmental interactions involved in disease are not fully understood. It is evident that dietary patterns are important factors in the etiology of several major chronic diseases and that dietary modifications can reduce such risks. Nevertheless, for most diseases, it is not yet possible to provide quantitative estimates of the overall risks and benefits.

Fats, Other Lipids, and High-Fat Diets

There is a substantial body of evidence pertaining to fats and other lipids and their impact on health. Most of this evidence concerns atherosclerotic cardiovascular diseases, several forms of cancer, and to a lesser extent, obesity. For atherosclerosis, the evidence is derived from decades of study, including extensive epidemiologic investigations in many parts of the world, laboratory experiments in different animal species, clinical studies, and intervention trials. In these studies, investigators have examined the effect of the type and amount of various dietary fatty acids, cholesterol, and other dietary components on blood lipid and lipoprotein profiles, on the development of atherosclerotic lesions, and on the occurrence of coronary events as well as the effects of dietary intervention alone or in combination with cholesterol-lowering drugs. Although most of these investigations have drawbacks, as discussed in Chapters 2, 7, and 19, overall they provide an extensive and reliable body of evidence from which to draw conclusions.

The information pertaining to fats and cancer risk (Chapters 7 and 22) pertains primarily to cancers of the colon, prostate, and breast is derived from ecological, case-control, and prospective studies in humans in many parts of the world and from extensive laboratory experiments on spontaneous and chemically induced cancers in rodents. The data base on fat and cancer is limited compared to that on coronary heart disease, especially with respect to the relative effects of different types and amounts of fats and because of the absence of intervention trials. Nonetheless, it is sufficient to serve as the basis for certain conclusions.

There have been relatively few studies in humans on the effect of fat intake per se on obesity (Chapters 6, 7, and 21), and these are compromised by the difficulty of separating the effect of fat from the effects of total calories and other macronutrients. In contrast, there is a substantial body of laboratory evidence on this subject.

The following conclusions derive from the committee's extensive review of the data described in Chapters 6 (Calories), 7 (Fats and Other Lipids), 19 (Atherosclerotic Cardiovascular Diseases), 21 (Obesity and Eating Disorders), 22 (Cancer), and 25 (Hepatobiliary Disease).

General Conclusion

- There is clear evidence that the total amounts and types of fats and other lipids in the diet influence the risk of atherosclerotic cardiovascular diseases and to a less well-established extent, certain forms of cancer, and possibly obesity. The evidence that the intake of saturated fatty acids and cholesterol are causally related to atherosclerotic cardiovascular diseases is especially strong and convincing.

Specific Conclusions

Total Fats

- In several types of epidemiologic studies, a high-fat intake is associated with increased risk of certain cancers, especially cancers of the colon, prostate, and breast. The epidemiologic evidence is not totally consistent, but it is supported by experiments in animals. The combined epidemiologic and laboratory evidence suggests that a reduction of total fat intake is likely to decrease the risk of these cancers.

- High-fat intake is associated with the development of obesity in animals and possibly in humans. In short-term clinical studies, a marked reduction in the percentage of calories derived from dietary fat has been associated with weight loss.

- Although gallbladder disease is associated with obesity, there is no conclusive evidence that it is associated with fat intake.

- Intake of total fat per se, independent of the relative content of the different types of fatty acids, is not associated with higher blood cholesterol levels and coronary heart disease (CHD). A reduction in total fat consumption, however, facilitates reduction of saturated fatty acid intake; hence in addition to reducing the risk of certain cancers, and possibly obesity, it is a rational part of a program aimed at reducing the risk of CHD.

Saturated Fatty Acids (SFAs)

- Clinical, animal, and epidemiologic studies demonstrate that increased intakes of saturated fatty acids (12 to 16 atoms in length) increase the levels of serum total and low-density-lipoprotein (LDL) cholesterol and that these higher levels in turn lead to atherosclerosis and increase the risk of CHD. Saturated fatty acid intake is the major dietary determinant of the serum total cholesterol and LDL cholesterol levels in populations and thereby of CHD risk in populations. Lowering saturated fatty acid intake is likely to reduce serum total and LDL cholesterol levels and, consequently, CHD risk.

- The few epidemiologic studies on dietary fat and cancer that have distinguished between the effects of specific types of fat indicate that higher intakes of saturated fat as well as total fats are associated with a higher incidence of and mortality from cancers of the colon, prostate, and breast. In general, these findings are supported by data from animal experiments.

Polyunsaturated Fatty Acids (PUFAs)

• Clinical and animal studies provide firm evidence that omega-6 PUFAs when substituted for SFAs result in a lowering of serum total cholesterol and LDL cholesterol and usually also some lowering of high-density-lipoprotein (HDL) cholesterol levels.

• Laboratory studies in rodents suggest that diets with high levels of vegetable oils containing omega-6 PUFAs promote certain cancers more effectively than diets with high levels of saturated fats, whereas there is some evidence that diets with a high content of omega-3 PUFAs may inhibit these same cancers. However, these findings are not supported by the limited number of epidemiologic studies that have distinguished between the effects of different types of fat. There are no human diets that naturally have very high levels of total PUFAs, and there is no information about the long-term consequences of high PUFA intakes.

• Fish oils containing large amounts of omega-3 PUFAs reduce plasma triglyceride levels and increase blood clotting time. Their effects on LDL cholesterol vary, and data on the long-term health effects of large doses of omega-3 PUFAs are limited. Limited epidemiologic data suggest that consumption of one or two servings of fish per week is associated with a lower CHD risk, but the evidence is not sufficient to ascertain whether the association is causal or related to the omega-3 PUFA content of fish.

Monounsaturated Fatty Acids (MUFAs)

• Clinical studies indicate that substitution of MUFAs for SFAs results in a reduction of serum total cholesterol and LDL cholesterol without a reduction in HDL cholesterol.

Dietary Cholesterol

• Clinical, animal, and epidemiologic studies indicate that dietary cholesterol raises serum total cholesterol and LDL cholesterol and increases the risk of atherosclerosis and CHD. There is substantial inter- and intraindividual variability in this response. High dietary cholesterol clearly seems to contribute to the development of atherosclerosis and increased CHD risk in the population.

Trans Fatty Acids (TFAs)

• Clinical studies indicate that TFAs and their cis isomers have similar effects on plasma lipids. Animal studies do not indicate that TFAs have a greater tumor-promoting effect than their cis isomers.

Carbohydrates, Vegetables, Fruits, Grains, Legumes, and Cereals and Their Constituents

The committee's conclusions on carbohydrates and foods containing complex carbohydrates—i.e., vegetables, fruits, grains, legumes, and cereal products—derive from a review of direct and indirect evidence. Many epidemiologic studies in different parts of the world have focused on diets high in plant foods in general or in green, yellow, and cabbage-family vegetables and citrus fruits in particular. They have concentrated on the incidence of or mortality from different forms of cancer (especially cancers of the lung, large bowel, stomach, and esophagus) and on coronary heart disease. In some of these studies, the diets of vegetarians and nonvegetarians have been compared. Many clinical metabolic studies have focused on the effects of refined sugars and specific starches on blood glucose and insulin sensitivity. In a series of experiments in animals, investigators have examined the effects of certain components of these foods (e.g., different fibers, vitamins, minerals, and nonnutritive components) on plasma cholesterol levels or on different types of cancer. The indirect evidence on plant foods and chronic disease risk is derived from epidemiologic studies that have focused on diets that are high in fat and animal proteins and that usually tend to be low in carbohydrates and plant foods. Both the direct and indirect evidence has been useful in drawing conclusions, although the committee notes the difficulty in comparing the results of epidemiologic studies, which generally pertain to foods, to metabolic studies or animal experiments, which often deal with single nutrients.

The following conclusions are based on a review of the evidence throughout the report, especially Chapters 7 (Fats and Other Lipids), 9 (Carbohydrates), 10 (Dietary Fiber), 11 (Fat-Soluble Vitamins), 12 (Water-Soluble Vitamins), and 22 (Cancer).

Conclusions

• Diets high in plant foods—i.e., fruits, vegetables, legumes, and whole-grain cereals—are associated with a lower occurrence of coronary heart disease and cancers of the lung, colon, esophagus, and stomach. Although the mechanisms underlying these effects are not fully understood, the inverse association with CHD may be largely explained by the usually low SFA and cholesterol content of such diets. Such diets are also low in total fat, which is directly associated with the risk of certain cancers, but rich in complex carbohydrates (starches and fiber) and certain vitamins, minerals, trace elements, and nonnutritive constituents, and these factors probably also confer protection against certain cancers and CHD.

• Compared to nonvegetarians, complete vegetarians and lacto-ovovegetarians have lower serum levels of total and LDL cholesterol and triglycerides. These lower levels may be the combined result of lower intakes of saturated fatty acids and total fat and higher intakes of water-soluble fiber (e.g., pectin and oat bran). In clinical and animal studies, such fiber has been found to produce small reductions in serum total cholesterol independently of the effect due to fat reduction.

• Populations consuming high-carbohydrate diets, which are high in plant foods, have a comparatively lower prevalence of NIDDM, possibly because of the higher proportion of complex carbohydrate intake and lower prevalence of obesity—a risk factor for NIDDM. In clinical studies, such diets have been shown to improve glucose tolerance and insulin sensitivity.

• Epidemiologic studies indicate that consumption of carotenoid-rich foods, and possibly serum carotene concentration, are inversely associated with the risk of lung cancer.

• Laboratory studies in animals strongly and consistently indicate that certain retinoids prevent, suppress, or retard the growth of chemically induced cancers at a number of sites, including the esophagus, pancreas, and colon, but especially the skin, breast, and bladder. However, most epidemiologic studies do not show an association between preformed vitamin A and cancer risk or a relationship between plasma retinol level and cancer risk.

• Epidemiologic studies suggest that vitamin C-containing foods such as citrus fruits and vegetables may offer protection against stomach cancer, and animal experiments indicate that vitamin C itself can protect against nitrosamine-induced stomach cancer. The evidence linking vitamin C or foods containing that vitamin to other cancer sites is more limited and less consistent.

• Some investigators have postulated that several other vitamins (notably vitamin E, folic acid, riboflavin, and vitamin B_{12}) may block the initiation or promotion of cancer, but the committee judged the evidence too limited to draw any conclusions.

• Epidemiologic and clinical studies indicate that a diet characterized by high-fiber foods may be associated with a lower risk of CHD, colon cancer,

diabetes mellitus, diverticulosis, hypertension, or gallstone formation, but there is no conclusive evidence that it is dietary fiber, rather than the other components of vegetables, fruits, and cereal products, that reduces the risk of those diseases. Although soluble fibers can decrease serum cholesterol and glucose levels, and certain insoluble fibers inhibit chemically induced tumorigenesis, it is difficult to compare the effects of specific dietary fibers tested in the laboratory with the effects of fiber-containing foods or of other potentially protective substances present in these foods.

• Although human and animal studies indicate that all fermentable carbohydrates can cause dental caries, sucrose appears to be the most cariogenic. The cariogenicity of foods containing fermentable carbohydrates is influenced by the consistency and texture (e.g., stickiness) of the food as well as by the frequency and sequence of consumption. Sugar consumption (by those with an adequate diet) has not been established as a risk factor for any chronic disease other than dental caries in humans.

Protein and High-Protein Diets

Compared to the association of fats and complex carbohydrates with chronic disease risk, the association between high-protein diets or protein per se with such risk has received little attention. Much of the evidence on protein and chronic diseases derives indirectly from epidemiologic studies that examined the effects of high fat diets on the risk of atherosclerotic cardiovascular diseases or cancer. In contrast, many animal experiments have measured the effect of high animal-protein intake on serum total cholesterol or on tumor yield. These studies are reviewed in Chapters 8 (Protein), 19 (Atherosclerotic Cardiovascular Diseases), and 22 (Cancer). The committee also examined the limited data on the effect of protein intake on urinary calcium excretion and its possible consequences for osteoporosis, as well as the basis for the more recent interest in the potential adverse effects of a high-protein intake on chronic renal disease. These topics are examined in Chapters 8 (Protein), 13 (Minerals), and 23 (Osteoporosis). Following are the committee's major conclusions.

Conclusions

• In intercountry correlation studies, diets high in meat—a major source of animal protein—have a strong positive association with increased atherosclerotic coronary artery disease and certain cancers, notably breast and colon cancer. Such diets are often characterized by a high content of SFAs and cholesterol, which probably accounts for a large part of the association with CHD, and by a high content of total fat, which is directly associated with the risk of these cancers. However, these diets also tend to have low levels of plant foods, the consumption of which is inversely associated in epidemiologic and animal studies with the risk of heart disease and certain cancers. Total serum cholesterol can be reduced in people with high blood cholesterol by replacing animal foods in their diet with plant foods.

• High protein intake can lead to increased urinary calcium excretion. The impact of this finding on the development of osteoporosis in the general population is unclear.

• The data linking elevated intakes of animal protein to increased risk of hypertension and stroke are weak, and no plausible mechanisms have been posited for either effect.

Energy

The associations among intake of energy-yielding foods, energy expenditure, and obesity and their relation to chronic diseases have been studied for decades, as evidenced by a voluminous literature on these topics. More recently, investigators have been examining the relationship between genetic factors and energy balance. These topics are reviewed in Chapters 6 (Calories) and 21 (Obesity). There are extensive data from epidemiologic, clinical, and animal studies concerning the effect of modifying caloric and nutrient intake on body weight and adiposity. The clinical data pertain to over- and underfeeding of nonobese and obese individuals and the effect of starvation on body weight and body composition. Numerous animal experiments have been conducted in nonobese and spontaneously obese rodents. Studies in both humans and animals demonstrate the difficulty of accurately measuring total food and caloric intake, assessing energy balance, and separating the effects of caloric intake per se from the effect of specific macronutrients on body weight. The committee has analyzed the association between energy balance (energy intake and energy expenditure) and body weight and obesity and has examined obesity as an independent risk factor for atherosclerotic cardiovascular diseases, hypertension, NIDDM, and certain cancers.

The following conclusions are based on this assessment.

Conclusions

• Positive energy balance can result from increased energy intake, reduced energy expenditure, or both, and over the long term can lead to obesity and its associated complications.

• Although data from clinical and animal studies demonstrate that overfeeding leads to obesity, increased body weight in cross-sectional and longitudinal population surveys of adults cannot be accounted for by increased energy intake. Thus, it is likely that obesity develops in adult life either because of reduced physical activity, or overfeeding, or both. Obesity is enhanced not only by this energy imbalance but also by a genetic predisposition to obesity and altered metabolic efficiency.

• Epidemiologic studies indicate that increased energy expenditure is inversely associated with the risk of CHD.

• Epidemiologic and clinical studies and some experiments in animals demonstrate that obesity is associated with an increased risk of NIDDM, hypertension, gallbladder disease, endometrial cancer, and osteoarthritis. It may also be associated with a higher risk of CHD and postmenopausal breast cancer.

• Studies in humans suggest that fat deposits in the abdominal region pose a higher risk of NIDDM, CHD, stroke, hypertension, and increased mortality than do fat deposits in the gluteal or femoral regions.

• Experience in long-term management of obesity indicates that neither frequent fluctuations in body weight nor extreme restrictions of food intake are desirable.

• Long-term follow-up studies indicate that extreme leanness is associated with increased mortality and that the causes of that mortality are different from those associated with excess weight.

• The specific causes of obesity are not well known, although some obese people clearly consume more energy compared to people of normal weight, whereas others are very sedentary or may have increased metabolic efficiency. Compared to maintenance of stable weight, weight gain in adult life is associated with a greater risk of cardiovascular disease, NIDDM, hypertension, gallbladder disease, and endometrial cancer. Certain risk factors—e.g., high serum cholesterol, elevated serum glucose, and high blood pressure—can be curtailed by weight reduction in overweight adults.

Alcoholic Beverages

The extensive data on the health effects of alcohol consumption are examined in Chapters 16 (Alcohol), 19 (Atherosclerotic Cardiovascular Diseases), 20 (Hypertension), 22 (Cancer), and 25 (Hepatobiliary Disease). In these chapters, special note is made of the high incidence of alcoholism in the United States and the difficulty of obtaining accurate measures of alcohol intake. Attention is given to separating the effects of mild and moderate levels of alcohol consumption from those of excessive intake or alcohol abuse. The effects of alcohol consumption have been studied in relation to malnutrition, obesity, carcinogenesis, hypertension, cardiovascular diseases, total mortality, cirrhosis of the liver, several diseases of the nervous system, and adverse pregnancy outcome.

Following are the committee's major conclusions related to alcohol.

Conclusions

• When consumed in excess amounts, alcohol replaces essential nutrients including protein and micronutrients and can lead to multiple nutrient deficiencies.

• Sustained heavy intake of alcoholic beverages leads to fatty liver, alcoholic hepatitis, and cirrhosis. It also increases the risk of cancers of the oral cavity, pharynx, esophagus, and larynx, especially in combination with cigarette smoking, whereupon the effects on cancer risk become synergistic. There is some epidemiologic evidence that alcohol consumption is also associated with primary liver cancer and that moderate beer drinking is associated with rectal cancer. The association of alcohol consumption with increased risk of pancreatic or breast cancer is less clear.

• Excessive alcohol consumption is associated with an increased incidence of CHD, hypertension, stroke, and osteoporosis.

• Alcohol consumption during pregnancy can damage the fetus, cause low infant birth weight, and lead to fetal alcohol syndrome. No safe level of alcohol intake during pregnancy has been determined.

Salt and Related Compounds

Most studies pertaining to salt and human health have focused on hypertension or gastric cancer. The epidemiologic evidence pertaining to hypertension is extensive and comes from longitudinal and cross-sectional studies in large and varied populations throughout the world and from clinical metabolic studies among smaller groups. These data are complemented by a considerable body of evidence derived from studies of animals. In contrast, the data on salt and gastric cancer derive primarily from correlation studies in different parts of the world and a limited number of case-control studies of cancer risk in migrants. These have generally been assessments of the role of salt-pickled and salt-cured foods rather than of sodium chloride intake per se on cancer risk. The effects of several other dietary elements (e.g., potassium, calcium, magnesium, and PUFA) on hypertension have also been examined, but these data are limited compared to those on sodium chloride.

The following conclusions are based on the evidence concerning salt and related compounds and their relation to chronic diseases. This evidence is reviewed in Chapters 15 (Electrolytes), 20 (Hypertension), and 22 (Cancer).

Conclusions

• Blood pressure levels are strongly and positively correlated with the habitual intake of salt. In populations with a sustained salt intake of 6 g or more per day, blood pressure rises with age and hypertension is frequent, whereas in populations consuming less than 4.5 g of salt per day, the age-related rise in blood pressure is slight or absent and the frequency of hypertension is uniformly low. Clinical studies demonstrate that once hypertension is established, it cannot always be fully corrected by resumption of a moderately low (<4.5 g/day) salt intake.

• Although clinical and epidemiologic studies indicate that some people are more susceptible to salt-induced hypertension than others, there are no reliable markers to predict individual responses. Epidemiologic evidence suggests that blacks, people with a family history of hypertension, and all those over age 55 are at a higher risk of hypertension.

• Epidemiologic and animal studies indicate that the risk of stroke-related deaths is inversely related to potassium intake over the entire range of blood pressures, and the relationship appears to be dose dependent. The combination of a low-sodium, high-potassium intake is associated with the lowest blood pressure levels and the lowest frequency of stroke in individuals and populations. Although the effects of reducing sodium intake and increasing potassium intake would vary and may be small in some individuals, the estimated reduction in stroke-related mortality for the population is large.

• A high salt intake is associated with atrophic gastritis in epidemiologic and animal studies, and there is also epidemiologic evidence that a high salt intake and frequent consumption of salt-cured and salt-pickled foods are associated with an elevated incidence of gastric cancer. The specific causative agents in these foods have not been fully identified.

Minerals and Trace Elements

The association of calcium, and to a lesser extent phosphorus and magnesium, with human health has received considerable attention in recent years. Most of the attention has been directed to the role of calcium and magnesium in regulation of blood pressure, the association of calcium and phosphorus intake with peak bone mass and development of osteoporosis, and the relationship of calcium to colon cancer. This evidence derives from epidemiologic studies, cross-sectional studies, many clinical metabolic studies, a few recent intervention trials with calcium supplements, a large number of animal experiments pertaining to calcium intake and bone diseases, and a few experiments on calcium intake and carcinogenesis. These studies are reviewed in Chapters 13 (Minerals), 20 (Hypertension), 22 (Cancer), and 23 (Osteoporosis).

Trace element nutrition has also received much attention in the past decade, especially the role of iron, zinc, selenium, and fluoride intake in human health (see Chapter 14, Trace Elements). With the exception of epidemiologic and laboratory studies on selenium and cancer and on fluoride and dental caries and a few studies on zinc and tumorigenesis, the data pertaining to trace element ingestion and chronic diseases are extremely limited and thus limit the committee's ability to arrive at conclusions. Of particular importance in the committee's assessment were potential antagonistic and synergistic interactions, which occur often among trace elements but about which knowledge is incomplete.

The following conclusions are based on this review.

Conclusions

• Epidemiologic, clinical, and animal studies suggest that sustained low calcium intake is associated with a high frequency of fractures in adults, but the role of dietary calcium in the development of osteoporosis and the potential benefits of calcium supplements—in amounts that exceed the Recommended Dietary Allowances (RDAs)—in decreasing the risk of osteoporosis are unclear.

• Some epidemiologic studies have shown an association between calcium intake and blood pressure, but a causal association between low calcium intake and high blood pressure has not been established.

• A few data from epidemiologic and animal studies suggest that a high calcium intake may protect against colon cancer, but the evidence is preliminary and inconclusive.

• Unequivocal evidence from epidemiologic and clinical studies indicates that fluoridation of drinking water supplies at a level of 1 ppm protects against dental caries. Such concentrations are not associated with any known adverse health effects, including cancer.

• Low selenium intake in epidemiologic and animal studies and low selenium levels in human sera have been associated with an increased risk of several cancers. Moreover, some studies in animals suggest that diets supplemented with large doses of selenium offer protection against certain cancers. These data should be extrapolated to humans with caution, however, because high doses of selenium can be toxic.

• The data on most trace elements examined in this report (e.g., copper and cadmium) are too limited or weak to permit any conclusions about their effects on chronic disease risk.

Dietary Supplements

Claims for the health benefits of dietary supplements have drawn substantial attention in recent decades. Patterns of supplement use have been surveyed in small-scale studies as well as in recent nationwide surveys conducted by the Food and Drug Administration, the U.S. Department of Agriculture, and the National Center for Health Statistics (see Chapter 18). These surveys and other investigations have focused on the use of multiple vitamin–mineral supplements and individual nutrients in the general population and among population subgroups such as the elderly, children, medical students, and health professionals. Attempts have also been made to ascertain the motivation for supplement use and the contribution of supplements to total dietary intake of vitamins and minerals. In comparison to fairly extensive data on the patterns of supplement use, information on their health effects is meager, especially with regard to the long-term effects of multiple nutrient supplements. Several professional societies, notably the American Medical Association, the American Dietetic Association, the American Institute of Nutrition, and the American Society for Clinical Nutrition, have taken positions on the use of dietary supplements. The committee has based the following conclusion on the evidence reviewed in Chapter 18 (Dietary Supplements).

Conclusion

• A large percentage of people in the United States take dietary supplements, but not necessarily because of nutrient needs. The adverse effects of large doses of certain nutrients (e.g., vitamin A) are well documented. There are no documented reports that daily multiple vitamin–mineral supplements, equaling no more than the RDA for a particular nutrient, are either beneficial or harmful for the general population. The potential risks or benefits of the long-term use of small doses of supplements have not been systematically examined.

Coffee, Tea, and Other Nonnutritive Dietary Components

In the United States, nearly 3,000 substances are intentionally added to foods during processing. Another estimated 12,000 chemicals, such as vinyl chloride and acrylonitrile, which are used in food packaging and which inadvertently enter the food supply, are classified as indirect additives. Furthermore, minute quantities of many thousands of naturally occurring toxicants and environmental contaminants are found in foods. The health effects of these nonnutritive substances are reviewed in Chapter 17 (Coffee, Tea, and Other Nonnutritive Dietary Components) along with coffee and tea. The committee emphasizes the difficulty of assessing the long-term effects of this large group of substances. Many of them have not been tested or tested only in short-term experiments, and there are very few epidemiologic data. The committee also stresses the importance of considering dietary interactions (both synergistic and antagonistic), since many of these compounds occur simultaneously in foods. Chapter 17 includes a discussion of the potential health effects of mutagens in foods. Most of the evidence on nonnutritive components pertains to cancer risk.

The major conclusions pertaining to nonnutritive components are presented below.

Conclusions

• Coffee consumption has been associated with slight elevations in serum cholesterol in some epidemiologic studies. Epidemiologic evidence linking coffee consumption to the risk of CHD and cancer in humans is weak and inconsistent.

• Tea drinking has not been associated with an increased risk of any chronic disease in humans.

• The use of such food additives as saccharin, butylated hydroxyanisole, and butylated hydroxytoluene does not appear to have contributed to the overall risk of cancer in humans. However, this lack of evidence may be due to the relatively recent use of many of these substances or to the inability of epidemiologic techniques to detect the effects of additives against the background of common cancers from other causes. The association between food additives and cancer is also complicated by the long latency period between initial exposure to a carcinogen and the subsequent development of cancer.

• A number of environmental contaminants (e.g., some organochlorine pesticides, polychlorinated biphenyls, and polycyclic aromatic hydrocarbons) cause cancer in laboratory animals. The committee found no evidence to suggest that any of these compounds *individually* makes a major contribution to the risk of cancer in humans; however, the risks from simultaneous exposure to several compounds and the potential for adverse effects in occupationally exposed people have not been adequately investigated.

• Certain naturally occurring contaminants in food (e.g., aflatoxins and *N*-nitroso compounds) and nonnutritive constituents (e.g., hydrazines in mushrooms) are carcinogenic in animals and thus pose a potential risk of cancer in humans. Naturally occurring compounds shown to be carcinogenic in animals have been found in small amounts in the average U.S. diet. There is no evidence thus far that any of these substances *individually* makes a major contribution to cancer risk in the United States.

• Most mutagens detected in foods have not been adequately tested for carcinogenic activity. Although mutagenic substances are generally suspected of having carcinogenic potential, it is not yet possible to assess their contribution to the incidence of cancer in the United States.

• Overall, there is a shortage of data on the complete range of nonnutritive substances in the diet. Thus, no reliable estimates can be made of the most significant exposures. Exposure to non-nutritive chemicals individually, in the minute quantities normally present in the average diet, is unlikely to make a major contribution to the overall cancer risk to humans in the United States. The risk from simultaneous exposure to many such compounds cannot be quantified on the basis of current evidence.

REFERENCES

AHA (American Heart Association). 1982. Rationale of the diet-heart statement of the American Heart Association. Report of Nutrition Committee. Circulation 65:839A–854A.

AHA (American Heart Association). 1986. Dietary guidelines for healthy American adults: a statement for physicians and health professionals by the nutrition committee, American Heart Association. Circulation 74:1465A–1468A.

AHA (American Heart Association). 1988. Dietary guidelines for healthy American adults: a statement for physicians and health professionals by the nutrition committee, American Heart Association. Circulation 77:721A–724A.

Ahrens, E.H., Jr. 1985. The diet-heart question in 1985: has it really been settled? Lancet 1:1085–1087.

Ahrens, E.H., Jr., W.E. Connor, E.L. Bierman, C.J. Glueck, J. Hirsch, H.C. McGill, Jr., N. Spritz, L. Tobian, Jr., and T.B. Van Itallie. 1979. Symposium report of the task force on the evidence relating six dietary factors to the nation's health. Am. J. Clin. Nutr. 32:2621–2748.

American Diabetes Association. 1987. Nutritional recommendations and principles for individuals with diabetes mellitus: 1986. Nutr. Today 22:29–35.

Blackburn, H. 1979. Diet and mass hyperlipidemia: a public health view. Pp. 309–347 in R.I. Levy, B.M. Rifkin, B. Dennis, and N. Ernst, eds. Nutrition, Lipids, and Coronary Heart Disease: A Global View. Raven Press, New York.

CAST (Council for Agricultural Science and Technology). 1977. Dietary Goals for the United States: A Commentary. Report. No. 71. CAST, Ames, Iowa. 18 pp.

Connor, W.E. 1979. Too little or too much: the case for preventive nutrition. Am. J. Clin. Nutr. 32:1975–1978.

Council on Scientific Affairs. 1979. American Medical Association concepts of nutrition and health. J. Am. Med. Assoc. 242:2335–2338.

Dawber, T.R., R.J. Nickerson, F.N. Brand, and J. Pool. 1982. Eggs, serum cholesterol, and coronary heart disease. Am. J. Clin. Nutr. 36:617–625.

DHEW (U.S. Department of Health, Education, and Welfare). 1979. Healthy People: the Surgeon General's Report on Health Promotion and Disease Prevention. DHEW (PHS) Publ. No. 79-55071. Office of the Assistant Secretary for Health and Surgeon General, Public Health Service, U.S. Department of Health, Education, and Welfare. U.S. Government Printing Office, Washington, D.C. 177 pp.

DHHS (U.S. Department of Health and Human Services). 1988. The Surgeon General's Report on Nutrition and Health. DHHS (PHS) Publ. No. 88-50210. Public Health Service, U.S. Department of Health and Human Services.

U.S. Government Printing Office, Washington, D.C. 712 pp.

Goldstein, J.L., and M.S. Brown. 1984. Progress in understanding the LDL receptor and HMG-CoA reductase, two membrane proteins that regulate the plasma cholesterol. J. Lipid Res. 25:1450–1461.

Grobstein, C. 1983. Should imperfect data be used to guide public policy? Science 83 4:18.

Gussow, J.D., and P.R. Thomas. 1986. Dietary goals and guidelines: a progressive jump or jumping the gun? Pp. 110–155 in The Nutrition Debate: Sorting Out Some Answers. Bull Publishing, Palo Alto, Calif.

Habicht, J.P., H. Orlans, W.H. Stewart, D.M. Hegsted, R.N. Brandon, and M.R. McHugh. 1979. Symposium: translation of scientific and nutrition findings to social policy. Fed. Proc. 38:2551–2569.

Harper, A.E. 1978. Dietary goals—a skeptical view. Am. J. Clin. Nutr. 31:310–321.

Hegsted, D.M. 1978. Dietary goals—a progressive view. Am. J. Clin. Nutr. 31:1504–1509.

Levy, R.I., B.M. Rifkin, B.H. Dennis, and N. Ernst, eds. 1979. Nutrition, Lipids and Coronary Heart Disease: A Global View. Raven Press, New York. 566 pp.

Nichols, A.B., C. Ravenscroft, D.E. Lamphiear, and L.D. Ostrander. 1976. Daily nutritional intake and serum lipid levels: the Tecumseh Study. Am. J. Clin. Nutr. 29:1384–1392.

NIH (National Institutes of Health). 1984a. Health Implications of Obesity: National Institutes of Health Consensus Development Conference Statement. Ann. Intern. Med. 103:1073–1077.

NIH (National Institutes of Health). 1984b. Osteoporosis: Consensus Development Conference Statement, Vol. 5. Publ. No. 421-132:4652. National Institute of Arthritis, Diabetes, and Digestive and Kidney Diseases and the Office of Medical Applications of Research. U.S. Government Printing Office, Washington, D.C. 6 pp.

NIH (National Institutes of Health). 1985. Lowering blood cholesterol to prevent heart disease: consensus conference. J. Am. Med. Assoc. 253:2080–2090.

NRC (National Research Council). 1980. Toward Healthful Diets. Report of the Food and Nutrition Board, Division of Biological Sciences, Assembly of Life Sciences. National Academy of Sciences, Washington, D.C. 24 pp.

NRC (National Research Council). 1982. Diet, Nutrition, and Cancer. Report of the Committee on Diet, Nutrition, and Cancer, Assembly of Life Sciences. National Academy Press, Washington, D.C. 478 pp.

O'Connor, T.P., and T.C. Campbell. 1986. Dietary guidelines. Pp. 731–771 in C. Ip, D.F. Birt, A.E. Rogers and C. Mettlin, eds. Dietary Fat and Cancer. Alan R. Liss, New York.

Olson, R.E. 1979. The U.S. quandary: can we formulate a rational nutrition policy? Pp. 119–133 in M. Chou and D.P. Harmon, Jr., eds. Critical Food Issues of the Eighties. Pergamon Press, New York.

Page, I.H., E.V. Allen, F.L. Chamberlain, A. Keys, J. Stamler, and F.J. Stare. 1961. Dietary fat and its relation to heart attacks and strokes. Circulation 23:133–136.

Palmer, S. 1983. Diet, nutrition, and cancer: the future of dietary policy. Cancer Res. 43:2509s–2514s.

USDA (U.S. Department of Agriculture). 1985. Report of the Dietary Guidelines Advisory Committee on the Dietary Guidelines for Americans. Human Nutrition Information

Service, U.S. Department of Agriculture, Hyattsville, Md. 19 pp.

USDA/DHHS (U.S. Department of Agriculture/Department of Health and Human Services). 1980. Nutrition and Your Health: Dietary Guidelines for Americans. Home and Garden Bulletin No. 232. U.S. Department of Agriculture and Department of Health and Human Services, Washington, D.C. 20 pp.

U.S. Senate. 1977. Dietary Goals for the United States, 2nd ed. Report of the Select Committee on Nutrition and Human Needs. Stock No. 052-070-04376-8. U.S. Government Printing Office, Washington, D.C. 83 pp.

28

Recommendations on Diet, Chronic Diseases, and Health

The committee's overall recommendations on diet, chronic diseases, and health are presented in this chapter along with a discussion of the criteria, the process, and the factors considered in formulating them. There is also a discussion of the nature of the recommendations and the target populations and comparisons with recommendations of other expert groups in the United States and abroad. In addition, this chapter includes an assessment and some quantitative estimates of the potential benefits and adverse consequences of dietary modifications as they relate to chronic disease risk and recommendations for research to increase knowledge in this area.

CRITERIA AND PROCESS FOR FORMULATING DIETARY RECOMMENDATIONS

Absolute proof is difficult to obtain in any branch of science. As evidence accumulates, however, it often reaches the point of proof in an operational sense, even though proof in an absolute sense may be lacking. In law, proof beyond a reasonable doubt is generally accepted as a standard for making decisions and taking action. The degree of evidence as well as the severity of the crime are the bases for the relative intrusiveness of legal actions taken, e.g., issuing a warning for a misdemeanor compared to the imposition of severe

penalties for a felony. A similar paradigm can be applied to evidence on dietary patterns and associated health risks. For example, public education might be sufficient to warn against the potential hazard of excess caffeine intake, whereas evidence on the toxicity and carcinogenicity of aflatoxin warrants government regulation to curtail aflatoxin contamination of grains and milk. The strength of the evidence might not be the only relevant criterion for determining the course of action; other factors include the likelihood and severity of an adverse effect, potential benefits of avoiding the hazard, and the feasibility of reducing exposure.

The Committee on Diet and Health adopted this approach of gearing dietary recommendations—the proposed level of action—to such critical features as the level of certainty, the potential for public health benefit, and the likelihood of minimal risk. Thus, although much remains to be learned before firm conclusions and recommendations can be made regarding the total impact of diet on chronic disease risk, in the committee's judgment it would be derelict to ignore the large body of evidence while waiting for absolute proof of benefit from dietary change. The committee concluded that the overall evidence regarding a relationship between certain dietary patterns (e.g., a diet high in saturated fat and total fat) and chronic diseases (e.g., cardiovascular diseases or certain cancers) supports (1) a comprehensive effort to inform the public about the likelihood of certain risks and the possible benefits of dietary modification and (2) the use of technological and other means (e.g., production of leaner meat) to facilitate dietary change.

The process of arriving at dietary recommendations, rather than the recommendations themselves, previously has received little attention. One relevant attempt is the development of the *Public Health Objectives for the Nation* by the Office of Disease Prevention and Health Promotion of the U.S. Department of Health and Human Services (DHHS, 1983). That office proposed 17 priority objectives for improving nutrition during the 1990s as well as an implementation plan for meeting these objectives. A midcourse review of the status of these objectives documented the process of developing the objectives and suggested that substantial progress has been made in achieving certain nutrition-related objectives (DHHS, 1986). The logic, criteria, and philosophy for formulating dietary recommendations are also discussed in reports by the Health Education Council in the United Kingdom (NACNE, 1983), the American Heart Association in its *Dietary Guidelines for Healthy American Adults* (AHA, 1986), the National Research Council's Committee on Diet, Nutrition, and Cancer (NRC, 1982), and a Food and Nutrition Board report entitled *Toward Healthful Diets* (NRC, 1980b).

Several individual attempts to define or analyze the process of developing dietary recommendations also provide insights into the philosophy underlying recommendations issued in different countries (e.g., Grobstein, 1983; Langsford, 1979; Molitor, 1979; Palmer, 1983). The committee hopes to contribute to this nascent field through the discussions that follow.

A special feature of the present study is its attempt to develop recommendations and strategies for risk reduction across the entire spectrum of major diet-related chronic diseases. Several factors were considered in this process: risks and benefits; the advantages of making recommendations by nutrient, by food, or by dietary pattern; the basis for proposing quantitative as opposed to qualitative recommendations; recommendations for individuals as opposed to populations; and the feasibility of implementation. These are discussed in the following sections.

Assessment of Risks and Benefits

To develop dietary recommendations for reducing the overall risk of diet-related chronic diseases,

it is essential to analyze and compare recommendations pertaining to individual diseases. For example, recommendations to increase calcium intake to provide possible protection against osteoporosis might in isolation be viewed as conflicting with recommendations for coronary heart disease (CHD) prevention, because dairy products—which contribute the most calcium to the U.S. diet—are also major sources of saturated fatty acids (SFAs), which are known to increase plasma cholesterol levels and CHD risk. Thus, recommendations for maintaining adequate bone mass and for preventing CHD would both have to stress consumption of low-fat dairy products.

Other important considerations are dietary interactions and their synergistic or antagonistic effects. For example, the potential benefits of enhanced trace element intake for certain cancers might be offset by increasing the intake of vegetables and cereals in an attempt to reduce risk for colon cancer, because such foods are also high in fiber, which could in principle initially inhibit intestinal absorption of certain trace elements.

As exemplified systematically at the end of this chapter, the committee considered such potential risks as well as dietary interactions and dose-response relationships in assessing the probable impact of dietary modification on risk factors across the range of chronic diseases. To some extent, this task was simplified by the inherent concordance in dietary risk and protective factors. For example, a recommendation to lower fat intake would be consistent with evidence that low-fat intake may reduce the risk of certain cancers and with stronger evidence that decreased SFA and cholesterol intakes reduce cardiovascular disease risk.

Recommendations by Nutrients, Foods, or Dietary Patterns

The committee discussed whether to base its recommendations on individual nutrients, single foods or food groups, or the overall pattern of dietary intake. Nutrient-based recommendations (e.g., fluoridation of water for the general population or iron fortification to reduce the risk of iron deficiency) might be easy for public health personnel to interpret and implement (e.g., through supplementation or food fortification); however, they may fail to take into account needs that arise from interactions among nutrients (e.g., increased selenium requirements for those on a high-vitamin C diet or enhanced iron absorption in the presence of vitamin C). Furthermore, such recommendations may be difficult for the public to interpret or translate into diets, e.g., understanding how to plan diets to obtain at least 800 mg of calcium—the Recommended Dietary Allowance (RDA) per day. Thus, recommendations pertaining to nutrient intake would usually need to be translated by professionals into guidance about food choices for the public.

Recommendations based on single foods or food groups are easier to implement when only a few foods serve as the major sources of an essential dietary component (e.g., dairy products, which are the primary source of calcium in the U.S. diet). However, such guidance can be misleading. Rich sources of nutrients are not necessarily good dietary sources unless the food is eaten frequently or in large amounts and the nutrient is bioavailable. For example, although the calcium content of spinach is higher than that of dairy products, dairy products are better sources of calcium because of greater bioavailability and more frequent consumption. Furthermore, such recommendations may ignore food group commonalities (i.e., foods with similar nutrient profiles can be exchanged for each other).

As summarized later in this chapter, guidelines issued by other expert groups, including the American Diabetes Association (1987), the American Heart Association (AHA, 1988), the National Research Council's Committee on Diet, Nutrition, and Cancer (NRC, 1982), the U.S. Department of Agriculture and the Department of Health and Human Services (USDA/DHHS, 1985), and the U.S. Surgeon General (DHHS, 1988), are in general based on overall dietary patterns. Furthermore, epidemiologic evidence on chronic diseases pertains more often to foods or diets and less often to single nutrients or other nonnutritive substances (e.g., coffee and tea). Therefore, nutrient-based recommendations must be derived often from the epidemiologic data on dietary patterns. For example, the statement that diets with a high plant-food and low fat content are associated with reduced rates of certain cancers more accurately reflects present knowledge than do conclusions that diets high in selenium or isothiocyanates are likely to reduce cancer risk. The latter requires an inference about cause and effect that is not yet justified by the data.

Recommendations about overall dietary patterns may be difficult to implement, however, if they are too general, devoid of quantification, or provide quantitative information that the average person cannot interpret. For example, the basic five food groups recommended by the USDA are repre-sented in the average fast-food cheeseburger, but not in the desirable proportions (i.e., only a small proportion from the fruit and vegetable group, but high proportions of salt and fat). Alternatively, few people would be able to translate a recommendation to consume a "lower-fat" diet or only "30% of calories from fat" into appropriate food choices. In light of these considerations, the committee concluded that dietary guidelines to prevent chronic diseases and improve the health of the general U.S. population should emphasize overall dietary patterns but should also incorporate relevant information about food groups, foods, and nutrients.

Quantitative Versus Qualitative Recommendations

The committee considered the extent to which its recommendations could be quantified. In general, its decisions were based on the strength of the evidence. The need for quantification also depended on whether dietary effects have a threshold and whether the effects seem to be linear or curvilinear in nature. Quantitative guidelines can take into account nutrient interactions, they are less susceptible to misinterpretation when translated into food choices, and they can be presented as single numbers or as ranges. Furthermore, they are more likely to result in dietary modification because they provide specific targets.

The committee weighed these advantages against the possibility that specifying quantities might in some cases give the appearance of greater certainty than is justified by the evidence. Overall, the committee found the arguments for quantification compelling.

Recommendations for Individuals as Opposed to Populations

There are two approaches to reducing dietary risk factors for chronic diseases: the first is the individual-based approach aimed at identifying and treating individuals at high risk and the second a more global population-based or public health approach aimed at the general population (Blackburn and Jacobs, 1984; Goldbourt, 1987; Olson, 1986). These two approaches are complementary to each other (Rose, 1985; WHO, 1982).

Recommendations tailored to special needs of individuals based on age, sex, physiological status (e.g., pregnancy and lactation), genetic background, and body build, as well as to special conditions such as occupational exposures and metabolic defects, would be ideal. Recommendations to individuals or special population subgroups could also take into consideration thresholds for nutrient requirements (e.g., upper limits or ranges of nutrient intake set to avoid deficiency or toxicity) or specify an optimal average nutrient intake over time. Recommendations suited to individual needs are desirable because every person is genetically unique, and genetic determinants influence the etiology and pathogenesis of practically all chronic diseases associated with nutritional factors. For example, high blood pressure, obesity, hyperlipidemia and atherosclerosis, and certain cancers appear to aggregate in families because of interaction of genetics and a shared environment. Public health recommendations to modify undesirable dietary patterns are unlikely to apply equally to everyone because genetic–environmental interactions as well as dietary exposures contribute to the outcome in specific individuals.

For conditions such as the hyperlipidemias, we can identify some persons at high risk and concentrate specific preventive efforts in this subpopulation. For other conditions, where specific tests are lacking, a strong family history of the disease may suggest that special preventive approaches are needed. It is usually not feasible, however, to identify people at high risk or to screen the entire population. Moreover, people at only moderate or slightly increased risk—e.g., those with borderline-high blood cholesterol levels—will also benefit greatly from the dietary recommendations given to high-risk individuals (National Cholesterol Education Program, 1988).

For most diseases, we are prevented from making individually based recommendations because of a lack of knowledge about susceptible genotypes or risks to particular individuals and about the distribution of dietary requirements in the population. Nevertheless, dietary recommendations aimed at reducing the risk in the general population can have a major benefit for the nation's health. This is because even a relatively small reduction in risk for a disease that occurs in a large number of people who are at moderate risk could lead to a larger reduction in risk for the total population than a large reduction in risk for a smaller number of people at higher risk. For example, the majority of CHD deaths occurs not among those at high risk because of high serum cholesterol levels, but in people who have only moderate elevations in serum cholesterol (i.e., <240 mg/dl; National Cholesterol Education Program, 1988). Thus, any reduction in the intake of saturated fatty acids,

total fat, and cholesterol in this segment of the population could result in a large absolute decrease in CHD deaths. Similarly, for the general population, decreased salt intake may substantially reduce the risk of hypertension and a reduced fat intake may curtail the risk of certain cancers, although the effects on many individuals may be small or absent. Furthermore, although genetic factors can affect individual susceptibility, they appear to account for only a small part of the observed variation in disease incidence among populations, as exemplified by the tendency of migrants to acquire the disease rates of their adoptive countries (see Chapter 5).

Thus, a major focus of any preventive strategy should be to shift the distribution of risk factors (including adverse dietary exposures) in the entire population, thereby decreasing overall disease risk. This is best accomplished through recommendations for the general population. This public health approach requires special strategies, including support of the media, the food industry, nutritionists, public health personnel, the medical profession, educators, and government. Such a policy has many merits if it is feasible to implement without harm to individuals, since it may benefit many people, is simpler to implement, and the overall costs to society are usually low. Examples of such policies in other arenas are mass vaccinations against poliomyelitis despite a wide range of genetic susceptibility to paralysis, fluoridation of the entire water supply to prevent caries despite differences in caries susceptibility (see Chapters 14 and 26), or iron fortification of cereals, even though only children and adult women are at risk of iron deficiency and such fortification may adversely affect those few with hemochromatosis (see Chapters 4 and 14). With advances in knowledge of genetic variability and its interaction with the environment, in the future we will be increasingly able to supplement general recommendations for the population with more sophisticated, individually based dietary intervention.

The committee also considered the relationship between public health goals and dietary recommendations aimed at individuals. Dietary recommendations for individuals are derived almost entirely from data on benefit or risk in certain populations and thus require considerable discretion and clinical judgment in their application. Goals or guidelines for the general population attempt to consider the wide variation in the distribution of dietary or nutrient requirements in the population, but they fail to consider individual

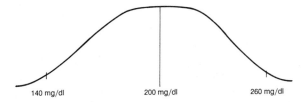

FIGURE 28–1 Hypothetical distribution of serum total cholesterol levels (mean ± 2 SD) in a population associated with a public health goal of 200 mg/dl.

needs and are therefore not identical to guidelines for the individual.

For example, the recommendation that individuals limit SFA intake to less than 10% of total calories derives mainly from evidence that populations with mean intakes of less than 10% of calories as SFA have low mean serum total cholesterol levels and are relatively free of atherosclerotic diseases. However, this recommended goal for individuals is different from the goal for a *population*. Figures 28–1 and 28–2 illustrate the different bases of recommendations for individuals and for the population as a whole. In the hypothetical example in Figure 28–1, serum cholesterol levels in a population range from 140 to 260 mg/dl with a mean of 200 mg/dl. This distribution—i.e., the mean ± 2 standard deviations (SD)—is compatible with a goal of 200 mg/dl for the general population (National Cholesterol Education Program, 1988). In contrast, Figure 28–2 shows the population serum cholesterol distribution that might be associated with a recommendation that *all individuals* lower their serum total cholesterol to 200 mg/dl or less. To achieve this goal (i.e., where very few individuals would have levels above 200 mg/dl) would require a much lower *population average* of serum total cholesterol levels (i.e., approximately 150 mg/dl).

The dietary recommendations in the following section are directed to individuals, but they incorporate public health goals for the general population as well.

Feasibility of Implementation

Should the feasibility of implementation affect dietary recommendations? For example, if an expert committee concludes that the population would be healthier if fat consumption were reduced from an average of 40% to no more than 10% of total calories, should it consider not only the feasibility of designing nutritionally balanced diets with only 10% of calories from fat but also the

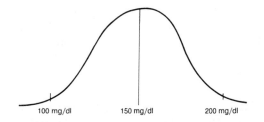

FIGURE 28–2 Hypothetical distribution of serum total cholesterol levels (mean ± 2 SD) in a population associated with a public health goal that all individuals lower their serum total cholesterol to 200 mg/dl or less. The range of cholesterol levels is assumed to be narrower than that shown in Figure 28-1.

feasibility of achieving such dietary change? If such a recommendation would fit within a balanced diet, it could be made in principle, despite the recognition that fat consumption would decline gradually at best and that a more readily attainable goal may encourage more change.

The committee carefully considered the feasibility of designing nutritionally balanced diets based on its recommendations and, to a limited extent, the factors involved in the implementation of its recommendations. In general, however, its recommendations are based on the scientific principles described above.

THE COMMITTEE'S DIETARY RECOMMENDATIONS

The dietary recommendations of the Committee on Diet and Health, given below, are directed to healthy, North American adults and children. Wherever evidence permits, the committee attempts to identify the special dietary needs of population subgroups at high risk for specific diseases or with different dietary requirements because of age, sex, or physiological status. The special dietary needs of the elderly are largely unknown.

As discussed above, the quantities proposed in the committee's recommendations are goals for intake by *individuals*. To achieve these goals, the mean intake by the *population* (the public health goal) would have to be higher or lower than the recommended intake for individuals, depending on the direction of the proposed dietary modification. For example, a recommendation that all *individuals* should reduce their fat intake to 30% or less of calories can be expected to lead to a population mean intake substantially *below* 30% of calories from fat. Similarly, a recommendation that individuals increase their carbohydrate intake to more than 55% of total calories can be expected to lead to a population mean intake clearly above 55% of calories from carbohydrates. Thus, the guidelines for individuals differ somewhat from the public health (population) goals, which need to be more stringent in order to achieve the goals for individuals.

The extent to which the public health goal for a nutrient differs from the goal for individuals in the population will depend on the distribution of intake for that nutrient in the population. In most cases, however, the variation in nutrient intakes in the population is not well known.

The recommendations in this report are the product of a systematic and extensive analysis of the literature by a multidisciplinary committee that considered the criteria and the process for arriving at recommendations and documented the extensive literature on which they are based. They are generally in agreement with the advice provided by other expert panels in the United States and abroad, although in most cases they include more specific quantitative recommendations. These recommendations are appropriate for current patterns of dietary intake and disease morbidity and mortality in the United States and are based on conclusions regarding the association of dietary factors with the entire spectrum of chronic diseases. They take into account competing risks for different diseases as well as nutrient interactions. These recommendations should be reexamined as new knowledge is acquired and as the patterns of morbidity and mortality change over the next decades.

The committee's recommendations are presented in a logical sequence that also reflects a general order of importance. For example, all dietary macrocomponents are addressed first. Among these, highest priority is given to reducing fat intake, because the scientific evidence concerning dietary fats and other lipids and human health is strongest and the likely impact on public health the greatest. Lower priority is given to recommendations on other dietary components, because they are derived from weaker evidence or because the public health impact is likely to be comparatively less. Where the evidence is strongest, the committee presents quantitative recommendations. It recognizes that setting specific quantitative goals is somewhat arbitrary and is based on informed judgment rather than on scientifically derivable formulas; however, quantification facilitates translation of goals into dietary patterns and food choices. Goals are needed to develop and evaluate programs aimed at achieving dietary changes and serve as

the basis for regulatory actions such as those relating to food labeling and the validity of health claims for foods and nutrients.

The committee's recommendations derive from an assessment of the evidence on chronic diseases, but should be used in combination with the RDAs to achieve an optimal and highly desirable dietary pattern for the maintenance of good health. In the committee's judgment, these recommendations have the potential for a substantial reduction in the risk of diet-related chronic diseases in the general population.

- *Reduce total fat intake to 30% or less of calories. Reduce saturated fatty acid intake to less than 10% of calories and the intake of cholesterol to less than 300 mg daily. The intake of fat and cholesterol can be reduced by substituting fish, poultry without skin, lean meats, and low- or nonfat dairy products for fatty meats and whole-milk dairy products; by choosing more vegetables, fruits, cereals, and legumes; and by limiting oils, fats, egg yolks, and fried and other fatty foods.*

A large and convincing body of evidence from studies in humans and laboratory animals shows that diets low in saturated fatty acids and cholesterol are associated with low risks and rates of atherosclerotic cardiovascular diseases. High-fat diets are also linked to a high incidence of some types of cancer and, probably, obesity. Thus, reducing total fat and saturated fatty acid intake is likely to lower the rates of these chronic diseases. Fat intake should be reduced by curtailing the major sources of dietary fats rather than by eliminating whole categories of foods. For example, by substituting fish, poultry without skin, lean meats and low- or nonfat dairy products for high-fat foods, one can lower total fat and saturated fatty acid intake while ensuring an adequate intake of iron and calcium—two nutrients of special importance to women. Dietary fat can also be reduced by limiting intake of fried foods, baked goods containing high levels of fat, and spreads and dressings containing fats and oils.

Different types of fatty acids have different effects on health. SFAs and dietary cholesterol tend to increase total and LDL serum cholesterol and, consequently, the risk of cardiovascular disease. The extent of this activity differs among SFAs; palmitic, myristic, and lauric acids have the greatest cholesterol-raising effect. The main dietary sources of these cholesterol-raising SFAs are dairy and meat products and some vegetable oils, such as coconut, palm, and palm-kernel oils. Dietary cholesterol is found mainly in egg yolks, certain shellfish, organ meats, and, to a lesser extent, in other meats and dairy products. Thus, the intake of these foods should be curtailed. MUFAs are found in a variety of foods but are especially abundant in olive oil and canola oil. PUFAs are of two types—omega-6 and omega-3; both are essential nutrients and cannot be synthesized endogenously. Omega-6 PUFAs are common in several plant oils, including corn, safflower, soybean, and sunflower oils. Omega-3 PUFAs are found in cold-water marine fish (such as salmon and mackerel) and in some plant oils (e.g., soybean and canola oils). Omega-6 PUFAs and MUFAs (and carbohydrates) lower LDL cholesterol when substituted for saturated fatty acids. Omega-3 PUFAs also lower LDL cholesterol when substituted for SFAs, but they are more effective in lowering elevated serum triglyceride levels. Although consumption of fish one or more times a week has been associated with a reduced risk of CHD, the committee does not recommend the use of concentrated fish oil supplements, because there is insufficient evidence that they are beneficial and the absence of long-term adverse effects has not been established.

The evidence linking high-fat diets to increased cancer risk is less persuasive than that associating saturated fatty acids and dietary cholesterol to CHD, but the weight of evidence indicates that high-fat diets are associated with a higher risk of several cancers, especially of the colon, prostate, and breast. Most evidence from studies in humans suggests that total fat or saturated fatty acids adversely affect cancer risk. No studies in humans have yet examined the benefits of changing to low-fat diets; however, such evidence exists from experiments in animals. The combined evidence from epidemiologic and laboratory studies suggests that reduction of total fat is likely to reduce the risk of these cancers.

Epidemiologic data on the possible association of low serum cholesterol levels with an increased incidence of and mortality from cancer in general or colon cancer in men in particular are inconsistent and do not suggest a causal association. Rather, they indicate that the lower serum cholesterol levels in some of these studies were in part the consequence of undetected cancers. The overall evidence indicates that dietary modification to lower serum total cholesterol and CHD risk is likely to reduce the risk of colon cancer without increasing the risk of other cancers.

Animal studies also suggest that high-fat diets may lead to obesity, possibly because dietary fat is converted to body fat more efficiently than are other sources of calories. Short-term clinical studies in humans indicate that a substantial reduction in fat intake may be accompanied by weight loss; however, reduced caloric intake was observed in some of these reports and although not specifically noted is likely to have occurred in others. This indicates that a substantial reduction in fat intake may result in overall caloric reduction, perhaps because of the caloric density of dietary fat. From a public health perspective, this phenomenon may be important, regardless of whether fat reduction per se results in weight loss or whether weight loss results from an overall reduction in caloric intake.

In the committee's judgment, concerns that reduced fat intake may curtail intake of meats and dairy products and thus limit intakes of adequate iron and calcium in women and children or that young children on reduced-fat diets might not obtain adequate calories to support optimal growth and development are not justified. Fat intake can be reduced to approximately 30% of calories without risk of nutrient deficiency, and this level of fat intake after infancy has not been associated with any detrimental effects. Furthermore, adequate caloric intake can readily be maintained in children on diets containing 30% of calories from fat.

Although the committee recommends that the total fat intake of individuals be 30% or less of calories, there is evidence that further reduction in fat intake may confer even greater health benefits. However, the recommended levels are more likely to be adopted by the public because they can be achieved without drastic changes in usual dietary patterns and without undue risk of nutrient deficiency. Furthermore, they permit gradual adaptation to lower-fat diets as more lower-fat foods become available on the market. The committee recommends that people who should not lose weight should compensate for the caloric loss resulting from decreased fat intake by consuming greater amounts of foods containing complex carbohydrates (e.g., vegetables, certain fruits, legumes, and whole-grain cereal products).

Although the committee recommends that SFA intake be maintained at less than 10% of total calories by individuals, it is highly likely that further reduction, to 8 or 7% of calories or lower, would confer greater health benefits. Such further reductions can best be achieved by substituting additional complex carbohydrates and MUFAs for SFAs in the diet. Larger reductions in cholesterol intakes—e.g., to 250 to 200 mg or even less per day—may also confer health benefits.

The committee recommends that the PUFA

intake of individuals not exceed 10% of total calories and that PUFA intake in the population be maintained at current levels in the U.S. diet, i.e., an average of approximately 7% of total calories. (The requirement for omega-6 PUFAs can be met by 1 to 2% of calories as linoleic acid.) Concern that an increase in PUFA intake may increase risk of certain cancers derives primarily from studies of animals on very-high-PUFA diets. Given the absence of human diets naturally very high in total PUFAs and the lack of information about the long-term consequences of high PUFA intake (see Chapter 7), it seems prudent to recommend that PUFA intake not be increased above the current average in the U.S. population. However, since most of the PUFAs in the current U.S. diet are of the omega-6 rather than the omega-3 type, and since the committee's recommendation is directed mainly at omega-6 PUFAs, any increase in total PUFA resulting from an increase in foods containing omega-3 PUFAs (e.g., by eating more fish containing such fatty acids) is reasonable.

• *Every day eat five or more servings** of a combination of vegetables and fruits, especially green and yellow vegetables and citrus fruits. Also, increase intake of starches and other complex carbohydrates by eating six or more daily servings of a combination of breads, cereals, and legumes.*

The committee recommends that the intake of carbohydrates be increased to more than 55% of total calories by increasing primarily complex carbohydrates. Fats and carbohydrates are the two major sources of calories in the diet. National food consumption surveys indicate that the content of the average U.S. diet is high in fat and low in complex carbohydrates (e.g., starches, vegetables, legumes, breads, cereals, and certain fruits). Green and yellow vegetables, fruits, especially citrus fruits, legumes, and whole-grain cereals and breads, which constitute a small portion of the present U.S. diet, generally contain low levels of fat; thus, they are good substitutes for fatty foods and good sources of several vitamins, minerals, complex carbohydrates, and dietary fiber. The recommended number of servings is derived from experience in planning nutritionally balanced diets that would meet the committee's dietary recommendations. The amounts recommended would facilitate an increase in the total carbohydrate and

complex carbohydrate content of the diet, make up for the calorie deficit due to fat reduction, and supply sufficient quantities of essential vitamins and minerals. The committee does not recommend increasing the intake of added sugars, because their consumption is strongly associated with dental caries and although they are a source of calories for those who may need additional calories, they provide no nutrients. Furthermore, foods high in added sugars (e.g., desserts and baked goods) are generally also high in fat.

Studies in various parts of the world indicate that people who habitually consume a diet high in plant foods have low risks of atherosclerotic cardiovascular diseases, probably largely because such diets are usually low in animal fat and cholesterol, both of which are established risk factors for atherosclerotic cardiovascular diseases. Some constituents of plant foods, e.g., soluble fiber and vegetable protein, may also contribute—to a lesser extent—to the lower risk of atherosclerotic cardiovascular diseases. The mechanism for the link between frequent consumption of vegetables and fruits, especially green and yellow vegetables and citrus fruits, and decreased susceptibility to cancers of the lung, stomach, and large intestine is not well understood because the responsible agents in these foods and the mechanisms for their protective effect have not been fully determined. However, there is strong evidence that a low intake of carotenoids, which are present in green and yellow vegetables, contributes to an increased risk of lung cancer. Fruits and vegetables also contain high levels of fiber, but there is no conclusive evidence that the dietary fiber itself, rather than other nutritive and nonnutritive components of these foods, exerts a protective effect against these cancers. The committee does not recommend the use of fiber supplements.

Vegetables and fruits are also good sources of potassium. A diet containing approximately 75 mEq of potassium (i.e., approximately 3.5 g of elemental potassium) daily may contribute to reduced risk of stroke, which is especially common among blacks and older people of all races. Potassium supplements are neither necessary nor recommended for the general population.

• *Maintain protein intake at moderate levels.*
Protein is an essential nutrient, and protein-containing foods are important sources of essential amino acids in the diet. However, because there are no known benefits and possibly some risks in consuming diets with a high animal protein content, the committee recommends that protein

---

*An average serving is equal to a half cup for most fresh or cooked vegetables, fruits, dry or cooked cereals and legumes; one medium piece of fresh fruit; one slice of bread; or one roll or muffin.

intake not be increased to compensate for the caloric loss that would result from the recommended reduction in fat intake. In general, average protein intake by adults in the United States considerably exceeds the RDA, which is 0.8 g/kg of desirable body weight for adults.

The committee recommends maintaining total protein intake at levels lower than twice the RDA for all age groups (e.g., less than 1.6 g/kg body weight for adults).

Increased risks of certain cancers and CHD have been associated in some epidemiologic studies with diets high in meat and, as a consequence, in animal protein and with high protein intake alone in laboratory studies. It is not known whether these adverse effects are due solely to the usually high total-fat, saturated-fatty acid, and cholesterol content of diets that are rich in meat or animal protein, or to what extent protein per se or other factors also contribute. High protein intake may also lead to increased urinary calcium loss.

The committee is aware of concerns among some scientists that animal protein restriction might curtail the ability of some population subgroups with habitually lower protein intakes (e.g., women and the elderly) to meet the RDA for certain other essential nutrients such as iron. However, the recommendation to maintain intake below twice the RDA for all age groups would require no reduction of current average intakes in the United States. The committee does not recommend against eating meat; rather, it recommends consuming lean meat in smaller and fewer portions than is customary in the United States.

• *Balance food intake and physical activity to maintain appropriate body weight.*

Excess weight is associated with an increased risk of several chronic disorders, including NIDDM, hypertension, CHD, gallbladder disease, osteoarthritis, and endometrial cancer. The risks appear to decline following a sustained reduction in weight. Increased abdominal fat carries a higher risk for these disorders than do comparable fat deposits in the hips and thighs. New standards for healthy body composition take into account such differences in regional body fat distribution as well as weight-to-height ratios. Neither large fluctuations in body weight nor extreme restrictions in food intake are desirable.

In the U.S. population and other westernized societies, body weight and body mass index are increasing while the overall caloric intake of the population is decreasing. These trends as well as the association of moderate, regular physical activity with reduced risks of heart disease lead to the committee's recommendation that the U.S. population increase its physical activity level and that all healthy people maintain physical activity at a moderately active level, improve physical fitness, and moderate their food intake to maintain appropriate body weight. For adult men and women of normal weight, this will also allow the ingestion of adequate calories to meet all known nutrient needs. Overweight people should increase their physical activity and reduce their caloric intake, and people with a family history of obesity should avoid calorically dense foods and select low-fat foods.

• *The committee does not recommend alcohol consumption. For those who drink alcoholic beverages, the committee recommends limiting consumption to the equivalent of less than 1 ounce of pure alcohol in a single day. This is the equivalent of two cans of beer, two small glasses of wine, or two average cocktails. Pregnant women should avoid alcoholic beverages.*

Excessive alcohol drinking increases the risk of heart disease, high blood pressure, chronic liver disease, some forms of cancer, neurological diseases, nutritional deficiencies, and many other disorders. Even moderate drinking carries some risk in circumstances that require neuromotor coordination and judgment, e.g., driving vehicles, working around machinery, and piloting airplanes or boats. Consumption of even small amounts of alcohol can lead to dependence. Approximately 10% of those who consume alcoholic beverages in the United States are alcoholics. Pregnant women and women who are attempting to conceive should avoid alcoholic beverages because there is a risk of damage to the fetus and no safe level of alcohol intake during pregnancy has been established.

Although several studies show that moderate alcohol drinking is associated with a lower CHD risk, it would be unwise to recommend moderate drinking for those who do not drink because, in the committee's judgment, a causal association has not been established and because even moderate drinking poses certain other risks, including the risk of alcohol addiction.

• *Limit total daily intake of salt (sodium chloride) to 6 g or less. Limit the use of salt in cooking and avoid adding it to food at the table. Salty, highly processed salty, salt-preserved, and salt-pickled foods should be consumed sparingly.*

Studies in human populations in different parts of the world show that a diet containing more than

6 g of salt per day is associated with elevated blood pressure, and many Americans habitually exceed this level. It is probable that susceptibility to salt-induced hypertension (salt sensitivity) is genetically determined, but no reliable genetic marker has yet been identified. Thus, those who are most susceptible to developing salt-induced hypertension, and therefore likely to benefit most from this recommendation, cannot yet be identified. In salt-sensitive people, the recommended level of salt intake is unlikely to contribute to blood pressure elevation and may even lead to blood pressure reduction. In the general population, the recommended level will have no detrimental effect. The committee is aware that a greater reduction in salt intake (i.e., to 4.5 g or less) would probably confer greater health benefits than its present recommendation, but chose 6 g as an initial goal that can be achieved more readily. This does not preclude a subsequent recommendation for further reduction.

The evidence linking salt intake per se to stomach cancer is less persuasive than that for salt and hypertension. There is consistent evidence, however, that frequent consumption of salt-preserved or salt-pickled foods increases the risk of stomach cancer. The specific causative agents in those foods have not been identified.

● *Maintain adequate calcium intake.*

Calcium is an essential nutrient; it is necessary for adequate growth and skeletal development. Certain segments of the population, especially women, because of their low caloric intake, and adolescents, because of their higher nutrient requirements, need to make careful food choices to obtain adequate calcium from the food supply. The committee recommends consumption of low- or nonfat dairy products and dark-green vegetables, which are rich sources of calcium and can assist in maintaining calcium intake at approximately RDA levels. Although low calcium intake is associated with a higher frequency of fractures and possibly with high blood pressure, the potential benefits of calcium intakes above the RDAs to prevent osteoporosis or hypertension are not well documented and do not justify the use of calcium supplements.

● *Avoid taking dietary supplements in excess of the RDA in any one day.*

A large percentage of the U.S. population consumes some vitamin or mineral supplement daily. The supplements are often self-prescribed and not based on known nutrient deficiencies. It is not known what, if any, benefits or risks accrue to individuals or the general population from taking small doses of supplements. Some population subgroups (e.g., those suffering from malabsorption syndromes) may require supplements, but they should take them only under professional supervision. A single daily dose of a multiple vitamin–mineral supplement containing 100% of the RDA is not known to be harmful or beneficial; however, vitamin–mineral supplements that exceed the RDA and other supplements (such as protein powders, single amino acids, fiber, and lecithin) not only have no known health benefits for the population but their use may be detrimental to health. The desirable way for the general public to obtain recommended levels of nutrients is by eating a variety of foods.

Thus, the committee supports the general scientific opinion and the opinions of several other expert panels that have recently commented specifically on supplement use. It emphasizes, however, that the long-term health effects (risks and benefits) of supplements have not been adequately studied.

● *Maintain an optimal intake of fluoride, particularly during the years of primary and secondary tooth formation and growth.*

There is convincing evidence that consumption of optimally fluoridated water (i.e., 0.7 to 1.2 ppm fluoride, depending on ambient temperature) significantly reduces the risk of dental caries in people of all ages, especially in children during the years of primary and secondary tooth formation and growth. There is no evidence that such fluoride concentrations have any adverse effects on health, including cancer risk. In the absence of optimally fluoridated water, the committee supports the use of dietary fluoride supplements in the amounts generally recommended by the American Dental Association, the American Academy of Pediatrics, and the American Academy of Pediatric Dentistry.

IMPLICATIONS OF RECOMMENDATIONS FOR FOOD CHOICES

What do the committee's recommendations imply with regard to selection of foods and food groups? To some extent, this issue is addressed under each recommendation. Therefore, only a synthesis is provided here. Principles of food selection will also be explained in more detail in the committee's forthcoming report to the general public.

In summary, the diet recommended by the committee should contain moderately low levels of fat, with special emphasis on restriction of saturated fatty acids and cholesterol; high levels of complex carbohydrates; only moderate levels of protein, especially animal protein; and only low levels of added sugars. Caloric intake and physical activity should be balanced to maintain appropriate body weight. The recommendation to maintain total fat intake at or below 30% of total caloric intake and saturated fatty acid intake at less than 10%, combined with the recommendation to maintain protein intake only at moderate levels, means that for most North Americans it will be necessary to select leaner cuts of meat, trim off excess fat, remove skin from poultry, and consume fewer and smaller portions of meat and poultry. Fish and many shellfish are excellent sources of low-fat protein. By using plant products (e.g., cereals and legumes) instead of animal products as sources of protein, one can also reduce the amount of saturated fatty acids and cholesterol in the diet.

Dairy products are an important source of calcium and protein, but whole milk, whole-milk cheeses, yogurt, ice cream, and other milk products are also high in saturated fatty acids. Therefore, low-fat or skim milk products should be substituted. Furthermore, it is desirable to change from butter to margarine with a low SFA content, to use less oils and fats in cooking and in salad dressings, and to avoid fried foods.

For most people, the recommended restriction of fat intake, coupled with the recommendation for moderation in protein intake, implies an increase in calories from carbohydrates. These calories should come from an increased intake of whole-grain cereals and breads rather than from foods or drinks containing added sugars. For example, bakery goods, such as pies, pastries, and cookies, although they provide complex carbohydrates also tend to contain high levels of total fat, saturated fatty acids, and added sugars, all of which need to be curtailed to meet the committee's recommendations.

In general, vegetables and fruits are unlikely to contribute substantially to caloric intake but are major sources of vitamins, minerals, and dietary fiber. The committee places special emphasis on increasing consumption of green and yellow vegetables as well as citrus fruits, particularly since their consumption in North America is relatively low. The committee's recommendations would lead to a substantial increase in consumption frequency and portion sizes, especially of vegetables, for the average person. Thorough washing of fresh vegetables (especially leafy ones) and fruits will minimize the consumption of pesticide residues in the diet.

The need for restriction of certain dietary components—such as egg yolks; salt; salty, smoked, and preserved foods; and alcoholic beverages—is clearly explained in the recommendations. Further considerations include methods of preparation, cooking, and processing, which can have important effects on the composition of foods. The committee emphasizes the need to read the labels on prepared, formulated, and other processed foods to identify their contribution of nutrients in general and of salt, fats and cholesterol, and sugars in particular. With regard to the risk of chronic diseases, maximum benefit can be attained and any unknown, potentially harmful effects of dietary constituents minimized by selecting a variety of foods from each food group, avoiding excessive caloric intake (especially excessive intake of any one item or food group), and engaging regularly in moderate physical exercise.

COMPARISON OF THE COMMITTEE'S RECOMMENDATIONS WITH THOSE BY OTHER EXPERT GROUPS

Recommendations to the General Population

In the recent history of dietary recommendations for overall health, an expert group from Sweden, Norway, and Finland was among the first to propose in 1968 that the general population should avoid excessive caloric intake, reduce fat intake from 40 to 25–30% of calories, reduce saturated fatty acid intake while increasing dietary polyunsaturated fatty acids, reduce consumption of sugar and sugar-containing foods, and increase the consumption of vegetables, potatoes, skim milk, fish, lean meat, and cereal products (Anonymous, 1968). The next two decades were characterized by a proliferation of dietary recommendations by authoritative groups in the United States, Canada, many western European countries, Japan, Australia, and New Zealand.

In the past decade alone, more than a dozen expert committees, voluntary health organizations, and government agencies in the United States have issued dietary guidelines to promote good health in general or to lower the risk of specific chronic diseases (see Table 28–1). The recommendations for general health maintenance include *Dietary Goals for the United States*, issued in 1977 by a select committee of the U.S. Senate (1977); the Surgeon General's report on *Health Promotion and Disease Prevention* in 1979 (DHEW, 1979); a joint statement by the American Medical Association and the Food and Nutrition Board in 1979 (Council on Scientific Affairs, 1979); *Dietary Guidelines for Americans*, issued jointly by the Departments of Agriculture and Health and Human Services in 1980 and revised in 1985 (USDA/DHEW, 1980, 1985); and the *Surgeon General's Report on Nutrition and Health* (DHHS, 1988). Tables 28–1 and 28–2 summarize recent recommendations for overall health maintenance by official bodies in the United States and several other industrialized countries.

Many expert groups have focused on specific diseases. In the early 1960s, the American Heart Association was the first U.S. organization to recommend dietary modifications for reducing cardiovascular disease risk (Page et al., 1961). The AHA has periodically revised its recommendations, most recently in 1988 (AHA, 1988). The Inter-Society Commission for Heart Disease Resources (1970, 1984) has also periodically proposed dietary recommendations to lower the risk of heart disease in the United States. More recently, a Consensus Conference of the National Institutes of Health resulted in recommendations to lower blood cholesterol (NIH, 1985). Recent recommendations on diet and atherosclerotic cardiovascular diseases in the United States and abroad are summarized in Table 28–3.

Guidelines to lower cancer risk in the United States were first issued by the National Cancer Institute in 1979 and revised by that institute in 1984 and 1987 (NCI, 1984a,b, 1987; Upton, 1979). The National Research Council's Committee on Diet, Nutrition, and Cancer and the American Cancer Society also proposed interim dietary guidelines aimed at lowering cancer risk (ACS, 1984; NRC, 1982). Dietary guidelines on cancer risk in the United States and abroad are summarized in Table 28–4.

Several voluntary health organizations and other expert groups have periodically issued other disease-specific recommendations. For example, the American Diabetes Association (1987) has made recommendations aimed at dietary management of noninsulin-dependent diabetes mellitus (NIDDM), and the National Institutes of Health have recommended weight reduction for overweight individuals and those with obesity-related

chronic conditions (NIH, 1984a) and have also proposed dietary modification to prevent osteoporosis (NIH, 1984b).

Tables 28–1 to 28–4 show that there are many similarities among dietary recommendations in the United States and other industrialized countries. Most sets of recommendations deal with the type and amount of fat and cholesterol in the diet; body weight and exercise; complex carbohydrates, fiber, and refined sugars; sodium, salt, or salty foods; alcoholic beverages; and variety in the diet. Some also address avoidance of toxic substances, and two recent statements specifically focus on the intake of dietary supplements (Callaway et al., 1987; Council on Scientific Affairs, 1987). Some of the recommendations specify quantities (e.g., percentage of calories from fat or grams of salt per day), whereas others are general in nature, suggesting that people should eat more of or avoid too much of some dietary component. Most recommendations are directed to the general population, although several expert groups (e.g., the National Cholesterol Education Program, 1988) also highlight the needs of certain high-risk population subgroups. Other organizations (e.g., Council on Scientific Affairs, 1979; NRC, 1980b) have cautioned against aiming broad, sweeping dietary recommendations at the general population.

The general agreement among dietary recommendations from different sources is striking. The vast majority of expert panels have recommended maintenance of appropriate body weight, and on the basis of actuarial data, some have also proposed weight/height standards. These recommendations are aimed at curtailing the prevalence of obesity—a major contributor to several chronic disorders, including hypertension, NIDDM, hyperlipidemia, cardiovascular disorders, some hepatobiliary diseases, and some types of cancer. New standards for health with regard to height, weight, and body composition take into account differences in regional body fat distribution as well as weight/height ratios.

The committee supports the recommendation to maintain appropriate body weight, made by practically all organizations listed in Tables 28–1 to 28–4, and it emphasizes that physical activity and food intake should be balanced in order to avoid obesity. The recommendation to avoid frequent fluctuations in weight and extreme dieting is in accord with similar recommendations from the American Dietetic Association (ADA, 1986).

Perhaps the most common and consistent recommendation for the general population is to limit the intake of total fat, usually to approximately 30% of total calories. This is usually intended to reduce the risk of cardiovascular diseases, certain cancers, and possibly obesity. Most expert panels also suggest a reduction in saturated fatty acid intake, usually to ≤10% of total calories (see, e.g., AHA, 1986, 1988; Department of National Health and Welfare Canada, 1977; DHEW, 1979; NCI, 1984a,b, 1987; NIH, 1985; USDA/DHHS, 1985; WHO, 1982). There is less general agreement about the proportional intake of PUFAs. The American Heart Association has previously recommended that PUFAs partially replace saturated fatty acids in the diet to make up about 10% of total calories (AHA, 1982); however, their recent guidelines (AHA, 1986, 1988) and those of the National Institutes of Health (NIH, 1985) suggest instead that PUFAs should not exceed 10% of total calories.

Recommendations on dietary cholesterol are also inconsistent, although the most widely accepted recommendation is to limit cholesterol intake to ≤300 mg/day. Recent suggestions that cholesterol intake be limited to ≤100 mg/1,000 kcal per day (e.g., AHA, 1986; WHO, 1982) have been reviewed recently by the American Heart Association, which has again recommended that cholesterol intake should be less than 300 mg/day (AHA, 1988)—a dietary goal that can be readily achieved by U.S. adults.

The committee's quantitative limits on the intake of total fat, saturated fatty acids, and cholesterol are consistent with advice from other expert panels in the United States as well as international expert groups on heart disease and cancer (e.g., ACS, 1984; AHA, 1988; Department of National Health and Welfare, Canada, 1977; DHSS, 1984; ECP/IUNS, 1986; NIH, 1985; NRC, 1982; WHO, 1982). The committee points out, however, that the recommended diet would only be "moderately" low in fat, whereas evidence indicates that further reductions in fat, saturated fat, and cholesterol intake might confer additional benefits; for PUFAs, however, it proposes maintaining intake at the average levels currently consumed by the U.S. population.

Most organizations have also advised increasing complex carbohydrate intake, and some have specified dietary fiber (e.g., Commonwealth Department of Health/National Health and Medical Research Council, 1983; Department of National Health and Welfare, Canada, 1982; NACNE, 1983; National Advisory Committee, New Zealand, 1982; NCI, 1984a,b, 1987), usually with a concomitant decrease

in consumption of refined sugars. These guidelines generally stem from concern about diabetes, obesity, dental caries, or cancer. However, they are less often stated in quantitative terms, perhaps because the evidence linking these components to specific diseases is (with the exception of sugars and dental caries) less clear or convincing than for fats. Complex carbohydrates are generally recommended in preference to refined sugars, even though there is only minimal evidence linking sugar intake per se to specific health problems (except for dental caries). Addition of refined sugars to the diet contributes calories without providing any essential nutrients. As discussed in Chapter 24, recent studies have focused on the glycemic index of different foods in subjects with NIDDM, but no clear and clinically significant conclusions can yet be drawn from such studies, especially for individuals without the disease.

Recommendations on dietary fiber intake are less consistent within the United States, although as shown in Table 28–3, increased fiber intake has been recommended by expert groups from the United Kingdom, Canada, Australia, and New Zealand. In the United States, recommendations on fiber range from suggestions to increase intake to 20 to 35 g/day (LSRO, 1987; NCI, 1984a,b, 1987) to recommendations simply to consume more fiber (USDA/DHHS, 1985) or to increase consumption of high-fiber vegetables, fruits, and whole-grain cereal products (NRC, 1982). In some cases, dietary fiber is subsumed under complex carbohydrates. The absence of definitive data has precluded recommendations on specific types of dietary fibers (e.g., soluble and insoluble).

The Committee on Diet and Health agrees with most other expert groups in proposing that the intake of vegetables, fruits, and other sources of complex carbohydrates should be increased and that the intake of added sugars should be limited (e.g., ACS, 1984; AHA, 1988; DHEW, 1979; DHSS, 1984; NIH, 1985; NRC, 1982; USDA/DHHS, 1985). The committee's recommendations extend beyond those of most other groups because they specify the minimum number of servings per day and propose a quantitative goal for total carbohydrate intake. However, unlike some expert panels (e.g., LSRO, 1987; NCI, 1984a,b, 1987), the committee believes that the strength of the evidence does not justify making specific recommendations pertaining to dietary fiber at this time. The committee's recommendation to emphasize the consumption of vegetables, fruits, and other sources of complex carbohydrates would, however,

TABLE 28-1 Dietary Recommendations to the U.S. Public, 1977 to 1989

Type of Recommendation Reference	Maintain Appropriate Body Weight, Exercise	Limit or Reduce Total Fat (% kcal)	Reduce Saturated Fatty Acids (% kcal)	Increase Polyunsaturated Fatty Acids (% kcal)	Limit Cholesterol (mg/day)	Limit Simple Sugars	Increase Complex Carbohydrates (% kcal from *total* carbohydrates)	Increase Fiber	Restrict Sodium Chloride (g)	Moderate Alcohol Intake	Other Recommendations
General Health Maintenance											
U.S. Senate (1977)	Yes	27–33	Yes	Yes	250–350	Yes	Yes	Yes	8	Yes	Reduce additives and processed foods
Council on Scientific Affairs (AMA) (1979)	Yes	No	No	No	No	Yes	NC	NC	12	Yes	Consider high-risk groups
DHEW (1979)	Yes	Yes	Yes	NS	Yes	Yes	Yes	NS	Yes	Yes	More fish, poultry, legumes; less red meat
NRC (1980b)	Yes	For weight reduction only	No	No	No	For weight reduction only	No	No	3–8	For weight reduction only	Variety in diet; consider high-risk groups
USDA/DHHS (1980; 1985)	Yes	Yes	Yes	No	Yes	Yes	Eat adequate starch and fiber		Yes	Yes	Variety in diet; consider high-risk groups
DHHS (1988)	Yes	Yes	Yes	No	Yes	Yes	Yes	Yes	Yes	Yes	Fluoridation of water; adolescent girls and women increase intake of calcium-rich foods; children, adolescents, and women of childbearing age increase intake of iron-rich foods

Diet and Health (1989)	Balance energy intake and expenditure	≤30	<10 for individuals and 7–8 population mean	Up to 10 for individuals and ~7 population mean	<300	Yes	(At least 55); ≥five daily servings of vegetables and fruits; ≥six daily servings of cereals, breads, and legumes	Directly through vegetables, fruits, and cereals	≤6 g/day with a goal of 4.5 g/day	If you drink, limit to <1.0 oz alcohol or <2 drinks/day	Avoid dietary supplements, especially in excess of RDAs; drink fluoridated water; limit protein intake to moderate levels (less than twice the RDA)
Heart Disease											
Inter-Society Commission for Heart Disease Resources (1984)	Yes	<30	8	10	<250	NC	Increase to make up caloric deficit	NC	5 g/day	NC	NS
NIH (1985)	Yes	<30	<10	Up to 10	250–300	Endorsed recommendations of AHA (1982) and Inter-Society Commission for Heart Disease Resources (1984)			NC	NC	Specific recommendations for high-risk groups; also physicians, public, and food industry
AHA (1988)	Yes	<30	<10	Up to 10	<300	NS	(50 or more)	NS	≤3 g/day of sodium	1–2 oz ethanol/day	Protein to make up remainder of calories; wide variety of foods
Cancer											
NRC (1982)	NC	~30	Yes	No	NC	NC	Through whole grains, fruits, and vegetables	NS	By limiting intake of salt-cured, pickled, smoked foods	Yes	Emphasize fruits and vegetables; avoid high doses of supplements; pay attention to cooking methods
ACS (1984)	Yes	~30	Yes	No	NC	NC	Same as NRC (1982)	Yes	Same as NRC (1982)	Yes	Same as NRC (1982)
NCI (1987)	Yes	Yes	Yes	No	NC	NC	Yes, more whole grains, fruits, and vegetables	To 20–35 g	NC	Yes	Variety in diet; avoid fiber supplements

TABLE 28–1 *Continued*

Type of Recommendation Reference	Maintain Appropriate Body Weight, Exercise	Limit or Reduce Total Fat (% kcal)	Reduce Saturated Fatty Acids (% kcal)	Increase Poly-unsaturated Fatty Acids (% kcal)	Limit Cholesterol (mg/day)	Limit Simple Sugars	Increase Complex Carbohydrates (% kcal from total carbohydrates)	Increase Fiber	Restrict Sodium Chloride (g)	Moderate Alcohol Intake	Other Recommendations
Osteoporosis											
NIH (1984b)	Exercise	NC	NC	NC	NC	NC	NC	NC	NC	NC	Raise calcium to 1,000 mg/day (premenopausal), 1,500 mg/day (postmenopausal); use calcium supplements if needed; use vitamin D for calcium absorption
Diabetes											
American Diabetes Association (1987)	Yes	<30	Yes	No	<300	Yes	(55–60)	Yes	Yes	Yes	Nonnutritive sweeteners permitted but not recommended; limit protein to RDA level; avoid supplements except in special cases

NOTE: NC = No comment; NS = Not specified.

indirectly result in increased consumption of dietary fiber.

Recommendations on protein intake have seldom been included among dietary guidelines by expert groups in the United States, and protein intake per se has received little attention compared to calories, fats, or carbohydrates. However, an expert panel in Ireland (Department of Health, Ireland, 1984) proposed reducing protein intake to 1 g/kg body weight—i.e., approximately the RDA level (NRC, 1980a)—and a panel in the Netherlands suggested that only 30 to 50% of protein should come from animal sources (Food and Nutrition Council, Netherlands, 1983–1984). Furthermore, protein-containing foods have been highlighted by several international expert panels who suggest selection of lean meats, more poultry and fish, and foods with more vegetable and less animal protein (e.g., Department of Health, Ireland, 1984; Food and Nutrition Council, Netherlands, 1983–1984; National Advisory Committee, New Zealand, 1982; WHO, 1982). In the United States, an earlier Surgeon General's Report (DHEW, 1979) recommended consumption of less red meat and more poultry and fish, while the 1988 report (DHHS, 1988) recommends selection of lean meats in addition to poultry and fish.

The Committee on Diet and Health proposes maintaining protein intake at moderate levels (i.e., <1.6 g/kg body weight for adults). This reflects its judgment that there is no benefit from consuming amounts of protein that are higher than the RDA and that there is some evidence that diets excessively high in animal protein may be harmful to health.

With few exceptions, experts recommend a reduction in salt intake generally or to a specific level to reduce the risk of hypertension in the population. Several expert groups concerned with cancer risk also suggest limiting salt-cured and salt-pickled foods to lower the risk of stomach cancer (ACS, 1984; NRC, 1982; Panel on Nutrition and Prevention of Diseases, 1983). The Panel on Nutrition and Prevention of Diseases (1983) in Japan singled out salt as a possible causative agent for stomach cancer. No concrete recommendations have been made concerning calcium, magnesium, or chloride to reduce the risk of hypertension.

The committee's recommendation to limit salt intake to 6 g/day or less is similar to the recommendations of other expert groups and pertains both to hypertension and to stomach cancer. However, the committee specifically acknowledges the existence of genetic predisposition to salt-induced hypertension and also makes a specific quantitative recommendation for potassium intake.

Even though consumption of alcoholic beverages has been addressed by only about half the expert groups, their recommendations are fully consistent. There is general agreement that excessive alcohol intake should be avoided; moderation is usually recommended for those who drink, but it is often not defined. This recommendation stems from concern about the risk of chronic liver disease, hypertension, some forms of cancer, and cardiovascular diseases.

The committee's overall recommendation on alcoholic beverages is in agreement with others (e.g., ACS, 1984; DHHS, 1988; NACNE, 1983; NCI, 1984a,b, 1987; NRC, 1982; Swedish National Food Administration, 1981; USDA/DHHS, 1985). It makes a specific mention of the need to avoid alcohol intake in pregnancy—an issue still not fully resolved in the judgment of some experts (NIAAA, 1986). The committee supports the general opinion that a recommendation that would encourage moderate drinking for the general population to lower the risk of coronary events would not be prudent, since the data do not establish a causal association (Castelli, 1979; Hennekens et al., 1979).

Nutrient adequacy has been primarily the focus of the RDAs, which are developed by the Food and Nutrition Board (NRC, 1980a). The USDA/DHHS *Dietary Guidelines for Americans* (USDA/DHHS, 1985) addressed adequate nutrient intakes in its recommendation to "Eat a variety of foods." The American Dietetic Association's recommendations for women emphasized the need for adequate consumption of calcium and, during the years of menstruation, also of iron (ADA, 1986). The statement on osteoporosis issued by the NIH Consensus Development Conference recommends intake of 1,000 to 1,500 mg of calcium daily, which exceeds the current RDA of 800 mg (NIH, 1984b). Most discussions of nutrient adequacy continue to use the RDAs as the standard for adequate nutrient intakes.

The Committee on Diet and Health does not specifically address nutrient adequacy in its report; however, in its overall recommendations, it takes into account the adequacy of certain nutrients whose intake might be curtailed (e.g., calcium or iron) or greatly exceeded (e.g., protein) as a result of the recommendations. Furthermore, it emphasizes that in planning optimal diets to attain

TABLE 28-2 General Dietary Recommendations in Other Industrialized Countries, 1978–1987

Country (Reference)	Maintain Appropriate Body Weight	Limit or Reduce Total Fat (% kcal)	Reduce Saturated Fatty Acids (% kcal)	Increase Polyunsaturated Fatty Acids (% kcal)	Limit Cholesterol (mg/day)	Limit Simple Sugars	Increase Complex Carbohydrates (% kcal from total carbohydrates)	Increase Fiber	Restrict Sodium Chloride	Moderate Alcohol Intake	Other Recommendations
Sweden (Swedish National Food Administration, 1981; Expert Group for Diet and Health, 1985)	Yes	25–35	Yes	P/S = 0.5[a]	Yes	<10% of energy	Yes (50–60)	>30 g/day	~7–8 g/day	Yes	Varied diet; exercise; regular meals
France (Dupin et al., 1981)	Yes	30–35	Yes	NS	NS	Yes	(50–55)	Yes	Yes	<10% kcal	Water fluoridation
Norway (Royal Ministry of Health and Social Services, 1981–1982)	NC	<35	Yes	P/S = 1:2	NS	<10% of energy	Yes (50–60)	Yes	NC	NC	Maintain adequate nutrient intake
Canada (Department of National Health and Welfare, 1982)	Yes	35	Yes	Yes	No	Yes	Yes	Yes	Yes	Yes	Exercise
New Zealand (National Advisory Committee, 1982)	Yes	Yes	Yes	NS	NS	Yes	Yes	Yes	Yes	Yes	Variety; less animal protein; water fluoridation
Australia (Commonwealth Department of Health/National Health and Medical Research Council, 1983, 1987)	Yes	33	NC	NC	NC	<12% of energy	Indirectly	To 30 g/day	To 100 mmol/day	<5% kcal/day	Promote breastfeeding; variety; Year 2000 targets; water fluoridation

————— Year 2000 targets —————→

									Variety
Netherlands (Food and Nutrition Council, 1983–1984)	Yes	30–35	Yes	Max. 10%	Yes	NS	NC	NC	Yes	Variety
United Kingdom (NACNE, 1983)	Yes	30	NS	No	To 20 kg/year	Through whole grains, vegetables, and fruits	To 30 g/day	Decrease by 3 g/day	≤4% of calories	Exercise; food labeling; nutrition education
Federal Republic of Germany (German Society of Nutrition, 1985)	Yes	Yes	NS	NS	Avoid excess	Fresh fruits and vegetables, whole-grain cereals	Yes	Yes	Yes	Variety; small, frequent meals; proper cooking; sufficient protein
Ireland (Department of Health, 1984)	Yes	≤35	Yes	NC	Moderation ≤70 g/day after weight reduction	Yes	To 20–35 g/day	<9 g/day	<5% kcal	Reduce protein to 1 g/kg body weight; more vegetable protein
Japan (Japanese Ministry of Health and Welfare, 1985)	Yes	20–25	Yes	Use vegetable and fish oils	NC	NC	NC	<10 g/day	NC	Varied diet (at least 30 foods daily); home cooking; pleasant eating environment

aRatio of polyunsaturated to saturated fatty acids.
NOTE: NC = No comment; NS = Not specified.

maximal benefit, it is advisable to use the RDAs in combination with its dietary recommendations.

The absence of supportive data precluded a specific recommendation about the need for variety in the diet or the number of meals per day. Nevertheless, the committee supports the concepts of eating a variety of foods to ensure nutrient adequacy and eating meals regularly in a pleasant environment as proposed by the Japanese Ministry of Health and Welfare (1985).

In the United States, three recent statements have specifically addressed the use of vitamin–mineral supplements (ADA, 1987; Callaway et al., 1987; Council on Scientific Affairs, 1987). In general, these groups and others listed in Tables 28–1 through 28–4 consider supplementation to be warranted only under special conditions when nutrient needs cannot be or are not being met by diet alone. These conditions include nutrient malabsorption (resulting, for example, from gastrointestinal tract damage or drug–nutrient interactions), nutrient depletion (e.g., in chronic diarrhea), or increased physiological requirements (e.g., during pregnancy and lactation). These same organizations usually warn against megadoses of supplements (although megadoses are seldom defined), usually because of the risk of toxicity from fat-soluble vitamins and the more recently recognized toxicity of certain water-soluble vitamins (e.g., pyridoxine). The committee supports these recommendations. It stresses, however, that although the acute toxicity of many nutrients is well documented, the long-term health effects (risks or benefits) of low levels of supplements have not been adequately studied (see Chapter 18). The committee supports fluoridation of water to prevent dental caries.

In summary, the few differences of opinion on dietary recommendations stem largely from incomplete data on diet and chronic diseases. The absence of clearly defined and universally accepted criteria for interpreting the evidence and formulating dietary recommendations to the public has also hampered the achievement of consensus. Expert groups also sometimes differ about the target population, i.e., whether recommendations should be directed to the general population or only to high-risk groups (e.g., Council on Scientific Affairs, 1979; DHEW, 1979; NRC, 1980b). Sometimes a comparison of recommendations tends to highlight inconsistencies, because not all expert panels address all dietary components or diseases and their recommendations may be focused on a single chronic disease such as cancer or heart

disease rather than on overall health (e.g., AHA, 1988; NRC, 1982; USDA/DHHS, 1985). Furthermore, there is often a difference of opinion about the importance of diet in comparison to other environmental and genetic risk factors for specific chronic diseases and, consequently, about the potential impact of dietary modification on these risk factors. The Committee on Diet and Health recognizes the importance of genetic variation for dietary recommendations. Its recommendations are intended to improve the health of the total population without harming anyone, although not every individual may benefit equally.

Recommendations Pertaining to Age, Sex, and Physiological Status

Most of the dietary recommendations summarized in Tables 28–1 through 28–4 are directed to the general population (i.e., to adults), although several expert groups have also commented on their applicability to children, the elderly, and women (e.g., ADA, 1986; NIH, 1985). Because nutrient and dietary needs often vary by age, sex, and physiological status, there is often a question about whether one set of dietary recommendations can be justified for the whole population. Following are the specific reasons for concern:

• Are the data pertaining to the pediatric diet and the subsequent risk of adult chronic diseases complete or convincing enough to justify modifying diet in childhood? (See Chapters 7, 19, and 20.)

• Will fat-restricted or calorie-restricted diets curtail growth and lead to protein or micronutrient deficiency in young children? (See Chapter 7.)

• Do the general recommendations address the special needs of all women or of pregnant and lactating women in particular? (See following section, Potential Adverse Consequences of Dietary Recommendations.)

• Will restriction of dietary fats, calories, and other nutrients place elderly people, whose caloric intake is often low, at special risk of nutrient deficiency? (See following section, Potential Adverse Consequences of Dietary Recommendations.)

The Inter-Society Commission for Heart Disease Resources (1970) was the first to recommend that infants and children should also modify their diets with the objective of preventing atherosclerotic diseases in later life. The American Academy of Pediatrics (AAP, 1983) believed that the relationship of childhood arterial lesions to clinically significant lesions in adults had not been proven, that the effectiveness of dietary modification in preventing CHD had not been established, and that it might be hazardous to tamper with a diet that has been successful in promoting growth and preventing other diseases in children. However, the AAP agreed that children at high risk, usually defined as those with more than 230 mg/dl serum total cholesterol, should be advised to modify their diets or possibly to begin drug therapy (AAP, 1983).

In the 1970s, evidence increasingly indicated that U.S. children had higher plasma cholesterol levels than did children in other countries and that they might thus be at higher risk of CHD in adulthood. In 1983, the American Heart Association recommended that all children over 2 years of age reduce total fat intake to 30% or less of calories, with 10% or less from saturated fatty acids and not more than 10% from polyunsaturated fatty acids and that they should reduce cholesterol intake to 100 mg/1,000 kcal (AHA, 1983). Similar recommendations were made by the American Health Foundation (1983) and at the NIH Consensus Development Conference in 1984 (NIH, 1985). The AAP Committee on Nutrition stated, however, that "current dietary trends in the United States toward a reduced consumption of saturated fats, cholesterol and salt and an increased intake of polyunsaturated fats should be followed with caution. Diets that avoid extremes are safe for children" (AAP, 1983).

The recent recommendations of these expert groups are remarkably similar, despite the sharp division in opinion in previous years about the appropriateness of fat-modified diets for children. In the United States, dietary intakes of fat and cholesterol by children and adults have declined in recent years; continued reductions would bring actual intakes very close to those recommended by the American Heart Association (AHA, 1983). Thus, the only major difference between the recommendations of the American Heart Association, the American Health Foundation, and the National Institutes of Health and those of the American Academy of Pediatrics is the absence of quantitative targets in the recent American Academy of Pediatrics' statement (AAP, 1983). These issues are discussed in more detail in Chapter 7.

Relatively little attention has been given to the role of the pediatric diet in modifying the risk of such other diseases in adults as hypertension and obesity. In general, short-term intervention trials have not provided impressive data to suggest that sodium intake affects blood pressure in normotensive children, but the data from observational studies concerning sodium intake and blood pressure are more consistent and more impressive. It is well established that populations that maintain low sodium intake from birth do not experience a rise in blood pressure with age, nor do they develop clinical hypertension. It is not clear, however, whether there is a threshold for the effect of salt on clinical hypertension. In general, populations consuming 1,200 mg of sodium or less per day (≤3 g of salt) have very low rates of hypertension, whereas salt intakes above 3 g/day from a young age appear to show a direct, linear relationship with the risk of hypertension in adults (MacGregor, 1985). There is less convincing evidence about the effect of childhood intakes of potassium, calcium, and polyunsaturated fatty acids on hypertension in adulthood (Miller et al., 1987, 1988).

Data on the effects of diet in infancy or early childhood on the development of cancer in adults are extremely limited. Therefore, no specific dietary recommendations have been aimed at reducing cancer risk from childhood. On the basis of the overall evidence on dietary factors and carcinogenesis, however, particularly the changes observed in migrant populations (see Chapter 22), it is reasonable to conclude that childhood eating patterns are important determinants of adult risk of certain diet-related cancers, most notably breast cancer and stomach cancer. This important area requires additional study.

Considerably more is known about the correlation between diet in infancy and childhood and the development of obesity in adults (see Chapters 6 and 21). It is generally recognized that overeating and obesity in infancy are not good predictors of obesity in adulthood but that the correlation between the two improves with age and that adiposity in later childhood is an increasingly better predictor of obesity in adolescence and adulthood (Garn and LaVelle, 1985; Shapiro et al., 1984).

There is little doubt about the importance of dietary patterns (especially patterns of sugar consumption) in children and the development of dental caries (see Chapter 26). On the other hand, there is little information pertaining to childhood eating patterns and NIDDM in adults.

The committee's review of the limited evidence on the role of the pediatric diet in predisposition to chronic diseases in adulthood suggests that its dietary recommendations to the general public are

TABLE 28-3 Dietary Recommendations to Lower Coronary Heart Disease Risk in the United States and Abroad

Country (Reference)	Target Population[a]	Body Weight/ Exercise	Total Fat (% kcal)	Saturated Fatty Acids (% kcal)	Polyunsaturated Fatty Acids (% kcal)	Cholesterol (mg/day)	Complex Carbohydrates and Fiber	Simple Sugars	Sodium Chloride	Alcohol Intake	Other Recommendations
Sweden, Finland, Norway (Anonymous, 1968)	GP	Reduce calories to avoid obesity; exercise	Reduce to 25–35	Reduce	Increase	NC	Increase vegetables, fruits, potatoes	Decrease	NC	NC	10–12% of calories from protein, of which 30–50% should be of animal origin
United States (American Health Foundation, 1972)	GP	Avoid obesity	Reduce to 35	Isocaloric amounts of SFAs, PUFAs, and MUFAs		300	Increase	NC	Reduce to 5 g/day	NC	NC
Netherlands (Netherlands Nutrition Council, 1973)	GP	Maintain appropriate body weight	33	Restrict	10–13	250–300	Increase to make up caloric needs	Use little	NC	NC	NC
Federal Republic of Germany (Pahlke, 1975)	GP	NC	Reduce	Reduce	Increase	Reduce	NC	NC	NC	NC	NC
New Zealand (National Heart Foundation of New Zealand, 1976)	GP HR	Maintain appropriate body weight	35	Reduce, especially for HR	HR should substitute for SFA	Reduce	NC	Restrict to reduce weight	NC	Restrict to reduce weight	NC
Canada (Department of National Health and Welfare, 1977)	GP	Maintain appropriate body weight	Reduce to 35	10	10	NC	Increase	NC	Restrict	NC	Variety of foods
Australia (National Heart Foundation of Australia, 1979)	HR	Avoid obesity	Reduce to 30–35	P:S[b] = 1:0		Restrict	Eat enough	Use less	Restrict	Moderation	Focus on HR groups, food labeling
United Kingdom (Ad Hoc Working Group on Coronary Prevention, 1982)	GP	Avoid obesity; increase exercise	30	<10	NC	NC	Increase	NC	NC	NC	Special attention to children
World Health Organization (WHO, 1982)	GP	Avoid obesity	Reduce to 20–30	<10	Up to 10	<300	Increase	NC	<5 g/day	Drink less	Emphasis on plant foods, fish, poultry, lean meats, low-fat dairy products, and fewer whole eggs

Source	Population										Other
Japan (Panel on Nutrition and Prevention of Diseases, 1983)	GP	NC	20–25	NC	Cook with vegetable oil	NC	Increase	Reduce	Limit to <10 g/day	Avoid too much	Variety; eat enough protein, half from vegetables and half from animal sources; eat enough potassium, especially from green vegetables. Eat lean meat and fish; eat fewer confections
United Kingdom (DHSS, 1984)	GP	Avoid obesity; exercise	Reduce to 35	Reduce to 15	NS; P/S ~0.45	NS	Increase breads, cereals, fruits, vegetables	NC	Decrease	<90 ml/day for males; <65 ml/day for females	Special recommendations to government, professionals, industry
United States (Inter-Society Commission for Heart Disease Resources, 1984)	GP	Control obesity	<30	8	10	<250	Increase to make up caloric loss	NC	5 g/day	NC	NS
United States (NIH, 1985)	GP HR	Maintain appropriate body weight	<30	<10	Up to 10	250–300	Endorsed earlier recommendations of AHA (1982) and the Inter-Society Commission for Heart Disease Resources (1984)	NC	NC	NC	Special recommendations for high-risk groups; guidelines for health professionals, industry, and public
Finland (Finnish Heart Association, 1987)	GP HR	Avoid excess weight; exercise	<30	Reduce	P/S >0.5	Reduce	NC	NC	Reduce for HR <5 g/day	Moderation	Avoid trace element deficiencies; food labeling; focus on HR groups
Canada (Canadian Consensus Conference on Cholesterol, 1988)	GP HR	Adjust caloric intake and expenditure	<30	<10	<10	Restrict through less organ meats and egg yolks; for HR <300 mg	Increase	NC	Limit	Limit	Focus on HR groups; limit protein
United States (AHA, 1988)	GP	Maintain appropriate body weight	<30	<10	Up to 10	<300	Increase to derive ≥50% kcal from total carbohydrates	NS	≤3 g/day of sodium	1–2 oz ethanol/day	Protein to make up remainder of calories; wide variety of foods

aGP = General population; HR = High-risk population.
bP:S = Ratio of polyunsaturated to saturated fatty acids.

NOTE: NC = No comment; NS = Not specified.

TABLE 28-4 Dietary Recommendations to Lower Cancer Risk in the United States and Abroad

Country (Reference)	Maintain Appropriate Body Weight	Limit or Reduce Total Fat (% kcal)	Modify Ratio of Dietary Fats	Emphasize Fruit and Vegetable Intake	Increase Complex Carbohydrate Intake	Restrict Sodium Chloride	Food Preparation Methods	Food Additives and Contaminants	Alcohol Intake	Other Recommendations
United States (NRC, 1982)	NC	To ~30	NC	Especially citrus fruits, green and yellow and cruciferous vegetables	Whole-grain products	Indirectly	Minimize cured, pickled, and smoked foods	Monitor, test, and reduce exposure	Drink less, if at all	Monitor and test mutagens and carcinogens; recommendations made to government, scientists, and industry
Japan (Panel on Nutrition and Prevention of Diseases, 1983)	NC	Avoid excess	NC	Especially green and yellow vegetables, oranges, carotene, and fungi	Unrefined cereal, seaweed, fiber-rich legumes	Yes	Avoid hot drinks and burned food	NC	Same as NRC (1982)	Varied diet; chew food well
United States (ACS, 1984)	Yes	To ~30	NC	Especially vitamin A- and C-rich foods and cruciferous vegetables	High-fiber foods, whole-grain cereals	NS	Same as NRC (1982)	NS	Same as NRC (1982)	NC
Canada (Canadian Cancer Society, 1985)	Yes	Reduce	Decrease saturated fatty acids and cholesterol	Yes	More fiber-containing foods	NS	Same as NRC (1982)	Same as NRC (1982)	Two or fewer drinks per day, if any	NC
Europe (ECP/IUNS, 1986)	Yes	To <30	NC	Yes	Yes	To <5 g/day	Same as NRC (1982) and NCI (1987)	Same as NRC (1982) and NCI (1987)	Same as NRC (1982)	Varied diet; recommendations made to government, scientists, and industry
United States (NCI, 1987)	Yes	To ~30	NC	Vitamin A-rich green and yellow and cruciferous vegetables, citrus fruits	Whole-grain products; eat 20–30 g fiber/day	NS	Same as NRC (1982); avoid frying and high-temperature cooking	NC	Same as NRC (1982)	Balanced diet; read labels; follow USDA/DHHS (1985) guidelines

NOTE: NC = No comment; NS = Not specified.

TABLE 28-5 Studies Demonstrating an Inverse Relationship Between Serum Cholesterol and Cancer Mortality[a]

Study, Year (Reference)	Number in Study Male	Number in Study Female	Age (years) Male	Age (years) Female	Years Followed	Site-Specific Inverse Relationships	Variables Controlled in Statistical Analysis	Mean Cholesterol Level of Study Population (mg/dl)	Comments
Six studies pooled, 1974 (Rose et al., 1974)	36,211	—	35–64	—	5–23	Colon[b]	NR	NR	Study of colon cancer only (90 colon cancer deaths)
Evans County, Georgia, 1980 (Kark et al., 1980)	948[c] 537[d]	970[c] 647[d]	15–74	15–74	12–14	All except pancreas, ovary, and basal cell	Age, race, overweight, social class, smoking	White male: 213 Black male: 206 White female: 229 Black female: 219	Statistical significance of inverse relationships in males only; low serum cholesterol correlated with low vitamin A levels (166 cancer cases; 103 cancer deaths)
Honolulu Heart Study, 1980 (Kagan et al., 1981)	8,006	—	45–64	—	9	Colon[b]	Age, systolic blood pressure, cigarette smoking, alcohol, relative weight	218 (survivors)	Greatest risk at cholesterol ≤180 (185 cancer deaths)
Paris Prospective Study of Coronary Heart Disease, 1980 (Cambien et al., 1980)	7,603	—	43–52	—	6.6 (average)	All except bronchus and lungs	NR	223 (survivors)	Study suggests low cholesterol levels secondary to preexisting disease (134 cancer deaths)
New Zealand Maoris, 1980 (Beaglehole et al., 1980)	319	311	25–74	25–74	11	NR	Age, systolic blood pressure, Quetelet body mass index	Male: 225 Female: 212	Effect of preexisting disease not considered; numbers small; total of 30 cancer deaths
Puerto Rico Heart Health Program, 1980 (Garcia-Palmieri et al., 1981)	9,824	—	45–64	—	8	NR	Relative weight, heart rate, physical activity, hematocrit, education, cigarette smoking	Rural: 196 Urban: 205	After multivariate analysis, inverse relationship only in rural men; greatest risk at serum cholesterol ≤165 (179 cancer deaths)
Whitehall Study, 1980 (Rose and Shipley, 1980)	17,716	—	40–64	—	7.5	Lung, stomach, and colon	NR	197 (plasma)	Study suggests low cholesterol levels secondary to preexisting disease (353 cancer deaths)
Framingham Heart Study, 1981 (Williams et al., 1981)	2,336	2,873	35–64	35–64	24	Men: colon and all other sites combined[e]	Age, alcohol, cigarette smoking, education, systolic blood pressure, relative weight	Male: 235 Female: 241 (measurement at fourth visit only)	Inverse relationship only in males; greatest risk at serum cholesterol ≤190; inverse relationship for LDL cholesterol and cancer (691 incident cancers)

[a] Adapted from Sidney and Farquhar, 1983.
[b] p < .05.
[c] White.
[d] Black.
[e] p < .01.

NOTE: NR = Not reported.

also suitable for children after infancy. It is well recognized that there are critical stages in life when eating habits are formed. Although additional research is needed to clarify the interrelationship between childhood eating patterns and most chronic diseases in adults, there is sufficient basis for assuming that the proposed recommendations will be beneficial to children and unlikely to adversely affect their growth and development.

POTENTIAL ADVERSE CONSEQUENCES OF DIETARY RECOMMENDATIONS

The committee considered the potential benefits (see next section on Public Health Impact) and adverse consequences of its dietary recommendations by using several approaches: examining concordance among trends in life expectancy and the rates and trends of mortality from cardiovascular disease, cancer, and other major causes of death, both within and among countries; assessing concordance between dietary patterns and mortality rates; estimating risk in the population attributable to dietary factors; examining concordance of the habitual diet with diet-related risk factors; estimating the potential for nutrient deficiency or toxicity in some population subgroups or individuals at the ranges of intake recommended for the general population; and examining the evidence on clustering of diseases, risk factors, and precursors of diseases in the same individuals.

Concordance Between Life Expectancy and Causes of Death

Concordance between death rates for cardiovascular and noncardiovascular chronic diseases (including cancer) would provide evidence that a common environmental factor, such as habitual diet, might influence both these major causes of death. Discordant death rates would suggest that an environmental variable (e.g., dietary pattern) that promotes one disease might inhibit another and, for example, that dietary contributors to certain cancers and cardiovascular diseases are not the same. Similarly, concordance of diet with diet-related risk factors or disease precursors (e.g., between a diet low in total fat and saturated fat and low serum cholesterol levels or reduced prevalence of colonic polyps, or among energy intake, relative body weight, and blood pressure) would also suggest possible common dietary risk factors for several diseases and, thus, little likelihood of adverse

effects from a recommended action, for example, to lower blood cholesterol levels in the population. In contrast, lack of concordance would lead to concerns about increasing the susceptibility of population subgroups to one disease while decreasing the susceptibility to other chronic conditions.

The same logic applies to parallel time trends in incidence or mortality rates and to clustering of several major diseases, risk factors, or high-risk behaviors. For example, it would be important to learn whether people with cardiovascular diseases also often have precursor states for cancer (e.g., bronchial metaplasia).

Similarly, concordance between longer life expectancy and low death rates from cardiovascular diseases and cancer would indicate that effective prevention of one or the other major causes of death has no hidden adverse consequences for the population. In fact, countries having among the lowest death rates from cardiovascular diseases (i.e., Japan and Greece) have substantially greater life expectancy at all ages compared to countries with the highest CHD death rates (i.e., the United Kingdom, Finland, and the United States) (WHO, 1987).

Patterns of Mortality from Major Chronic Diseases

A thorough review of the evidence presented in Chapters 7, 19, and 22 suggests that there is concordance between mortality from heart diseases and certain cancers and that high fat intake is a risk factor for both diseases. Furthermore, dietary fat is not established as a protective factor for any major cause of death or for any of the chronic diseases examined in this report. Cited below are examples (from Chapter 7) indicating that the committee's recommendation to reduce intake of total fat and SFAs should lead to a reduction in the incidence of heart disease as well as certain cancers.

In many countries, correlational data indicate parallel trends in mortality from heart disease and cancers of several sites, including the colon and breast. Sidney and Farquhar (1983) demonstrated a positive ecological correlation ($R = .74$) between death rates from CHD and colon cancer for 49 countries (Figure 28–3) that reported such data to the World Health Organization. Similarly, T. Thom (National Heart, Lung, and Blood Institute, personal communication, 1989) plotted change in mortality from heart disease, stroke, and cancer in 27 countries from 1970 to 1983 and showed that heart disease, stroke, and total cancer deaths (other than from lung cancer) declined in parallel

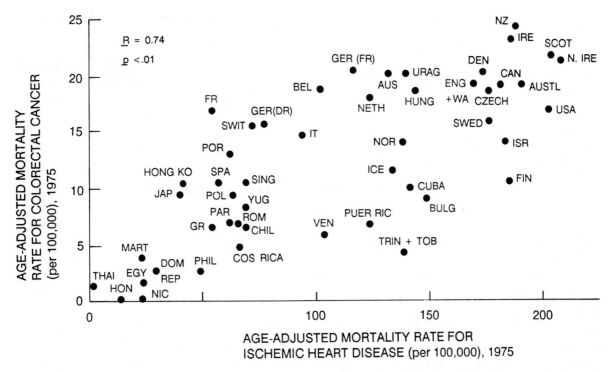

FIGURE 28–3 International comparison of 1975 age-adjusted mortality rates from ischemic heart disease and colorectal cancer, 49 countries. From Sidney and Farquhar (1983).

in the majority of countries surveyed, also presumably due to some common environmental risk factors.

Comparisons of deaths from heart disease and certain cancers require further consideration, however. For example, the substantial decline in CHD mortality from 1970 to 1983 observed in these 27 countries by T. Thom and the decline in CHD incidence observed in several large cohorts, as well as data from other sources, indicate that improved treatment methods as well as a reduction in risk factors account for these effects. During the same period, however, although mortality from colon cancer has decreased in some countries, its incidence has remained largely unchanged—probably reflecting improved therapy, early diagnosis, or both. If dietary fat exerts a major influence on the risk of both CHD and colon cancer, the lack of concordance in the *incidence* (but not the mortality) might be due to the long latency period for colon cancer and the finding in several epidemiologic studies that a diet high in total fat (both saturated and unsaturated) rather than saturated fat alone is associated with high colon cancer risk. This interpretation is further supported by dietary survey data (see Chapter 3), which indicate that, although over the last few decades saturated fat intake in the United States has declined substan-

tially, the intake of total fat has remained stable or increased somewhat. Nevertheless, there is no increase in the incidence of colon cancer.

Finally, the U.S. vital statistics (DHHS, 1987) show clear parallels in death rates for all the major chronic diseases for men and women in the United States. Between 1950 and 1978, for example, all major causes of death (heart disease, cerebrovascular disease, and cancers other than lung) declined in parallel, whereas lung cancer death rates rose steeply during that period. This observation is consistent with other evidence suggesting that certain dietary components are common risk factors for several major causes of death but are not the primary risk factors for lung cancer. Although cigarette smoking is a risk factor for many diseases, it is a much more powerful contributor to lung cancer risk than to the risk of other diseases.

DIETARY FAT INTAKE, SERUM CHOLESTEROL LEVELS, AND MORTALITY FROM CARDIOVASCULAR DISEASES AND CANCER

A major goal of the committee's recommendation to reduce the intake of total fat, SFAs, and dietary cholesterol is to lower the population mean and distribution of serum total and low-density

TABLE 28-6   Studies Not Demonstrating an Inverse Relationship Between Serum Cholesterol and Cancer Mortality[a]

Study, Year (Reference)	Number in Study		Age (years)		Years Followed	Mean Cholesterol Level of Study Population (mg/dl)
	Male	Female	Male	Female		
Norwegian workers, 1972 (Westlund and Nicolaysen, 1972)	3,751	—	40–49	—	10	270
American Heart Association Pooling Project, 1980 (NHLBI, 1980)	8,503	—	30–65+	—	8.3–12.0	235
Chicago Heart Association Detection Project in Industry, 1980 (Dyer et al., 1981)	6,890	5,750	45–64	45–64	5 (average)	214
Chicago Peoples Gas Study, 1980 (Dyer et al., 1981)	1,233	—	40–59	—	18	236
Chicago Western Electric Company, 1980 (Dyer et al., 1981)	1,899	—	40–55	—	17	248
WHO Clofibrate Trial, 1980 (Oliver et al., 1978, 1980)	10,414	—	30–59	—	9.6 (average)	Group II: 247 Group III: 181
Yugoslavia Cardiovascular Disease Study, 1980 (Kozarevic et al., 1981)	11,121	—	35–62	—	7	205
Israel Ischemic Heart Disease Study, 1981 (Yaari et al., 1981)	10,059	—	40–64	—	7	209

[a]From Sidney and Farquhar (1983).

lipoprotein (LDL) cholesterol. In several prospective studies, however, serum cholesterol levels at entry were observed to be inversely related to subsequent risk of colorectal cancer in men (Table 28–5), but this relationship was not found in other studies (Table 28–6) (Sidney and Farquhar, 1983). Subjects in some studies that showed a statistically significant inverse association had intrinsically low blood cholesterol levels, despite their consumption of a relatively high-fat diet. In some studies, the relationship was no longer significant after excluding those who died a short time after entry into the study, i.e., subjects with a low serum total cholesterol presumably due to preclinical cancer. In some other studies, the inverse association disappeared when other risk characteristics were taken into consideration (McMichael and Potter, 1984; Sidney and Farquhar, 1983).

The evidence reviewed in Chapter 7 does not support a causal relationship between low serum cholesterol levels and colon cancer. Nevertheless, the committee considered a worst-case estimate of the effect of reducing dietary SFAs and cholesterol and consequently serum cholesterol, using data

from 18 years of follow-up in the Framingham study (Williams et al., 1981). A downward shift of 10% in serum cholesterol levels in each category of men was associated with a 6% estimated increase in colorectal cancer incidence. If the men in the Framingham study during the 1960s and 1970s are assumed to be representative of all U.S. men, a serum cholesterol decrease of 10% would mean an additional 2,840 colon cancer cases in addition to 105,000 cases estimated for the United States in 1988 (Silverberg and Lubera, 1988). As noted above, however, this extreme estimate of colon cancer risk is not supported by the detailed review of evidence presented in Chapter 7. Furthermore, as discussed later in this chapter, a conservative estimate of the number of CHD deaths prevented (approximately 100,000) in the population from a 10% reduction in serum cholesterol levels suggests that the net effect of serum cholesterol reduction would be a major benefit.

In fact, many comparisons within and among populations (reviewed in Chapter 7) suggest that reduced intakes of saturated fatty acids and total fat to <10% and <30% of calories, respectively, would lead to a *decrease* in the incidence of several cancers, including colon cancer. For example, a case-control study by Jain et al. (1980) indicated a population-attributable risk of 42%, suggesting that a notable reduction in colon cancer incidence might result from reducing fat intake to the lowest level found in that study (<30% of calories daily). Even when the hypothetical, and unlikely, adverse effects of a downward shift in serum cholesterol levels are considered, the overall evidence indicates a net reduction in colon cancer rates. Moreover, ecological studies in 20 countries show that per capita intake of total fat and saturated fatty acids is directly correlated with mortality from colon cancer and all cancer sites (Sidney and Farquhar, 1983). Despite their limitations, data from such studies provide no support for a causal relationship between a low-fat diet, low serum cholesterol, and cancer.

Further evidence is provided by Sidney and Farquhar (1983), who plotted the mean total serum cholesterol against cancer mortality in seven countries (Keys, 1980) geographically remote from each other. These data show a highly positive correlation ($R = .73$) between the average serum cholesterol levels and cancer mortality in the population. Phillips (1975) reported that in Seventh-Day Adventists, who consume vegetarian diets (i.e., low-fat, high-carbohydrate diets), the rates of cardiovascular disease and all cancers, including colon cancer, are low as are their average serum cholesterol levels.

Thus, several lines of evidence indicate that lowering total fat, SFA, and cholesterol intake and a resultant decrease in mean serum cholesterol levels would not increase cancer risk. Other assessments of competing risks, described below, also indicate that reduced intake of total fat, SFAs, and cholesterol is associated with overall reduction in the risk of both cardiovascular diseases and certain cancers.

Commonality in Risk and Protective Factors for Major Chronic Diseases

The literature reviewed in this report provides strong evidence that major diet-related chronic diseases have common environmental causes and thus justify a common approach to prevention. Other evidence comes from the application of risk profiles derived from longitudinal studies of one disease to predict the risk of another. For example, the profile for CHD risk in the Seven Countries Study accurately predicted the long-term risk of stroke, cancer, and all causes of death (Farchi et al., 1987). Such commonality can also be discerned in the protective factors for major diseases. For example, the Alameda County Index of "seven healthy daily habits" correlated positively with a lower risk of CHD, cancer, and other major causes of death (Breslow and Enstrom, 1980). In the Göteborg Study, several of the same social attributes were related to the risk of mortality from all causes (Wilhelmsen et al., 1986). In the United Kingdom, an inverse gradient was found between social class of civil servants and mortality from CHD and other major causes of death (Marmot et al., 1978). The evidence reviewed in Chapter 14 suggests that a low selenium intake may be a risk factor for heart disease as well as for cancer.

Long-term intervention trials, especially those using dietary modification, also provide evidence of commonality in risk and protective factors for the major causes of death and suggest that the dietary changes recommended by the committee are unlikely to have adverse health effects. In some of the cholesterol-lowering trials, there was a tendency for an increase in mortality from neoplasms in the groups treated with diet and drugs; however, this finding was not confirmed in other trials and was not statistically significant in any trial or when data from all trials were combined (R. Peto, University of Oxford, personal communication, 1987). A few studies noted an increase in the rates of death due to trauma in the treated groups when compared to the control groups. However, a statistical summary of all the trials suggests that although there is a tendency toward increased mortality, there is no real excess of trauma deaths in the treated groups. Furthermore, there is no plausible mechanism to explain why interventions that reduce serum cholesterol levels would increase the risk of trauma. Similarly, in the North Karelia community intervention program involving dietary modification throughout the 1970s, mortality from cardiovascular diseases and cancer tended to decrease in parallel (Tuomilehto et al., 1986).

Low Serum Total Cholesterol and the Risk of Stroke in Hypertensives

As discussed in Chapters 7 and 19, epidemiologic observations in Japan and Honolulu (Reed et al., 1986) and Framingham (Kannel and Wolf, 1983), as well as findings from the large cohort screened in the Multiple Risk Factor Intervention Trial (MRFIT) (Iso et al., 1988), show a consistent pattern of increased deaths from hemorrhagic stroke among hypertensives who have low serum cholesterol values. In contrast, as the ability to distinguish hemorrhagic and thrombotic stroke has improved, a linear, positive relationship has been found consistently between serum total cholesterol and thrombotic stroke risk.

Hemorrhagic stroke risk is concentrated among those with the lowest cholesterol levels, usually below 160 to 170 mg/dl, and the excess risk is largely confined to hypertensive individuals, i.e., those with greater than 90 mm Hg diastolic pressure (Iso et al., 1988). The strength, consistency, and temporal nature of the relationship between serum cholesterol levels and cerebral hemorrhage suggest causality, but no plausible pathophysiological mechanism has been established for such an effect, and confounding factors such as low dietary and plasma protein, high salt intake, alcohol consumption, liver disease, and bleeding disorders have not been ruled out. Even if the association were causal, it would not indicate that reduction of the relatively high serum cholesterol levels in most industrial societies would increase the risk of hemorrhagic stroke in the population. Moreover, it would be possible to identify high-risk people by their combined high blood pressure and low serum cholesterol values and to reduce their risk by controlling their hypertension.

In contrast, the estimated reduction in thrombotic stroke and coronary disease risk in the population from reducing serum cholesterol levels would vastly counterbalance any small (and thus far entirely hypothetical) possibility that the risk of hemorrhagic stroke would be increased. Furthermore, the committee's recommendations to control weight, avoid or moderate alcohol intake, reduce the intake of sodium chloride, and increase potassium intake are likely to reduce the number of hypertensives in the population and, thus, the number of those at increased risk for stroke associated with low serum cholesterol (if in fact low serum cholesterol levels among hypertensives are causally associated with the risk of stroke).

Decreased Saturated Fatty Acid and Cholesterol Consumption

Evidence from epidemiologic, clinical, and metabolic studies reviewed in Chapter 7 indicates that SFA and cholesterol intake are the major dietary determinants of serum total and LDL cholesterol levels in populations and, thereby, of CHD risk. The committee's recommendation to reduce SFA intake to less than 10% of calories along with

reducing cholesterol intake is therefore likely to reduce serum cholesterol levels and, consequently, CHD risk in the population. The few epidemiologic studies on dietary fat and cancer that have distinguished among the effects of specific types of fat suggest that reduction of SFA intake to the levels recommended by the committee will also lead to a reduction in the incidence of and mortality from cancers of the colon, prostate, and breast. The committee found no evidence to suggest that the recommended reduction in SFA intake will increase the risk of any other chronic disease.

Increased Polyunsaturated Fatty Acid Consumption

The committee's dietary recommendations would not increase the average intake of PUFAs in the U.S. population (now approximately 7% of calories). Animal studies consistently show an increase in colon or mammary cancers at very high PUFA intake (see Chapter 7). Observations in human populations and in animal experiments in which PUFAs were partially substituted for SFAs suggest that PUFA intake of up to 10% of calories does not increase the population risk of cancer. However, human populations have seldom been observed to increase their PUFA consumption dramatically, and few populations regularly consume high levels (>10% of calories) of PUFAs. Thus, the current U.S. average PUFA intake combined with the committee's recommended decrease in total fat and SFA consumption is likely to lead to an overall decrease in the risk of diet-related cancers.

Increased Monounsaturated Fatty Acid Consumption

The committee's recommendations on saturated, polyunsaturated, and total fats might indirectly result in a relative increase in the consumption of MUFAs. Evidence within populations is not strong but suggests that substitution of MUFAs for SFAs may decrease cancer risk. For example, a case-control study of colorectal cancer showed a lower risk in those with a high intake of olive oil (Macquart-Moulin et al., 1986). Cross-cultural population studies suggest that an increased intake of MUFAs should reduce rates of colorectal cancer when SFA and total fat consumption are also reduced. For example, low colon cancer rates are found in southern Europe where olive oil is a staple but where SFA intake is low in comparison to western or northern Europe (Keys, 1980; Waterhouse et al., 1982).

Increased Carbohydrate Consumption

A substantial amount of data indicates that diets with high levels of plant foods and complex carbohydrates are associated with reduced risk of several chronic diseases, but a positive association between carbohydrate intake and gastric cancer risk reported in two studies (Hakama and Saxén, 1967; Risch et al., 1985) may raise questions about the consequences of increasing carbohydrate intake in the U.S. diet. Since other studies have not found increased gastric cancer risk, it is likely that the association is attributable to the frequent consumption of such dietary components as salted, pickled, and smoked foods, which is common in some populations on high-carbohydrate diets (Miller, 1982). In contrast, Seventh-Day Adventists, who generally consume high-carbohydrate diets that are low in salted or pickled foods, have a low cancer risk (Phillips, 1975). In the committee's judgment, any hypothetical increase in gastric cancer risk from high complex carbohydrate intake would be substantially less than the overall reduction in risk likely to occur with decreases in fat and nitrite intake and increases in vegetable and vitamin C consumption. The net effect of the committee's recommendations is likely to be a reduction in gastric and colon cancer rates.

Increased Consumption of Vegetables and Other Sources of β-Carotene

The evidence reviewed in Chapter 11 indicates that low consumption of carotenoid-containing foods is consistently associated with a higher risk of several cancers, especially lung cancer, although some evidence suggests an increased risk of prostate cancer in elderly men who consume higher levels of carotenoids. However, prostate cancer risk has been much more consistently associated with high-fat than with high-carotenoid consumption. Nevertheless, the committee does not recommend use of carotene supplements.

Pesticide Residues on Vegetables and Fruits

Increased consumption of vegetables and fruits can be expected to result in increased ingestion of residues of herbicides and pesticides used in agriculture. Therefore, the committee emphasizes the need to wash all raw fruits and vegetables thoroughly. Although some of these chemicals are carcinogenic in animals, there are very few studies pertaining to their carcinogenicity in humans. A few epidemiologic studies of agricultural workers and others exposed to phenoxyacetic acid and herbicides have reported increased risk of non-Hodgkin's lymphoma and possibly soft tissue sarcomas (Hardell et al., 1981; Hoar et al., 1986). Inhalation was the route of exposure in those studies, however, and limited data suggest that no adverse effects result from the ingestion of small amounts of these agents in foods. Furthermore, the potential small increased risk of these somewhat uncommon tumors that might result from increased exposures in the general population would be greatly outweighed by the potential benefits (i.e., reduced risk of cancers of the lung, stomach, colorectum, and other sites and reduced risk of other chronic diseases) to be expected from greater fruit and vegetable consumption. Thus, the committee concluded that the recommendation to consume liberal amounts of fruits and vegetables is appropriate and poses no undue competing risk.

Alcoholic Beverages and Human Health

Would the committee's decision not to recommend alcohol for those who do not drink deprive some people who are at risk of myocardial infarction of any potential benefits of alcohol? The association between moderate alcohol intake and lower CHD risk is consistent, but not strong, and not established as causal. Furthermore, the potential benefits of moderate alcohol intake itself have not been differentiated from the effects of other healthy behaviors generally found among people who control their alcohol intake. The relationship also appears to be independent of the absolute amount of alcohol intake. Even if very moderate alcohol intake were shown to be causally associated with lower CHD risk, the potential benefits of recommending alcohol for nondrinkers would be far outweighed by the well-established health risks and accidents associated with alcohol consumption.

Potential for Nutrient Deficiency or Toxicity

The use of optimal nutrient thresholds offers another approach to assessing public health benefits or risks of dietary modification. What is the impact of the committee's recommendations on the adequacy of nutrient intakes, especially for population subgroups that may be at risk of deficiency or toxicity? The effects of most, if not all, of the dietary factors examined by the committee vary directly and continuously with the level of intake; some relationships are curvilinear. Recommended nutrient thresholds are therefore arbitrary, and arbitrary cutpoints are proposed with the aim of reducing the population risk and facilitating individual choices. They are not true thresholds below or above which benefit or risk is absent or great.

Nutrient requirements vary among individuals. Thus, a recommended range of nutrient intake that meets most people's requirements may exceed a toxic threshold for a few. For example, the recommended intake of iron may lead to iron deficiency anemia in a small segment of the population at one end of the spectrum and hemochromatosis at the other. In general, however, the recommendations take into account the dietary needs of most individuals and are likely to be beneficial to the general population without posing significant risks. For example, could decreased red-meat consumption, which is likely to result from attempts to lower fat intake, lead to decreased iron intake among those vulnerable to iron deficiency (i.e., women in their reproductive years and children)? The committee recommends that fatty meats be replaced with lean meats, poultry (skin removed), fish, and sources of plant protein, such as dried beans. This recommended dietary pattern would continue to furnish adequate sources of heme iron, which is more readily absorbed than inorganic iron in plant foods. The committee also advocates increased consumption of vegetables and fruits (sources of vitamin C), which improve absorption of inorganic iron when consumed at the same time. Furthermore, the relatively low iron intake of women in their reproductive years is due partly to their low caloric intakes; increased energy expenditure through more physical exercise would permit a higher caloric intake without resulting in obesity (if exercise and caloric intake are properly balanced) and would increase the intake of many nutrients, including iron.

The committee's recommendation to balance physical activity and food intake in such a way as to maintain appropriate body weight should not result in nutrient deficiencies, which might occur if caloric intakes were substantially reduced. In fact, increased activity and caloric intake should improve the nutrient quality of the diet, if calories are provided by a variety of nutrient-dense foods.

The committee recommends limiting, not eliminating, egg yolks. Would decreasing the intake of eggs result in a decline in protein intake among children and the elderly? In the 1977–1978 Nationwide Food Consumption Survey (USDA, 1984), the mean percentage of protein intake from eggs was 4% in the adult population in contrast to 3% supplied by nuts, seeds, and legumes as a group. Eggs furnished an average of 4.3% of the protein intake from infancy to 5 years of age and 2.4% for children between the ages of 6 and 8. For men and women 65 to 74 years old, eggs furnished an average of 5 and 4% of the protein intake, respectively. For men and women 75 years and over, they supplied 6 and 4.3%, respectively. A recent survey by the U.S. Department of Agriculture indicated that children 1 to 5 years of age obtained 2.7% of their protein from eggs (USDA, 1987). Therefore, eggs do not appear to be a major protein source for any sex-age group in the U.S. population.

Similarly, decreased salt intake (and consequently decreased iodized salt intake) should not be detrimental to iodine status because the average U.S. diet is considered to be excessively high in iodine content. As discussed in Chapters 3 and 14, a National Research Council committee in 1980 recommended that steps be taken to lower dietary sources of iodine (NRC, 1980a).

The Committee on Diet and Health recommends increased consumption of foods such as whole grains, legumes, vegetables, and fruits—a practice that would increase dietary fiber intake. Is increased dietary fiber intake likely to result in decreased absorption of calcium and other minerals? A recent review indicates that mineral absorption and metabolism are not adversely affected when total dietary fiber, provided by a variety of traditional foods, is as high as 35 g/day (Kelsay, 1986). The committee does not advocate increasing dietary fiber intake by adding purified components of fiber, such as bran or guar gum. Many communities have adapted well to high fiber intakes without apparent detrimental effects on mineral status (Jenkins, 1988). Although continued research on the influence of dietary fiber on mineral absorption is needed, current evidence does not indicate that the general public will experience adverse effects (that might counteract the anticipated beneficial effects) from the kind of diet recommended by the committee.

PUBLIC HEALTH IMPACT (POTENTIAL BENEFITS) OF DIETARY RECOMMENDATIONS

What would be the impact on public health if the committee's dietary recommendations are fully adopted? Data on diet and disease risk for individuals are appropriate for estimating the effects in the population under certain conditions—when the observations are population-based, extensive, and long term so that population-attributable risk can be calculated; when the congruence of evidence permits a strong inference of causality; and when the observations are reasonably current. These conditions are especially relevant to studies of the relationship between dietary and serum total cholesterol and CHD risk and experimental reduction in serum total cholesterol and subsequent CHD risk. The excess of coronary events attributable to elevated serum cholesterol can be calculated from data on several populations. Moreover, the Hegsted and Keys equations (Hegsted, 1986; Keys, 1984) described in Chapter 7 can be used to predict the downward shift in the population mean and distribution of serum cholesterol that might result from large-scale implementation of the committee's recommendations. The population risk attributable to elevated serum cholesterol could then be used to estimate the number of cases of CHD prevented or the percentage reduction in disease rates.

Lower Serum Cholesterol and Estimated Reduction in CHD Mortality

Amler and Dull (1987) report that the population-attributable risk fraction (PARF) for cardiovascular diseases due to elevated serum total cholesterol levels ($\geq$220 mg/dl) is approximately 10% and that reduction of these levels to below 220 mg/dl could prevent more than 100,000 deaths annually. A widespread reduction in other diet-related risk factors (e.g., reduced blood pressure and improved glucose tolerance in the population in addition to lower serum cholesterol levels) could lead to an even greater reduction in mortality. These rough estimates are based on single-factor correlations within populations that have a high CHD incidence and may underestimate the potential for reducing atherosclerosis and other cardiovascular diseases through relatively modest downward shifts in the population mean and distribution of major risk factors, particularly in the levels of atherogenic serum lipoproteins.

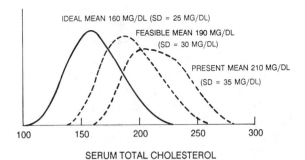

FIGURE 28–4 These idealized smoothed curves portray the present distributions of serum total cholesterol found in samples of the U.S. population (right); distributions believed to be attainable by a continuation of current changes in U.S. eating patterns over the next 10 years (middle); and distributions believed to be ideal for reducing the large population burden of atherosclerotic cardiovascular diseases (left). These curves also display the phenomena that skewness and the relative excess of individuals having high values tend to diminish as the population mean is lowered. From the American Health Foundation (1979).

Figure 28–4 shows three distribution curves for total serum cholesterol—one represents the U.S. adult population during the late 1970s with a mean of 210 mg/dl and is associated with the relatively high CHD mortality of that period; another represents populations with a mean of 160 mg/dl in which the incidence of atherosclerosis is low and CHD is rare; the intermediate curve, with a mean serum cholesterol of approximately 190 mg/dl, represents a feasible reduction of about 10% in average serum cholesterol values for the U.S. adult population (i.e., from the current mean of 210 mg/dl). This corresponds to distributions found in populations (e.g., in southern Europe) that have substantially lower cardiovascular disease rates than the United States. Thus, a reduction of approximately 10% in mean serum cholesterol levels for the whole population to approximately 190 mg/dl could lead to a large reduction in coronary disease rates (American Health Foundation, 1979). Moreover, populations that have 10 to 20% lower average serum cholesterol levels than the current U.S. average consistently are found to have extremely low rates of CHD. These observations indicate that there is a potential for substantial reduction of atherosclerotic CHD and stroke in the entire population and for a continued favorable downward trend in the United States.

The reduction in all-cause mortality and CHD mortality can be roughly estimated by applying the committee's dietary recommendations for reduced intake of total fat, saturated fatty acids, and cholesterol and using 6-year death rates in men from the MRFIT study (Iso et al., 1988). On the basis of the Keys equation (Keys, 1984), one could estimate that the committee's recommendations— i.e., a 4% reduction in calories from saturated fatty acids (from 14 to 10% of calories with no change in PUFA intake) and a reduction in dietary cholesterol from 420 to 300 mg daily (a reduction of 120 mg, or 40 mg/1,000 kcal, assuming an intake of 3,000 calories/day)—may lead to a 20-mg/dl reduction in mean serum cholesterol levels. The reduction in 6-year mortality in MRFIT screenees could then be estimated to be approximately 21% for CHD, approximately 16% for all cardiovascular diseases, and approximately 2% for all deaths. These would be underestimates of the effects of overall dietary modification because they do not consider the independent effects of reducing dietary cholesterol on CHD risk or the effects of reduced salt intake and reduced body weight on hypertension.

Similarly, the proportionate reduction in CHD incidence that would result from a reduction in serum cholesterol can be estimated from the graded risk observed in very-long-term cohort studies, i.e., an approximately 3% reduction in incidence for each 1% difference in the average serum cholesterol level at entry (R. Peto, University of Oxford, personal communication, 1987). Such estimates are reasonable in light of the reduced mean serum cholesterol levels in the population and the decline in coronary deaths documented in the United States over the past 20 years, as well as results of clinical trials among high-risk people.

All these estimates have severe limitations. For example, the data on disease risk are based on the level of risk at entry and relatively short periods of observation. There are no appropriate models for considering *postponed* rather than *prevented* events; some people saved from early cardiovascular deaths will surely die from other causes. Also, continuous changes in multiple risk factors affect people of different ages, sex, and cultures in different ways.

Diet-Related Risk Factors and CHD Risk

As suggested above, systematic population data on the decline in diet-related risk factors (e.g., blood cholesterol or blood pressure) and the observed decline in deaths from cardiovascular diseases over the past 20 years in the United States can serve as one basis for estimating the public health impact of a recommended dietary change.

Estimates based on such data suggest that a reduction in blood cholesterol alone may have been responsible for approximately 25 to 30% of the overall decline in reported CHD deaths in the United States since 1967 (Byington et al., 1979; Goldman and Cook, 1984). Because the average population blood cholesterol levels are determined predominantly by the composition of the average diet, the approximately 10% reduction in average serum cholesterol levels in the United States since the 1960s is comparable to the change that might be anticipated from large-scale implementation of the committee's recommendations. A further substantial decline in CHD mortality is therefore possible.

Other limitations of these estimates stem from the uncertainties in the cross-sectional data on which they are based, i.e., misclassification of causes of death; failure to consider cohort effects; lack of data on true incidence in the population; lack of systematic, parallel determinations of serum cholesterol data in population samples during the same period as the observed decline in coronary deaths; and confounding due to changes in the levels of other risk factors, especially blood pressure and cigarette smoking.

Variations in Dietary Lipid Profiles and Estimated CHD Risk

Another basis for estimating the effects of dietary change are data from comparative studies of different populations, especially the Seven Countries Study (Keys, 1980), which over 15 years included systematic observations of a wide range of dietary intakes in several countries, some intakes comparable to the current U.S. diet, and others comparable to that now recommended by the committee. In such comparisons, numerous confounding factors may contribute to differences in disease incidence among populations. Nevertheless, in the Seven Countries Study, differences in dietary composition and in average blood cholesterol explained a major part of the population variance in coronary disease rates (Keys, 1980). Without exception, populations consuming the levels of saturated fatty acids recommended by the committee—i.e., <10% of calories—have had little burden of atherosclerotic disease (see Chapter 7). These observations suggest that atherosclerotic diseases could be confined to a much smaller and older segment of the population. Such a projection is also supported by the observed 30 to 50% decline (depending on age, sex, and race) in U.S. coronary death rates in the past 20 years.

Dietary Intervention and Estimated Reduction in CHD Risk

Data from intervention trials to lower serum cholesterol by diet alone or by a combination of diet and drugs strongly confirm the long-term observations reported above and reviewed in detail in Chapter 7. These data indicate that CHD incidence is related proportionately to reduced serum cholesterol levels and the duration of exposure to low serum cholesterol levels. They also show a relatively rapid effect on coronary disease risk, i.e., a reduction of risk after approximately 2 years of reduction in blood lipoprotein levels. Moreover, when the data from the cholesterol-lowering trials are taken together, there is no statistically significant excess of neoplastic or all-cause mortality among the treated groups.

Dietary Modification and Potential Reduction in Cancer Risk

As discussed in Chapter 7, there have been few long-term observations and few intervention trials for cancer and other noncardiovascular causes of death. Thus, there is much less certainty about the public health impact of dietary recommendations for reducing risk of these diseases than for reducing risk of CHD. Nonetheless, estimates have been made of the proportion of cancer incidence attributable to diet and, by extrapolation, the potential effect of dietary recommendations in reducing cancer rates. Higginson and Muir (1979) estimated the proportion of cancers related to various environmental factors. They stated that although cancer incidence due to diet could not be precisely estimated, dietary factors are among the general "lifestyle" factors estimated to be responsible for approximately 90% of all cancers. Wynder and Gori (1977) were more specific. On the basis of international and national comparisons of cancer incidence, reported differences between U.S. mortality rates and the lowest reported worldwide mortality rates for each cancer site, and results of case-control studies, they concluded that a little more than 40% of cancers in men and almost 60% of cancers in women in the United States could be attributed to dietary factors.

Using a similar approach, Doll and Peto (1981) were somewhat more cautious. They agreed that a substantial proportion of cancers in both sexes in the United States was likely to be attributable to dietary factors, but from a survey of the literature, they provided a wide range of estimates (i.e., 10 to 70%) for the proportion of cancer deaths that could be reduced by practical dietary means. They stated that it might not be possible to achieve a large reduction in the near future but suggested that dietary modifications might eventually result in a 35% reduction of cancer deaths in the United States. This reduction was estimated to include a 90% reduction in deaths from cancers of the stomach and large bowel; a 50% reduction in deaths from cancers of the endometrium, gallbladder, pancreas, and breast; a 20% reduction in deaths from cancers of the lung, larynx, bladder, cervix, mouth, pharynx, and esophagus; and a 10% reduction in deaths from cancer at other sites. These investigators placed a greater degree of confidence in the projected 35% reduction in overall mortality than in the estimated contribution of diet to specific cancer sites. More recently, the National Cancer Institute's Committee on Prevention suggested that of NCI's goal of a 50% reduction in cancer mortality, about 8% might be achieved by dietary modification (Greenwald and Sondik, 1986).

Two case-control studies of dietary factors and cancer in Canada, which were based on reasonably representative population controls, enabled the authors to estimate the proportion of the cancers that might be attributable to dietary factors. One of the studies pertained to breast cancer and showed a weak positive association with total dietary fat. On the basis of those data, Miller (1978) estimated that 27% of the breast cancer risk for these women might be attributable to total dietary fat intake. The second study showed a moderately increased risk for colorectal cancer associated with a high saturated fatty acid intake in both men and women. On the basis of those data, Jain et al. (1980) estimated that 41% of the risk for males and 44% of the risk for females might be attributable to saturated fatty acid intake. Both estimates, which were based on the observed degrees of association in these representative studies, may be low because artifacts in the dietary data tend to lead to low estimates of relative risk (Marshall et al., 1981). This is particularly true for breast cancer, because estimated effects of dietary factors based on current intake are likely to be substantially below the true effect for a factor that is operational earlier in life, possibly during adolescence.

Amler and Dull (1987) estimated that a 20% reduction in both colon cancer and breast cancer rates could result from changes in the habitual diet; they considered this to be a conservative estimate.

TABLE 28-7 Health Impact of Major Cancers Associated with Dietary and Other Interventions in the United States in 1980[a]

Cancer Sites	Risk Factor (AR %)[b]	Total Number of Cancer Deaths in 1980	Number of Cancer Deaths in 1980 Attributed to the Risk Factor[c]
Lung	Smoking (75.9)	67,140	50,959
	Occupation (12)	10,615	1,274
Colon and Rectum	Diet (20)	11,444	2,289
Breast	Diet (20)	7,504	1,501
Pancreas	Smoking (25.8)	5,931	1,530
Bladder	Smoking (39.0 M) (16.4 F)	4,347	[d]
	Occupation (23)	2,530	582
Larynx	Smoking (74)	2,552	1,888
	Alcohol (16.9)	583	99
Cervix	Smoking (24.1)	1,320	318
Total		113,966	
% of all cancers		28	

[a]Adapted from Amler and Dull (1987).
[b]AR = attributable risk.
[c]Number of attributable deaths in 1980 = attributable risk (as a percentage) × total number of cancer deaths in 1980.
[d]Cannot calculate using combined male and female deaths.

Table 28–7 provides estimates (column 2), by cancer site, of the percentage of total risk attributable to major risk factors. Multiplying these attributable risks by the total number of 1980 cancer deaths (column 3) gives the number of cancer deaths for each site (column 4) attributable to each risk factor. Although attributable risk estimates are only approximate, Table 28–7 suggests that dietary recommendations similar to those of the Committee on Diet and Health could prevent more than 2,000 deaths from colorectal cancer and approximately 1,500 from breast cancer annually. These calculations also probably underestimate the real potential of dietary change, because these apparently diet-related tumors are very rare in some populations.

All these estimates about the extent of cancer attributable to diet should be interpreted cautiously, since they are based on data that are subject to considerable error and require making a number of assumptions about which opinions might reasonably differ.

Overview and Summary of Risks and Benefits of Dietary Modification

In summary, the committee used several approaches and various lines of evidence to assess possible adverse consequences of its dietary recommendations for the general population. For example, it examined the degree of concordance in death rates and mortality trends among the major diet-related causes of death (i.e., coronary heart disease and cancers) to determine the commonality in dietary risk factors and protective characteristics. It also analyzed the possible consequences of reducing the intake of total fat, SFAs, and cholesterol—actions that would reduce serum cholesterol and CHD risk but that in some studies are also associated with increased risk of colon cancer mortality. Furthermore, it considered the effect of reducing serum total cholesterol in the population on the risk of hemorrhagic stroke in hypertensives, the possible adverse effects of increased PUFA or MUFA intake, increased carbohydrate intake, increased intake of vegetables and carotene, possible increased exposure to pesticides, moderate alcohol intake versus avoidance, and the potential for nutrient deficiency or toxicity among population subgroups. Using worst-case scenarios, the committee concluded that the potential for adverse effects (e.g., increased colon cancer risk due to a reduction in the population mean for serum total cholesterol) is minimal at best and is far outweighed by the many potential benefits. Various lines of evidence indicate that risk factors and protective factors for the major diet-related chronic diseases and causes of death run in parallel and that, in general, dietary intervention to reduce the risk of one disease (e.g., CHD) is likely also to reduce the risk of other diseases (e.g., several cancers).

Central to the committee's deliberations was the extent to which the overall risk of chronic diseases in the U.S. population might be reduced by dietary modification. Because the extent to which dietary factors are involved in the etiology of different chronic diseases varies considerably (see Chapter 27), the impact of dietary modification on the risk of different diseases will also vary.

The committee used several approaches for developing quantitative estimates of the expected public health impact if its dietary recommendations were to be fully adopted by the public. The accuracy of such an estimate is determined by the availability of strong, consistent, and congruent evidence from a variety of sources, especially from extensive, long-term observations of dietary interventions in human populations. Such data are most extensive for serum cholesterol levels and the risk of CHD and much less extensive for dietary factors and CHD, cancer, and other major causes of death.

Estimates for the reduction in CHD risk were derived by extrapolating the effects of a downward shift in average serum cholesterol levels, by comparing CHD risk in populations with substantially different diets and mean serum cholesterol levels, and by examining the results of cholesterol-lowering trials on cardiovascular disease incidence. There are many drawbacks to using any of these approaches, as explained above. Taken together, however, these approaches strongly suggest that following the committee's recommendations for reducing intake of SFAs, cholesterol, and total fats and a consequent modest (at least 10%) reduction in serum cholesterol levels should lead to at least a 20% reduction in CHD risk in the United States beyond the 1987 levels. More stringent dietary modification provides the potential for even greater reduction in coronary disease in the future. This underestimates the benefits of dietary modification because it only focuses on certain lipids and does not take into account the potential benefits of reductions in body weight and blood pressure in the population.

The picture is less clear for the risk of cancer. The committee's conclusions are generally in agreement with those of the National Research Council's Committee on Diet, Nutrition, and Cancer, which in 1982 concluded that cancers of most major sites are influenced by dietary patterns (NRC, 1982). The data are not sufficient, how-

ever, to quantitate the contribution of diet to overall cancer risk or to determine the quantitative reduction in risk that might be achieved by dietary modifications. The committee notes that several countries (e.g., Mediterranean countries) with dietary patterns similar to those recommended here have about half the U.S. rates for diet-associated cancers (see Chapter 22). This suggests that the committee's dietary recommendations could also have a substantial impact on reducing the risk of cancers in the United States.

For the other chronic diseases and conditions considered in this report (i.e., hypertension, obesity, osteoporosis, diabetes mellitus, hepatobiliary disease, and dental caries), the magnitude of risk reduction expected through full implementation of the committee's guidelines on diet and health cannot be reliably estimated due to limitations in the data. Nevertheless, the committee concluded that implementation of its dietary recommendations through readily available natural diets is likely to result in considerable reductions in the overall risk of these chronic diseases without a discernible increase in the risk of any cause of death or disability.

The committee also categorized dietary factors according to the strength of the evidence relating each to the risk of chronic diseases and the potential public health impact of dietary modification. In the committee's judgment, modification of the total diet along the lines of its recommendations is necessary to achieve the maximum public health benefit, and among dietary factors, modifications in the intake of total fat, SFAs, and dietary cholesterol are likely to have the greatest impact.

IMPLEMENTATION OF DIETARY RECOMMENDATIONS

What strategies are needed to implement the committee's dietary recommendations, and what are their implications for society? These questions are the subject of a separate study by the Food and Nutrition Board. Therefore, these issues are considered only briefly in this report.

As summarized in Tables 28–1 through 28–4, a comparison of dietary guidelines from diverse, authoritative sources in the United States and abroad suggests that scientists and public health agencies now widely agree on general nutrition principles to promote good health, but the best way to implement these principles has not been determined. It is apparent to the committee and the Food and Nutrition Board that if one of our national goals is to reduce the risk of chronic diseases and if dietary modification is likely to assist in achieving that goal, then various sectors of society need to collaborate in implementing dietary recommendations. The committee is aware that a number of efforts to implement dietary recommendations are already under way both within and outside the U.S. government. The U.S. Department of Health and Human Services, for example, has developed implementation plans to coincide with 17 priority objectives for improving nutrition during the decade 1980 to 1990. These plans include measures to improve health, reduce risk factors, increase public and professional awareness, and improve services and surveillance (DHHS, 1983), and many of them are consistent with implementing dietary changes. Voluntary health organizations, health professionals, and the food industry are also taking actions that pertain to implementation of nutrition policies. Nevertheless, the committee wishes to draw special attention to the following general issues pertaining to implementation.

A concerted effort will be needed to make changes in the food supply and in nutrition policy and programs to increase the availability of low-fat, low-saturated fat, and low-salt foods in supermarkets and in public eating facilities such as school cafeterias and restaurants. Consideration may need to be given to the most effective means of achieving such modification: through technological changes, massive public education efforts, legislative measures such as food labeling, or a combination of such strategies. Although the committee's report to the public, which will follow this report, will explain its major conclusions and recommendations in lay terms, leaders in government agencies, the health professions, the food industry, and the mass media face the challenge of interpreting the committee's nine dietary recommendations for the general public and their implications for high-risk groups. They will need to convey in practical terms the concept of certainty or uncertainty of benefit, competing risks, dietary interactions, and target populations. There is a need to develop adequate educational tools and to identify the best means of educating and motivating the public. Health professionals, government agencies, and the food and agriculture industries must also undertake additional research to identify ways of effecting dietary change.

Health professionals specifically need to undertake more definitive research to determine the suitability of traditional nutrition education tools

such as the *Basic Four Food Guide* (Page and Phipard, 1957) for use with the current recommendations and to consider new food guidance systems, such as the ones discussed by Cronin et al. (1987), that take into account the proposed changes in the macronutrient composition of the average U.S. diet.

The food industry has traditionally exerted a major influence on eating patterns. Although producers of meat, poultry, fats, and oils have in the past taken issue with certain dietary recommendations, they have been increasingly responsive to dietary guidance. For example, there is an increasingly wide variety of diet menus in restaurants (Burros, 1985), and the food industry has undertaken research that attempts to implement current recommendations (e.g., the production of leaner animals) and has voluntarily adopted measures to control additives and contaminants of concern. The challenge to the private sector now is to undertake more scientifically based advertising, to develop suitable educational materials, and to make more nutritionally desirable and affordable foods more widely available in grocery stores, restaurants, hospitals, and other public eating facilities.

Food marketing research suggests that the public is now better informed and more intensely interested in matters pertaining to diet, chronic diseases, and health and that it actively seeks nutrition guidance (Jones and Weimer, 1981; Louis Harris & Associates, Inc., 1978, 1979; Mark Clements Research, Inc., 1980). However, food marketing surveys also demonstrate that the general public does not necessarily apply the advice it seeks. The multiple forces that compete for the public's attention in the marketplace and the absence of criteria for separating fact from fallacy underscore the need for a coordinated approach to implementing dietary recommendations—a strategy that involves cooperation among government agencies, professionals, and the private sector.

It is apparent to the Food and Nutrition Board and its Committee on Diet and Health that many actions within and outside the federal government directly or indirectly influence the development and implementation of dietary recommendations. However, these actions appear fragmented, often pertain to a single disease or a single dietary recommendation, and are not necessarily consistent. Furthermore, their effectiveness is unclear. In view of these concerns, another Food and Nutrition Board committee is developing a strategy for implementing the dietary recommendations proposed in this report.

The committee is confident that it is feasible to implement its recommendations within the framework of the current U.S. lifestyle, and it is encouraged by knowledge that dietary habits in the United States already have changed markedly—in many ways that are consistent with current recommendations. Thus, it seeks the collaboration of government agencies, the food industry, health professionals (physicians, nutritionists, dietitians, and public health personnel), educational institutions, leaders in mass media, and the general public in interpreting and implementing the proposed dietary modifications.

RESEARCH DIRECTIONS

Fundamental scientific discoveries generally occur in completely unexpected ways. Thus it is impossible to predict where the major discoveries will be made or which research directions will prove to be the most fruitful. Therefore, the committee does not wish to stifle creativity by specifying experimental protocols or directing research. Nevertheless, it is possible and desirable to propose a scheme for organizing research to seek more definitive data on the associations between diet and chronic diseases. The committee's conclusions and dietary recommendations reflect its assessment of current knowledge and actions justified now; they can be made more definitive only through additional research of the kind recommended below.

The seven categories of research proposed below are not presented in order of priority. Rather, taken together, they reflect a conceptual framework for interdisciplinary collaborative research that encompasses different kinds of investigations: short- and long-term experiments in vitro and in vivo, food consumption surveys, food composition analyses, descriptive and analytical epidemiologic studies, metabolic studies and clinical trials in humans, and social and behavioral research. More detailed and specific research recommendations are summarized in Chapters 4 and 6 through 26.

Identification of Foods and Dietary Components That Alter the Risk of Chronic Diseases and Elucidation of Their Mechanisms of Action

Much needed research falls in this category. Many dietary constituents are already known to play a role in the etiology of chronic diseases, but additional and more specific knowledge, especially concerning mechanisms of action, will lead to more definitive conclusions and provide more precise guidance about the ways to reduce the risk of different chronic diseases.

With regard to macroconstituents, the committee recommends that additional research focus on the following issues.

- Separating the effects of energy intake per se from those of specific sources of calories, e.g., fats, on disease risk, especially the risk of certain cancers, obesity, and noninsulin-dependent diabetes mellitus (NIDDM).
- The effects of increasing the proportion of carbohydrates in the diet on CHD morbidity and mortality among individuals with diabetes.
- The mechanism for regional fat accumulation, the feedback signals for regulation of fat stores, the means to modify body fat distribution, and the relative risks associated with regional fat deposits.
- The role of postprandial lipoproteins and their remnants in atherogenesis and in the risk of coronary heart disease and their relationship to dietary fat intakes.
- The nature and the regulation (including regulation by dietary intake) of heterogeneity within each major class of lipoproteins and the role of different lipoprotein subclasses in atherosclerosis and CHD.
- The major dietary determinants of plasma HDL and the role of HDL in preventing coronary heart disease.
- The mechanism whereby the type and amount of dietary fat influence different stages of carcinogenesis, e.g., PUFA (omega-3 and omega-6) and cancer risk, or MUFA intake and breast cancer risk.
- The relative importance of different types of proteins (animal and vegetable) compared to different types and amounts of fats in chronic disease etiology and their mechanisms of action (e.g., in coronary heart disease, different cancers, hypertension, and stroke).
- The relative effects of different types and amounts of fibers in chronic disease etiology and the mechanisms whereby they may affect serum lipid levels, CHD, different cancers, NIDDM, and gallstones.
- The influence of dietary factors other than fats on serum lipids, the atherosclerotic process, and cardiovascular diseases.
- The nutritional, environmental, behavioral, and genetic factors in the etiology of obesity associated with NIDDM.

• The potential link between the intake of total carbohydrates, different types of carbohydrates, and stomach cancer.

• Further identification of eating patterns that are protective against dental caries and the contributory role of sugars in the pathogenesis of caries versus the effect of fluoride in caries prevention.

• The mechanisms whereby chronic alcohol ingestion increases the risk of hypertension and possibly that of breast cancer.

With regard to research directions for foods and their microconstituents, the committee wishes to draw attention to the following topics.

•. Further identification of the constituents in plant foods (vegetables, whole-grain products, and citrus fruits) that may modify the risk of different chronic diseases and elucidation of their mechanisms of action.

• The specific dietary and other environmental factors associated with vegetarian lifestyles and their relative contribution to the overall maintenance of health and reduction of the risk of specific chronic diseases.

• The mechanisms whereby various ions (e.g., sodium, potassium, chloride, and possibly calcium) affect blood pressure.

• The potential role of specific B vitamins in carcinogenesis and of carotenoids as potential chemopreventive agents for specific neoplasms.

• The mechanism whereby vitamin E deficiency combined with a high PUFA intake may enhance carcinogenesis.

• The mechanisms, other than nitrosamine-inhibition, whereby vitamin C may influence carcinogenesis and the specific effects of vitamin C versus those of other substances in plant foods that are associated with a lower cancer risk.

• The potential role of calcium and vitamin D in the etiology and prevention of osteoporosis.

• The relative role of different types of coffee and constituents of coffee and tea in altering cancer risk and in affecting serum cholesterol levels and heart disease risk.

• Further identification of nutritive and nonnutritive dietary constituents that may cause, or protect against, various chronic diseases.

• Evaluation of the carcinogenic potential of suspect carcinogens in common foods, e.g., certain mycotoxins, polycyclic aromatic hydrocarbons, and naturally occurring constituents such as flavonoids.

• The effect of diet on the endogenous formation of mutagens, such as nitrosamines and fecal and urinary mutagens, and the carcinogenicity of such mutagens.

Improvement of the Methodology for Collecting and Assessing Data on the Exposure of Humans to Foods and Dietary Constituents That May Alter the Risk of Chronic Diseases

Methodological shortcomings limit the interpretation of data and often prevent the derivation of precise conclusions about the association of diet and chronic diseases. Thus, the committee recommends that high priority be given to the following types of research.

• Development of better methods to monitor and quantify dietary exposures in human populations. This includes improvement in food composition data for both nutritive and nonnutritive substances (especially fiber and microconstituents), methods for more frequent and long-term monitoring of dietary intake, and better methods to quantify dietary intake, especially for energy and alcohol. In particular, the methodology of USDA's Nationwide Food Consumption Surveys and the National Center for Health Statistics' Health and Nutrition Examination Surveys should be improved to permit assessment of the long-term health effects of dietary factors, both nutritive and nonnutritive.

• Development of better methods for data analysis from epidemiologic studies, for example, statistical methods that take into account collinearity and multiple interactions among dietary variables and that permit simultaneous analysis of the association between specific foods, food classes and food constituents, and disease end points.

• Additional techniques for assessing the mutagenic effects of chemicals on human cells in vivo and application of such techniques to assess mutagenicity of diets that are believed to present a high or a low risk for cancer.

Identification of Markers of Exposure and Early Indicators of the Risk of Various Chronic Diseases

This category of research is designated for two purposes: first, to circumvent the shortcomings of using the disease itself as the sole end point, i.e., because of the long latency period of many chronic diseases, evidenced by the delay between dietary exposure and disease expression; and second, to circumvent problems of exposure misclassification when dietary recall methods are used. In the committee's judgment, there is a pressing need to identify biochemical/biological markers of dietary exposure, early biological markers that can forecast the emergence of clinical disease, and genetic markers that can identify high-risk subgroups in the population. In addition, the committee proposes further use of molecular biology techniques to study gene-nutrient interactions that can help characterize individual variability in nutrient requirements and susceptibility to various chronic diseases. The following are examples of specific topics that deserve attention.

- Additional and better biochemical markers of exposure to dietary fats and early biological markers of neoplasia.
- Genetic control of response to dietary fats, the interaction of genetic factors and dietary fats, and their impact on specific chronic diseases, especially cardiovascular diseases, cancer, and gallbladder disease.
- The role of gene–nutrient interactions in the etiology of NIDDM, alcohol dependence, hypertension, osteoporosis, certain cancers, food intake and obesity, and dental caries.
- Simpler methods for identifying high-risk groups.

Quantification of the Adverse and Beneficial Effects of Diet and Determination of the Optimal Ranges of Intake of Dietary Macro- and Microconstituents That Affect the Risk of Chronic Diseases

Although most dietary constituents are known to have some effect on the risk of certain chronic diseases, much less is known about the magnitude of this effect. The committee believes that there is a strong need to quantify these effects in order to estimate the contribution of diet to the risk of chronic diseases. These efforts should include a study of nutrient interactions, competing risks, and dose–response relationships. The ultimate aim of such research should be to determine the optimal ranges of intake of various dietary components for health maintenance, keeping in mind the desirability of identifying their effects and the shape of the dose–response curve. The following are examples of specific areas that deserve attention.

- More discriminating data on the effect of the type and amount of fat on the risk of cardiovascular diseases and cancers of the breast, colon, and prostate and on the levels of fat intake associated with the maximum risk reduction. Special attention is needed to determine the effects on cancer and cardiovascular disease risk of very high intakes of polyunsaturated fats (e.g., of the kind found in fish oils) and to determine the optimal proportion of polyunsaturated, monounsaturated, and saturated fatty acids in the diet.
- The optimal range of protein intake by identifying the effects of the amounts and types of protein on chronic diseases including atherosclerosis, certain cancers, hypertension and stroke, and osteoporosis.
- The long-term effects of excessive protein intake on renal function in humans and its relationship to the risk of end-stage renal disease.
- The role of specific amino acids or combinations of amino acids in augmenting chronic disease risk.
- The nature of interaction between protein and different carcinogens in experimentally induced carcinogenesis.
- The long-term effects of increasing the proportion of complex carbohydrates (starches and fibers) in the diet on the risk of, and biochemical markers for, several diseases, especially stomach and pancreatic cancers, NIDDM, and atherosclerotic cardiovascular diseases, and the specific roles of individual fibers in disease onset.
- The potential beneficial or adverse effects of mild to moderate alcohol consumption on coronary heart disease risk.
- The optimal range of intake of water-soluble vitamins for prevention of chronic diseases, especially cancer and liver disease at all stages of the life cycle.
- Dose–response curves for trace elements with the potential for reducing chronic disease risk (e.g., selenium and copper).
- Interactions among nutrients or among nutrients and other environmental risk factors at ranges of exposure that have the potential for modifying chronic disease risk. These would include interactions of physical activity, fat intake, and obesity; alcohol and vitamin A or alcohol and the B vitamins and cancer; fiber and micronutrients such as calcium, zinc, or vitamin C and various diseases; vitamin E, polyunsaturated fatty acids, and CHD; vitamin E, selenium, and cancer; sodium, potassium, and their anions, alcohol, lipids, proteins, and hypertension, or dietary electrolytes and calcium and hypertension; fluoride, the spectrum of carbohydrate intake, and dental caries; diet, phys-

ical fitness, and blood pressure; and synergistic and antagonistic interactions among food additives, contaminants, nutrients, and cancer risk.

Through Intervention Studies, Assessment of the Potential for Chronic Disease Risk Reduction

Carefully designed intervention studies should be conducted to assess the public health impact of dietary modification. Although many such studies have been conducted for heart disease, hypertension, dental caries, and obesity, and a few have focused on osteoporosis, no such long-term studies have yet been completed for cancer. The committee has considered whether priority should be given to large-scale trials or whether current knowledge is sufficient to undertake interventions in the population and subsequently to assess their effectiveness by careful monitoring of trends in disease incidence and mortality.

Intervention trials should be undertaken only when a substantial body of data indicates a high likelihood of benefit without discernible risk. A few such trials (e.g., fat-reduction for breast cancer risk; a trial to examine multiple risk factors to test multiple disease end points; a trial with sodium restriction, potassium supplementation, and weight control for hypertension; β-carotene supplements for the risk of cancers of the lung, gastrointestinal tract, and cervix; increased dietary fiber for the risk of colon cancer; and especially trials that can simultaneously measure the impact of dietary modification on multiple disease end points) might be justified to obtain more definitive data, but they should not be used as a basis for delaying prudent dietary modifications warranted by current knowledge. Any intervention studies should be accompanied by effective monitoring to assess disease incidence, prevalence, and mortality rates.

Application of Knowledge About Diet and Chronic Diseases to Public Health Programs

Social and behavioral research should be undertaken to achieve a better understanding of factors that motivate people to modify their food habits. This knowledge is indispensable for designing effective public health programs to reduce the risk of chronic diseases. Furthermore, improved technologies are needed to enhance the availability of foods that conform to the committee's dietary

recommendations. Examples of the type of research are listed below.

- Comparisons of the behavior and motivations of people who have changed their food habits with those who have not.
- Natural history of dietary change in humans to identify periods of vulnerability to change in eating habits.
- Methods for reducing obesity and maintaining weight loss.
- Methods for controlling alcohol abuse and alcohol dependence.
- Methods for monitoring and evaluating the impact of dietary recommendations on chronic disease risk.
- Ethnic and cultural differences in response to dietary modification and means of incorporating these differences in strategies for risk reduction.
- Animal husbandry and food technology research to produce leaner animals, plant foods with less pesticide or toxic chemical residues, and a greater variety of processed foods with less fat, modified fatty acid composition, less salt, more complex carbohydrates, and less refined sugars.

Expansion of Basic Research in Molecular and Cellular Nutrition

The six categories described above focus on research to enhance knowledge of the interrelationship among dietary factors, chronic diseases, and health, and this research includes an understanding of the underlying mechanisms. The committee emphasizes the need for such fundamental research to further advance our knowledge of basic cellular and molecular mechanisms. Research in disciplines ranging from the physical sciences to biochemistry, physiology, applied biology, nutrition, medicine, epidemiology, biophysics, cellular and molecular biology, and genetics is needed to fill the gaps in our understanding of how dietary, environmental, and genetic factors interact to influence the risk of chronic diseases.

REFERENCES

AAP (American Academy of Pediatrics). 1983. Toward a prudent diet for children. Pediatrics 71:78–80.
ACS (American Cancer Society). 1984. Nutrition and Cancer: Cause and Prevention. American Cancer Society Special Report. American Cancer Society, New York. 10 pp.
ADA (American Dietetic Association). 1986. The American Dietetic Association's nutrition recommendations for women. J. Am. Diet. Assoc. 86:1663–1664.

ADA (American Dietetic Association). 1987. Recommendations concerning supplement usage: ADA statement. J. Am. Diet. Assoc. 87:1342–1343.

Ad Hoc Working Group on Coronary Prevention. 1982. Prevention of coronary heart disease in the United Kingdom. Lancet 1:846–847.

AHA (American Heart Association). 1982. Rationale of the diet–heart statement of the American Heart Association: Report of Nutrition Committee. Circulation 65:839A–854A.

AHA (American Heart Association). 1983. Diet in the healthy child: task force committee of the Nutrition Committee and the cardiovascular disease in the young council of the American Heart Association. Circulation 67:1411A–1414A.

AHA (American Heart Association). 1986. Dietary guidelines for healthy American adults: a statement for physicians and health professionals by the Nutrition Committee, American Heart Association. Circulation 74:1465A–1468A.

AHA (American Heart Association). 1988. Dietary guidelines for healthy American adults: a statement for physicians and health professionals by the Nutrition Committee, American Heart Association. Circulation 77:721A–724A.

American Diabetes Association. 1987. Nutritional recommendations and principles for individuals with diabetes mellitus: 1986. Diabetes Care 10:126–132.

American Health Foundation. 1972. Position statement on diet and coronary heart disease. Prev. Med. 1:255–286.

American Health Foundation. 1979. Conference on the health effects of blood lipids: optimal distributions for populations. Prev. Med. 8:580–759.

American Health Foundation. 1983. Summary and recommendations of the conference on blood lipids in children: optimal levels for early prevention of coronary artery disease. Prev. Med. 12:728–740.

Amler, R.W., and H.B. Dull, eds. 1987. Closing the Gap: The Burden of Unnecessary Illness. Oxford University Press, New York. 210 pp.

Beaglehole, R., M.A. Foulkes, I.A.M. Prior, and E.F. Eyles. 1980. Cholesterol and mortality in New Zealand Maoris. Br. Med. J. 280:285–287.

Blackburn, H., and D. Jacobs. 1984. Sources of the diet-heart controversy: confusion over population versus individual correlations. Circulation 70:775–780.

Breslow, L., and J.E. Enstrom. 1980. Persistence of health habits and their relationship to mortality. Prev. Med. 9:469–483.

Burros, M. 1985. Dining choices for healthier food. New York Times, May 11, p. 52.

Byington, R., A.R. Dyer, D. Garside, K. Liu, D. Moss, J. Stamler, and Y. Tsong. 1979. Recent trends of major coronary risk factors and CHD mortality in the United States and other industrialized countries. Pp. 340–380 in R.J. Havlik, M. Feinleib, T. Thom, B. Krames, A.R. Sharrett, and R. Garrison, eds. Proceedings of the Conference on the Decline in Coronary Heart Disease Mortality. DHEW Publ. No. (NIH) 79-1610. National Heart, Lung, and Blood Institute, National Institutes of Health, Public Health Service, Department of Health, Education, and Welfare, Bethesda, Md.

Callaway, C.W., K.W. McNutt, R.S. Rivlin, A.C. Ross, H.H. Sandstead, and A.P. Simopoulos. 1987. Statement on vitamin and mineral supplements. The Joint Public Information Committee of the American Institute of Nutrition and the American Society for Clinical Nutrition. J. Nutr. 117:1649.

Cambien, F., P. Ducimetiere, and J. Richard. 1980. Total serum cholesterol and cancer mortality in a middle-aged male population. Am. J. Epidemiol. 112:388–394.

Canadian Cancer Society. 1985. Facts on Cancer & Diet: Your Food Choices May Help You Reduce Your Cancer Risk. Canadian Cancer Society, Toronto. 23 pp.

Canadian Consensus Conference on Cholesterol. 1988. Preliminary Report. A Conference on the Prevention of Heart and Vascular Disease Through Altering Serum Lipids and Lipoprotein Risk Factors, March 9–11, 1988. Government Conference Centre, Ottawa, Ontario, Canada. 16 pp.

Castelli, W.P. 1979. How many drinks a day? J. Am. Med. Assoc. 242:2000.

Commonwealth Department of Health/National Health and Medical Research Council. 1983. Nutrition Policy Statements. C.J. Thompson, Commonwealth Government Printer, Canberra, Australia. 39 pp.

Council on Scientific Affairs. 1979. American Medical Association concepts of nutrition and health. J. Am. Med. Assoc. 242:2335–2338.

Council on Scientific Affairs. 1987. Vitamin preparations as dietary supplements and as therapeutic agents. J. Am. Med. Assoc. 257:1929–1936.

Cronin, F.J., A.M. Shaw, S.M. Krebs-Smith, P.M. Marsland, and L. Light. 1987. Developing a food guidance system to implement the dietary guidelines. J. Nutr. Educ. 19:281–302.

Department of Health, Ireland. 1984. Guidelines for Preparing Information and Advice to the General Public on Healthy Eating. Food Advisory Committee, Department of Health, Dublin, Ireland. 26 pp.

Department of National Health and Welfare, Canada. 1977. Recommendations for Prevention Programs in Relation to Nutrition and Cardiovascular Disease. Report of the Committee on Diet and Cardiovascular Diseases, Bureau of Nutritional Sciences, Health Protection Branch, Ottawa, Ontario, Canada. 46 pp.

Department of National Health and Welfare, Canada. 1982. Canada's Food Guide Handbook (revised). Report of the Committee on Diet and Cardiovascular Diseases. Ottawa Supply and Services, Ottawa, Ontario, Canada. 52 pp.

DHEW (U.S. Department of Health, Education, and Welfare). 1979. Healthy People: the Surgeon General's Report on Health Promotion and Disease Prevention. DHEW (PHS) Publ. No. 79-55071. Office of the Assistant Secretary for Health and Surgeon General, Public Health Service, U.S. Department of Health, Education, and Welfare. U.S. Government Printing Office, Washington, D.C. 177 pp.

DHHS (U.S. Department of Health and Human Services). 1983. Public health service implementation plans for attaining the objectives for the nation: improved nutrition, summary of the problem. Public Health Reports 98:132–155.

DHHS (U.S. Department of Health and Human Services). 1986. The 1990 Health Objectives for the Nation: A Midcourse Review. Office of Disease Prevention and Health Promotion, Public Health Service. U.S. Government Printing Office, Washington, D.C. 253 pp.

DHHS (U.S. Department of Health and Human Services). 1987. Monthly Vital Statistics Report, Vol. 36: The Advance Report of Final Mortality Statistics, 1985. DHHS Publ. No. (PHS) 87-1120. National Center for Health

Statistics, Public Health Service, U.S. Department of Health and Human Services, Hyattsville, Md. 48 pp.

DHHS (U.S. Department of Health and Human Services). 1988. The Surgeon General's Report on Nutrition and Health. DHHS (PHS) Publ. No. 88-50210. Public Health Service, U.S. Department of Health and Human Services. U.S. Government Printing Office, Washington, D.C. 712 pp.

DHSS (Department of Health and Social Security). 1984. Diet and Cardiovascular Disease. Report on Health and Social Subjects No. 28. Report of the Panel on Diet in Relation to Cardiovascular Disease, Committee on Medical Aspects of Food Policy. Her Majesty's Stationery Office, London. 32 pp.

Doll, R., and R. Peto. 1981. The causes of cancer: quantitative estimates of avoidable risks of cancer in the United States today. J. Natl. Cancer Inst. 66:1191–1308.

Dupin, H., et al. 1981. Apports Nutritionnels Conseillés pour la population française. Technique et Documentation, Lavoisier, France. 101 pp.

Dyer, A.R., J. Stamler, O. Paul, R.B. Shekelle, J.A. Schoenberger, D.M. Berkson, M. Lepper, P. Collette, S. Shekelle, and H.A. Lindberg. 1981. Serum cholesterol and risk of death from cancer and other causes in three Chicago epidemiological studies. J. Chronic Dis. 34:249–260.

ECP/IUNS (European Organization for Cooperation on Cancer Prevention Studies/International Union for Nutritional Sciences). 1986. Proceedings of a joint ECP–IUNS workshop on diet and human carcinogenesis (Århus, Denmark; June 1985). Nutr. Cancer 8:1–40.

Farchi, G., A. Menotti, and S. Conti. 1987. Coronary risk factors and survival probability from coronary and other causes of death. Am. J. Epidemiol. 126:400–408.

Finnish Heart Association. 1987. Prevention of Coronary Heart Disease in Finland. National Board of Health, National Public Health Institute, Finnish Cardiac Society. Finnish Heart Association, Helsinki, Finland. 96 pp.

Food and Nutrition Council, Netherlands. 1983–1984. Food Policy Note (Nota Voedingsbeleid). Ministry of Health, Welfare, and Culture, Ministry of Agriculture, and the Ministry of Economics. The Hague. 94 pp.

Garcia-Palmieri, M.R., P.D. Sorlie, R. Costas, Jr., and R.J. Havlik. 1981. An apparent inverse relationship between serum cholesterol and cancer mortality in Puerto Rico. Am. J. Epidemiol. 114:29–40.

Garn, S.M., and M. LaVelle. 1985. Two-decade follow-up of fatness in early childhood. Am. J. Dis. Child. 139:181–185.

German Society of Nutrition. 1985. Ten Guidelines for Sensible Nutrition. Deutsche Gesellschaft für Ernährung e.V. Frankfurt, Federal Republic of Germany. 6 pp.

Goldbourt, U. 1987. High risk versus public health strategies in primary prevention of coronary heart disease. Am. J. Clin. Nutr. 45 suppl. 5:1185–1192.

Goldman, L., and E.F. Cook. 1984. The decline in ischemic heart disease mortality rates. An analysis of the comparative effects of medical interventions and changes in lifestyle. Ann. Intern. Med. 101:825–836.

Greenwald, P., and E.W. Sondik, eds. 1986. Cancer control objectives for the nation: 1985–2000. J. Natl. Cancer Inst. Monogr. 2:1–105.

Grobstein, C. 1983. Should imperfect data be used to guide public policy? Science 83 4:18.

Hakama, M., and E.A. Saxén. 1967. Cereal consumption and gastric cancer. Int. J. Cancer 2:265–268.

Hardell, L., M. Eriksson, P. Lenner, and E. Lundgren. 1981. Malignant lymphoma and exposure to chemicals, especially organic solvents, chlorophenols and phenoxy acids: a case-control study. Br. J. Cancer 43:169–176.

Hegsted, D.M. 1986. Serum-cholesterol response to dietary cholesterol: a re-evaluation. Am. J. Clin. Nutr. 44:299–305.

Hennekens, C.H., W. Willett, B. Rosner, D.S. Cole, and S.L. Mayreut. 1979. Effects of beer, wine, and liquor in coronary deaths. J. Am. Med. Assoc. 242:1973–1974.

Higginson, J., and C.S. Muir. 1979. Environmental carcinogenesis: misconceptions and limitations to cancer control. J. Natl. Cancer Inst. 63:1291–1298.

Hoar, S.K., A. Blair, F.F. Holmes, C.D. Boysen, R.J. Robel, R. Hoover, and J.F. Fraumeni, Jr. 1986. Agricultural herbicide use and risk of lymphoma and soft-tissue sarcoma. J. Am. Med. Assoc. 256:1141–1147.

Inter-Society Commission for Heart Disease Resources. 1970. Primary prevention of the atherosclerotic diseases. Circulation Suppl. 42:A55–A95.

Inter-Society Commission for Heart Disease Resources. 1984. Optimal resources for primary prevention of atherosclerotic diseases. Circulation 70:153A–205A.

Iso, H., D.R. Jacobs, Jr., D. Wentworth, J.D. Neaton, and J. Cohen. 1988. Relationship of serum cholesterol to risk of different types of stroke: 28th conference on cardiovascular disease epidemiology. CVD Epidemiol. Newsletter (AHA) 43:40.

Jain, M., G.M. Cook, F.G. Davis, M.G. Grace, G.R. Howe, and A.B. Miller. 1980. A case-control study of diet and colo-rectal cancer. Int. J. Cancer 26:757–768.

Japanese Ministry of Health and Welfare. 1985. Dietary Guidelines for Health Promotion, Vol. 29. Health Promotion and Nutrition Division, Health Services Bureau. Ministry of Health and Welfare, Tokyo. 6 pp.

Jenkins, D.J.A. 1988. Carbohydrates (B) dietary fiber. Pp. 52–71 in M.E. Shils and V.R. Young, eds. Modern Nutrition in Health and Disease, 7th ed. Lea & Febiger, Philadelphia.

Jones, J.L., and J. Weimer. 1981. Health-related food choices. Fam. Econ. Rev. Summer:16–19.

Kagan, A., D.L. McGee, K. Yano, G.G. Rhoads, and A. Nomura. 1981. Serum cholesterol and mortality in a Japanese-American population: the Honolulu Heart Program. Am. J. Epidemiol. 114:11–20.

Kannel, W.B., and P.A. Wolf. 1983. Epidemiology of cerebrovascular disease. Pp. 1–24 in R.W.R. Russell, ed. Vascular Disease of the Central Nervous System, 2nd ed. Churchill Livingstone, Edinburgh.

Kark, J.D., A.H. Smith, and C.G. Hames. 1980. The relationship of serum cholesterol to the incidence of cancer in Evans County, Georgia. J. Chronic Dis. 33:311–322.

Kelsay, J.L. 1986. Update on fiber and mineral availability. Pp. 361–372 in G.V. Vahouny and D. Kritchevsky, eds. Dietary Fiber: Basic and Clinical Aspects. Plenum Press, New York.

Keys, A. 1968. Official Collective Recommendation on Diet in the Scandinavian Countries. Nutr. Rev. 26:259–263.

Keys, A. 1980. Pp. 345–359 in Seven Countries: A Multivariate Analysis of Death and Coronary Heart Disease. Harvard University Press, Cambridge, Mass.

Keys, A. 1984. Serum cholesterol response to dietary cholesterol. Am. J. Clin. Nutr. 40:351–359.

Kozarevic, D., D. McGee, N. Vojvodic, T. Gordon, Z. Racic, W. Zukel, and T. Dawber. 1981. Serum cholesterol and mortality: the Yugoslavia Cardiovascular Disease Study. Am. J. Epidemiol. 114:21–28.

Langsford, W.A. 1979. A food and nutrition policy. Food Nutr. Notes Rev. 36:100–103.

Louis Harris & Associates, Inc. 1978. Health Maintenance. Pacific Mutual Life Insurance Co., Newport Beach, Calif. 88 pp.

Louis Harris & Associates, Inc. 1979. The Perrier Study: Fitness in America. Great Waters of France, Inc., New York. 59 pp.

LSRO (Life Sciences Research Office). 1987. Physiological Effects and Health Consequences of Dietary Fiber. Federation of American Societies for Experimental Biology, Bethesda, Md. 236 pp.

MacGregor, G.A. 1985. Sodium is more important than calcium in essential hypertension. Hypertension 7:628–640.

Macquart-Moulin, G., E. Riboli, J. Cornée, B. Charnay, P. Berthezène, and N. Day. 1986. Case-control study on colorectal cancer and diet in Marseilles. Int. J. Cancer 38: 183–191.

Mark Clements Research, Inc. 1980. Trends in Nutrition, I. The Benchmark Survey, February, 1980. Self Magazine, New York. (various pagings)

Marmot, M.G., A.M. Adelstein, N. Robinson, and G.A. Rose. 1978. Changing social-class distribution of heart disease. Br. Med. J. 2:1109–1112.

Marshall, J.R., R. Priore, S. Graham, and J. Brasure. 1981. On the distortion of risk estimates in multiple exposure level case-control studies. Am. J. Epidemiol. 113:464–473.

McMichael, A.J., and J.D. Potter. 1984. Parity and death from colon cancer in women: a case-control study. Comm. Health Study 8:19–25.

Miller, A.B. 1978. An overview of hormone-associated cancers. Cancer Res. 38:3985–3990.

Miller, A.B. 1982. Risk factors from geographic epidemiology for gastrointestinal cancer. Cancer 50 suppl. 11:2533–2540.

Miller, J.Z., M.H. Weinberger, and J.C. Christian. 1987. Blood pressure response to potassium supplementation in normotensive adults and children. Hypertension 10:437–442.

Miller, J.Z., M.H. Weinberger, S.A. Daugherty, N.S. Fineberg, J.C. Christian, and C.E. Grim. 1988. Blood pressure response to dietary sodium restriction in healthy normotensive children. Am. J. Clin. Nutr. 47:113–119.

Molitor, G.T. 1979. National nutrition goals: how far have we come? Pp. 135–141 in M. Chou and D.P. Harmon, Jr., eds. Critical Food Issues of the Eighties. Pergamon Press, New York.

NACNE (National Advisory Committee for Nutrition Education). 1983. A Discussion Paper on Proposals for Nutritional Guidelines for Health Education in Britain. Health Education Council, London. 40 pp.

National Advisory Committee, New Zealand. 1982. Nutrition goals for New Zealanders. Health 34:11–12.

National Cholesterol Education Program. 1988. Report of the National Cholesterol Education Program Expert Panel on Detection, Evaluation, and Treatment of High Blood Cholesterol in Adults. Arch. Intern. Med. 148:36–69.

National Heart Foundation of Australia, Committee on Diet and Heart Disease. 1979. Diet and coronary heart disease: a review. Med. J. Aust. 2:294–307.

National Heart Foundation of New Zealand. 1976. Coronary Heart Disease: A Progress Report, 1976. Report by a Committee Convened by the Scientific Committee of the National Heart Foundation of New Zealand. National Heart Foundation of New Zealand, Dunedin, New Zealand. 132 pp.

NCI (National Cancer Institute). 1984a. Cancer Prevention: Good News, Better News, Best News. NIH Publ. No. 84-2671. National Institutes of Health, Public Health Service, U.S. Department of Health and Human Services. U.S. Government Printing Office, Washington, D.C. 20 pp.

NCI (National Cancer Institute). 1984b. Diet, Nutrition, and Cancer Prevention: A Guide to Food Choices. NIH Publ. No. 85-2711. National Institutes of Health, Public Health Service, U.S. Department of Health and Human Services. U.S. Government Printing Office, Washington, D.C. 52 pp.

NCI (National Cancer Institute). 1987. Diet, Nutrition, and Cancer Prevention: A Guide to Food Choices. NIH Publ. No. 87-2878. National Institutes of Health, Public Health Service, U.S. Department of Health and Human Services. U.S. Government Printing Office, Washington, D.C. 39 pp.

NHLBI (National Heart, Lung, and Blood Institute). 1980. Summary Report of the NHLBI Cholesterol Workshop, February 26–27, 1980. Division of Heart and Vascular Disease, National Institutes of Health. U.S. Government Printing Office, Washington, D.C.

NIAAA (National Institute on Alcohol Abuse and Alcoholism). 1986. Toward a National Plan to Combat Alcohol Abuse and Alcoholism: A Report to the United States Congress. National Institutes of Health, Public Health Service, U.S. Department of Health and Human Services, Rockville, Md. 81 pp.

NIH (National Institutes of Health). 1984a. Health Implications of Obesity: National Institutes of Health Consensus Development Conference Statement. Ann. Intern. Med. 103:1073–1077.

NIH (National Institutes of Health). 1984b. Osteoporosis: Consensus Development Conference Statement, Vol. 5. Publ. No. 421-132:4652. National Institute of Arthritis, Diabetes, and Digestive and Kidney Diseases and the Office of Medical Applications of Research. U.S. Government Printing Office, Washington, D.C. 6 pp.

NIH (National Institutes of Health). 1985. Lowering blood cholesterol to prevent heart disease: consensus conference. J. Am. Med. Assoc. 253:2080–2086.

NRC (National Research Council). 1980a. Recommended Dietary Allowances. 9th ed. A Report of the Committee on Dietary Allowances, Food and Nutrition Board, Assembly of Life Sciences, National Academy of Sciences. National Academy Press, Washington, D.C. 185 pp.

NRC (National Research Council). 1980b. Toward Healthful Diets. Report of the Food and Nutrition Board, Division of Biological Sciences, Assembly of Life Sciences. National Academy of Sciences, Washington, D.C. 24 pp.

NRC (National Research Council). 1982. Diet, Nutrition, and Cancer. Report of the Committee on Diet, Nutrition, and Cancer, Assembly of Life Sciences, National Academy Press, Washington, D.C. 496 pp.

Oliver, M.F., J.A. Heady, J.N. Morris, and J. Cooper. 1978. A co-operative trial in the primary prevention of ischaemic heart disease using clofibrate: report from the Committee of Principal Investigators. Br. Heart J. 40:1069–1118.

Oliver, M.F., J.A. Heady, J.N. Morris, and J. Cooper. 1980. W.H.O. cooperative trial on primary prevention of ischaemic heart disease using clofibrate to lower serum cholesterol: mortality follow-up. Report of the Committee of Principal Investigators. Lancet 2:379–385.

Olson, R.E. 1986. Mass intervention vs screening and selective intervention for the prevention of coronary heart disease. J. Am. Med. Assoc. 255:2204–2207.

Page, I.H., E.V. Allen, F.L. Chamberlain, A. Keys, J. Stamler, and F.J. Stare. 1961. Dietary fat and its relation to heart attacks and strokes. Circulation 23:133–136.

Page, L., and E.F. Phipard. 1957. Essentials of an Adequate Diet. Home Economics Research Report No. 3. Agricultural Research Service, U.S. Department of Agriculture. U.S. Government Printing Office, Washington, D.C. 21 pp.

Pahlke, G. 1975. Dietary fat and degenerative vascular diseases. Nutr. Metab. 18:113–115.

Palmer, S. 1983. Diet, nutrition, and cancer: the future of dietary policy. Cancer Res. 43 suppl. 5:2509s–2514s.

Panel on Nutrition and Prevention of Diseases. 1983. Dietary guidelines and nutrition policies in Japan. Ministry of Health and Welfare, Public Health Bureau. Japan Dietetic Association, Tokyo. 168 pp.

Phillips, R.L. 1975. Role of life-style and dietary habits in risk of cancer among Seventh-Day Adventists. Cancer Res. 35: 3513–3522.

Reed, D., K. Yano, and A. Kagan. 1986. Lipids and lipoproteins as predictors of coronary heart disease, stroke, and cancer in the Honolulu Heart Program. Am. J. Med. 80: 871–878.

Risch, H.A., M. Jain, N.W. Choi, J.G. Fodor, C.J. Pfeiffer, G.R. Howe, L.W. Harrison, K.J. Craib, and A.B. Miller. 1985. Dietary factors and the incidence of cancer of the stomach. Am. J. Epidemiol. 122:947–959.

Rose, G. 1985. Sick individuals and sick populations. Int. J. Epidemiol. 14:32–38.

Rose, G., and M.J. Shipley. 1980. Plasma lipids and mortality: a source of error. Lancet 1:523–526.

Rose, G., H. Blackburn, A. Keys, H.L. Taylor, W.B. Kannel, O. Paul, D.D. Reid, and J. Stamler. 1974. Colon cancer and blood-cholesterol. Lancet 1:181–183.

Royal Ministry of Health and Social Affairs. 1981–1982. On the Follow-up of Norwegian Nutrition Policy. Report No. 11 to the Storting (1981–1982). Oslo. 79 pp.

Shapiro, L.R., P.B. Crawford, M.J. Clark, D.L. Pearson, J. Raz, and R.L. Huenemann. 1984. Obesity prognosis: a longitudinal study of children from the age of 6 months to 9 years. Am. J. Public Health 74:968–972.

Sidney, S., and J.W. Farquhar. 1983. Cholesterol, cancer, and public health policy. Am. J. Med. 75:494–508.

Silverberg E., and J.A. Lubera. 1988. Cancer statistics, 1988. CA Mag. 38:5–22.

Swedish National Food Administration. 1981. Swedish Nutrition Recommendations. National Food Administration, Uppsala. 11 pp.

Tuomilehto, J., J. Geboers, J.T. Salonen, A. Nissinen, K. Kuulasmaa, and P. Puska. 1986. Decline in cardiovascular mortality in North Karelia and other parts of Finland. Br. Med. J. 293:1068–1071.

Upton, A.C. 1979. Statement on Diet, Nutrition, and Cancer. Hearings of the Subcommittee on Nutrition of the Senate Committee on Agriculture, Nutrition, and Forestry, October 2, Washington, D.C.

U.S. Senate. 1977. Dietary Goals for the United States, 2nd ed. Report of the Select Committee on Nutrition and Human Needs. Stock No. 052-070-04376-8. U.S. Government Printing Office, Washington, D.C. 83 pp.

USDA (U.S. Department of Agriculture). 1984. Nationwide Food Consumption Survey. Nutrient Intakes: Individuals in 48 States, Year 1977–78. Report No. I-2. Consumer Nutrition Division, Human Nutrition Information Service, Hyattsville, Md. 439 pp.

USDA (U.S. Department of Agriculture). 1987. Nationwide Food Consumption Survey. Continuing Survey of Food Intakes by Individuals. Women 19–50 Years and Their Children 1–5 Years, 4 Days, 1985. Report No. 85-4. Nutrition Monitoring Division, Human Nutrition Information Service, U.S. Department of Agriculture, Hyattsville, Md. 182 pp.

USDA/DHHS (U.S. Department of Agriculture/Department of Health and Human Services). 1980. Nutrition and Your Health: Dietary Guidelines for Americans. Home & Garden Bulletin No. 228. U.S. Department of Agriculture and Department of Health and Human Services, Washington, D.C. 20 pp.

USDA/DHHS (U.S. Department of Agriculture/Department of Health and Human Services). 1985. Nutrition and Your Health: Dietary Guidelines for Americans, 2nd ed. Home & Garden Bulletin No. 228. U.S. Government Printing Office, Washington, D.C. 24 pp.

Waterhouse, J., C. Muir, K. Shanmugaratnam, and J. Powell, eds. 1982. Cancer Incidence in Five Continents, Vol. IV. International Agency for Research on Cancer, Lyon, France. 812 pp.

Westlund, K., and R. Nicolaysen. 1972. Ten-year mortality and morbidity related to serum cholesterol. Scand. J. Clin. Lab. Invest. 30 suppl. 127:1–24.

WHO (World Health Organization). 1982. Prevention of Coronary Heart Disease. Report of a WHO Expert Committee. Technical Report Series No. 678. World Health Organization, Geneva. 53 pp.

WHO (World Health Organization). 1987. World Health Statistics Annual 1987. World Health Organization, Geneva. 455 pp.

Wilhelmsen, L., G. Berglund, D. Elmfeldt, G. Tibblin, H. Wedel, K. Pennert, A. Vedin, C. Wilhelmsson, and L. Werkö. 1986. The multifactor primary prevention trial in Göteborg, Sweden. Eur. Heart J. 7:279–288.

Williams R.R., P.D. Sorlie, M. Feinleib, P.M. McNamara, W.B. Kannel, and T.R. Dawber. 1981. Cancer incidence by levels of cholesterol. J. Am. Med. Assoc. 245:247–252.

Wynder, E.L., and G.B. Gori. 1977. Contribution of the environment to cancer incidence: an epidemiologic exercise. J. Natl. Cancer Inst. 58:825–832.

Yaari, S., U. Goldbourt, S. Even-Zohar, and H.N. Neufeld. 1981. Associations of serum high density lipoprotein and total cholesterol with total, cardiovascular, and cancer mortality in a 7-year prospective study of 10,000 men. Lancet 1:1011–1015.

Index

A